LIPPINCOTT WILLIAMS & WILKINS'

Comprehensive Dental Assisting

LIPPINCOTT WILLIAMS & WILKINS'
Comprehensive Dental Assisting

. Wolters Kluwer | Lippincott Williams & Wilkins
Health

Philadelphia · Baltimore · New York · London
Buenos Aires · Hong Kong · Sydney · Tokyo

Senior Publisher: Julie K. Stegman
Senior Acquisitions Editor: Peter Sabatini
Product Director: Eric Branger
Senior Managing Editor: Heather A. Rybacki
Developmental Editor: Tom Lochhaas
Marketing Manager: Shauna Kelley
Manufacturing Coordinator: Margie Orzech-Zeranko
Design Coordinator: Steve Druding
Compositor: SPi Global
Printer: Command Digital

First Edition

Copyright © 2012 Lippincott Williams & Wilkins, a Wolters Kluwer business.

351 West Camden Street	**Two Commerce Square**
Baltimore, MD 21201	**2001 Market Street**
	Philadelphia, PA 19103

Printed in The United States of America

Library of Congress Cataloging-in-Publication Data
Lippincott Williams & Wilkins' Comprehensive dental assisting
     p. ; cm.
  Lippincott Williams and Wilkins' comprehensive dental assisting
  Comprehensive dental assisting
  Includes index.
  ISBN 978-1-58255-815-8 (hardback)
  1. Dental assistants. 2. Dentistry. I. Lippincott Williams & Wilkins. II. Title: Lippincott Williams and Wilkins' comprehensive dental assisting. III. Title: Comprehensive dental assisting.
  [DNLM: 1. Dental Assistants. 2. Dentistry. WU 90]

RK60.5.L58   2011
617.6'0233—dc22

                                          2011007546

To purchase additional copies of this book, call our customer service department at **(800) 638-3030** or fax orders to **(301) 223-2400.** International customers should call **(301) 223-2300.**

Visit Lippincott Williams & Wilkins on the Internet: http://www.LWW.com. Lippincott Williams & Wilkins customer service representatives are available from 8:30 am to 5:00 pm, EST.

5 6 7 8 9 10

Meet the Editorial Advisory Board

In an effort to create resources that align with the needs of dental assisting instructors, Lippincott Williams & Wilkins enlisted the help of many industry experts in writing, editing, and reviewing *Lippincott Williams & Wilkins' Comprehensive Dental Assisting*, *Lippincott Williams & Wilkins' Comprehensive Dental Assisting Workbook*, and *Lippincott Williams & Wilkins' Certification Preparation for Dental Assisting*. We are pleased to introduce these board members, as follows.

Barbara Bennett, CDA, RDH, has been actively involved in dentistry for over thirty years as both a clinician and educator. She is a DANB-Certified Dental Assistant and a Registered Dental Hygienist. She served as an instructor in the dental assisting and dental hygiene programs at Parkland College in Champaign, IL, for ten years, as well as coordinating and presenting continuing education programs. She was instrumental in the development and accreditation of the dental assisting and dental hygiene programs at Texas State Technical College in Harlingen, TX, where she continues to teach in both programs. She has served as program chair of the dental assisting program, and currently holds the position of Program Chair of the Dental Hygiene Program, and Division Director of Allied Health Programs.

Barbara has served as a curriculum consultant for the American Dental Association Council on Dental Accreditation for both dental hygiene and dental assisting. She is a contributing author for several textbooks for dental assisting and dental hygiene, and speaks at the national level on topics of interest to health professionals such as infection control, communicable diseases, and periodontology. She received her Master's of Education degree from Eastern Illinois University in Adult Technical Education.

Barbara contributed to the development of *LWW's Certification Preparation for Dental Assisting*.

Carolyn Breen, Ed.D, CDA, RDA, RDH, is the Chair of the Department of Allied Dental Education and Director of the Dental Assisting and Dental Hygiene Programs at the University of Medicine and Dentistry of New Jersey (UMDNJ), School of Health Related Professions (SHRP). She received a Certificate in Dental Assisting from Union County Vocational Technical Institute in Scotch Plains, NJ, and holds an Associate's degree in Applied Science degree from Middlesex County College, Edison, NJ, Bachelor of Science degree from Montclair State College, Montclair, NJ, Master of Education degree from Rutgers University, New Brunswick, NJ, Doctor of Education degree from Nova Southeastern University, Fort Lauderdale, FL, and a Management Certificate from Middlesex County College, Edison, NJ.

Dr. Breen's teaching responsibilities have included multiple courses in allied dental education and in the dental component of the Bachelor of Science in Health Science (BSHS) program at the University. She participates in the development and provision of continuing education courses and has presented multiple educational programs as an invited speaker on both state and national levels. Dr. Breen currently serves as a consultant to dental hygiene and dental assisting education programs for the American Dental Association (ADA) Commission on Dental Accreditation, (CODA) and recently completed a four-year term as a member of the ADA - CODA Dental Assisting Review Committee, participates as a state delegate to the American Dental Assistants Association (ADAA) annual meeting. In addition to her involvement in several dental hygiene associations in the state of New Jersey, Dr. Breen also serves on the Board of Directors of the Dental Assisting National Board (DANB). She has received multiple recognitions and awards for her dedication and contributions to both dental assisting and dental hygiene. Dr. Breen is a current member of the editorial board of *Inside Dental Assisting*.

Dr. Breen contributed to the development of *LWW's Comprehensive Dental Assisting*.

Alison Collins, CDA, MS, is the program director of the Dental Assistant Program at Northwestern Michigan College in Traverse City, Michigan. She has been teaching dental assisting courses at NMC for over 30 years. Alison is a certified dental assistant. Her educational background includes an associate degree in Dental Assisting from Northwestern Michigan College, a bachelor's degree in Allied Health Teacher Education from Ferris State University and a master's degree in Occupational and Technical Education from Ferris State University. Alison has practiced as a clinical dental assistant in a prosthodontic and an oral surgery office and also helped establish and manage a low-income community-based dental clinic.

Alison contributed to the development of *LWW's Comprehensive Dental Assisting* and *LWW's Comprehensive Dental Assisting Workbook*.

Denise Campopiano, CDA, RDH, BS, graduated from Old Dominion University with a BS in Dental Hygiene. She worked in private practice for 25 years, and has over 10 years of experience as a Dental Assisting Program Director/Instructor in several states, including Georgia, New Jersey, and, now, North Carolina. She has served as an ADA CODA curriculum consultant and was a committee member of the ADA CODA Dental Assisting Review Committee. Currently, Denise is the Dental Assisting Program Director and an instructor at Miller-Motte College in Raleigh, NC.

Denise contributed to the development of *LWW's Comprehensive Dental Assisting*, *LWW's Comprehensive Dental Assisting Workbook*, and *LWW's Certification Preparation for Dental Assisting*.

Mary R. Costello, CDA, has a BS in Health Administration from Governors State University, Illinois. She has over 45 years experience in the dental field, serving as an Expanded Duties Dental Auxiliary for the U.S. Army, a Dental Coordinator for a hospital-based dental center, and a Dental Dam Instructor lecturing throughout the United States and Canada on Dental Dam Dentistry. Mary developed the Dam-It, It's Easy!℠ Educational Programs and is currently Manager of Continuing Education and Professional Relations-Hygienic Products for Coltene Whaledent, Inc.

Mary contributed to the development of *LWW's Comprehensive Dental Assisting*.

Professor **Sharon K. Dickinson, CDA, CDPMA, RDA,** has been actively involved in the dental profession as a chairside assistant, office manager, consultant, and educator. Since 1981, Professor Dickinson has held the position of Director of the Dental Assisting Program at the El Paso Community College. She is considered a curriculum expert for the Texas Coordinating Board, infection control expert serving on the infection control test development committee for the Texas State Board of Dental Examiners. With more than 35 years of clinical and practical experience in dentistry, Professor Dickinson speaks and consults extensively on OSHA, infection control, the practice and delivery of four-handed dentistry, ergonomics, and dental team communications. In addition, Professor Dickinson has published numerous articles and continuing education courses nationally and internationally.

Sharon contributed to the development of *LWW's Certification Preparation for Dental Assisting*.

Jessica L. Fisher, CDA, has been an advocate of formal education for dental assistants for many years. She began her career as a dental assistant by attending Professional Careers Institute in 2000. Once she graduated from PCI, she decided to become a Certified Dental Assistant and then took the Expanded Functions Course at Indiana University-Purdue University Indianapolis. She worked in a dental office until 2005 and then became a dental assisting instructor. In 2009, she was promoted to Dental Assisting Program Director at FORTIS College in Indiana. In 2007, Jessica returned to school at Troy University while continuing to work full-time as a Dental Assisting Program Director. In 2010, she earned her associate degree in Science in Criminal Justice. In 2011, she began taking classes at Indiana Wesleyan to complete her bachelor's degree. When asked how she feels about education she stated, "I respect my students and try to model my beliefs. I value learning and still get excited from teaching. Every single day is new, exciting and greatly rewarding for all."

Jessica contributed to the development of *LWW's Comprehensive Dental Assisting* and *LWW's Certification Preparation for Dental Assisting*.

Mari Frohn, CDA, CDPMA, EFDA, has been in the dental profession for more than 40 years, with a career that began in the dental office and has since included roles as an educator at five Boston-area colleges. She received her Dental Assisting Certificate, an AS in Business Administration, and a BS in Management from Northeastern University, where she graduated Magna Cum Laude. She is currently involved in graduate work in Curriculum Design. She holds a Certificate in Dental Public Health from Harvard School of Dental Medicine and completed Expanded Functions Training for Dental Educators at the University of Pennsylvania Dental School.

Mari, a former local and state President of the MDAA, as well as a former Dental Assistant Advisor to the Massachusetts Board of Dental Registration, has received many awards, including the 2003 Massachusetts Dental Society "Dental Educator of the Year" and a National "Excellence In Teaching Award" at the National Institute for Staff and Organization Development Conference in 2001.

Mari has authored pieces in various journals and has been a frequent textbook reviewer and practicing consultant in Dental Education and Dental Office Management. A busy local and national speaker on numerous and varied dental and medical topics, Mari is currently teaching at Tri-County RVTHS in Franklin, MA.

Mari contributed to the development of *LWW's Comprehensive Dental Assisting* and *LWW's Comprehensive Dental Assisting Workbook*.

Marie Varley Gillis, RDH, MS, is a graduate of Forsyth School for Dental Hygienists, Northeastern University, and the University of Maryland. She is currently a doctoral student at Nova Southeastern University, majoring in Healthcare Education. She was Dental Hygiene faculty, program director, and Infection Control officer at Howard University, College of Dentistry. In addition, she has over 20 years of clinical practice in periodontal settings.

Marie served as past president of Maryland Dental Hygienists' Association and a member of the ADHA/ Advanced Dental Hygiene Practitioner Curriculum Task

Force. She is the author of many scholarly articles and the recipient of multiple research grants and awards. She has written a chapter for a key dental hygiene textbook and authored an online review course for the National Board in Dental Hygiene titled *Clinical Dental Hygiene I and II*.

Currently employed by Education Affiliates, she is the National Dean of Dental Programs for 28 dental assisting and 7 dental hygiene programs.

Marie contributed to the development of *LWW's Comprehensive Dental Assisting*.

Heidi Gottfried-Arvold, BA, CDA, has been the Dental Assistant Program Director and Chairperson at Gateway Technical College since 2003. She is a graduate of the Dental Assistant program at Madison Area Technical College and is also a Certified Dental Assistant through the Dental Assistant National Board. She holds a BA in Healthcare Administration and is looking forward to graduating with a Master's Degree in Education in December 2011. Heidi has worked in the dental field for over 20 years and finds dentistry more and more exciting every year.

Heidi contributed to the development of *LWW's Comprehensive Dental Assisting*.

Teresa A. Macauley is the program chair of dental assisting at Ivy Tech Community College in Anderson, IN. She previously taught in the dental assisting program at Indiana University School of Dentistry. Before becoming an educator, Teresa spent six years as a chairside assistant in the pediatric dental clinics at Indiana University School of Dentistry and James Whitcomb Riley Hospital for Children. She also worked in private practice as an Expanded Functions Dental Assistant and Office Manager in a pediatric dental practice in Indianapolis, IN. A graduate of Indiana University Purdue University at Indianapolis, Teresa has baccalaureate and master's degrees in Health Occupations Education from the School of Health and Rehabilitative Sciences. Teresa is also a consultant for the Commission on Dental Accreditation of the American Dental Association.

Teresa contributed to the development of *LWW's Certification Preparation for Dental Assisting*.

Tracy Marsh, CDA, RDH, BS, brings an abundance of knowledge to her chosen profession, with 25 years of experience of on-going practice as a dental assistant and dental hygienist, and, for the past 12 years, serving as an educator at The University of Medicine and Dentistry of New Jersey. Active in both her state professional associations, Tracy is the Legislative and Education Chair for the New Jersey Dental Assisting Association and a Past President for the New Jersey Dental Hygienists association, positions that require her to keep current with all aspects of her field. Demonstrating a true passion for dentistry, Tracy has created and presented numerous lectures, serves as a volunteer, and has provided feedback for other dental publications. Tracy currently teaches at Fortis Institute in Wayne, NJ, where she is the Dental Assisting Clinical Coordinator. She resides in northern New Jersey with her very supportive husband and two children.

Tracy contributed to the development of *LWW's Comprehensive Dental Assisting* and *LWW's Comprehensive Dental Assisting Workbook*.

Adela E. Mills, CDA, RDH, BASDH, began her dental career as a formally trained dental assistant in 1980 and has clinical experience in general and specialty care. Mrs. Mills has over thirty years of combined occupational experience as a clinical dental assistant, dental insurance administrator, dental office administrator, clinical hygienist and educator. She is an Expanded Functions Dental Assistant in the State of Florida, concentrating her areas of expertise in Orthodontics and Periodontics. She holds an AA degree in Dental Science from Miami-Dade College, a baccalaureate degree in Dental Hygiene with special focus on educational methodologies from St. Petersburg College, and is a candidate to the Masters Degree in Higher Education Administration from Florida International University.

Mrs. Mills subscribes to the comprehensive and relationship-centered philosophy of care shared by her mentor, the late Dr. Lindsey D. Pankey, Jr. She holds a current Registered Dental Hygienist license and is presently Program Director of the Dental Assisting Program at Fortis College-Miami. She is a member of several professional organizations and has served as volunteer director of several open-door clinics to meet the dental needs of the underserved. Adela and her husband of 28 years, Steve, reside in Cutler Bay, FL, and have a son Marcus, 20, and a daughter Krystel, 17.

Adela contributed to the development of *LWW's Comprehensive Dental Assisting Workbook*.

Diana L. Graham Olsen, CDA, is the coordinator of the Expanded Functions Dental Assistant Program at York County Community College in Wells, Maine. With more than thirty years of teaching experience, Diana served as Associate Professor and Chair of the Dental Health Programs at University College of Bangor, University of Maine at Augusta. Her educational background includes: a Certificate in Dental Assisting from Beth Israel Hospital, Boston University; Certificate in Expanded Functions Dental Assisting from York County Community College; Associates Degree in Dental Hygiene from the University of Maine; Bachelors Degree in Health and Family Life Education from the University of Maine; and Masters Degree in Public Health and Healthcare Management from Boston University.

Before becoming a dental assisting and dental hygiene educator, she practiced chairside dental assisting and clinical dental hygiene in private practice. A Certified Dental Assistant since 1969, Diana has been a member of local, state, and national Dental Assistants Associations and Dental Hygienists' Associations for nearly forty years, holding offices as Vice President of the Maine Dental Hygienists' Association from 2004-2006 and President, Secretary and Treasurer of the Maine Dental Assistants Association between 1970 and 1990. Diana has been a member of the American Association of Women in Community and Junior Colleges, American Association of Dental Schools, and National Association of Dental Assisting Educators, and served on task force studies and legislative committees for the Maine Dental Association specific to EFDA education and credentialing, infection control recommendations for dental professionals, and education and licensure of dental radiographers. Diana has served as a consultant in dental assisting education to the Commission on Dental Accreditation. She has presented numerous continuing education programs at local and state meetings.

Diana contributed to the development of *LWW's Certification Preparation for Dental Assisting*.

Helene A. Pizzuta, CDA, RDA, is the Dental Program Director at the American Institute in Clifton, New Jersey, where she is developing the dental assisting program. Helene began her education studying General Education at Los Angeles City College, and then later graduated from the Dental Assisting Program at Berdan Institute in Totowa, NJ, where she was the Valedictorian and made the Dean's list. She went on to earn credit towards a Bachelor's of Science degree through the Prior Learning Assessment program at Thomas Edison State College, and is currently pursuing her BS in Allied Health from Montclair State University.

Before becoming a dental assisting educator, Helene practiced as a Certified Dental Assistant in private practice, after which she taught clinical dental assisting and eventually served as the Dental Program Director at Berdan Institute in Totowa/Wayne, NJ. She is also a Registered Dental Assistant through the New Jersey State Board of Dentistry and x-ray-licensed through the New Jersey Department of Environmental Protection.

Helene contributed to the development of *LWW's Comprehensive Dental Assisting* and *LWW's Certification Preparation for Dental Assisting*.

Vaishali Singhal, DMD, MS, is an Associate Professor at the University of Medicine and Dentistry of New Jersey's (UMDNJ) School of Health Related Professions, Department of Allied Dental Education. She teaches Dental Radiology, Local Anesthesia, Pharmacology, Medical Emergencies and Nitrous Oxide Sedation. Dr. Singhal recently completed a Master of Science in Heath Systems degree and is also pursuing a PhD. She is a graduate of UMDNJ's New Jersey Dental School located in Newark, NJ.

Dr. Singhal contributed to the development of *LWW's Comprehensive Dental Assisting*.

Reviewers

Nicole Abbott, RDA, BSTM
Dental Assisting Program Director
Carrington College California
Sacramento, CA

Kimberly G. Bastin, CDA, EFDA, RDH, MS
Dental Assisting Program Director
University of Southern Indiana
Evansville, IN

Heidi Denson, CDA, BA
Dental Assisting Instructor
Ogden Weber Applied Tech College
Ogden, UT

Teresa Desrosiers
Program Manager/Department Head, Dental Assisting
Anthem College
Orlando, FL

J. Victor Duran, DDS, DMD
Dental Assisting Program Director
Burlington County Institute of Technology
Westampton, NJ

Che' Evans, CDA, QDA, DRT
Dental Assistant Program Director
Medix School
Towson, MD

Gabriele M. Hamm, RDA, CDA, CDPMA, AS
Dental Assisting Instructor/Coordinator
Hudson Valley Community College
Troy, NY

Deb Jennings, DMD
Dental Services Faculty
Trident Technical College
North Charleston, SC

Kay Jukes, CDA, RDA, BS
Dental Assisting Program Instructor and Clinical Coordinator
Coleman College for Health Sciences
Houston, TX

Paulette S. Kehm, CDA, EFDA, MPA
Dental Assisting Program Director
Northeast State Community College
Blountville, TN

Marina Klebanov
Medical Assisting Chairperson
Mandl Allied Health School
New York, NY

Janice Lewis, AAHCA, BSHA
Dental Assistant Instructor
Pima Medical Institute
Houston, TX

Ninette Lyon, RDA, CDA, EFDA
Dental Assistant Program Director
Carrington College
Portland, OR

Martha L. McCaslin, CDA, MA
Dental Assisting Program Director
Dona Ana Community College
Las Cruces, NM

Deedee McClain, RDH, BS, MS
Former Instructor, Dental Assisting
Dental Assistants College of Saint John, Inc.
Saint John, NB
Canada
Former Program Director of Dental Hygiene/Assisting
York Technical College
Rock Hill, SC

Melanie Mitchell, CDA-Emeritus, BGS
Dental Assistant Program Instructor
Wichita Area Technical College
Wichita, KS

Stephanie Olson, CDA, BA
Dental Assisting Program Coordinator
University of Alaska Anchorage
Anchorage, AK

Robert Pruitt, CDA, BS
Dental Assistant Program Director
Concorde Career College
Kansas City, MO

Craig A. Shecter, DMD
Dental Assistant Program Director
Sanford-Brown Institute
Trevose, PA

Angela E. Simmons, CDA, CPDA, BS
Dental Assisting Department Chair
Fayetteville Technical Community College
Fayetteville, NC

Deborah J. Smith, CDA, BS
Dental Assisting Program Coordinator
Milwaukee Area Technical College School of Health Sciences
Milwaukee, WI

Diana Macalus Sullivan, CDA, LDA, BS, MS
Dental Assisting Program Director
Dakota County Technical College
Rosemount, MN

Gail Vasilenko
Allied Dental Education Assistant Professor
University of Medicine and Dentistry/School of Health Related
    Professions
Scotch Plains, NJ

Rose White
Dental Assisting Instructor
Mid-Plains Community College
North Platte, NE

Publisher's Preface

The dental office represents a whirl of activity. From the moment a patient enters the door to the time he or she leaves, their care is the responsibility of a team that needs to function smoothly and in an expert manner. The dental assistant is a critical member of that team, whether ensuring the visit and the office is run efficiently and with patient care in mind, or assisting at the chairside setting with the dentist and the dental hygienist. In a dental assisting course, students are taught how to work as part of a larger team to provide patients with optimal care and to create a thriving and well-run dental practice.

Lippincott Williams & Wilkins has been a publisher for the dental professions since 1846, publishing the original textbook for dental hygiene (*Mouth Hygiene: A Text-book for Dental Hygienists* by Dr. Alfred C. Fones) under the Lea and Febiger imprint in 1916. We have a long history of providing our customers, instructors, and students with quality, accurate, and comprehensive textbooks for teaching and learning the dental professions. With this emphasis on publishing excellence, and with the team-based approach, we have developed a new textbook for the Dental Assisting profession.

From front office to chairside, *Lippincott Williams & Wilkins Comprehensive Dental Assisting* provides the dental assisting instructor and student with a comprehensive, yet approachable, textbook to teach and learn the skills needed to succeed as a dental assistant. Understanding that dental assisting students represent a myriad of different learners—from adults pursuing a new occupation to students fresh out of high school—we have worked to develop a textbook that allows the student to easily engage with the content, providing a simpler, more direct and less obtuse writing style.

Unique features such as Voice of Experience and the Dentist's Perspective emphasize the criticality of the team-based approach to the office setting. These features also give students practical, real-life tips for how they can apply what they have learned and what they will encounter in the dental office. The Extra Patient Care and Check Your Ethics boxes prepare students for the real world, where optimal patient care is critical and ethics consistently factor into responding to and caring for patients appropriately.

In addition to these unique features, we have also worked to develop application scenarios through the Apply It feature and easy-to-follow, step-by-step Procedures. An engaging art program features hundreds of photographs, illustrations, and diagrams that illustrate key dental assisting concepts including dental anatomy, dentition, disease, pathology, radiographs, instruments and equipment, dental and laboratory materials, and procedures. Finally, at the end of each chapter we help the student prepare for the certifying exam by outlining the chapter topics that are on the Dental Assisting National Board (DANB) exam.

Recognizing that our world is becoming increasingly "electronic"—in our teaching, in our learning, and in our professions—Lippincott Williams & Wilkins has developed electronic resources for both the instructor and student. Accompanying our textbook is an educational version of Dentrix G4, the Dentrix G4 Learning Edition, provided courtesy of Henry Schein Practice Solutions, American Fork, UT. The Dentrix G4 Learning Edition is designed to give students the opportunity to learn software skills using a market-leading dental practice management system. In addition, students have access to animations and videos depicting skills, clinical simulations, anatomical concepts, and more; interactive dental instrument flash cards; interactive tray set-ups; charting exercises; a database of dental materials; crossword puzzles, quizzes, and other activities for self-study; Dentrix G4 practice management learning activities; a study guide map to the DANB exam; a Spanish-to-English translation guide; and a sign language chart. To help dental assisting instructors make the best use of their limited time, we have provided instructors with comprehensive resources to help them prepare for their class, including PowerPoint slides with integrated images; an image bank with PDF and JPG images of all of the figures from the book; a test generator; lesson plans; and a CODA Accreditation content map.

The development of *Lippincott Williams & Wilkins Comprehensive Dental Assisting* ran the same way as the dental office: with a team-based approach where every member served a critical role. We could not have developed this book without the contributions of the Editorial Advisory Board (listed on pages v–viii). The members of the Board took on many roles: Some painstakingly worked with us to create and develop each chapter and the chapter features to ensure the content was comprehensive, approachable, and relevant for students; others participated in the creation of the art; all were there to answer questions and queries as they arose to ensure that the textbook was on target. Our Reviewers provided the extra care to ensure that that the content in each chapter was complete and appropriate. We thank both our Editorial Advisory Board and Reviewers for their expertise and contributions. Much gratitude is also given to Tom Lochhaas, who worked with the Lippincott Williams & Wilkins team to craft our vision and guide its safe passage. We are also indebted to Heather Rybacki, Senior Product Manager, who knows the importance of this undertaking and delivered with her customary excellence. Finally, as with any Lippincott Williams & Wilkins publication, we must thank you, our reader. We appreciate all of the input and suggestions we have received in the past, including the suggestion to create this textbook, and thank you for your continued support.

Julie K. Stegman
Senior Publisher

Pete Sabatini
Senior Editor, Dental Assisting

Lippincott Williams & Wilkins Comprehensive Dental Assisting
Lippincott Williams & Wilkins | Wolters Kluwer Health
Baltimore, Maryland

Preface to the Student and Instructor

Preparing for a career in dental assisting means preparing to become part of a team. Dental assistants play an important role in the dental office, from helping to ensure that patients have a positive experience, to keeping the office running smoothly, to working chairside with the dentist and hygienist.

At Lippincott Williams & Wilkins, we want to provide dental assistants with the background, knowledge, skills, and confidence to be a valuable and valued member of the dental office team. To this end, we are pleased to introduce *Lippincott Williams & Wilkins' Comprehensive Dental Assisting*, a fully comprehensive dental assisting textbook that is the first in an exciting new series published by Lippincott Williams & Wilkins in the field of dental assisting. This series will:

- provide *students* with user-friendly textbooks, workbooks, and support materials that better prepare them to step into a dental assisting career
- provide *faculty* with texts and support materials that make it easy to create a robust curriculum that adheres to accreditation standards and produces qualified dental assistants

This engaging new textbook reflects the strength found in teams by garnering the knowledge and experience from dental assistants and other dental professionals across the country to create a better learning experience and a better teaching experience.

About this Book

LWW's Comprehensive Dental Assisting uses a student-friendly approach to provide coverage of the core dental assisting topics and skills students must master in their studies. Students will notice:

- a more straightforward writing style that makes reading and learning easier
- an emphasis on ease of use, with boxed features, bulleted and numbered lists, an open attractive design, and lots of artwork

- features that focus on real-world applicability and allow them to translate their experiences in the classroom to the dental setting

In addition to priming students for the dental office, *LWW's Comprehensive Dental Assisting* also equips students with the knowledge and standards needed for Dental Assisting National Board (DANB) Certification.

Unique Features of this Book

Special features throughout *LWW's Comprehensive Dental Assisting* guide students in their study and provide helpful tips and insight along the way. Two unique features found in *LWW's Comprehensive Dental Assisting* bring the dental setting into focus through the words and wisdom of other dental team members. They are:

- **"Voice of Experience"**
  Insider tips from seasoned dental assistants about aspects of dental assisting learned from experience on the job.

- **"From the Dentist's Perspective"**
  A dentist's point of view about actions or characteristics desirable in a dental assistant, designed to build self-esteem and self-confidence in a student studying to be a dental assistant.

Two other elements found in *LWW's Comprehensive Dental Assisting* emphasize critical thinking and applying information to direct patient care. They are:

- **"Check Your Ethics"**
  Brief scenarios involving ethical dilemmas that prepare dental assistants to address difficult situations commonly encountered in practice. Each scenario is related to its chapter's content and is followed by critical thinking questions.

- **"Let's Apply It"**
  Short patient care scenarios, followed by questions requiring students to apply the knowledge they have gained from the chapter.

Other Special Features

Additional special features found in *LWW's Comprehensive Dental Assisting* make learning more enjoyable, and help students fully understand and retain what they have learned. They include:

- **"Extra Patient Care"**
  Advice on how to go the extra mile to create a better patient experience, including tips on patient education and patient-centered care.

- **"Procedures"**
  Special displays portraying clinical skills performed step-by-step, often using photos or line art to enhance the numbered directions. A list of equipment and supplies stated at the beginning of the directions helps focus the student's attention on details presented in the directions.

- **"Dental Facts"**
  Fun dental factoids or statistics, with topics ranging from historical developments to interesting beliefs about the teeth or past dental curiosities appropriate to the content of that chapter.

- **"From Classroom to Clinic"**
  Information and attributes that will help students successfully apply the knowledge obtained in school to their experiences in an internship or in clinical practice.

- **"Cultural Diversity"**
  Interesting details and tips about diverse backgrounds that prime students for the variety of patients they will interact with in the dental office.

Standard Features in All Chapters

In addition to all of the special features mentioned above, each chapter in this book includes the following standard features:

- **Chapter Outline**
  Allows students and faculty to know, at a quick glance, which topics are to be covered in that chapter.

- **Chapter Checklist**
  A list of objectives that the student will be able to do upon completion of that chapter. The chapter checklist can also be used as a self-check on completion of the chapter to ensure that the student understands the key concepts.

- **Key Terms**
  Need-to-know terms introduced in the chapter that students should be able to define upon completion of the chapter. They are boldfaced in the text at first use, listed and defined at the beginning of the chapter, and included in the Glossary at the end of the text.

Pronounciations of difficult terms are provided in the Key Terms list and in the Glossary.

- **Checkpoints**
  Several student learning self-checks are found throughout each chapter, each with a few short-answer, recall questions about content covered in the preceding section of the chapter. These are designed to help ensure that students grasp the material presented so far before moving on.

- **Chapter Highlights**
  A chapter summary, in the form of a bulleted list at the end of each chapter, that students can use to ensure that they fully comprehend all the major components of that chapter.

- **Review Questions**
  Multiple choice questions that students can use to review chapter content and to assess their learning. The answers are provided with the Instructor Resources.

- **Active Learning Exercises**
  Critical thinking questions at the end of each chapter that require the student to draw on what they have learned in the preceding pages.

- **Application Activities**
  Activities the students may do that require them to apply the knowledge they have gained from the chapter. These activities may include internet research projects, professional phone interviews, journaling activities, group projects, and personal evaluation and planning exercises. These activities are designed to help students fulfill one or more of the objectives listed at the beginning of the chapter.

- **Preparing for Certification**
  Boxes at the end of applicable chapters that highlight which topics students can expect to find on the Dental Assisting National Board (DANB) certification exam.

In addition to the features listed above, this book also includes many other boxed features and tables throughout the chapters, a Glossary alphabetically listing and defining bolded key terms found throughout the book, an Appendix listing various dentistry-related organizations, a list of references and resources for further reading and development, and a comprehensive index.

Supplementary Materials

Student Resources

In addition to the text and a student workbook that coincides with the text chapter by chapter, the interactive learning activities provided on the Student Resource CD-ROMs packaged with this text and online at **thePoint** ✳ www.thepoint.lww.com/LWWsCompDA1e deliver a variety of activities to reinforce and expand upon what has been learned in the text, including:

On CD 1 and on thePoint:

- Videos and animations of skills, clinical simulations, anatomical concepts, and more
- Interactive dental instrument flash cards
- Interactive tray set-ups
- Charting exercises
- A database of dental materials
- Crossword puzzles, quizzes, and other activities for self-study
- Dentrix G4 practice management learning activities
- A study guide map to the DANB exam
- Spanish-to-English translation guide
- Sign language chart

On CD 2:

- Educational version of Dentrix G4 practice management software (Dentrix G4 software courtesy of Henry Schein Practice Solutions, American Fork, UT)
- Dentrix G4 practice management User's Guide
- Dentrix G4 practice management Installation Guide

Faculty Resources

An Instructor Resource CD-ROM and a Faculty Resource Site at **thePoint** ✳ http://thepoint.lww.com/LWWsCompDA1e deliver resources designed specifically to help instructors teach more effectively and save time. There you will find:

- PowerPoints with integrated images
- Image bank with PDF and JPG images of all of the figures from the book
- Test generator with ready-to-go multiple choice questions
- Lesson plans for each chapter
- A CODA Accreditation content map
- Access to all student resources
- Customized course content for use with your learning management system, such as WebCT, Blackboard, or Angel

Thank you!

Thank you for choosing *Lippincott Williams & Wilkins Comprehensive Dental Assisting*, the book designed to make the study of dental assisting approachable and effective. We are confident that this book and all of its supplemental resources will lead to student success!

Acknowledgments

The creation of a textbook is not unlike a dental office—in order for each to be successful, both require a team of diverse people who share their knowledge, strengths and talents in pursuit of a common goal. In a dental practice, the goal is to provide patients with optimal care, and in developing *Lippincott Williams & Wilkins' Comprehensive Dental Assisting*, our goal has been to provide a key member of the dental team - the dental assistant - with the skills, knowledge, and confidence needed to thrive in a dental practice. We at Lippincott Williams & Wilkins extend our heartfelt gratitude to the many wonderful people who became part of *our* team through the creation of this textbook, sharing with us their voice, their vision, and their passion for the profession. Our deepest appreciation goes out to:

- The members of our Editorial Advisory Board, introduced on pages v-viii, each of whom contributed to this book in a unique but meaningful way, sharing not only their time and experiences to shape the development of the text, but also expressing their love of the profession and dedication to their students in everything that they did.
- The members of our Review Board, listed on pages ix-xii, who meticulously reviewed manuscript pages and provided us with feedback and guidance through every chapter.
- Tom Lochhaas, Developmental Editor, who set forth the plan and then made sure we stuck to it. We are eternally indebted to him for his clear vision and careful eye.
- The editorial team who worked tirelessly behind the scenes, including editors, artists, photographers, copyeditors, and others dedicated to producing the best Dental Assisting textbook possible.
- Carolyn Breen, EdD, EdM, Chair of the Allied Dental Education program at University of Medicine and Dentistry of New Jersey, Scotch Plains, who graciously opened the doors of her facility to us for the photo shoot, and Vaishali Singhal, DMD, MS, Associate Professor at University of Medicine and Dentistry of New Jersey, Scotch Plains, who worked tirelessly to make sure we had everything - and everyone - we could possibly need.

- The faculty, staff, and students at the University of Medicine and Dentistry of New Jersey, Scotch Plains, who served as models, subject matter experts, and tray setup specialists, and in a multitude of other ways during the photography sessions. They are:

Sonia Baker	Lucilene Goncalves	Edna Paul
Zakia Brown	Charlotte Haldy	Laura Read
Leanne Burns	Karen Kulikowski,	Jennifer
Zeneta Casado	DDS	Rodriguez
Brianna	Luis Lugo	Lisa Seubert
Catapano	Liam McArdle	Vaishali Singhal,
Lisa Cordova	Kim McMahon,	DMD, MS
Renee	CDA, RDA	Ileanet Soler
Creekmur	Marcelia Mesquita	Angela Swandrak
Erin DeVries	Amy Moiseyev	Paula Valencia
Ana Paula Ferri	Trudy Nguyen	Eliana Vanegas
Patricia	Badal Patel	Erin Walsh
Francisco		

- Special thanks also go out to Park Avenue Dental Laboratory and Perfection Dental Studio, both located in Scotch Plains, NJ, for providing some of the materials and prostheses used in our photographs.
- Finally, we extend our gratitude to Mary R. Costello, CDA, who shared her abundant knowledge of dental procedures and materials to guide the creation of the accompanying videos; to Bruce W. Small, DMD, PA, for allowing us to film the ancillary procedural videos in his clinic; and to Dr. Small's wonderful staff, especially Sharon Clawges, CDA, RDA, who was an invaluable asset during the video shoot.

Thank you to each and every person who lent their voice to this project! We are indebted to you for your kindness and assistance, and consider each of you part of the Lippincott Williams & Wilkins family.

Julie K. Stegman, Sr. Publisher
Peter Sabatini, Sr. Acquisitions Editor
Heather A. Rybacki, Sr. Product Manager

Contents

part i

Introduction to Dental Assisting   1

part ii
Dental Sciences 51

part iV

Basic Skills   233

Part VIII

Dental Materials 617

Part IX

Assisting in Dental Procedures   681

Procedures

How to Use This Text

Lippincott Williams & Wilkins' Comprehensive Dental Assisting is the ideal core text to prepare you for your career as a dental assistant. The text is organized into ten parts comprising 48 chapters. Each chapter has many elements designed to help you learn and retain the core material and learn skills that you will need to succeed as a dental assistant. Read this User's Guide before starting the book so you will understand how what of these features can do for you.

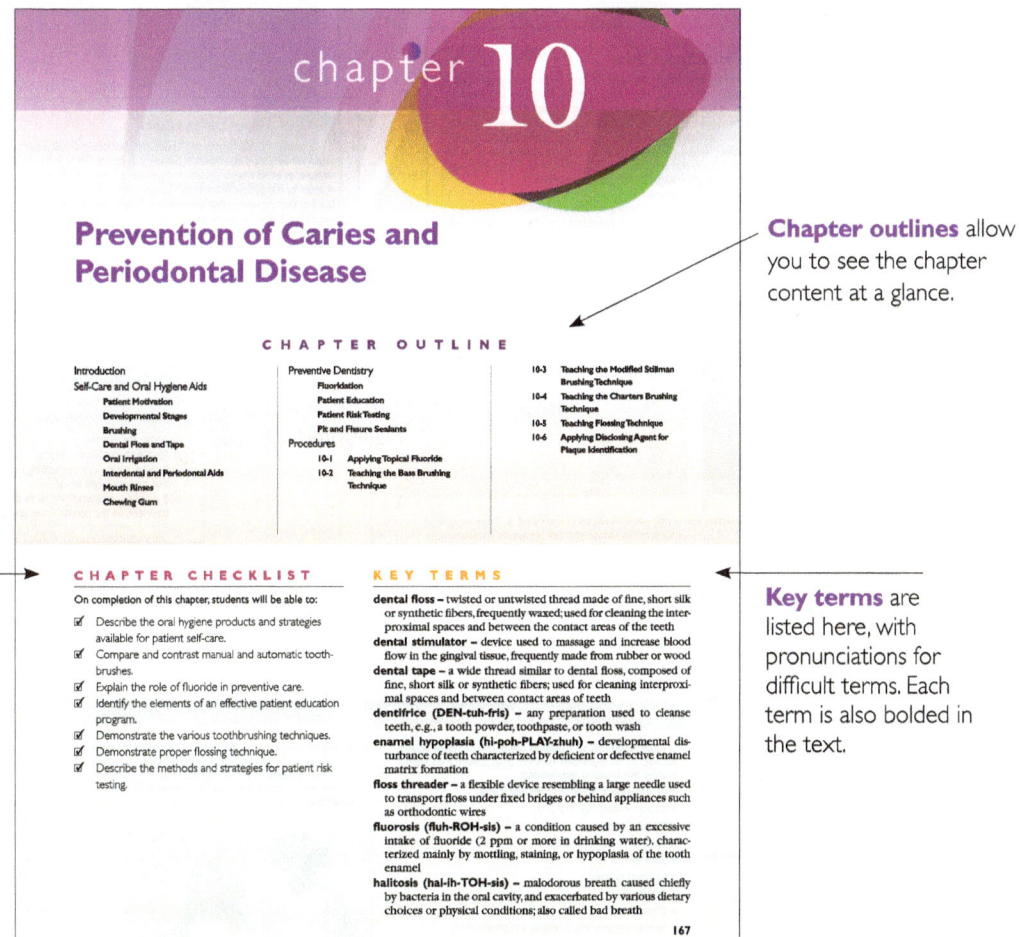

Chapter outlines allow you to see the chapter content at a glance.

Chapter objectives highlight what you will learn, and can be used as a review tool when you've finished the chapter.

Key terms are listed here, with pronunciations for difficult terms. Each term is also bolded in the text.

From Classroom to Clinic helps you to bridge your knowledge from school to your internship or clinical practice.

Cultural Diversity boxes provide interesting information about and tips for working with patients from diverse backgrounds.

Voice of Experience includes helpful advice from practicing dental assistants.

Dental Facts boxes give you interesting and little known facts about dentistry and dental care.

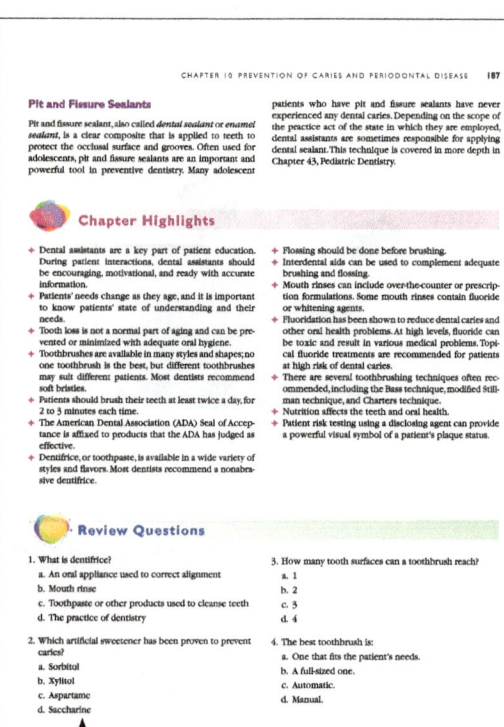

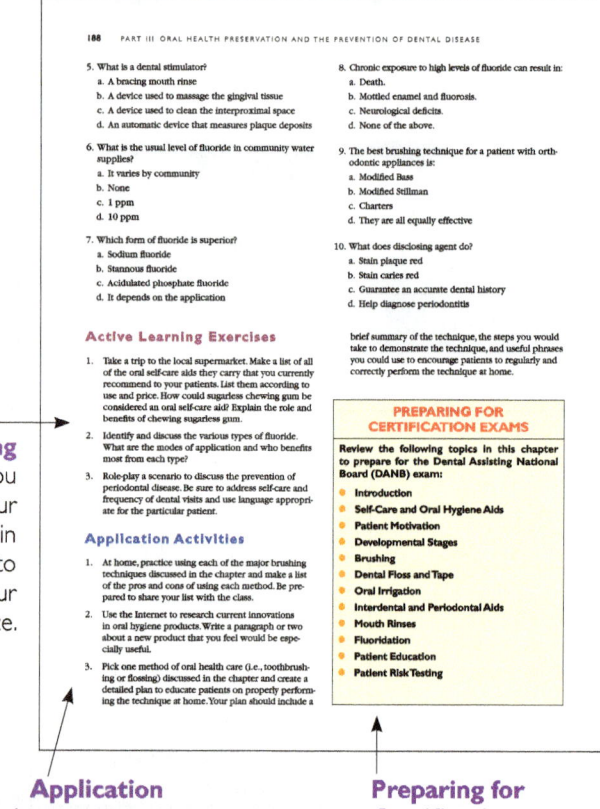

Chapter Highlights list the most important content from the chapter. Use it as a tool for reviewing what you have read.

Review Questions help you access the information you have learned.

Active Learning Exercises get you working with your classmates or out in the community to help broaden your experience.

Application Exercises encourage you to experience dental assisting tasks.

Preparing for Certification Exams highlight the topics you can expect to find on the DANB exam.

A **Student Resource CD-ROM and thePoint site** delivers videos, a variety of engaging activities, a study guide map to the DANB exam, Spanish-to-English translation guide, crossword puzzles, sign language chart, and other valuable resources. Plus, a **BONUS DVD** features Dentrix G4 Learning Edition Software, a practice management software that helps you learn the software skills you'll need to be successful in the office setting using a market-leading interactive dental office management system.

Introduction to Dental Assisting

The Dental Assisting Profession

CHAPTER OUTLINE

CHAPTER CHECKLIST

On completion of this chapter, students will be able to:

- ☑ Discuss the contributions various ancient civilizations made to the field of dentistry.
- ☑ Identify the major figures in the history of dentistry and describe their key achievements.
- ☑ Identify the educational requirements for the various members of the dental team.
- ☑ Identify major professional organizations in the field and describe their functions.
- ☑ Identify the requirements for becoming a certified dental assistant (CDA).

KEY TERMS

Albucasis (al-byuh-KA-sis) – noted Islamic physician (936–1013). In addition to his accomplishments as a surgeon, he identified tartar on the teeth as a major cause of gingival disease and wrote detailed instructions on how dentists could effectively scrape it away using special dental instruments he had designed

American Dental Assistants Association (ADAA) – professional organization representing dental assistants on a national level

American Dental Association (ADA) – the world's largest and oldest professional organization dedicated to dentistry and dental health issues

The American Dental Hygienists Association (ADHA) – largest professional organization representing the interest of dental hygienists

cosmetic dentistry – branch of dentistry that deals with improving the appearance of otherwise healthy teeth

dental assistant – dental professional trained to provide support to a dentist by performing a multitude of tasks ranging from clerical work and assistance at chairside to laboratory work, infection control, and possibly additional enhanced functions

Dental Assisting National Board (DANB) – agency that administers the national examination to certify dental and orthodontic assistants

dental hygienist (hi-JEN-ist) – licensed, professional auxiliary in dentistry who is both an oral health educator and clinician, and who uses preventive, therapeutic, and educational methods for the control of oral diseases

dental implant – a metal fixture typically made of titanium which is surgically embedded into the jaw. The implant acts as the root and allows for an abutment or prosthesis to be attached to it, such as a crown, bridge, or denture attachment

dental laboratory technician – dental professional who provides support to dental practices by filling prescriptions from dentists for crowns, bridges, dentures, and other dental prosthetics

dentistry – the science and art concerned with the prevention, diagnosis, and treatment of deformities, diseases, and injuries to the teeth, gingiva, oral cavity, and jaws

Pierre Fauchard (pee-AIR foe-SHARD) – 18th-century French physician who is known as "the Father of Modern Dentistry." He described advanced techniques for cleaning the teeth and filling caries in his comprehensive textbook on dentistry, *Treatise on the Teeth* (1723)

Isaac Greenwood – first American-born dentist

Hippocrates – ancient Greek physician (500 BCE) who is considered the father of modern medicine. Many fundamental concepts of modern medicine, including patient confidentiality and the ethical obligation to do no harm, can be traced to his early writings and teachings

Ambroise Paré (AME-brohz pah-RA) – 16th-century French surgeon who is considered the Father of Surgery. He wrote extensively on dental procedures, particularly extraction and reimplantation, in his *Complete Works*

restorative dentistry – branch of dentistry that deals with restoring or replacing damaged or missing teeth

veneer (vuh-NERE) – a thin layer of acrylic, composite, or porcelain used to cover the facial (front) surface of badly stained teeth or to improve the shape of highly visible front teeth

whitening – lightening of teeth to a whiter color by the use of dental bleaching materials

Introduction

Dentistry is one of the world's oldest medical arts. For thousands of years, people have tried to care for their teeth well enough to keep their mouths healthy and pain-free for a lifetime. The concerns of people through the ages have remained surprisingly similar, whereas the technology available for modern dental care continues to advance and better address those needs. As the profession has grown over the years, the roles and responsibilities for the various members of the dental team, including dental assistants, have become better defined. Formal education and a structured certification process ensure that patients receive quality care. A number of professional organizations exist to promote professional standards, advocate sound oral health care practices, and support members of the dental profession.

History of Dentistry

Early History

Some early dental practices were strikingly similar to our own and continue into the present day. For example, to help prevent tooth decay, or caries, the people in many early civilizations were urged to rinse their mouths after every meal. Some cultures even included the practice in religious rituals. Toothbrushes took many forms and were made of a wide assortment of materials, including animal hair and twigs. A surprising number of early dentists and doctors around the world explained caries and pain as products of a mysterious "toothworm." Nearly all early civilizations frowned on pulling, or extracting, teeth, especially the cuspid, or "eye" teeth, and reserved the practice for a last resort. Each region of the world had its favorite materials for constructing the dentures used to replace lost teeth. Dentistry developed steadily as early peoples used whatever resources and knowledge were available to them. (See Table 1-1.)

Egypt

As early as 5,000 years ago, physicians in Egypt began to move from treating the entire human body into specializing in healing and treating specific parts of it. Some doctors specialized in the eyes, others in the stomach or head. Records remain of a physician named Hesi-Re, who was known to his colleagues as "chief of the toothers" and is recognized as the first known dentist. Evidence from Egyptian graves of that era shows that his patients suffered tooth and bone loss from gingival disease and had surgery to drain dental abscesses.

Greece

The ancient Greek physician **Hippocrates**, who lived around 500 BCE, raised the art of medicine to a high level. The ideals of modern medicine, including patient confidentiality and the ethical obligation to do no harm, can be traced to his early writings and teachings. Hippocrates is perhaps best-known for the Hippocratic Oath, which outlines the standards and ethical responsibilities of health care providers. A version of the Hippocratic Oath is still taken by many medical practitioners today (see Chapter 4, Ethics and Law). Like his predecessor, the famous Greek physician Aesculapius, Hippocrates appreciated the importance of teeth and devoted many pages of his writings to them. He rejected the use of magic to treat toothache and dental

Hebrews

The Jewish scripture, the Talmud, written between 300 and 400 CE, describes false teeth made of gold, silver, and wood, and blames the mysterious "toothworm" for dental caries. Surviving Hebrew writings describe little more about dentistry.

China

The toothbrush as we know it today, with bristles sideways to the handle, was invented by the Chinese in the 1490s, but advanced treatments and practices began much earlier in China. Ancient manuscripts describe the repair of a cleft palate around 250 BCE. Dentists later combined mercury with silver to fill dental caries more than a thousand years before dentists in the West, and developed full dentures as early as the 12th century CE. In the 13th century, the explorer Marco Polo describes Chinese who, whether for cosmetic or treatment purposes, adorned their teeth with carefully fitted thin pieces of gold.

Japan

The earliest Japanese dentures were carved from a single piece of wood, usually a sweet-smelling variety, such as box, cherry, or apricot. Treatments for toothache included cautery and acupuncture as well as occasional use of charms and magic incantations. Extraction remained a last resort.

Islamic World

Physicians of the Islamic world, which, after the 8th century CE, included the Middle East, North Africa, and Spain, wrote widely on medicine, including dentistry. During Europe's Middle Ages, they rejected magic and superstition as cures, and helped keep alive the rational approaches of the Greek physicians who had come before them. The noted Islamic physician **Albucasis** (936–1013) of the Spanish city of Córdoba understood that the accumulation of tartar on the teeth was a major cause of gingival disease and wrote detailed instructions on how dentists could effectively scrape it away using special dental instruments he had designed. Illustrations of these and other instruments, including forceps for surgery, cautery irons, and dental saws and files, were featured in his famous book on medicine and surgery, *The Method*.

The most famous Islamic physician, known in the West as Avicenna, stressed the importance of keeping the teeth clean and recommended various tooth powders for this purpose, including salt and powdered snail shells.

Popular toothbrushes called *siwaks* were made from twigs of the evergreen tree *Salvadora persica* (Figure 1-2). They retained the sodium bicarbonate, tannic acid, and other astringents found in the tree's wood and proved beneficial to the gingiva. Using the toothbrush, as well as rinsing the mouth after meals and before prayer, was an important part of the cleanliness ritual advocated by

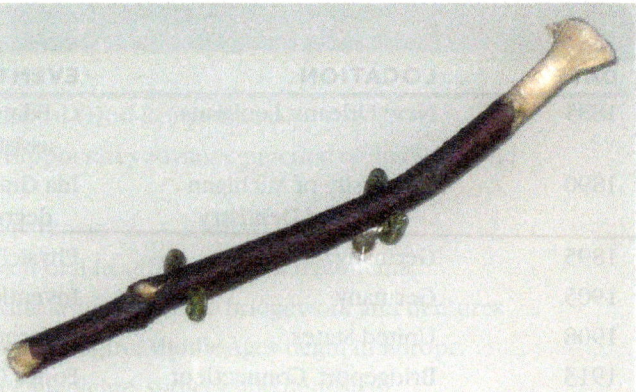

Figure 1–2 The *siwak*, a toothbrush stick still used in parts of the world today. (Courtesy of National Museum of Dentistry, Baltimore, MD.)

Islamic religious authorities. Siwaks continue to be used in parts of the world today.

> **CHECKPOINT**
> **1-1** Which ancient Greek physician is credited with establishing fundamental ideals that are still used in medical professions today?

Middle Ages

After the Roman Empire fell in 410 CE, most Europeans adopted the practice of using magic and superstition to treat dental disease and pain and rejected the medically based approaches of the Greeks, Romans, and others. Sound European medical knowledge became the property of the monasteries, where monks became practicing doctors and dentists. Barbers acted as their assistants. When medieval Christian religious authorities in the 10th century declared that priests and monks must not participate in the cutting of the body and the shedding of blood during surgery, barbers took over the practice of surgery. Known as **barber surgeons**, these practitioners included tooth extraction among their surgical duties; outside the monastery walls, they were joined by "tooth drawers," who traveled from one medieval town to another providing their services. Among the most famous of barber surgeons was **Ambroise Paré**, the 16th-century French surgeon considered the Father of Surgery, who wrote extensively on dental procedures, particularly extraction and reimplantation, in his *Complete Works*.

Renaissance

With the arrival of the Renaissance period in 16th-century Europe, magic and superstition began to fall out of favor as approaches to medicine and dentistry. Physicians and dentists returned to the respect for science and learning that had characterized earlier periods and civilizations. Their careful observations of medical and dental techniques brought many new ideas to preventive care and innovations to dental surgery. The study of human anatomy took on more importance at universities and medical schools. Renaissance artists, such as Italy's Leonardo da Vinci, drew the skeletal and muscular details of the human body with great accuracy. He studied the skull and all external and internal structures of the body very carefully. Though not trained as a doctor or dentist, he was the first anatomist to distinguish between premolars and molars.

Pierre Fauchard (Figure 1-3), an 18th-century French physician, became known as "the Father of Modern Dentistry." He disputed the long-held belief that caries was caused by a "toothworm" and described advanced techniques for cleaning the teeth and filling caries in his comprehensive textbook on dentistry, *Treatise on the Teeth*, published in 1723. Led by his example, other dentists in Europe began describing and sharing their discoveries on dental surgery and care in articles and books published for their colleagues. Despite other advances in his thinking, Fauchard continued to advocate for the practice of people rinsing their mouths each morning with several tablespoons of their own fresh urine. Once widely practiced, this hygienic ritual continues today in some isolated regions of the world.

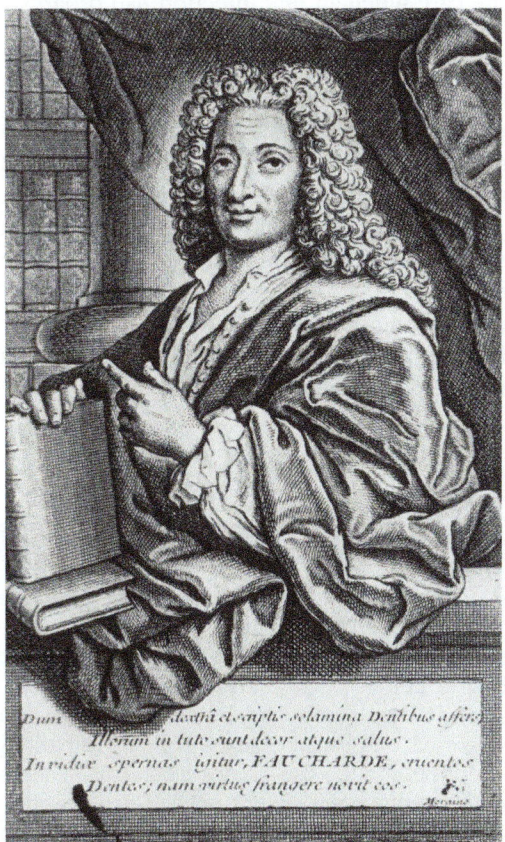

Figure 1–3 **Pierre Fauchard**, French physician and the "Father of Modern Dentistry."

CHECKPOINT

1-2 When monks in 10th-century Europe were no longer able to practice surgery, which group became responsible for performing surgery and basic dental procedures?

Dentistry in America

Early American Dentistry

Robert Wooffendale, a British-trained dentist, arrived in North America in 1766 and traveled throughout the American colonies. He offered surgical procedures and reconstruction of missing teeth. Wooffendale was followed by John Baker, an Irish physician who chose to practice dentistry. Baker set up practices in numerous colonial cities, including Philadelphia, New York, and Boston. He included George Washington among his patients.

Though he practiced a relatively short time, the most famous dentist of early America was undoubtedly the patriot and silversmith Paul Revere of Boston. Revere studied dentistry as an apprentice under John Baker in Boston. In 1768, when Baker moved to New York, Paul Revere took over his dental practice. His primary interest in dentistry, however, was the use of his skills as a silversmith to produce pontics and dental instruments. Despite eventually tiring of his practice, Revere left his mark on dental history by making the first forensic identification of a corpse using dental records. He identified the anonymous remains of a man killed at the Battle of Bunker Hill as a former patient for whom he had constructed a dental bridge some years earlier.

Isaac Greenwood, born in 1730, is considered the first American-born dentist. Like Paul Revere, he studied under John Baker in Boston. His son, John Greenwood, entered dental practice in New York following the Revolutionary War and served as another of George Washington's dentists.

Evolution of Modern Dentistry

Dentistry as we know it today in the United States began to take shape in the early part of the 19th century. A patient of the New York dentist John Greenwood, Horace H. Hayden was inspired to become a dentist himself. He lectured to medical school students on dentistry and wrote dental textbooks and articles for professional journals. He and his student, Chapin A. Harris, established the first professional organization for dentists in the United States. In 1840, they founded the world's first dental college, the Baltimore College of Dental Surgery, now the School of Dentistry at the University of Maryland.

G. V. Black

Born in 1836, Dr. Green Vardiman Black (Figure 1-4) became known worldwide as a dental reformer and

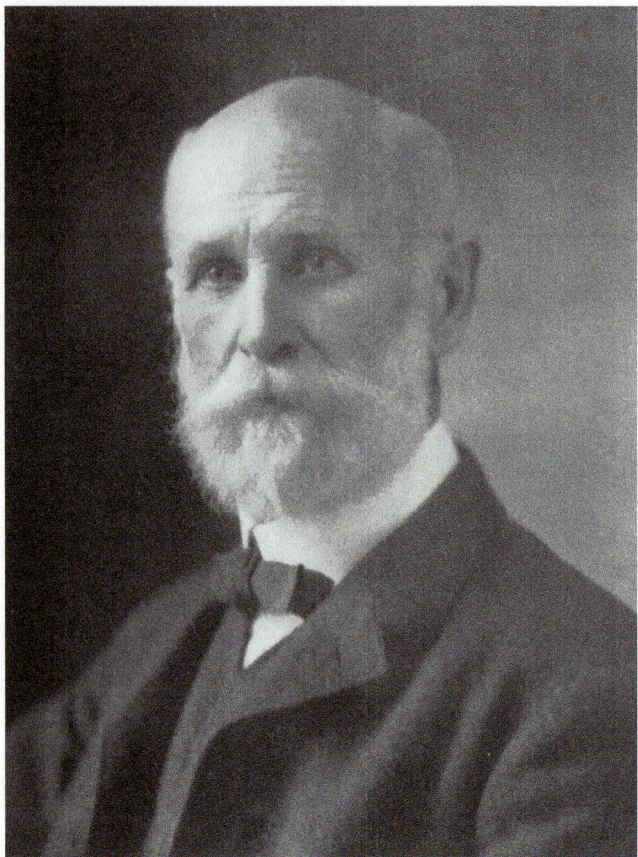

Figure 1–4 **G.V. Black,** the "Grand Old Man of Dentistry." (Courtesy of University of Maryland Health Sciences & Human Services Library, Baltimore, MD.)

educator. He championed dentistry as a profession separate from medicine. He invented numerous dental instruments and machines. Along with serving as a professor and dean, he wrote more than 500 articles and several books on dentistry, including *Operative Dentistry* in 1908. Black stressed the importance of preserving healthy teeth with preventive care, rather than simply waiting to restore them following disease or damage.

Inhalation Anesthesia
Horace Wells, a Connecticut dentist, first used nitrous oxide as an inhaled anesthetic, or painkiller, in 1844. His discovery revolutionized all surgeries, including dental surgery, which had previously relied on alcohol or opium or other equally troubling and ineffective methods to dull pain during surgery.

Wilhelm Conrad Roentgen (1845–1923)
Another of the most important discoveries in modern dentistry occurred just at the end of the 19th century when the German physicist Willhelm Conrad Roentgen discovered the mysterious x-ray, or radiograph, in 1895. His discovery revolutionized medicine and forever changed how dental disease was detected and diagnosed. For a detailed look at Roentgen and his discovery, see Chapter 29, Basics of Dental Radiography.

CHECKPOINT
1-3 Which American dentist is credited with first using nitrous oxide as an inhaled anesthetic during surgeries?

Dentistry Around the World

Dental care and oral hygiene practices vary widely around the world. They may even vary between people who live in cities and towns and those in the countryside and among people from different economic backgrounds in the same country.

Many people around the world continue to practice habits first introduced by traditional healers or medical and religious authorities in the distant past. Basic preventive care, such as cleaning and regular examination, is not available everywhere. When dental caries and pain appear, professional dentists may not be locally available or treatment may be beyond the financial reach of some. American and British dentists working in Africa have described patients who had to travel more than 1,000 miles to reach adequate care when an oral infection had progressed into the bones of the jaw. Despite care, one patient lost all her lower teeth.

Getting access to dental care is harder in countries where the number of dentists is very low compared to the number of residents. In industrialized countries, such as the United States, Britain, Japan, and Australia, there may be 1 dentist for every 1,600 people. In countries with scarcer economic resources, such as many in Africa and Southeast Asia, there may be 1 dentist for every 119,000 people. To make matters worse, most professionally trained dentists in developing countries have settled in large urban population centers, although many residents continue to live in distant rural areas.

Dental Facts India

In many areas of India, toothbrushes made from fresh twigs, with the ends frayed into fibers, are favored for daily brushing. Twigs are selected from specific trees according to the season of the year and the individual user's temperament. Most brushes have a bitter taste and an astringent quality believed to be beneficial to the gingiva. After brushing their teeth, Indians traditionally use a curved silver instrument to scrape the tongue free of accumulated coatings and then rinse the mouth with water combined with specially selected herbs and spices.

Dental Facts China

A longstanding shortage of professionally trained dentists persists in China, particularly in rural areas. As the Chinese government works to increase the number of university-trained professional dentists, the gap in care in rural areas is filled by young, specially trained technicians, known as "barefoot dentists." They offer various kinds of basic dental care, including simple restorations, extractions, and treatment of some gingival ailments. They have some medical resources available to them, such as anesthetics to kill pain during procedures, but they commonly lack x-ray machines and other specialized equipment. For dental emergencies, they must refer their patients to large dental facilities in major Chinese cities and provincial capitals.

To help provide as much access to dental care as possible, some countries have begun using community health nurses and other appropriately trained health care providers to provide a basic package of oral health care to people regardless of where they live. Ingredients of basic care may include pain relief, fluoride treatments, dental health education, and basic restorative treatments to fix caries and broken or damaged teeth.

Contemporary Trends in Dentistry

Patients today are more active participants in their own medical and dental treatment. Many make it a point to keep current on new developments in dental treatment, especially opportunities to maintain oral health and prevent dental disease from developing in the first place. Some patients have a particular interest in improving the appearance of otherwise healthy teeth, or they want to put the finishing touches on restorative dental work by seeking out the latest techniques in **cosmetic dentistry**. Cosmetic dentistry includes many techniques and procedures already practiced in dental offices, but begins by examining the patient's entire oral cavity—including the shape, color, and structure of teeth—and working to improve overall appearance, or aesthetics. Television, advertising, and other visual media have a powerful influence over the expectations of many patients. Along with questions about brushing, flossing, rinsing, and other preventive measures for better dental health, you can expect to answer numerous patient questions about treatment options that have a purely cosmetic or aesthetic purpose.

Whitening

As we age, our teeth may appear increasingly stained or worn. Habits such as drinking tea or coffee and chewing or smoking tobacco can increase this appearance. **Whitening**, or bleaching, has become one of the most requested services provided in dental offices and is often performed by dental assistants. Whitening materials penetrate the tooth's enamel into the dentin. A light source or heat is used to speed up the lightening process. Patients not interested in undergoing whitening treatments in the dental office may instead ask you about commercially available home whitening treatments. For more information on tooth whitening, see Chapter 46, Cosmetic Dentistry.

Veneers

Veneers are thin layers of acrylic, composite, or porcelain placed on the outer surface of the teeth to improve their appearance or shape. Their placement requires little if any removal of existing tooth structure, but may require some surface preparation before they are bonded in place. Some veneers require routine polishing and regular maintenance after they are placed; others are more durable. Resin and porcelain are two of the materials frequently used for veneers. For more information on veneers, see Chapter 38, Fixed Prosthodontics.

Implants

Dental implants are a popular method of replacing one or more missing teeth. Implants are metal devices surgically placed into the jaw bone and allowed to bond with the surrounding bone tissue over a period of 6 months. After successful bonding, the implant may be used to anchor in place a single crown, a bridge, or a partial or full denture. For a detailed look at dental implants, see Chapter 38, Fixed Prosthodontics.

History of Dental Assisting

Before the late 19th century, dentists sometimes hired men and boys to assist them in their practices. In 1885, a New Orleans dentist, C. Edmund Kells (1856–1928) (Figure 1-5),

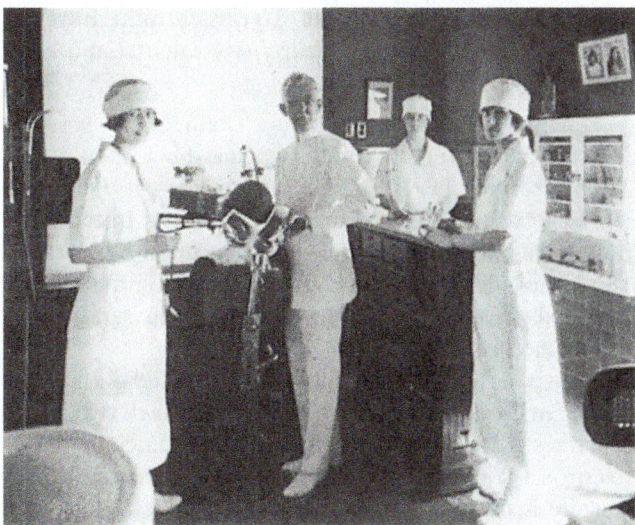

Figure 1–5 C. Edmund Kells, the first dentist to hire female dental assistants, shown with his assistants. (Courtesy of Bird DL, Robinson DS. *Torres and Ehrlich Modern Dental Assisting*, 9th ed. Philadelphia, Saunders: 2009.)

became the first dentist to employ a female dental assistant. The public responded positively to his decision and other dentists followed his example. The first "lady assistants," as they were originally known, made it more comfortable and respectable for women patients to visit a dental practice alone. The assistants began by helping with office duties and gradually moved into helping dentists chairside. This made it possible for dentists to increase the number of patients they saw and the amount of dentistry that their practice could perform. More and more dentists saw the value in employing assistants and began to train their own. In the 1930s, an accepted curriculum to train dental assistants began to emerge. In 1948, what is now the **Dental Assisting National Board (DANB)** was formed to recognize the professional competence and qualifications of trained dental assistants. In the 1950s, colleges and other institutions increased the number of programs available to train professional dental assistants.

History of Dental Hygiene

A dental assistant in Connecticut was the first person to be trained as a dental hygienist. In the early 1900s in Bridgeport, Irene Newman began to provide preventive care services under the supervision of Dr. Alfred C. Fones, who wanted to allow time in his practice for other procedures. Dr. Fones went on to found the School of Dental Hygiene that bears his name at the University of Bridgeport in 1913. Irene Newman became the first licensed dental hygienist in 1917.

Women and Minorities in Dentistry

Though women in the 18th century and early 19th century were not allowed to formally study for a career in dentistry, they nonetheless found ways to enter the profession and paved the way for the nearly 50% of dental students today who are women.

Emeline Roberts of Danielson, Connecticut, was the first woman to practice dentistry in the United States. After observing her husband practice dentistry, she studied basic science on her own and, in 1859, became her husband's partner in his dental office. Upon his death in 1864, she took over his practice, supporting herself and her small children, and continued practicing dentistry for the next 60 years.

Lucy B. Hobbs-Taylor originally apprenticed with a male dentist in Cincinnati, Ohio. She later established two dental practices of her own. She remained determined, however, to enroll as a student at the Ohio College of Dental Surgery. Despite many obstacles, she persisted in her efforts and finally graduated in 1866, the first woman in the world to graduate from a dental school.

Robert Tanner Freeman earned a doctor of medical dentistry degree from Harvard University's School of Dental Medicine in 1869, becoming the first African American to graduate from dental school. From the 1870s until educational desegregation in the 1950s, most African American dentists were educated at traditionally black Howard University in Washington, D.C., or at Meharry Medical College, a private medical school for black physicians in Nashville, Tennessee.

In 1890, Ida Gray became the first African American woman to graduate from a U.S. dental college. After her graduation from the University of Michigan's School of Dentistry, she went on to practice dentistry in Chicago until her retirement in 1928.

Education in Dental Professions

Dentists

To practice dentistry in the United States, a dentist must graduate from an accredited dental school approved by the American Dental Association's (ADA) Commission on Dental Accreditation (CODA). Dental education accreditation began in the early part of the 20th century and is intended to ensure the quality and continuous improvement of dental and dental-related education in the United States. Typically, a dentist completes an undergraduate education and goes on to study at a dental school, which includes both coursework and clinical practice on patients. When the dentist graduates, he or she receives either a doctor of dental surgery (DDS) or a doctor of medical dentistry (DMD) degree. Many dentists go on to additional specialist training. In addition to these requirements, dentists need to take and pass a national written exam and written and clinical exams in the states in which they plan to practice.

After obtaining a license to practice, most dentists go into general dentistry where they handle a wide variety of situations and patients. Other dentists choose to specialize in one of nine specialties. For more information about dental specialists, see Chapter 3, The Dental Office Team. Additional coursework and written and practical

From the Dentist's Perspective

I've been practicing for 10 years, and every year my practice gets busier. New families move into town. My colleagues retire and refer their patients to me. I'm glad, but it does keep me busier than I expected. I know one thing: I could not do everything I do without my terrific staff. Just last year I hired a new dental assistant, Daniel. He graduated from the program at our community college, got an associate degree, and passed his Certification Exam to become a certified dental assistant. He is wonderful with the patients and really great with all of us here in the office. I can really see the difference from other assistants I hired over the years. When I started out, I wanted to train my own assistants. I felt I could do a better job of letting them know what I needed. It did not turn out that way. I just did not have enough time to do a good job. Sometimes I skipped over the most important details, just because I thought I had already gone over them. Daniel came prepared. He completed the practical experience he needed for his degree at a big clinic downtown. He saw everything there and worked with children, older adults, people from other countries, people with less money, people with more money. He is comfortable with everyone and really knows how to get people to open up and talk with him. He knows what to expect and how to prepare for each type of procedure I do. I always know he will have everything ready before we start. He also keeps up on things. Last time he brushed up on his Continuing Education credits, he got to use what he had learned right away when I worked on a patient who had recently gone through a whole series of cosmetic procedures at another office. Daniel got the best training he could and set out to succeed at his job; he helps all the rest of us at the office succeed, too.

examinations are required for dentists to specialize in any of these areas.

Dentists today are more involved than ever with their patients' overall general health. While treating the gingiva and teeth, many detect early signs of other health conditions that require referral to a physician. Dentists may employ dental assistants, dental hygienists, and dental laboratory technicians in their offices.

Dental Assistants

Most **dental assistants** acquire their training in community college, trade school, or technical institute training programs. Some dental assistants are trained in schools associated with the armed forces. ADA's CODA accredits more than 260 formal training programs across the country. An accredited training program for dental assistants includes both classroom and laboratory instruction in dental assisting skills. Students also gain practical experience in dental offices, clinics, and schools before they graduate. Completion of a 2-year program at a community or junior college may lead to an associate's degree; most schools, including trade schools and technical institutes, offer a certificate or the ability to obtain licensure. Regulations regarding programs and degrees differ by state, so be sure to check the regulations in your area. Students may search for dental assisting programs accredited by CODA at www.ada.org/prof/ed/programs/search_index.asp.

American Dental Association
Commission on Dental Accreditation
211 East Chicago Avenue
Suite 1900
Chicago, Illinois 60611
telephone: 800-621-8099 or 312-440-4653
e-mail: accreditation@ada.org

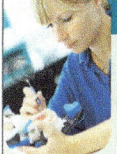

Voice of Experience

The best part of my job is meeting people. Sometimes that is the most challenging part, too, but it is always interesting. My patients come from all over the country and all over the world. No matter where they are from, I try to see them all as individuals. I tell myself I am helping to treat somebody's grandmother or somebody else's dad. When I work with people from another country, who are new to my town, I try to make them as comfortable as possible. I do not ask endless questions about where they are from and what the government is like there, for example. I do not ask them about their accents. But I do try to find out how they feel about their teeth, how they take care of them, and whether they have pain and where. I try to find out how they brush their teeth, whether they floss, and if they are comfortable with mouthwash and what they use. I have gotten some strange answers from people, believe me. One person told me he preferred to keep brushing his teeth with the twigs and sticks he had grown up using. He did not like plastic and synthetic bristle tooth brushes. They felt too big and clumsy in his mouth and he missed the bittersweet taste of the wood twigs. I selected a smaller toothbrush for him that fit his mouth better and suggested he might like to try an herbal-flavored toothpaste. Whatever people tell me, I try to make them comfortable enough so that they'll tell me more. When I suggest ways they could improve their care, I do it quietly and calmly. Working together, we can both feel more at home.

Dental Hygienists

Dental hygienists provide preventive dental care by removing calculus, stains, and plaque from teeth, and by teaching patients about good oral hygiene. Additional responsibilities can include developing dental radiographs, applying fluoride treatments, and performing other patient care tasks.

In nearly all states, dental hygienists become licensed by graduating from a dental hygiene program accredited by the ADA's CODA, and passing written and clinical examinations. Most accredited programs, such as many at junior or community colleges, lead to an associate degree. Others lead to a certificate or a bachelor's degree. Some lead to a master's degree. Graduates of 2- and 4-year programs who successfully complete their licensing examinations use the title registered dental hygienist (RDH) after their name (some states use the title LDH, which stands for licensed dental hygienist).

Dental Laboratory Technicians

Dental laboratory technicians, also known as *dental technicians*, provide support to dental practices by filling prescriptions from dentists for crowns, bridges, dentures, and other dental prosthetics. They customize each prescription according to models of the individual patient's oral cavity, bite, and adjoining teeth. Dental technicians are skilled artisans whose work is detailed and demanding. They may work for individual dentists or for dental laboratories. Some technicians train in business and management and go on to establish their own dental laboratories.

Formal training to become a dental technician varies greatly in length and in the level of skill acquired. Training programs are available through community and junior colleges, vocational-technical institutes, and through the armed forces. Some programs are accredited by CODA. These programs combine classroom and laboratory instruction with supervised practical work experience. Becoming a fully trained dental technician may take 3 to 4 years, but more on-the-job experience is required to become an accomplished technician. Dental laboratory technicians seeking credentials to reflect their qualifications and professional competence take and pass an examination to become certified dental technicians (CDTs).

Professional Organizations

Founded in 1859, the **American Dental Association (ADA)** is the world's largest and oldest professional organization dedicated to dentistry and dental health issues. Made up of dentists from all over the United States, the group works to advance professional standards and to promote good oral health practices for the public. Involved in the testing and rating of dental products, the ADA awards a seal of approval to items that it considers safe and effective. The ADA is also involved in establishing educational standards for dentists and other dental professionals. In addition, the group produces a monthly publication called the *Journal of the American Dental Association*. For more information, go to the ADA's website at www.ada.org.

The **American Dental Assistants Association (ADAA)** is the oldest and largest organization in the United States representing professional dental assistants. It promotes the advancement of the profession in matters of education, legislation, credentialing, and professional activities and seeks to enhance the delivery of quality health care to the public. Statewide chapters exist in many states. See Chapter 2, Professionalism, for more information about the ADAA and its role in the education and professional development of dental assistants.

The **American Dental Hygienists Association (ADHA)** is the largest professional organization representing the interests of dental hygienists. It offers professional support and educational programs to advance the art and science of dental hygiene and to promote the highest standards of education and practice in the profession. Publications and other information are available at www.adha.org.

Certification

Dental assistants who have graduated from an ADA-accredited educational program, or those who have completed 2 years of full-time or 4 years of part-time work experience as a dental assistant, may apply to take the certification examination to become a certified dental assistant (CDA) or certified orthodontic assistant (COA). Successful completion of the certification examination, given by the DANB, recognizes the dental assistant's qualifications and professional competence. More than 30 states recognize or require DANB certification. Some states allow dental assistants to perform special expanded functions in the dental office, such as taking radiographs and performing other special procedures. These special tasks can only be performed by dental assistants who have completed additional training and passed a certification examination. Some states also require the dental assistant to obtain a license from the state radiological board or equivalent to perform additional procedures. Requirements and expanded functions vary from state to state. DANB administers examinations that qualify dental assistants to perform these expanded functions according to the regulations in their home state. For a list of requirements and allowed functions for your state, visit www.danb.org/main/statespecificinfo.asp.

All applicants for DANB certification must hold and maintain up-to-date certification in cardiopulmonary resuscitation (CPR). After successful completion of the examination, they must also complete Continuing Education credits each year to qualify for annual recertification. Certification examination schedules and other information are available at www.danb.org.

Check Your Ethics

You are assisting the dentist while he performs a radiographic procedure on a patient. The patient is correctly positioned, and the dentist is getting ready to take the radiograph when he is interrupted by the news that a patient has arrived who needs emergency dental care. The dentist asks you to finish taking the radiograph. You've been taking a class in radiography, and you know exactly what to do, but you also know that state law prevents you from performing this procedure without certification.

1. What would you do?
2. How do you explain your actions to the dentist?
3. What are the possible consequences if you perform the procedure?

CHECKPOINTS

1-4 Name the division of the American Dental Association responsible for accrediting dental education programs.

1-5 What does "DANB" stand for?

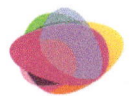 ## Chapter Highlights

+ Dentistry is one of the world's oldest medical arts. Some early dental practices were strikingly similar to our own, including rinsing the mouth and using a toothbrush.

+ The Egyptian physician Hesi-Re is believed to be the first dentist.

+ The ancient Greek physician Hippocrates developed many concepts that are fundamental to medical practice today, including patient confidentiality and the ethical obligation to do no harm.

+ Early Roman dentistry combined the medicine of the Greeks with the restorative dentistry of the Etruscans. Among the many advances during this time were the classification of teeth, the invention of the dental drill, and the use of narcotics to ease dental pain.

+ In Europe in the 10th century, barbers took over the practice of surgery. Known as *barber surgeons*, these practitioners included tooth extraction among their medical duties.

+ In the Renaissance period, beginning in the 16th century, European physicians and dentists returned to the respect for science and learning that had characterized earlier periods and civilizations. Their careful observations of medical and dental techniques brought many new ideas to preventive care and innovations to dental surgery.

+ In the United States, dentistry as we know it today began to take shape in the early part of the 19th century. The first professional organization for dentists was founded, and the first dental college was established. The use of nitrous oxide as a painkiller and discovery of the x-ray further advanced the practice of dentistry.

+ Dental care and oral hygiene practices vary widely around the world. Basic preventive care, such as cleaning and regular examination, is not available everywhere. Getting access to dental care is harder in countries where the number of dentists is very low compared to the number of residents.

+ Cosmetic (or aesthetic) dentistry emphasizes improving the appearance of otherwise healthy teeth. Whitening, veneers, and implants are among the techniques used in this branch of dentistry.

+ In the 19th century, dentists began hiring assistants to help them in their practices. By the 1930s an accepted curriculum to train dental assistants began to emerge. In 1948 what is now the Dental Assisting National Board (DANB) was formed to recognize the professional competence and qualifications of trained dental assistants.

+ Dentists must pass written and practical licensing examinations and have a degree from a dental school accredited by the American Dental Association's (ADA) Commission on Dental Accreditation (CODA).

+ Most dental assistants acquire their training in community college, trade school, or technical institute training programs. Dental assistants who have graduated from a program accredited by the American Dental Association, or those who have completed 2 years of full-time or 4 years of part-time work experience as a dental assistant, may apply to take the certification examination to become a certified dental assistant (CDA) or certified orthodontic assistant (COA).

+ In nearly all states, dental hygienists become licensed by graduating from a dental hygiene program accredited by the American Dental Association's (ADA) Commission on Dental Accreditation (CODA) and passing written and clinical examinations.

+ Formal training to become a dental technician varies greatly in length and in the level of skill acquired. Training programs are available through community and junior colleges, vocational-technical institutes, and through the armed forces. Dental laboratory technicians can take an examination to become certified dental technicians (CDTs).

+ Professional organizations in the field of dentistry include the American Dental Association (ADA), American Dental Assistants Association (ADAA), and the American Dental Hygienists Association (ADHA).

 ## Review Questions

1. The first known dentist, Hesi-Re, lived in

   a. Ancient Rome.

   b. Ancient Greece.

   c. Ancient Egypt.

   d. Medieval Paris.

2. Which of the following tasks is the responsibility of a dental lab technician?

   a. Making crowns

   b. Polishing teeth

   c. Removing calculus from teeth

   d. Processing test results

3. Thin layers of acrylic, composite, or porcelain used to cover the front surface of stained teeth are called
   a. *Sawiks*.
   b. Veneers.
   c. Lacquers.
   d. Bleachings.

4. The first toothbrush as we know it today, with bristles sideways to the handle, was invented in the 1490s by
   a. The Italian explorer Marco Polo.
   b. The Japanese.
   c. The Chinese.
   d. Renaissance artists.

5. Albucasis, one of the best known physicians of Spain and the Islamic world, believed that the accumulation of tartar on the teeth was a major cause of
   a. Discoloration of the teeth.
   b. Gingival disease.
   c. "Toothworm" infestation.
   d. Mouth sores.

6. A primary role of a dental hygienist is
   a. Removing calculus from teeth.
   b. Designing dentures.
   c. Updating patient records.
   d. Assessing a patient's bite.

7. The two most important discoveries of the 19th century to impact the practice of modern dentistry were
   a. Fluoridation of water and fluoride toothpastes.
   b. The invention of Novocaine and the rubber dental dam.

   c. Inhalation anesthesia and the radiograph.
   d. Amalgam restorations for dental caries and toothbrushes with synthetic bristles.

8. Which of the following has *the least* effect on access to dental care in developing countries?
   a. The number of residents versus dentists available
   b. Whether dentists tend to reside in the cities or the countryside
   c. Whether trained individuals other than dentists can provide basic care
   d. The attitudes of traditional healers toward professionally trained dentists

9. Which of the following is *not* used to speed up the process of tooth whitening?
   a. Lasers
   b. Low-intensity heat
   c. Sealants on the surface of the teeth
   d. High-intensity light

10. In addition to graduation from an accredited program in dental assisting, a certified dental assistant (CDA) must have completed
    a. 50 hours of community service in a neighborhood dental clinic.
    b. The certification examination administered by the Dental Assisting National Board (DANB).
    c. The certification examination administered by the assistant's home state.
    d. Additional training in one of the nine dental specialties.

Active Learning Exercises

1. Make a list of the professional dental organizations. Identify each organization's founder and which profession's members belong to each organization. Are these organizations still operating today?

2. Go online and research the necessary credentials for at least five surrounding states. Identify and list the requirements for Registration, Certification, Licensure or other credentialing.

3. What role does the dental laboratory technician play with regard to the dental office? Locate several technicians in your area and find out if they work independently or within a dental office.

Application Activities

1. Visit the website for the Dental Assisting National Board (DANB) to gather what information you can about your state's requirements for dental assistants. List the dental assisting job titles that are available in your state and write a short summary listing the requirements for obtaining a license in each of the positions.

2. Select one of the professional organizations discussed in the chapter and locate several journals or other items published by the organization. Read the material and write a paragraph or two summarizing what you've learned. Be sure to consider how the organization could be used to expand your career opportunities. Be prepared to discuss your findings during the next class period.

Professionalism

CHAPTER CHECKLIST

On completion of this chapter, students will be able to:

- ☑ Discuss the idea of professionalism and identify how a profession differs from a job.
- ☑ Identify the most important personal characteristics of a professional dental assistant.
- ☑ Identify the most important components of a dental assistant's professional appearance.
- ☑ Discuss the importance of maintaining patient confidentiality and identify the most important set of federal regulations governing it.
- ☑ Explain the importance of continuing education and professional development for dental assistants.

KEY TERMS

accuracy – being true, correct, or exact

adaptability – the quality of being adaptable; able to adjust oneself to changing circumstances

administrator – one who manages a business or agency

advocate – one who defends or acts on behalf of an individual or cause

certified dental assistant (CDA) – designation earned by dental assistants who have successfully completed the Dental Assisting National Board certification examination and complete continuing education offerings annually as required

certified orthodontic assistant (COA) – designation earned by orthodontic assistants who have successfully completed the Dental Assisting National Board certification examination and complete continuing education offerings annually as required

clinician – health professional who examines and helps care for patients

commitment – the act of promising to engage in a particular act or course of action

dependable – worthy of trust; reliable

educator – trained teacher or other individual who plans, directs, or engages in education

empathy – identifying with and understanding another person's situation or feelings

HIPAA – Health Insurance Portability and Accountability Act of 1996; specific regulations that ensure privacy and confidentiality of patient health care information

hygiene – practices that promote or preserve health

initiative – possessing the readiness and ability to take action of one's own

maturity (muh-CHUR-uh-tee) – the state of being mature or fully developed

pathogen (PATH-uh-jin) – an agent, such as a bacterium or fungus, that causes disease

personal characteristic – a trait that characterizes a person, such as honesty, tactfulness, adaptability, or compassion

professional – an individual whose knowledge, training, skills, and conduct meet the standards of a chosen profession

responsibility – being obliged to certain actions or outcomes

Standard of Care (SOC) – the diagnostic and treatment process that a health care provider should follow for a particular type of patient, illness, or circumstance

tactfulness – avoiding giving offense; being considerate in dealing with others

Introduction

Dental assistants are trained, multiskilled professionals who are valuable members of the dental team. During the course of a day, they may perform a wide range of tasks. They may function as **clinicians** who care for patients and see to their well-being, as **educators** for better patient dental health, as patient **advocates** who respond to the needs and concerns of their patients, and as **administrators** who help run and maintain the dental practice. Some are very versatile and can run an office from the business end. Making and scheduling appointments, managing inventory, and keeping up with insurance submissions and the accounts receivable and payable are just a few other areas in which a dental assistant can be skilled. A wide range of skills and knowledge make for a truly valued dental professional.

Regardless of the type of practice where they are employed, dental assistants perform their tasks with professionalism and attention to detail and continually remember their own importance to the dental team.

Characteristics of a Professional

A profession is much more than a job. It is an occupation or career that requires preparation, including specialized study and considerable training. You *practice* a profession as opposed to *working* at a job. **Professionals** possess a specialized body of knowledge and offer a specific set of skills. Members of a profession, such as dental assisting, have a group identity and sense of mission; that is, they are all working toward the same goal. Many health professionals, such as dental assistants, share a service orientation. They want to help people, and they practice a profession that allows them to do so.

The members of a profession hold one another to standards of behavior and standards of practice. They may be held to a formal code of conduct as well as to state and federal laws that govern the practice of their profession. Institutions where they practice may also have rules of conduct. Many health professions have a formal **Standard of Care (SOC)** that spells out the obligations of health care providers while caring for individual patients. Professionals never stop learning about the profession they practice. They take pride in being lifelong learners.

As a dental assistant, your salary, benefits, and hours may vary depending on your work setting and where in the United States you live and practice your profession. Regardless of these distinctions, however, a career as a dental assistant calls for maintaining professionalism at all time.

Personal Characteristics

Personal characteristics, such as honesty and dependability, are the foundation of our personal character. If you do not already possess the following important personal characteristics, work toward making them a part of who you are both as a person and as a professional dental assistant. In some cases, your success as a dental assistant will depend on it.

Dependability and Punctuality

- Your team members and patients expect you to be there to help them.
- If you miss work or are late, someone else must be found to do your work in your absence.

Adaptability

- As you move through your day, be willing to take on unexpected roles or duties when necessary.
- If the clinic or office where you work remains open some evenings or weekends, be willing to work your share of those hours.

Maturity

- Remain calm in emergencies and do what you can to help.
- Listen to constructive criticism without becoming defensive. See it as an essential part of learning to do a better job.

Accuracy

- Your patients and the dentist you assist depend on your accuracy and close attention to detail.
- Mistakes can be costly to patient health and to the reputation of the practice. Some may even result in legal action.

Honesty

- If you make a mistake, admit it immediately.
- Do not blame your mistakes on others.
- Refrain from using office resources or time for personal business.

Empathy

- Even in difficult situations, try to see things through your patient's eyes.
- If you can, imagine how you might feel in a similar situation.
- Help ensure patients get the care they need, even if they are frightened or in pain.

Courtesy and Patience

- Graciously welcome all patients and families who come to you for care.
- Exercise patience in your interactions with all those who come to you for care and with your colleagues.
- When asked to explain procedures to patients, speak slowly and remember to use words and explanations the patient is likely to understand (Figure 2-1).
- Patiently repeat yourself if necessary, or choose new words to explain.

Tactful Communication

- Do not discuss your personal problems with patients or with colleagues in the dental office.

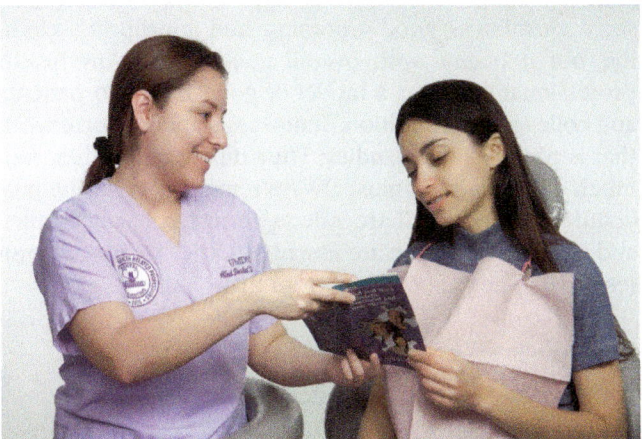

Figure 2–1 Displaying patience and courtesy leads to positive communication between the assistant and the patient.

- Choose your words carefully, whether in casual conversation or difficult treatment situations.
- Choosing the right words at the right time can make a great deal of difference to your patients and colleagues.
- In some cases, you may be able to reassure a nervous patient or redirect an unsettling discussion.

Positive Attitude

- Be confident in your abilities as a trained health professional.
- You have the responsibility to provide quality care and the training and ability to do so.
- Become and remain a team player. Successful patient care depends on a team effort.

Initiative

- Work with a minimum of instruction or supervision.
- Do whatever is expected of you by your fellow team members.
- When your own duties permit, volunteer to help others who may need it.

Extra Patient Care

As a professional dental assistant, you have the opportunity to reassure patients who are anxious or apprehensive about procedures. Showing concern, communicating clearly, and answering questions patiently are part of your professional responsibility and will help any procedure go more smoothly. The opportunity to reassure patients does not end when the procedure does.

When a patient has experienced a particularly complicated procedure or undergone surgery, consider placing a post-care phone call later that day to check on her. Patients will appreciate the time you take with them, and will probably have questions they forgot to ask or were hesitant to call the office about. Allow a few hours for the patient to begin to recover from the procedure and call in the late afternoon or evening. Following procedures or surgery on a Friday, you might call to check how recovery is going over the weekend. Taking patient phone numbers home with you for this purpose is not a breach of patient privacy or confidentiality. Remember, however, not to discuss patients or their care with anyone outside the office. That includes members of your own family and household and also members of the patient's family and household. Remember, no medical information should be discussed with anyone other than the patient. If you call a patient at home and someone else answers the phone, ask for the patient and offer no other comments. If the patient is not available, say, "Please say I called."

Trustworthiness

The most important personal characteristic of a professional dental assistant is trustworthiness. You must be able to keep confidential all patient information, whether personal, financial, medical, or dental, of which you become aware. Information that must be kept confidential includes the following:

- Identity of patients
- Procedures completed
- Conversations
- Financial arrangements

Always respect patient confidentiality. Safeguarding confidentiality goes back to the earliest traditions of medical care.

- Failing to maintain patient confidentiality is against the law.
- Betraying patient confidentiality can ruin the reputation of the practice where you work and your own professional reputation.
- A breach of confidentiality can result in legal action against all parties involved.

Cultural Diversity

Though respecting patient confidentiality is paramount, be aware that in Russia and other Eastern European cultures, some believe that if something is wrong with the patient, the family must know first. It is only after a family discussion that they will decide when and how much to tell the patient. They may believe that knowing too much about a condition can make the patient anxious and diminish the patient's spirits, making the illness worse.

HIPAA Regulations

The Health Insurance Portability and Accountability Act of 1996 (HIPAA) is a set of federal regulations governing patient privacy. You will give a great deal of thought to HIPAA regulations during your training and your time as a professional dental assistant.

- HIPAA regulations are intended to make it possible for health care providers to share important information about patients without infringing on patient privacy.
- Health information regarding medical histories, previous procedures, drug allergies, and other concerns must often be shared among health providers to prevent mistakes and ensure safe and effective treatment.
- HIPAA regulations protect patient privacy to ensure that this knowledge is never abused.

Finally, as a professional dental assistant, always hold yourself to the highest moral and ethical standards of behavior both at work and away. Remember that you represent your profession and are a model for it. (See Chapter 4, Ethics and Law, for more details about ethical and legal considerations, including a closer look at HIPAA regulations.)

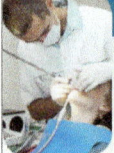

Voice of Experience

I know that patients expect a great deal of me as a professional dental assistant. They trust that I will do nothing to hurt them and that I'll look out for them whenever they're here. Part of looking after patients is safeguarding their confidential information. They trust that I'm not going to go all over town talking about what I know about them— what I know about their medical history, their financial arrangements, their dental work. For starters, violating patient confidentiality is against the law and can get me and the practice I work for in legal trouble. Beyond that, no one would trust us again. Patients have to trust us in order to sit in a dental chair and let us care for them. Violating confidentiality does not just destroy trust; it can end up denying patients the care they need.

CHECKPOINT

2-1 Patient confidentiality is protected by which set of federal regulations?

Professional Appearance

Numerous details may go into maintaining a professional appearance, but they are not time consuming or particularly difficult to keep in mind. Remember that maintaining a professional appearance shows your patients and colleagues that you take your work seriously and value the role you play on the office team.

A messy or unkempt appearance, on the other hand, gives coworkers and patients the idea that you might not care about the work you are doing. In addition, personal cleanliness in a dental office carries implications for infection control and prevention of disease. Your appearance is the first thing patients and coworkers notice about you, and judgments regarding you and the quality of your work will quickly follow.

Maintaining a professional appearance includes personal cleanliness, good grooming, and appropriate clothing, but it begins with overall good health. Any health professional serves as a model of good health to patients and colleagues. In addition, dental assistants perform work that is physically demanding. They must stay on their feet much of the day and must always remain alert during procedures and patient care. Adequate rest, a balanced diet, and sufficient exercise are essential. Other basics of a professional appearance follow from this.

Hygiene

- Take a daily bath or shower.
- Use deodorant.
- Maintain good oral **hygiene** of your own, including fresh breath.

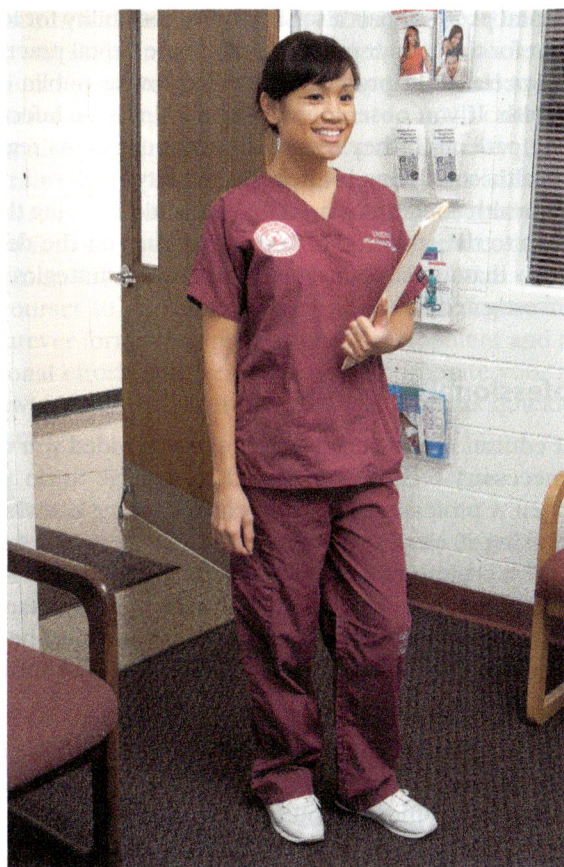

Figure 2–2 Maintaining a professional appearance in the dental office includes wearing professional attire.

Clothing

- If you wear a uniform to the office, make sure it is freshly washed and ironed (Figure 2-2). Clean, but wrinkled, uniforms are not acceptable.
- Unclean garments can harbor **pathogens** (germs and bacteria) that can pass along illness and disease.
- If you do not wear a uniform, avoid choosing clothing that is too trendy or suggestive.
- Make sure to wear appropriate undergarments under all clothing.
- Repair or replace any clothing that is torn or stained.
- Make sure to sew on any missing buttons.
- Shoes should be clean and polished. Make sure laces, if any, are clean and are the proper length.
- If your office allows sneakers to be worn to work, wear all-white ones.
- Check for runs or snags in any nylon hosiery that is part of your outfit or uniform, and replace as needed.

Hair

- Wash your hair regularly to make sure it looks and smells clean.
- Use clips or ponytail holders to style long hair back and away from your face.

Makeup and Fragrance

- If you wear makeup, keep it to a minimum and use lighter colors appropriate for daytime.
- Keep scented products, such as scented body lotions or sprays, to a minimum, or avoid them altogether. Limit use of perfume, because it may be offensive to others. Some patients or coworkers may not be able to tolerate strong scents and can experience allergic reactions.
- Avoid using tobacco products of any kind. Their odor permeates clothing and lingers in your hair.

Fingernails

- Keep fingernails short.
- Long fingernails interfere with dental procedures and can rip protective gloves.
- Long fingernails are difficult to keep clean. They are one of the main spots on the body to harbor pathogens that can pass along illness or infection to you or your patients.
- Nails should be neatly manicured, and any polish should be clear or light-colored.

Jewelry

- Keep jewelry tasteful and to a minimum.
- Limit earrings to a single pair of small studs.
- Remove or conceal any body jewelry.
- Wear rings with caution. Some can puncture protective gloves or interfere with procedures.

From the Dentist's Perspective

I take my time hiring a dental assistant. Through the years, I have learned how important they are to the success of the practice. If they are trustworthy, patients open up to them in ways they might not to me. They do have to look the part, though. When I interview, I make sure the dental assistant understands the importance of a professional appearance. It has to be there from the very beginning. When dental assistants are professionally trained, you do not have to explain how clothing, jewelry, fingernails—even shoelaces—can present problems with germs and bacteria. They already know to be careful and keep cleanliness in mind at all times. Along with appearance comes professional attitude. Professionally trained assistants make it a priority to get along with patients and with everyone here. We are a very busy practice. I do not have time to settle disputes or listen to needless complaints. But I do want somebody I can trust to come to me if something is really wrong.

Commitment

You and your colleagues on the dental team share a **commitment** to the success of the entire dental practice. Some dental assistants perform primarily administrative tasks in the reception and office areas of the practice. Others work mostly chairside with the dentist, assisting with procedures and patient care. Ideally, dental assistants would

5. Showing commitment to the success of the entire dental practice involves

   a. Focusing only on clinical tasks.

   b. Putting your best effort into all assigned tasks.

   c. Placing administrative duties ahead of all others.

   d. Performing only tasks that you truly enjoy.

6. Professional responsibility for patient well-being begins with

   a. Doing nothing to harm the patient.

   b. Educating the patient about proper care and hygiene.

   c. Notifying the dentist about any concerns you may have regarding the patient.

   d. Keeping examination rooms stocked and clean.

7. Professional standards of behavior require that you refrain from treating patients

   a. Who cannot pay for services.

   b. Who refuse certain procedures.

   c. If you are impaired by drugs or alcohol or by mental illness.

   d. Who are overly anxious.

8. Demonstrating compassion and empathy for patients includes

   a. Discussing your personal life with those you have known a long time.

   b. Becoming personally involved with them outside the office.

   c. Trying to talk them into treatments or procedures they are hesitant about.

   d. None of the above.

9. Continuing Dental Education (CDE) credits can be earned by completing any of the following *except*

   a. Home study courses.

   b. Audio and video seminars.

   c. Hours worked in a clinical setting.

   d. College courses.

10. The Dental Assisting National Board (DANB) outlines the ethical obligations of dental assistants to patients, employers, professional colleagues, and the public in a

    a. Code of Professional Conduct.

    b. Statement of Disciplinary Policies and Procedures.

    c. Standard of Care.

    d. Professional Development Examination Program.

Active Learning Exercises

1. Think about the ideal dental professional. What personal characteristics would be most important to you when working with your peers?

2. What kind of continuing education is required by the Dental Assisting National Board (DANB) in your home state? List how many credentials are required each year and indicate how you keep track of your credits.

Application Activities

1. If you are a dental assisting student in a formal program, consider a Student Membership in the American Dental Assistants Association (ADAA). Visit the ADAA website and find information on ADAA activities and benefits at www.dentalassistant.org.

2. Visit the American Dental Assistants Association (ADAA) website and look up the state chapter of the ADAA for your home state. When was the chapter established? Who serves as its president? Does it have an annual meeting near you that you can attend? What will be included on the meeting's educational agenda? Check whether the ADAA has a local chapter in your immediate area that might also offer opportunities for networking and education.

PREPARING FOR CERTIFICATION EXAMS

Review the topic "Professional Characteristics" in this chapter to prepare for the Dental Assisting National Board (DANB) exam.

The Dental Office Team

CHAPTER CHECKLIST

On completion of this chapter, students will be able to:

- ☑ Describe the characteristics of a dental office team.
- ☑ List the requirements to practice dentistry.
- ☑ Identify and describe the areas of emphasis of the nine dental specialties.
- ☑ Describe the general responsibilities of a dental assistant.
- ☑ Name and describe the various roles of a dental assistant.
- ☑ Describe the responsibilities of an expanded functions dental assistant.
- ☑ Describe the responsibilities of other members of the dental office team.

KEY TERMS

armamentarium – the instruments, equipment, and materials used for a procedure

chairside dental assistant – works on the opposite side of the chair from the dentist; mixes materials, exchanges instruments, and manages oral evacuation during procedures

circulating assistant – assists in whatever ways are needed in the office

certified dental technician (CDT) – credentialed by passing written and clinical examinations offered through the Dental Assisting National Board

dental equipment technician – repairs and maintains dental equipment

dental public health – dental specialty emphasizing prevention and control of dental diseases and promotion of dental health through community efforts

dental supply person – representative of one or more dental supply companies; takes orders and provides product information

detail person – representative of a specific company; takes orders and provides information about that company's services and products

endodontics (en-doh-DON-tiks) – dental specialty concerned with diseases of and injuries to the pulp

expanded functions dental assistant (EDFA) – a dental assistant who is able to provide additional specific chairside duties after meeting state requirements, which typically include taking additional course work in a state-approved program or a program accredited by the American Dental Association's Commission on Dental Accreditation (CODA) and passing an examination

general dentist – dentist practicing all phases of dentistry; often refers cases to specialists for specific treatment

oral and maxillofacial (mak-sihl-oh-FAY-shul) pathology – dental specialty concerned with diagnosis, causes, and treatment of diseases of the oral cavity

oral and maxillofacial radiology – dental specialty using imaging techniques to locate tumors, disorders, and other conditions affecting the head, jaw, and neck

oral and maxillofacial surgery – dental specialty concerned with diagnosis and surgical correction of defects, injuries, and diseases of the head, jaws, and teeth

orthodontics (or-thoh-DON-tiks) and dentofacial orthopedics (den-toh-FAY-shul or-thoh-PEE-diks) – dental specialty concerned with diagnosing and recommending treatment for all forms of poor alignment and malocclusion of the teeth or jaws

pediatric dentistry – dental specialty concerned with the dental care and treatment of children

periodontics (per-ee-oh-DON-tiks) – dental specialty concerned with the treatment of abnormal conditions of the tissues surrounding the teeth

prosthodontics (pros-thoh-DON-tiks) – dental specialty concerned with providing substitutes for missing, damaged, and malformed teeth

team – group working toward a common goal; members see themselves and their work as interdependent and are committed to each other's success

work group – group working toward a common goal; members generally focus on their own assigned tasks

Introduction

Think about times when you have worked with others toward a common goal, either in school or on the job. In some cases, you might have been part of what is called a **work group**: In working toward a common goal, group members' responsibilities and tasks might overlap, but much of each person's work is done independently. Although work groups can be very effective, the focus of each member is on completing his or her own tasks effectively and efficiently. As a result, the success of a work group is the sum of each person's individual contributions. Effective work groups need two more ingredients to become a **team**: a sense of interdependence and a commitment to each other's success.

From Classroom to Clinic

The staff of a dental office must function like a team, and knowing what role each member plays is important. Familiarize yourself with your role as dental assistant and carry out your particular duties to be a valuable member of the team!

When a group of people is working as a team, each member of the team is focused on common organizational goals. In addition, each team member is aware of how his or her special skills connect with and support the work of others. Team members are committed to each other's success. Team members pitch in and help others as needed so that together they can produce better results than if they focused on accomplishing just their own tasks. Being a member of a dental office team means that you understand your office's commitment to meeting client needs in the most professional and effective way. It means that you are willing to help out other team members. For example, you may help with instruments or charting to deliver quality service on time and in a client-friendly manner. It also means that you are willing to focus your efforts toward achieving the common goals of your office.

Dentists

Dentists diagnose and treat diseases of the teeth and oral cavity and repair fractured and disfigured teeth. In order to obtain a license to practice in the United States, dentists must graduate from a dental school accredited by the American Dental Association's Commission on Dental Accreditation (CODA) and pass a national written exam and written and clinical licensing examinations in the state they are going to practice in. Typically, a dentist completes an undergraduate education and goes on to study at a dental school, which includes both coursework and clinical practice on patients. When the dentist graduates, he or she receives either a doctor of dental surgery (DDS) or a doctor of medical dentistry (DMD) degree.

Along with the rest of the team in the office, dentists are responsible for following state regulations as defined in each state's dental practice act. Part of the dentist's role is to make sure all team members know and follow the legal requirements and regulations that affect their work. The dentist also plays a major role in establishing and maintaining office teamwork.

Dental Facts

In earlier centuries, barbers were also surgeons and dentists. Gradually, the professions separated; in 1745 the British Parliament dissolved the combination of surgeons and barbers.

Dental Specialties

General dentists are those who practice all phases of dentistry; however, general dentists often refer cases requiring more specialized treatment to a dental specialist. The American Dental Association (ADA) recognizes nine dental specialties, described in Table 3-1.

CHECKPOINTS

3-1 What is the main difference between a work group and a team?

3-2 What are the requirements to become a dentist?

3-3 How many dental specialties are recognized by the American Dental Association (ADA)?

TABLE 3-1 ADA Recognized Dental Specialties

SPECIALTY	MAJOR EMPHASIS	EXAMPLES
Dental public health	Focuses on preventing and controlling dental disease through community-wide efforts	Public health dentists might be involved in developing local health programs, providing dental screening programs, and promoting education programs.
Endodontics	Identifies and treats diseases and injuries to the pulp and surrounding structures	Endodontists perform all aspects of root canal therapy, including endodontic surgery.
Oral and maxillofacial pathology	Diagnoses and treats diseases of the oral cavity and surrounding structures	An oral pathologist might work with an oral surgeon to perform biopsies and provide diagnostic information.
Oral and maxillofacial radiology	Uses imaging techniques to locate tumors, disorders, and other conditions affecting the head, jaw, and neck	A dental radiologist interprets results from radiographs, magnetic resonance imaging, and ultrasound to recommend appropriate next steps.
Oral and maxillofacial surgery	Diagnoses and treats defects; injuries; and diseases of the mouth, jaw, teeth, neck, gingiva, and other soft tissues of the head	Oral surgeons commonly deal with wisdom teeth removal, facial pain, temporomandibular joint disorders, dental implants, and the removal of tumors and cysts. They are also able to offer reconstructive facial surgery.
Orthodontics and dentofacial orthopedics	Diagnoses and recommends treatment for all forms of malocclusion (poor alignment of the teeth or jaws)	Although an orthodontist is usually associated with fitting braces, he or she also addresses wider issues that might affect the bone structure of the face and jaw.
Pediatric dentistry	Focuses on the oral health of children from birth through adolescence	Pediatric dentists teach young people about the importance of oral hygiene. They specialize in helping children feel comfortable about visiting the dentist.
Periodontics	Diagnoses and treats diseases affecting the tissues that surround the tooth	Periodontists often treat patients who have plaque and calculus buildup, gingival disease, or who may have lost bone around a tooth.
Prosthodontics	Provides simple to complicated restorations of the whole mouth as well as treating facial deformities and aiding facial reconstruction using prosthetics	A prosthodontist may restore or replace natural teeth with crowns, bridges, dentures, and more.

Dental Assistants

Some who enter the dental assistant profession may have little or no formal training. More and more, however, those entering the profession complete a dental assistant training program. Educationally qualified dental assistants (DAs) in the United States graduate from a school accredited by the ADA Commission on Dental Accreditation. Accredited programs are usually 1 year long and include classroom, laboratory, and clinical content. Most states require dental assistants to have this kind of formal education. Certified dental assistants (CDAs) have completed an additional course of study and passed written and clinical exams offered through the Dental Assisting National Board (DANB) and must complete the required number of Continuing Dental Education (CDE) hours and examination annually to retain certification. In most cases, a formally educated dental assistant with credentials can perform all aspects of dental assisting consistent with state regulations.

Dental Assistant Responsibilities

As the name indicates, a dental assistant supports the dentist in various phases of the practice. In addition to caring for patients and assisting chairside, most dental assistants perform some administrative tasks during the course of the day. Whether you are a DA or a CDA, your responsibilities may include many or all of the following:

- Greeting patients and office visitors
- Answering the phone
- Instructing new patients on customary office practices
- Handling patient insurance forms
- Helping patients feel comfortable about their dental treatment
- Managing confidential patient medical, dental, personal, and financial information
- Maintaining examining rooms
- Keeping examining rooms properly supplied
- Assuming overall responsibility for infection control, including preparing and sterilizing instruments and equipment
- Scheduling patient appointments
- Communicating with suppliers and other team members about supplies, billing, and administrative matters
- Screening sales representatives
- Screening other office visitors
- Paying bills
- Billing patients and others

For additional information on working with patients and maintaining patient records, see Chapter 23, Communication, and Chapter 21, The Patient Record.

Extra Patient Care

It's the little things that count. For example, it's critical to check lab cases the day before a patient is to come in for a crown, denture, or other type of prosthetic insertion. It would be so inconvenient for the patient to travel all the way to the office only to find out that their crown or other insertion is not there. Imagine how you would feel if that happened to you. Let the patient know when you confirm her appointment that the crown or other device is in the office. That shows you are efficient and care about patient needs.

Dental Assistant Roles

Depending on licensing requirements and local practices, you may also take on certain specific roles. As you carry

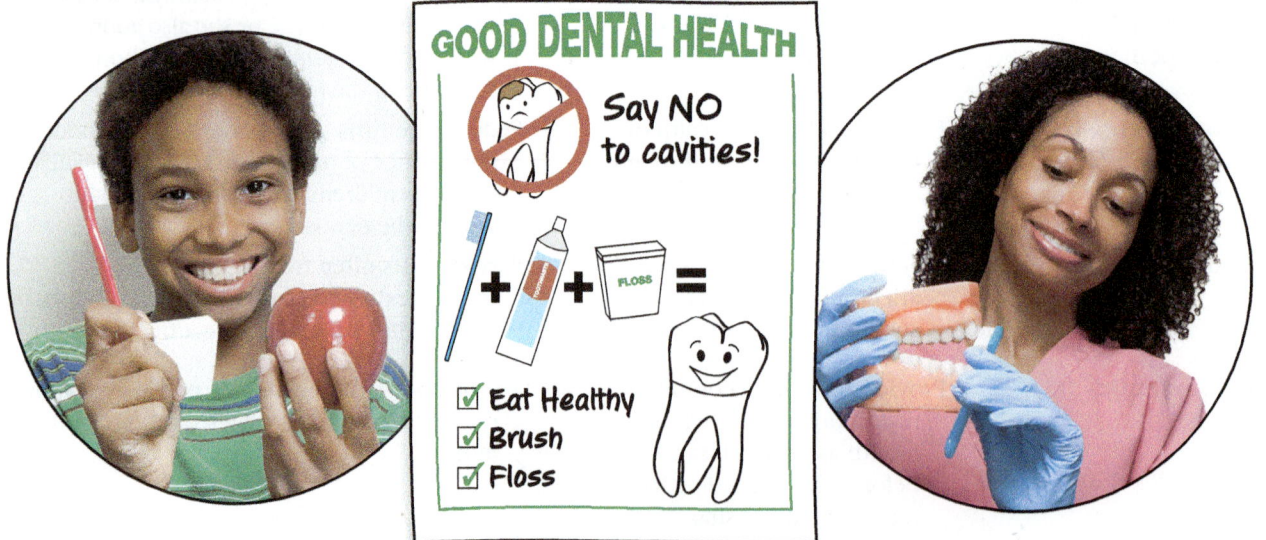

Figure 3–1 A dental assistant participates in a school education program.

out your work, you may find yourself in the role of **chairside assistant**. In this case, you and the dentist sit on either side of the patient's chair. Some roles may include these responsibilities:

- Obtaining and recording patient medical history and vital signs
- Preparing patients for examinations or treatment
- Sterilizing instruments
- Selection and preparation of **armamentarium** (the instruments, equipment, and materials used for a procedure)
- Administering medications or injections
- Maintaining the patient's chart
- Mixing dental materials
- Managing infection control procedures
- Pouring and trimming models
- Providing oral evacuation during dental procedures
- Exposing and processing radiographs
- Ensuring compliance with other safety regulations
- Recognizing and responding to medical emergencies

You may also serve as a **circulating assistant**, or floater. In this situation, you may help out anywhere in the practice where your assistance is needed, from preparing instruments to providing patient education.

Depending on the practice, you may become responsible for community work and participate at community health fairs or in school education programs (Figure 3-1). You might be responsible for managing infection control through the sterilization procedures and activities in your office (Figure 3-2) (see Chapter 14, Disease and Infection Control, for more information). You may also assume the role of business assistant and oversee the financial and record-keeping functions of the office (Figure 3-3; see also Chapter 47, Office Management). You may also have the opportunity to fill the role of dental hygiene assistant, supporting the work of the dental hygienist (Figure 3-4).

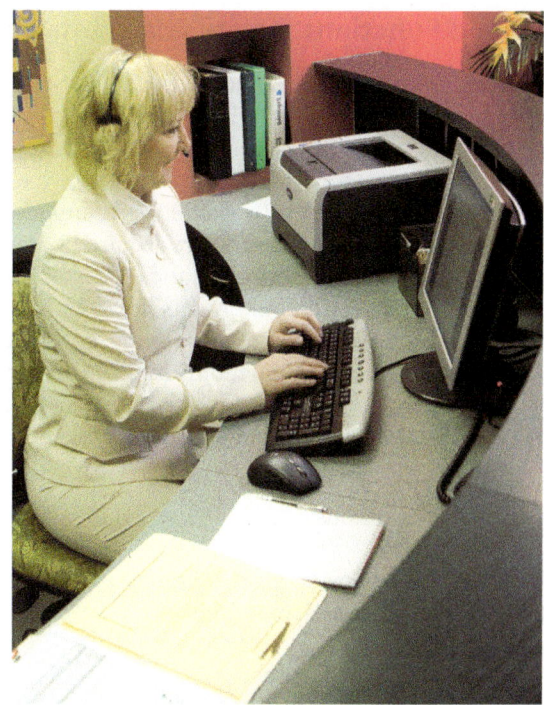

Figure 3–3 Updating computer records may be a task performed by the dental assistant.

Voice of Experience

When I first became a dental assistant, I wasn't sure that I would be able to perform all the roles in the office. I quickly learned that the best approach was to observe, ask questions, and listen carefully to suggestions. I started at the front desk, a great place to begin. By making patient appointments, becoming familiar with patient records, meeting suppliers, and observing the flow of activity in the office, I learned how the office responsibilities fit together. I then became a circulating assistant, helping out wherever I was needed and improving my skills at the same time. Taking continuing education courses has helped me become more versatile, boosting my skills and my ability to contribute to the team.

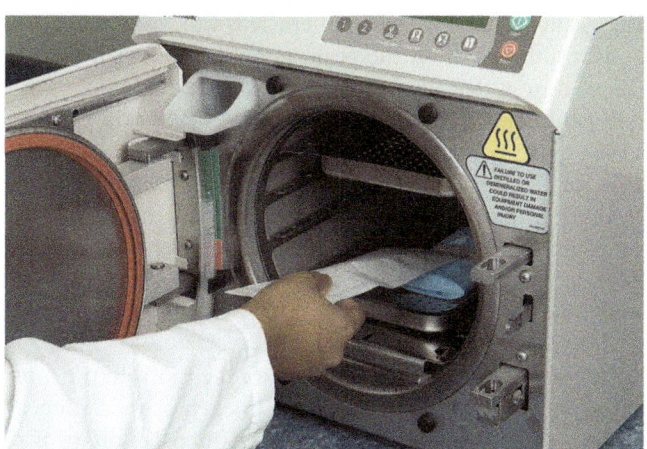

Figure 3–2 A dental assistant performs sterilization duties.

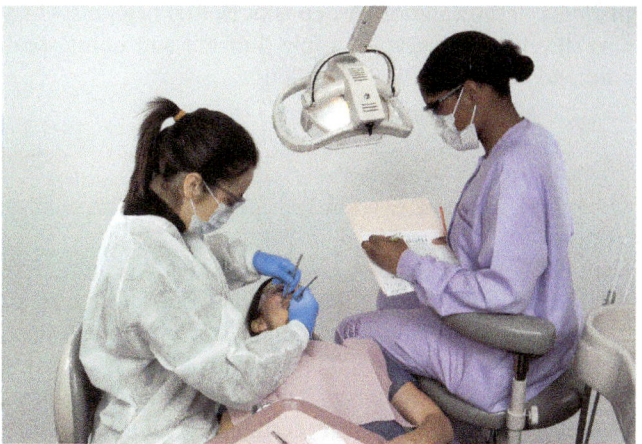

Figure 3–4 At times, the assistant may give support to the dental hygienist.

Expanded Functions Dental Assistants

Some states recognize and allow dental assistants to perform a number of other clinical care tasks, known as *expanded functions*. To become an **expanded functions dental assistant (EFDA)**, you must pass a state- or CODA-approved program offering EFDA training; complete a written examination; and, where required, complete a clinical examination or perform duties to demonstrate competency. Once these requirements are met, you may apply for licensure. Education and training requirements vary from state to state, as do definitions of the expanded duties. Depending on the state and your qualifications, as an EFDA, you might perform the following procedures:

- Placing dental sealants
- Obtaining impressions
- Removing sutures
- Placing and removing surgical dressings
- Placing and removing dental dams
- Applying fluoride
- Applying topical anesthetics
- Creating temporary crowns or bridges

Some dental assistants begin with a goal to fulfill a certain role in the office; others work in many different roles during their careers. A wide variety of roles is available to you as a dental assistant. See Chapter 48, Employment and Career Issues, for information about employment options and career planning.

Dental Hygienists

Most registered dental hygienists (RDH) have attended 2- or 4-year schools, received at least an associate's degree in an ADA-accredited program, and passed state written and clinical examinations. Although responsibilities vary from state to state, a dental hygienist usually provides patient education about oral health along with removing plaque, calculus, and other deposits. Dental hygienists may also develop radiographs, apply fluoride and dental sealants, and administer oral anesthetics.

Dental Laboratory Technicians

Dental laboratory technicians, also known as *dental technicians*, follow written prescriptions from the dentist to make crowns, bridges, and dentures from impressions taken by the dentist. Dental technicians may have learned these skills on the job or may have graduated from a 2-year, ADA-accredited program. A certified dental technician (CDT) has passed an additional examination to receive that credential. Although dental laboratory technicians usually work in a separate dental lab, they may occasionally come to the dental office to meet with the dentist and the patient. Their work is important to the success of the whole dental team. As a dental assistant, you will likely communicate regularly with the technicians to provide special instructions and information about the time requirements for a particular case.

Office Staff and Supporting Services

The dental office staff may include a receptionist, administrative assistant, and others who provide a variety of support services, including scheduling patient appointments, assisting with computer technology, and processing insurance claims. Others who are not in the office provide valuable services as well. A **dental supply person** represents one or more dental supply companies and will regularly call on your office to take orders or explain products. In contrast, a **detail person** represents a specific company, usually a pharmaceutical company or manufacturer, who will visit your office to discuss his or her company's products. **Dental equipment technicians** maintain and repair dental equipment.

CHECKPOINTS

3-4 What additional requirements must a candidate for certified dental assistant (CDA) certification meet?

3-5 What requirement must an expanded functions dental assistant (EFDA) meet?

Functioning as a Team

An effective dental office team is key to providing the highest quality patient care. A patient may not understand the responsibilities of all the team members, but that patient does know when his or her situation is handled smoothly and professionally. Are waiting patients taken on time for treatments? Are patient records up to date and readily available for the dental assistant, hygienist, or dentist? Is all the needed equipment sterilized and ready for the procedure or treatment? Is the treatment or procedure completed correctly? Are patient concerns addressed promptly and with the correct information? Is any follow-up or referral handled promptly?

When all members of the team do their jobs in the most effective way and are committed to each other's success, willing to help each other out, and focused on providing the best possible patient care, the answer to all of the above questions will be "Yes."

From the Dentist's Perspective

When I think of my office as a team, what comes to mind is how critical each person is in providing the level of service our clients expect. Purchasing quality products, creating well-fitting crowns, maintaining accurate patient records, providing patient-focused chairside care—these all are important to our success. I want people in my practice who appreciate the value other team members provide.

Check Your Ethics

Your coworker asks you to punch his time card for him tomorrow so that he can come in late. He has never asked before and has what seems to be a good reason for being late. You want to keep a good team relationship in the office but are concerned about his request. How will you respond to this request? Why?

Chapter Highlights

- When a group of people works as a team, each member is focused on common organizational goals, has a sense of interdependence, and is committed to each other's success.
- To practice dentistry in the United States, a dentist must complete an undergraduate education, graduate from an accredited dental school, and pass national and state examinations.
- The American Dental Association recognizes nine dental specialties: dental public health, endodontics, oral and maxillofacial pathology, oral and maxillofacial radiology, oral and maxillofacial surgery, orthodontics and dentofacial orthopedics, pediatric dentistry, periodontics, and prosthodontics.
- Educationally qualified dental assistants graduate from schools accredited by the American Dental Association's Commission on Dental Accreditation.
- Certified dental assistants have completed additional courses of study and passed written and clinical exams.

- A dental assistant supports the dentist in all phases of the dental practice. Duties vary depending on state regulations and the needs of the practice.
- Dental assistants often work chairside, mixing dental materials, managing infection control procedures, charting, and assisting with patient care.
- Circulating assistants help out in all areas of the practice as needed.
- A registered dental hygienist removes plaque and other deposits and educates patients regarding oral health care.
- A dental laboratory technician makes crowns, bridges, and dentures.
- A dental supply person represents one or more dental products supply companies.
- A detail person represents a specific pharmaceutical company or product manufacturer.
- A dental equipment technician maintains and repairs dental equipment.

Review Questions

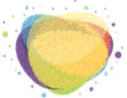

1. Which dental specialty performs root canals?

   a. Endodontics

   b. Pediatric dentistry

   c. Periodontics

   d. Prosthodontics

2. Which dental specialty interprets radiographs and magnetic imaging results results?

   a. Dental public health

   b. Oral and maxillofacial radiology

   c. Orthodontics and dentofacial orthopedics

   d. Prosthodontics

3. Which dental specialty would restore the oral cavity after an accident?

   a. Endodontics

   b. Oral and maxillofacial pathology

   c. Oral and maxillofacial radiology

   d. Prosthodontics

4. Which dental specialty would your community use to help create a dental screening program for children?

   a. Periodontics

   b. Endodontics

   c. Pediatric dentistry

   d. Dental public health

5. Which organization offers national certification examinations for dental assistants?
   a. Dental Assisting National Board
   b. Division of Dental Public Health
   c. American College of Dentists
   d. Commission on Accreditation

6. Which dental office position is most likely responsible for infection control?
   a. Dental assistant
   b. Dental hygienist
   c. Dental laboratory technician
   d. All of the above

7. Which is a responsibility of a chairside dental assistant?
   a. Removes calculus from the teeth
   b. Processes radiographs
   c. Manages patient financial records
   d. Maintains office dental equipment

8. Which dental office position follows prescriptions to create bridges and crowns?
   a. Dentist
   b. Dental assistant
   c. Dental hygienist
   d. Dental laboratory technician

9. What is the primary role of the dental hygienist?
   a. Plaque removal and patient education
   b. Ordering supplies
   c. Managing office finances
   d. Fabricating dental prostheses

10. Which person would provide information on a variety of dental products from several companies?
    a. Detail person
    b. Dental supply person
    c. Administrative assistant
    d. Dental equipment technician

Active Learning Exercises

1. Make a list of five dental supply companies that can be used for ordering dental supplies. Then list 10 critical supplies that would be ordered most often. Which companies have better prices?

2. Identify the roles and responsibilities of the dental assistant. List the differences between the expanded duty assistant and the assistant who does not have an expanded duty credential.

Application Activities

1. Select one of the dental assistant roles identified in this chapter. Make two lists. In the first list, write down the qualities, skills, and knowledge you have at this point that would help you succeed in that role. In the second list, include questions you have about that role for discussion with your instructor or classmates.

2. Visit a dental specialty office or research that specialty on the Internet. Make a list of criteria that makes that practice different from general dentistry. Based on research or observation, make a list of the roles and responsibilities of dental assistants in that office.

3. Research expanded functions dental assistant programs. What programs are offered and where?

Create a chart detailing specifics about each program: What are their requirements? What is the program content?

4. As a dental assistant, you will interact with all the other members of the dental office team. Think about how the way you do your job could help each of the other team members succeed in his or her job. For example, keeping accurate, legible charts helps the dentist and other dental assistants do their work more effectively. For each of the dental team members below, give at least one example of how the way you do your job could help that team member.

   Dentist
   Office administrative assistant
   Registered dental hygienist
   Dental laboratory technician

PREPARING FOR CERTIFICATION EXAMS

Review the topic "Dental Assistant Responsibilities" in this chapter to prepare for the Dental Assisting National Board (DANB) exam.

Ethics and Law

CHAPTER OUTLINE

CHAPTER CHECKLIST

On completion of this chapter, students will be able to:

- ☑ Define *ethics*.
- ☑ Identify four ethical principles and give examples of how they apply in a dental office.
- ☑ Explain the purpose of a professional code of ethics.
- ☑ Describe the steps involved in resolving an ethical dilemma.
- ☑ Define *civil law*.
- ☑ Give examples of express and implied contracts in dental practice, including how to document informed consent.
- ☑ Define *tort* and give examples of torts that might occur in a dental practice.
- ☑ Define *criminal law* and give examples of criminal behaviors that might occur in a dental practice.
- ☑ Explain the purposes of a state dental practice act, including scope of practice.
- ☑ Explain the "four Ds" of malpractice.
- ☑ List the key requirements of the Health Insurance Portability and Accountability Act (HIPAA) Privacy Rule.
- ☑ Define *risk management* and describe ways in which dental office staff behaviors can positively affect risk management in a dental practice.

KEY TERMS

abandonment – to withdraw protection, support, or help

Americans with Disabilities Act (ADA) – enacted in 1990; prohibits discrimination against those with disabilities and ensures equal access to employment, education, public accommodations, transportation, telecommunications, and all levels of government service

autonomy (aw-TON-ah-mee) – ethical principle of a patient's personal independence

beneficence (buh-NIHF-ih-senz) – ethical principle of the habit, intention, or practice of doing good

code of ethics – a set of rules or principles to be followed voluntarily by members of a profession; often based in part on a moral code of right and wrong

civil law – includes laws that address wrongful acts that are not crimes, for which the guilty party may have to pay a monetary amount

commission (act of) – the act of professional negligence and performing a treatment incorrectly on a patient or committing a wrongful act on a patient

confidentiality – legally protected right and responsibility of health professionals not to disclose information gained during consultation with or treatment of a patient

contract – voluntary agreement between two parties from which each party benefits

criminal law – includes laws that address wrongs committed against a person or society as a whole for which the guilty party may go to jail

dental practice act – title given to each set of state laws that regulate the dental profession

ethics – principles or guidelines for determining proper behavior or conduct and standards of practice

Good Samaritan law – state laws protecting people from being sued if they help an injured victim in an emergency

jurisprudence (juh-ris-PROO-denz) – the law as it relates to dentistry, professional malpractice, or the dental practice act

implied consent – principle that patient's consent has been given (implied) because the patient's action indicates he or she is accepting treatment (for example, opening the mouth when the dentist sits down)

informed consent – principle that patients have the right to know about and understand any procedure that is to be performed; usually obtained in writing

law – set of rules established and enforced by local, state, and national officials

malpractice – mistreatment of a patient through ignorance, carelessness, neglect, or criminal intent; professional negligence

memorandum of understanding (MOU) – a legal document describing an agreement between two or more parties

negligence – failure to perform duties or activities with due diligence and attention or to meet the standards of regular care; the failure to use due care or the lack of due care (omission and commission)

nonmaleficence (non-mah-LEF-uh-senz) – ethical principle of doing no harm

omission (act of) – the failure to perform a service that should be performed on a patient

protected health information (PHI) – includes all records that have information that could link their contents to a specific patient

reciprocity (res-ih-PROS-uh-tee) – agreement between two states in which each agrees to grant a license to practice dentistry to any person licensed by the other state

res gestae (REEZ JES-tee) – "things done"; the facts that may be used in evidence in a legal case, such as words or statements said by the assistant during treatment (for example, "Oops!"); these statements can be admitted as legal evidence against the dentist

respondeat (rih-SPON-dee-uht) superior – legal principle that means the head of an organization can legally be held responsible for the actions of those who report to him or her; the dentist is responsible for any harm caused the patient by an employee (dental assistant, registered dental hygienist, etc.) while carrying out the requests or expectations of the dentist/employer

risk management – practices in an office or business that minimize the potential for errors or legal action

tort (TORT) – wrongful acts or breach of contract for which damages can be obtained

Introduction

How do you decide the right way to behave in a given patient care or office situation? How do you obtain patient consent for a specific treatment? How do you know which types of patient communications are legal and which are not? What do you do if you suspect child abuse?

Each of these questions concerns common situations dental professionals deal with every day. The daily decisions you make as a dental assistant may involve your understanding of legal issues, ethical considerations, and local practice—and your personal experience. The more you are aware of the federal and state laws governing dental care and the ethics involved in making decisions about how you practice your role as a dental assistant, the more effective you will be for the patient, for your team members, and for yourself.

Ethics

Ethics are usually defined as guidelines for determining proper behavior. Personal ethics include the moral values and the understanding of right and wrong you have learned throughout your life. Professional ethics involve standards of behavior and practice that are generally expected of people in a career field.

At the very minimum, health care ethics require that you:

- Protect the privacy of patient information.
- Follow all state and federal laws.
- Be honest in all your actions.

You must always follow ethical standards as you perform your duties. Health care ethics require that your concern should always be for the rights, welfare, and concerns of your patients first. This means you should show *all* patients the same quality of care, kindness, and respect.

Ethical issues, though, are not always clear cut. Unlike legal issues, which are governed by laws that you must

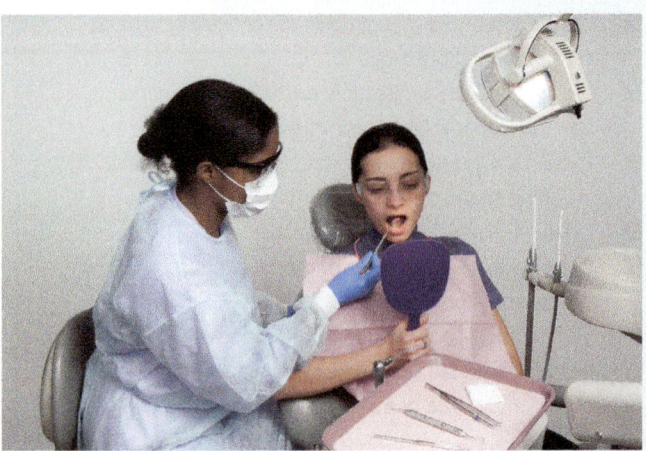

Figure 4–1 A dental assistant provides proper care to a patient.

follow, ethical issues often involve interpretation or "gut feeling." That is because ethics refers to what you *should* do, not what you *must* do by law (see later sections of this chapter on laws and legal requirements). However, dental ethical principles and codes of conduct provide guidance for making decisions about how you do your work and how you care for your patients (Figure 4-1).

Basic Ethical Principles

The basis for all health care ethics is the Hippocratic Oath, traditionally taken by medical practitioners. As one modern translation says, "May I always act so as to preserve the finest traditions of my calling and may I long experience the joy of healing those who seek my help." The themes of the Hippocratic Oath form the basis of the basic principles of dental ethics that will help you identify, clarify, and make ethical choices.

Nonmaleficence

The key idea in the Hippocratic Oath is to "do no harm." This is exactly what **nonmaleficence** means: Do no harm. In dentistry, this means everyone in the profession is bound by the ethical principle to do no harm. If a patient has an allergy to a specific kind of medication, you have an ethical obligation to note that in the patient's chart and work as a team to find an alternative.

Beneficence

Beneficence means to actually "do good." Acting according to this principle means going beyond not causing harm. It means taking responsibility for doing good—perhaps through community service work or treating an extremely nervous patient with extra care and patience.

Autonomy

Every patient has the right to be treated as an independent person. The principle of **autonomy** is based on the idea that people have freedom of choice and also have responsibility for their actions. In dental practice, this means patients have the right to participate in decisions related to their dental care and the right to refuse treatment, assuming that they have been properly informed on all the benefits and risks of treatment as well as any possible side effects.

Right to Privacy

The right to privacy or **confidentiality** is central to the conduct of dental professionals. Patients have the right to have their conversations with dental professionals kept confidential. Dental professionals have legally protected rights to keep those conversations private as well. The right to privacy of medical records is a key component of the Health Insurance Portability and Accountability Act (HIPAA) requirements, discussed later in this chapter.

Health care professionals have to be very careful to never reveal personal information about a patient, whether at work or not. Dental staff must be mindful not to have conversations about patients at any time, especially at the front desk or in other areas where other patients may hear what is being said. Remember, HIPAA also mandates that no information about a patient may be released unless by direct authority of the patient. Conflicts can arise regarding confidentiality, however. For example, most states have laws requiring health professionals to report suspected cases of abuse. In these cases, a patient's right to have personal information kept confidential may give way to legal mandates, such as in cases of child or older adult abuse. In addition, although not legally required to do so, dental professionals may feel the ethical obligation to assist in cases of suspected spousal or partner abuse.

Professional Code of Ethics

A professional **code of ethics** refers to the voluntary principles of conduct governing an individual or group within a particular career field. These principles of conduct usually develop over time and are often written down as codes of conduct. Codes of conduct are developed for many reasons:

- To make known the standard of care patients can expect
- To encourage ethical behavior as a responsibility among the organization's members
- To guide members in making informed ethical decisions
- To establish standards for professional conduct

The American Dental Association has its own *Principles of Ethics and Code of Conduct*. Just reading the *Preamble* will give you a good idea of the ethical goal of your profession: Knowledge, skills, and personal qualities are focused on providing care that benefits the patient.

American Dental Association

Principles of Ethics and Code of Conduct: Preamble

The American Dental Association calls upon dentists to follow high ethical standards which have the benefit of the patient as their primary goal … The Association believes that dentists should possess not only knowledge, skill and technical competence but also those traits of character that foster adherence to ethical principles. Qualities of honesty, compassion, kindness, integrity, fairness and charity are part of the ethical education of a dentist and practice of dentistry and help to define the true professional. As such, each dentist should share in providing advocacy to and care of the underserved. It is urged that the dentist meet this goal, subject to individual circumstances. The ethical dentist strives to do that which is right and good.

Reprinted with permission from the American Dental Association.

These overall principles are echoed in the American Dental Assistants Association's *Principles of Ethics and Professional Conduct*.

American Dental Assistants Association

Principles of Ethics and Professional Conduct

The member shall refrain from performing any professional service which is prohibited by state law, and has the obligation to prove competence prior to providing services to any patient. The member shall constantly strive to upgrade and expand technical skills for the benefit of the employer and consumer public. This member should additionally seek to sustain and improve the local organization, state association, and the American Dental Assistants Association through active participation and personal commitment.

Reprinted with permission from the American Dental Assistants Association.

CHECKPOINTS

4-1 Explain the difference between nonmaleficence and beneficence.

4-2 What are professional ethics?

Ethical Dental Business Practices

Ethical behavior includes all areas of dental practice.

Advertising

Traditionally, dentists and dental services did not advertise. Advertising is not illegal when the advertisements are truthful and not misleading; however, many once thought advertising a professional service was not ethical. These attitudes have changed. The current thinking is that advertising is a way of communicating with potential patients. When advertising is truthful about services, treatments, and the dental practice in general, it is now viewed as acceptable. You will find advertising for dental offices and services in phone books, on television, on the radio, and even on billboards. It is important to remember that no matter how many advertisements a dental office creates, the best advertisement is the quality care and the satisfied client that may lead to referrals.

Fees

Dental fees and charges are also guided by ethical decisions. It is appropriate for dental offices to charge for the services provided. Professional fees are based on what is common in that particular locale. Charges should reflect the level of difficulty of the service being provided. Dental offices can also charge for processing insurance paperwork and for a missed appointment when the patient has been reminded of the appointment day and time. It is good customer relations—and good business practice—for dental staff members to make sure patients

are aware of charges or fees before they occur. Think about how you feel when a service provider charges you for something you did not expect. Providing patients with information about charges and fees is another way of respecting the ethical principle of autonomy.

Patient Treatment

Dentists and all dental office staff have an ethical responsibility to treat all patients regardless of race, color, religion, country of origin, sexual preference, or current medical condition. It is unethical to refuse to treat someone whose background is different from yours or whose value system conflicts with your own. For example, you may have concerns about the way a patient dresses or the political views a patient discusses. Nevertheless, you need to put those concerns aside and provide the patient the same level of courtesy and care you provide to any other patient.

Ethical Situations in Dentistry

Because ethics involves generally accepted standards for behaviors and practices, rather than the rule of law, they are not as clear cut. Personal ethics and professional ethics can sometimes clash. When ethics and law—or ethical standards—differ, a dilemma can result. A dilemma is a problem caused by a conflict between choices. Often the choice is not between right and wrong but between several possible alternatives. In an ethical dilemma, the conflict is between rights, responsibilities, and values.

Resolving Ethical Dilemmas

Here is an example of an ethical dilemma: Suppose you work for a family dentist in a small town. The dentist has been serving the community for more than 40 years. He is now in his late 70s and is beginning to show signs of dementia. He forgets to review patient charts and has seemed disoriented and confused on several occasions. You respect the dentist and are hesitant to question his abilities. However, at the same time, you know that patients deserve high-quality care. You are concerned that the dentist's behavior may be affecting patient health and safety. Do you protect the dentist's reputation and license by keeping your thoughts to yourself? Do you ensure patient safety by talking about your concerns with the dentist or reporting your concerns to the state board?

The following is a way to think about this situation, or any ethical dilemma, in a way that will help you decide what to do:

1. Make sure you fully understand the situation that is causing the dilemma.
2. List your range of choices for action and examine each one. For each choice, first determine if it is legal. If it is not, eliminate it as a choice.
3. Determine the likely result of each action on each of the parties affected by the situation. For example, you

might decide to speak with the dentist first before contacting the state board.

4. For each choice, ask yourself if the harm done to some of the parties will be greater than the good done for others.

5. Chose a course of action that takes into consideration what should or should not be done ethically and professionally.

Following these steps will make the ethics of each choice clearer and the best decision much easier to identify.

Dealing with ethical dilemmas is not always easy, but experiencing them is a fact of life in any profession. Keeping in mind the ethical principles of nonmaleficence, beneficence, autonomy, and privacy will help you think through possible courses of action. Following the behaviors outlined in the American Dental Assistants Association's *Principles of Ethics and Professional Conduct* will help you resolve the inevitable ethical dilemmas that will occur.

CHECKPOINT

4-3 Under what condition is dental advertising considered to be ethical?

The Law

Governments have responsibility for protecting the welfare, safety, and health of all citizens. To do so, governments propose and pass **laws**, the set of rules established and enforced by local, state, and national officials. Laws often regulate certain kinds of behaviors for the general good. For example, laws regulate the legal age for smoking or drinking alcohol. Although there are many reasons why the ages are set where they are, one reason is health related: Smoking cigarettes and drinking alcohol at a young age may have negative physical effects on growing bodies. It is in the interest of society that such effects not happen.

Legal requirements may or may not exactly match up with ethical principles. For example, cheating on a certification examination is unethical and unprofessional, but it may not be illegal. On the other hand, illegal behaviors or actions in the health care context are usually also unethical. Practicing a dental function that may be performed only by certified dental assistants when you are not certified, for example, is illegal and also unethical.

Dental practice is governed by a combination of federal, state, and local laws. For this reason, it is important to know how laws affect the way you and your team members practice dentistry.

Types of Law

Laws passed by the U.S. Congress or state legislatures are called *statutes*. Laws passed at a local level—for example,

by a city council—are called *ordinances*. Taken together, statutes and ordinances form a body of law known as *statutory law*.

A government agency creates *administrative law*. Because administrative laws are not passed by legislatures, they are not statutes. Instead, they are called *administrative rules* or *regulations*. Violation of these rules or regulations can be considered as serious an offense as breaking a statutory law. The main purpose of administrative law is to provide details that make statutes clearer. For example, a state's dental practices statute may require a dentist to be a graduate of an accredited dental school. What exactly does that mean? Accredited by whom? Many groups rate and approve dental schools. In this case, the state dental board would create an administrative rule, or regulation, specifying the accreditation needed for a dental school's graduates to be licensed in that state.

The courts of the judicial branch are the third source of law. When judges decide cases, they first look at previous cases tried under the same law to determine how the law was applied. Those earlier decisions become *precedents*, or guides, that the judge applies in deciding the current case. Because this type of law comes from past court cases rather than from legislatures or government agencies, it is known as *case law*. It is also called *common law*, because it applies in all situations for which the facts are the same.

These three types of law—statutory, administrative, and case—depend on which group has made the law. There is another way of looking at the law: to whom or what it applies rather than where it began. Looked at this way, there are two broad divisions of law: civil law and criminal law.

Civil Law

Civil law involves relationships between individuals or between a person and the government. Civil law covers wrongful acts that are not crimes. Under civil law, such charges arise when one party (the plaintiff) claims to have been injured by the actions of another party (the defendant) and sues the defendant. Most civil suits fall into one of three categories: family issues (including divorce, child support, or custody issues), contract disputes, and torts. The last two types of civil suits are the ones you would experience as a dental professional.

Contract Law

A **contract** is a voluntary agreement between two parties from which each party benefits. If the agreement is spoken or put into writing, it is called an *express contract*. Contracts also can result from the behavior or actions of each party. This type of agreement is called an *implied contract*.

Here is an example of how express and implied contracts might occur in a dental office. Your first patient comes in to have a tooth pulled. You explain the procedure and the possible complications. You ask the patient to sign

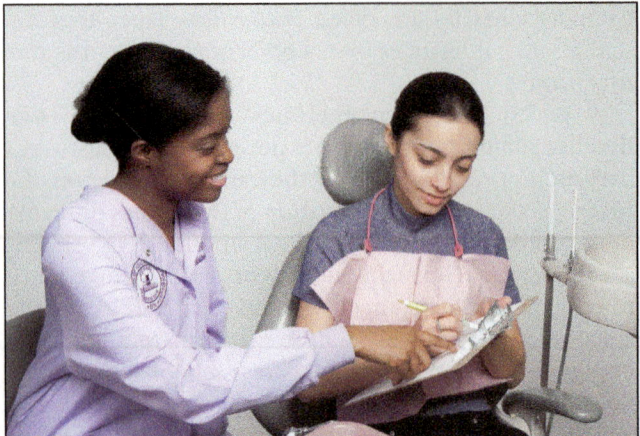

Figure 4–2 A signed consent form is also referred to as an *informed consent* or *express contract*.

an agreement indicating that he or she understands the procedure, is aware of possible complications, and agrees that the procedure should be done (Figure 4-2). This agreement is an express contract: a written agreement between the dentist as the service provider and the patient as the recipient of the service, also called **informed consent**. Your second patient has a toothache and wants to find out if he or she needs a root canal. The fact that the patient came in and allows the dentist to conduct an examination implies treatment is wanted. No written contract is needed in this case; this is an example of an implied contract, also called **implied consent**.

Another situation involving consent can arise when a parent calls the dental office to make a hygienist appointment for a child who is a minor. The calling and arranging of the appointment implies consent. However, a problem arises if, for example, after the hygienist completes that work, the dentist finds that the child needs a restoration and completes the restoration without calling or asking permission from the parent. In this case there is no consent, and the parent has the legal right to refuse to pay for the treatment, because consent to have a restoration done was not obtained.

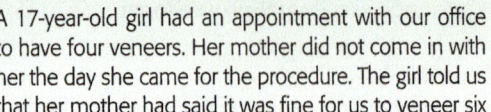

Voice of Experience

A 17-year-old girl had an appointment with our office to have four veneers. Her mother did not come in with her the day she came for the procedure. The girl told us that her mother had said it was fine for us to veneer six teeth. We went ahead and did the procedure. The mother threatened to sue the office because, despite what her daughter had told us, she had never given her consent to work on the other two teeth. This was a lesson for us: It is important to make sure to get signed consent and to make sure a minor is accompanied by an adult when getting treatment. At the time, the office did not have signed releases—we have them now.

Tort Law

Torts are wrongs committed against a person or property that do not involve violation of a contract. Intentional torts involve deliberate misconduct. There are several kinds of intentional torts; some may result in criminal charges as well as civil lawsuits.

- Slander: speaking lies about another person that harm the person's reputation. For example, if you tell your coworkers that you have heard one of the assistants is an alcoholic—even though you do not know for sure that this is true—then you have slandered the assistant.
- Libel: damaging a person's reputation in writing. If you make the same accusation about the other assistant in an email or in writing, the assistant can sue you for libel.
- Assault: threatening a person or acting in a way that causes the person to fear harm. For example, suppose you are trying to examine a squirming child. If you threaten to strike the child if he or she does not remain still, you have just committed assault.
- Battery: unlawful touching, whether or not the touching causes bodily harm. To avoid the tort of battery, you should never touch a patient without his or her consent. This does not necessarily mean that you have to ask permission, however. For example, if you approach a patient with a dental mirror and pick in your hands ready to begin an examination, and the patient opens his or her mouth, the patient has indirectly given consent.
- Invasion of privacy: in a dental office, this most often involves disclosing patient information. For example, if you were to discuss the details of an interesting case with friends at a party, you would be invading the patient's privacy.
- Fraud: any dishonest practice that is intended to deceive another person. In a dental setting, trying to convince a patient to accept a certain treatment when that treatment is not necessary would be an example of fraud.

One way to deny charges of wrongdoing is to show that it never took place. In such situations, the best defense may be the patient's chart or record. This is one reason why it is important that all contact with a patient be accurately recorded in the chart.

Criminal Law

The second division of law is **criminal law**. Although crimes are committed against individuals, criminal law exists to protect all members of society. Crimes are violations that can occur in two ways:

- Performing an action that has been banned such as driving while drunk
- Failing to perform an action that is required such as failing to stop for a red light at an intersection

Laws address two types of crimes:

- Felonies are serious crimes that are punishable by long prison sentences or even by death. Some of the more notorious felonies include murder, rape, kidnapping, robbery, and arson.
- Misdemeanors are less-serious crimes that are punishable by fines or short jail sentences. Examples include traffic offenses, stealing something worth a small amount of money, and disturbing the peace.

Some examples of criminal behavior that might involve a dental practice include abuse, embezzlement, fraud, and battery.

- Child abuse is a felony and one of the leading causes of death in children under 5 years of age. According to federal law, child abuse is any act or failure to act by a parent or caregiver that results in the death or serious harm to the emotional or physical health of a child, including sexual abuse and exploitation. As a dental assistant, you are professionally and ethically responsible for reporting any suspected abuse to the dentist (see Suspected Abuse Reporting Laws later in the chapter for more information).
- Embezzlement is wrongfully taking money or property that you are responsible for and using it for your own personal needs. An employee who steals money from his or her employer is committing embezzlement, which is a felony.
- Fraud can be a criminal offense as well as a civil one. Submitting a claim that you know to be false to a patient's health insurance plan is one example of fraud. Falsifying patient records can also be considered fraud in some cases. Fraud is a felony, too. A patient who has lost his or her job and dental insurance may ask the dental assistant to submit an insurance claim using a date when the patient was still employed; this is also fraud.
- Battery can be a criminal offense as well as a civil one. Examples of battery can range from acts such as striking an employee or a patient to various kinds of sexual contact. All such acts are felonies. If a pediatric or special needs patient needs to be restrained for dental treatment to be performed, the dentist must be very clear to the parent or guardian what they are doing so no misconceptions occur.

If you are aware of a crime and do nothing about it, your lack of action is also a criminal act. In this case, you would be considered an accessory: someone who does not actually commit the crime but who directly or indirectly contributes to it. Here are some behaviors that could cause someone to be charged as an accessory to a crime:

- Encouraging another person to commit a crime
- Witnessing a crime and doing nothing
- Helping cover up a crime after it has been committed

CHECKPOINTS

4-4 What is the basic difference between ethics and laws?

4-5 What is the difference between express and implied contracts?

4-6 Define and give an example of a tort.

4-7 List three ways someone could be an accessory to a crime.

State Practice Acts

Each state has drafted and passed a **dental practice act** that provides specific legal requirements and regulations governing those in dental practice. Although each state's act is specific to that state, each typically addresses the following issues:

- Requirements for obtaining and maintaining a license
- Requirements for continuing education
- Specific duties each member of the dental team may perform
- Recommendations for infection control
- Requirements for the use of radiation, anesthesia, and sedation

These acts also address which procedures can be performed by a dental assistant under general supervision and which must be performed only under the direct supervision of a dentist.

From Classroom to Clinic

Dental assistants must know the statutes and regulations in their particular states—and they must also be familiar with what they can and cannot do as part of their clinical internships outside of school. Many schools set up a **memorandum of understanding (MOU)** with their clinical affiliates. The MOU outlines students' limitations during their rotations. Find out if your school has a MOU and what it says about your role as an intern.

Scope of Practice

Dental practice acts define the *scope of practice*, or the tasks each dental practitioner is qualified to perform. In most cases, being "qualified" depends on the employee's level of education and training. For some, such as dentists, the scope of practice is determined by the laws governing the type of license held. States may also specify the scope of practice for dental assistants. Make sure you are familiar with your state's definitions and requirements.

State Board of Dentistry

A dental practice act also creates a state board of dentistry, whose responsibility is to interpret and implement state regulations. Members of these boards are usually appointed by state governors. Although the size and membership of the board may be different in each state, the board usually includes practicing dental assistants, dentists, and dental hygienists as well as members of the public.

Licensure/Registration

One of the most significant features of any state dental practice act is the licensing requirements. The state dental practice act spells out the requirements that dental assistants, dentists, and dental hygienists need to meet in order to obtain and maintain licenses or registration within that state. The act sets up requirements for state board examinations and for continuing education. Each state's act also explains the conditions under which a license can be renewed, suspended, or revoked.

Dentists, dental hygienists, and, in many cases, dental assistants must be registered or have certification or specialty permits in the state in which they practice. Some states also have **reciprocity** agreements with other states. Such an agreement allows a dentist or other licensed team member to practice in another state, usually without taking an additional exam. Reciprocity agreements often exist between states that share boarders or that have similar licensing requirements.

Respondeat Superior

Within a dental practice, the dentist is viewed as ultimately responsible for the work of all others in the practice. This responsibility is called *respondeat superior*, a Latin legal term that means "let the master answer" in situations that involve civil law. It is not a defense for your employer, but it can be an important legal protection for you if you are ever accused of a tort. For example, if you were to perform a procedure for which you had been trained and something went wrong, the dentist is ultimately responsible for your actions and their results.

This legal principle applies when the actions you take are within your scope of practice. You should always be on guard against acting outside your scope of practice. If you do, your employer generally will not be legally responsible for your actions. If the result is a tort, you could be personally sued, and *respondeat superior* would not protect you. For example, if, as a dental assistant, you administered local anesthesia to a patient, *respondeat superior* will not protect you in a court of law.

Even under *respondeat superior*, you are still responsible for your own actions, and an injured patient may file suit against you. For this reason, you might choose to have your own liability or malpractice insurance.

Some states allow the dentist to delegate certain tasks to a dental assistant or dental hygienist. How the dentist delegates these tasks is usually included in the state's dental practice act.

- Direct supervision: When direct supervision is required, the dentist can delegate specific tasks to a legally qualified dental assistant or hygienist or assistant, but the dentist must be physically present in the office when the task or procedure is performed.
- General supervision: Under the principle of general supervision, the dentist has authorized specific tasks to be done whenever needed by legally qualified members of the office staff. Under these conditions, the dentist does not need to be physically present in the dental office. General directions have been provided to the staff in advance. Exposing radiographs or re-cementing a temporary crown are examples of tasks that might come under general supervision.
- Immediate supervision: Under this principle, the dentist can delegate procedures to qualified members of the staff, but the procedures must be supervised by a licensed dentist who remains in the dental facility, personally diagnoses the condition to be treated, personally authorizes the procedures, and evaluates the performance of the assistant before the patient leaves.

Expanded Functions

Some states' dental practice acts include expanded functions (see Chapter 3, The Dental Office Team). These are specific tasks delegated to dental assistants who have advanced training or certification. The requirements for such additional training or certification—and the tasks that person may then be authorized to do—may be specified in the state's dental practice act.

Take time to become familiar with your state's dental practice act—it provides the legal foundation for your profession.

Patient Care Laws and Concepts

In addition to the general kinds of laws that regulate the dental profession, there are several specific laws or legal principles that directly affect the delivery of dental care, specifically issues related to patient care. These include the Americans with Disabilities Act, informed consent, standard of care, and Good Samaritan laws.

Americans with Disabilities Act

The **Americans with Disabilities Act (ADA)** of 1990 prohibits discrimination against those with disabilities and ensures equal access to employment, education, public accommodations, transportation, telecommunications, and all levels of government service. You can see many of the effects of this act in your office: A ramp or other method of access allows people access to your office; doors are wide enough to accommodate wheelchairs; and treatment rooms are large enough and are arranged to accommodate people with a wide range of disabilities. The ADA protects you and other employees as well: Your employer cannot make hiring and firing decisions based on a disability as long as the person is capable of doing the job.

Informed Consent

A patient must be aware of the risks of having a dental procedure, the risks of not having the procedure, and any alternatives that may exist. A patient's agreement to a treatment after being educated is called **informed consent**. The patient will be asked to sign a form indicating that he or she understands the treatment and possible risks. Obtaining informed consent is the dentist's responsibility. As a dental assistant, you owe a duty of care to the dentist to make sure that properly signed and dated consent forms are in the patient's chart before the treatment or procedure is performed. The dentist may also ask you to witness the patient's signature if that is needed.

If the patient is a child, the parent, custodial parent, or legal guardian must give consent. One approach is to ask in advance for the responsible adult's blanket consent for emergency treatments; obtaining written consent prevents a delay should a minor need emergency care when the responsible adult is not present. This can be of particular importance for children who are in school and may be transported to a dental office for emergency care. With this method, consent is already obtained in case of an emergency. Note, however, that this applies only to emergency care. For routine care, many legal advocates and dental insurance companies recommend that a dentist should not treat a child who is a minor without a parent or an adult guardian present.

Extra Patient Care

It is always important to make sure a patient has understood what will happen during treatment. This is especially true if the patient is having a critical procedure, such as anesthesia, extraction, or surgery—or when the patient is a minor. Take the time to double check to make sure everything was clearly communicated. Providing information or reassurance is an important part of the care you give to your patients.

Standard of Care

The **standard of care** is the ordinary level of skill and care that any dental care practitioner would be expected to observe in caring for patients. Like scope of practice, standard of care is closely linked to education and training.

For example, dentists are held to a higher standard of care than are dental assistants; this is because dentists have more training than dental assistants.

The dental assistant standard of care does not depend on your own skills and training. Regardless of your own background, the standard of care expected from you depends on what is reasonable to expect from most dental assistants.

Duty of Care

Duty of care is a part of standard of care. It refers to the legal obligation you have to your patients. For example, you have a legal obligation to keep a patient's health information private and confidential.

Abandonment

The relationship between a patient and a dentist is a contractual one. Although patients may sign agreements for receiving specific services, the ongoing relationship between the dentist and the patient is more of an implied contract: The patient comes in for regular appointments, and the dentist and dental staff perform needed services. Usually, the contract ends when services are completed. There are times, though, when a patient ends a relationship with your dental office by not returning to complete services. In cases like this, legally, the dentist should send a letter to the patient to confirm that the patient wants to end the relationship. It is important to record these efforts in the patient's file.

There are also times when a dentist decides to end a relationship with a patient. This can happen when the patient refuses to follow recommendations for dental care, does not keep appointments, or fails to pay bills. In each of these cases, the dentist must attempt to make contact with the patient; records of these attempts need to be included in the patient's record.

Ending the relationship with a patient without proper notice while the patient still needs treatment is called **abandonment**, and the patient can take legal action against the dentist. The proper, legal approach is to send a letter to the patient. As a dental assistant, you may be responsible for preparing the letter or making sure the patient's file includes all correspondence. The letter must contain the following:

- A statement that the dentist intends to end the relationship
- The reasons for this action
- A termination date at least 30 days from the date on the letter
- A statement that the patient's records will be transferred to another dental office at the patient's request
- A recommendation urging the patient to seek any additional care that may be required
- A statement that if a dental emergency occurs in the interim, the dentist will provide only emergency services until a new dental practitioner is engaged

The termination letter must be sent by certified mail with a return receipt requested. Make sure to keep copies of all correspondence and the returned receipt as part of the patient's record.

Malpractice

Negligence results from failing to act with reasonable care, causing harm to another person. Negligence can occur in either of two ways:

- **Commission (act of):** doing something a reasonable person would not do
- **Omission (act of):** not doing something that a professional person would do

When a professional person is negligent in his or her duties, this is known as **malpractice**: mistreatment of a patient through ignorance, carelessness, neglect, or criminal intent. As with negligence, harm or injury must result for malpractice to occur.

For a health professional to be sued successfully for malpractice, the plaintiff (the accuser or injured person) usually must prove four things:

- Duty—the responsibility to provide a reasonable standard of care to the patient
- Dereliction of duty—not providing a reasonable standard of care to the patient
- Direct or proximate cause—the direct or indirect cause of the patient's injury
- Damages—the harm suffered by the patient

Here is an example that illustrates the difference between negligence and malpractice: A patient arrived for an appointment to have a cavity treated and filled. This patient was previously identified as having a jaw shape that requires the dentist to inject a local anesthetic in a place that is different from the usual location. Although the patient's file includes notes about this unique situation, neither the dentist nor the dental assistant reviewed the notes. As a result, the patient received two injections, but neither one had the effect of numbing the patient's jaw. The dentist then reviewed the patient's chart, found and read the previous notes, apologized to the patient, and set up a new appointment for the work to be done.

In this case, the dentist and the dental assistant may have been negligent for not reviewing past notes in the patient chart. However, although the patient spent time in the dental office with no treatment being accomplished, no harm was done. Therefore, this would not be a case of malpractice. (It was, however, an oversight on the part of the dentist.)

Malpractice could have been an issue if the dentist had injected the patient with an anesthetic to which the patient had a known, life-threatening allergy; this would have been an act of commission, or performing an act that a reasonable professional would not do. If the dentist had not taken radiographs of the affected tooth or had ignored the patient's concern about the tooth, resulting later in an unnecessary root canal, that would have also been an act of omission, or not performing an act that a reasonable professional would do. In either case, a malpractice suit could have been the result.

Dentists and dental team members do everything they can to minimize the potential for malpractice. Doing so starts with understanding and abiding by the ethical principles described earlier in this chapter, following professional standards of care, adhering to all applicable laws and regulations, and establishing effective communication with other team members and patients. Minimizing malpractice possibilities can be traced back to the "little things": quality patient relations, accurate and complete charting, and communication among all members of the dental team (see Risk Management later in this chapter).

Good Samaritan Laws

In most states, the laws that regulate health care include a Good Samaritan act (a "Good Samaritan" is someone who unselfishly helps others). Good Samaritan laws protect people—including health care providers—from being sued for negligence if they help an injured victim in an emergency.

For example, suppose you are going to lunch, and you come upon someone who has been hit by a car. Your state's Good Samaritan act does not require you to help the person (except in Vermont). But if you do try to assist, the person usually cannot sue you if your aid does not help or causes more harm. In general, emergency care provided under a Good Samaritan law must meet a reasonable person's standard. This standard will be higher for a Good Samaritan who has medical training than it will be for someone with no medical training. Because these laws vary state to state, make sure you know the content of the Good Samaritan laws for the state in which you practice.

CHECKPOINTS

4-8 What is scope of practice?

4-9 Explain how *respondeat superior* applies to dental practice.

4-10 What is standard of care?

4-11 Explain how the "four Ds" of malpractice apply to dentistry.

HIPAA and Patient Records

In 1996, the U.S. Congress passed the Health Insurance Portability and Accountability Act (HIPAA), which sets standards for the way that patient information is recorded and handled. It also contains provisions designed to protect patient confidentiality. HIPAA requirements apply to all direct and indirect health care providers. Direct providers include hospitals, medical facilities, and dental offices. Indirect providers include laboratories and any services that deal with patient information.

This law has brought sweeping changes to the health care industry. Its original purpose was to

- Improve health benefits for workers who change jobs
- Reduce costs by streamlining the health care system
- Simplify the processing of health insurance claims

Standardized Code Sets and Claims Procedures

Code sets are the codes dental providers use for billing. Under HIPAA requirements, these standardized codes are revised every 2 years. The Current Dental Terminology (CDT) includes 12 categories; for example, Preventive (D1000–D1999) and Restorative (D2000–D2999) list the codes to use when billing for a variety of services in each category.

HIPAA also introduced other standardized procedures, such as submission of Medicare claims in an electronic format. If a dental provider files a Medicare claim, that filing would fall under this requirement.

HIPAA Privacy Rule

Over time, concerns about privacy and confidentiality became central to the way HIPAA was applied. As computers began to be used more widely for billing, keeping track of patient accounts, scheduling appointments, and entering and storing patients' medical information, concerns grew about the privacy and confidentiality of computerized records. In response, Congress added protections for patients' privacy when it passed HIPAA.

The law itself contains only a few privacy requirements. Instead, Congress empowered the U.S. Department of Health and Human Services (HHS) to issue rules that set standards for patient privacy. Because administrative rules have the same authority as statutes, they must be obeyed.

The HHS privacy rule greatly affects how a dental office must operate. Here are some of the rule's key provisions that are important for you to know.

- All records containing any items (called "patient identifiers") that could link their contents to a specific patient must be treated as **protected health information (PHI)**.
- Except as required by law or allowed by the privacy rule, PHI may not be disclosed to others without the patient's written permission.
- Only the information that is needed should be supplied in response to a request. For example, if an insurance company is being billed for a specific treatment, only the parts of the patient's medical record related to that treatment should be disclosed.
- Patients have a right to view and receive copies of their own medical records, except in very limited and specific circumstances.

- Patients have a right to know to whom their PHI has been disclosed, except in very limited circumstances.
- Each health care provider must have a privacy notice—a document that states its privacy policies and practices.
- Each health care provider must train its employees about the HHS privacy rule and appoint a privacy officer to be in charge of its enforcement.

HIPAA-Required Privacy Notice

- Must be provided to any patient who starts with your office
- States policies and procedures for protecting confidentiality and handling protected health information (PHI)
- Explains how the office handles PHI (for example, using patient's phone number to call with appointment reminders)
- Defines circumstances in which the office may disclose PHI without obtaining the patient's consent
- Outlines patients' legal rights regarding PHI and rights to object to its uses
- Provides contact information for the practice's privacy officer

Patient Identifiers

To completely protect a patient's identity, if any of these appear in a patient's record, the record must be treated as private protected health information.

- Name
- Address
- Zip code
- Phone/fax number
- Email address
- Date of birth
- Birth certificate
- Social Security number
- Medical record number
- Health plan number
- Driver's license number/photo
- Vehicle identification number
- Website address
- Fingerprints/voiceprints
- Photos

Check Your Ethics

You're at a party and meet a relative of one of your patients. He asks you how the patient's oral surgery went because he knew how nervous the patient was about it and is concerned. What do you say?

Confidentiality Exceptions

There are some exceptions to the rules governing privacy and confidentiality of records. The privacy rule lets health providers release PHI without the patient's permission in these circumstances:

- To a family member who is directly responsible for the patient's care; for example, if a mentally incompetent adult is cared for by an adult relative

■ To other health care providers who become involved in the patient's care; for example, to a dental specialist to whom the patient is referred

■ To attorneys, public health officials, and law enforcement authorities if required by court order or state law

Patients are required to sign a consent form that allows the dental office to release PHI to insurance companies for payment. This consent form is signed once and is valid for all following visits and treatments.

Dental Charts

Because the dental chart is the key document in the patient's record, it is critical that charts be accurate and complete—and that they be kept confidential. The patient's chart includes all the records of the patient's care and treatment except for financial records. Technically, the records included in the patient chart, including radiographs and prescriptions, are the dentist's property; in many states, however, patients have the right to review their records. Because patient records are acceptable in court, they must be accurate and complete.

■ Complete chart entries legibly and in ink.

■ Correct chart errors promptly and properly. To make corrections on a dental chart or record, do not erase any material or use correction fluid (such as, Wite-Out®). Instead, make corrections by drawing a single line through the error. Add the date and a description that an error occurred, and then write the corrections. Make sure the updated material is dated and signed (not initialed) by the dentist (Figure 4-3).

Keep charts for the proscribed amount of time for your state. Note that it is best to keep records indefinitely, because, in certain legal proceedings, the dental office may still need to produce records after the state time requirements have elapsed (Figure 4-4).

Some dental offices are now using computerized patient charts. An excellent storage option for these records is to have all the information placed on a disc or memory card, with one backup, and saved until the practice is dissolved and patients are contacted and asked if they would like their records. Computerized records are legal documents, too, and must be securely maintained and kept confidential. (See Chapter 21, The Patient Record, for detailed information on dental charts and other forms of patient records.)

HIPAA Privacy Rule Effects on Dental Office Practices

Think about what happens when a patient is waiting in the lobby to be called in for an appointment. As the dental assistant, you might open the door and call out the patient's name; doing so is not a violation of privacy under HIPAA, as long as no other patient information is spoken in the public area. But what if your patient is a child—can you go to the reception area and tell the child's parent that the dentist will need more time to complete the procedure? No, this is not allowed under privacy regulations because it would involve the potential for personal information to become public. In this case, ask the parent to come with you to the child's treatment room or find another private place for the conversation.

What if your patient wants to discuss paying the bill? Your office should be arranged so that the patient can talk with the person handling accounts without the potential for that conversation to be overhead by others in the waiting room (Figure 4-5). If no private space is available, use the dentist's private office.

How do you handle phone messages? You can call a patient's home and leave a message reminding the patient of an appointment scheduled the next day. However, you

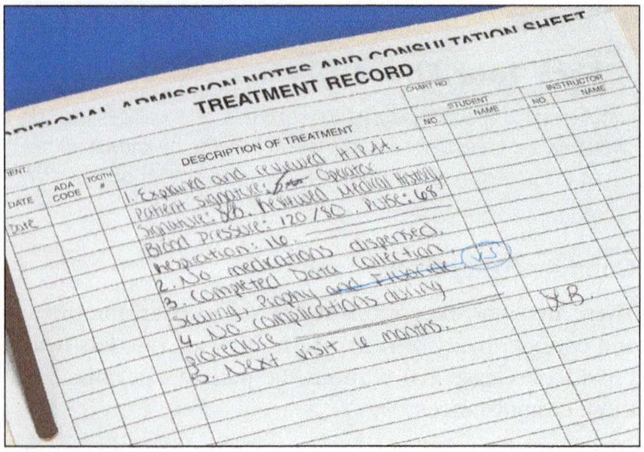

Figure 4–3 The patient record is a legal document and must be accurate.

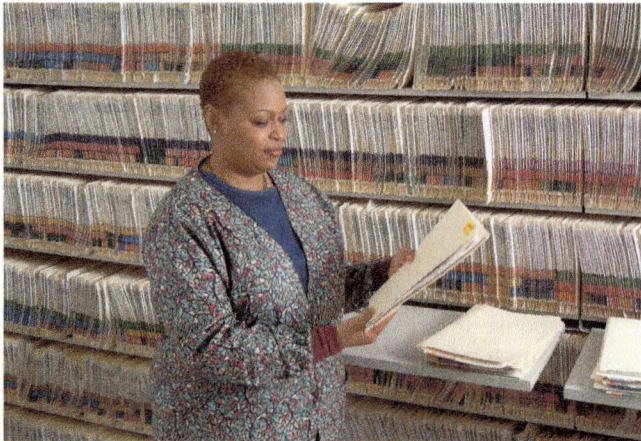

Figure 4–4 Patient records should be kept indefinitely for legal reasons.

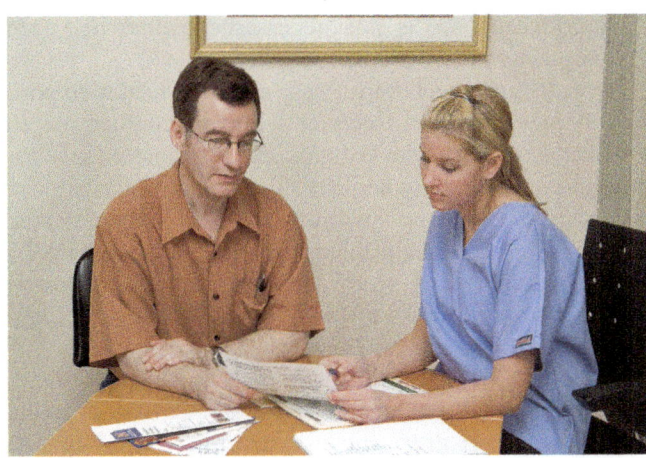

Figure 4–5 The business and waiting areas of a dental office should be clearly distinguished.

cannot say what the appointment is for or what treatment is needed. You also cannot leave information about the results of an examination or treatment on an answering machine. Additionally, you should never repeat a patient's phone number or any other PHI out loud if someone else can hear it.

How do you handle the patient records? Your office needs to be arranged so that the sheet showing the daily appointment schedule is not visible for everyone to see. Charts must be kept where they could not be seen by someone passing by. Many offices post a daily schedule within each treatment room that is covered with a blank piece of paper so that the information is out of view of a passerby. Copy and fax machines need to be located so that individuals passing by cannot see materials being copied or faxed. Cabinets or drawers where patient records are kept need to be locked whenever patient records are left unattended.

Enforcement and Penalties

The HHS Office of Civil Rights oversees enforcement of HIPAA requirements. The dental office staff, under the leadership of the privacy officer, is responsible for making sure all office practices are in compliance. If there is a complaint—and anyone, including employees, can make a complaint—you or your employer can be fined up to $25,000 for each offense. If you deliberately violated a patient's right to privacy, you could also be liable for a fine up to $50,000 and 1 year in jail.

Training

Complying with HIPAA is a demanding responsibility. You can easily see the value of having a staff member with the responsibility of being the privacy officer to make sure all office practices meet HIPAA requirements. The HIPAA administrative rules, your office practices, and your job

assignments change over time. For these reasons, ongoing review, in-service training, and additional classes for all employees regarding HIPAA, patient privacy, and confidentiality are critical. Additional training or disciplinary measures may be needed with employees who are not following privacy policies. Office disciplinary procedures should be part of the office HIPAA manual.

Suspected Abuse Reporting Laws

As health care providers, dental practice members are required by state law to report suspected abuse or neglect. Dental practitioners may be among those who see the results of physical abuse, because injuries to the neck or head are common; dental professionals may also observe behaviors that might suggest abuse.

- Child abuse: Suspected or validated child abuse must be reported by phone or in person at once, followed by a written report, usually within 72 hours, although laws vary from state to state.
- Spousal abuse: Most states do not require the reporting of spousal abuse unless the patient states his or her injuries were the result of abuse. However, all states have laws to protect victims of domestic violence. Some dental practitioners place spousal and partner abuse information and protective referral information in the ladies' room where the patient may receive this information privately, away from the partner.
- Older adult abuse: Most states require health care practitioners to report suspected abuse of older adults.
- Evidence of violence: In all states, health care professionals must report injuries that appear to have been caused by gunshots, stabbing, rape or evidence that suggests rape, or assault.

If you suspect abuse, your responsibility is to document what you have observed or been told, inform your supervisor, and report the suspected abuse or have your employer report the abuse based on the requirements in your state's laws.

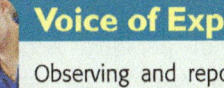
Voice of Experience

Observing and reporting suspected abuse is one responsibility of dental professionals. This can be especially difficult in cases of suspected abuse of older adults, which can be physical, sexual, emotional, and often financial. Everyone in our office has been trained to look for certain signs: physical injuries around the head, neck, and mouth; poor personal hygiene; withdrawal; and other kinds of behavior changes. In these cases, the older person is often reluctant to bring charges because the abuser may be a relative, and very often the older adult will deny it. In most states, reports of older adult abuse can be made to state agencies that help older adults. It's very important to know the abuse reporting requirements in your state.

Regulatory Agencies

In addition to the state and federal agencies and regulatory groups discussed in this chapter, other federal agencies also regulate aspects of dental practice.

- Occupational Safety and Health Administration (OSHA): This federal agency can issue standards and mandates that must be followed. Although there are currently no specific standards for dentistry, many OSHA requirements designed to protect safety and health also apply to dentistry. These include exposure to bloodborne pathogens, such as hepatitis and acquired immunodeficiency syndrome (AIDS); requirements for hazard communication; use of personal protective equipment; and sanitation procedures. In one specific instance, OSHA has determined that "since the ends of orthodontic wires can penetrate the skin, their contamination with blood can reasonably be anticipated. OSHA believes that they must be classified as 'sharps' … and disposed of accordingly." Orthodontic brackets are also classified as sharps, as is any broken or sharp instrument or piece of equipment. A broken glass vial, for example, should be disposed of in a sharps container.
- National Institute for Occupational Safety and Health (NIOSH): This research agency pays particular attention to preventing injuries in the workplace. For example, because dental offices and dental labs may use workplace chemicals, office staff members need to be aware of warnings and requirements for substances such as nitrous oxide.

See Chapter 14, Disease and Infection Control, and Chapter 15, Safety Regulations, for additional information about agencies such as these.

Risk Management

Risk management includes all those professional and office practices designed to reduce the risk of injury to patients and employees—and, therefore, the risk of lawsuit.

Personal Behavior

Risk management starts with personal behavior and responsibility. One of the best ways to manage potential risk is to know and follow professional codes and standards (see Professional Code of Ethics, discussed earlier). Being ethical and thoughtful in how you work with patients goes a long way toward developing positive relationships. Not only is this the right approach, it also helps to reduce the risk of patient dissatisfaction and possible legal action.

Treatment errors and other "bad acts" that harm patients can lead to lawsuits. These are three of the major reasons people file lawsuits:

- Poor outcomes: Sometimes, despite everyone's best efforts, the result is not what was hoped for or expected.

A bad outcome is not necessarily malpractice (see malpractice discussion earlier).

- Unrealistic expectations: These are often related to poor outcomes. Medical treatments and technology are so advanced that some patients expect more than what is possible. Then, when the outcome is not what was expected, patients can think they have been treated poorly. You can help manage patient expectations by explaining exactly what will happen during a procedure, what the risks might be, and what results could realistically be expected.
- Poor quality of care: Sometimes, a dental practitioner may not meet the duty or standard of care owed to the patient. Other times, the attitude and behavior of staff members may cause the patient to think acceptable care has not been provided. Following the ethical principles of nonmaleficence and beneficence will help you provide the best quality of care you can.

In all these cases—and sometimes with actual malpractice, too—the attitude of the people who work in the practice can make the patient more or less likely to contact an attorney. Sometimes, just acknowledging you have made a mistake—and saying you're sorry—is all the patient really wants to hear.

When You Make a Mistake

Everyone makes mistakes. When your mistake affects someone else—patient or coworker—this is the best way to proceed:

- Admit the mistake.
- Apologize specifically. Saying "I'm sorry" does not always sound sincere. Instead, say something like, "I'm sorry I forgot to process that payment right away."
- If possible, do something to fix the mistake. In the case of the payment, let the person know you are handling it right away.

Think about a time you were a patient and were not treated with the respect and consideration you deserved. How did that make you feel? Often, it is not what was done but how it was done that makes the difference. You can also think of this as, "It's not what you said, but the way you said it." Often the dental staff may be under stress, but it is never appropriate to take it out on the patients by speaking sharply to them.

- Scheduling appointments. Patients have no idea how crowded your schedule is. It helps to manage their expectations by offering one or two available appointment times. Many offices keep appointment times open for emergencies or build in to the schedule some time to catch up. It helps if you keep a positive attitude when trying to manage difficult schedules with patients.
- Waiting. When a patient has an appointment, he or she expects to be taken at that time. Although there may be valid reasons why the dentist or hygienist is

behind schedule, being made to wait makes the patient feel unimportant and inconvenienced. Keep patients updated about the status of their appointments and be realistic about the time. Offer the patient options, if available, when the dentist is running behind. If possible, contact the patient before he or she leaves work or home to let him or her know the dentist is running behind. This allows the patient to come in later or reschedule. Otherwise, let the patient know the situation as soon as he or she arrives. It might be possible for the patient to return at a later time. When you offer patients options, they are less likely to become upset, because they are taking part in the decision-making process.

- Overbooking. Some offices "double book" two patients in the same time slot or schedule patients very tightly. This can cause long delays for some patients. It can also lead to a very crowded waiting room. If this happens frequently in your office, the staff might want to consider more effective ways to schedule patient appointments.
- Patient records. Many patients feel that they "own" their records. Legally, the dentist must keep possession of the record. The office can make copies of a patient record if the patient is moving or being referred to a specialist, or if the patient is simply changing dentists. The dentist is allowed by law to charge a "reasonable" fee to do so. If there is a lawsuit against the dentist involving a patient, the dentist must surrender the original records and all parts of that legal record, including radiographs, study models, prescriptions, letters, mailing receipts, and, of course, the dental chart. Anything the doctor writes in the chart may be subject to subpoena, although this varies from state to state.

Documentation

Another way to practice effective patient care and avoid legal action is to document patient treatments and consent. As discussed in the section on Dental Charting, make sure all procedures, treatments, and referrals are documented in the patient's chart. All patient appointments and missed or cancelled appointments should also be noted in the chart. In addition, make sure each patient's chart includes signed and dated consent forms necessary for treatment. If a patient refuses an examination, treatment, or test, document the refusal in the chart. If possible, ask the patient to sign a statement indicating that he or she is refusing treatment and keep that statement in the chart.

Updating a patient's medical history is another role the dental assistant may assume under the direction of the dentist. In general, medical history should be updated every visit, even if the patient was seen last week. Always ask patients when you are seating them if there have been any changes in their medical history or the medications that they take. Then document this on the patient record and have the patient sign and date it in ink. This last technique could prevent a possible malpractice suit against the doctor.

There may be times when a patient's actions—such as not returning for scheduled appointments—negatively impact treatment outcomes. In these situations, contributory negligence can be used as a defense that claims the patient's own actions contributed to an injury or lack of treatment progress. Even if the health provider admits to negligence, if he or she can prove the patient was also partly at fault, the patient cannot collect damages.

Because patient charts are legal documents, keeping them updated and accurate is a necessity.

Professional Competence

Maintaining an appropriate level of professional competence also helps you manage risks. There are several ways you can keep up with current developments and demonstrate your professional competence:

- Read journals and newsletters
- Interact with other dental assistants and learn from them
- Obtain or maintain credentials through continuing education courses
- Participate in staff training if it is offered
- Attend professional meetings, conferences, and noncredit classes

> **Dental Assistant Behaviors That Reduce Risk**
> - Always act within your scope of practice
> - Treat all patients with courtesy and respect
> - Thoroughly document all patient contact
> - Maintain the confidentiality of all patient information
> - Never promise a recovery or cure
> - Keep equipment in working order and ready to use
> - Dispose of hazardous waste properly
> - Keep floors clean and clear
> - Open doors carefully
> - Acknowledge long waiting times and give patients reasons for the wait

In addition to maintaining confidentiality about patients and their records at all times, it is important to keep critical comments or concerns about treatment of office practices to yourself. Under the legal concept of *res gestae*, "things done," any comments made at the time of an allegedly negligent act can be admitted as evidence and may be damaging to you or to the dentist. Even seemingly innocuous statements, such as "oops" or "uh-oh," made by the dentist or the dental assistant while performing a procedure may cause the patient to lose confidence and believe that a serious wrong has occurred. These statements may also be used as legal evidence against the dentist in court.

From the Dentist's Perspective

Some years ago, a dental assisting student was working in our office as part of a clinical externship. The patient in the chair suffered a collapse. In the midst of the confusion and concern, this student told me she would go outside to meet the ambulance when it arrived and direct the ambulance crew through the dental office to the patient in the correct treatment room to help prevent any delay in emergency treatment. Because this student kept her head and reacted quickly to help the patient, I hired her when she graduated even though I didn't need an additional assistant at that time.

Preventing Malpractice

You can help your employer prevent malpractice lawsuits by following the "four Cs" of malpractice prevention:

- Provide *care* for patients
- Practice effective *communication* skills
- Make sure *charting* is thorough and accurate
- Achieve and improve *competence* by continuing to update skills and follow proper procedures

CHECKPOINTS

4-12 Explain and give an example of protected health information.

4-13 What must you do if you suspect child abuse?

4-14 Define and give an example of risk management.

Chapter Highlights

- Ethics are usually defined as guidelines for determining proper behavior. Medical ethics require that your concern should always be for the rights, welfare, and concerns of your patients.
- Ethical considerations in dentistry include nonmaleficence, beneficence, autonomy, and the right to privacy.
- Professional ethics refers to the voluntary principles of conduct governing an individual or group within a particular career field.
- Ethical behavior needs to govern all areas of dental practice, including advertising, fees, and patient treatment.
- Laws tell you what you must do; ethical principles tell you what you should do.
- Civil laws cover wrongful acts that are not crimes.
- Contracts are voluntary agreements between parties; contracts may be explicit or implied.
- Torts are wrongs committed against a person or property that do not involve a contract violation.
- Criminal laws protect all of society by banning harmful actions and requiring other actions to prevent harm.
- Examples of criminal behavior that might involve a dental practice include abuse, embezzlement, fraud, and battery.
- A state dental practice act provides specific legal requirements and regulations governing those in dental practice, including licensing requirements. It also defines the scope of practice, or the tasks each dentistry practitioner is qualified to perform.
- A patient's agreement to a treatment after being educated is called *informed consent*.
- The standard of care is the ordinary level of skill and care that any dental care practitioner would be expected to observe in caring for patients.
- If the dentist ends the relationship with a patient without proper notice while the patient still needs treatment, it is considered abandonment, and the patient can sue.
- Malpractice is mistreatment of a patient through ignorance, carelessness, neglect, or criminal intent.
- The Health Insurance Portability and Accountability Act (HIPAA, 1996) ensures the privacy and confidentiality of patient health care information.
- All records containing any items (called "patient identifiers") that could link their contents to a specific patient must be treated as protected health information (PHI).
- Because patient records are acceptable in court, they must be accurate and complete.
- As health care providers, dental practice members are required by state law to report suspected abuse or neglect.
- Risk management includes all those professional and office practices designed to reduce the risk of injury to patients and employees—and, therefore, the risk of lawsuit.

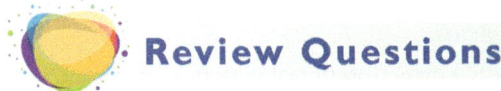
Review Questions

1. Which is the ethical principle to do no harm?
   a. Autonomy
   b. Beneficence
   c. Nonmaleficence
   d. Right to privacy

2. Which is the best first step to take to resolve an ethical dilemma?
   a. Consider if harm will be done by each choice for action.
   b. Determine the likely result of each choice for action.
   c. List your alternatives and examine each one.
   d. Make sure you understand the situation.

3. Which type of law is created by a government agency?
   a. Case
   b. Common
   c. Statutory
   d. Administrative

4. An implied contract can exist between two people when both
   a. Sign a document in which each promises to do something.
   b. Act in a way that indicates they agree to do something.
   c. Swear to their agreement in front of a judge.
   d. State their agreement in front of witnesses.

5. Which tort involves speaking lies about another person that harm the person's reputation?
   a. Libel
   b. Fraud
   c. Battery
   d. Slander

6. The range of activities a dental professional is qualified to perform is called
   a. Duty of care.
   b. Standard of care.
   c. Scope of practice.
   d. Code of conduct.

7. Which legal principle protects a dental assistant who has used a procedure he or she has been trained to use and something went wrong?
   a. *Res gestae*
   b. Autonomy
   c. Nonmaleficence
   d. *Respondeat superior*

8. Which law protects those who provide assistance in an emergency without expecting payment?
   a. Good Samaritan act
   b. Dental practice act
   c. Common law
   d. Civil law

9. A dental record is legally owned by the
   a. Dentist.
   b. Patient.
   c. State legal system.
   d. Dental association.

10. Which is true about patient charts?
    a. They cannot be used in court.
    b. They must be updated weekly.
    c. They must be kept confidential.
    d. They cannot be viewed by patients.

11. If you know that a crime has been committed and do nothing about it, your lack of action
    a. Protects you in a court of law.
    b. Is a violation of implied consent.
    c. Prevents anyone from getting in trouble.
    d. Is also a criminal act.

12. Behaviors that are unethical
    a. May not be against the law.
    b. Are acceptable to most people.
    c. Always lead to ethical dilemmas.
    d. Are usually still proper.

13. Unethical behavior in a dental office is likely to lead to

    a. Poor customer service.

    b. Fewer patients for the practice.

    c. Lawsuits.

    d. All of the above.

14. You can call a patient at home and leave a message

    a. To report the results of a medical test.

    b. To remind the patient of a scheduled appointment.

    c. To detail a scheduled procedure.

    d. With the patient's sister, explaining that the patient has an appointment for a root canal procedure the next day.

15. What should you do if you notice an error in a patient's chart?

    a. Write the correction in red pencil so everyone will quickly notice the new entry.

    b. Transfer all the patient information to a new chart and throw away the old chart.

    c. Draw a single line through the error, add the date and a description of the error, write the correction, and have the dentist date and sign the updated chart.

    d. Carefully erase the incorrect information and add the correct material.

Active Learning Exercises

1. Go to your state's Board of Dentistry website and look up its statutes and regulations (state dental practice act). Identify the legally delegated functions for your state. Make a list of the functions that both credentialed and noncredentialed assistants may perform.

2. Role-play the following scenario: Explain to a patient how the Health Insurance Portability and Accountability Act (HIPAA) is incorporated in the dental office and explain the office policy regarding confidentiality, privacy, and patient records. Have someone facilitate the scenario, take notes, and give feedback regarding the event.

Application Activities

1. Write a paragraph or two about how never leaving a patient alone in a room or alone with a dentist will help you prevent malpractice issues.

2. Research your state's chapter of the American Dental Assistants Association. Does your state association have its own professional code of ethics? If so, obtain a copy of the code and bring it with you to the next class period.

3. Think of a time when you had to make a decision that involved weighing several possible courses of action. Think about the process you used to come to your decision. Then, using the steps described in this chapter for resolving an ethical dilemma, explain to a partner how you would approach this same decision following those steps. Would your approach now be different? If so, how?

4. Assume that you are responsible for your dental office's compliance with the Health Insurance Portability and Accountability Act (HIPAA) privacy rule. You have been asked to develop the HIPAA-required privacy notice for your office. Using what you have learned about the HIPAA requirements, develop the privacy notice for the dentist to review.

5. As a dental assistant, you can help manage risk in your office. Based on your reading and experience, what is one key thing you could do to make sure you are practicing each of the "four Cs" of risk management and malpractice prevention?

PREPARING FOR CERTIFICATION EXAMS

Review the following topics in this chapter to prepare for the Dental Assisting National Board (DANB) exam:

- **The Law**

- **State Practice Acts**

- **Health Insurance Portability and Accountability Act (HIPAA) and Patient Records**

Dental Sciences

General Anatomy and Physiology

CHAPTER CHECKLIST

On completion of this chapter, students will be able to:

☑ Identify and define the terminology used to locate and describe different locations in the body.

☑ Identify and describe the four structural levels of the body.

☑ Name each of the body systems.

☑ Identify and describe the basic structures of each system.

☑ Explain the purpose and major function of each system.

☑ Identify common disorders of each system.

KEY TERMS

abdominal cavity – part of the ventral cavity; contains the digestive tract and related organs and structures

alveolar (al-VEE-uh-lur) sacs – grapelike clusters of alveoli within the lungs

alveoli (al-VE-oh-lie) – small, thinly walled sacs within the lungs that facilitate respiration and the exchange of oxygen and carbon dioxide

anatomical position – the position the body assumes when discussing bodily planes and directions

anterior – located toward the front of the body

atrophy – to decrease in size and strength and deteriorate in condition

autoimmune disorder – a mistaken destructive response by the immune system to the body's own organs and tissues

autoimmune response – the immune system's response to foreign cells, bacteria, viruses, and other substances

axial skeleton – one of the two main divisions of the skeleton; corresponds to the axial region of the body and includes the bones of the cranium, face, ribs, spinal column, and sternum

basal cell carcinoma – one of the two most common types of skin cancer

bronchi (BRONG-kee) – also known as *bronchial tubes*; connect the trachea, or "windpipe," to the lungs

bronchioles (BRONG-kee-ole) – small tubes that funnel air from the bronchi into the alveolar sacs of the lungs

cancellous (KAN-suh-luhs) bone – meshlike networks of light-weight intersecting bone called *trabeculae*; also called *spongy bone*

cartilage – a particularly strong kind of connective tissue that lacks any blood vessels; found where bones join and in parts of the nose and ears

cerebellum – region of the brain coordinating unconscious and conscious movement

cerebrum – region of the brain known as the "seat of consciousness"; origin of uniquely human reasoning and thought

compact bone – the hardest bone found in the body; also known as *dense bone*

condyloid (KON-duh-loyd) joint – one of six types of synovial joints

cranial nerves – operate between the brain and organs and structures of the head and neck

dorsal – toward the back half of the body

epidermis – the topmost layer of skin

fibromyalgia – a chronic condition characterized by widespread pain and stiffness of connective tissues

Hodgkin disease – also known as *Hodgkin lymphoma*; a cancer of the lymph nodes

homeostasis – the proper balance of conditions within the body necessary for its survival

hyperthyroidism – overactive thyroid

hypothyroidism – underactive thyroid

hypertension – high blood pressure

hypotension – low blood pressure

inferior – located below the transverse plane of the body, toward the legs and feet

Langerhans (LANG-er-hanz) cells – found in the upper layer of the skin, they protect the body against invasive pathogens

malignant melanoma – a particularly dangerous form of skin cancer

mastication – the act of chewing

metabolism – refers to the body's creation and use of energy

myelin sheath (MI-uh-lihn) – soft white material, made up of protein and fatty substances, that surrounds and protects some nerves in the peripheral nervous system

osseous (AW-see-us) tissue – the connective tissue that makes up bone

peripheral nervous system – nerves outside the brain and spinal cord that transmit and receive stimuli from inside and outside the body.

pharynx – the throat

posterior – toward the back half of the body

rheumatoid arthritis – an autoimmune disorder characterized by swollen, painful, stiff, and sometimes degenerating joints

squamous (SKWAY-mus) cell carcinoma – one of the two most common types of skin cancer

superior – located above the transverse plane of the body, toward the head

temporomandibular joint (TMJ) – articulation between the temporal and mandible bones

temporomandibular joint dysfunction (TMJD) – joint inflammation and dysfunction caused largely by stress-induced clenching and grinding of the teeth

tonsillitis (ton-suh-LIE-tihs) – an infection of the tonsils common in children

trabeculae (truh-BEK-yoo-lee) – the interior substance of spongy or cancellous bone; meshlike in structure and spongelike in appearance

ventral – toward the front of the body

ventral cavity – made up of the thoracic, abdominal, and pelvic cavities

Introduction

The work of a professional dental assistant goes far beyond an individual patient's oral cavity and teeth. While working chairside, the dental assistant considers the patient's entire health history, discusses any special needs or preferences the patient may have, and helps alleviate discomfort and pain. In order to address these issues adequately, you must communicate effectively with both patients and other members of the dental team. As nearly as possible, all must speak the same language. A professional dental assistant needs to know how the human body is structured and how its various systems work. An awareness of the numerous common disorders that might influence treatment, or be encountered during the course of treatment, is also essential.

Medical professionals acquire knowledge of the body and its systems through the study of anatomy and physiology. Anatomy refers to the structures and individual organs of the body; it is the "what." Physiology refers to the functions and purpose of structures and organs; it is the "why" and "how." This chapter explores both.

The Body

Learning about the structures and functions of the body means that we need to look at the body from a variety of perspectives. Breaking the body down into planes, directions, cavities, and regions can help us learn to locate and identify the different parts of the body. As we discuss these anatomical perspectives, we can picture a person standing in an upright position, facing toward us, with arms at the side, palms facing forward, feet slightly apart. This is referred to in medicine as the **anatomical position** (Figure 5-1).

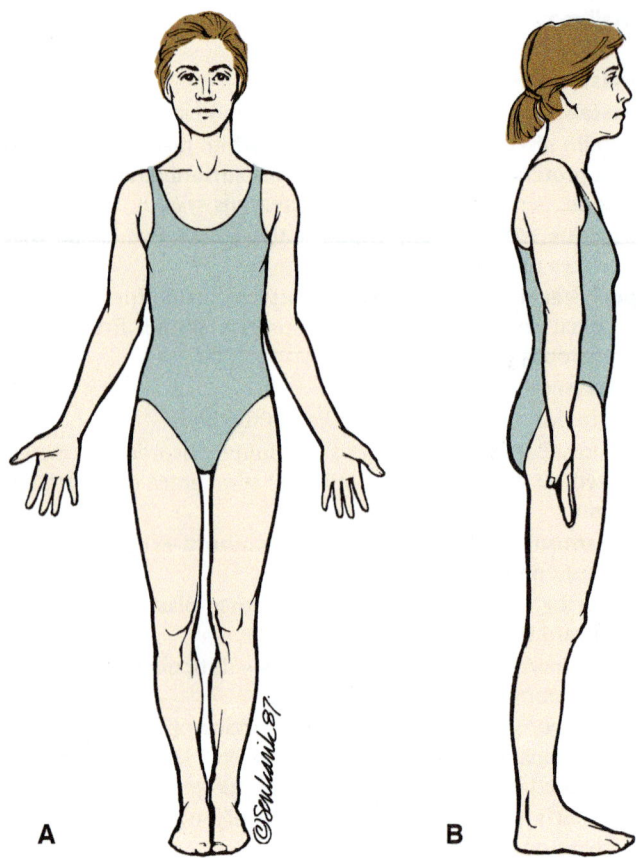

A   **B**

Figure 5–1 Correct anatomical position. A. Frontal view.
B. Lateral view.

Planes

Three lines, or planes, run through the body and divide it
into vertical and horizontal sections (Figure 5-2). The sagittal
plane, running down the middle from head to toe, divides the
body into left and right halves. The transverse plane, running

through the body horizontally, at about hip level, divides the
body into upper and lower sections. The frontal, or coronal,
plane runs from the middle of the top of the head to the
feet, dividing the body into front and back halves.

Directions

We use these planes to divide the body into pairs of opposite
directions, as outlined in Table 5-1 and shown in Figure 5-2.

When discussing patient care with other professionals
on the dental team, you may have to describe to colleagues
a particular tooth, physical characteristic, or abnormality.
Sometimes you may need to locate one of these features
yourself. The terms used to locate characteristics accurately and precisely, so as to avoid confusion, are listed in
Table 5-2.

Body Cavities

Body cavities are spaces within the body that contain
and hold secure its vital organs and related structures.
The body cavities are divided into two main sections in
front of and behind the frontal plane (Figure 5-3). The dorsal cavity is located toward the back of the body and is
made up of the spinal canal, which contains the spinal
cord, and the cranial cavity, which contains the brain. The
ventral cavity is located toward the front of the body
and is made up of three cavities of its own: the thoracic
cavity, containing the lungs and heart; the **abdominal
cavity**, containing the stomach, liver, intestine, and associated structures for digestion; and the pelvic cavity located
below, or inferior to, the abdominal cavity. The pelvic cavity contains the urinary bladder and reproductive organs,
including the uterus and ovaries in women and the prostate gland in men.

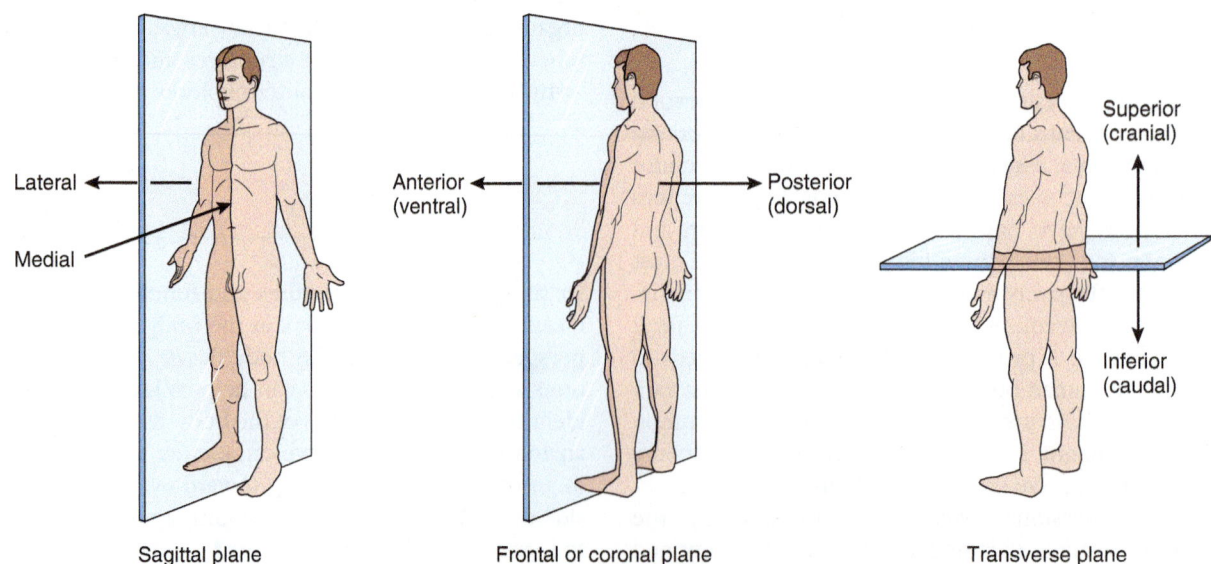

Sagittal plane   Frontal or coronal plane   Transverse plane

Figure 5–2 Planes are used to divide the body into pairs of opposing directions.

TABLE 5-1	Planes and Directions of the Body	
PLANE	**DIRECTION**	**DIRECTION**
Sagittal plane	Left half	Right half
Transverse plane	**Superior** or cranial (toward the head)	**Inferior** or caudal (toward the feet)
Frontal plane	**Anterior** or **ventral** (toward the front)	**Posterior** or **dorsal** (toward the back)

Body Regions

The body has two main regions. The first region, known as the *axial portion*, consists of the head (cranial region), neck (cervical region), and trunk. The second region, called the *appendicular portion*, consists of the appendages— the arms and legs.

Experts in anatomy (anatomists) divide these main regions of the body even further (see Table 5-3). For example, the top and back of the head is further divided into the cranial, parietal, and occipital regions. The front of the head is divided into the temporal (the temple, located just below the forehead on the side of the face), frontal (forehead), orbital (eye socket), nasal (nose), and buccal (mouth) regions. Anatomical regions of the head and neck are of particular interest to dental assistants and will be explored further in Chapter 6, Head and Neck Anatomy.

Nearby bodily structures, such as blood vessels or nerves, are often named after the region where they are found. For example, the occipital sinus is located near the lower back of the head; the superficial temporal vein is at the side of the head; and the supraorbital vein is just above the eye.

The arms and legs are also divided into smaller, more specific regions. The patellar region, for example, refers to the front of the knee; the femoral region refers to the upper leg or thigh.

Each vital organ of the body, and the major structures associated with it, also has its own special descriptive term or adjective (see Table 5-4). The term *pulmonary*, for example, describes anything associated with the lungs. The term *cutaneous* describes anything associated with the skin.

TABLE 5-2 Terminology Used to Locate and Describe		
DESCRIPTIVE TERM	**DEFINITION**	**ANATOMICAL EXAMPLE**
Inferior	Below, or lower than	The knee is inferior to the thigh.
Superior	Above, or higher than	The nose is superior to the mouth.
Posterior	Nearer to or toward the back	The tongue is posterior to the lips.
Anterior	Nearer to or toward the front	The heart is anterior to the spine.
Dorsal	Toward the back of the body	The shoulder blade (scapula) is on the dorsal side of the body.
Ventral	Toward the front of the body	The patella (kneecap) is on the ventral side of the leg.
Medial	Toward or nearer to the middle of the body or a structure	The heart is medial to the lungs.
Lateral	Away from the middle of the body	The arms and hands are lateral to the trunk.
External	Outside	The vertebrae of the "backbone" are external to the spinal cord.
Internal	Within	The lungs are internal to the ribs.
Deep	Within or toward the inside	The tonsils are deep to the pharynx.
Superficial	On or toward the surface	Gloves can help protect the hands from superficial injury.
Peripheral	Away from the main part	Peripheral arterial disease develops in blood vessels away from the heart.
Central	The main part	The central nervous system consists of the spinal cord and brain.
Proximal	Near or nearer to	The submandibular lymph nodes are proximal to the mandible bone (lower jaw).
Distal	Farther away from	The distal clavicle is the part of the collarbone farthest away from the neck.

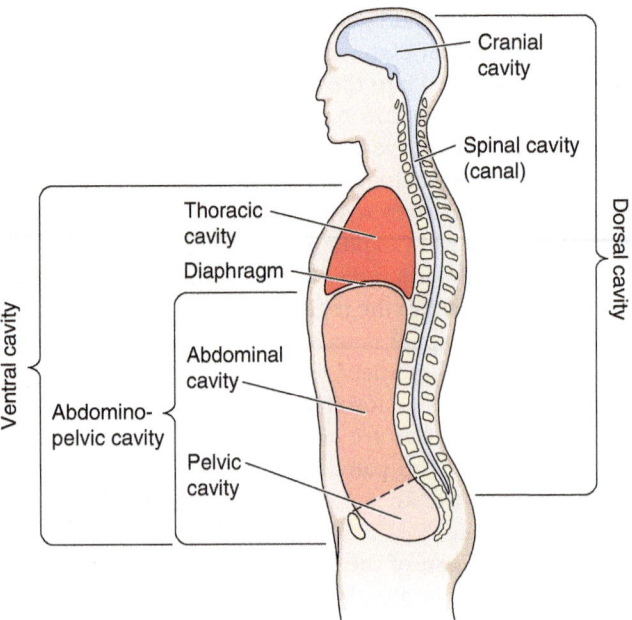

Figure 5–3 Body cavities, lateral view. Shown are the dorsal and ventral cavities with their subdivisions.

CHECKPOINTS

5-1 What is the meaning of the word *inferior* in anatomy?

5-2 What is the difference between something located in the patellar region and something located in the plantar region?

5-3 Cardiology is the study of what?

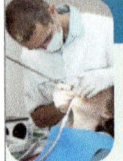

Voice of Experience

The teeth and oral cavity make up just one small arena of our amazing bodies. I was a little overwhelmed by my introduction to anatomy and physiology in my dental assisting classes. I wondered why I had to know about all these details. Directions, regions, body systems … The truth is, nothing in our bodies is separate from everything else. When I examine patients and note details about their self-care, the state of their teeth and gingival tissue, and their overall health, I can do it in a way that makes sure everyone understands what I am seeing and hearing. The language of medicine and professional dentistry is exact. By learning to use it, we can make sure the dentist looks at the same chipped or cracked tooth we do or notices the same skin change or swelling in the knee. Knowing something about anatomy and the way our bodies work keeps us all on the same page.

Also, I have known patients who began developing a disorder after we had been treating them for several years. One man developed Parkinson disease. The first sign of it was a tremor in his hands. Once someone in a business office had thought he was extremely nervous and asked him to calm down. He always felt comfortable interacting and talking with me, however. I knew about Parkinson disease and how it might affect him. Because he was comfortable coming to see us, we were able to keep helping him, and we still see him today.

TABLE 5-3 Major Regions of the Body

ANATOMICAL REGION	REFERS TO
Antebrachial	Forearm
Antecubital	Front of elbow
Axillary	Armpit
Brachial	Upper arm
Buccal	Mouth
Cervical	Neck
Cranial	Head
Deltoid	Shoulder
Femoral	Thigh
Frontal	Forehead
Gluteal	Buttocks
Iliac	Hip
Inguinal	Groin
Lumbar	Small (middle) of back
Mammary	Breast
Nasal	Nose
Occipital	Back of head
Orbital	Eye socket
Parietal	Crown of head
Patellar	Kneecap
Pectoral	Chest
Pedal	Foot
Plantar	Sole of foot
Popliteal	Back of knee
Sacral	Lower back
Scapular	Shoulder blade
Sternal	Breastbone
Temporal	Side of head
Umbilical	Navel (belly button)
Volar	Palm of hand

TABLE 5-4 Major Bodily Organs

ADJECTIVE USED	ORGAN DESCRIBED
Cardiac	Heart
Cutaneous	Skin
Gastric	Stomach
Hepatic	Liver
Pulmonary	Lungs
Renal	Kidneys

Structural Levels of the Body

When we look at a person, whether at ourselves in a mirror, a friend, or a patient in the dental chair, we usually see that person as one moving, functioning whole. All the anatomical regions described above blend into one another, and we see the person we recognize as our friend or patient. Rarely do we stop and think about the building blocks of life, and how we are actually put together. The body systems that enable us to live are built from three successively larger elements. Cells, the smallest functioning unit of the body, group together to form tissues, and tissues grow large enough to form organs. These organs and their interactions form our body's various systems. When these systems function properly together, they maintain what is known as **homeostasis**, or the proper balance of conditions necessary for the body's survival.

Cells

All structures and systems of the body begin with specialized cells. Cells differ in appearance and structure according to their function, but nearly all have similar basic features. A cell wall, or membrane, surrounds the cell and separates it from surrounding cells. The cell membrane controls how gases, such as oxygen and carbon dioxide, and other substances leave and enter the cell, and how hormones, such as insulin, interact with the interior of the cell.

The interior of the cell is composed of cytoplasm, a watery solution containing minerals, gases, and other materials. Some types of cell cytoplasm contain small, specialized structures called *cell organelles*. The organelles and other contents of the cytoplasm enable the cell to carry on all the processes essential to life. At the center of the cell is the nucleus. Each cell nucleus in our body contains the 46 chromosomes that both make us human and distinguish us from one another. Among the various types of human cells, only mature red blood cells lack a nucleus.

Tissues

Cells organize themselves according to their specialized structure and function into various types of tissues. To form the tissue, individual cells are bound to one another by an intracellular matrix or natural "glue." The human body contains four distinct types of tissue. Epithelial tissue forms the coverings and linings of the body, such as skin; connective tissue includes blood, bones, ligaments, and tendons; nervous tissue forms the brain and spinal cord. Muscle tissue takes three forms. Skeletal, or striated, muscle is attached to the skeleton and enables voluntary motion, such as lifting, running, and throwing. Smooth muscle is found in interior structures of the body, such as the walls

of arteries, where it helps maintain blood pressure, and the esophagus and intestine, where it helps move food and digestive products along. Smooth muscle normally functions involuntarily. Cardiac muscle is the muscle specific to the chambers of the heart, where it pumps blood to supply the rest of the body.

Organs

An organ may be defined as a group of tissues designed to accomplish a specific task. Among our body's most vital organs are the kidneys, heart, lungs, liver, and stomach. More than one of the four main types of tissue may help form an organ. The stomach, for example, is lined with epithelial tissue, but has walls of smooth muscle. Both types of tissue are essential to the stomach as it processes food.

Body Systems

Organs are organized into body systems. Each system has a specific purpose and uses specially equipped organs to accomplish it. Some organs are part of two body systems, where they may perform different functions.

CHECKPOINT
5-4 What are the three types of muscle?

Body Systems

Skeletal System

Like the body, the skeletal system (Figure 5-4) is divided into axial and appendicular portions. The bones of the cranium (skull), face, spinal column, ribs, and sternum (breastbone) make up the **axial skeleton**. The appendicular skeleton is made up of bones from the appendages—the arms and legs. These include leg, arm, foot, hand, hip, and shoulder bones.

Functions

The skeleton supports the body and sustains its shape. It provides a framework for the skeletal muscles that enable the body to move. Red bone marrow in the bones of the skeletal system manufactures red blood cells, white blood cells, and platelets. Children have the greatest amount of red bone marrow. In adults, marrow is found in the ends of long bones—such as the femur or thigh bone—and in the middle of other bones. As people age, yellow bone marrow, which is mostly fat and does not produce blood cells, slowly replaces much of the body's red bone marrow. Minerals, such as calcium, are stored in the bones themselves.

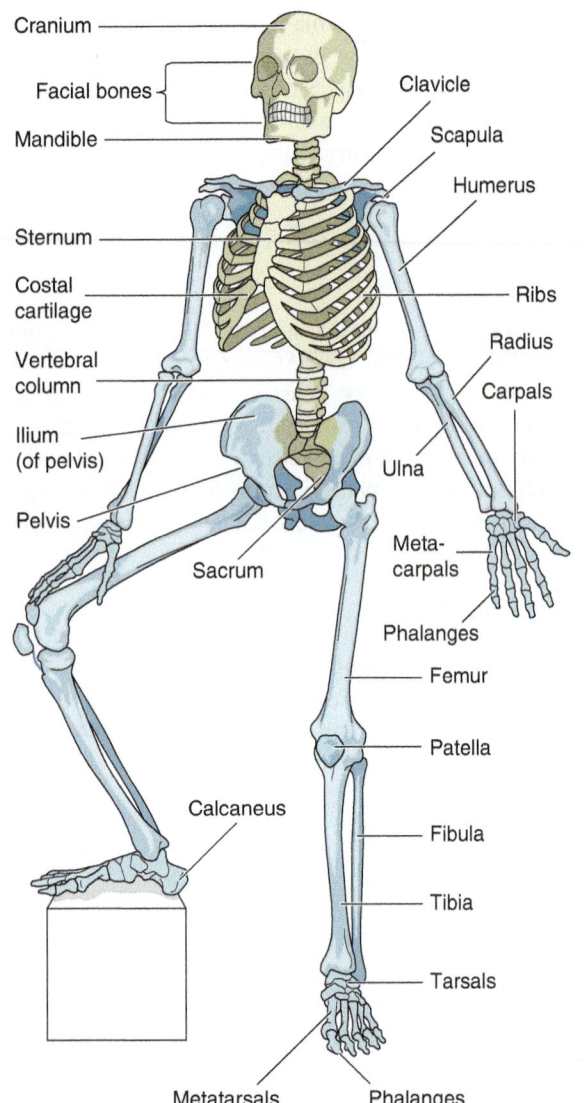

Figure 5–4 **The skeletal system is divided into two portions.** The axial system, shown in yellow, consists of the skull, spinal column, ribs, and sternum. The appendicular system, shown in blue, is made up of all the bones that are suspended from the axial system, known as the *appendages*, and consists of the arms, legs, hips, and shoulders.

Basic Structures

The skeletal system includes bones, ligaments, cartilage, and joints. Bone is made of a connective tissue called **osseous tissue** (Figure 5-5). Osseous tissue takes two forms: **cancellous bone** (also called *spongy bone*) and **compact bone** (also called *dense bone*). Cancellous bone consists of networks of intersecting bone called **trabeculae** that appear spongelike. The thin, interconnecting trabeculae of cancellous bone add strength to the bone without adding weight. Cancellous bone is found in the ends of long bones and in the middle of other bones. Red bone marrow is found within the meshwork of cancellous bone.

Compact, or dense, bone is the hardest section of bones. It forms the shaft, or long middle section, of long bones

and the outer layer of other bones. The center shafts of long bones contain yellow bone marrow.

The vertebrae of the spinal column (Figure 5-6), some of the most important bones in the body, are divided into five sections. Moving inferiorly from the base of the skull, they are the cervical, thoracic, and lumbar vertebrae, followed by the sacrum (sacral) and coccyx, or tailbone. Familiarity with the structure and proper positioning of the spinal column aids dental assistants as they position themselves chairside and seek to make their patients comfortable in the dental chair.

Cartilage is a particularly strong kind of connective tissue that lacks any blood vessels. It is found where bones join and in parts of the nose and ears.

Joints are found where two or more bones meet or form a junction. Joints are usually made of cartilage and other types of connective tissue. There are three types of joints: fibrous joints, cartilaginous joints, and synovial joints. Fibrous joints are made of fibrous connective tissue and do not move. The tissue that fills in and connects the skull plates of children as they age is an example of fibrous joints. Cartilaginous joints, on the other hand, are made of cartilage and can move slightly. The joints found between the vertebrae of the spinal column are examples of cartilaginous joints. Synovial joints take six forms and are the most familiar to us: ball and socket, hinge, pivot, gliding, saddle, and **condyloid** (Figure 5-7). They take their name from the synovial fluid within them, a transparent fluid that eases the joint's movement. Most of the familiar joints in the body, such as knees and elbows, are synovial joints.

A joint of particular interest to dental assistants is the **temporomandibular joint** (Figure 5-8). This is a gliding joint that helps open and close the mouth, and joins the mandible, or lower jaw, to the temporal bone above it. Also known as the *TMJ*, it is often the site of pain and tenderness when it becomes inflamed or dysfunctional. Some dentists specialize in the treatment of TMJ disorders, head and neck pain, and sports injuries to the TMJ area.

Common Disorders in the Skeletal System

One of the most common disorders in the skeletal system is **temporomandibular joint dysfunction (TMJD)**. The disorder limits jaw movement and causes significant pain and tenderness, sometimes accompanied by a clicking or popping sensation or sound in the jaw. Headaches and earaches as well as aches of the facial muscle, shoulder, back, and neck may accompany the joint pain. Muscle tension or spasm in the muscles surrounding the jaw can cause the pain, as can dysfunction or derangement of the joint itself. See Chapter 6, Head and Neck Anatomy, for more information about TMJD, including a detailed description of the TMJ.

Fractures are breaks in the bone or cartilage and are often referred to as "broken bones." Fractures are usually treated by immobilizing the broken bone, sometimes in a cast, sling,

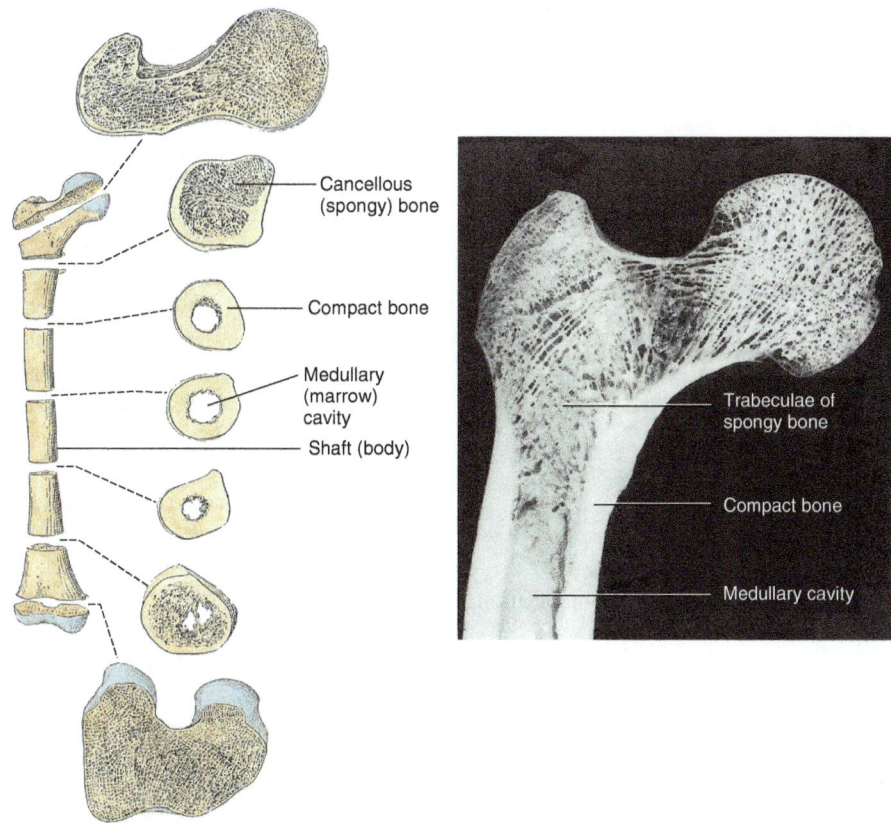

Figure 5–5 **Bone or osseous tissue is found in two forms:** cancellous bone and compact bone.

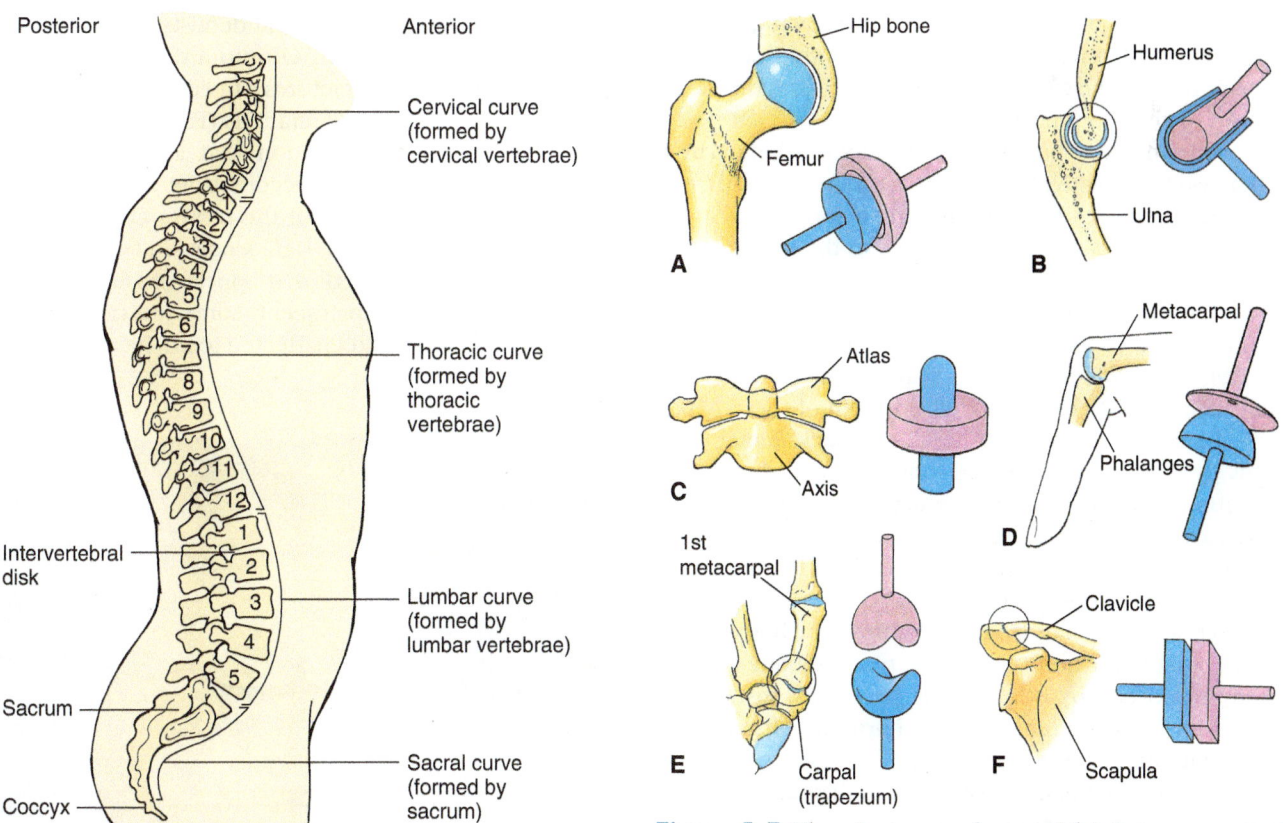

Figure 5–6 Vertebrae of the spinal column.

Figure 5–7 **The six types of synovial joints are named for the movement they allow. A.** Ball and socket. **B.** Hinge. **C.** Pivot. **D.** Condyloid. **E.** Saddle. **F.** Gliding.

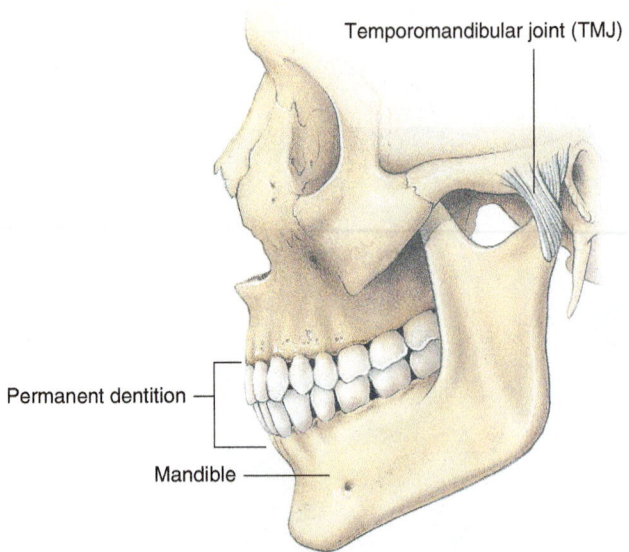

Temporomandibular joint (TMJ)

Permanent dentition —

Mandible —

Figure 5–8 The temporomandibular joint is a combination hinge and glide type of synovial joint.

or brace. Displaced fractures, where the pieces of broken bone have shifted out of position, must often be treated surgically. Patients who visit a dental office while in treatment for a fracture may require special consideration for positioning in the dental chair. When updating the patient's health history prior to treatment, it is appropriate to inquire about any medication the patient may be using to address pain.

Cleft palate is a congenital condition, meaning that it is present at birth. Cleft palate occurs when the sections of densely fused bone called *maxillae*, which form the palate or roof of the mouth, fail to unite properly. A cleft palate can occur on one or both sides of the mouth. Cleft palate is often associated with cleft lip, which results from failure of the nasal processes to unite properly before birth. A cleft lip may appear as only a slight notch in the lip, or it may be a complete split that extends all the way to the base of the nose. Current access to modern medicine usually enables these conditions to be repaired by age 1 year or even younger. Nonetheless, you may encounter both adult and pediatric patients with either or both of these conditions. Some individuals may hesitate to seek dental treatment or may experience self-consciousness about their condition when they do. As with all patients, a professional dental assistant uses communication skills to reassure and help patients with cleft lip or palate feel at ease, regardless of physical conditions or limitations.

Osteoporosis results from the failure of the body to produce enough new bone to take the place of bone that has been reabsorbed by other bodily processes. Insufficient dietary intake of calcium as well as hormonal changes that occur with menopause can make osteoporosis more likely. Though most common in women older than age 50, osteoporosis can occur in either gender and at any age. One of its symptoms is low back pain, sometimes as the result of fractured vertebrae. Exercising caution while positioning

patients with osteoporosis in the dental chair and remaining aware of the potential for fracture in unusually brittle and fragile bones can help dental assistants avoid causing unnecessary discomfort or even injury.

Osteomyelitis is an acute or chronic bone infection normally caused by bacteria. The infection that causes it usually originates in another part of the body and reaches the bone through the blood supply. In children, osteomyelitis most often occurs in the long bones; in adults, it is more likely to occur in pelvic bones and vertebrae. Dental assistants should note that the disease can alter the results of radiographs taken of joints, such as the TMJ. Osteomyelitis is normally treated with antibiotics, although surgery is sometimes necessary.

Osteogenesis imperfecta (OI) is a genetically acquired condition present at birth. It is usually caused by a defect in a gene that produces type 1 collagen, an important component of developing bone. OI varies in severity, and, depending on its type, signs of it may not appear for years. Like osteoporosis, OI causes weak and brittle bones but for different reasons. Whether pediatric or adult, patients with OI may be unusually short in stature; have a blue tint to the whites of their eyes; have legs that appear bowed; use assistive devices, such as crutches, canes, or walkers to get around; and experience early hearing loss. Recognizing signs of hearing loss as well as other signs of OI can help you communicate more effectively with patients. Among other concerns in the dental office, the condition may affect the ability of patients to readily adjust to seating requirements. Dental assistants, hygienists, and dentists must never force the limbs of patients with OI into a desired position for treatment or imaging. Fractures can very easily occur.

Dentinogenesis imperfecta (DI) (Figure 5-9) is another genetically acquired condition that accompanies some cases of OI and can also occur on its own. Dentin, the material that forms much of the tooth's crown and root, is rich in type 1 collagen. Deficiencies in type 1 collagen production result in teeth that appear misshapen, brown, purple, or thin and opalescent. Some individuals have a mixture of affected and unaffected teeth. Teeth affected by

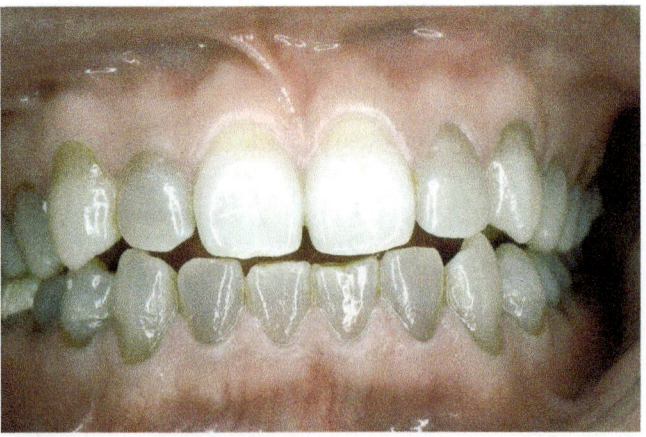

Figure 5–9 Dentinogenesis imperfecta is a genetic disorder.

DI chip, break, and decay easily. Radiographs may reveal narrow roots and narrow or absent pulp chambers. Children as young as age 6 months who are known to have OI may visit dentists to be screened for DI. Treatments for DI are largely cosmetic or restorative and depend on the severity of the condition and the age of the patient.

Muscular System

The more than 600 muscles found throughout the body make up 30% to 40% of our body weight. Muscles differ in appearance according to their function and purpose. Muscle fibers (about the thinness of a human hair) are organized into sheets of fiber and connective tissue called *fascia*. Muscles remain toned with use and deteriorate (**atrophy**) with inactivity. All muscular movement is controlled from the brain and spinal column. Some muscles are under voluntary or conscious control. Other muscles function independently and are controlled by the autonomous nervous system. These include the muscles of the heart and the digestive organs.

Functions

External or skeletal muscles, such as those in the arms and legs, enable the body, including the face, to move (Figures 5-10 and 5-11). Internal muscles move food along

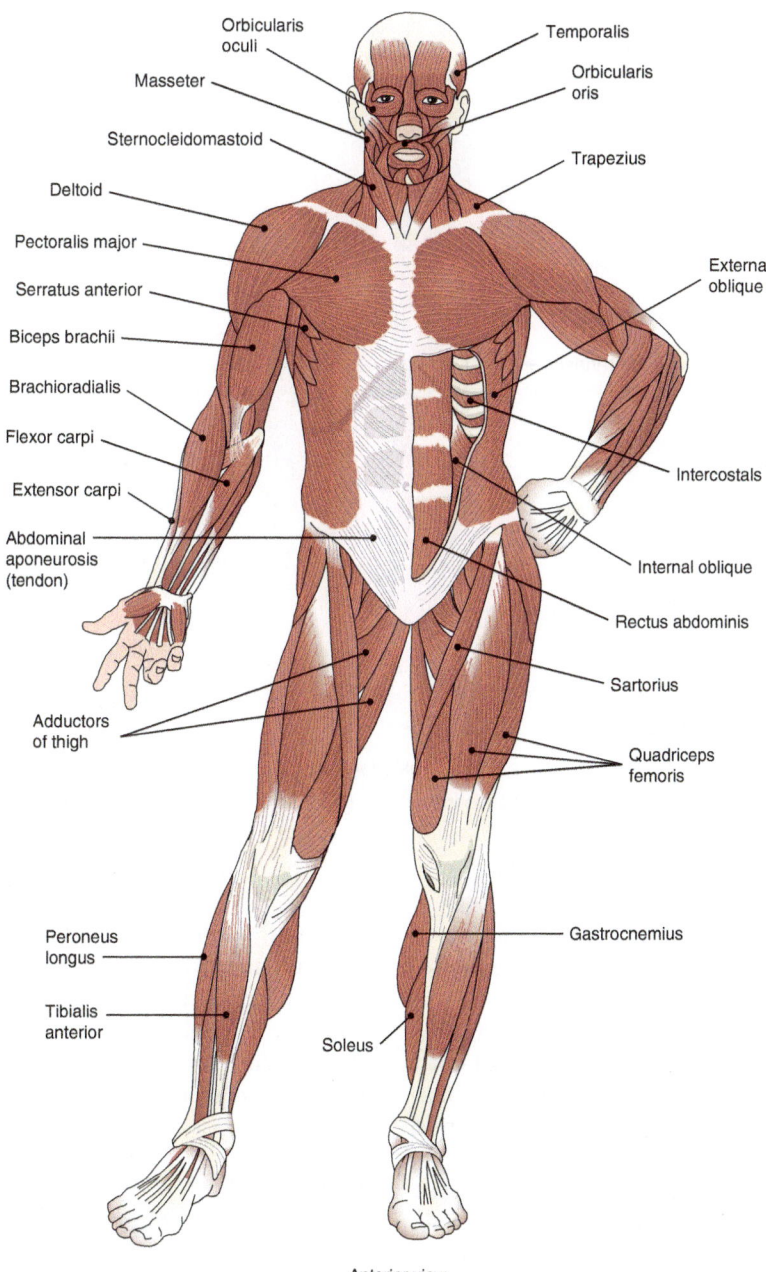

Anterior view

Figure 5–10 An anterior view of the superficial muscles of the body.

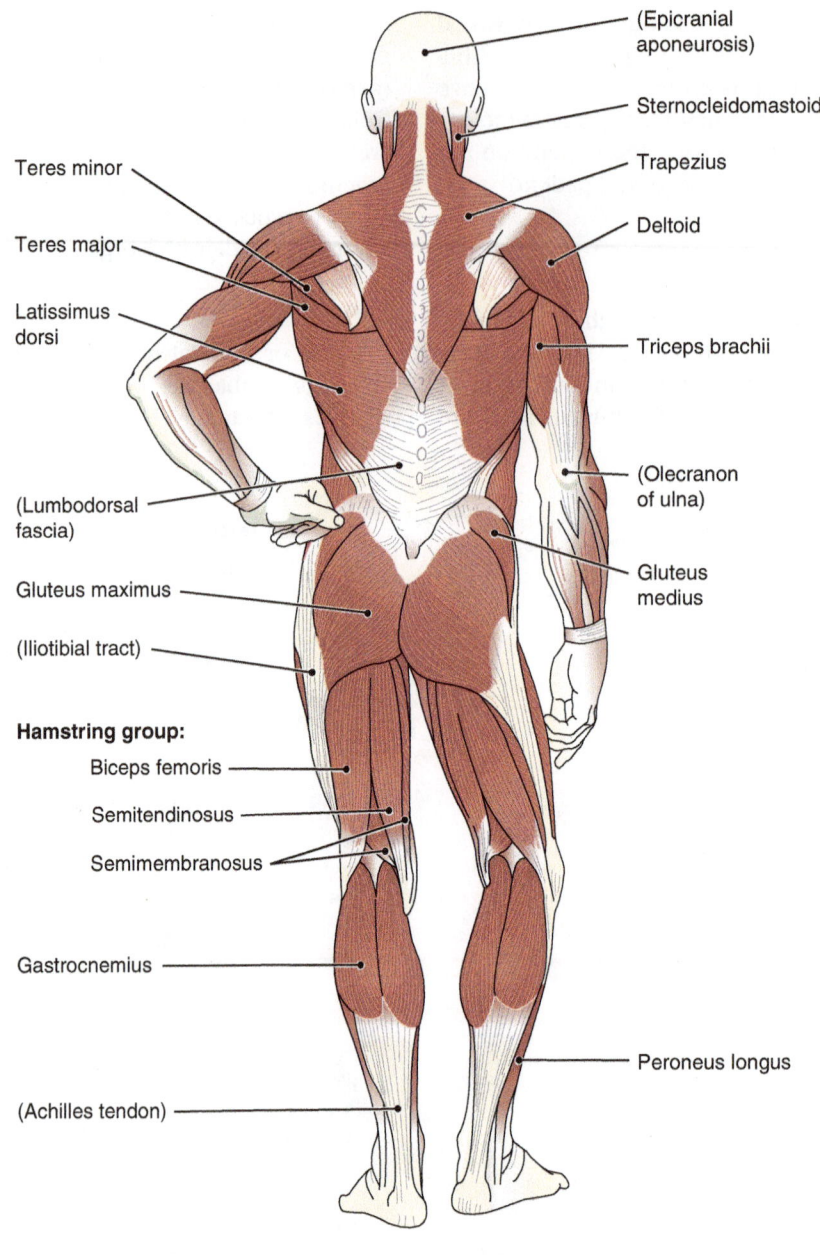

Teres minor

Teres major

Latissimus
dorsi

(Lumbodorsal
fascia)

Gluteus maximus

(Iliotibial tract)

Hamstring group:

Biceps femoris

Semitendinosus

Semimembranosus

Gastrocnemius

(Achilles tendon)

(Epicranial
aponeurosis)

Sternocleidomastoid

Trapezius

Deltoid

Triceps brachii

(Olecranon
of ulna)

Gluteus
medius

Peroneus longus

Posterior view

Figure 5–11 A posterior view of the superficial muscles of the body.

the digestive tract or, in the case of the heart, pump blood throughout the body. The energy produced by muscles produces body heat.

Muscles work by contracting and relaxing according to impulses they receive from the brain and spinal cord. They shorten when contracting and return to their normal length when relaxing. Most striated muscles function in opposing pairs called *antagonistic pairs*. While one set of muscles contracts, another corresponding set relaxes. These coordinated movements enable the body to move.

Dental assistants will be most conscious of patients' facial, head, and neck muscles, such as those that allow

chewing, swallowing, smiling, or speaking. While treating patients and assisting the dentist, dental assistants use neck and lower back muscles. Inactive muscles deteriorate and lose strength. Keeping your back and neck muscles flexible and strong will allow you to maintain a healthy posture and avoid unnecessary strain.

Basic Structures

Muscles come in three types: striated, or skeletal muscles; cardiac, or heart muscle; and smooth, or internal muscle (Figure 5-12).

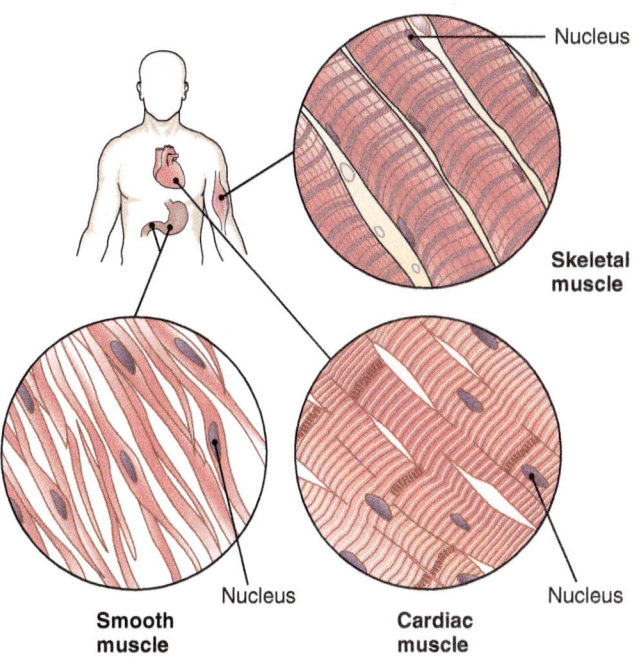

Figure 5–12 The three types of muscles.

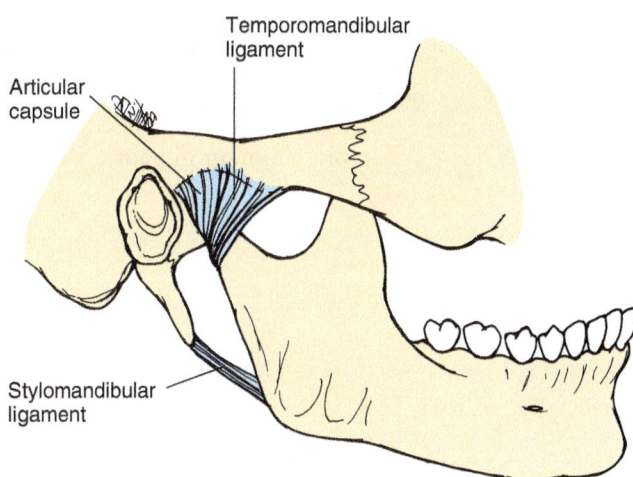

Figure 5–13 Ligaments attach bone to bone.

Striated muscle is also known as *skeletal* or *voluntary muscle*. It is named after the stripes or bands that appear across its long, thin cells. It is attached to the skeleton and moves with it under voluntary control.

Cardiac muscle is only found in the heart. Cardiac muscle has the same striated appearance as skeletal muscle but is controlled involuntarily. It keeps the heart beating by responding to impulses sent to the muscle by the brain.

Smooth muscle is not striated and moves involuntarily under control of the body's autonomous nervous system. Smooth muscle is found in internal organs other than the heart.

Muscles attach to the skeleton in a variety of ways. Tendons consist of specialized connective tissue that extends beyond the muscle to allow it to attach to bone. Ligaments are bands or sheets of fibrous connective tissue that connect or support two or more bones (Figure 5-13).

Common Disorders in the Muscular System

Muscle cramps, spasms, strains, and inflammation, along with ligament sprains, commonly occur as a result of overexertion, dehydration, or accidental injury. If a patient presents with a recent history of such injuries, it is appropriate for the dental assistant to inquire about any medication the patient may be using to address pain.

Fibromyalgia is a chronic condition characterized by widespread pain and tenderness in muscles, joints, tendons, and associated soft tissues. Numbness may occur in the hands and feet. Sleep disturbance, fatigue, headache, depression, and anxiety typically complicate the condition. Fibromyalgia can develop on its own

or may be associated with other conditions, such as **rheumatoid arthritis** or systemic lupus erythematosus. The cause of fibromyalgia is unknown. Physical or emotional trauma may play a role in its development, as may sleep disturbances or unidentified viruses. Some researchers consider abnormal responses to the transmission of pain or changes in skeletal muscle metabolism to be root causes. You should note any patient complaints of chronic pain (especially in the aftermath of other illness or trauma), recording them in an updated medical history and bringing them to the attention of other members of the dental team.

Muscular dystrophy refers to a group of disorders that are usually inherited and commonly recognized in early childhood. Each is characterized by progressively worsening deterioration of skeletal muscle. Other symptoms vary with the particular type of muscular dystrophy. Mental retardation is present with some types, along with delayed development of motor skills, trouble walking, and difficulty using one or more muscle groups. Some types of muscular dystrophy affect specific muscles only.

Fascioscapulohumeral muscular dystrophy, for example, mainly affects the facial, shoulder, and upper arm muscles. Early symptoms are usually mild and worsen gradually. They may include drooping eyelids, decreased facial expression, and difficulty pronouncing words. Individuals may have trouble raising their arms because of shoulder and arm weakness. Fascioscapulohumeral muscular dystrophy normally becomes apparent between the ages of 10 and 26 years. You should take note of any patient complaints regarding these or similar symptoms.

Myasthenia gravis is an **autoimmune disorder** characterized by progressively weaker and fatigued skeletal muscles. It results when nerve impulses from the brain to skeletal muscles are interrupted by an erroneous autoimmune response and rendered inadequate. Weakness may first appear in facial and swallowing muscles. The dental assistant and dental team should take note of any patient complaints regarding such symptoms. Patients with myasthenia gravis are at increased risk of having other autoimmune disorders, such as rheumatoid arthritis and systemic lupus erythematosus. Myasthenia gravis can occur at any age but is more common in young women and older men.

CHECKPOINTS

5-5 What are the names of the five sections of bone found along the spinal column?

5-6 Which is the only type of muscle under voluntary control?

Respiratory System

We hardly ever think about breathing, yet it is the most essential activity we engage in. Deprivation of oxygen for even a short period of time can irreversibly damage tissues and organs. The respiratory system has two main parts. The upper respiratory tract is located outside the chest cavity and includes the nose, pharynx, larynx, and upper trachea. The lower respiratory tract is located within the chest cavity and includes the lower trachea and the lungs themselves (Figure 5-14).

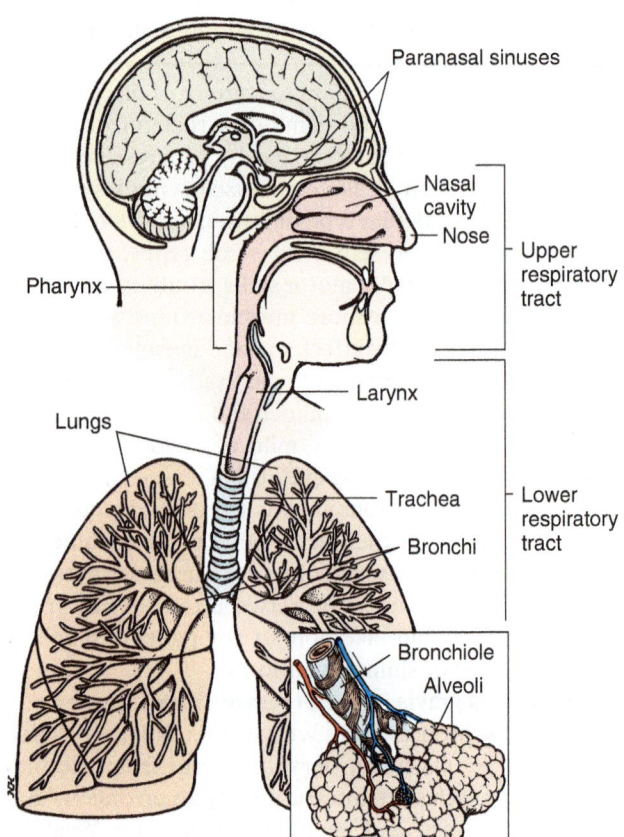

Figure 5–14 The upper and lower respiratory tracts.

A dental assistant's knowledge of the respiratory system can prove life saving. Patients may experience reactions to anesthesia during treatment, chronic respiratory disease may not allow the use of certain medications, or patients may unexpectedly choke on foreign substances that reach the throat and windpipe. You should remain alert for signs of respiratory distress or unusually shallow breathing.

Functions

The respiratory system enables breathing and the exchange of oxygen and carbon monoxide.

Basic Structures

The respiratory system consists of the nose, pharynx, larynx, trachea, bronchi, and lungs. Outside air enters the body through the nose. The lining of the nose, called the *nasal mucosa*, warms and moistens the air as it enters. The nose also contains receptors for the sense of smell. **Pharynx** is another word for throat. Air flows down its various sections until it reaches the larynx, or voice box. Inside the larynx, the vocal cords are positioned to produce sound and speech. The trachea, also known as the *windpipe*, sits inferior to the larynx. Its 5 or so inches of length are the final path for air to reach the lungs. (These structures of the upper respiratory tract will be discussed further in Chapter 6, Head and Neck Anatomy.)

Two branching **bronchi,** also known as *bronchial tubes*, connect the trachea to the lungs. Bronchi end in **bronchioles**, or smaller tubes that funnel air into the **alveolar sacs** of the lungs. The alveolar sacs resemble clusters of grapes. Exchange of carbon dioxide for newly arrived oxygen happens in the individual "grapes," or **alveoli**, of the lungs.

Common Disorders in the Respiratory System

Asthma occurs when the lining of the bronchi—the tubes leading from the trachea to the lungs—becomes inflamed and swollen. Muscles around the bronchi tighten in response, and breathing becomes difficult. Wheezing sounds may be heard as the person tries to catch a breath. Typical symptoms of asthma include breathing difficulty and wheezing, coughing, and tightness in the chest. These symptoms sometimes resolve on their own over time, but, in most cases, some kind of treatment is warranted. An asthma attack can last from minutes to days; it becomes an emergency if the swelling and inflammation restrict air flow severely. Asthma attacks can be triggered by allergens, such as pet dander, dust, respiratory infections, and tobacco smoke, and even powerful emotions, such as anxiety. Nonsteroidal anti-inflammatory drugs (NSAIDs) can provoke asthma attacks in some people.

A variety of medications are used to prevent and treat asthma. Some people with asthma carry medicinal inhalers containing bronchodilators to use in case of an attack. For information about caring for a patient suffering from an asthma attack, see Chapter 18, Responding to Medical Emergencies.

Tuberculosis (TB), also known as *pulmonary tuberculosis*, is a bacterial infection of the lungs. It is transmitted from one person to another through inhaling airborne droplets when an infected person sneezes, talks, or coughs. Symptoms include fever, night sweats, cough, fatigue, and unintentional weight loss. Older adults, infants, the homeless, and those with weakened immune systems are most at risk for developing active TB. Risk factors for active infection include poor nutrition and crowded or unsanitary living conditions. TB is usually treated with powerful antibiotics. Infected individuals must finish the course of treatment for it to be effective.

Though outbreaks of TB are closely monitored by public health authorities, a professional dental assistant should remain aware of the possibility of encountering patients with active TB. Dental teams who specialize in public health dentistry are at an increased likelihood of encountering these patients, but all dental health professionals should be familiar with the symptoms of TB and exercise appropriate measures to prevent its spread and encourage its treatment.

Chronic obstructive pulmonary disease (COPD) is a common health concern and takes various forms, including emphysema and chronic bronchitis. Chronic bronchitis causes long-term swelling and large amounts of mucus in the main bronchial airways. Emphysema gradually destroys the alveoli or air sacs of the lungs. Patients with COPD may have symptoms of both of these diseases. Cigarette smoking is the leading cause of COPD. Secondhand smoke, allergies, air pollution, and infection are also potential causes.

Symptoms of COPD include shortness of breath that worsens with activity, wheezing, fatigue, a mucus-producing cough, and headaches. Ankles and feet may swell. Some individuals may develop respiratory acidosis, a condition in which blood tests reveal higher-than-normal levels of carbon dioxide and lower-than-normal levels of oxygen. Treatments for COPD include bronchodilators, like those used for asthma, and steroids to reduce lung inflammation.

You may encounter patients whose COPD may not allow for common treatment methods, or for certain types of anesthesia. In such situations, procedures must be adjusted accordingly.

Digestive System

Dental assistants and other members of the dental team play an active role in maintaining the health of their

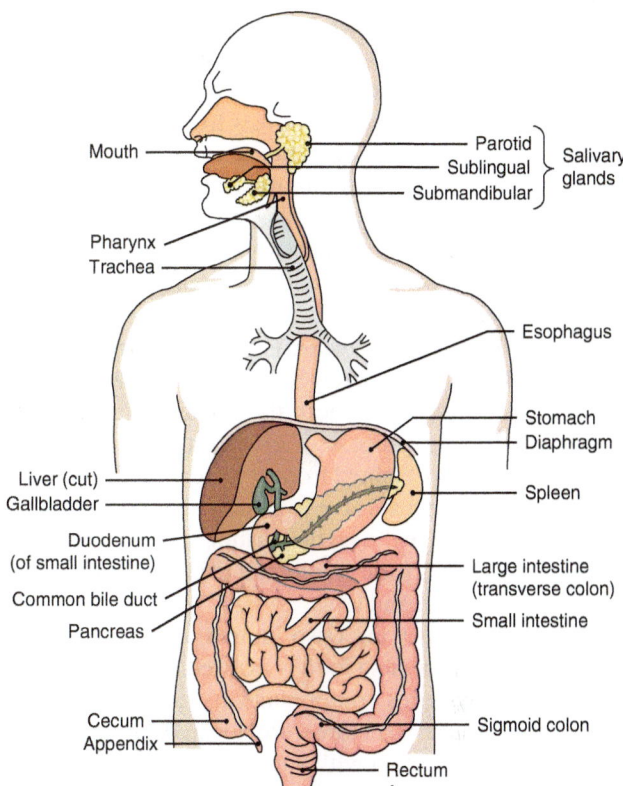

Figure 5–15 **The digestive system.** Saliva from the salivary glands, mixed with food, begins the digestive process.

patients' digestive systems (Figure 5-15). Healthy teeth and gingival tissue are essential to the process of chewing and ingesting food. Adequate dental health allows individuals to eat the foods they prefer and to maintain the variety that is part of a healthful diet.

Functions

Through digestion and absorption, the digestive system converts solid foods into nutrients that enable the body to maintain and repair itself as well as fuel the activities of daily living. After obtaining all the nutrients it can from food, the digestive system eliminates solid wastes from the body.

Basic Structures

The digestive system has two main components. The first of these, the alimentary canal, can be thought of as a tube that runs nearly the length of the body, from the mouth to the anus. In between these two points, food travels through a network of organs that systematically process it into smaller bits, nutrients, and, finally, leftover waste.

We are conscious of the alimentary canal's work only at the very beginning and the very end of the digestive cycle. In between, its work is controlled by the autonomous nervous system.

The process of tasting and chewing takes place in the mouth, where the sense of taste can greatly increase our enjoyment of food. Chewed food moves from the oral cavity into the pharynx, where it is swallowed into the esophagus. The pharynx is where the respiratory and digestive systems diverge. Air moves from the mouth and pharynx into the larynx and thorax to be taken into the lungs, whereas food moves into the esophagus to be transported to the stomach. A sac-like organ, the stomach is capable of holding up to a half gallon of food. The gastric juices it produces, together with peristalsis, the powerful movements of its smooth muscle, churn and mix food into a semifluid mass called *chyme*. The digestive work of the stomach takes approximately 3 hours. Below the stomach lies the small intestine, where the chyme formed in the stomach is further processed. It is from the small intestine that nutrients obtained from the processed food enter the bloodstream and are able to nourish the body. Leftover waste products leave the small intestine and enter the large intestine, where they are stored and eventually eliminated through the rectum and anus.

The work of chewing (also known as **mastication**), digesting, and processing food is assisted by the second of the digestive system's components, its accessory organs. These organs and structures are located along the alimentary canal and help with such tasks as softening food and contributing special fluids to the digestive process. The first accessory organs are found in the mouth. They include the teeth, tongue, and salivary glands. The salivary glands, which release saliva to soften food as it is being chewed, will be discussed further, along with the teeth and the tongue, in Chapter 6, Head and Neck Anatomy.

The liver, located roughly to the right of the stomach, produces bile to aid in the digestion of fats. The gallbladder, sitting just adjacent to the liver, stores bile, which it releases when needed into the small intestine. The pancreas also lies along the route of the small intestine and injects additional digestive juices into it.

Common Disorders in the Digestive System

Gastroesophageal reflux disease (GERD) involves the upward flow of gastric juices from the stomach into the esophagus. This action irritates the esophagus, causing heartburn and other symptoms. Depending on how far up the alimentary canal gastric juices travel, some people may experience a sore throat, coughing, hoarseness, or difficulty swallowing with GERD. Dental assistants may observe such symptoms during treatment.

Ulcers most commonly occur along the digestive tract in either the stomach or the duodenum, the uppermost part of the small intestine. The linings of the stomach and duodenum are normally protected against the enzymes and acids that help digest food. Ulcers develop when these safeguards break down. Bacteria living in the digestive tract may make some people more prone to ulcers, as can excessive use of alcohol, tobacco, and NSAIDs.

Dental caries, commonly known as *tooth decay*, may be seen as a disorder of the digestive system, because the teeth are one of the digestive system's accessory structures. In addition, nutrition and a proper diet play an important role in maintaining the health of the teeth and gingiva. See Chapter 11, Nutrition, for more information about how food and diet play a role in dental caries.

CHECKPOINTS

5-7 Where in the lungs does the actual exchange of carbon dioxide for oxygen take place?

5-8 Mastication is another word for what?

Cardiovascular System

All our vital organs, along with the farthest reaches of our feet and hands, require a healthy, adequate blood supply. Blood provides fuel to the body, and the heart delivers blood via the cardiovascular system (Figure 5-16).

Functions

The purpose of the cardiovascular system is to circulate oxygen and nutrients to organs and tissues while removing waste products, including carbon dioxide and cellular wastes.

Basic Structures

The cardiovascular system includes the heart, blood, arteries, veins, and capillaries. One of the most vital parts of the body, the heart is a muscular organ roughly the size of a fist. It sits nestled between the lungs and is surrounded by the pericardium, a double-walled protective membrane. Heart valves open and close with each heartbeat and ensure that blood travels in only one direction through the heart (see Figure 5-16).

The heart's work begins when two major veins deliver oxygen-poor blood to be circulated through the lungs and replenished with oxygen. The superior vena cava delivers blood from the head and upper body, whereas the inferior vena cava brings blood up from the legs, abdomen, and pelvis. Both veins empty into the upper right chamber of the heart, the right atrium. From there, the blood passes through the tricuspid valve and into the lower right chamber of the heart, the right ventricle. The blood then enters the pulmonary artery, the only artery in the body to transport oxygen-poor blood. The pulmonary artery carries the blood to the lungs, where carbon dioxide is exchanged for fresh oxygen.

The blood returns to the heart via the pulmonary vein, the only vein in the body to carry freshly oxygenated blood, and enters the upper left chamber of the heart, the left atrium. From there, blood flows through the bicuspid valve into the lower left chamber of the heart, the left ventricle. It exits that fourth and final chamber through the aortic valve and enters the body's main artery, the aorta. From

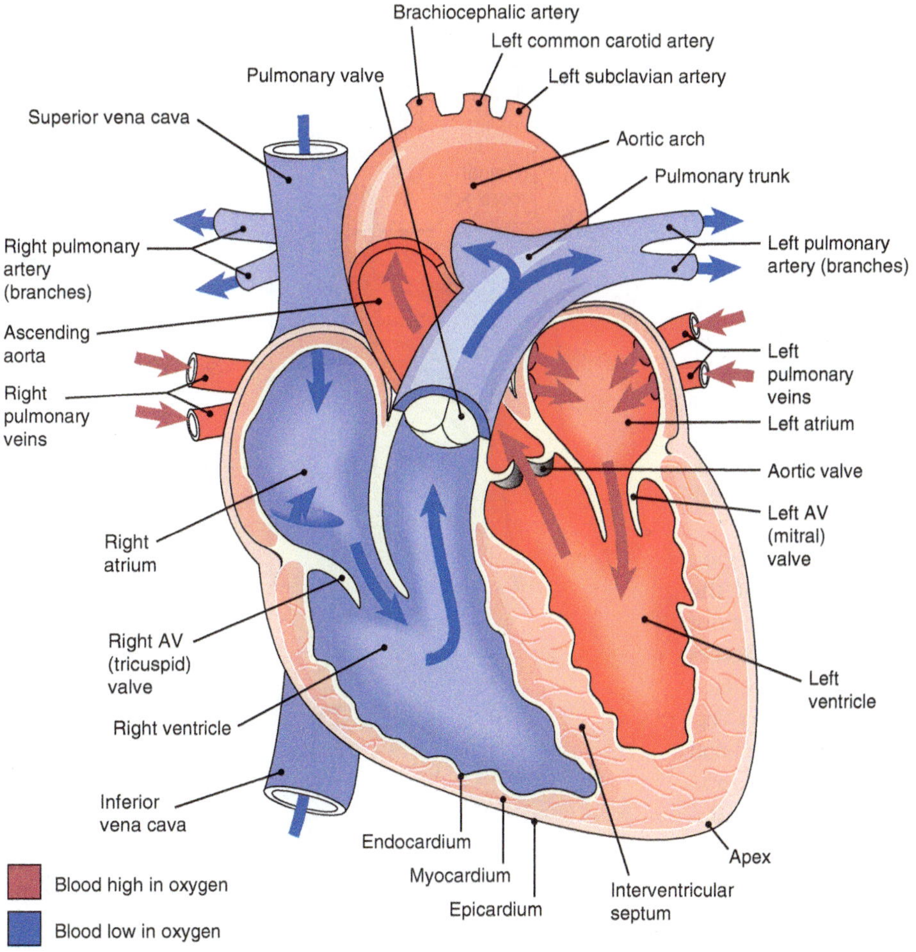

Figure 5–16 The heart and great vessels. The abbreviation AV means atrioventricular.

Brachiocephalic artery
Left common carotid artery
Left subclavian artery
Pulmonary valve
Aortic arch
Pulmonary trunk
Superior vena cava
Right pulmonary artery (branches)
Left pulmonary artery (branches)
Ascending aorta
Left pulmonary veins
Right pulmonary veins
Left atrium
Aortic valve
Left AV (mitral) valve
Right atrium
Right AV (tricuspid) valve
Left ventricle
Right ventricle
Inferior vena cava
Endocardium
Apex
Myocardium
Interventricular septum
Epicardium

Blood high in oxygen
Blood low in oxygen

there it will flow via arteries and capillaries throughout the body.

Although they are the smallest blood vessels in the body, the capillaries are the sites of life-sustaining exchanges. Oxygen, along with nutrients, hormones, and antibodies, enter the cells adjacent to the capillaries. In exchange, carbon dioxide and waste products enter the blood stream for delivery back to the lungs, where they will be exchanged for fresh oxygen.

Approximately 4 to 6 quarts of blood flow through the body of an average adult. Blood itself is composed of a watery substance called *plasma* into which various types of blood cells, known as *corpuscles*, are integrated. There are three types of corpuscles:

- Erythrocytes—also known as *red blood cells*—carry oxygen and nutrients. They have a short lifespan, after which they are destroyed by the liver and spleen. New erythrocytes are formed in the red bone marrow. Erythrocytes, with their oxygen-carrying capacity, are far more numerous than the other corpuscles.
- Leukocytes—also known as *white blood cells*—come in five different types. The main task of each type of white blood cell is the protection of the body against disease.

- Thrombocytes—also known as *platelets*—are the blood's clotting factor by which it controls bleeding following a wound or injury.

Each of us possesses one of four types of blood: A, B, O, or AB. Blood typing becomes important when individuals are ill or injured and require blood transfusions. Some of us can donate to any of the other three types, but others are limited in their donor capabilities; similarly, some of us can receive blood from anyone else, but others are strictly limited in who can donate to them.

Each of us also has blood that is either Rh negative or Rh positive. The Rh factor is an antigen found on the surface of blood cells. Its presence is most consequential when babies with the Rh factor are born to mothers who do not possess it.

Common Disorders in the Cardiovascular System

Atherosclerosis, also known as *hardening of the arteries*, is among the most familiar disorders of the cardiovascular system. It refers to the clogging of arteries by a mixture of cholesterol and other byproducts. With considerable blockage, the organ or affected part of the body becomes starved of oxygen. Only then do symptoms most commonly first occur. Risk factors for developing atherosclerosis include obesity, diabetes, smoking, lack of exercise, and a family history of the condition.

Myocardial infarction, commonly known as a *heart attack*, usually occurs when a blood clot, formed of the same material that causes atherosclerosis, blocks one of the arteries in the heart, depriving the heart of oxygen. Signs and symptoms usually appear suddenly and may include chest pain, numbness in the left arm, dyspnea (shortness of breath), nausea, excessive sweating, and dizziness. If these symptoms appear during dental treatment, medical assistance should be summoned immediately. Although anxiety can cause some of these symptoms, heart disease is widespread enough that patients should be examined and treated immediately. For more information about what to do if a patient has a heart attack, see Chapter 18, Responding to Medical Emergencies.

Untreated **hypertension**, or chronically high blood pressure, can damage internal organs and is one of the risk factors for heart disease. Most of the time, there is not one single identifiable cause for the condition. Risk factors for developing it, however, include heredity, obesity, lack of exercise, a diet heavy in salt and low in fruits and vegetables, and excessive alcohol consumption. Hypertension is a risk factor for a stroke, also known as a *cerebrovascular accident*. For more information about what to do if a patient has a stroke, see Chapter 18, Responding to Medical Emergencies. Hypertension should be recorded on a patient health history, along with any medications being used.

Many people have blood pressure that is lower than the average. It is most likely normal for them and not of any concern. However, an individual whose blood pressure drops unexpectedly has developed **hypotension**. Hypotension can result from blood loss, widened blood vessels, heart failure, dehydration, and some drugs, including those used to treat hypertension. Symptoms include frequent lightheadedness, especially when rising from a seated position. Some individuals experience nausea, vomiting, and even fainting. Hypotension is usually treated by addressing the underlying cause. Persistent cases may require medication. After being positioned in a reclining (supine) position, dental patients may experience "postural hypotension," a feeling of dizziness or lightheadedness, upon rising from the dental chair.

Nervous System

Functions

The nervous system gathers and interprets sensory information from inside and outside the body. It also initiates involuntary and voluntary movement and regulates basic bodily functions (Figure 5-17).

Basic Structures

The central nervous system consists of the brain and spinal cord. The **peripheral nervous system** consists of the

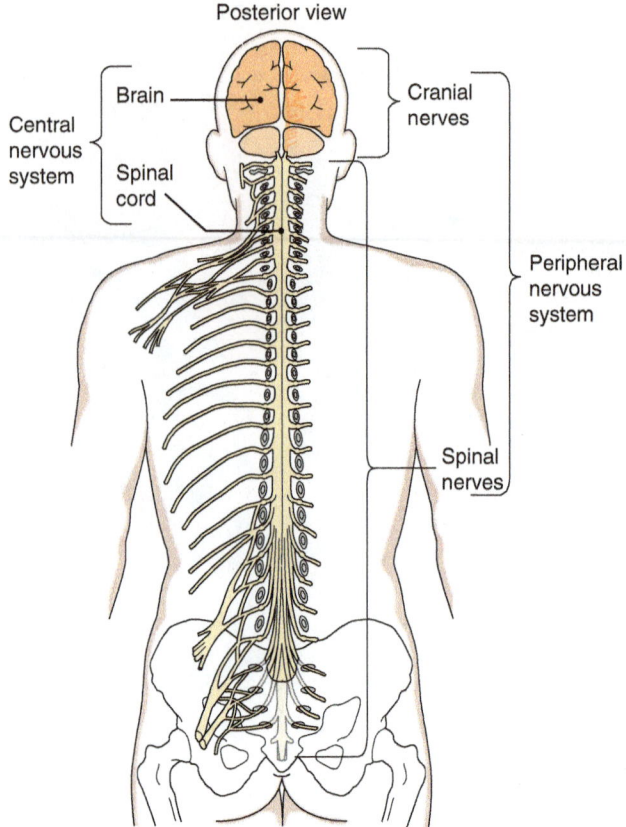

Figure 5–17 The nervous system is broken down into two systems: The central nervous system (CNS) consists of the brain and the spinal cord. The peripheral nervous system (PNS) consists of all of the nerves.

nerves that transmit and receive stimuli from inside and outside the body. The autonomous nervous system consists of a specialized network of nerves that transmit stimuli to regulate heartbeat, digestion, respiration, and other bodily processes that are not normally under conscious control.

Neurons are specialized nerve cells that serve as the basic functioning unit of the nervous system (Figure 5-18). Like most cells, neurons contain a nucleus and are surrounded by a cell wall. They differ from other cells in that special nerve fibers extend away from and to the cell to receive and respond to stimuli. Nerve fibers that transmit impulses to the cell body are called *dendrites*. Nerve fibers that conduct impulses away from the nerve cell are called *axons*. Nerve fibers move impulses through a kind of junction called a *synapse*. Here axons release chemicals to help impulses move along to the next dendrite and nerve cell. Some nerve cells in the peripheral nervous system are insulated by a layer of protective cells that form a **myelin sheath**. The myelin sheath allows rapid and efficient transmission of impulses between nerve cells. Damage to the myelin disrupts these impulses and can result in diseases such as multiple sclerosis.

Sensory organs such as the eyes, ears, nose, mouth, and skin use sensory neurons to transmit stimuli to the brain

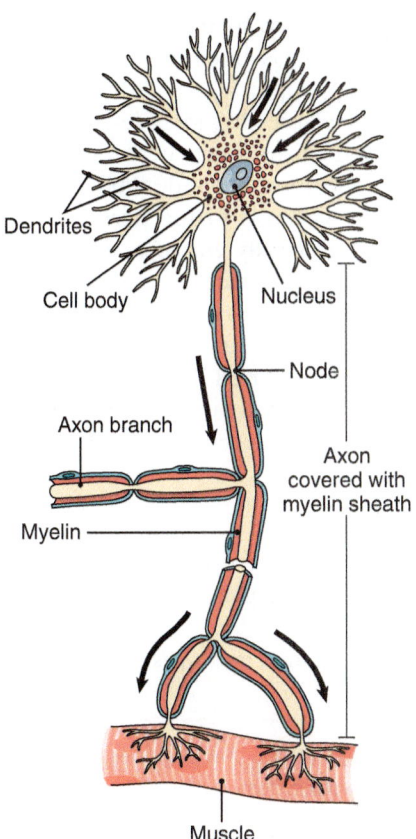

Figure 5–18 The neuron is a specialized cell; its basic function is to direct communication or nerve impulses.

Dendrites

Cell body

Nucleus

Node

Axon branch

Axon covered with myelin sheath

Myelin

Muscle

for interpretation. Motor neurons transmit any information needed for a physical reaction back to appropriate muscle cells. The spinal cord serves as a center for reflex or involuntary actions to stimuli. Stimuli that call for an immediate response, such as a finger touching a burning stove, are routed to the spinal cord, which responds with stimuli for a reflexive action. In less urgent situations, the spinal cord also transmits stimuli to the brain for interpretation and transmits any response back to muscles via motor neurons.

Twelve **cranial nerves,** numbered I through XII, operate between the brain and facial structures such as the tongue, eyes, and nose. These nerves are particularly important to the dental assistant when providing anesthesia and patient care. They will be discussed at length in Chapter 6, Head and Neck Anatomy.

The brain itself can be divided into three parts: the brainstem, **cerebellum**, and **cerebrum** (Figure 5-19). These separate regions function interdependently and together produce a wide range of abilities, both physical and mental. The brainstem, located just above the spinal column, regulates much of the autonomous nervous system and the basic functions of life. The brainstem is divided into the reticular formation, which controls whether we are awake or asleep; the medulla, which controls heart and breathing rate; and the midbrain, from which posture and involuntary movement are controlled. The cerebellum, located posterior to the brain stem, coordinates conscious and unconscious movement. It is where we store information on learned movement, such as exercise and athletic routines. The cerebrum, the large, outermost region of the brain, coordinates our conscious and voluntary responses. It is known as the "seat of consciousness" from which language, logic, and self-awareness originate. The cerebrum is divided into left and right halves, or cerebral hemispheres (this is the origin of such terms as "right-brain thinking"). Each hemisphere is divided into four separate lobes.

Common Disorders in the Nervous System

Alzheimer disease is a degenerative brain disease that grows progressively worse over time. It affects behavior; memory; and thought processes, such as decision-making, judgment, and attention span. Alzheimer disease causes

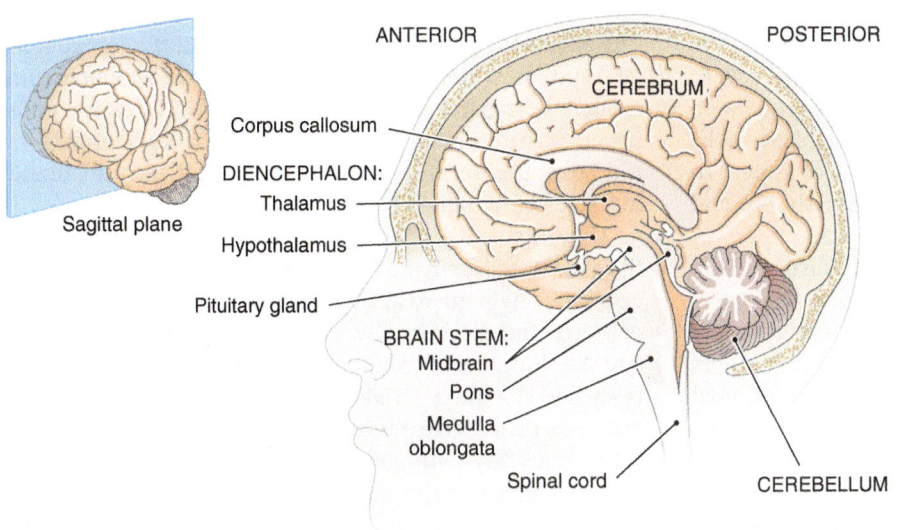

Figure 5–19 The brain is the primary control center for regulating and coordinating all body activities.

Sagittal plane

ANTERIOR

POSTERIOR

CEREBRUM

Corpus callosum

DIENCEPHALON:
Thalamus
Hypothalamus

Pituitary gland

BRAIN STEM:
Midbrain
Pons
Medulla oblongata

Spinal cord

CEREBELLUM

structural and chemical changes and disconnects portions of the brain that would normally function well together. Early symptoms of Alzheimer disease include personality changes, repeating statements, losing or misplacing items, and losing interest in familiar or favorite activities. Symptoms worsen with time and may come to include agitation, memory loss regarding current events or personal history, arguments, and even aggressive behavior. Dental assistants who have long cared for the same patient are in a position to note any such behavioral changes and should bring them to the attention of other members of the dental team. Remaining aware of the medical history of patients who have already been identified as having Alzheimer disease will help the dental team treat these patients with patience as well as with an awareness of how their condition may affect behavior. See Chapter 22, Patients with Special Needs, for more information.

Multiple sclerosis (MS) is a progressively worsening autoimmune disease that affects the brain and spinal cord. The disease usually appears between the ages of 20 and 40 years and affects women more frequently than men. MS is caused by degeneration or destruction of the myelin sheath that surrounds the nerve fibers of the brain and spinal cord. Loss of myelin slows down or stops nerve impulses, impeding communication between the brain and the rest of the body. Attacks of MS occur sporadically and can last for days, weeks, or months. Symptoms of an attack differ according to which nerves and parts of the body are involved but may involve muscle weakness or pain, rapid involuntary eye movement, facial pain, and incontinence. For information about providing dental care to patients who have MS, see Chapter 22, Patients with Special Needs.

Parkinson disease is a progressively worsening disease of the brain that causes tremors and difficulty with walking and muscle coordination. Parkinson disease results from a failure of brain cells to manufacture sufficient dopamine, a brain chemical necessary for accurate and reliable muscle movement. Early symptoms may include mild tremors in the hands or feelings of stiffness in the feet and legs. The type and severity of symptoms vary from one patient to another. Dental assistants may encounter patients with Parkinson disease who exhibit a masklike or blank facial expression, blink more slowly than expected, or appear to drool uncontrollably. They may walk with a shuffle and speak unusually slowly or in a monotone voice.

Epilepsy is not a disease, but rather a seizure disorder caused by abnormally excited electrical signals in the brain. These malfunctioning signals cause a variety of types of seizures, ranging from simple staring spells, during which the person appears to be unaware of what is going on around him or her, to an abrupt loss of consciousness and violent convulsions. Many different conditions and diseases are known to cause epileptic seizures. These include brain damage, use or abuse of certain drugs, chronic diseases such as diabetes, and acute infections anywhere in the body. In many cases, the cause of an individual's epilepsy is unknown. A family history may predispose some people.

An epileptic seizure that includes violent convulsions and loss of consciousness may occur suddenly and unexpectedly. It may be upsetting or difficult for others to watch but is normally harmless to the person experiencing it. The seizure will normally end after about 30 seconds to 2 minutes. Prolonged seizures, or a series of seizures during which the person does not regain consciousness, constitute a medical emergency; help should be summoned immediately. See Chapter 18, Responding to Medical Emergencies, for information about what to do if a patient experiences a seizure while receiving dental care.

CHECKPOINTS

5-9 Where in the circulatory system does the exchange of carbon dioxide for oxygen take place?

5-10 What are the three main types of blood cells, also known as *corpuscles*?

5-11 Which region of the brain regulates most of the autonomous nervous system?

Integumentary System

The major component of the integumentary system, the skin, is the body's largest organ and its first line of defense against disease and invasive bacteria (Figure 5-20).

Functions

The skin protects the body from pathogens, prevents dehydration, regulates body temperature, excretes liquids and salts, and provides the sense of touch.

Basic Structures

The skin is the most important structure of the integumentary system, which also includes hair, nails, subcutaneous tissue, sweat glands, and sebaceous glands. The skin is composed of three main layers of tissue: the **epidermis**, or top layer; the dermis, or middle layer; and the subcutaneous layer of fat beneath them.

The epidermis is thickest on the soles of our feet and the palms of our hands. Two important functions of the epidermis help guard against disease and infection. As skin cells age and die, they rise to the surface of the epidermis and are sloughed off. Microorganisms on the surface of the body are sloughed off along with them. In addition, special cells called **Langerhans cells**, also called *dendritic cells*, attack any pathogens that attempt to enter the body through breaks in the skin. The Langerhans cells first form in red bone marrow and are very mobile. After capturing the invading pathogen in the epidermis, they transport

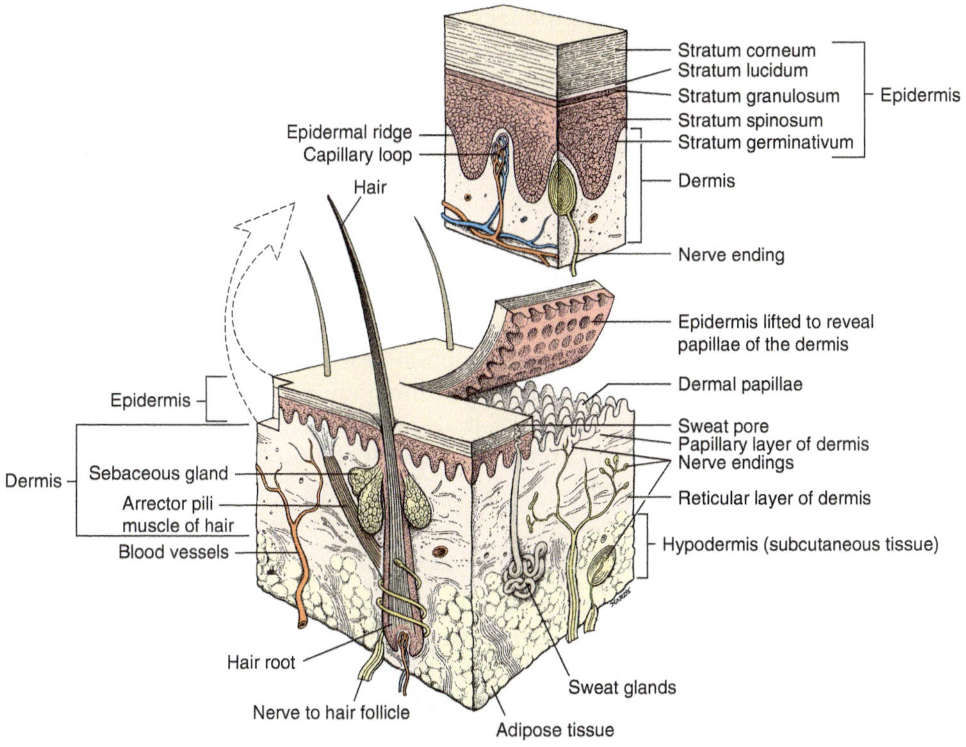

Figure 5–20 Skin is the body's largest organ.

it to nearby lymph nodes where they present it to white blood cells (lymphocytes) for destruction.

The thicker dermis layer below the epidermis is composed of connective tissue and gives the skin its bulk. It also contains sensory nerve endings and receptors, which allow for the sense of touch, along with sensations of pain and temperature.

The bottommost subcutaneous fat layer of the skin attaches the skin to underlying organs and, with its bulk, helps maintain body temperature and prevent dehydration.

Hair, fingernails, toenails, and certain glands are also part of the integumentary system. Sweat glands are important in regulating body temperature. Sebaceous glands, or oil glands, release sebum, an oily substance that inhibits the growth of skin bacteria and keeps the skin supple and less prone to breakage.

Common Disorders in the Integumentary System

Fluid-filled blisters form in the epidermis when friction separates it from the dermis below.

Calluses form when the epidermis thickens in response to pressures placed on it. Calluses are most common on the feet and hands but can occur anywhere on the body.

Burns to the skin are classified as superficial, partial thickness, and full thickness (Figure 5-21). Superficial, or first-degree, burns affect only the most superficial layers of the epidermis and are painful but do not blister. Partial-thickness, or second-degree, burns affect the lower layers of the epidermis; blisters form when tissue fluid collects

at the burn site. Full-thickness, or third-degree, burns are the most serious and result in the destruction of the entire layer of epidermis. Some full-thickness burns extend into the dermis and subcutaneous fat layer. Full-thickness burns are particularly serious because the destruction of the epidermis leaves the living tissue below exposed to infection and susceptible to dehydration.

Exposure to sunlight is the most important factor in developing skin cancer (Figure 5-22). People with lighter complexions are most susceptible to the sun damage that leads to skin cancer, but anyone can develop it. The most common forms are **squamous cell carcinoma** and **basal cell carcinoma**. They appear as surface changes in the appearance of the skin. They are biopsied to confirm a diagnosis and then excised. Both types are usually slow to metastasize—that is, to spread to lymph nodes or other organs. A rarer and more dangerous form of skin cancer is **malignant melanoma**. It may metastasize rapidly to the lungs, liver, or other vital organs. Although the most common forms of skin cancer are readily curable, prevention, through the use of sunscreen, clothing, and shade, remains the best defense.

As a dental assistant, you are in a position to notice changes or unusual developments on the skin surface of patients. This is particularly important if the change is in an area not readily visible to the patient. Inquiring about a particularly noticeable skin change is appropriate. The most common types of skin cancer are readily curable if treated early. Encourage a patient to consult a dermatologist regarding any sudden or unusual change.

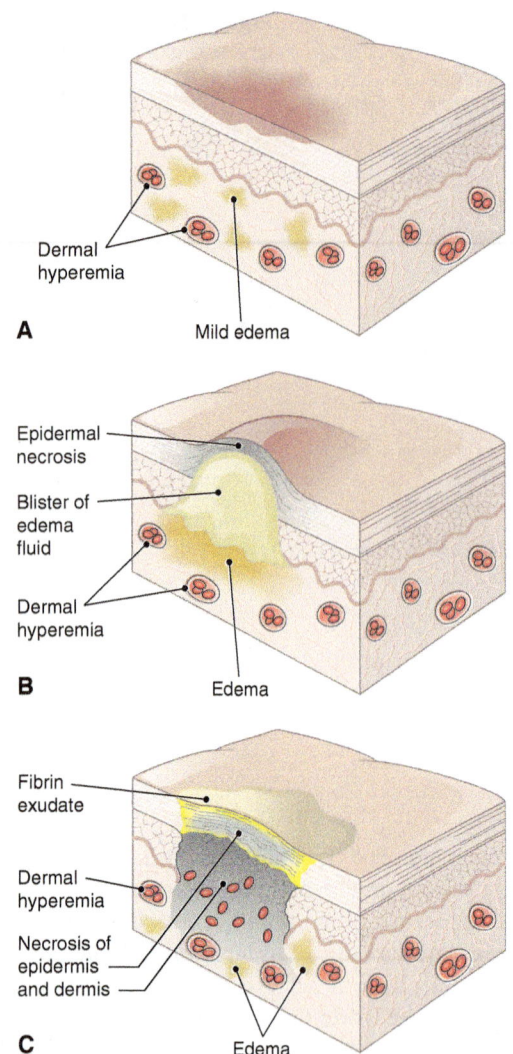

A

Dermal hyperemia

Mild edema

Epidermal necrosis

Blister of edema fluid

Dermal hyperemia

B

Edema

Fibrin exudate

Dermal hyperemia

Necrosis of epidermis and dermis

C

Edema

Figure 5–21 Skin burns are classified as superficial, partial thickness, or full thickness. A. Superficial burns affect only the outer layer of epidermis. **B.** Partial-thickness burns affect the lower layers of epidermis. **C.** Full-thickness burns destroy the entire layer of epidermis.

Endocrine System

The endocrine system, like the autonomous nervous system, helps regulate the body's natural processes. Endocrine glands are found throughout the body (Figure 5-23).

Each produces a specific hormone and releases it into the closest capillaries. Each hormone has one or more target organs or tissues. Once released, hormones circulate through the blood until they are picked up by special chemical receptors on the cell walls of their target organ or organs.

Functions

Almost like a bodily thermostat, the endocrine system controls the body's home environment. It regulates growth, reproduction, reaction to stress, use of calcium, fluid levels within the body, and **metabolism**. Through the pancreas, it also produces the insulin necessary for maintaining appropriate blood glucose (blood sugar) levels.

Basic Structures

Glands of the endocrine system include the pancreas, thyroid gland, parathyroid gland, pituitary gland, adrenal gland, testes, and ovaries. The pituitary serves as a kind of "lead gland," regulating the behavior of other glands in the system. It signals the ovaries, for example, to release estrogen and progesterone; correspondingly, in males, it signals the testes to release testosterone. The thyroid gland, located within the neck on the front and sides of the trachea just below the larynx, regulates growth and metabolic rates through the release of thyroxin and other hormones.

Common Disorders in the Endocrine System

Diabetes mellitus (diabetes) is a chronic disease characterized by high blood glucose levels. Under normal circumstances, glucose is removed from the blood by insulin. Insulin transports glucose from the bloodstream to cells, where it is used as energy. In diabetic patients, however, glucose builds up in the bloodstream, because there is either not enough insulin to remove it or the cells have become resistant to insulin. Symptoms of diabetes include increased thirst, frequent urination, unusual hunger, unexplained weight loss, fatigue, blurred vision, slow-healing sores, and frequent infections of the gingiva or skin.

Figure 5–22 Skin cancer. A. Basal cell carcinoma. **B.** Squamous cell carcinoma. **C.** Malignant melanoma.

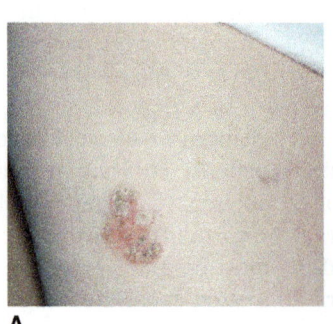

A

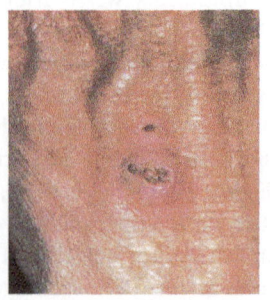

B

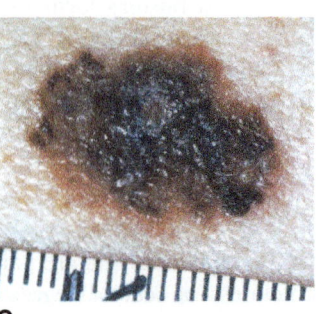

C

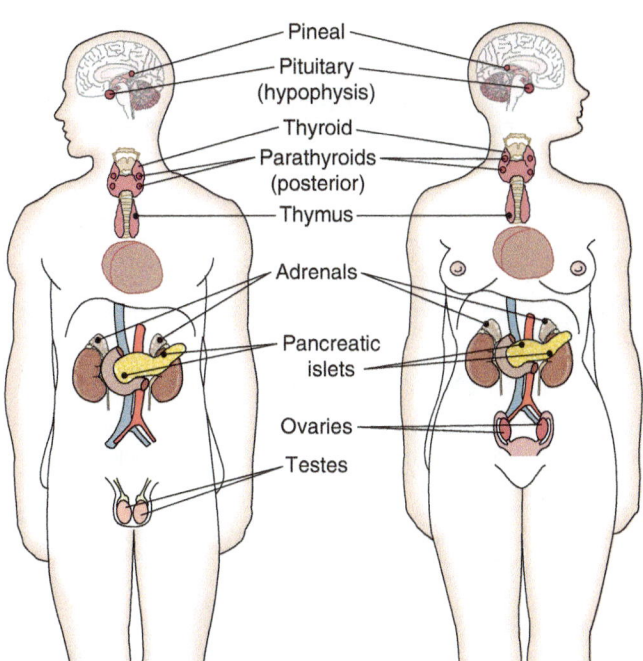

Figure 5–23 The endocrine glands secrete hormones directly into the bloodstream of the body.

There are two main types of diabetes:

- *Type 1 diabetes.* Formerly known as *juvenile-onset diabetes*, type 1 diabetes appears in childhood or early adulthood and is preceded by insufficient insulin production by the pancreas. Type 1 diabetic patients must inject insulin daily to prevent serious complications.
- *Type 2 diabetes.* In this type of diabetes, insulin levels may be normal or even elevated, but the insulin receptors on the body's cells become resistant to insulin. In response, the body manufactures even more insulin, and the cells raise their resistance until, eventually, both insulin and glucose levels are extremely high. Most diabetes is type 2 diabetes, which appears in adulthood and is preceded by the body's developing resistance to insulin. The chief risk factor is obesity, and the incidence of type 2 diabetes is increasing as obesity rates rise. Type 2 diabetes is treated largely by dietary changes and exercise. Some cases may require treatment with insulin and other medications.

Pregnant women may experience a disorder known as *gestational diabetes*. Unlike type 1 and type 2 diabetes, gestational diabetes is not a chronic condition. It appears during pregnancy in women experiencing high blood glucose levels. It is treated through diet and careful monitoring of the baby's development.

See Chapter 18, Responding to Medical Emergencies, for information about special considerations when providing dental care to diabetic patients.

Hyperthyroidism occurs when the thyroid gland produces too much of the hormone thyroxin.

Hypothyroidism occurs when the thyroid gland does not produce enough hormones. Both conditions affect metabolic rate.

With the release of excess thyroxin, individuals may develop hyperthyroidism, sometimes known as an *overactive thyroid*. Symptoms of hyperthyroidism include sweating, weight loss, rapid heartbeat, and nervousness. Hyperthyroidism is commonly treated with medication to slow the production of thyroxin. Surgery or radiation treatment is required in some cases.

Hypothyroidism, sometimes known as an *underactive thyroid*, is characterized by weight gain and symptoms such as cold intolerance, depression, and fatigue. This chronic condition is more common in women, especially those who are older than age 50 years. If untreated, hypothyroidism can cause a chemical imbalance. The condition is treated with medication to supplement the low levels of thyroxin.

CHECKPOINTS

5-12 What is the uppermost layer of skin called?

5-13 Insulin is produced by which gland in the endocrine system?

Lymphatic and Immune Systems

Lymphatic System

The lymphatic system is a circulatory system with its own set of capillaries and vessels (Figure 5-24). Rather than circulating blood, the lymphatic system transports tissue fluid.

Functions

The lymphatic system circulates and filters lymphatic fluid, also known as *tissue fluid*, which is important in fighting disease.

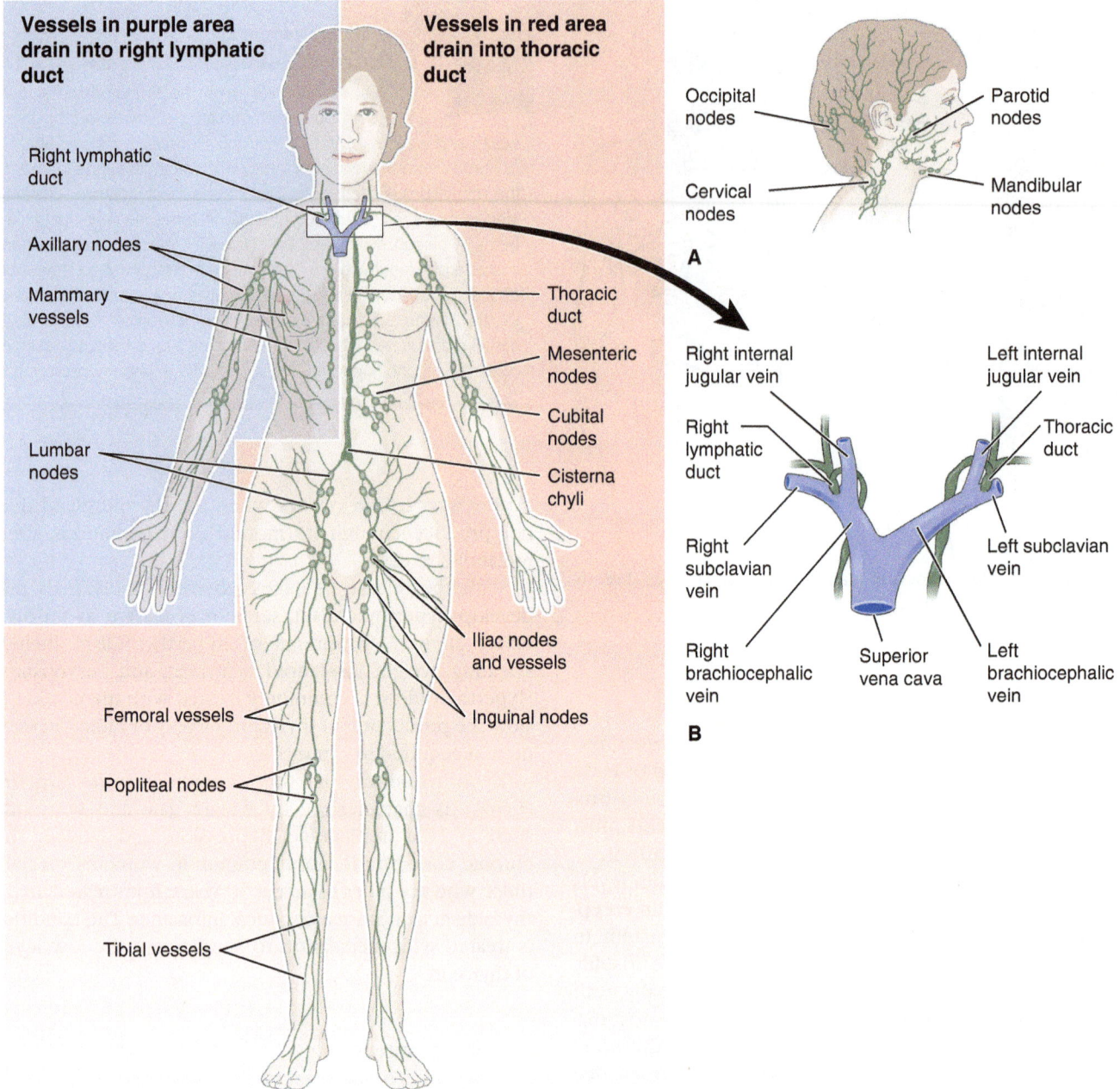

Figure 5–24 The **(A)** lymph nodes and **(B)** lymph vessels of the body.

Basic Structures

The lymphatic system is composed of the spleen, lymph nodes and nodules, lymph fluid, and thymus gland. Although it filters blood rather than lymph, the spleen is the system's chief filtering organ. It removes old red blood cells, bacteria, and other invasive foreign material and maintains a rich blood supply of its own for use in case of blood loss. Lymph nodes and nodules are masses of lymphatic tissue found along the route of the lymph vessels. The best known lymph nodes are in the neck, armpit, and groin, but others are found throughout the body. Each lymph node drains the particular region of tissue surrounding it.

Lymph nodes commonly swell when infection is present in the surrounding tissue. A dental assistant may encounter patients whose cervical or submaxillary lymph nodes, located in the neck and face, are swollen in response to infection. The tonsils, a special collection of lymphatic tissue at the base of the throat, help guard the body against bacteria that may enter from the respiratory or digestive tract. (Chapter 6, Head and Neck Anatomy, will discuss the lymphatic system of the head and neck, including the tonsils, in greater detail.)

The thymus gland, located inferior to the thyroid gland, is part of the lymphatic system. It produces T lymphocytes, also known as *T cells*, which are essential for a healthy immune system.

Common Disorders in the Lymphatic System

Tonsillitis, an infection of the tonsils, is common in children and is frequently encountered among pediatric dental patients.

Hodgkin disease, also known as Hodgkin lymphoma, is a cancer of the lymph nodes and other lymphatic tissue. The earliest sign of the disease is usually a lymph node that swells for no apparent reason. The cancer can then spread to other nearby lymph nodes and later to the liver, lungs, or bone marrow. Hodgkin disease is most common among people between 15 and 35 years of age and those between 50 and 70 years of age.

As a dental assistant, you should report any suspicious swelling in the neck or jaw to the dentist and bring it to the attention of the patient. Early diagnosis of Hodgkin lymphoma is extremely important to the patient's life and future health. If a patient mentions unexplained swelling in other areas, such as the armpit or groin, report this to the dentist also.

From the Dentist's Perspective

The dental assistants who work with me know that I want to hear from them. This is especially helpful when we are treating new patients or those who are usually reluctant to talk about themselves. One day a patient we had not seen for quite a while came in for us to take a look at a broken tooth. The dental assistant took an updated history, and nothing very unusual came up. The patient gave one-word responses to most of the questions. When the dental assistant went chairside, however, to begin examining the patient's oral cavity, she noticed a scar under the turtleneck the woman was wearing. Without hesitating for a minute, she asked the patient about it. It turned out the woman had recently undergone treatment for a malignant tumor and was receiving follow-up radiation. This had been a very difficult and frightening time for her and she was reluctant to talk about it. She told my dental assistant that she had not thought it necessary to mention it, thinking it had nothing to do with her dental care and treatment. My dental assistant, however, knew to ask about any change she noticed. Recent radiation therapy is just one of many things that can potentially affect treatment. Our knowledgeable and professional dental assistant helped both me and my patient that day.

Immune System

Numerous organs, tissues, and specialized cells participate in the immune system (Figure 5-25). The immune system functions by recognizing each cell, tissue, and organ in the human body as the body's very own. When it senses a foreign tissue, bacteria, virus, or toxin, the immune system employs various methods to destroy it, called **auto-immune responses**. These invasive bacteria and other substances are referred to as antigens.

In addition to foreign antigens, the immune system recognizes mutated cells as antigens and usually destroys them before they can develop into cancer. Organ transplants are challenging, because the immune system recognizes transplanted organs as foreign and attempts to destroy them. Transplant patients are typically given medications to suppress their immune system for as long as necessary.

Functions

The immune system destroys pathogens that enter the body and protects the body from foreign substances, cells, and tissues.

Basic Structures

The immune system includes many different types of cells, including blood cells; tissues, including lymphatic tissues; organs, including the spleen; and body systems, including the lymphatic circulatory system. Our immunity is perhaps best understood through its various levels and approaches.

The first line of defense is the innate immunity, or nonspecific immunity, that we possess from the time we are born. This protects us against any harmful agent in general. Examples of innate immunity include our cough reflex, the formation of mucus, our skin, the tears in our eyes, stomach acid, and fever.

The second line of defense is acquired immunity, or the immunity to a specific disease that we develop by repeated exposure to that disease. This includes immunity to diseases such as chickenpox, which do not recur after we have had them once. (The varicella-zoster virus

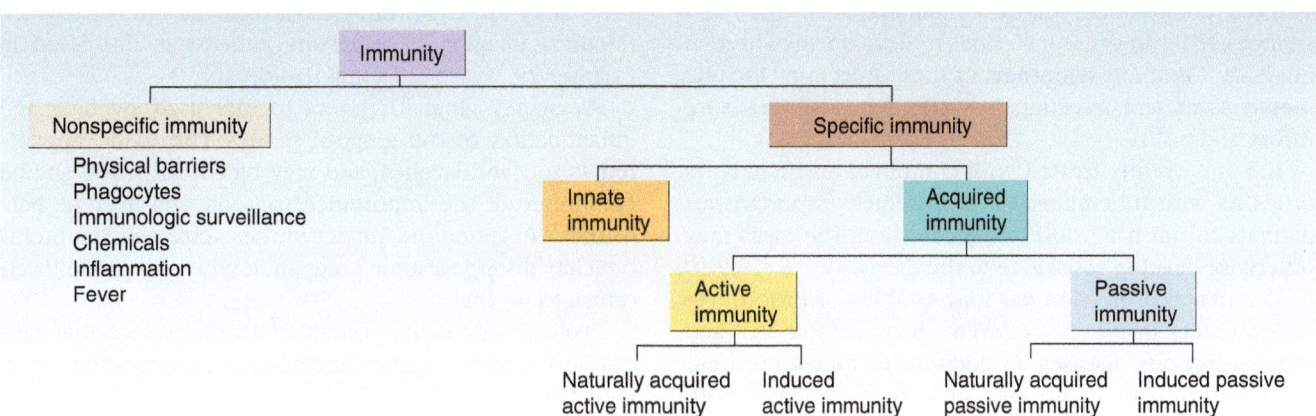

Figure 5–25 Various levels of immunity.

that causes chickenpox remains in the body, however, and may later become active, resulting in shingles.) Vaccination, which produces antibodies to an illness, is a form of acquired immunity.

Of all the parts of our body involved in the immune response, blood cells are the most important. White blood cells, or leukocytes, include the B cells, which produce antibodies, and the T cells, which attack antigens directly.

Inflammation, such as the swelling that occurs after injury or in response to bacteria or toxins, is another form of immune response. Swelling works by creating fluid that isolates the offending injury or substance from the rest of the body.

Other types of immunity include passive immunity, which is passed from mothers to infants in the womb, and genetic immunity, which is built into our chromosomes and prevents us from catching or developing diseases that occur in species other than human beings.

Common Disorders in the Immune System
Autoimmune disorders occur when the immune system mistakenly identifies part of its own body as foreign and begins attacking it. There are more than 80 types of autoimmune disorders. Common ones include:

- Rheumatoid arthritis, characterized by swelling, pain, stiffness, and, sometimes, degeneration in the joints
- Systemic lupus erythematosus, characterized by inflammation in the skin, joints, kidneys, heart, or other organs
- Multiple sclerosis
- Type 1 diabetes
- Graves disease

Allergies occur when the immune system reacts to a harmless substance it would normally ignore. Common allergies involve dust, pet dander, and pollen.

Human immunodeficiency virus (HIV) is caused by an infection that seriously weakens and can destroy the immune system. It is spread by contaminated blood products and transfusions, intimate sexual contact with an infected person, and use of contaminated needles and syringes. HIV can cause infections to develop anywhere in the body. Common symptoms of these infections include mouth sores and infections, swollen lymph nodes, sore throat, and rash.

HIV is currently treated with combinations of antiviral drugs. As with tuberculosis, it is extremely important for patients to finish all doses of medication. The virus may otherwise develop resistance to the drugs.

The dental profession has long-established procedures and practices in place to prevent the spread of HIV and other infectious diseases. In addition to following these scrupulously, dental assistants should ask patients about the history of any unusual mouth sores.

Reproductive System

The main purpose of both male and female reproductive systems is the creation of life and the continuance of the human species. Both male and female reproductive systems have external and internal structures, called *genitalia*, which are related to sexual intercourse and reproduction. Dental assistants should keep in mind that both the female and male reproductive systems are consequential to health in ways that extend beyond sexuality and reproduction.

Female Reproductive System

Most female patients experience hormonal influence, pregnancy, puberty, menopause, and menstruation at one time or another. Some of these can influence dental care in surprising ways. The reproductive organs of both female and male patients must be shielded during dental radiographs. These procedures are discussed fully in Section VII, Dental Radiography.

Functions
The female reproductive system produces eggs, provides an environment for fertilization of eggs during intercourse, and provides an environment for development of the embryo and fetus until birth.

Basic Structures
Internal female genitalia include the ovaries, which release one or more eggs for possible fertilization each month; the fallopian tubes, which transport eggs between the ovaries and uterus; the uterus, which provides a nurturing environment for development of the embryo and fetus after fertilization; and the vagina, which leads from the uterus to the external opening of the female reproductive system, the vulva.

Common Disorders in the Female Reproductive System
Though not a disorder, pregnancy in dental patients merits special mention. The hormonal changes that occur in pregnancy can cause or aggravate changes in oral tissues. (Medical imaging of pregnant patients is discussed in Chapter 29, Basics of Dental Radiography.)

Pregnancy gingivitis refers to increased swelling and inflammation of the gingival tissues. The tissue appears red, is soft and swollen, and may bleed easily. You should communicate the importance of good oral hygiene habits that can lessen the impact of these changes. Symptoms typically disappear after pregnancy, when hormone levels return to normal.

Pyogenic granuloma refers to an oral tumor that may develop in both pregnant and nonpregnant women and in men. The result of local irritation and hormonal imbalance, it grows rapidly but is usually painless and easily removed (excised). Once removed, it may return if hormonal imbalance continues. In pregnant patients, a pyogenic granuloma is usually removed only after the pregnancy is over.

Female patients in their teens may also develop gingival conditions related to hormonal changes during puberty. These conditions resemble pregnancy gingivitis, with red, swollen gingival tissue that may bleed easily. Although male patients in their teens may also develop this puberty-related condition, it is more common in females.

Other disorders of the female reproductive system include toxic shock syndrome, a potentially serious complication associated with menstruation and tampon use. Symptoms are flulike and include fever, headache, vomiting, rash, and hypotension.

Pelvic inflammatory disease (PID) is an infection of the fallopian tubes and ovaries. Its symptoms include abdominal pain, fever, and vaginal discharge. A leading cause of female infertility, its early diagnosis is essential. If symptoms such as these are noted during a health history, the patient should be advised to seek medical care immediately.

Male Reproductive System

Life stages, such as puberty and aging, can influence the dental care of male patients in surprising ways. The male reproductive system also shares organs with the male urinary tract. Some common disorders may interfere with the functioning of one or both systems.

Functions

The male reproductive system produces and transports sperm, which can fertilize the female's egg.

Basic Structures

The internal genitalia of the male reproductive system include the prostate gland, which produces and releases one of the fluid components of male ejaculate, the fluid released during ejaculation; the seminal vesicles, which produce and release a different fluid; and the ejaculatory duct, which transports fluids to the urethra for ejaculation. External genitalia include the testes, which produce sperm; the scrotum, which contains the testes; and the penis, which provides for fertilization of eggs during intercourse.

Common Disorders in the Male Reproductive System

Pyogenic granuloma refers to an oral tumor that may develop in both women and men. The result of local irritation and hormonal imbalance, it grows rapidly but is usually painless and easily removed. Once removed, it may return if hormonal imbalance continues.

Male patients in their teens may develop gingival conditions related to hormonal changes during puberty. These conditions resemble pregnancy gingivitis among women, with red, swollen gingival tissue that may bleed easily. You should communicate the importance of good oral hygiene habits that can lessen the impact of this condition. Symptoms related to these conditions typically disappear after hormone levels return to normal.

Urinary System

The body produces waste products as a result of the daily demands of living. These accumulate in the bloodstream and must be removed before they reach toxic levels. The kidneys gather these waste products and form urine that excretes them from the body. In this process, the kidneys perform other important tasks to keep fluid levels and composition in check. In a sense, the remaining structures of the urinary system, such as the bladder and urethra, exist to carry out the work begun by the kidneys (Figure 5-26).

Functions

The urinary system maintains fluid volume and appropriate composition of bodily fluids, regulates the volume of blood by excreting or conserving water, removes waste products from the blood, and excretes or conserves minerals in the blood.

Basic Structures

The basic structures of the urinary system include the two kidneys, where urine forms; the two ureters, which carry urine to the bladder; the bladder, which stores urine until it can be eliminated; and the urethra, which transports urine from the bladder for elimination outside the body.

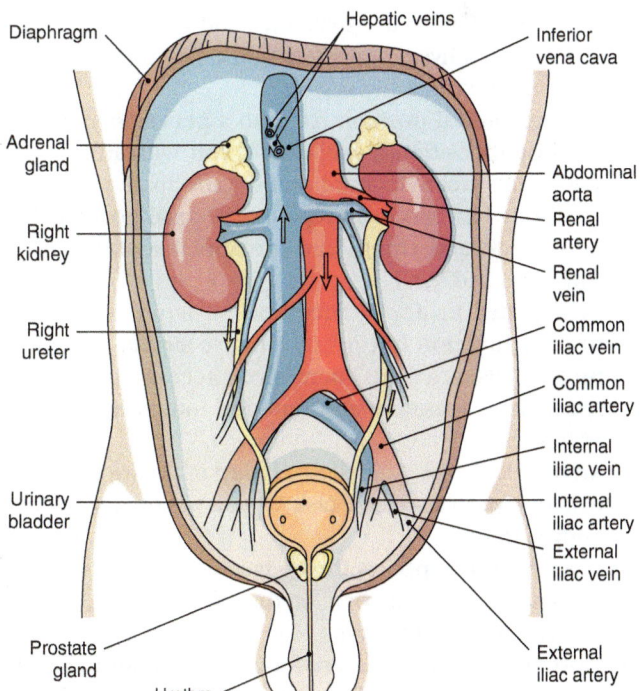

Figure 5–26 The male urinary system, showing blood vessels.

Common Disorders in the Urinary System

Urinary incontinence is the inability to control the passage of urine from the bladder. Urinary incontinence takes three forms: stress incontinence, which can occur during laughter, sneezing, or other abrupt activity; urge incontinence, which is characterized by insufficient warning of the need to urinate; and mixed incontinence, which contains elements of both types. Incontinence is most common among older women. Resources are available to treat incontinence, but it remains embarrassing and concerning to patients. Depending on the cause, it may be treated with medications, exercise, or weight loss and dietary changes. You can lessen the embarrassment caused by incontinence by remaining calm and supportive of patients who experience it. Including incontinence in a health history can encourage patients to view it as a health concern, instead of a personal weakness or an inevitable result of aging.

Renal failure, or kidney failure, is a serious disorder of the urinary system and has two main causes: diabetes and hypertension, which damage blood vessels within the kidneys themselves. Other causes include inadequate blood flow to the kidneys, exposure to toxins, or damage to organs and structures farther along the urinary tract. Acute kidney failure may be treated by discovering and treating the original cause. Chronic, or permanent, kidney failure is treated with hemodialysis—the use of an artificial kidney machine.

CHECKPOINTS

5-14 Lymph nodes frequently swell in response to what?

5-15 Coughing is an example of what type of immunity?

5-16 Where might a dental assistant notice the effects of fluctuating hormone levels in both men and women?

5-17 Chronic kidney failure is treated how?

Interrelatedness of Body Systems

Body systems complement one another. The endocrine system and the nervous system interact through the pituitary gland, for example. From its position deep within the brain, the pituitary gland receives signals from the autonomous nervous system that help it regulate the release of hormones from all other glands in the endocrine system. The respiratory and circulatory systems work together to enable the exchange of oxygen and carbon dioxide within the lungs. The marrow of bones in the skeletal system produces blood cells. Together and separately, all body systems work to maintain health and life.

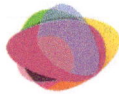

Chapter Highlights

+ Anatomy refers to the structures and individual organs of the body. Physiology refers to the functions and purpose of structures and organs.
+ The anatomical position refers to a person standing in an upright position, facing toward you, with arms at the side, palms facing forward, feet slightly apart.
+ The body has two main regions: the axial portion (the head, neck, and trunk) and the appendicular portion (the arms and legs).
+ Cells differ in appearance and structure according to their function but nearly all have similar basic features. Cells organize themselves according to their specialized structure and function into various types of tissues.
+ An organ may be defined as a group of tissues designed to accomplish a specific task. Organs are organized into body systems.
+ The skeleton supports the body and sustains its shape. It provides a framework for the skeletal muscles that enable the body to move.
+ More than 600 muscles are found throughout the body Muscles come in three types: striated (or skeletal); cardiac (or heart); and smooth (or internal).

+ The respiratory system enables breathing and the exchange of oxygen and carbon monoxide.
+ The digestive system converts solid foods into the nutrients that the body uses to maintain and repair itself and to fuel the activities of daily living. The digestive system then eliminates the waste products from the body.
+ The cardiovascular system is made up of the heart, blood, arteries, veins, and capillaries. The heart circulates blood throughout the body, which provides oxygen and nutrients to organs and tissues while removing waste products, including carbon dioxide and cellular wastes.
+ The nervous system gathers and interprets sensory information from inside and outside the body, initiates involuntary and voluntary movement, and regulates basic bodily functions.
+ The skin is the body's largest organ and its first line of defense against disease and invasive bacteria. The skin protects the body from pathogens, prevents dehydration, regulates body temperature, excretes liquids and salts, and mediates the sense of touch.
+ The endocrine system helps regulate the body's natural processes by producing specific hormones.

◆ The lymphatic system is a circulatory system with its own set of capillaries and vessels that transport tissue fluid, which is important in fighting disease.

◆ The immune system functions by recognizing each cell, tissue, and organ in the human body as the body's very own. When it senses a foreign tissue, bacteria, virus, or toxin, the immune system employs various methods to destroy it.

◆ The female reproductive system produces eggs, provides an environment for fertilization of eggs during intercourse, and provides an environment for development of the embryo and fetus until birth. The male reproductive system produces and transports sperm, which may fertilize the female's egg during intercourse.

◆ The urinary system maintains fluid volume and appropriate composition of bodily fluids, regulates the volume of blood by excreting or conserving water, removes waste products from the blood, and excretes or conserves minerals in the blood.

◆ Together and separately, all body systems work to maintain health and life.

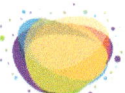 ## Review Questions

1. What are the three planes into which anatomists divide the body to study it?

   a. Posterior, inferior, and dorsal

   b. Sagittal, transverse, and frontal

   c. Cranial, abdominal, and plantar

   d. Medial, proximal, and distal

2. When anatomists describe something as superficial, they mean that it is

   a. Close to the surface.

   b. Unnecessary.

   c. An early symptom.

   d. Alongside something else.

3. The word "buccal" is used to indicate which part of the body?

   a. Hip

   b. Mouth

   c. Lungs

   d. Heart

4. The four main structural levels of the human body are

   a. Respiratory, cardiovascular, urinary, and digestive.

   b. Bone, muscles, skin, and blood.

   c. Cells, tissues, organs, and body systems.

   d. Planes, sections, regions, and cavities.

5. The temporomandibular joint (TMJ) is which type of joint?

   a. Ball and socket

   b. Gliding

   c. Pivot

   d. Condyloid

6. Muscles of the face are which type of muscle?

   a. Skeletal

   b. Smooth

   c. Involuntary

   d. Fascia

7. What canal is the anatomical "tube" running from the mouth to the anus?

   a. Sagittal

   b. Fascial

   c. Dorsal

   d. Alimentary

8. The part of the digestive tract that handles the absorption of nutrients into the bloodstream is the

   a. Small intestine.

   b. Large intestine.

   c. Esophagus.

   d. Stomach.

9. The bottom chambers of the heart, from which blood is pumped to the lungs or to the aorta, are the

   a. Right atrium and left atrium.

   b. Superior and inferior vena cava.

   c. Tricuspids.

   d. Left and right ventricles.

10. Thrombocytes are the part of the blood responsible for

    a. Transporting oxygen.

    b. Fighting disease.

    c. Gathering carbon dioxide.

    d. Clotting blood to stop bleeding.

11. The part of the brain known as the "seat of consciousness" is the
    a. Brainstem.
    b. Cerebellum.
    c. Cerebrum.
    d. Medulla.

12. Which gland is the "lead gland" of the endocrine system, and regulates the behavior of other glands in the system?
    a. Thyroid
    b. Pancreas
    c. Pituitary
    d. Prostate

Active Learning Exercises

1. Name the three planes and the two primary cavities that clinicians use to divide and describe the human body. What is the significance of understanding body planes and cavities even though dentistry primarily deals with the head and neck?

2. List three diseases of the nervous system. Consider how these conditions could affect dental care and treatment.

Application Activities

1. Practice using the terminology outlined in Table 5-2 to locate common body parts. Get a set of index cards and write down the names of 20 body parts, one on each card. Draw two cards and use the terms presented in the table to describe the relationship between the two body parts. For example if you select the terms *lungs* and *brain* you could say, "The lungs are inferior to the brain" and "The brain is superior to the lungs."

PREPARING FOR CERTIFICATION EXAMS

Review the following topics in this chapter to prepare for the Dental Assisting National Board (DANB) exam:

- **Common Disorders in the Skeletal System**
- **Common Disorders in the Digestive System**

Head and Neck Anatomy

CHAPTER OUTLINE

CHAPTER CHECKLIST

Upon completion of this chapter, students will be able to:

☑ Locate and identify the bones of the cranium and face.

☑ Describe the action of the temporomandibular joint and identify its components.

☑ Identify and describe the major muscles of mastication and facial expression.

☑ Identify and describe the nerves innervating the maxillary and mandibular areas of the oral cavity.

☑ Describe how blood circulates throughout the head and neck.

☑ Locate and identify major salivary glands.

☑ Explain the importance of lymph nodes in extraoral examination.

☑ Identify and describe the nine main regions of the face.

☑ Identify and describe landmark features of the face.

KEY TERMS

ala (A-luh) – rounded outside tip of each nostril

alveolar process – bony ridge on either side of the upper and lower jaw; contains sockets for teeth

angle of the mandible – lower portion of the mandibular ramus nearest the ear

aorta – major artery ascending from the heart with blood to supply branch arteries throughout the body

bruxism (BRUK-sihz-uhm) – the habit of grinding or gritting the teeth; particularly during sleep or times of stress

buccinator (BUK-suh-nay-ter) muscle – a thin, broad muscle of facial expression; forms the wall of the cheek

canthus (KAN-thus) (inner) – fold of tissue at the inner corner of the eyelid

canthus (outer) – fold of tissue at the outer corner of the eyelid

common carotid artery – branches from the aorta to supply blood to the head

carotid artery (external) – branches from the common carotid artery to supply blood to the face and mouth

carotid artery (internal) – branches from the common carotid artery to supply blood to the brain

cranium – the portion of the skull that encloses the brain

digastric muscle – one of the muscles of the floor of the mouth; assists in swallowing

ethmoid (ETH-moid) bone – thinly walled bone with a honeycomb-like structure; sits in the center of the skull between the eye sockets and helps form parts of the nasal and orbital cavities

foramen magnum – the natural opening in the base of the occipital bone through which the spinal cord passes

frena (FREE-nuh) (singular: frenum) – folds of skin or a mucous membrane that are positioned between a more stationary and a more flexible part or organ, which restricts movement

frontal bone – the forward-most bone of the cranium; shapes the forehead and forms most of the top of the eye sockets, or orbits

genioglossus (jee-nee-oh-GLAW-sus) muscle – one of the extrinsic muscles of the tongue; depresses the tongue and enables it to protrude

geniohyoid muscle – one of the muscles of the floor of the mouth; draws the hyoid bone and tongue forward

gingiva – the tissue that surrounds the necks of the teeth and covers the alveolar processes; also called *gums*

hard palate – the bony anterior portion of the palate; forms the roof of the mouth

hyoid (HI-oyd) bone – suspended between the mandible and larynx; supports the tongue and other nearby muscles

hyoglossus muscle – one of the extrinsic muscles of the tongue; retracts and pulls down the tongue

labial commissures (KOM-ih-shorz) – corners of the mouth

lacrimal (LAK-rih-muhl) bones – two small, thin bones at the corner of each orbit at the inner angle of the eye socket

lymph node – part of the lymphatic system; produces lymphocytes in response to disease and infection

lymph node (cervical) – lymph node in the neck; may be palpable when swollen

lymphadenopathy (lim-fad-uh-NAP-uh-thee) – swollen and enlarged lymph nodes that last for several months

mandible – long, strong bone that forms the lower jaw

mandibular ramus (man-DIB-yoo-ler RAY-mus) – the vertical portion on either side of the lower jaw that articulates with the skull

masseter (mah-SEE-ter) muscle – one of four pairs of muscles of mastication

maxillae (mak-SIL-ee) – bones that form the upper part of the jaw and a part of the hard palate

maxillary tuberosity – large, rounded protuberance situated on the outer surface of the maxillary bones near the posterior teeth

mental protuberance – a tuberosity of the mandible or lower jaw; commonly known as the chin

meatus (mee-AY-tus) – the external opening of a bodily canal

mentalis (men-TAY-lus) – muscle of facial expression that moves the chin and lower lip

mylohyoid muscle – one of the muscles of the floor of the mouth; forms the floor itself

naris (NAY-rihs), anterior – facial landmark; refers to the nostril

nasal bone – forms the bridge of the nose

nasal conchae (KONG-kee) – three bony projections that scroll inward from the ethmoid bone and form the nasal cavity; known as the *inferior*, *medial*, and *superior* nasal conchae

nasal septum – the bony and cartilaginous partition between the two nasal passages

nasion (NAY-zee-on) – facial landmark lying midway between the eyes, just below the eyebrows

nasolabial groove – runs from the ala of the nose to the corners of the mouth

occipital bone – the lower-most bone of the skull; forms the back and base of the cranium

orbicularis oris (or-bik-yoo-LAR-is OR-is) muscle – one of the muscles of facial expression; encircles and helps move the mouth

palatine (PAL-uh-tine) bone – facial bone important to the structure of the mouth; forms the posterior portion of the roof of the mouth and the floor of the nose, along with the side walls of the nasal cavity

palatoglossus (pal-uh-toe-GLAW-sus) – one of the two major muscles of the soft palate

palatopharyngeus (pal-uh-toe-fa-RIHN-jee-us) – one of the two major muscles of the soft palate

parietal bone – found on each side of the cranium; forms its rounded back and upper sides

parotid (pah-ROT-id) duct – duct that carries saliva from the parotid gland to the mouth; also known as Stensen duct

parotid gland – the largest of the salivary glands; located on each side of the head just below and in front of the ear

philtrum (FILL-trum) – the ridge running from just under the nostrils to the middle of the upper lip

process – a raised portion or projection along the surface of a bone; sometimes called a prominence

pterygoid (TER-ih-goyd) muscle (external) – one of four pairs of muscles of mastication

pterygoid muscle (internal) – one of four pairs of muscles of mastication

septum – facial landmark; connective tissue that divides the nasal cavity into two passages

sialolith (SIGH-uh-loe-lith) – salivary gland stone

sinus – in head and neck anatomy, an air-filled cavity within any of a number of the bones of the skull; usually communicates with the nostrils

sphenoid (SFEE-noyd) bone – forms the anterior, or forward-most part, of the base of the skull

styloglossus (sti-loe-GLO-sus) muscle – one of the extrinsic muscles of the tongue; retracts the tongue

stylohyoid (sti-lo-HI-oyd) muscle – one of the muscles of the floor of the mouth; assists in swallowing

sublingual duct – duct that transports saliva from the sublingual glands to the oral cavity; also known as Bartholin duct

sublingual gland – major salivary gland; located under the mucous membrane between the tongue and the mandible

submandibular duct – duct that transports saliva from the submandibular gland to the oral cavity; also known as Wharton duct

submandibular gland – major salivary gland; located on each side of the mouth inside and near the lower edge of the mandible

suture – the jagged articulation where bones, for example, of the skull, meet and form a fibrous joint that does not move

temporal bone – found on each side of the cranium and surrounding the ear

temporal muscle – one of the four pairs of muscles of mastication

temporomandibular joint (TMJ) – articulation between the temporal and mandible bones

temporomandibular joint dysfunction (TMJD) – joint inflammation and dysfunction caused largely by stress-induced clenching and grinding of the teeth

tragus – portion of the external ear lying anterior to the acoustic meatus

trigeminal nerve – cranial nerve V; serves as the primary source of innervation for the oral cavity

vermilion border – the border of the lips

vermilion zone – reddish portion of the lips

vestibule (of the oral cavity) – space between the teeth and the inner lining of the cheeks and lips

vomer (VOE-mer) – a single, flat bone that forms the base of the nasal septum

zygomatic bone – also known as malar bone; helps form the prominence, or highest part, of each cheekbone and the side and bottom of each eye socket

zygomatic major – a muscle of facial expression that extends along the cheek to the mouth; important in laughter

Introduction

Major anatomical structures within the head and neck—whether bones, muscles, nerves, blood vessels, or glands—are very important in the daily work of dental assistants. Many structures take their name from the anatomical areas they support, move, innervate, supply, or drain.

While working chairside, the dental assistant considers the patient's entire oral health history, discusses any special needs or preferences the patient may have, and helps alleviate discomfort and pain. To address these issues adequately, the dental assistant must communicate effectively both with patients and other members of the dental team. As nearly as possible, they must all speak the same language—the language of anatomy. To provide quality patient care, you need to know how the human head and neck are structured and how the various systems of the body interact within the oral cavity.

Bones

Although we often think of the skull as one unit, it is actually composed of separate bones, each of which provides the underlying structure that supports and protects the significant organs and tissues located within the head. The skull is divided into two main sections: the **cranium**, which covers and protects the brain, and the face, which underlies and supports our most familiar features (Figure 6-1).

Bones of the Cranium

The bones of the cranium are the frontal, occipital, sphenoid, and ethmoid bones, which occur singly, and the paired parietal and paired temporal bones, one of which appears on either side of the head (Figure 6-2). The bones of the cranium are joined together by immovable articulations called **sutures**.

Ethmoid Bone

The **ethmoid bone** sits in the center of the skull between the orbits, or eye sockets, and helps form parts of the nasal and orbital cavities. This thinly walled, complex bone has a honeycomb-like structure and contains numerous small spaces, known as the *ethmoid sinuses*. The *medial concha* and *superior concha* are bony processes that extend out from the ethmoid bone and help form the meatuses, or outer openings, of the nasal cavity.

Frontal Bone

The **frontal bone** is the forwardmost bone of the cranium. It shapes the forehead and forms part of the floor of the cranium and most of the roof of the orbits, or eye sockets.

Occipital Bone

The **occipital bone** is the lowest bone of the skull and forms the back and base of the cranium. It is joined on either side by the parietal bones. Just before it attaches to the brain stem, the spinal cord passes through a small round opening, called the **foramen magnum**, in the base of the occipital bone (Figure 6-3).

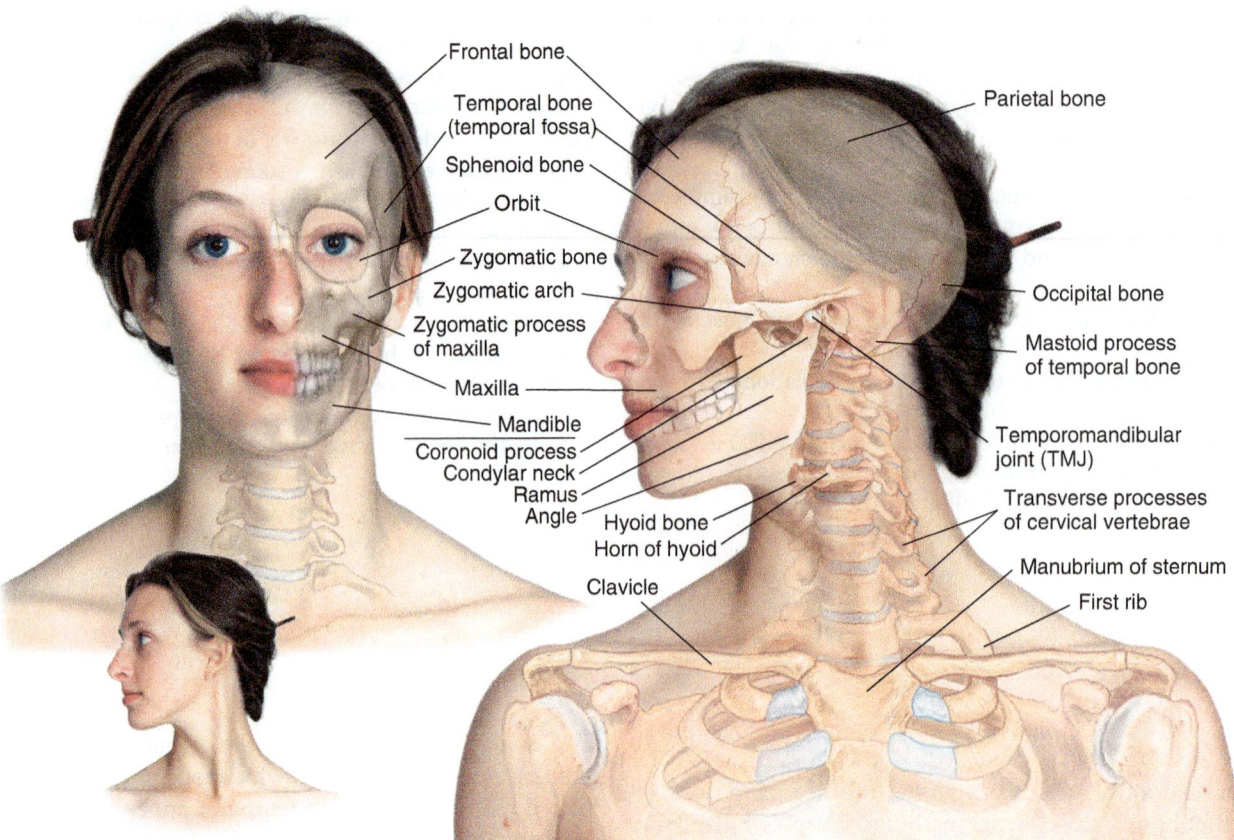

Figure 6–1 Bones of the skull are divided into cranial bones and facial bones.

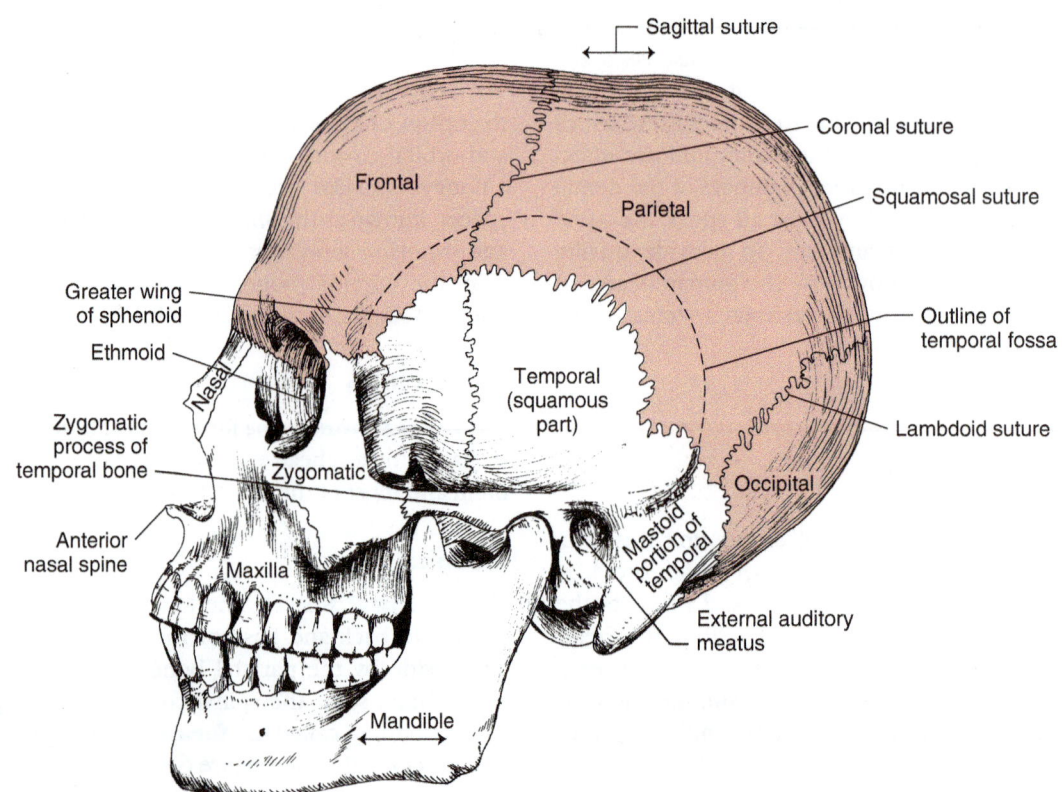

Figure 6–2 The bones of the cranium include the frontal, occipital, sphenoid, ethmoid, parietal, and temporal bones.

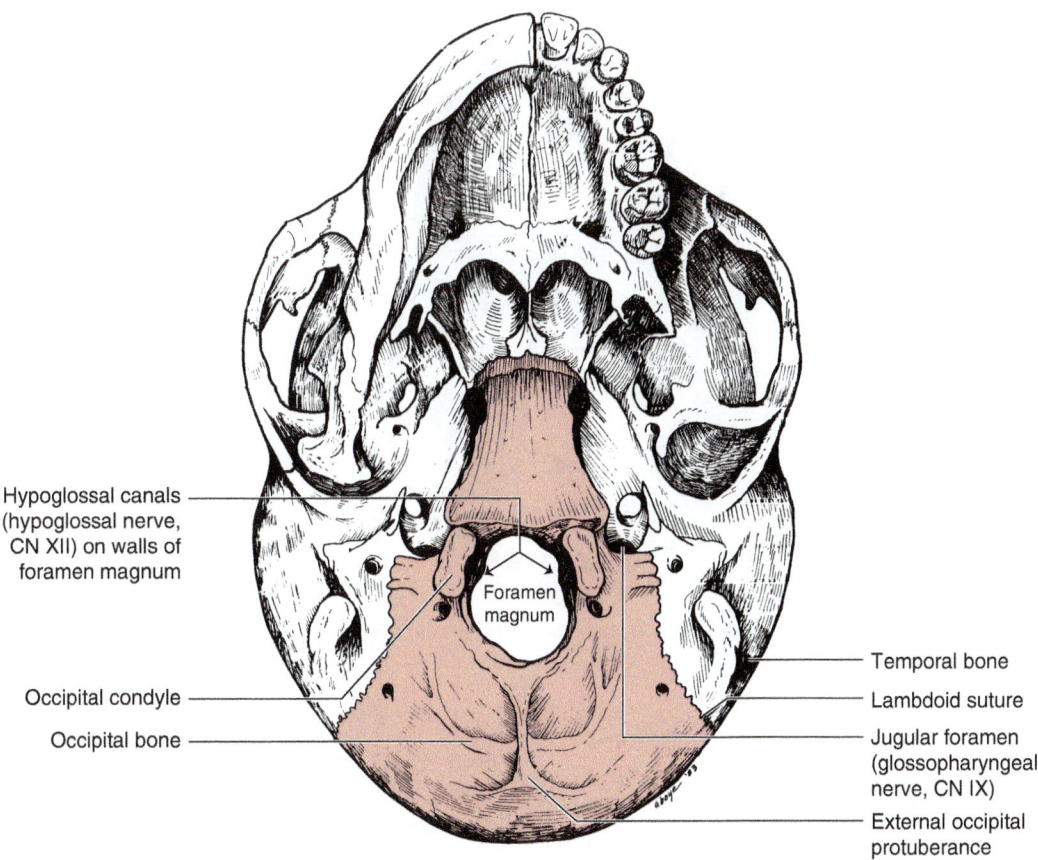

Hypoglossal canals
(hypoglossal nerve,
CN XII) on walls of
foramen magnum

Foramen
magnum

Occipital condyle

Occipital bone

Temporal bone

Lambdoid suture

Jugular foramen
(glossopharyngeal
nerve, CN IX)

External occipital
protuberance

Figure 6–3 The back and base of the cranium, the occipital bone, contains the foramen magnum through which the spinal cord passes. CN, cranial nerve.

Parietal Bones

The two **parietal bones** form the rounded back and upper sides of the cranium. They join together at the sagittal suture at the middle of the back of the skull (Figure 6-4). At their top they are joined to the frontal bone at the coronal suture near the crown of the skull. In newborn babies, this suture is not yet closed and its site is occupied by a "soft spot," known as the *anterior fontanelle*, where the bones will later join together (Figure 6-5).

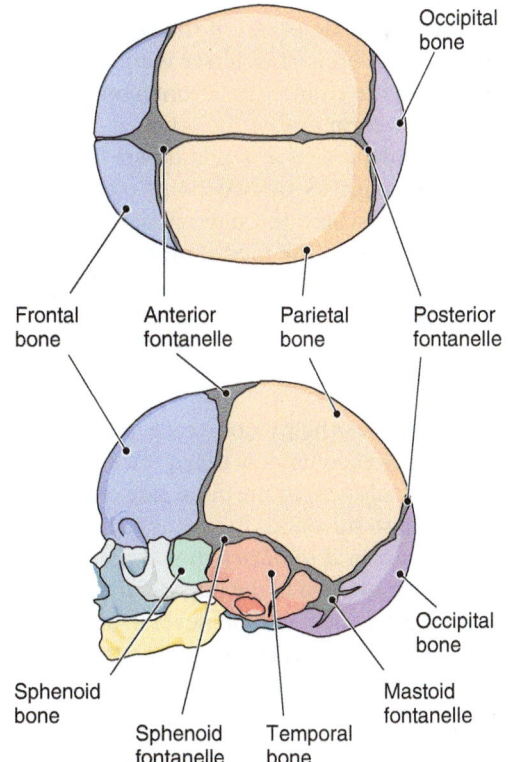

Occipital
bone

Frontal
bone

Anterior
fontanelle

Parietal
bone

Posterior
fontanelle

Sphenoid
bone

Sphenoid
fontanelle

Temporal
bone

Occipital
bone

Mastoid
fontanelle

Figure 6–5 "Soft spots," known as *fontanelles*, are where the cranial bones will later join together by sutures.

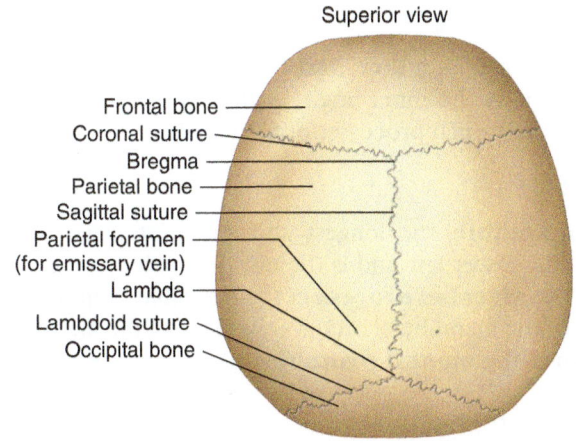

Superior view

Frontal bone
Coronal suture
Bregma
Parietal bone
Sagittal suture
Parietal foramen
(for emissary vein)
Lambda
Lambdoid suture
Occipital bone

Figure 6–4 Sutures join the bones of the cranium together.

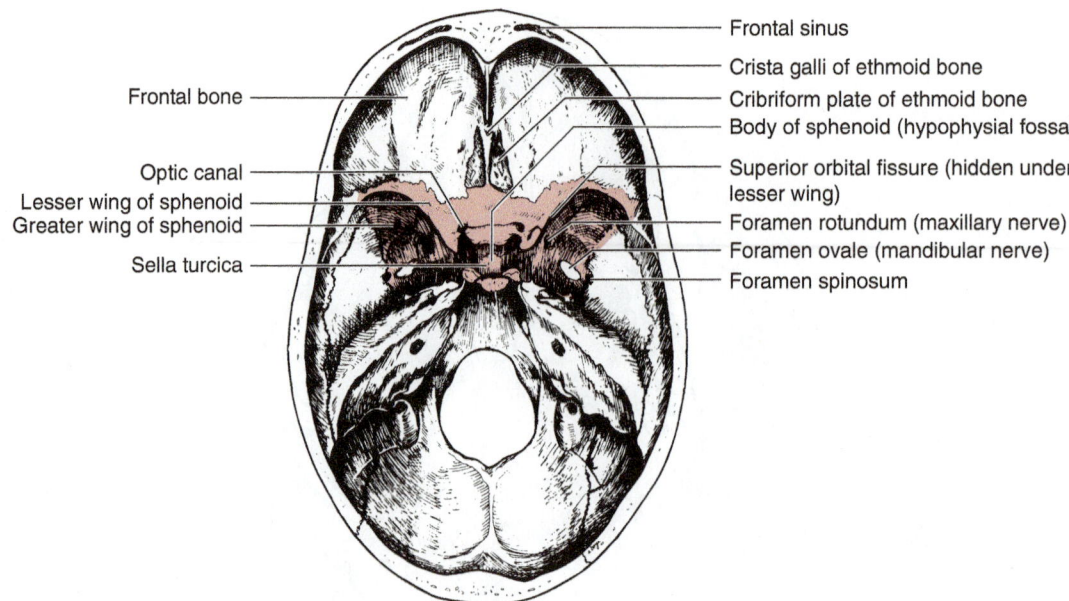

Frontal sinus
Crista galli of ethmoid bone
Cribriform plate of ethmoid bone
Body of sphenoid (hypophysial fossa)
Superior orbital fissure (hidden under lesser wing)
Foramen rotundum (maxillary nerve)
Foramen ovale (mandibular nerve)
Foramen spinosum

Frontal bone
Optic canal
Lesser wing of sphenoid
Greater wing of sphenoid
Sella turcica

Figure 6–6 The sphenoid is a butterfly- or bat-shaped bone that forms the anterior part of the base of the skull and acts as an anchor.

Sphenoid Bone

The **sphenoid bone** (Figure 6-6) is composed of a main body and paired greater and lesser wings. It forms the anterior part of the base of the skull. The sphenoid bone forms important attachments with other bones of the face and skull. At key points, the greater wing of the sphenoid bone attaches to the temporal and frontal bones of the skull, and with the zygomatic bones of the face, where it helps to form part of the orbits. The lesser wing of the sphenoid bone attaches to the ethmoid and frontal bones of the skull and also helps to form part of the orbit.

The pterygoid process extends down from the sphenoid bone and consists of two bony plates. The lateral pterygoid plate is where the internal and external pterygoid muscles originate. The medial pterygoid plate ends in the hook-shaped pterygoid hamulus, which supports the soft palate's tensor veli palatini muscle.

Temporal Bones

The **temporal bones** help to form each side of the cranium, including the region commonly called the *temple* along the side of the head adjacent to the distal side of the orbits. The temporal bone also surrounds the ear, and, through an opening called the *external auditory meatus*, allows the outer ear canal passage to open to the outside of the skull.

The temporal bones include several other structures of anatomical importance. These include the mastoid process, a projection of bone located just behind the ear. The mastoid process contains spaces that open up into the adjoining middle ear.

The glenoid fossa is a grooved depression on the lower part of the temporal bone that allows it to articulate, or move together, with the upper jaw or mandible. The gle-

noid fossa forms part of the temporomandibular joint, which is of particular importance in dentistry and will be discussed in detail later in this chapter.

Auditory Ossicles

Each middle ear contains three auditory ossicles, or bones of the middle ear: the malleus, the incus, and the stapes.

Bones of the Face

The 14 bones of the face are the lacrimal bones, the nasal bones, the vomer, the nasal conchae, the zygomatic bones, the maxillae, and the mandible. Although made of many bones, the face's skeletal structure is connected through **processes** and other bony structures that allow its various components to support neighboring bones as well as move and function together when necessary.

Lacrimal Bones

The two small, thin **lacrimal bones** sit at the corner of each orbit at the inner angle of the eye socket, directly behind the frontal processes of the maxillae.

Mandible

The **mandible**, the longest and strongest facial bone, forms the lower jaw and is the only movable bone in the skull. The **alveolar process** of the mandible supports the teeth of the mandibular arch. A tuberosity of the mandible, known as the **mental protuberance**, forms the chin.

Maxillary Bones

The maxillary bones, or the **maxillae**, form the upper part of each jaw and a part of the hard palate (Figure 6-7). They

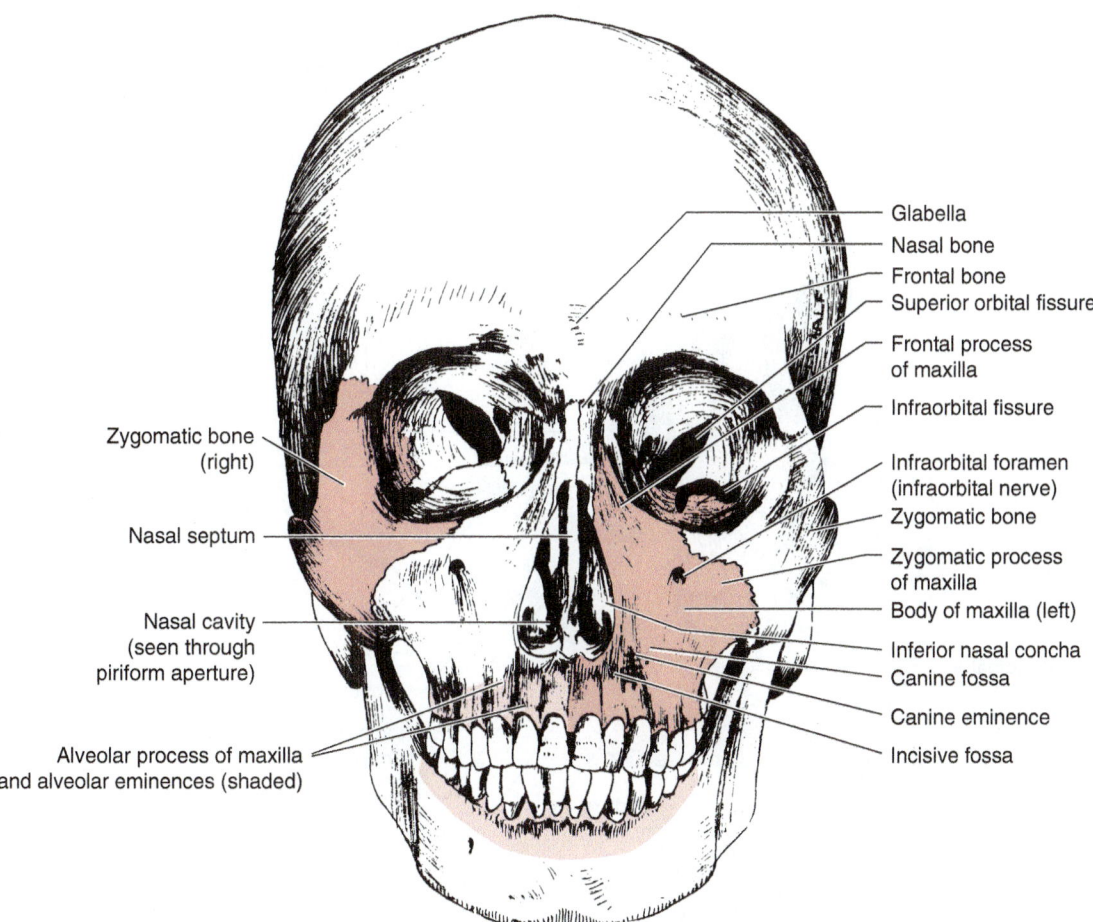

Figure 6–7 The zygomatic and maxillary bone and their parts.

provide the supporting structure for most of the upper teeth and join together at their midline at the maxillary suture. The zygomatic process of the maxillary bones rises up to articulate with the zygomatic bone. As with the mandible below, the alveolar process of the maxillae forms the support for the teeth of the maxillary arch. The large, rounded **maxillary tuberosity**, situated on the outer surface of the maxillary bones near the posterior teeth, provides a useful landmark when mounting maxillary radiographs.

Nasal Bones

The two **nasal bones** form the bridge of the nose. Superiorly, they articulate with the frontal bone and help to form the **nasal septum**, which separates the two nasal passages.

Nasal Conchae

On each side, the nasal cavity consists of three bony projections that scroll inward from the ethmoid bone. These are called the *inferior*, *medial*, and *superior* **nasal conchae**.

Vomer

A single, flat bone, the **vomer** forms the base of the nasal septum.

Zygomatic Bones

Also known as the *malar bones*, the two **zygomatic bones** (see Figure 6-7) help form the prominence of the cheekbone and the side and bottom of the orbit. A frontal process of the zygomatic bone extends upward to articulate with the frontal bone of the skull. The temporal bones of the skull join with the zygomatic bones at the zygomatic arch (Figure 6-8), which forms the prominence of the cheekbone.

Palatine Bones

Though they are not considered facial bones like those discussed above, the two **palatine bones** (Figure 6-9) are important to the structure of the oral cavity. The horizontal plate of the palatine bones forms the posterior of the mouth's hard palate and the floor of the nose; the vertical plate of the palatine bones forms the lateral walls of the nasal cavity. Anteriorly, both articulate with the maxillae.

Bones of the Neck

Hyoid Bone

Shaped like a horseshoe and suspended between the mandible and larynx, the **hyoid bone**'s important and sole

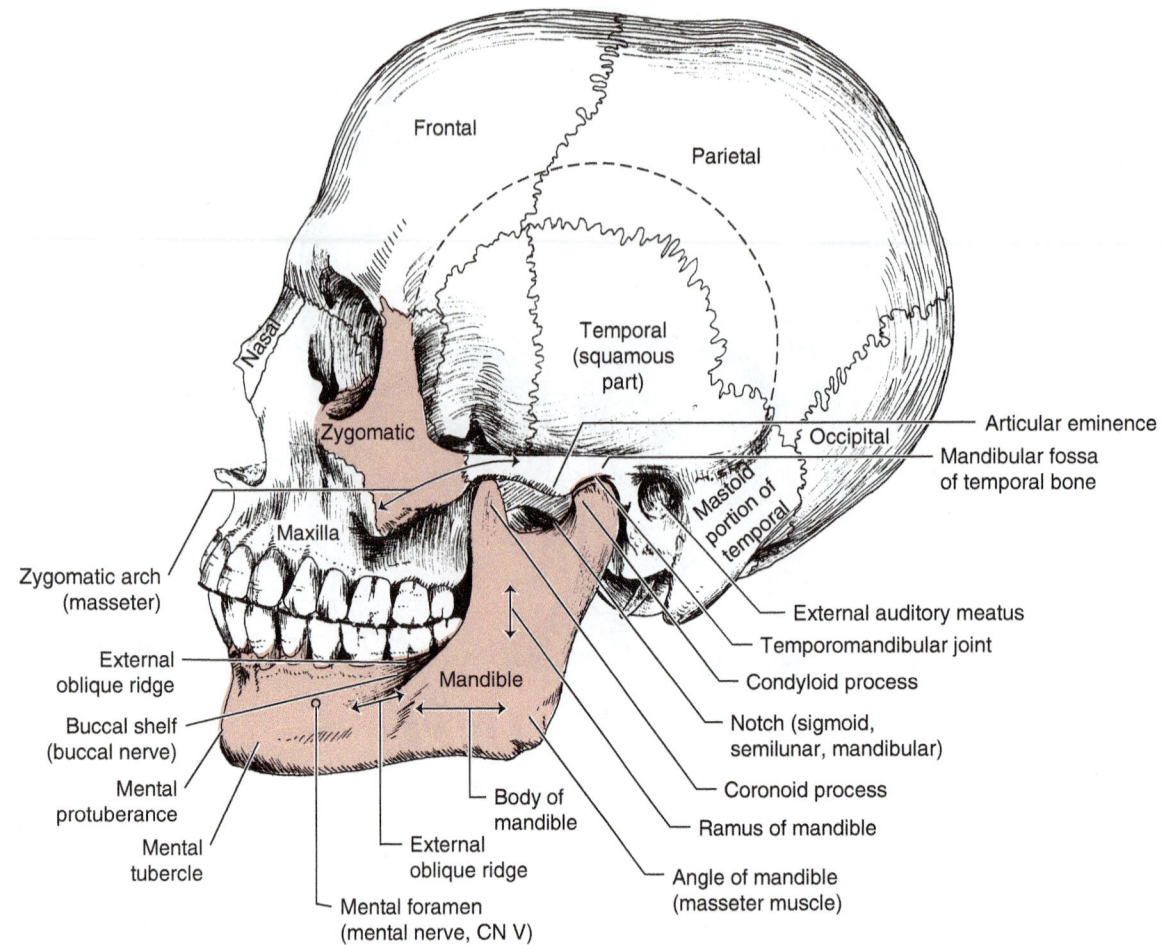

Figure 6–8 Landmarks of the mandible and the zygomatic arch. CN, cranial nerve.

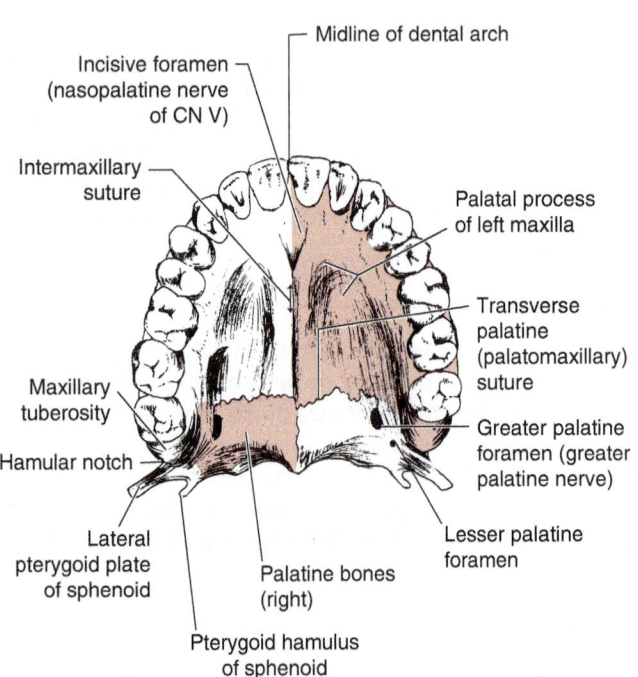

Figure 6–9 The palatine bones form the hard palate and floor of the nose. CN, cranial nerve.

function is to support the tongue and other nearby muscles. It does not join or articulate with any other bones.

Sinuses

A **sinus** is an air-filled space within a bone. Sinuses reduce the weight of the bone, produce mucus, and help to produce sound. Frontal sinuses are located in the frontal bone above each eye. Sphenoid sinuses are located in the sphenoid bone posterior to each eye. The ethmoid sinuses are located within the complex honeycomb structure of the ethmoid bone. Maxillary sinuses are located within the maxillary bones (Figure 6-10).

CHECKPOINTS

6-1 What are the two main sections of the skull?

6-2 The frontal bone shapes which part of the face?

6-3 Which is the only movable bone in the skull?

6-4 Which bone of the head and neck does not articulate with any other bones?

Paranasal Sinuses

Anterior View

Lateral View
(Conchae Removed)

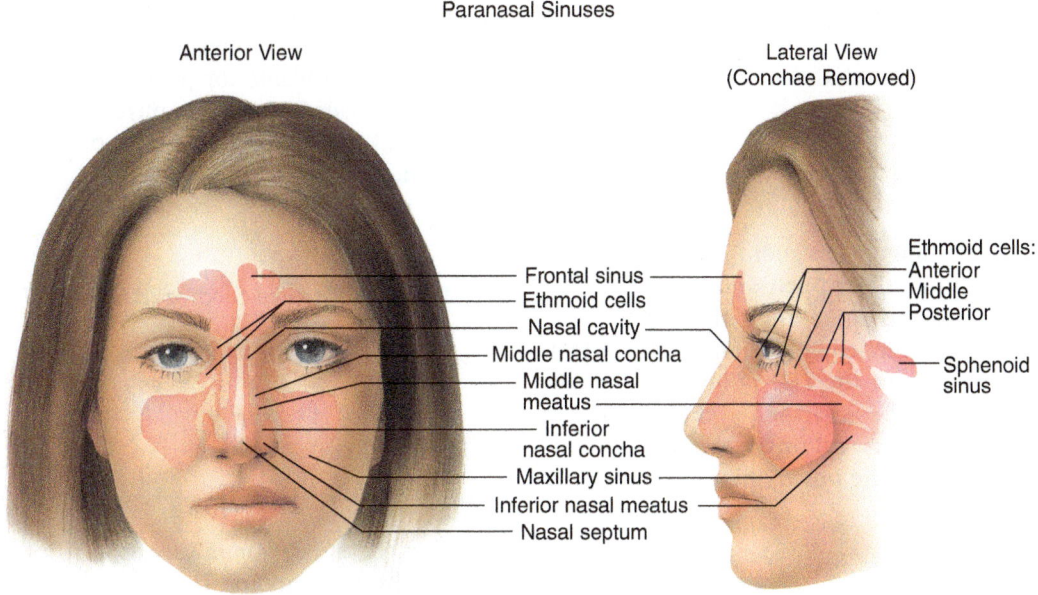

Frontal sinus
Ethmoid cells
Nasal cavity
Middle nasal concha
Middle nasal meatus
Inferior nasal concha
Maxillary sinus
Inferior nasal meatus
Nasal septum

Ethmoid cells:
Anterior
Middle
Posterior
Sphenoid sinus

Figure 6–10 Sinuses within the skull.

Temporomandibular Joint

The most significant joint in dentistry, the **temporomandibular joint (TMJ)** is a gliding joint that joins the mandible to the temporal bone above it (Figure 6-11). Located on either side of the head, toward the posterior end of the jaw, it allows the mandible, the only movable bone of the skull, to move. This allows the mouth to open and close, making the TMJ essential for mastication and speech.

The temporomandibular joint is composed of three main parts: (1) The glenoid fossa is an oval depression in the temporal bone and is located just anterior to the external auditory meatus. (2) The articular eminence is a raised spot on the temporal bone, located just anterior to the glenoid fossa. (3) The condyloid process of the mandible fits into the glenoid fossa, with the articular disc situated

Figure 6–11 The main components of the temporomandibular joint.

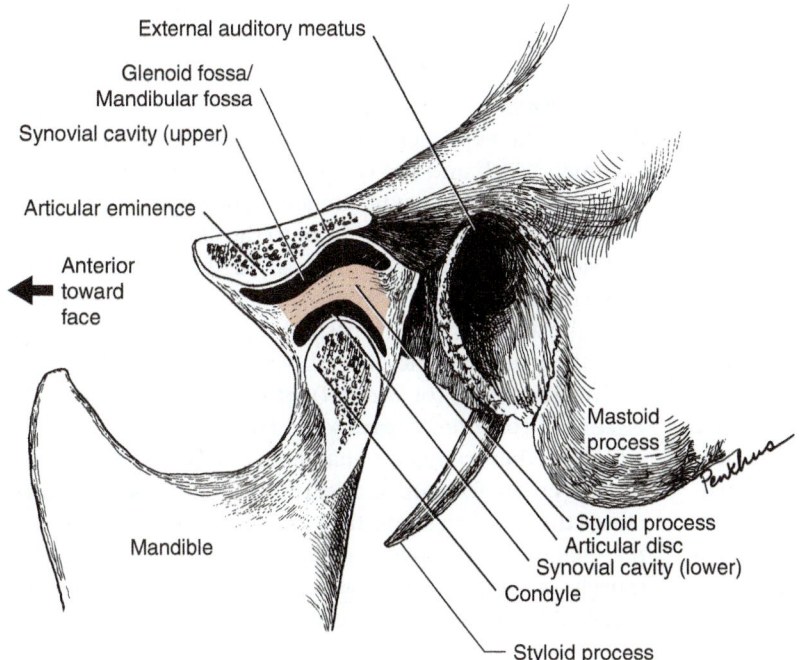

External auditory meatus

Glenoid fossa/
Mandibular fossa

Synovial cavity (upper)

Articular eminence

Anterior
toward
face

Mandible

Mastoid process

Styloid process
Articular disc
Synovial cavity (lower)
Condyle

Styloid process

between the two parts to act as a shock absorber. Often the articular disc is the cause of joint pain since it can become folded over or displaced due to trauma or grinding (bruxism).

Jaw Movement

The TMJ makes both hinged and gliding motions. These motions enable the mouth to open and close and the jaw to shift from side to side. When the mouth first opens, it does so with a hinged movement from the TMJ. Only the lower portion of the TMJ is involved in this motion. As the mouth opens farther, a gliding motion allows the jaw to move forward or backward. This gliding motion involves both the lower and upper portions of the joint.

Temporomandibular Joint Dysfunction

Temporomandibular joint dysfunction (TMJD) can cause the TMJ to become painful and tender. Pain and tenderness may occur in both joints or in only one. TMJD results from a complex of factors, beginning with *bruxism*—the stress-induced clenching and grinding of the teeth. Some people with TMJD have a history of clenching their teeth for prolonged periods during the day. Others may clench and grind their teeth while asleep. TMJD can also be caused by a history of trauma to the jaw, misalignment of the teeth, the aging process, and osteoarthritis and other systemic diseases.

TMJD can result in *crepitus*, the sound or sensation of grating or clicking under the skin and joints, in the TMJ. Other common ailments associated with TMJD include *trismus*—spasms that occur in the muscles of the jaw—and joints that pop or click.

The diagnosis and treatment of TMJD may require input from several different medical disciplines. Along with dentists, physicians, psychologists, and neurologists may also be included. If bruxism is the underlying cause of the TMJD, patients will often wear special splints at night to keep their top and bottom teeth apart.

Bruxism

Bruxism is the habit of grinding or clenching the teeth, particularly during sleep or times of stress. Clenching and grinding the teeth puts pressure on the muscles, tissues, and other structures around the jaw. TMJD can develop. In some individuals, intense grinding leads to a characteristic pattern of wear on the teeth, and, in more severe cases, this grinding can fracture the enamel off at the gingival margin, a condition known as *abfraction*. Symptoms of uncontrolled bruxism include earache, headache, and sore and painful jaws. Some instances of nocturnal bruxism may be loud enough to disturb sleeping partners.

Though not in itself a dangerous disorder, bruxism can cause permanent damage to the teeth. Various types of splints are available for patients to wear at night, and some individuals find relief in physical therapy for the jaw or in self-hypnosis, biofeedback, or other stress reduction techniques.

> **CHECKPOINT**
> **6-5** The stress-induced clenching and grinding of teeth is known as what?

Muscles

Locating the six major muscle groups of the head and neck and understanding the function of each is important to assessing the dental health of patients and recognizing potentially troubling developments. Muscles of the head and neck, like muscles in the rest of the body, move by expansion and contraction. Each muscle is attached on one end to a fixed point of origin—usually on a bone—and at the other end to a movable insertion point—again usually on a bone or joint—that helps to move the muscle.

Muscles of Mastication

All four muscles of mastication—for the chewing, grinding, and crushing of food—are attached in pairs to the mandible and work with the TMJ to make movement of the mandible possible. The **temporal muscles** originate from the temporal fossa of the temporal bone and attach to the coronoid process and anterior border of the mandibular ramus. The temporal muscles raise the mandible and close the jaw.

The **masseter muscles** (Figure 6-12) have two points of origin, the superficial origin on the lower border of the zygomatic arch and the deep origin on the posterior and medial side of the zygomatic arch. The superficial part of the masseter muscle attaches onto the angle and lower lateral side of the mandibular ramus. The deep portion of the masseter muscle attaches onto the upper lateral ramus and mandibular coronoid process. The masseter muscles also raise the mandible and close the jaw.

The **internal** (or *medial*) **pterygoid muscles** and **external** (or *lateral*) **pterygoid muscles** (Figure 6-13) work together to pull the mandible to one side or to bring the lower jaw forward. On its own, the internal pterygoid closes the jaw; also alone, the external pterygoid depresses the mandible to open the jaw. The internal pterygoid muscle originates from the medial surface of the lateral pterygoid plate of the sphenoid bone, the palatine bone,

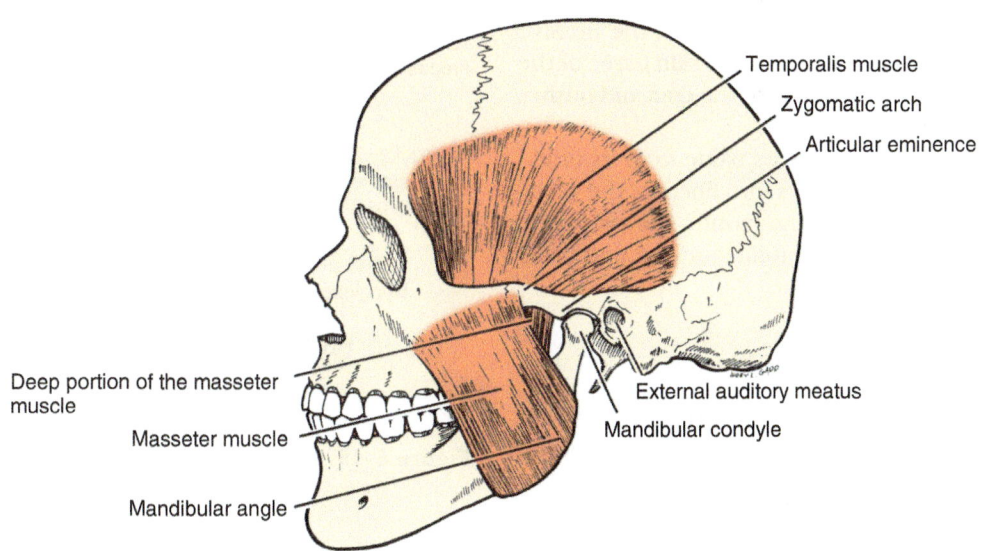

Figure 6–12 The temporalis and masseter muscles of mastication.

and the tuberosity of the maxillary bone. It attaches onto the medial surface of the ramus and the angle of the mandible. The external pterygoid muscle originates from the greater wing of the sphenoid bone and from the outer surface of the lateral pterygoid plate. It attaches onto the neck of the condyle of the mandible and onto the articular disc and capsular ligament of the TMJ.

Muscles of Facial Expression

Muscles of facial expression originate from a bone or other point of origin and insert onto skin tissue. The **orbicularis oris muscle**, which encircles the mouth, originates from muscle fibers around the mouth and has no skeletal attachment. It attaches onto itself and the surrounding skin tissue. The orbicularis oris has many functions: it closes, compresses, and puckers the lips; aids in chewing; and aids in speaking by helping press the lips against the teeth.

The **buccinator muscle** is a thin, broad muscle that forms the wall of the cheek. It originates at the posterior portion of alveolar processes of the maxillary bone and mandible. It attaches onto the fibers of the orbicularis oris muscle at the angle of the mouth. The buccinator muscle compresses the cheek wall against the teeth and retracts the angle of the mouth.

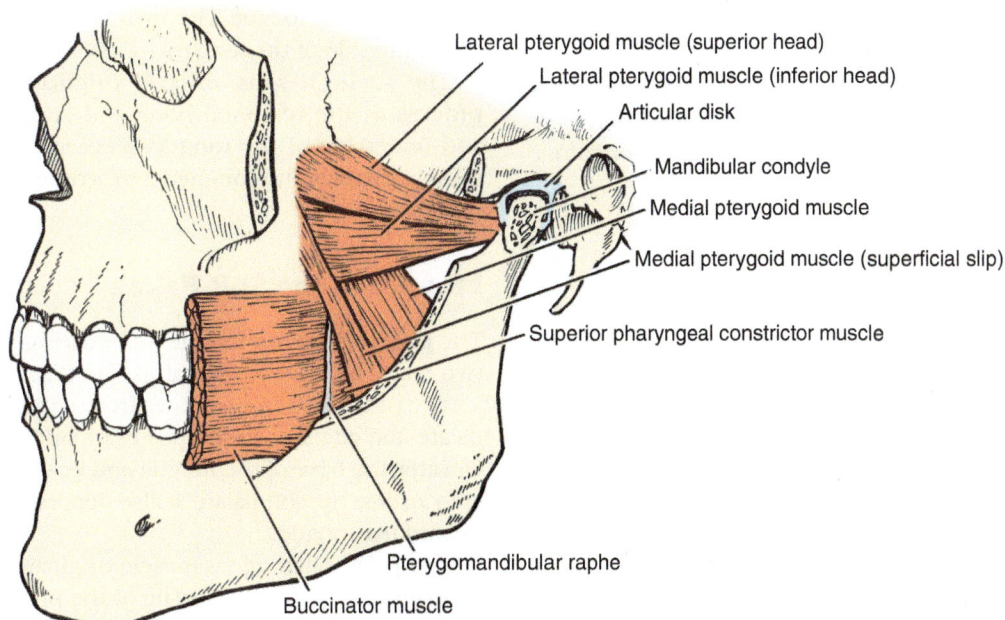

Figure 6–13 The internal (medial) and external (lateral) pterygoid muscles of mastication.

The **mentalis** is a muscle originating at the incisive fossa of the mandible that attaches to the skin tissue of the chin. It raises and wrinkles the skin of the chin and pushes up the lower lip.

The **zygomatic major** takes its name from its origin on the zygomatic bone. It attaches into fibers of the orbicularis oris muscle surrounding the mouth. The zygomatic major draws the angles of the mouth upward and backward during, for example, laughter.

Muscles of the Floor of the Mouth

The muscles of the floor of the mouth (Figure 6-14) are located between the mandible and the hyoid bone of the throat.

One branch, or *belly*, of the **digastric muscle** originates at the mandible, the other at the temporal bone. Both bellies attach at the hyoid bone—one at the body and the other at the great horn. The digastric muscle depresses the jaw and raises the hyoid bone, especially during swallowing.

Each of the two points of the **mylohyoid muscle** originates on the mylohyoid line of the mandible. After joining at the midline, both portions attach to the body of the hyoid bone. The mylohyoid muscle forms the floor of the mouth, elevates the tongue, and depresses the jaw.

The **stylohyoid muscle** originates at the styloid process of the temporal bone. It attaches to the body of the hyoid bone. The stylohyoid elongates the floor of the mouth while raising the hyoid bone during swallowing.

The **geniohyoid muscle** originates at the medial surface of the mandible and attaches to the body of the hyoid bone. It draws the tongue and hyoid bone forward and retracts and depresses the lower jaw.

Muscles of the Tongue

Muscles of the tongue are classified as either *intrinsic* (within the tongue) or *extrinsic* (outside of the tongue).

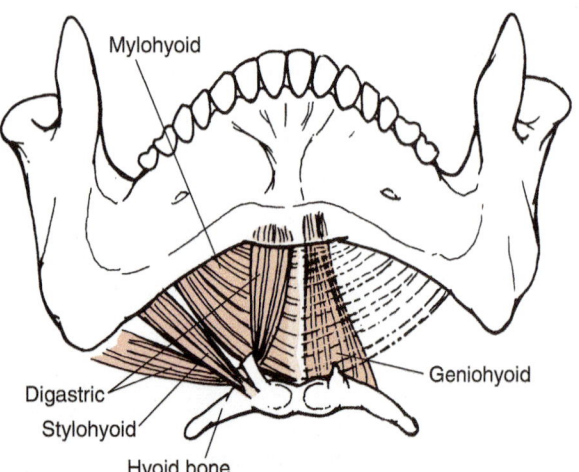

Figure 6-14 Muscles of the floor of the mouth.

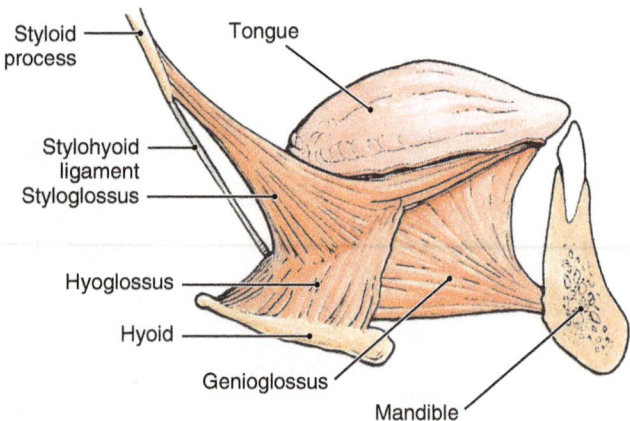

Figure 6-15 Extrinsic muscles of the tongue.

Intrinsic Muscles of the Tongue

Intrinsic muscles of the tongue shape the tongue during speech, mastication, and swallowing.

Extrinsic Muscles of the Tongue

Extrinsic muscles (Figure 6-15) enable the tongue's movement and functioning.

The **genioglossus muscle** originates at the medial surface of the mandible. It attaches to the hyoid bone and the inferior surface of the tongue. The genioglossus muscle depresses the tongue and enables it to protrude.

The **hyoglossus muscle** is unusual in that it originates at the hyoid bone, where the other muscles of the tongue and mouth floor attach, and ascends to attach to the side of the tongue. The hyoglossus retracts and pulls down the side of the tongue.

The **styloglossus muscle** originates at the styloid process of the temporal bone and attaches to the side and underside of the tongue. Whereas the genioglossus muscle enables the tongue to protrude, the styloglossus retracts it.

Muscles of the Soft Palate

The **palatoglossus** and the **palatopharyngeus** are the two major muscles of the soft palate (Figure 6-16).

The palatoglossus originates from either side of the soft palate and attaches to the posterior side of the tongue. It elevates the base of the tongue and enables the tongue to arch against the soft palate. It also depresses the soft palate toward the tongue.

The palatopharyngeus muscle originates at the thyroid cartilage and connective tissue of the pharynx. It attaches to the thyroid cartilage and the wall of the pharynx. The palatopharyngeal muscle forms the palatopharyngeal arch, also known as the *pillar of fauces*.

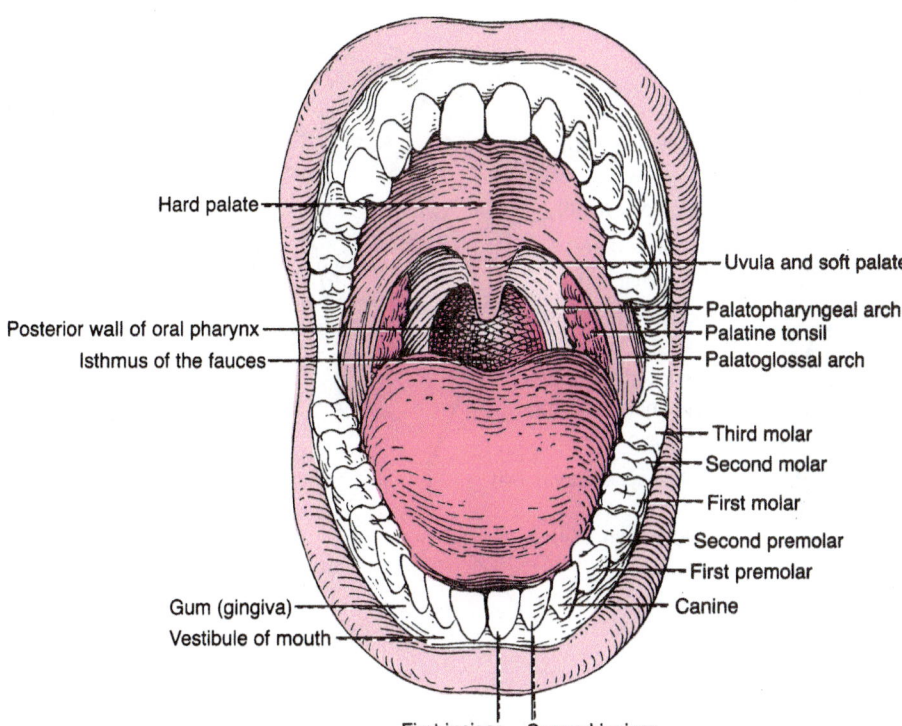

Hard palate

Posterior wall of oral pharynx

Isthmus of the fauces

Uvula and soft palate

Palatopharyngeal arch

Palatine tonsil

Palatoglossal arch

Third molar

Second molar

First molar

Second premolar

First premolar

Canine

Gum (gingiva)

Vestibule of mouth

First incisor   Second incisor

Figure 6–16 The two major muscles of the soft palate: the palatoglossus and the palatopharyngeus.

Muscles of the Neck

Both major muscles of the neck (Figure 6-17) may be easily *palpated* (located by touch) by either patients or dental assistants. Patients may experience pain in either of these muscles if dental assistants neglect proper patient positioning during treatment.

The sternocleidomastoid muscle originates from the clavicle and scapula. It attaches to the external auditory meatus, the canal leading from the external ear to the eardrum. The sternocleidomastoid muscle bends, extends, rotates, and flexes the head.

The trapezius muscle is a large triangular muscle located on either side of the upper back. It originates from the occipital bone at the base of the skull and from spinous processes of the last of the cervical and all the thoracic vertebrae. The trapezius attaches to the outer part of the clavicle, the acromion, and the spine of the scapulae. It lifts the clavicle and scapula when the shoulders are shrugged.

CHECKPOINT
6-6 Which facial muscle draws the mouth upward and backward during laughter?

Nerves

The successful application of local anesthesia during dental treatment depends on a thorough knowledge of the locations and functions of the nerves innervating the head and neck. Treating patients who have experienced nerve damage or disorders of the nervous system also requires a thorough understanding of nerves in the face, head, and neck.

Cranial Nerves

Cranial nerves are numbered I to XII (Figure 6-18) and generally are named for the area or function they serve. The **trigeminal nerve** (cranial nerve V) is the primary source of innervation for the oral cavity. It is subdivided into three divisions: maxillary, mandibular, and ophthalmic. Of

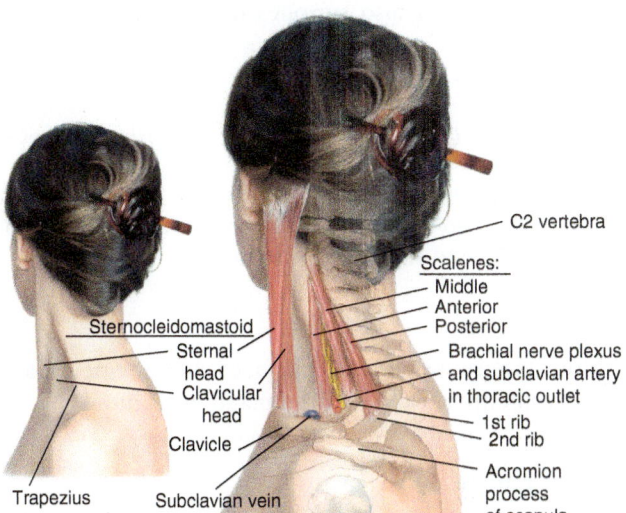

C2 vertebra

Scalenes:
Middle
Anterior
Posterior

Brachial nerve plexus and subclavian artery in thoracic outlet

1st rib
2nd rib

Acromion process of scapula

Sternocleidomastoid

Sternal head

Clavicular head

Clavicle

Trapezius   Subclavian vein

Figure 6–17 Major muscles of the neck, the sternocleidomastoid and the trapezius.

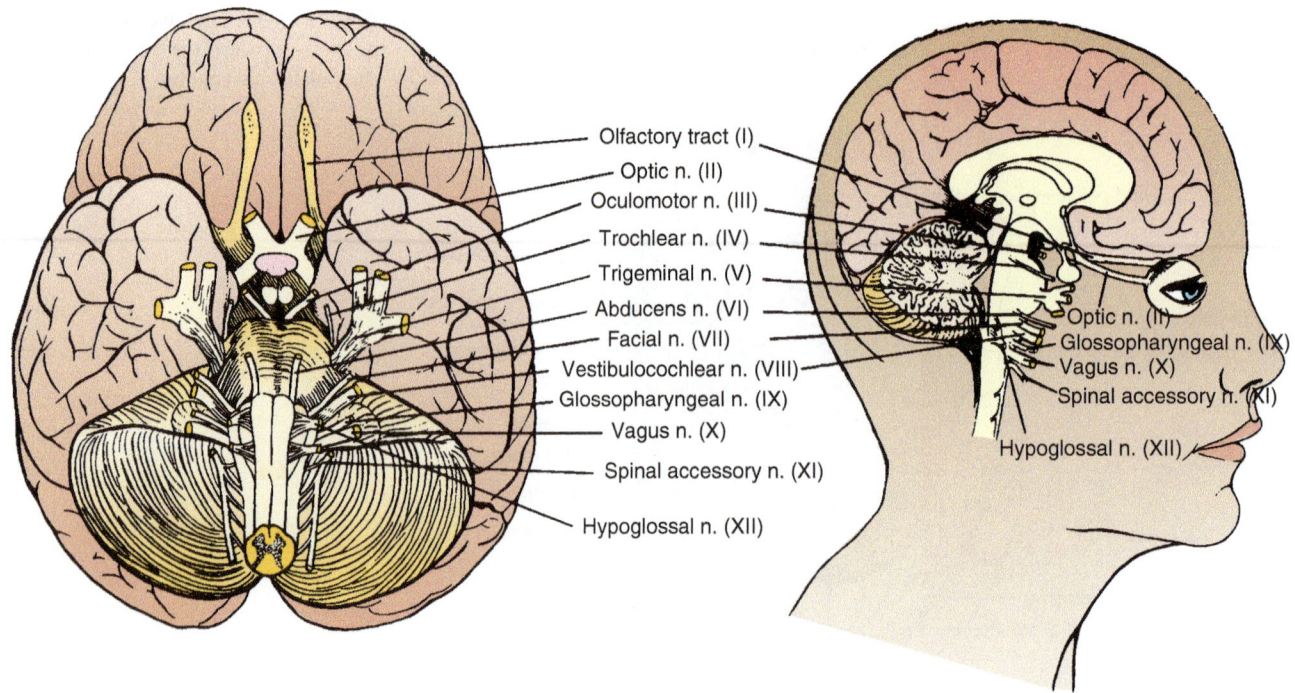

Figure 6–18 The 12 cranial nerves, numbered I to XII. n., nerve.

these three divisions, the maxillary and mandibular are of particular interest to dental professionals. The maxillary division innervates dental and oral structures along the upper jaw, upper lip, and face above the chin. The mandibular division innervates dental and oral structures along the lower jaw.

Maxillary Division of the Trigeminal Nerve

The maxillary division of the trigeminal nerve innervates the maxillary teeth, periosteum, mucous membranes, maxillary sinuses, and soft palate. The maxillary division further subdivides into five nerves that supply individual parts of the oral cavity.

Nasopalatine Nerve

The nasopalatine nerve passes through the incisive foramen and supplies the mucoperiosteum palatal to the maxillary anterior teeth.

Greater Palatine Nerve

The greater palatine nerve passes through the posterior palatine foramen and over the palate. It supplies the mucoperiosteum and intermingles with the nasopalatine nerve.

Anterior Superior Alveolar Nerve

The anterior superior alveolar nerve innervates the maxillary sinus. It also supplies the maxillary, central, lateral, and cuspid teeth, including the periodontal membranes—the connective tissue that holds teeth in their place in the socket—and

the gingiva—the soft tissue that surrounds the base of the teeth and covers the alveolar process, also known as *gums*.

Middle Superior Alveolar Nerve

The middle superior alveolar nerve innervates the maxillary first and second premolars, the mesiobuccal root of the maxillary first molar, and the maxillary sinus.

Posterior Superior Alveolar Nerve

The posterior superior alveolar nerve innervates the other roots of the maxillary first molar and the maxillary second and third molars. It also supplies the lateral wall of the maxillary sinus.

Mandibular Division of the Trigeminal Nerve

The mandibular division of the trigeminal nerve (Figure 6-19) also subdivides to supply individual parts of the oral cavity and surrounding structures.

Buccal Nerve

The buccal nerve innervates the buccal mucous membrane and the mucoperiosteum of the mandibular molars.

Lingual Nerve

As indicated by its name, the lingual nerve innervates the anterior two-thirds of the tongue and branches out to supply the lingual mucous membrane and the mucoperiosteum.

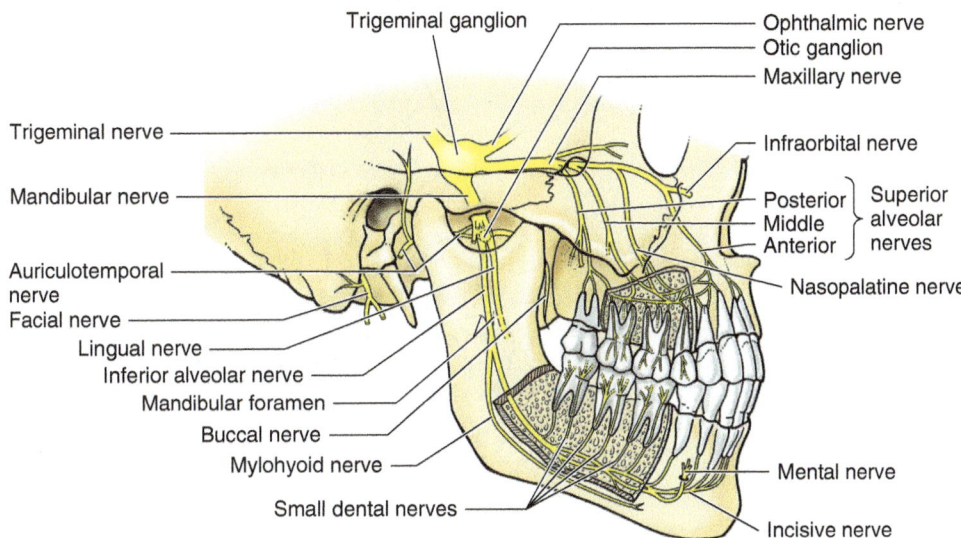

Figure 6–19 The maxillary division of the trigeminal nerve subdivides into five nerves that innervate parts of the oral cavity. The mandibular division of the trigeminal nerve subdivides into nerves that supply individual parts of the oral cavity and surrounding structures.

Inferior Alveolar Nerve

The inferior alveolar nerve passes through the mandibular canal and further divides into four smaller divisions:

- The mylohyoid nerve innervates the mylohyoid muscles and the anterior belly of the digastric muscle.
- The mental nerve continues outward and anteriorly through the mental foramen and supplies the chin and mucous membrane of the lower lip.
- As its name suggests, the incisive nerve continues anteriorly and divides into smaller branches to supply the incisor teeth.
- Smaller nerves continue on to supply the inferior molar and premolar teeth, alveolar process, and periosteum.

CHECKPOINTS

6-7 How are cranial nerves numbered?

6-8 The mental nerve supplies which region of the face?

Blood Vessels

Properly locating major blood vessels of the head and neck (Figure 6-20) is essential to anticipating potential circulatory or bleeding problems. Dental assistants should also be able to recognize how vessels can become compromised during dental treatments or injection of anesthetics.

Major Arteries of the Face and Mouth

The **aorta** arises from the left ventricle of the heart with oxygen-rich blood to supply branch arteries that will distribute it throughout the body. The **common carotid artery** arises from the aorta and carries blood to the upper portions of the body. It divides into the **internal carotid artery**, which supplies blood to the brain and eyes, and the **external carotid artery**, which supplies blood to the face and mouth.

The four main branches of the external carotid artery supply the tongue, face, ears, and wall of the cranium.

Lingual Artery

As its name suggests, the lingual artery consists of several branching blood vessels that supply the entire tongue, the floor of the mouth, lingual gingiva, and part of the soft palate and tonsils.

Facial Artery

The facial artery branches off from the external carotid artery and passes anteriorly and superiorly across the cheek toward the corner of the mouth. It continues upward along the side of the nose, and ends at the inner corner of the eye. The facial artery's six branches supply the pharyngeal muscles, the soft palate, the tonsils, the posterior tongue, the submandibular gland, and various facial muscles.

Maxillary Artery

The maxillary artery is the larger of the two branches of the external carotid artery. It arises behind the angle of the mandible from where it branches out to supply the deep structures of the face. It divides into three branches: the mandibular artery, the pterygoid artery, and the pterygo-palatine artery.

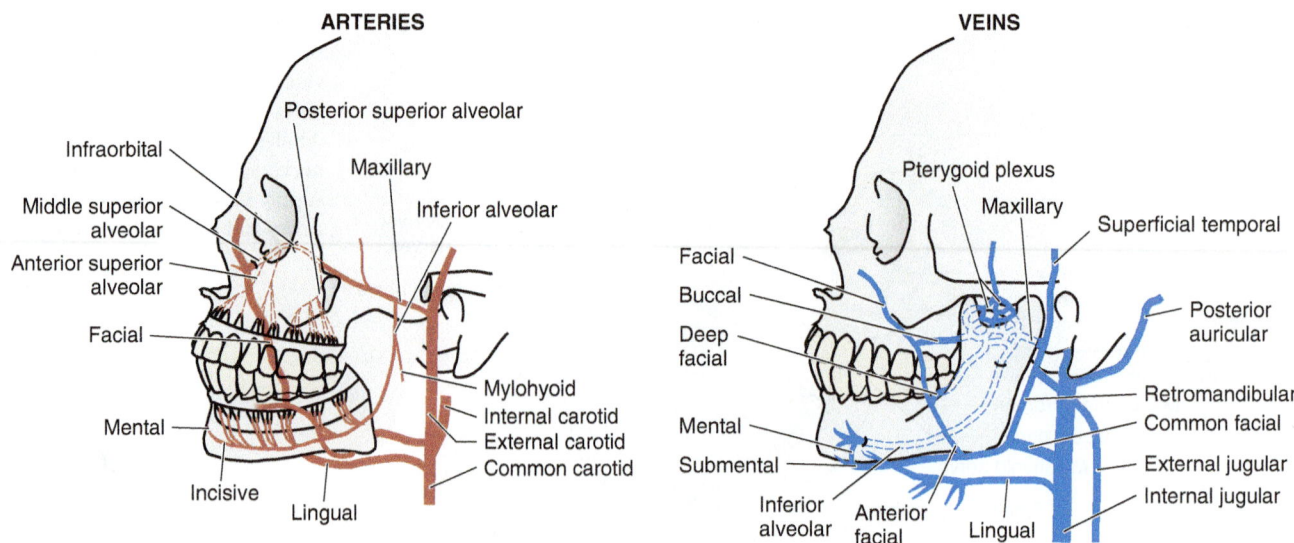

Figure 6–20 Major arteries and veins of the face and oral cavity.

Mandibular Artery

The mandibular artery is located behind the **mandibular ramus**. It branches into five smaller arteries:

- Lingual artery: supplies the surface of the tongue.
- Inferior alveolar artery: descends into the ramus, enters the mandibular foramen, and separates into the incisive and mental arteries at the first premolar.
- Mylohyoid artery: a branch of the inferior alveolar artery that supplies the mylohyoid muscle.
- Incisive arteries: the branch of the inferior alveolar artery that supplies the anterior teeth.
- Mental arteries: the branch of the inferior alveolar artery that supplies the chin and lower lip.

Pterygoid Artery

The five branches of the pterygoid artery supply the temporal, pterygoid, masseter, and buccinator muscles. The pterygoid artery has the following branches:

- Anterior and middle superior alveolar arteries: supply the maxillary incisors and cuspids and the maxillary sinuses.
- Posterior superior alveolar arteries: supply the maxillary premolars, molars, and gingiva.
- Infraorbital artery: supplies the face just below the eye.
- Greater palatine artery: supplies the hard and soft palates, the lingual gingiva, and the palatine glands.
- Anterior superior alveolar artery: supplies the anterior teeth.

Major Veins of the Face and Oral Cavity

Blood descends from the face and oral cavity in a manner corresponding to its ascension from the heart. The maxillary vein passes backward behind the mandible and gathers together blood that has first drained into the pterygoid plexus, a network of veins that drain the pterygoid muscles and face. The temporal vein and maxillary vein join to form the retromandibular vein. This descends through a parotid gland and divides into an anterior and posterior branch. The anterior branch descends to join the facial vein and eventually the internal jugular vein. The posterior branch joins with the posterior auricular vein to form the external jugular vein. The lingual veins drain the tongue and surrounding tissues and descend back along the route of the lingual artery, draining into the external jugular vein. The jugular veins empty into the superior vena cava, which transports blood to the heart and lungs for reoxygenation.

Salivary Glands

Important glands are found within the head and neck. The most significant for dental professionals are the major and minor salivary glands.

Salivary glands produce two types of saliva—the watery substance that lubricates food as we chew and ingest it. *Serous saliva* is thin, watery, and composed mainly of protein. *Mucous saliva* is thick and composed mainly of carbohydrates. The saliva produced by salivary glands in the mouth not only aids in food digestion, but also cleanses and lubricates the mouth. Among other effects, saliva helps maintain dental surfaces through a process called *remineralization*. Dental professionals are most familiar with saliva's role in the formation of dental plaque and its contribution of minerals to the process of calculus formation.

Salivary glands are classified according to their size as either *minor salivary glands* or *major salivary glands*. The major salivary glands are the parotid glands, submandibular glands, and sublingual glands (Figure 6-21).

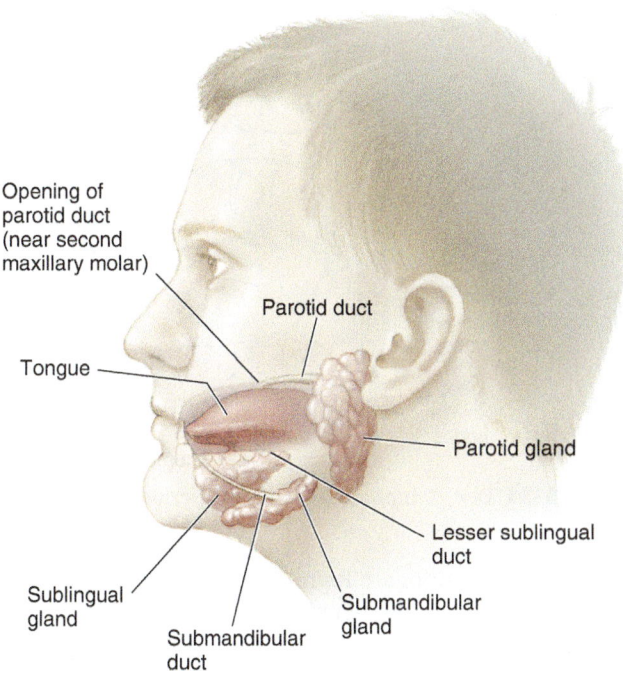

Figure 6–21 Major salivary glands.

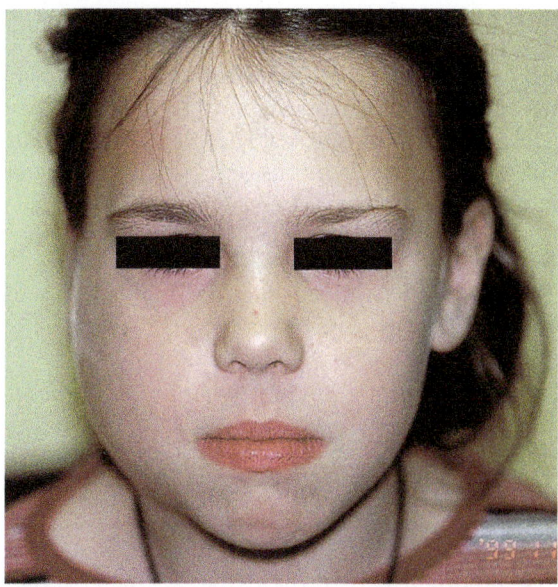

Figure 6–22 Mumps. (Courtesy of Dr. Martha Ann Keels.)

Parotid Glands

Parotid glands, like other major salivary glands, come in pairs, with one gland on each side of the mouth. The parotid glands are the largest of the salivary glands, and are located just below and in front of the ear. They produce about 25% of the total volume of saliva. Saliva travels from the parotid gland to the mouth via the **parotid duct**.

Mumps

The once familiar childhood disease mumps, medically termed *epidemic parotitis*, is a viral disease marked by fever and swelling of the parotid glands (Figure 6-22). Mumps also causes headache, muscle ache, fatigue, and loss of appetite. Patient appearance frequently resembles "chipmunk cheeks." Mumps is contagious, but cases are extremely rare in the United States since the introduction and use of the MMR (measles, mumps, rubella) vaccine for children.

Submandibular Glands

The **submandibular glands** are the second largest salivary glands. They produce about 65% of the total volume of saliva and are located in the submandibular fossa, under the mandible and just behind the sublingual glands. Saliva produced by these glands reaches the oral cavity through an adjacent **submandibular duct**.

Sialoliths

Sialoliths are salivary gland stones (calculi) made of crystallized minerals that sometimes develop in and block the salivary ducts that carry saliva from the glands to the mouth (Figure 6-23). Saliva that cannot flow freely backs up and accumulates in the gland, causing it to swell and become painful. Most sialoliths develop in the submandibular ducts. In some cases, dentists can palpate the stone and push it out of the duct. In other cases, sialoliths must be removed surgically.

Sublingual Glands

The **sublingual glands** are the smallest of the major salivary glands. They produce only about 10% of the total volume of saliva and are located in a fossa between the tongue and the mandible. Saliva reaches the oral cavity through the **sublingual duct**.

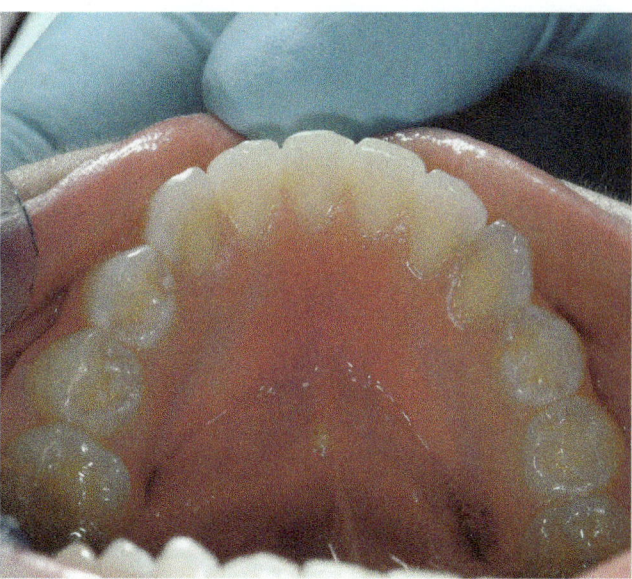

Figure 6–23 A sialolith calcification inside a salivary gland duct blocking saliva flow.

Minor Salivary Glands

Minor salivary glands are smaller than the sublingual glands and are scattered throughout the tissues of the buccal, labial, and lingual mucosa. They are also found in the soft palate, the lateral portions of the hard palate, and the floor of the mouth.

CHECKPOINT

6-9 What is another name for the calculus stones that sometimes form in and block salivary ducts?

Lymph Nodes

A very important part of the extraoral examination conducted by dental assistants is the palpation of lymph nodes located in the neck. **Lymph nodes** produce antibodies to fight disease as part of the body's immune response. Enlarged lymph nodes are a sign of disease process and could indicate infection or even cancer.

Location of Lymph Nodes

Lymph nodes in the neck are called **cervical lymph nodes** and include specific nodes that drain the oral cavity, including the teeth and gingiva. Lymph nodes in the neck also drain the eyes, ears, nasal cavity, and parts of the throat.

Lymph nodes in the head are classified as either *superficial* or *deep*. Superficial lymph nodes in the head are grouped as occipital, retroauricular, anterior auricular, superficial parotid, and facial nodes (Figure 6-24). Deep

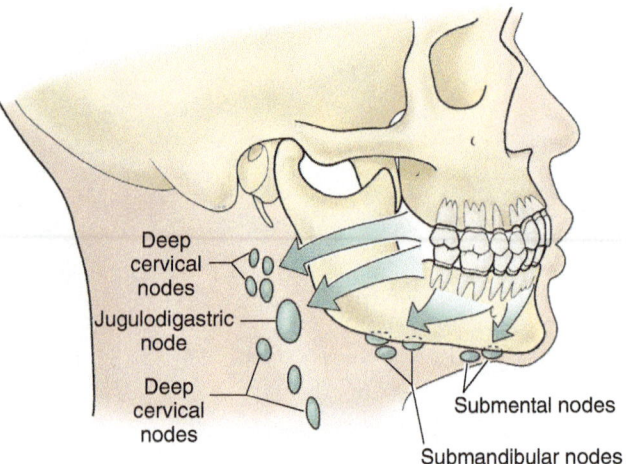

Figure 6–25 Deep lymph nodes drain the periodontium.

cervical lymph nodes are found along the internal jugular vein on each side of the neck (Figure 6-25).

Other lymph nodes in the body include axillary nodes (in the armpits) and inguinal nodes (in the groin).

Enlargement of Lymph Nodes

Lymph nodes swell and become palpable when sufficient numbers of lymphocytes grow larger and accumulate in greater numbers in response to disease or infection. This condition is known as **lymphadenopathy**. A patient with signs of lymphadenopathy could require immediate referral to a physician for evaluation.

CHECKPOINT

6-10 Lymph nodes swell in response to what?

Landmarks

Landmarks of the face and oral cavity are easily recognizable skeletal or soft tissue structures that provide important reference points for dental assistants as they examine patients and work with other members of the dental team. Landmarks, especially inside the oral cavity, also provide important reference points for dental radiography.

Regions of the Face

Anatomists define the face as the part of the head visible in a frontal view, anterior to the ears, and lying between the hairline and the chin. The face is divided into nine

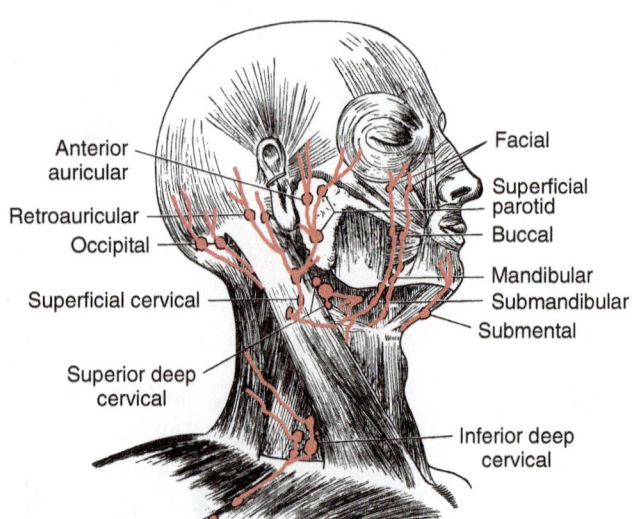

Figure 6–24 The superficial lymph nodes in the head.

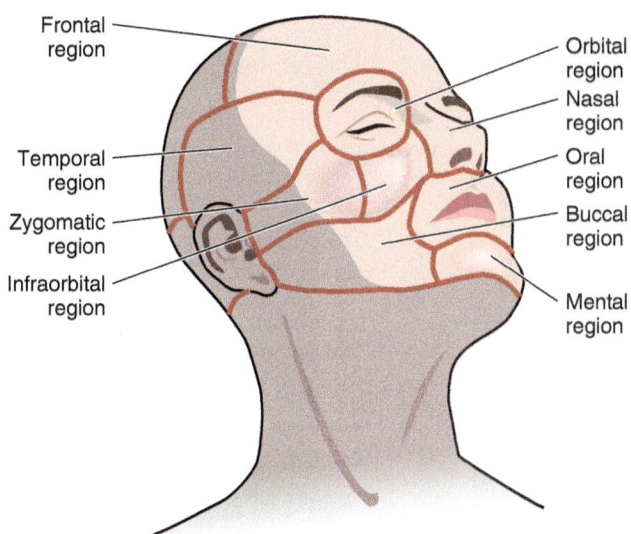

Figure 6–26 Regions of the face.

regions (Figure 6-26). The forehead extends from the hairline down to the eyebrows. The temples lie alongside the head directly posterior to the eyes. The orbital area is also known as the *eye and eye socket*. The area below the eye and eye socket is the infraorbital region. The external nose is one facial region. The zygomatic area refers to the cheekbone, or prominence of the cheek. The cheeks themselves constitute another facial region. The mouth and lips together constitute a facial region. Moving downward from the forehead, the chin constitutes the final facial region.

Landmarks of the Face

A more detailed examination of facial regions results in the designation of facial landmarks and features that provide important reference points for dental assistants. These landmarks can help reveal hidden abnormalities or mark the position of significant structures lying beneath the skin. They are also useful in accurately noting the exact location of sores, scars, and other changes and recording them on a patient health history.

You must be familiar with and be able to identify the following facial landmarks (Figure 6-27):

- The **outer canthus** of the eye is the fold of tissue at the outer corner of the eyelid; the **inner canthus** is the fold of tissue at the inner corner of the eye.
- The **ala** of the nose is the rounded outside tip of each nostril.
- The **philtrum** runs from just under the nostrils to the middle of the upper lip.
- From the ala of the nose to the corners of the mouth runs the **nasolabial groove**.
- The **tragus** is the portion of the external ear that lies anterior to the acoustic meatus.

- The **nasion** lies midway between the eyes, just below the eyebrows. Here the frontal bone joins to the nasal bones.
- The *glabella* is the smooth portion of the frontal bone located just above the top of the nose.
- The *root* is commonly known as the *bridge* of the nose.
- The **septum** divides the nasal cavity into two nasal passages.
- The **anterior naris** refers to the nostril.
- The reddish portion of the lips is known as the **vermilion zone**, and the reddish line that outlines the lips is called the **vermilion border** (Figure 6-28).
- On the lips themselves, the small enlargement at the center of the upper lip that sometimes thickens is called the *tubercle of the lip*.
- The corners of the mouth, where the upper and lower lip meet, are known as **labial commissures**.
- Just below the lower lip runs the horizontal *labiomental groove*, which separates the lip from the chin below.

The remaining facial landmarks refer to prominent bones. The *mental protuberance* of the mandible bone forms the chin. The **angle of the mandible** refers to the corner formed by the lowest point of the mandibular ramus. The zygomatic arch is what creates the prominence of the cheekbone.

From the Dentist's Perspective

I make it a practice to hire dental assistants whose education and training includes a thorough knowledge of anatomy, particularly of the oral cavity. Over the years, I have come to appreciate the importance of this. Obtaining a clinically acceptable dental impression, a diagnostic cast of a patient's oral cavity, is a very important step in treatment planning. Having a dental assistant who can be trusted to obtain a high-quality cast is very important. Treatment decisions based on an erroneous impression can be very costly, both professionally and financially. An assistant who knows which muscles and frenum attachments must be included in a given impression is invaluable to both me and my patients.

Landmarks of the Oral Cavity

Vestibule

The **vestibule** is the space between the teeth and the inner lining of the cheeks and lips (Figure 6-29). The deepest part of the vestibule is the vestibule fornix. This U-shaped pocket is continuous from the front around to the back of the mouth.

Frena

Frena (singular: frenum) are raised lines of mucosal tissue that become visible when the lips are pulled back. They serve to support or restrain teeth and other structures.

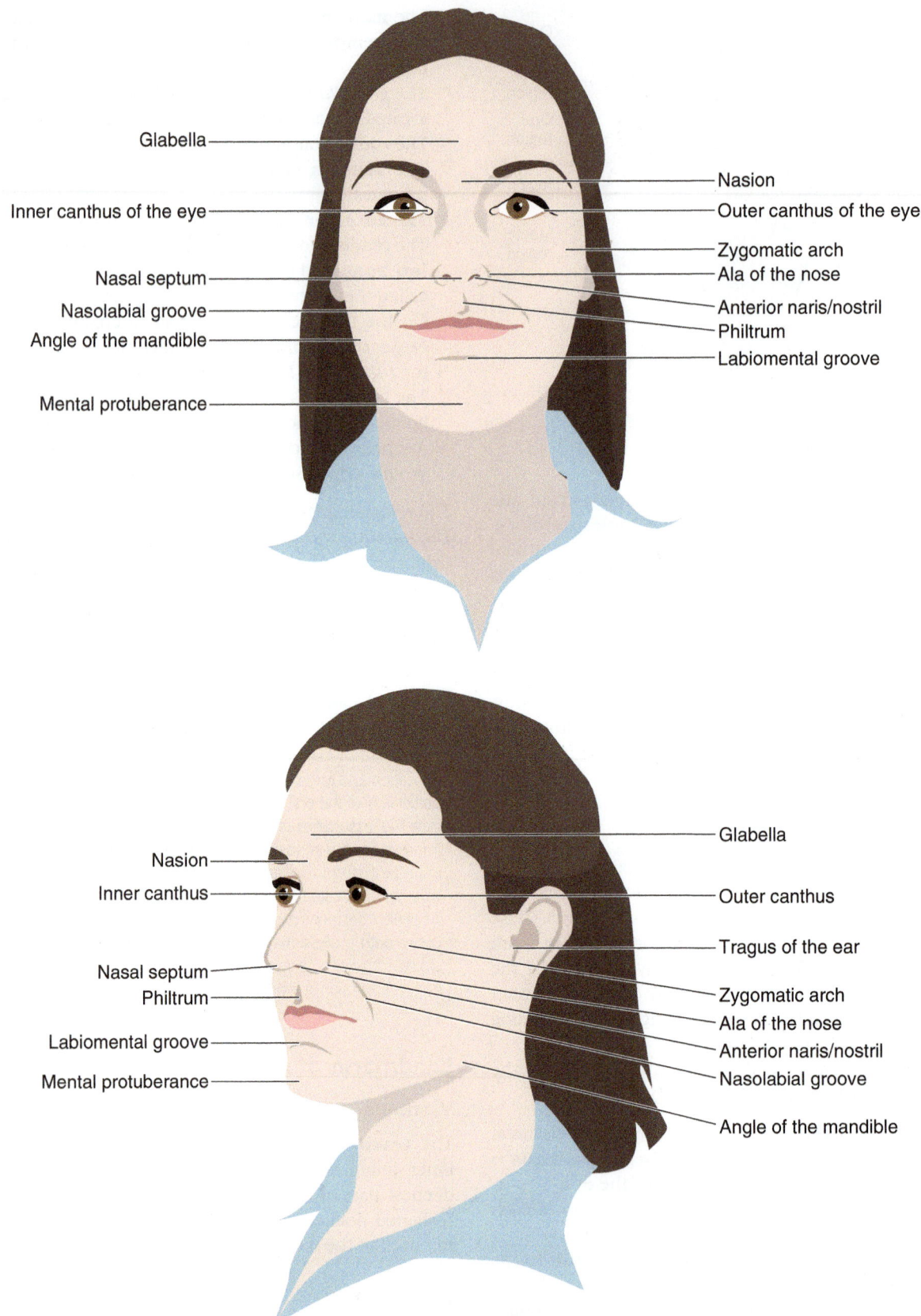

Figure 6–27 Landmarks of the face.

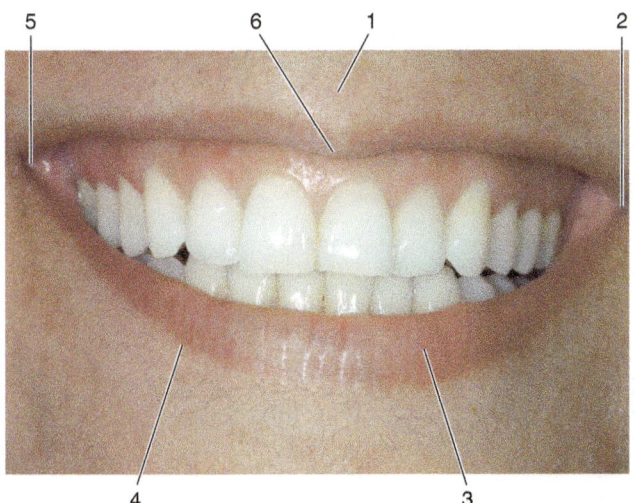

Figure 6–28 Anatomy of the lips and adjacent area. (1) Philtrum; (2) Commissural lip pit; (3) Vermillion zone; (4) Vermillion border; (5) Labial commissure; (6) Labial tubercle.

The most pronounced and visible frena are found between the mandibular and maxillary central incisors. Frena extend from the alveolar ridge into the labial and buccal mucosa around the inside of the mouth; these are called the *maxillary frenum* and the *mandibular frenum*.

Gingiva

The **gingiva**, commonly called the *gums*, are firmly attached to the alveolar ridge and vary in color from pale pink to brownish pink depending upon the individual's pigmentation (Figure 6-30). The area where the gingiva meet the teeth is called the *free gingiva* or *marginal gingiva*. This area is approximately 1 mm wide and is the first

to respond to inflammation. The groove found between the free gingiva and the tooth is called the *sulcus*. The mucogingival junction (MGJ), on the other hand, marks where the thick gingival tissue meets the soft mucous membrane. The thin line along the alveolar ridge where free gingiva ends and becomes attached is called the *gingival groove*. Interdental gingiva fill the space between adjacent teeth. Most gingiva is attached gingiva, which is firm and resistant and tightly adapts to teeth and bone. Attached gingiva is located from the base of the sulcus to the MGJ.

Palate Area

The palate area, which sits inside the curve of the maxillary teeth, is divided into the hard palate and the soft palate.

Hard Palate

The **hard palate**, a bony plate covered with keratinized tissue, sits toward the front of the mouth and forms the anterior portion of the palate (Figure 6-31). Raised areas mark and divide the hard palate. Just behind the maxillary incisors sits a raised area of tissue known as the *incisive papilla*. The ridged line that extends from behind the incisive papilla down the middle of the hard palate is called the *palatine raphe*. The horizontal ridges that run across the hard palate behind the incisive papilla are known as the *palatine rugae*.

Soft Palate

The soft palate is composed of muscle tissue rather than bone and sits toward the back of the mouth (Figure 6-32). Additional landmarks are associated with the soft palate and the oropharyngeal area behind it. The uvula, the projection visible when the mouth is opened wide, hangs from

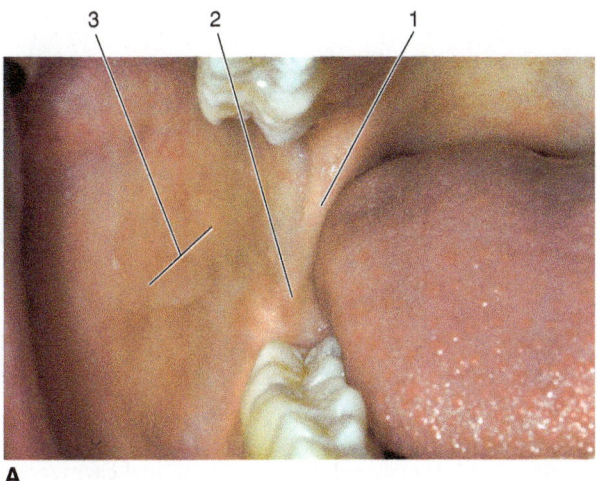

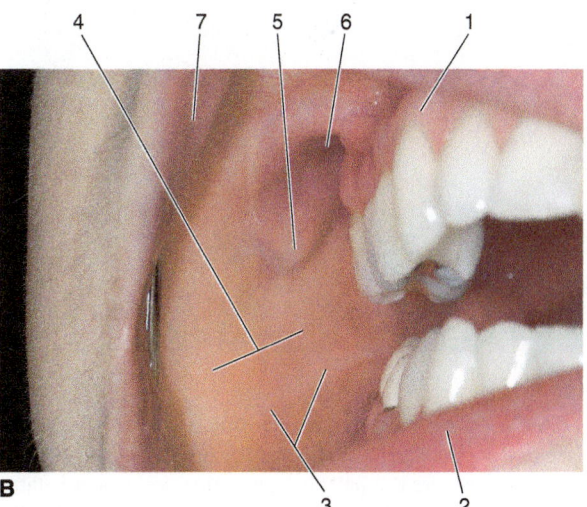

Figure 6–29 A. Buccal vestibule. Observe the pterygomandibular raphe and the retromandibular triangle. (1) Pterygomandibular raphe; (2) Retromolar pad; (3) Buccal vestibule. **B.** Buccal vestibule. Observe the linea alba and the parotid papilla. (1) Attached gingiva; (2) Lower lip; (3) Linea alba; (4) Buccal vestibule; (5) Parotid papilla; (6) Mucobuccal fold; (7) Fordyce granules.

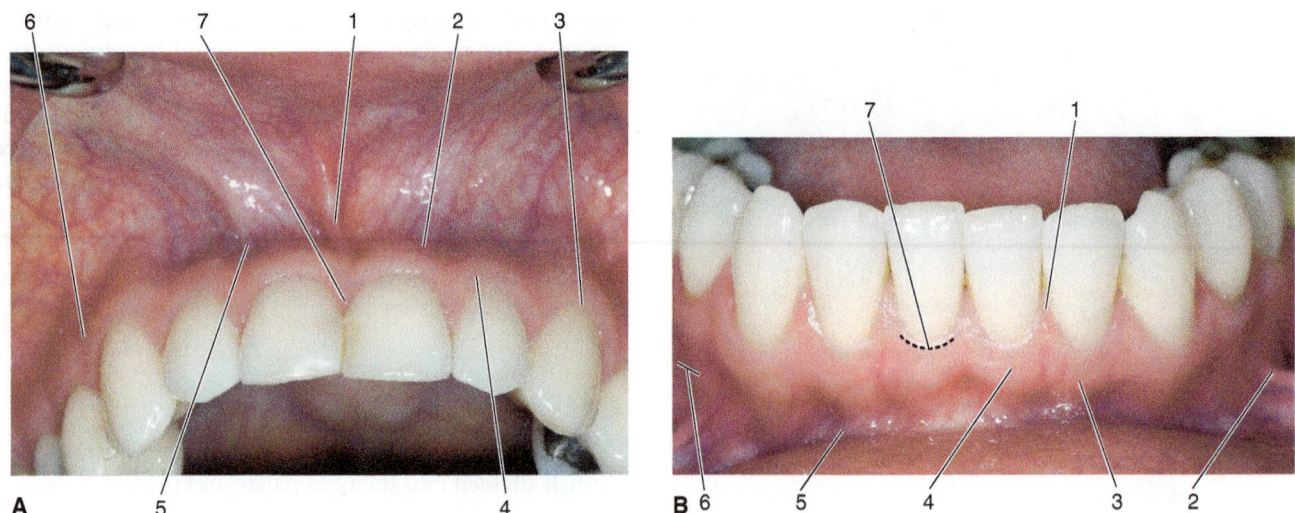

Figure 6–30 A. Superior labial vestibule indicating regionally named gingiva covering anatomic regions of maxillae. (1) Superior labial frenulum; (2) Mucogingival junction; (3) Marginal gingiva; (4) Attached gingiva; (5) Alveolar mucosa; (6) Canine fossa; (7) Interdental papilla. **B.** The lower jaw including the regional areas of the mucosa and gingiva. The free gingival groove represents the area above the dotted line. (1) Interdental papilla; (2) Labial frenulum; (3) Mucogingival junction; (4) Attached gingiva; (5) Mucolabial fold; (6) Canine eminence; (7) Free gingival groove.

the back of the soft palate. Extending from the uvula horizontally to the base of the tongue are folds of tissue called *anterior tonsillar pillars*, also known as *palatoglossal arches*. Another set of arches is found farther back in the throat. These are known as either the *posterior tonsillar pillars* or the *palatopharyngeal arches*. Between the two

sets of pillars or arches is a slightly depressed area where the palatine tonsils sit. The palatine tonsils may often appear to have deep grooves and reddish inflammation due to infection. The point at the back of the throat where food passes from the mouth into the pharynx is called the *fauces*.

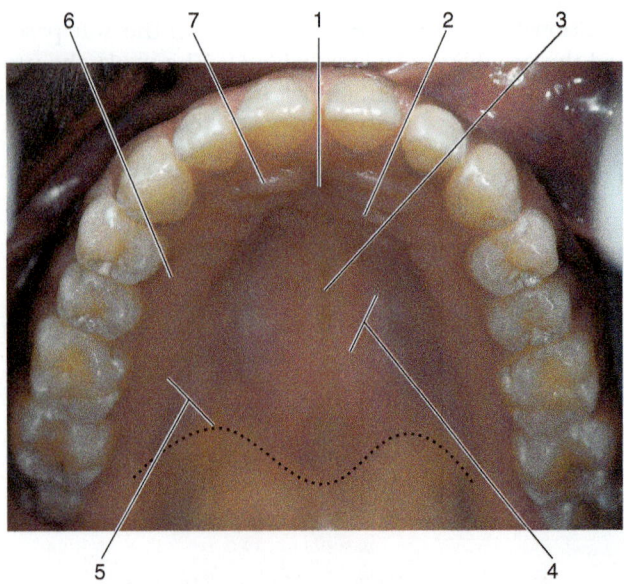

Figure 6–31 Palate. Most of the area shown is hard palate with its rugae and incisive papilla. The most posterior aspect behind the dotted line covers the palatine bone. Anterior aspect is fatty, giving way to a glandular region posteriorly. (1) Incisive papilla; (2) Palatine rugae (left side); (3) Median palatine raphe; (4) Anterior hard palate (glandular region); (5) Palatal gingiva; (7) Palatine rugae (right side).

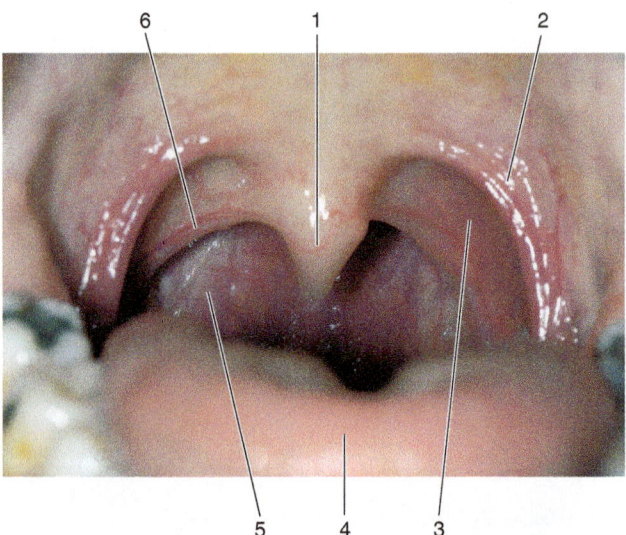

Figure 6–32 The shared anatomy of the oral cavity/oral pharynx with the tonsillar sinus separating the oral cavity from the oral pharynx. (1) Uvula; (2) Palatoglossal arch; (3) Palatine tonsil fossa; (4) Body of tongue; (5) Oropharyngeal wall; (6) Palatopharyngeal arch.

Tongue

Despite its seemingly uniform appearance, the tongue is itself a significant area of the mouth with many landmarks of its own (Figure 6-33). When the tongue is extended, the shallow V-shaped groove visible toward the back is called the *sulcus terminalis*. A depression known as the *median sulcus* runs from the base of the tongue to its tip and divides the dorsal surface of the tongue into halves.

Other landmarks are lined up along the ventral side of the tongue. A line of tissue called the *lingual frenum* extends from the underside of the tongue to the floor of the mouth. The lingual veins run the length of the tongue along either side of the lingual frenum. Folds of tissue called the *fimbriated folds* lie alongside the lingual veins.

Taste Buds

Taste buds allow us to enjoy the flavor of foods and to anticipate their temperature. Although there are multitudes of individual flavors, just a few primary tastes combine to create all of them. These are salty, sour, sweet, and bitter, and now scientists recognize a fifth taste called umami, or savoriness. Taste buds are found among the papillae—small raised projections along the tongue that hold taste buds. The dorsal surface of the tongue is covered with these. Other areas are anterior to the sulcus terminalis (the circumvallate papillae); anterior to the circumvallate papillae (the filiform papillae); along the lateral base of the tongue (foliate papillae); and the fungiform papillae along the dorsal surface.

Taste buds may become inactive in the aftermath of some medical procedures and drugs. New taste buds will generally replace the damaged ones and become active after 10 days.

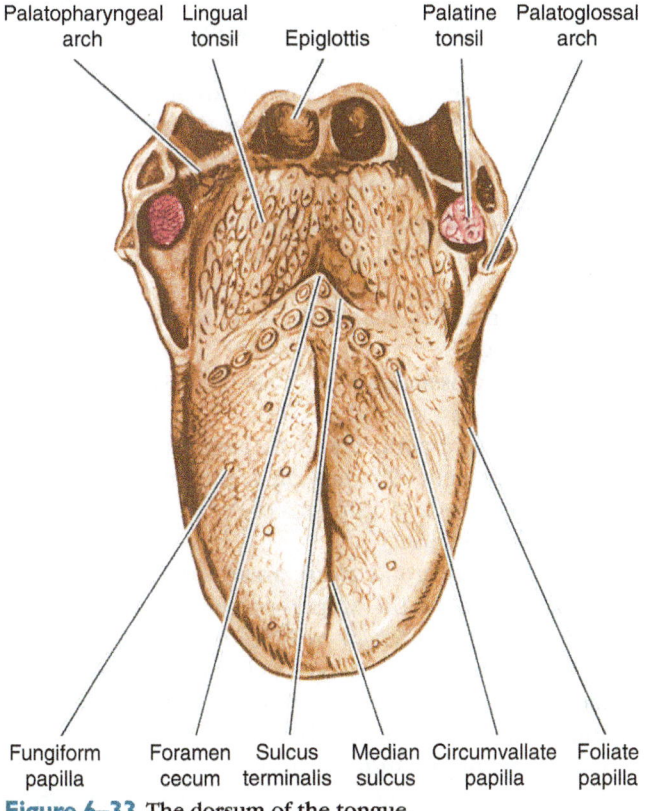

Palatopharyngeal arch   Lingual tonsil   Epiglottis   Palatine tonsil   Palatoglossal arch

Fungiform papilla   Foramen cecum   Sulcus terminalis   Median sulcus   Circumvallate papilla   Foliate papilla

Figure 6–33 The dorsum of the tongue.

Gag Reflex

The gag reflex is typically activated on the back wall of the throat. Its purpose is to prevent the entry of foreign objects into the windpipe. The strength of the gag reflex varies among individuals. For individuals who have a very sensitive and easily activated gag reflex, dental appointments and procedures may prove difficult.

If a patient expresses concern about a strong gag reflex, ask the patient if particular spots on the tongue are especially sensitive. Keeping instruments away from the soft palate may prove helpful. Observe whether the patient might be doing something to make the gagging response worse. Some patients, in an effort to prove helpful to the dentist, draw their tongue as far back in the mouth as possible, gagging themselves unintentionally in the process. Excessive worry about gagging can create tension and cause gagging.

Distracting patients from their worry and self-consciousness about gagging may prove helpful. Some may benefit from playing music on a personal stereo, meditating, or focusing on something else during dental procedures. Some dentists may use techniques such as deep breathing to help relax the patient's muscles. Commercial products are available to "numb" the gag reflex, but these must be used judiciously. Like many obstacles to dental care, concern about a gag reflex can be helped by good communication among patients, dental assistants, and other dental team members.

Floor of the Mouth

Landmarks along the floor of the mouth include the sublingual caruncles, two small, raised folds of tissue located where the lingual frenum attaches to the floor of the mouth (Figure 6-34). Salivary ducts lie on top of the caruncles. The sublingual folds originate at the caruncles and run backward along the tongue to its base. Alongside the sublingual folds is a horseshoe-shaped groove called the *sublingual sulcus*. The sulcus marks the end of the alveolar ridge and the beginning of the floor of the mouth.

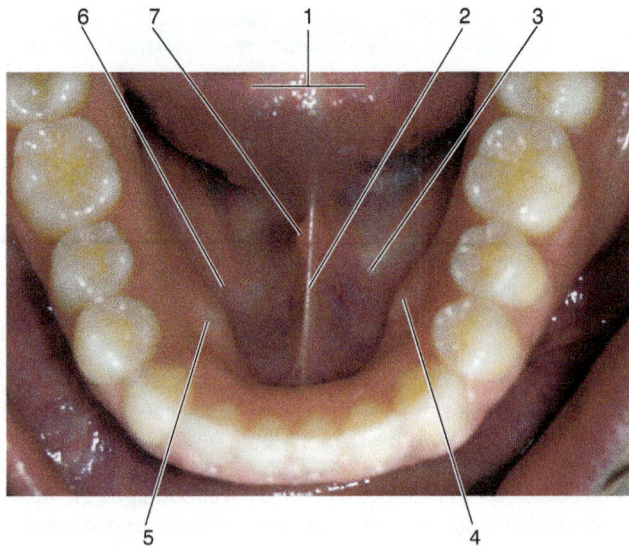

Figure 6–34 Floor of the mouth. Observe the sublingual caruncula indicating opening of the submandibular duct at the base of the lingual frenulum. Of special interest are the mandibular tori. (1) Tongue (ventral surface); (2) Lingual frenum; (3) Sublingual fold; (4) Mandibular torus (left side); (5) Mandibular torus (right side); (6) Sublingual sulcus; (7) Lingual caruncle.

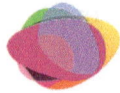

CHECKPOINTS

6-11 Which facial landmark divides the nasal cavity into two passages?

6-12 What is the purpose of the gag reflex?

Chapter Highlights

+ The skull is divided into two main sections: the cranium, which covers and protects the brain, and the face, which underlies and supports our most familiar features.
+ The bones of the cranium are the frontal, occipital, sphenoid, and ethmoid bones, which occur singly, and the paired parietal and paired temporal bones, one of which appears on either side of the head.
+ The bones of the cranium are joined together by immovable articulations called *sutures*.
+ The 14 bones of the face are the lacrimal bone, the nasal bone, the vomer, the nasal conchae, the zygomatic bone, the maxillae, and the mandible.
+ The hyoid bone is shaped like a horseshoe and sits suspended between the mandible and larynx. It supports the tongue and other nearby muscles.
+ Frontal sinuses are located in the frontal bone above each eye. Sphenoid sinuses are located in the sphenoid bone posterior to each eye. The ethmoid sinuses are located within the complex honeycomb structure of the ethmoid bone. Maxillary sinuses are located within the maxillary bones.
+ The temporomandibular joint (TMJ) is the most significant joint in dentistry. It joins the mandible to the temporal bone above it and is essential for mastication and speech.
+ Dysfunction or inflammation caused by temporomandibular joint dysfunction (TMJD) can cause the TMJ to become painful and tender.

+ Muscles of facial expression include the orbicularis oris muscle, the buccinator muscle, the mentalis muscle, and the zygomatic major.
+ Muscles of the floor of the mouth are located between the mandible and hyoid bone of the throat. They include the digastric muscle; the mylohyoid muscle; the stylohyoid muscle; and the geniohyoid muscle.
+ Muscles of the tongue are classified as either *intrinsic* or as *extrinsic*. Intrinsic muscles of the tongue shape the tongue during speech, mastication, and swallowing. Extrinsic muscles enable the tongue's movement and functioning.
+ The palatoglossus and the palatopharyngeus are the two major muscles of the soft palate.
+ The successful application of local anesthesia during dental treatment depends on a thorough knowledge of the locations and functions of the nerves innervating the head and neck.
+ The common carotid artery arises from the aorta and carries blood to the upper portions of the body. It divides into the *internal carotid artery*, which supplies blood to the brain and eyes, and the *external carotid artery*, which supplies it to the face and mouth.
+ Important glands of the head and neck include the *major* and *minor salivary glands*.
+ Lymph nodes produce antibodies to disease as part of the body's immune response. Enlarged lymph nodes are

a sign of disease process and could indicate infection or even cancer.

✦ The gag reflex is activated on the back wall of the throat. Its purpose is to prevent the entry of foreign

objects into your windpipe. For individuals who have a very sensitive and easily activated gag reflex, dental appointments and procedures may prove difficult.

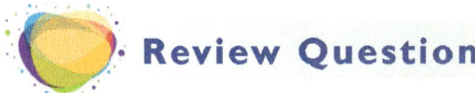

Review Questions

1. Which cranial bones appear singly?

   a. Lacrimal

   b. Temporal

   c. Parietal

   d. Occipital

2. Which of the following bones sits in the center of the skull between the eye sockets and helps form parts of the nasal and orbital cavities?

   a. Ethmoid bone

   b. Occipital bone

   c. Sphenoid bone

   d. Parietal bones

3. Teeth and structures of the upper jaw are referred to as

   a. Maxillary.

   b. Cranial.

   c. Palatine.

   d. Alveolar.

4. Teeth and structures of the lower jaw are referred to as

   a. Mental.

   b. Buccal.

   c. Lingual.

   d. Mandibular.

5. The main parts of the temporomandibular joint (TMJ) are

   a. The inferior, medial, and superior conchae.

   b. The maxillary arch and tuberosity.

   c. The alveolar process and the mental protuberance.

   d. The glenoid fossa, the articular eminence, and the condyloid process.

6. Which of the following is one of the muscles of mastication?

   a. Masseter

   b. Buccinator

   c. Trapezius

   d. Orbicularis oris

7. The muscle of facial expression that encircles the mouth and has no skeletal attachment is the

   a. Buccinator muscle.

   b. Zygomatic major.

   c. Orbicularis oris muscle.

   d. Mentalis muscle.

8. Which extrinsic muscle of the tongue *originates* at the hyoid bone?

   a. Hyoglossus

   b. Genioglossus

   c. Styloglossus

   d. Palatoglossus

9. Which *cranial* nerve is the primary source of innervation for the oral cavity?

   a. Maxillary nerve

   b. Mandibular nerve

   c. Trigeminal nerve

   d. Ophthalmic nerve

10. Blood vessels that supply the teeth and gingiva usually have which of the following terms in their name?

    a. Buccal

    b. Alveolar

    c. Lingual

    d. Palatine

Active Learning Exercises

1. Describe how the temporomandibular joint works. Draw a picture to describe the major parts of the joint.

2. Why is it important to palpate the glands and lymph nodes of a patient during a routine examination?

Application Activities

1. Use the Internet or the library to research temporomandibular joint dysfunction. Write a paragraph or two describing the condition, noting dental treatments that can help alleviate symptoms of this disorder.

2. Go back through the chapter and review the anatomical structures. How can knowledge of these structures make you a better dental assistant? List five situations in which your knowledge of the anatomy of the head and neck could be used to benefit a patient.

PREPARING FOR CERTIFICATION EXAMS

Review the following topics in this chapter to prepare for the Dental Assisting National Board (DANB exam):

- **Bones**
- **Temporomandibular Joint**
- **Muscles**
- **Nerves**
- **Blood Vessels**
- **Salivary Glands**
- **Landmarks**

chapter 7

Oral Embryology and Histology

CHAPTER OUTLINE

Introduction
Oral Embryology
    Development in Utero
    Development of the Face and Oral Cavity
    Developmental Anomalies

Life Cycle of the Tooth
    Initiation Stage
    Bud Stage
    Cap Stage
    Bell Stage
    Maturation
    Disturbances

Oral Histology
    Enamel
    Dentin
    Pulp
    Periodontium
    Oral Mucosa

CHAPTER CHECKLIST

On completion of this chapter, students will be able to:

- ☑ Distinguish between the three prenatal phases.
- ☑ Explain the development of the facial structures.
- ☑ Describe how developmental anomalies, such as cleft palate, occur.
- ☑ Describe the process of tooth development.
- ☑ Identify the structures present in each stage of tooth development.
- ☑ Identify the parts of the tooth.
- ☑ Explain the function of the components of the periodontium.
- ☑ Identify and describe the parts of the gingiva.
- ☑ Identify and describe the types of oral mucosa.

KEY TERMS

alveolar (al-VEE-uh-lur) bone – the bone that forms the sockets of the upper and lower jaw to support and protect the roots of the teeth

alveolar crest – the peak-like portion of the alveolar bone that is closest to the tooth crown

ameloblasts (uh-MEL-oh-blasts) – specialized cells of the enamel organ that produce enamel

anatomic crown – the part of the tooth covered by enamel

anatomic root – the part of the tooth covered by cementum

bell stage – the fourth stage of tooth development

bud stage – the second stage of tooth development

cap stage – the third stage of tooth development

cementoblasts – cells that produce cementum

cementoclasts – cells that resorb cementum

cementodentinal (sim-en-toe-DEN-tun-ul) junction – the area within the root of the tooth where the cementum lining meets the dentin

cementoenamel (sim-en-toe-ee-NAM-ul) junction (CEJ) – where the anatomic crown (enamel) joins the anatomic root (cementum)

cementum – the outer layer of the anatomic root

clinical crown – the part of the anatomic crown that is visible in the oral cavity (above the gingiva)

clinical root – the part of the anatomic root that is not visible in the oral cavity (below the gingiva)

cortical (KOR-tik-ul) bone – part of the alveolar bone that forms the hard outer wall of the upper and lower jaws, surrounds the lamina dura, and supports the sockets

dental lamina (LAM-uh-nuh) – specialized cell layer of the oral epithelium from which the tooth buds develop

dental papilla (puh-PIL-uh) – cells of the mesenchyme that form within the cap-shaped enamel organ

dental sac – an enclosure of the mesenchyme around the enamel organ and dental papilla

dentin – yellow-colored tissue that covers the pulp

dentinal (DEN-tun-ul) tubule – a tube or canal in the dentin that extends out from the pulp to the dentinoenamel and cementodentinal junctions

dentinoenamel (den-tuh-no-ee-NAM-ul) junction – where the enamel joins the dentin, on the inner surface of the tooth

ectoderm (EK-toe-durm) – the outermost layer of embryonic cells

embryo – the human organism from the second to eighth week of development

embryology – the study of an organism's development from conception to birth

enamel – the white outer surface of the anatomic crown

enamel lamellae (luh-MEL-ee) – leaf-like projections from the surface of the enamel to the dentinoenamel junction

enamel tuft – projection from the dentinoenamel junction into the enamel caused by a defect in mineralization

endoderm (EN-doe-durm) – the outermost layer of embryonic cells

fetus – the human organism from the ninth week of development until birth

fibroblasts – spindle-shaped cells that form the collagen fibers within the pulp

frontonasal process – area of facial development where the forehead, eyes, and nose form

gingival sulcus (jin-JIH-vul SUL-kus) – the small space between the tooth and the free gingiva

histology – the study of the relationship between the structure and function of cells, tissues, and organs

lamina dura – thin layer of bone that lines the tooth socket and surrounds the tooth roots.

mandibular process – process of the mandibular arch that forms the lower jaw and structures of the lower lip and lower cheeks

maxillary process – process of the mandibular arch that forms the upper jaw and structures of the upper lip and upper cheeks

mesoderm (MEZ-uh-durm) – the middle layer of embryonic cells

odontoblast (oh-DON-toe-blast) – cell that forms dentin

odontogenesis (oh-don-toe-JEN-uh-sis) – the process of tooth development

oral embryology – the study of the formation of the oral cavity and its structures

oral histology – the study of the structure and function of teeth and their connective tissues

osteoblast (OS-tee-oh-blast) – bone-forming cell

osteoclast(OS-tee-oh-klast) – bone-resorbing cell

periodontal ligament – the fibrous tissue that connects the roots of the teeth to the alveolar bone

periodontium (per-ee-oh-DON-she-um) – tissues that surround and support the tooth

primary dentin – dentin that begins forming during tooth development and continues until the root formation is finished

primary palate – triangle-shaped area of the palate located behind the upper four front teeth

pulp – the connective tissue at the center of the crown and root

pulp canal – the portion of the pulp cavity that extends into the root of the tooth

pulp cavity – the area of the tooth that contains the pulp

pulp chamber – the part of the pulp cavity that extends into the crown of the tooth

Retzius striae (RET-see-us STRY-ee) (lines) – darkened concentric lines visible in a cross-section of the tooth enamel that indicate variations in calcification

secondary dentin – dentin formed by the pulp of the tooth after root formation is finished

secondary palate – the area of the palate formed behind the primary palate by the fusion of the palatal shelves

stomodeum (stoh-muh-DEE-um) – primitive mouth of the embryo

tertiary dentin – dentin that forms in response to damage to or irritation of the tooth

zygote (ZIE-gote) – the fertilized egg

Introduction

An understanding of the development of oral structures throughout a patient's lifetime is essential for dental assistants. This knowledge provides the basis for understanding any developmental problems that may occur in these structures. Knowledge of the histology of the teeth, their supporting structures, and the oral mucosa is a vital tool you can use to better understand the disease processes that can occur and the clinical treatments required.

Oral Embryology

Embryology is the study of an organism's development from conception to birth. **Oral embryology**, in particular, is the study of the formation of the oral cavity and its structures.

Development in Utero

The average human gestation period (pregnancy) is 38 to 40 weeks, or a little over 9 months (Figure 7-1).

Prenatal Phases

The stages of pregnancy are commonly referred to as *trimesters*, which break the gestational period down into 3-month time periods. From an embryologic perspective, it is more useful to look at the three prenatal phases—the zygotic phase, the embryonic phase, and the fetal phase—to understand development.

Zygotic Phase

The zygotic phase represents the first week of pregnancy. A sperm cell joins with an egg cell to produce a fertilized egg, or **zygote**, with 46 chromosomes (23 pairs of chromosomes)—

half from the sperm and half from the egg. This process is known as *meiosis*. Shortly after the zygote forms, it begins to divide rapidly and becomes a cluster of cells. The growing cell cluster implants in the lining of the uterus.

Embryonic Phase

The embryonic phase begins in the second week, after the zygote implants in the uterus, and lasts until the eighth week. In its early stages, the human **embryo** looks much the same as the embryos of other mammals, such as cats, dogs, and even cows. By the end of the second month, however, the embryo more clearly resembles a human.

During this phase, cells continue to multiply and start to differentiate, or specialize, based on the structures they will form (e.g., brain, kidney, and heart). Because all body systems begin forming at this time, the embryonic phase is considered the most vulnerable stage of development. The heart and brain develop early and quickly become the most noticeable structures.

Fetal Phase

The fetal phase begins around the ninth week and lasts until birth. All of the systems have formed by this time, and this phase consists primarily of growth and maturation of those systems. The **fetus** grows most rapidly between the fourth and sixth months.

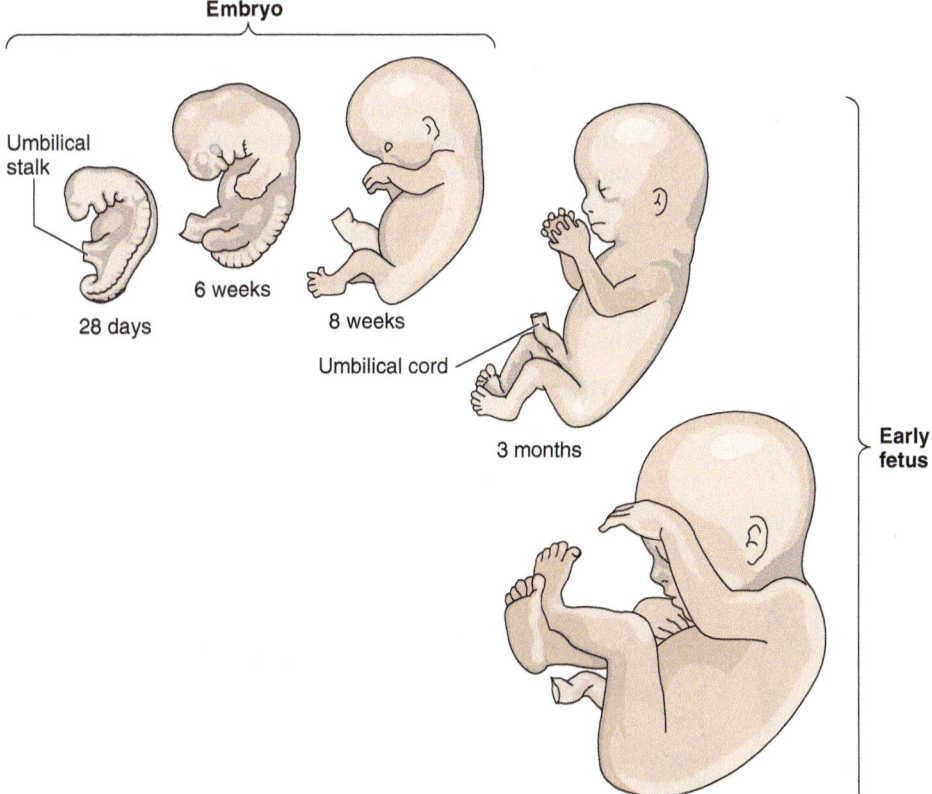

Figure 7–1 The development of an embryo and an early fetus.

Embryo

Umbilical stalk

28 days

6 weeks

8 weeks

Umbilical cord

3 months

5 months

Early fetus

Dental Facts Tetracycline Stains

Although the embryo is considered more vulnerable to developmental anomalies than the fetus, the fetus is still susceptible to what the mother consumes. For example, if the mother is given the antibiotic tetracycline, the drug can transfer through the placenta and into the fetus. The fetus's calcifying teeth and bones absorb the tetracycline, causing discoloration. The extent of the discoloration depends on the dosage, the length of use, the specific form of tetracycline, and the stage of tooth development at which the drug was administered. Only those teeth that have begun to calcify will be affected. The child's teeth can be stained a gray-brown or a light green to dark yellow color. In some cases, when exposed to ultraviolet light, the stained teeth will give off a bright glow.

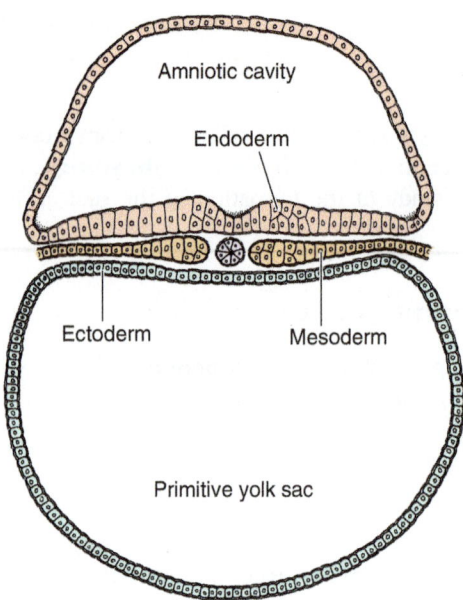

Figure 7–2 Primary embryonic layers form in the second stage of development.

Embryonic Layers

During the embryonic phase, the cells of the embryo multiply and differentiate into three embryonic layers according to the specific structures they will form (Figure 7-2):

- The **ectoderm** is the outermost layer of embryonic cells. These cells make up the nails, hair, tooth enamel, lining of the oral cavity, skin, spinal cord, and brain.
- The **mesoderm**, or middle layer of embryonic cells, forms all connective tissues; muscles; blood; cardiovascular and lymphatic systems; and the linings of the heart, lung, and abdominal cavities.
- The **endoderm** is the innermost embryonic cell layer that will form the lining of parts of the respiratory system, digestive tract, and certain glands.

CHECKPOINTS

7-1 During which prenatal phase are the heart and brain formed?

7-2 What are four of the structures formed by the embryonic ectoderm layer?

Development of the Face and Oral Cavity

The face begins to develop around the fourth week of pregnancy. At this time, the most notable features of the embryo are the bulges of the developing brain and heart and the indentation of the primitive mouth, or **stomodeum** (Figure 7-3).

Early Development

Between the fourth and fifth weeks, pouches and grooves develop in pairs across from each other along the area between the stomodeum and the bulge of the heart. The tissue of the pouches and grooves condense to form the branchial arches.

Development of the Branchial Arches

The structures of the face and oral cavity develop from the branchial arches (also known as *pharyngeal arches*), which form by the end of the fourth week:

- The first branchial arch, known as the mandibular arch, develops closest to the stomodeum. The *mandibular*

Figure 7–3 Structures of the face become more recognizable by the seventh week. (**A**) Fourth week. (**B**) Fourth to fifth week. (**C**) Fifth to sixth week. (**D**) Sixth to seventh week. Note how the nose develops and the eyes appear more anteriorly placed.

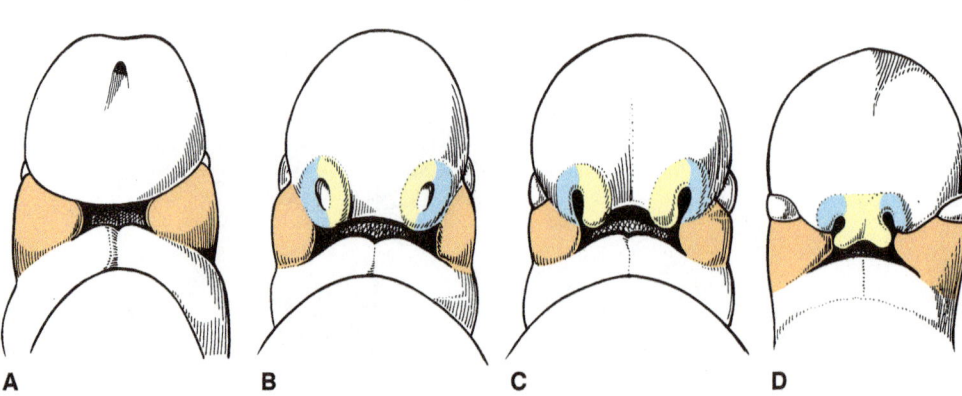

A   B   C   D

arch divides into the maxillary process and the mandibular process, which form the structures of the lips and cheeks as well as the muscles of mastication.

- The second branchial arch, the *hyoid arch*, forms structures in the frontal portion of the neck, part of the hyoid bone, the styloid process, the stylohyoid ligament, the lesser cornu, the stapes of the ear, and the muscles of facial expression.
- The third branchial arch, which is unnamed, forms the remainder of the hyoid bone, the greater cornu, and the stylopharyngeus muscle.
- The fourth through sixth arches are also unnamed and form the cartilages of the thyroid and larynx, the constrictor muscles of the pharynx, and the muscles of the larynx.

Development of the Palate

The **primary palate** is the triangle-shaped area of the palate located behind the upper four front teeth. The maxillary swellings (from the maxillary process) on either side of the stomodeum grow toward the middle of the face to become the upper jaw and fuse with the growth of the intermaxillary segment. As these areas come together, shelflike growths (palatal shelves) project from each swelling into the developing oral cavity. During the seventh week of development, the tongue drops into the oral cavity from the nasal cavity, and the palatal shelves move into position above the tongue and fuse along the midline, forming the **secondary palate**. The primary and secondary palates fuse to separate the oral cavity from the nasal cavity. Fusion of the primary and secondary palates creates the hard and soft palates (Figure 7-4).

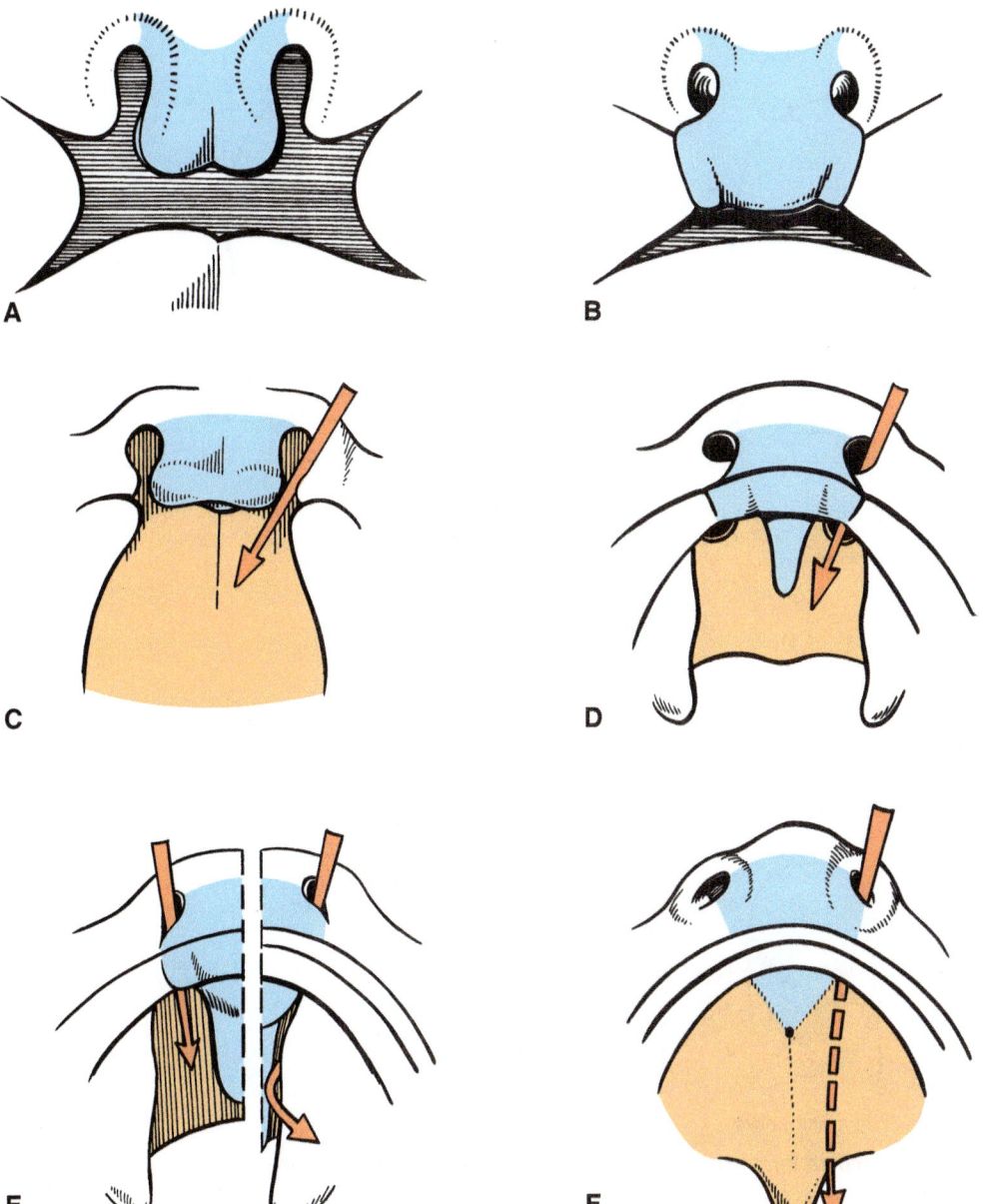

Figure 7–4 Development of the nose, mouth, and palate. (**A–B**) Formation of the nose and upper lip. (**C–F**) Formation of the philtrum, nose, and upper lip and the states of palate formation and closure. Observe the steps of developing separate oral and nasal cavities from the early common oronasal cavity.

Development of the Face

Portions of the face begin to form around the fourth week of development, and most of the facial development takes place from the fifth to eighth weeks (Figure 7-5). Between the fourth and sixth weeks, the nasal cavity opens, the tear ducts form, and the muscles of facial expression spread across the face.

There are essentially three areas of facial development: the frontonasal process, the maxillary process, and the mandibular process. The upper jaw and the structures of the upper lip and upper cheeks form in the **maxillary process**. The **mandibular process** forms the lower jaw and the structures of the lower lip and lower cheeks. As the maxillary and mandibular processes of the first branchial arch are growing toward the middle of the face, a bulge forms toward the front of the brain and moves down the middle of the face. This bulge grows into the **frontonasal process**, from which the forehead, eyes, and nose develop.

Nasal placodes develop as thick areas on either side of the frontonasal process, just above the stomodeum. Rims form and grow around the nasal placodes, leaving indentations called *nasal pits*—these rims and pits will eventually become the nostrils. As the rims of the nasal placodes grow toward each other, the inner parts of the rims fuse to form the intermaxillary segment, which will develop the following structures:

- nasal septum
- columella of the nose (the outer tissue between the nostrils)
- philtrum (groove between the nose and upper lip)
- primary palate
- anterior teeth with their supporting components and the gingiva

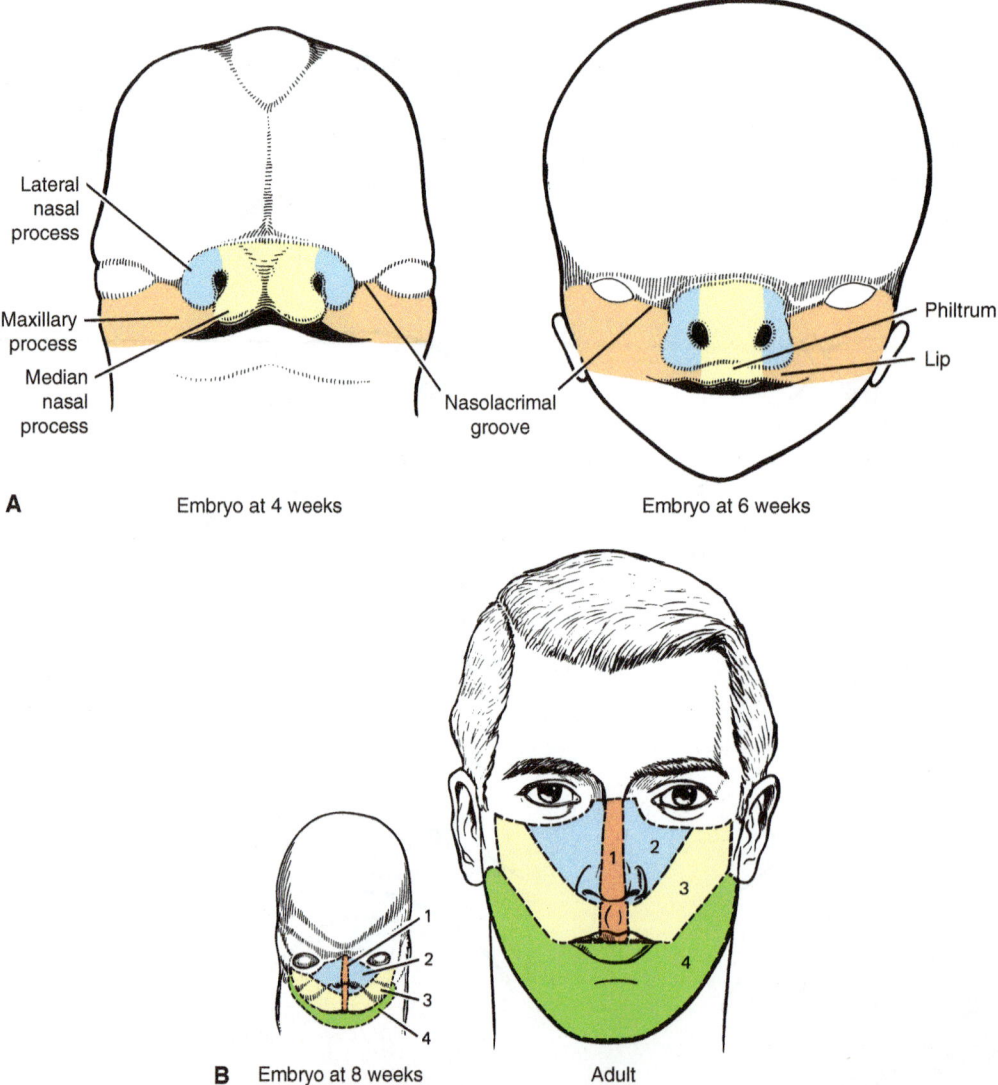

Figure 7–5 A. The nose, eyes, and mouth form between the fourth and sixth weeks of development. **B.** Development of the face illustrating derivatives of embryologic development. (1) Median nasal process; (2) Lateral nasal process; (3) Maxillary process; (4) Mandibular process.

As the developing areas of the face grow toward each other, the processes fuse as they meet:

- The intermaxillary segment and maxillary processes fuse on both sides of the philtrum.
- The maxillary processes fuse with the mandibular process at the corners of the mouth, known as the labial commissures.
- The frontonasal and maxillary processes fuse at the nasolacrimal groove.

Development of the Teeth

The embryonic ectoderm layer lines the stomodeum, which will become the oral cavity. As the cells of the ectoderm differentiate, they form the lining of the oral cavity known as the *oral epithelium*. Cells of the mesoderm layer differentiate to form the mesenchyme, the connective tissue beneath the oral epithelium. Both the mesenchyme and the oral epithelium serve an important function in tooth development: cells of these tissues will differentiate further to form specific parts of the tooth.

CHECKPOINTS

7-3 What are the three structures that develop from the frontonasal process?

7-4 What is the name of the first branchial arch?

7-5 Which part of the face is formed by the maxillary process?

Voice of Experience

Learning about the complex process of facial development in a human embryo has given me a better understanding of how the parts of the face fit together. With this knowledge, I can talk to patients about how a cleft lip is formed, or at what point the structures of the teeth start to develop. I also enjoy being able to share with pregnant patients some of the complex changes that are taking place as their child develops.

Developmental Anomalies

The development of a human from zygote to fetus is a delicate and complex process. Every part of this process is dependent on proteins regulating the expression of specific genes at the right time to coordinate the pattern of cell development. Even if a mother gets adequate nutrition and is careful to avoid anything that may harm the developing child, a protein may not bind properly, or a cell may not perform its necessary function. If a mother lacks proper nutrition or consumes a chemical that could be toxic (e.g., alcohol, cigarettes, cocaine, or even certain antibiotics), the risk of birth defects increases tremendously.

Cleft Lip

About 1 in every 900 babies is born with a cleft lip in the United States, and of these most are boys. Cleft lip forms when the maxillary process and the intermaxillary segment do not fuse completely (Figure 7-6). If only one side of the lip failed to fuse, the cleft is *unilateral*; if neither side fused, the cleft is *bilateral*. Cleft lip can be surgically corrected.

Cleft Palate

Cleft palate tends to be more common in girls than in boys, and occurs in about 1 in 2,500 births. A cleft palate results when the maxillae do not fuse with the primary palate. There are many varieties of cleft palate, all of which leave some degree of opening between the oral and nasal cavities. A baby born with a cleft palate will typically have trouble nursing because the baby will tend to suck in air rather than milk. Cleft palate can be surgically corrected, although it may take multiple surgeries depending on the severity of the cleft.

Other Developmental Disturbances

Torus

A bony cluster or mass, known as a *torus* (or *tori*, if plural), may be found along the midline of the hard palate (palatine torus) or along the inner surface of the jaw (mandibular torus),

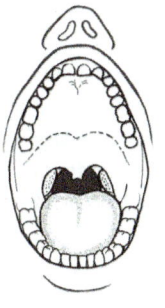 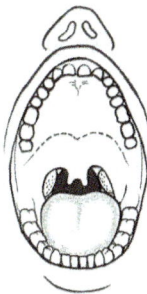 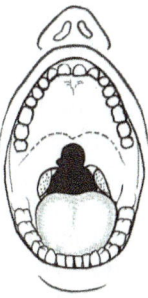 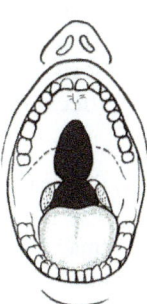 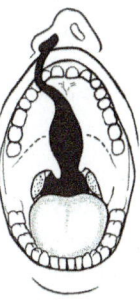 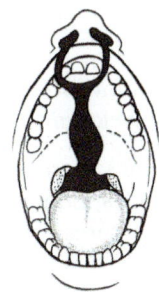

| Class 1 | Class 2 | Class 3 | Class 4 | Class 5 | Class 6 |

Figure 7–6 Classification of cleft lip and cleft palate.

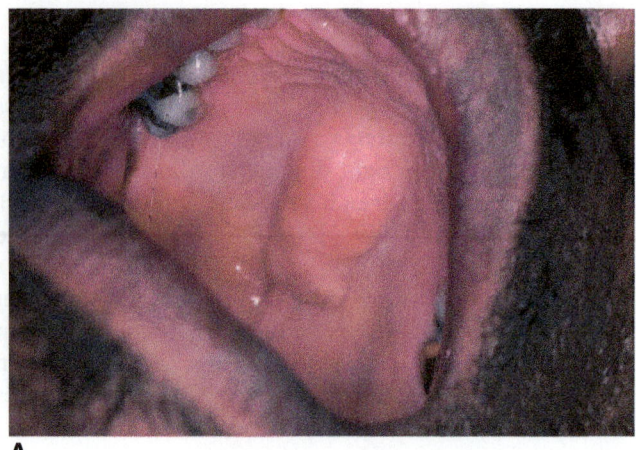

A

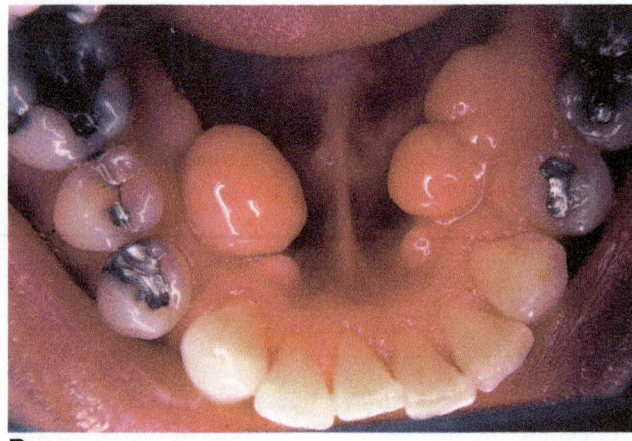

B

Figure 7–7 (**A**) Torus palatinus of the hard palate and (**B**) bilateral torus mandibularis.

near the tongue (Figure 7-7). Tori are relatively common and generally do not cause problems for the individual, except that the epithelium over the protrusions may be more likely to get scratched by the sharp edges of some foods. If the torus is large, however, it will need to be surgically removed to prepare for denture construction.

Fetal Alcohol Syndrome

Fetal alcohol syndrome (FAS) is a pattern of abnormal growth and development that results from prenatal exposure to alcohol, and is considered the most preventable birth defect. Alcohol is a teratogen (an agent that can cause birth defects) and may cause serious damage to the unborn child. Researchers have not been able to determine whether there is a "safe" amount of alcohol that can be consumed during pregnancy. Doctors recommend that no amount of alcohol be consumed at any time during pregnancy, because alcohol passes to the embryo or fetus freely across the placenta, which means that the developing child is essentially matching the mother drink for drink. As the alcohol passes through the placenta, it acts as a toxin that interferes with the developing structures of the embryo or the growth of the fetus.

Mothers who consume alcohol during pregnancy have an increased risk of miscarriages (spontaneous abortions) and stillbirths. Children with FAS have developmental disorders that range from mild to severe; these effects are known as *fetal alcohol spectrum disorders*. FAS affects all aspects of development:

- Major organs: increased risk of problems with the heart, liver, muscles, kidneys, and bones
- Facial structures: small head circumference, small eye opening, short nose, sunken nasal bridge, thin upper lip, poorly defined philtrum, small jaws
- Cognitive: difficulty with verbal and spatial learning; decreased ability to plan or organize

- Behavioral: short attention span and hyperactivity
- Functional: problems with vision and hearing; poor coordination

Down Syndrome

Down syndrome is a developmental anomaly generally caused by an extra chromosome transferred during meiosis. Remember that during fertilization the sperm's 23 chromosomes pair with the egg's 23 chromosomes to form the full 46-chromosome complement. Down syndrome typically results from a trisomy (i.e., three chromosomes), instead of a pair, at chromosome 21.

Although people with Down syndrome have a below-average IQ, they may be more socially advanced. They also tend to have weakened immune systems and are more likely to develop respiratory infections, leukemia, Alzheimer disease, and heart disease. People who have Down syndrome share similar physical characteristics:

- Short stature
- A round, flat face
- A short nose
- Wide-set, slanted eyes with thickened skin folds
- Poor muscle tone

In addition to these characteristics, children with Down syndrome are prone to particular abnormalities of the oral cavity. They have narrow palates and jaws, which tends to make the tongue appear larger than normal. Their tongue may also have deep fissures. Although the tongue may not be any larger on average, it is large for the space in the oral cavity, and children with Down syndrome usually hold their mouth open so that their tongue sticks out slightly. Their lips may be dry and cracked because of the excess saliva that collects while their mouth is open. Children with Down syndrome are more likely to have a cleft lip or palate, an irregular sequence of tooth emergence, and small teeth or fused teeth.

CHECKPOINTS

7-6 What chromosomal anomaly causes Down syndrome?

7-7 How does a cleft lip form?

Life Cycle of the Tooth

Teeth develop through the process known as **odontogenesis**, which begins around the sixth week of prenatal development (Figure 7-8). All primary teeth will have formed by the seventeenth week of gestation.

Initiation Stage

The first stage, called the *initiation stage*, is subject to the induction process. During the sixth to seventh weeks, the ectoderm lines the stomodeum. From there, the oral epithelium and, later, the **dental lamina** are created. Meanwhile, the neural crest cells influence the development of the ectomesenchyme. The basement membrane separates the ectomesenchyme and the oral epithelium.

Bud Stage

The **bud stage**, also known as *proliferation*, is the second stage of tooth development. Around the eighth week, a specialized layer of cells grows from the oral epithelium to form the dental lamina, from which the tooth buds develop. The dental lamina pushes into the mesenchyme beneath the oral epithelium as the tooth bud forms. Ten buds grow from the dental lamina on each arch, forming the primary teeth. As the tooth bud grows, it remains connected to the oral epithelium by a thin strand of the dental lamina. The epithelium of the tooth bud develops into the enamel organ, which is the first part of the tooth to form. The enamel organ will later become the tooth enamel.

Around the 17th week in utero, the first permanent molars begin to form in the dental lamina farther back along the jaw from the primary teeth. As the primary teeth develop, the tooth buds of the permanent teeth that will replace them form deeper within the dental lamina.

Cap Stage

During the third stage, the **cap stage**, cells of the tooth bud multiply (proliferate), and the growing enamel organ takes on a shape resembling a cap. This takes place

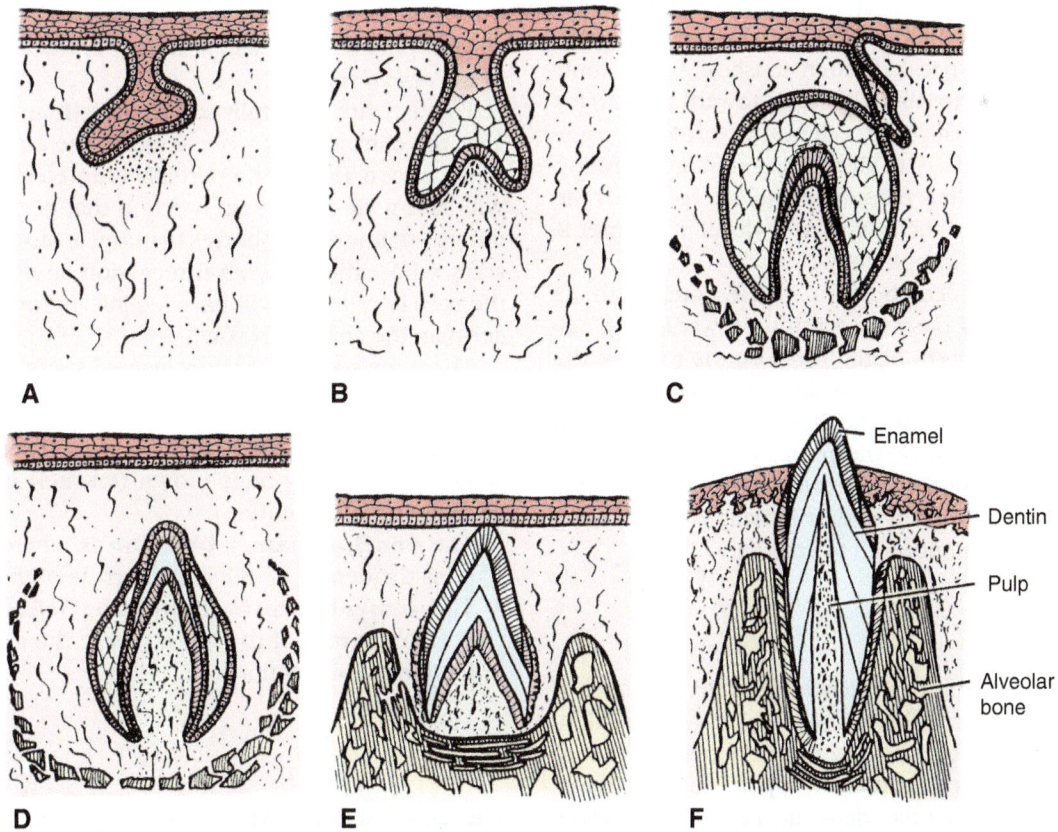

Figure 7–8 The life cycle in the development a tooth. (**A**) Bud stage. (**B**) Cap stage. (**C**) Bell stage. (**D**) Apposition stage. (**E**) Maturation stage. (**F**) Eruption.

around the ninth or tenth week. This cap formation can be seen in the earliest developing primary teeth by the 9th to 10th weeks in utero. Cells of the mesenchyme form the **dental papilla** inside the cap. Both the pulp and dentin are formed by specialized cells of the dental papilla. The mesenchyme closes around the enamel organ and dental papilla to form the **dental sac.**

Bell Stage

Cells continue to differentiate in the **bell stage** (the fourth stage, between the eleventh and twelfth weeks), and the developing tooth takes on a bell shape. The epithelial cells within the enamel organ differentiate into specialized cells that produce enamel, called **ameloblasts.** The outer cells of the dental papilla differentiate into **odontoblasts,** which form dentin. **Cementoblasts,** which produce cementum, differentiate from the cells of the dental sac. By the time the ameloblasts and odontoblasts are differentiating in the primary tooth, the bud of the permanent tooth has begun to form.

Maturation

Tooth crowns continue to form and calcify beneath the surface of the gingiva. The crowns of all primary teeth start calcifying between the fourth and sixth month in utero (the fetal phase), and calcification is completed within the first year after birth. Roots of the primary teeth begin to form after the crown calcification finishes. As the roots develop, they begin to push the tooth toward the surface of the gingiva. Eventually the tooth pushes through the gingiva and into the oral cavity. The roots continue to develop even after the tooth has emerged. (The emergence of the teeth, or eruption, will be discussed in detail in Chapter 8, Dentition and Tooth Morphology.)

The permanent teeth begin to calcify after birth. As their roots form and push the tooth up toward the gingival surface, **osteoclasts** begin to resorb the roots of the primary teeth. (Cells that specifically resorb cementum are called **cementoclasts.**) By the time the permanent tooth nears the gingival surface, the primary tooth roots have dissolved to the point that they cannot anchor the crown. The primary tooth loosens and eventually is lost, leaving room for the permanent tooth to emerge.

Disturbances

Throughout the course of the tooth life cycle, a number of disturbances can occur that cause problems in periodontal health, appearance, and regular development. These disturbances include anodontia, supernumerary teeth, macrodontia, microdontia, dens in dente, gemination, tubercles, and enamel and dentin dysplasia. The effects of these disturbances are varied, as is their severity.

✓ CHECKPOINTS
7-8 When does odontogenesis begin?

7-9 What are cementoblasts?

Oral Histology

Histology, in general, is the study of the relationship between the structure and function of cells, tissues, and organs. **Oral histology** is the study of the structure and function of teeth and their connective tissues.

There are essentially four components of the tooth: enamel, dentin, pulp, and the cementum (Figure 7-9), which is part of the periodontium. In a healthy tooth, the only two tissues visible are the enamel and cementum. Dentin and pulp are inner tissues that are normally not visible unless the tooth's outer layers are damaged.

The tooth consists of a crown and a root. The **anatomic crown** of the tooth is the part covered by enamel, and the term **clinical crown** specifically refers to the part of the crown that is *visible* in the oral cavity. Similarly, the **anatomic root** is the part of the tooth covered by cementum, and the **clinical root** refers only to the part of the root that is *not visible* because it is below the gingiva. Structures that are near the crown of the tooth are said to be *coronal,* and structures near the tip of the root (apex) are in the *apical* region.

For patients with fully erupted teeth and healthy gingiva, the clinical crown is essentially the same as the anatomic crown. However, a partially erupted tooth in a child will have a clinical crown (portion that is exposed in the mouth) that is much shorter than the anatomic crown. An adult who exhibits gingival recession, in which more of the root is exposed, will have a clinical crown that is longer than the anatomic crown.

There are several junctions named for the components of the tooth that join at that area:

- The **cementoenamel junction** (CEJ) marks the separation of the anatomic crown (enamel) from the anatomic root (cementum).
- The **dentinoenamel junction** is where the enamel joins the dentin, on the inner surface of the tooth.
- The **cementodentinal junction** refers to the area within the root of the tooth where the cementum lining meets the dentin.

Enamel

The **enamel** is the white outer surface of the anatomic crown. This protective layer of the tooth is the hardest substance in the body. Enamel develops from the ectoderm

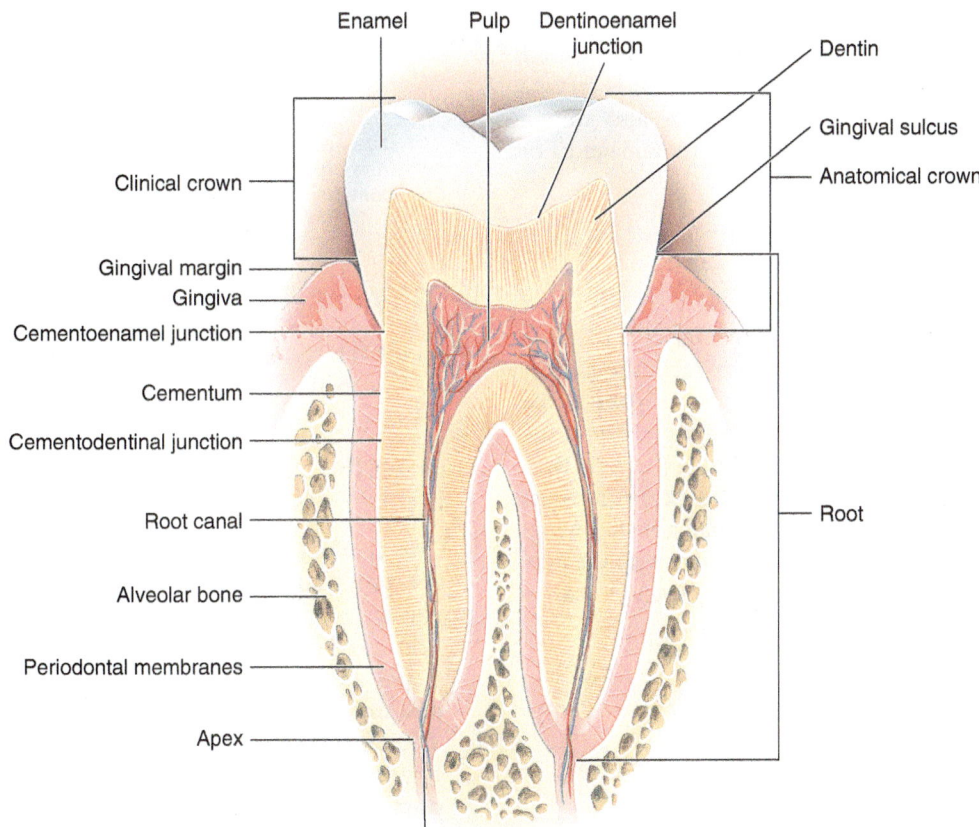

Figure 7–9 Structures of the tooth.

layer, which forms the enamel organ. Enamel is composed of microscopic, calcified rods that extend out from the dentinoenamel junction to the surface of the tooth. When examined under a microscope, the rods have a shape similar to a keyhole. The enamel is about 95% calcified (calcium hydroxyapatite). **Retzius striae** (lines) indicate variations in the calcification of tooth enamel. They appear as darkened concentric lines in a cross-section of the enamel, much like tree rings.

Sometimes defects occur in enamel formation. Two of the most common of these are enamel lamellae (an organic defect) and enamel tufts (a mineral defect). **Enamel lamellae** are leaflike projections from the surface of the enamel to the dentinoenamel junction. **Enamel tufts** project from the dentinoenamel junction into the enamel.

Dentin

Dentin is the yellow-colored tissue that covers the pulp, extending almost the full length of the tooth beneath the cementum and enamel. Because of its material composition, dentin is not quite as hard as enamel but is harder than cementum. Dentin is formed from the odontoblasts contained in the **dentinal tubules,** tubes or canals in the dentin that extend out from the pulp to the dentinoenamel and cementodentinal junctions (Figure 7-10).

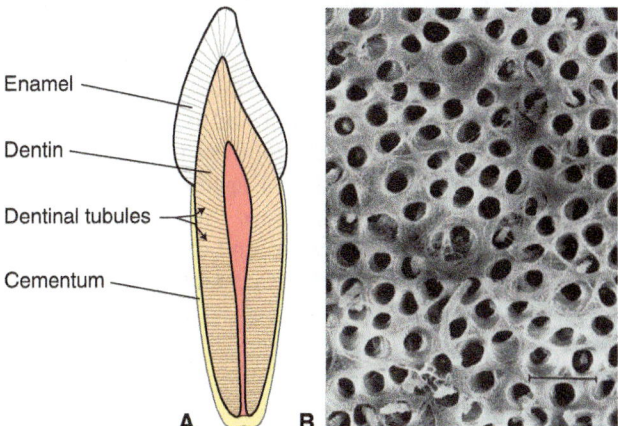

Figure 7–10 Dentinal tubules are microscopic canals that run through the dentin of a tooth. (**A**) Diagram of a dentinal tubule. (**B**) Scanning electron micrograph of dentinal tubules of a human tooth.

Primary dentin begins forming during tooth development and continues until the root formation is finished. After the root has formed, **secondary dentin** is formed by the pulp of the tooth. **Tertiary dentin**, also known as *reparative dentin*, forms in response to damage to or irritation of the tooth.

Pulp

Pulp is the connective tissue at the center of the crown and root. The area of the tooth that contains the pulp is known as the **pulp cavity**. The **pulp chamber** is the part of the pulp cavity that extends into the crown of the tooth, and the **pulp canal** is the portion in the root. Dentin surrounds the pulp cavity on all sides except for near the apex of the root, where there is a small hole known as the *apical foramen*. Collagen fibers that make up the connective tissue of the pulp are formed by spindle-shaped cells called **fibroblasts.**

✓ CHECKPOINTS

7-10 Describe the difference between the anatomic crown and the clinical crown.

7-11 What is the cementoenamel junction?

Periodontium

Periodontium refers to the tissues that surround and support the tooth and includes the cementum, alveolar bone, periodontal ligament, and gingiva (Figure 7-11).

Cementum

Cementum is the outer layer of the anatomic root. The cementum is a dull yellow color and is about as hard as bone. It protects the root of the tooth and acts as an anchor for the fibers of the periodontal ligament that keep the tooth in its place. The thickness of the cementum varies across the tooth; it is thinnest around the CEJ. The cementum is about 65% calcium hydroxyapatite, 23% collagen fibers, and 12% water.

Alveolar Bone

The **alveolar bone**, or *alveolar process*, forms the sockets of the upper and lower jaws to support and protect the tooth roots. The alveolar bone exists only when there is a tooth in the socket; it will not form if a tooth does not emerge, and if a tooth is removed, the bone is eventually

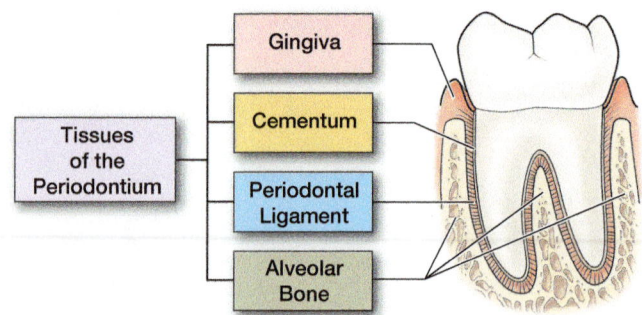

Figure 7–11 Periodontium, the tissue that makes up the support of the tooth.

resorbed. There are three main components of the alveolar bone:

- The **lamina dura** is the thin layer of bone that lines the tooth socket (alveolus) and surrounds the tooth roots.
- The **cortical bone** forms the hard outer wall of the upper and lower jaws that surrounds the lamina dura and supports the sockets.
- The cancellous (or spongy) bone is the spongy-looking bone found between the cortical bone and the lamina dura. The cancellous bone follows the contours of the tooth socket so that it gives extra support to the lamina dura.

The **alveolar crest** is the peaklike portion of the alveolar bone that is closest to the tooth crown.

The outer surface of the alveolar bone is covered by the periosteum, which is thick tissue made up of an inner layer of cells that generate new bone tissue and an outer layer of fibrous connective tissue that carries blood vessels and nerves.

Periodontal Ligament

The **periodontal ligament** is the fibrous tissue that connects the roots of the teeth to the alveolar bone (see Figure 7-11). The ligament surrounds the tooth in the area between the cementum and the alveolar bone. There are many fibers that make up the periodontal ligament. *Sharpey fibers* are the embedded ends of the fibers that connect to the cementum and the alveolar bone.

Two main fiber groups make up the periodontal ligament:

- The *gingival fiber groups* are located around the cervix (neck) of the tooth (where it tapers slightly at the CEJ) within the gingival tissues.
- The *principal fiber groups*, or dentoalveolar fibers, surround the root of the tooth. These collagen fibers are named according to their location on the root and their direction.

TABLE 7-1	Fiber Groups of the Periodontal Ligament	
NAME	**CONNECTION**	**FUNCTION**
GINGIVAL FIBER GROUPS		
Dentogingival fibers	From cervical cementum to free gingiva	Supports the free gingiva
Alveologingival fibers	From alveolar crest to free and attached gingiva	Provides support
Circumferential fibers	Surround the neck of the tooth	Maintains tooth position
Dentoperiosteal fibers	From cervical cementum, over alveolar crest, and into the alveolar bone	Provides support
Transseptal fibers	From cervix of one tooth to cervix of adjacent tooth	Resists tooth separation
PRINCIPAL FIBER GROUPS		
Apical fibers	From apex of root to adjacent surrounding bone	Resists vertical forces
Oblique fibers	From the root above the apical fibers at an upward slant to the alveolar bone	Resists vertical and unexpected strong forces
Horizontal fibers	From cementum mid-root to adjacent alveolar bone	Resists tipping of tooth
Alveolar crest fibers	From alveolar crest to just below the cementoenamel junction	Resists forces of intrusion
Irradicular fibers (only on multirooted teeth)	From the cementum of multirooted teeth to adjacent alveolar bone	Resists forces horizontally and vertically

Table 7-1 describes the different fibers that make up the two main fiber groups of the periodontal ligament.

Gingiva

The gingiva covers the cervix of the teeth and the alveolar bone. The coronal boundary of the gingiva is the gingival margin, and the apical boundary is the alveolar mucosa. The alveolar mucosa is easily distinguished from the gingiva because it tends to be a darker red and has a slick, shiny surface. There are four parts to the gingiva (Figure 7-12):

- Free gingiva is the portion of the gingiva that is not attached to the tooth or alveolar bone. It surrounds the area of the tooth near the CEJ like a freestanding collar.
- The **gingival sulcus** is the small space between the tooth and the free gingiva.
- The attached gingiva is bound tightly to the cementum and the periosteum of the alveolar bone by the periodontal ligament.
- Interdental gingiva (also called *interdental papilla*) is the gingival tissue between two adjacent teeth.

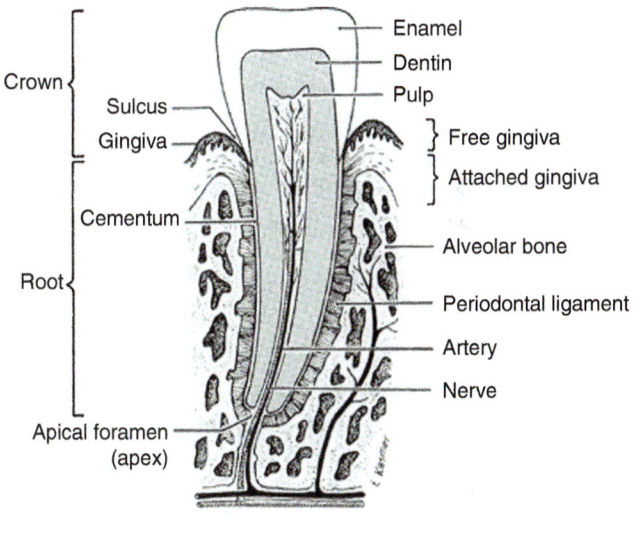

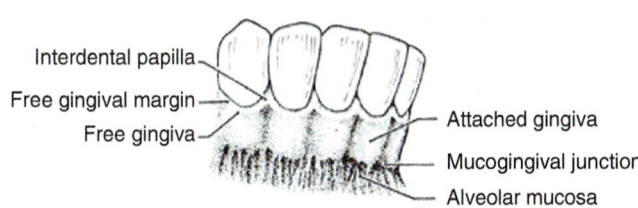

Figure 7–12 The parts of the gingiva.

CHECKPOINTS

7-12 What is the lamina dura?

7-13 What are Sharpey fibers?

7-14 What structures do the horizontal fibers connect, and what function do the fibers perform?

Oral Mucosa

Epithelial tissue covers the body's outer surface (skin) and lines the body cavities (mucosa). The epithelium of the oral cavity, the **oral mucosa**, is made up of stratified squamous epithelium—that is, layers of flat epithelial cells. Oral mucosa can be divided into three categories: lining mucosa, keratinized mucosa, and specialized mucosa.

Lining Mucosa

Lining mucosa is the soft, flexible epithelium that lines the inner lips and cheeks, the floor of the mouth, the underside of the tongue, the soft palate, and the alveolar mucosa. It provides a layer to cushion against stress and wear.

Keratinized Mucosa

Keratinized mucosa, sometimes called *masticatory mucosa*, covers the surfaces that receive the most wear and tear during food mastication: the gingiva and the hard palate. The keratinized epithelial cells provide a strong, protective surface layer.

Specialized Mucosa

Specialized mucosa covers the upper surface (dorsum) of the tongue and consists of papillae, or projections of the mucous membrane (Figure 7-13). Four kinds of papillae compose the surface of the tongue:

- Filiform papillae are thin, hairlike papillae that cover the dorsal surface. These papillae do not contain taste buds, and there are more of these than any of the other papillae.
- Fungiform papillae are mushroom-shaped papillae found on the tip and sides of the tongue, interspersed with filiform papillae. They are redder and shorter than the filiform, and they contain taste buds.
- Vallate (or circumvallate) papillae are the 8 to 14 circular papillae that form a V shape between the body of the tongue and the base. The walls of vallate papillae are lined with taste buds.
- Foliate papillae are vertical, leaflike folds along the rear edges of the tongue body. They contain some taste buds.

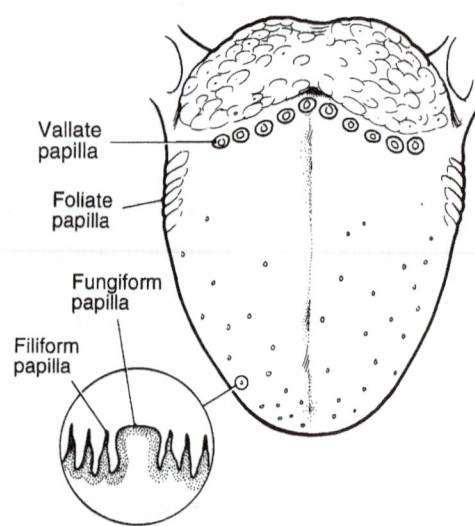

Figure 7–13 The four papillae found on the tongue include: filiform, fungiform, foliate, and the vallate papilla.

The fungiform, vallate, and foliate papillae all contain taste buds, which are the taste receptors. The taste buds are distributed across the surface of the tongue so that there are essentially taste clusters in different areas (Figure 7-14):

- Salty tastes are best experienced along the front edges of the tongue.
- Sweet tastes can be detected best toward the tip of the tongue.
- Sour tastes are most acute along the sides of the tongue.
- Bitter tastes are best detected by the V-shaped vallate papillae toward the back of the tongue.

From the Dentist's Perspective

As a dental assistant, you will encounter many abnormalities in the oral cavity, including those relating to the tongue. Knowing the placement and characteristics of the tongue papillae will help you better understand how a healthy tongue should look and which conditions may be cause for concern. Here are two of my favorite abnormal tongue conditions (discussed more fully in Chapter 12):

Geographic tongue refers to a condition in which the tongue loses filiform papillae, leaving red bare patches intermingled with the intact papillae. The patches create a maplike (geographic) pattern on the surface of the tongue. The condition is harmless and usually painless, although there may be some increased sensitivity.

Black hairy tongue is a condition in which the filiform papillae of the tongue lengthen abnormally, giving them a hairy appearance. The most common contributors to black hairy tongue are poor oral hygiene, tobacco products, and excessive coffee or tea consumption.

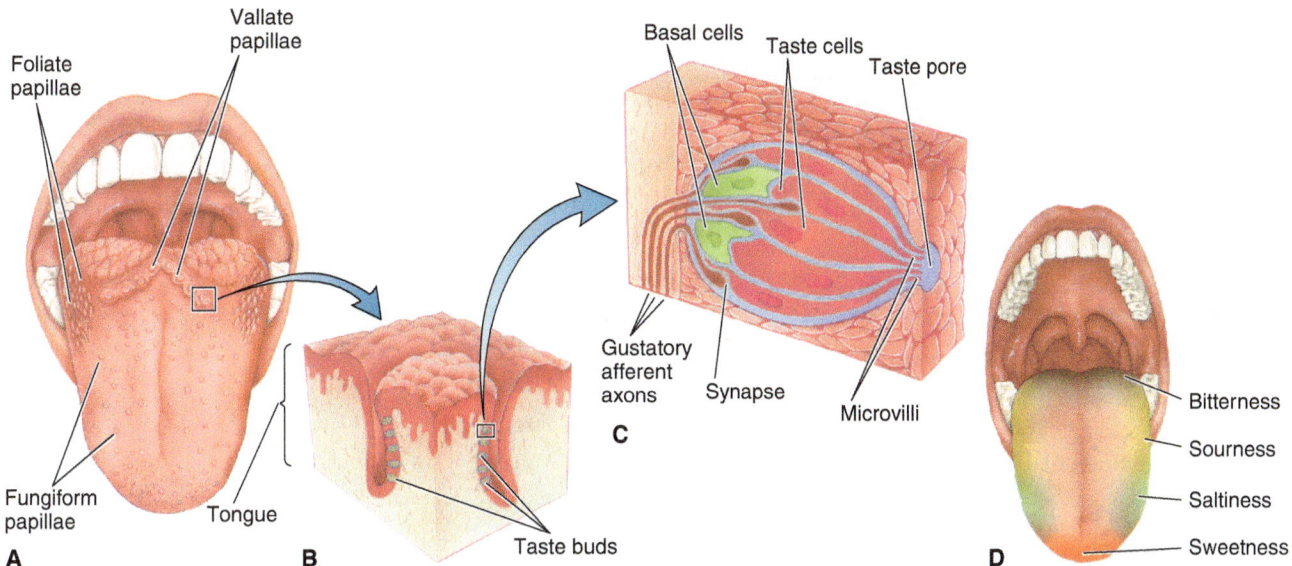

Figure 7–14 Taste buds and areas of taste on the dorsum of the tongue. (**A**) Papillae are the taste-sensitive structures. (**B**) Cross-sectional view of a vallate papilla showing the locations of taste buds. (**C**) A taste bud is a cluster of taste cells (receptor cells), gustatory afferent axons and their synapses with taste cells, and basal cells. (**D**) Areas of taste.

 ## Chapter Highlights

+ All body systems begin developing during the embryonic phase, and they grow and mature throughout the fetal phase.
+ All tissues and organs of the body develop from the differentiated cells of the embryonic ectoderm, mesoderm, and endoderm layers.
+ The stomodeum, or *primitive embryonic mouth*, is lined with the ectoderm layer.
+ The frontonasal, maxillary, and mandibular processes are the primary features of embryonic facial development.
+ The mandibular arch (the first branchial arch) is responsible for forming the structures of the upper and lower jaws, lips, and cheeks.
+ The intermaxillary segment forms the primary palate. Fusion of the palatal shelves forms the secondary palate. The hard and soft palates are formed by the fusion of the primary and secondary palates.

+ Each tooth is made up of enamel, dentin, cementum, and pulp. The *enamel* covers the anatomic crown of the tooth, and the *cementum* covers the anatomic root of the tooth.
+ The *clinical crown* of the tooth is the portion of the crown visible above the gingiva, whereas the *clinical root* is the portion of the root that is not visible.
+ Cementum, alveolar bone, periodontal ligament, and gingiva make up the periodontium.
+ Numerous fibers of the periodontal ligament connect the roots of the teeth to the alveolar bone. *Gingival fiber groups* and *principal fiber groups* are the two categories of fibers that make up the periodontal ligament.
+ There are three types of oral mucosa: lining mucosa, keratinized mucosa, and specialized mucosa.
+ Specialized mucosa, which is found on the upper surface of the tongue, consists of the filiform, fungiform, vallate, and foliate papillae.

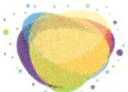 ## Review Questions

1. When does the fetal phase begin?
   a. Week 3
   b. Week 6
   c. Week 9
   d. Week 12

2. Which of these substances is the hardest?
   a. Dentin
   b. Cementum
   c. Enamel
   d. Bone

3. Which type of cell produces enamel?

    a. Odontoblast

    b. Ameloblast

    c. Osteoclast

    d. Cementoblast

4. What is the stomodeum?

    a. The primitive mouth

    b. The third branchial arch

    c. The innermost embryonic layer

    d. The point at which the enamel joins the cementum

5. When do the branchial arches form?

    a. Week 1

    b. Week 4

    c. Week 16

    d. Week 32

6. What is the second stage of tooth development?

    a. Cap stage

    b. Bell stage

    c. Pod stage

    d. Bud stage

7. Which of the following is *not* part of the periodontium?

    a. Gingiva

    b. Alveolar bone

    c. Pulp

    d. Lamina dura

8. What is a torus?

    a. The bony socket that surrounds the tooth root

    b. Bony mass or cluster that forms on the hard palate or inner jaw

    c. Tough outer layer of the enamel organ of the tooth

    d. The zygote cell cluster that implants in the wall of the uterus

9. Which of the papillae of the tongue do not contain taste buds?

    a. Filiform

    b. Fungiform

    c. Vallate

    d. Foliate

10. During which of the prenatal phases does odontogenesis begin?

    a. Fetal

    b. Zygotic

    c. Bud

    d. Embryonic

11. Which type of oral mucosa covers the surface of the hard palate?

    a. Keratinized

    b. Lining

    c. Mesenchyme

    d. Specialized

Active Learning Exercises

1. Identify two possible developmental disturbances. What are they, when do they occur, and what is the potential outcome of the disturbance?

2. What significant processes take place during the bud, cap, and bell stages?

3. Draw a picture of a tooth. Label the following: enamel, dentin, pulp, cementum, and gingiva. Describe what healthy, intact gingiva should look like.

Application Activities

1. Using the Internet or the library for research, write a paragraph or two about a developmental disturbance not covered in the text. How would this condition affect oral health care? Include some oral hygiene tips you would share with a patient suffering from the condition.

2. Write a paragraph or two describing how understanding the various stages of tooth development will make you a better dental assistant.

PREPARING FOR CERTIFICATION EXAMS

Review the topic "Oral Histology" in this chapter to prepare for the Dental Assisting National Board (DANB) exam.

Dentition and Tooth Morphology

CHAPTER CHECKLIST

On completion of this chapter, students will be able to:

- ☑ Describe the types of dentition and at what stage they occur.
- ☑ Explain the general schedule for eruption and exfoliation of primary teeth and eruption of permanent teeth.
- ☑ Identify and define the terminology used to describe the location of teeth in the oral cavity.
- ☑ Identify the characteristics and functions of each class of tooth.
- ☑ Describe the common systems of tooth numbering.
- ☑ Identify the divisions used to describe the surfaces of the teeth.
- ☑ Identify the anatomic structures and landmarks on the surfaces of the teeth.
- ☑ Identify and describe each tooth in the primary dentition.
- ☑ Identify and describe each tooth in the permanent dentition.

KEY TERMS

adjacent – directly next to

apex – the tip of the root

apical foramen (AP-ih-kul fuh-RAY-mun) – the small opening at the apex where nerves and blood vessels enter the root to connect with the tooth pulp

bicuspid (bi-KUS-pid) – a tooth with two cusps

bifurcated (BI-fur-kay-tid) – split into two

bifurcation (bi-fur-KAY-shun) – the area where the tooth roots separate into two

buccal (BUK-ul) – near the cheek

buccal surface – the facial surface of the posterior teeth that is near the cheek

canine (cuspid) – a sharply pointed anterior tooth distal to the lateral incisors

central groove – developmental groove at the center of the occlusal surface

cingulum (SING-you-lum) – a small bump located on the cervical third of the lingual surface of the anterior teeth

concave – a surface curved inward

contact area – where the proximal surfaces of adjacent teeth touch

convex – a surface curved outward

curve of Spee – anterior-to-posterior curvature that follows the line of the incisal edges and cusp tips

curve of Wilson – side-to-side curvature that follows the cusp tips of the posterior teeth

cusp – peak on the incisal surface of the canines or on the occlusal surface of premolars and molars

cusp of Carabelli – nonfunctional fifth cusp that often forms on the mesiolingual cusp of the maxillary first molar

cuspid (canine) – a sharply pointed anterior tooth distal to the lateral incisors

deciduous teeth – the primary teeth, which are lost or shed

dentition (den-TIH-shun) – the set of natural teeth on a dental arch

developmental groove – distinct linear depression formed while the tooth was developing that separates major features of the tooth or lobes on the occlusal surface of a posterior tooth

diastema (di-uh-STEE-muh) – space between adjacent teeth of the same arch that have no point of contact

distal (DIS-tul) – farther from the midline

distal surface – the side surface of a tooth that is farther from the midline

embrasure (em-BRAY-zhur) space – triangular spaces that surround the contact area of two adjacent teeth

exfoliation – the loss of the primary teeth

facial – toward the face

facial surface – the surface of the crown on the outer side of the dental arch, nearest to the face

fissure (FIH-shur) – narrow slit that forms deep within a groove during tooth development when enamel fails to fuse along the groove

fossa (FOS-uh) – a small depression located between the marginal ridges on the lingual surfaces of anterior teeth and on the occlusal surfaces of posterior teeth

furcal (FUR-kul) region – the area between two or more roots

furcation (fur-KAY-shun) – place where the root trunk branches off into separate roots

incisal (in-SI-zul) – toward the biting surface of an incisor or canine

incisal edge – the thin, flat incisal surface of an incisor

incisal surface – the biting surface of the incisors and canines

incisor, central – the tooth on either side of the midline at the front of the oral cavity

incisor, lateral – the tooth distal to the central incisors

interproximal space – embrasure space cervical to the contact area, just above the interdental papilla

labial – near the lips

labial surface – the facial surface of the anterior teeth that is near the lips

line angle – the intersection of two tooth surfaces along a line

lingual – near the tongue

lingual surface – the surface of the crown on the inner side on the dental arch that is near the tongue

malocclusion (mal-uh-KLOO-zhun) – a condition in which opposing teeth do not meet in normal occlusal contact

mamelons (MAM-uh-lunz) – three small bumps often present on the incisal surface of a newly erupted incisor

mandibular arch – dental arch of the lower jaw

marginal ridge – mesial and distal edges of the lingual surfaces of incisors and canines

maxillary arch – dental arch of the upper jaw

mesial (MEE-zee-ul) – closer to the midline

mesial surface – the surface of a tooth that is closer to the midline

midline – the imaginary line that splits a dental arch in half between the central incisors

mixed dentition – dentition consisting of both primary and permanent teeth

molar – a posterior tooth characterized by a broad crown, located at the back of the oral cavity

morphology – the anatomical form and structure of a tooth

oblique ridge – triangular ridges of the mesiolingual cusp and distobuccal cusp, which are diagonally across from each other, that meet along the occlusal surface

occlusal (uh-KLOO-zul) – toward the chewing surface of premolars or molars

occlusal surface – the chewing surface of premolars and molars

occlusion (uh-KLOO-zhun) – when the incisal and occlusal surfaces of opposing maxillary and mandibular teeth come together

palatal – near the palate

palatal surface – the lingual surface of the maxillary teeth that is near the palate

permanent dentition – the set of 32 teeth that are ordinarily present through a person's life

pit – pointed depression in the enamel surface caused by faulty enamel calcification deep within a fossa

point angle – the intersection of three tooth surfaces at a point

premolar (bicuspid) – a double-cusp tooth located between canines and molars

primary dentition – the first set of 20 teeth that erupt in a child's oral cavity

proximal – next to, adjacent

proximal surfaces – surfaces adjacent to other teeth

quadrant – the four identical sections of the oral cavity: upper right, upper left, lower left, lower right

sextant – the six parts of the dentition; there are three sextants on each arch

succedaneous (suk-sih-DAY-nee-us) teeth – the teeth that come after, or succeed, the primary teeth

sulcus (SUL-kus) – valley on the occlusal surface of a posterior tooth

supplemental groove – smaller, less distinctive groove that is not located between lobes or other notable features of the tooth

tooth morphology – study of a tooth's shape and structure

transverse ridge – two triangular ridges of cusps on opposite sides of the tooth that join at the depression in the occlusal surface

triangular ridge – a ridge that runs from the cusp tip to the center of the occlusal surface

trifurcated (tri-fur-KAY-tid) – split into three

trifurcation (tri-fur-KAY-shun) – the area where the tooth roots separate into three

Introduction

An understanding of dentition and the ability to identify teeth not only by their location in the oral cavity but also by their appearance is vital to the success of any dental assistant. Being able to accurately identify and number a patient's teeth help make the dental assistant a valued member of the dental team.

Types of Dentition

The complete set of natural teeth in an individual's oral cavity is called a **dentition.** There are three stages of human dentition: primary, mixed, and permanent (Figure 8-1).

Primary

Twenty teeth make up the **primary dentition,** which are the first teeth to emerge in a child's oral cavity. These are the only teeth a child has for about the first 6 years of

his or her life. Primary teeth are also called **deciduous teeth** because, like the leaves of deciduous trees, they eventually fall off the dental arches. Although the primary teeth are eventually lost, they perform important functions in a child's oral cavity. The primary teeth act as placeholders for the permanent teeth, and they help guide the permanent teeth into alignment. If primary teeth are not cared for and are lost before the permanent teeth are ready to replace them, the permanent teeth may not grow into their proper places. Because teeth play a role in pronouncing sounds in speech, primary teeth are essential to a child as he or she learns to talk. Children also need healthy primary teeth to chew food so that they receive adequate nutrition. Deciduous teeth were once called "milk teeth," because they are often much whiter than permanent dentition—something that has prompted many uninformed parents to question a dentist whether something is wrong with his or her child's incoming permanent teeth.

Mixed

Mixed dentition describes the presence of both primary and permanent teeth in a child's oral cavity. Children

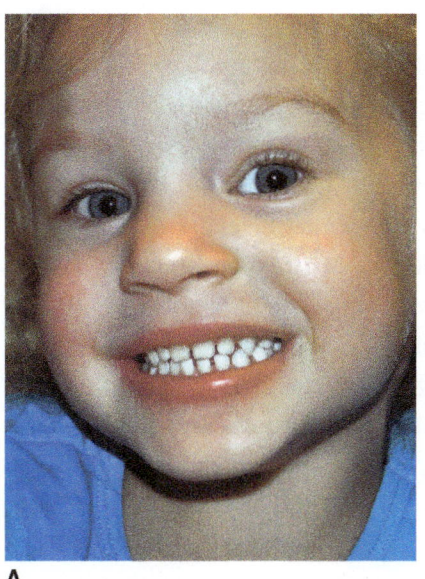 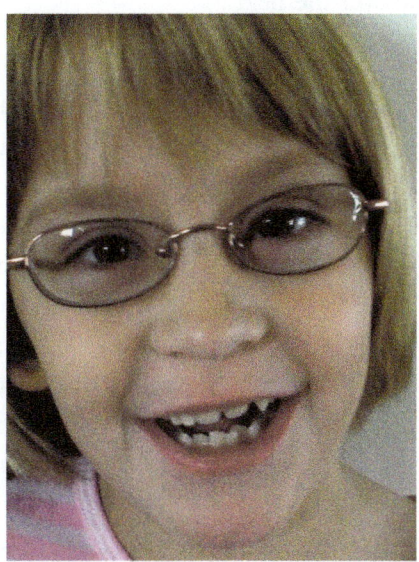 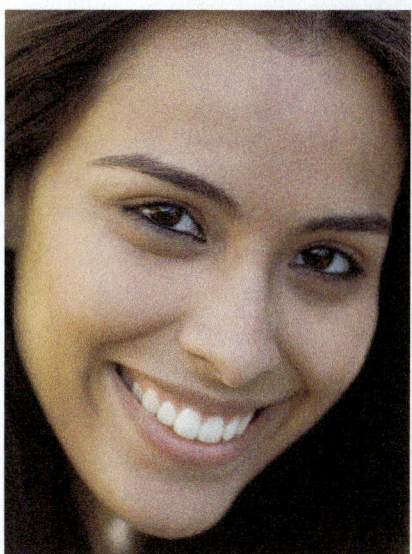

A   **B**   **C**

Figure 8–1 A. Child between the ages of 2 and 3 years old with primary/deciduous dentition. **B.** Child between the ages of 7 and 8 years old with mixed dentition. **C.** Adult with permanent dentition.

have mixed dentition beginning when the first permanent tooth emerges around age 6 years and continuing until the last primary tooth is lost, usually by age 12 years.

Permanent

There are 32 teeth in the **permanent dentition.** The teeth of the permanent dentition are also called **succedaneous teeth** because they replace or succeed (come after) the primary teeth. Technically, the third molars are not succedaneous teeth because they do not replace any of the primary teeth. Unlike primary teeth, permanent teeth do not have replacements. If a permanent tooth is lost, there will be a gap in the dentition.

Exfoliation and Eruption Schedules

Except in rare cases, children are born without any teeth visible in their oral cavity. The primary teeth first start to emerge between age 6 and 8 months. Over the next 2 years or so, all 20 primary teeth emerge, or erupt, into the child's oral cavity from beneath the gingiva, usually beginning with the mandibular central incisor (see Table 8-1). The roots of the primary teeth finish developing a little after the child's third year. Of course, though eruption follows a recognizable pattern, individual differences in children may cause them to experience eruption or exfoliation patterns ahead of or behind the norm. If any concerns arise due to a delay or acceleration of this pattern, they should be addressed by the dentist.

By this time, the crowns of the permanent first molars have finished developing, and crowns of other permanent teeth are well on their way to completion. As the roots of these permanent teeth develop and grow over the next 3 years, until they begin to erupt around age 6 years, the

crowns are pushed into the roots of the primary teeth, triggering resorption of the roots of the primary teeth. This action will eventually lead to the loosening and **exfoliation**, or loss, of the primary teeth.

Around age 6 years, the first permanent teeth erupt into the oral cavity: the first molars, also called the *6-year molars* (see Table 8-2). These teeth erupt distally to the primary second molars, so there is no exfoliation in this case. Shortly after the permanent first molars erupt, the first teeth exfoliated are usually the primary mandibular central incisors, which are, of course, replaced by the permanent mandibular central incisors.

The order for exfoliation of primary teeth and eruption of permanent teeth typically follows this pattern:

- Ages 6 through 9 years: all eight primary incisors are exfoliated and replaced by eight permanent incisors.
- Ages 9 through 12 years: all four canines and eight molars are exfoliated and replaced by four canines and eight *premolars*.
- Age 12 years: the permanent second molars (i.e., 12-year molars) erupt distally to the permanent first molars.
- Ages 17 to 21 years: permanent third molars (sometimes called "wisdom teeth") erupt distally to the second molars.

TABLE 8-1 Order of Primary Tooth Emergence

	ARCH	TOOTH	MONTH
1	Mandibular	Central Incisor	6
2	Mandibular	Lateral Incisor	7
3	Maxillary	Central Incisor	7 1/2
4	Maxillary	Lateral Incisor	9
5	Mandibular	First Molar	12
6	Maxillary	First Molar	14
7	Mandibular	Canine	16
8	Maxillary	Canine	18
9	Mandibular	Second Molar	20
10	Maxillary	Second Molar	24

TABLE 8-2 Order of Permanent Tooth Emergence

	ARCH	TOOTH	YEAR
1*	Mandibular	First Molar	6–7
1*	Maxillary	First Molar	6–7
1*	Mandibular	Central Incisor	6–7
2*	Mandibular	Lateral Incisor	7–8
2*	Maxillary	Central Incisor	7–8
3	Maxillary	Lateral Incisor	8–9
4	Mandibular	Canine	9–10
5*	Maxillary	First Premolar	10–11
5*	Mandibular	First Premolar	10–12
5*	Maxillary	Second Premolar	10–12
6*	Mandibular	Second Premolar	11–12
6*	Maxillary	Canine	11–12
7*	Mandibular	Second Molar	11–13
7*	Maxillary	Second Molar	12–15
8*	Mandibular	Third Molar	17–21
8*	Maxillary	Third Molar	17–21

* Denotes a tie, meaning one tooth or the other might come first.

Typically, by age 12 years, all primary teeth have been replaced by permanent teeth. As mentioned, third molars usually emerge sometime between ages 17 and 21 years; however, individuals may lack some or all of their third molars. In general, roots of the permanent dentition are completed 3 years after the tooth erupts.

Malocclusions and Anomalies

When teeth erupt in the correct positions, the incisal edges and buccal cusp tips follow a uniform curve around the U-shaped dental arches, and the lingual cusp tips follow a curve roughly parallel to it. In addition to the curve of the dental arch, the teeth generally follow two other patterns of curvature: the curve of Spee and the curve of Wilson. The **curve of Spee**, the curve of the teeth in occlusion, is best viewed along the buccal surface, and it follows the cusps from an anterior-to-posterior direction. The curve is convex on the maxillary arch and concave on the mandibular arch. The **curve of Wilson** follows the cusp tips from side-to-side across the posterior of the dental arches. It is convex on the maxillary arch and concave on the mandibular arch.

Proper alignment of teeth is important not only for the spatial relationships between the teeth within each arch but also for the opposing teeth of each arch. When you close your mouth, your mandibular teeth close, or occlude, against your maxillary teeth. Ideal **occlusion** occurs when the incisal and occlusal surfaces of opposing maxillary and mandibular teeth come together in best-fitting contact. In the early 1900s, Edward H. Angle defined this ideal relationship between teeth as class I ideal occlusion. Angle also classified bad (misaligned) occlusal relationships, called **malocclusion** (Figure 8-2). In malocclusion, some (or all) of the opposing teeth do not come into normal occlusal contact. For example, a mandibular molar may be too far lingual so that its occlusal surface does not fully contact the opposing maxillary molar. A mandibular central incisor may erupt so far to the labial side that it overlaps the front of the opposing maxillary incisor.

Sometimes malocclusion occurs because of skeletal relationships that affect how the jaws fit together (e.g., when one jaw protrudes too far past the other), but malocclusion can also result from dental misalignment. The following variations from the ideal alignment cause malocclusion:

- Labioversion: a tooth misaligned toward the labial (applies only to anterior teeth)
- Buccoversion: a tooth misaligned toward the buccal (applies only to posterior teeth)
- Linguoversion: a tooth misaligned toward the lingual
- Torsiversion: a tooth that is twisted along its vertical axis
- Supraversion: a tooth that is overerupted (i.e., supraerupted or extruded) to the point of being abnormally long
- Infraversion: an abnormally short tooth, which can occur if a primary tooth is carried over into permanent dentition or if the cementum of the tooth fuses to the alveolar bone

All of these types of dental malocclusion are a result of improper alignment during tooth eruption. Sometimes misalignment is caused by overcrowded teeth, which push the newly erupted tooth into misalignment; other times teeth may be missing or spaced too far apart. A **diastema** is the space between two adjacent teeth of the same dental arch that do not touch. When a total set of teeth is missing from birth (i.e., congenital), the condition is called *anodontia*. Partial anodontia refers to one or more teeth congenitally missing from a dentition, whereas total anodontia is the complete absence of both primary and permanent dentitions. The third molars are the most commonly missing teeth in the permanent dentition, with maxillary third

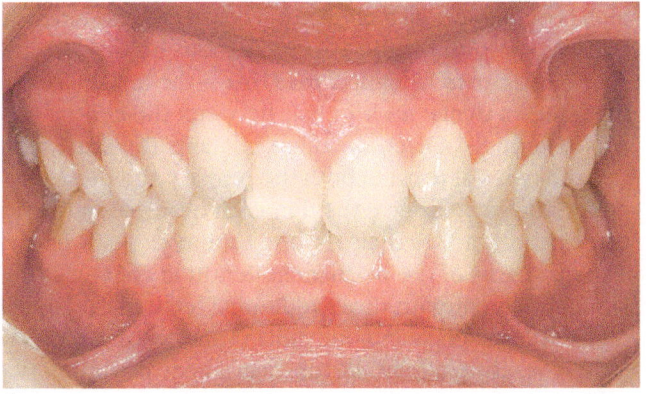
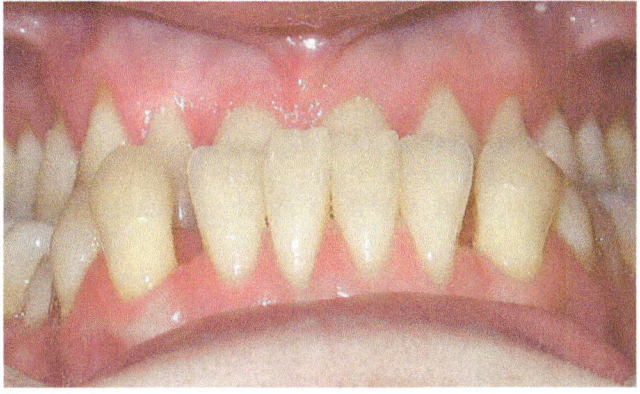

A **B**

Figure 8–2 Malocclusions. **A.** Angle class II center malocclusion. **B.** Angle class III center malocclusion.

Figure 8–3 **A.** Peg lateral. **B.** Marginal ridges on the mesial and distal of the mandibular incisors produce a shovel shape on the lingual surface of the teeth.

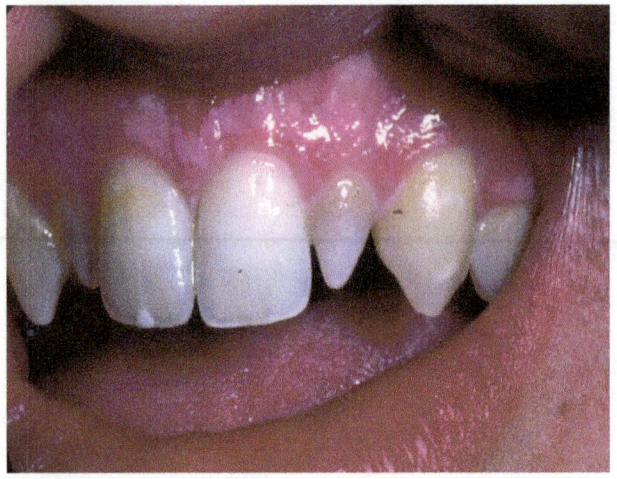
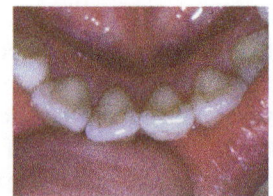
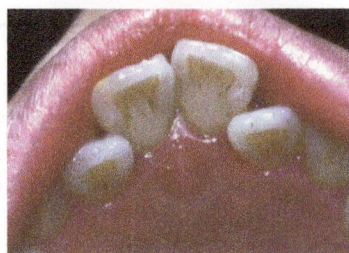

A

B

molars more frequently absent than mandibular third molars. Individuals may also have extra teeth erupt, known as *supernumerary teeth*.

Dental anomalies can also cause malocclusion. In such cases, the tooth may be properly aligned by not properly formed, preventing the opposing teeth from fitting together (Figure 8-3).

- *Peg-shaped lateral incisors* (pegged laterals) are peg- or cone-shaped incisors that occur in nearly 2% of the population. They are broadest near the cervix and taper to a blunt incisal point.
- *Shovel-shaped incisors* have prominent cingula and well-developed marginal ridges.
- *Microdontia* is a condition in which a tooth is normally shaped but abnormally small.
- *Macrodontia* is a condition in which a tooth is normally shaped but abnormally large.
- A single tooth bud may split so that a *twinned tooth* results. The crown of a twinned tooth is twice its normal size, but the tooth shares a single root and a single pulp canal.
- Similarly, a *fused tooth* results when adjacent tooth buds fuse along the dentin so that the crown formed appears to be one crown that is twice its normal width. However, the fused tooth does not share a single root—two roots are fused together with two distinct pulp chambers. (To distinguish between a twinned tooth and a fused tooth, count the twinned or fused tooth as two teeth; there will be one extra tooth on the arch if it is twinned and the normal number if it is fused.)

CHECKPOINTS

8-1 At which ages do each of the dentitions (primary, mixed, permanent) begin?

8-2 Which permanent teeth are usually the first to erupt?

Dental Arches, Quadrants, and Sextants

Teeth are located on both the **maxillary arch** (upper jaw) and the **mandibular arch** (lower jaw).

The upper jaw, or maxilla, is fixed, whereas the lower jaw, the mandible, moves up and down and slightly side to side. The movement of the mandible enables clear speaking as well as food chewing. Although the same number and types of teeth are found on both the maxillary and mandibular arches, there are necessary variances between the arches in the shapes and sizes of the teeth that allow the teeth to meet as the jaws close.

Sometimes groups of teeth are referred to according to their location toward the front or back of the oral cavity. **Anterior** teeth are the teeth at the front of the oral cavity. In both the primary and permanent dentition, the anterior teeth are the central incisors, lateral incisors, and canines of both dental arches. The **posterior** teeth are farthest to the back of the mouth. Primary posterior teeth are the first and second molars of both dental arches. Of the permanent teeth, the first and second premolars and the first, second, and third molars of both dental arches are all considered posterior.

The dentition on the two arches can be divided into four **quadrants** along the **midline**—the imaginary line that splits a dental arch in half between the central incisors (Figure 8-4). Each quadrant contains the same number and types of teeth in both the primary and permanent dentition. There are five teeth in each quadrant in the primary dentition: two incisors, one canine, and two molars. The quadrants of the permanent dentition contain a similar complement with three additional teeth in each quadrant: two premolars and one molar. This makes eight teeth total in each quadrant of the permanent dentition: two incisors, one canine, two premolars, and three molars.

Another way to subdivide the teeth of the dental arches is by **sextants** (six sections) (Figure 8-5). Unlike the

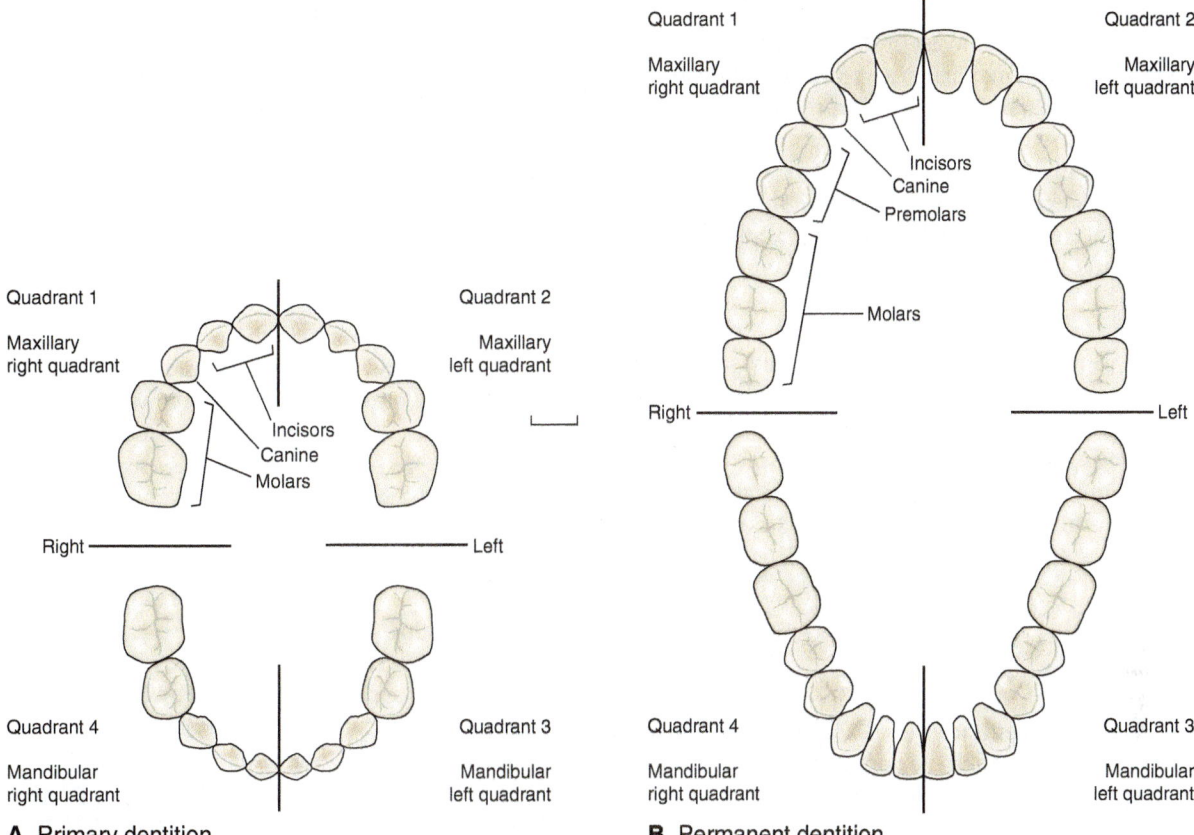

Figure 8–4 Primary dentition (**A**) and permanent dentition (**B**) are divided into four quadrants each.

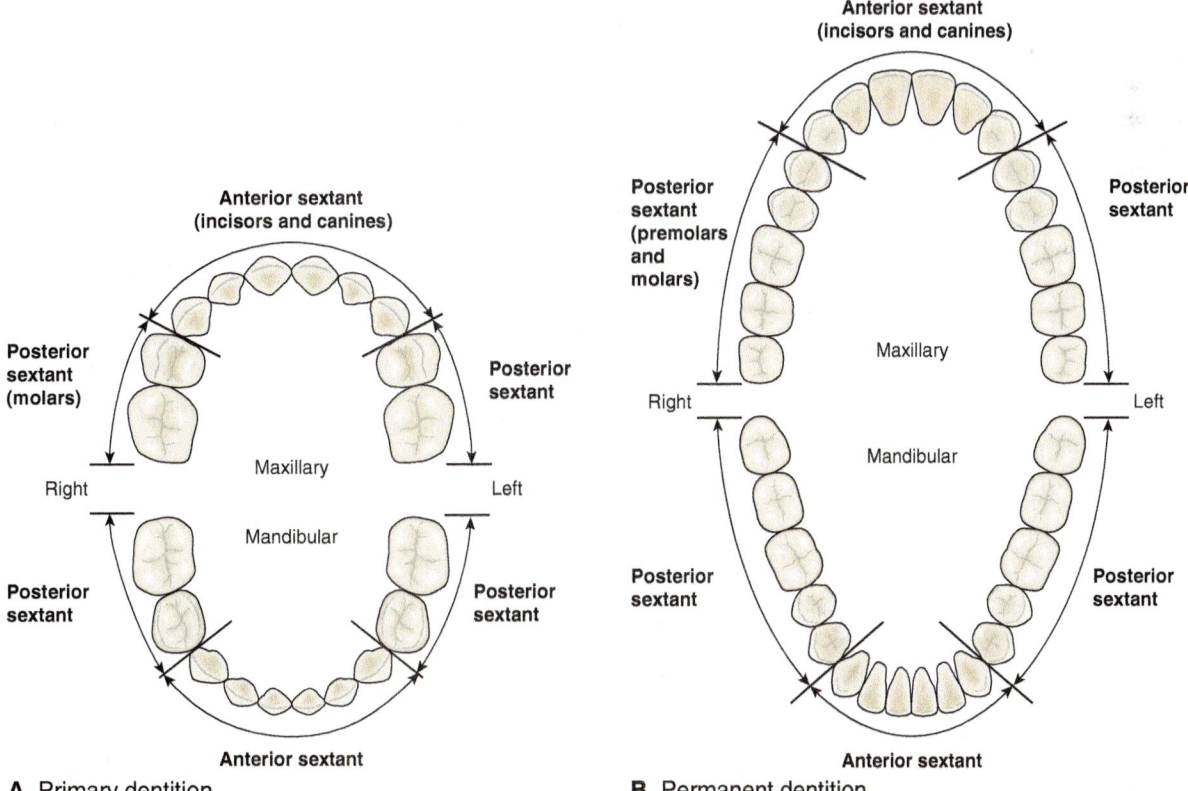

Figure 8–5 Primary dental arches (**A**) and permanent dental arches (**B**) are divided into sextants.

quadrants, however, the number of teeth in each sextant is not even. The sextants consist of the two sets of anterior teeth (mandibular and maxillary) and four sets of posterior teeth (two sets on each dental arch). In the primary dentition this breaks down to six teeth in each of the anterior sextants (the incisors and canines) and two teeth in each of the posterior sextants (only the molars). The permanent dentition has six teeth in each anterior sextant (incisors and canines) and five in each posterior sextant (premolars and molars).

Though these two subdivisions are different, they are both equally valid ways of organizing teeth. Regardless of which subdivision method is used, it allows dentists to stay organized by selecting a specific area to work on instead of arbitrarily choosing a tooth in one region and then moving on to another randomly selected tooth. Plus, there are ramifications in terms of anesthesia—it makes sense to focus on the anesthetized region until all dental work is completed there.

Tooth Classifications and Functions

The four classes of teeth are incisors, canines, premolars, and molars (Figure 8-6). Each type of tooth has special characteristics that aid its function in the oral cavity.

Molars

The primary function of the molars is food chewing, which is why molars have larger chewing surfaces than any of the other teeth on their arch. Molar crowns are shorter than those of other types of teeth because their purpose is grinding food rather than cutting. Molars also play a role in keeping teeth aligned on each arch and supporting the cheeks. There are two molars in each quadrant of the primary dentition and three molars in each quadrant of the permanent dentition.

Premolars

Premolars are found only in the permanent dentition. They replace the first and second molars of the primary dentition. Along with the molars, premolars help with food chewing. They also assist canine teeth in cutting food. Premolars provide an aesthetic function in that they support the cheeks and corners of the oral cavity to prevent sagging.

Canines

The term "canine" is derived from the Latin word for dog. With their sharp biting edges, canines are used to tear or cut food. They support the lips and the muscles around the oral cavity to maintain the facial profile. Because canines of both dental arches are long enough to overlap each other in the oral cavity, they help guide the jaws into proper occlusion, which protects the molars and premolars from wear caused by side-to-side motion while chewing. Canines are commonly used as anchors in dental procedures because of their thick, long roots. In both the primary and permanent dentition, there is only one canine tooth in each quadrant.

Figure 8–6 A. Occlusal view of primary dentition. **B.** Occlusal view of permanent dentition. Both are identified using the Universal Numbering System.

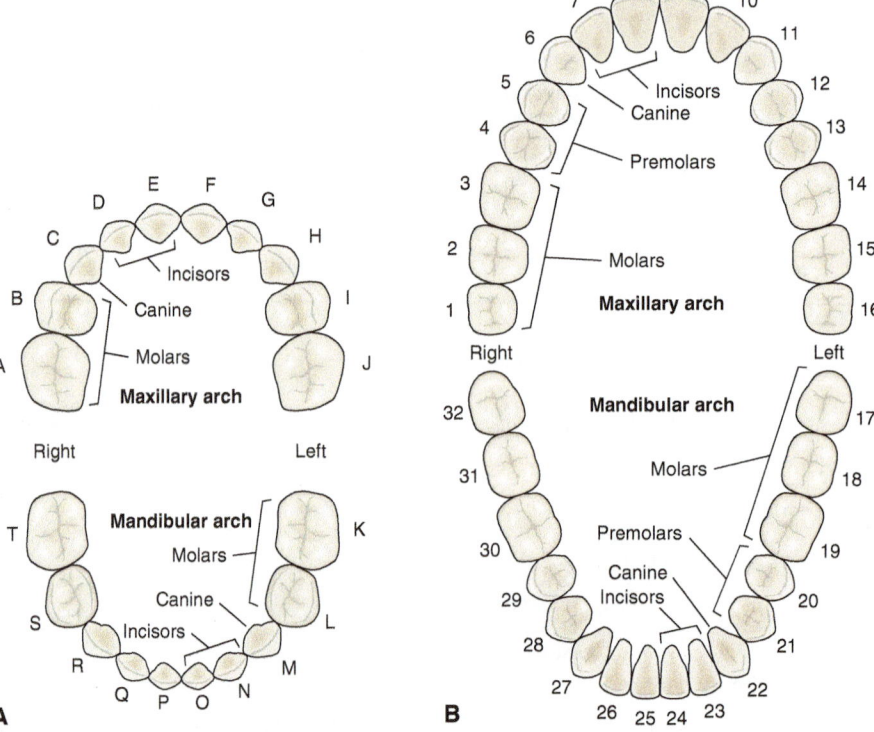

Incisors

Incisors cut food, support the lips, and aid in producing sounds when a person speaks (try pronouncing an "s" or a "t" without them). Incisors cut food with a flat biting surface rather than the more pointed surface of the canines. Even more so than the canines, the incisors are responsible for guiding the mandible into position as it closes. Both the primary and permanent dentition have two incisors in each quadrant.

Tooth Numbering Systems

Dental records are essential to providing care for patients. In order to make records as accurate and efficient as possible, you must be able to describe exactly which teeth need special attention. Imagine how much time it would take if you had to write out a full description of each tooth's location, for example, permanent mandibular right second premolar. Tooth numbering systems were devised as methods of shortened notation. The most common systems of notation are the Universal Numbering System, the International Standards Organization System (ISO), and the Palmer Notation System. (See Chapter 20, Oral Diagnosis and Treatment Planning, for a detailed look at using tooth numbering systems for charting and describing teeth.)

Universal Numbering System

This system begins tooth numbering with the upper right third molar as tooth 1 and counts to the upper left third molar as tooth 16, down to the patient's lower left third molar as tooth 17, and over to the lower right to the third molar as tooth 32 (see Figure 8-6).

Primary dentition for this system uses letters instead of numbers but also starts on the upper right with the second molar as tooth A and counts over to the upper left second molar as tooth J, down to the lower left second molar as tooth K, and over to the lower right second molar as tooth T (see Figure 8-6).

International Standards Organization System

The ISO system, used by the Fédération Dentaire Internationale (FDI), is a two-digit system that uses only numerals 1 through 8 for each digit. The first number indicates the quadrant where the tooth is found, and the second number identifies the individual tooth within that quadrant.

Palmer Notation System

The Palmer Notation System identifies the teeth by quadrant and number. This system is used by some orthodontists and

oral surgeons. With horizontal and vertical lines, it divides the dental chart into four lines of numbers representing the four quadrants of the intraoral cavity. When teeth are charted according to the Palmer method, vertical and horizontal brackets next to the number indicate the quadrant where the tooth is found. Arabic numerals (1–8) are used for permanent dentition, and letters are used for primary (A–E). Numbering in each quadrant begins at the midline (as with the ISO system) and moves to the rear of the oral cavity.

CHECKPOINT

8-3 Which numbering method numbers adult teeth 1 through 32?

Surfaces

The Five Surfaces

Each tooth has five surfaces exposed above the gingiva, and these surfaces are named according to their location in the oral cavity (Figure 8-7). Similar surfaces may have different names depending on the kind of tooth and its location in the oral cavity (e.g., posterior or anterior, maxillary or mandibular). It may be helpful to think about the clinical crown as a cube with five sides exposed and the last side resting on the gingiva.

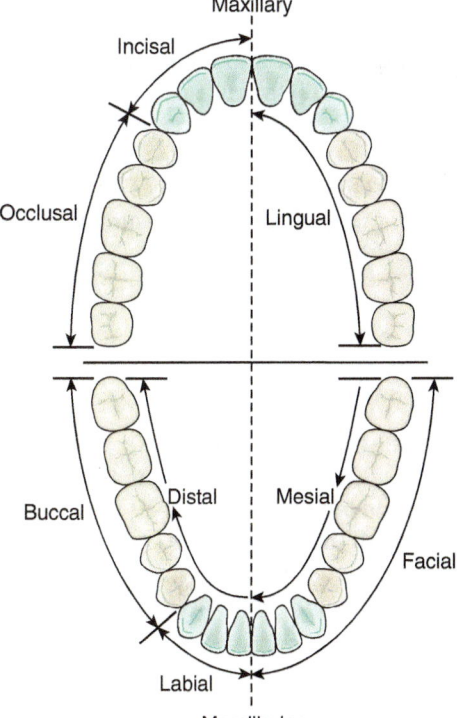

Figure 8–7 Tooth surfaces of the maxillary and mandibular arches. Anterior teeth are noted in blue.

Facial Surface

The **facial surface** of the tooth is the surface on the outer side of the dental arches, toward the face. This is the surface you see when someone flashes a big, toothy grin at you. Both posterior and anterior teeth are considered to have a facial surface.

If you want to refer specifically to the facial surface of *anterior* teeth, you would use the term **labial surface**, that is, near the lips. This term applies only to the canines and incisors. The facial surface of the *posterior* teeth can also be called the **buccal surface**, meaning the surface next to the cheek. This term may only be used to refer to the premolars and molars.

Lingual Surface

The tooth surface on the inner side of the dental arch is called the **lingual surface** because it is closest to the tongue. Although **lingual** applies to the inner surface on both dental arches, the inner surface of the maxillary arch may also be called **palatal**, because it is near the palate.

Incisal and Occlusal—The Biting Surfaces

The biting surfaces of the tooth are known either as **incisal** or **occlusal**. The anterior teeth have an **incisal surface**, which is the edge used for cutting or tearing food. The thin, flat incisal surface of an incisor is sometimes called an **incisal edge**. The **occlusal surface** refers to the surface of the posterior teeth used for chewing or grinding food.

Proximal Surfaces

Proximal surfaces of a tooth are the surfaces adjacent to other teeth. Most teeth will have adjacent teeth at both proximal surfaces, with the exceptions of the second molars in primary dentition and the third molars in permanent dentition. The proximal surfaces of the teeth can be specified according to whether the surface is on the side nearer to or farther from the midline:

- The **mesial surface** is the proximal surface of the tooth that is nearer to the midline.
- The **distal surface** is the proximal surface more distant from the midline.

Typically the distal surface of one tooth contacts the mesial surface of the adjacent tooth. There are two notable exceptions: the central incisors meet at their mesial surfaces, and there are no teeth that contact the distal surface of the third molars. The only points where two mesial surfaces meet are between teeth 8 and 9, and between teeth 24 and 25.

Contours

Each surface of a tooth has some degree of contour, or curvature, so that food pieces are guided away from the

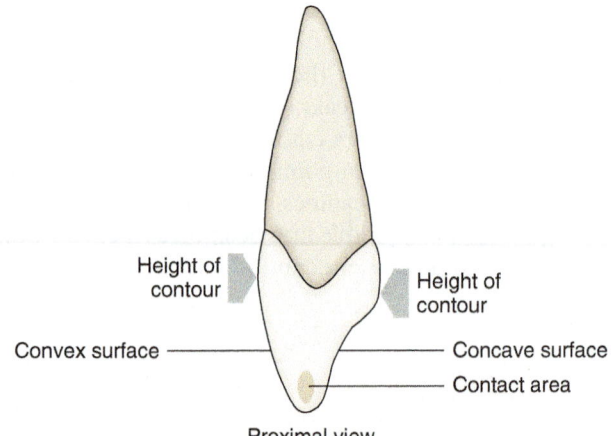

Height of contour

Height of contour

Convex surface

Concave surface

Contact area

Proximal view

Figure 8–8 Height of contour and contact area are shown on a permanent anterior tooth.

gingiva and toward the tongue and palate. These contours also promote self-cleaning of the teeth because the inner surface of the cheeks and lips rub across the facial surface contours of the teeth, and the tongue rubs across the lingual surface contours. Contours of the tooth surfaces are usually convex or concave, and sometimes a surface has a little of both. **Convex** surfaces curve outward, and **concave** surfaces curve inward.

The height of contour (also called the *crest of curvature*) is the point of greatest convexity from the root axis line (Figure 8-8)—the imaginary line that runs vertically from the apex to roughly the center of the cervix, dividing the root into mesial/distal halves and facial/lingual halves. On the facial and lingual surfaces of a tooth, the height of contour is easiest to see when viewing the tooth crown from the mesial or distal perspective. The height of contour is typically located on

- The facial surface of all crowns near the cervical third
- The lingual surface of the anterior teeth at the cervical third (on the cingulum)
- The lingual surface of the posterior teeth in the middle third

Contacts

The heights of contour on the mesial and distal surfaces of the crowns are the same as the contact areas of the teeth, in normal alignment. **Contact areas** are the places where the proximal surfaces of adjacent teeth touch (this applies only to adjacent teeth of the same arch). Contact areas begin as *contact points* on teeth that have just erupted. The contact point flattens into a contact area as the adjacent teeth rub together over time. Because teeth taper somewhat near the cervix, a contact area never occurs in the cervical third of the crown. Contact areas help keep teeth in place on the dental arches and protect the interdental papillae

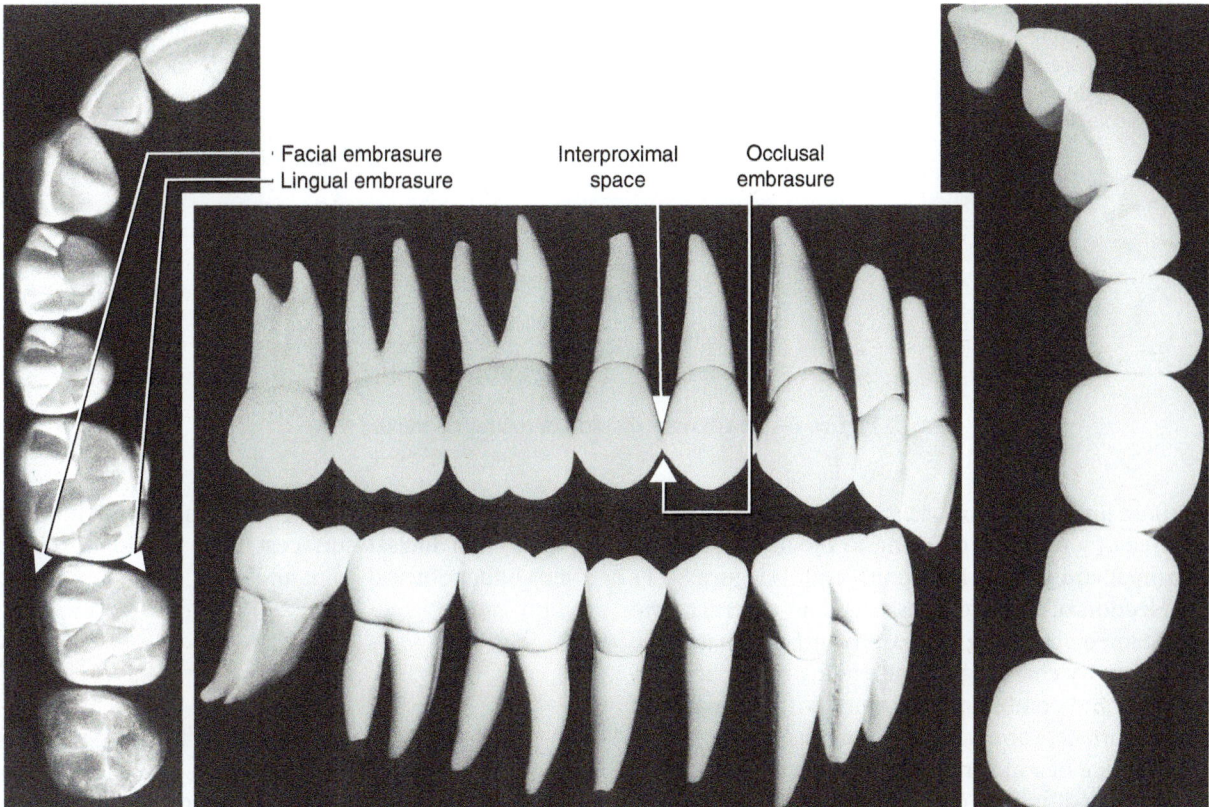

Facial embrasure
Lingual embrasure
Interproximal space
Occlusal embrasure

Figure 8–9 Embrasure and interproximal spaces. Photographs of large plastic tooth models show the contact points between teeth and the embrasure and interproximal spaces.

(gingiva between adjacent teeth) during food chewing. If teeth are not properly aligned on the dental arches, there may be instances of adjacent teeth that do not contact. The space between adjacent teeth that have no point of contact is called a *diastema*.

Embrasures

Embrasure spaces are the triangular spaces that surround the contact area of two adjacent teeth (Figure 8-9). There are four embrasure spaces, each of which narrow closest to the contact area and widen in the facial, lingual, occlusal or incisal, and cervical directions. The embrasure space cervical to the contact area, just above the interdental papilla, is called the **interproximal space.** The facial embrasure space tends to be smaller than the lingual embrasure because the facial side of most teeth is wider than the lingual.

CHECKPOINTS

8-4 What is the difference between the incisal surface and the occlusal surface?

8-5 What is the relationship between the height of contour and a contact area?

Divisions

In addition to being able to specify a tooth's location in the oral cavity, you will also need to refer to locations on the tooth itself as you learn about specific anatomic features of the tooth. For example, if you are looking at the ridges on a molar, you may want to refer to a ridge in a particular area of the tooth's surface. By considering the surfaces of the teeth in terms of divisions into horizontal and vertical thirds, you can more precisely refer to areas of the tooth (Figure 8-10).

Horizontal lines can divide the facial, lingual, mesial, or distal surface of the crown into thirds: cervical, middle, and occlusal (or incisal). The root of the tooth can also be divided by horizontal lines into cervical, middle, and apical thirds.

From the facial or lingual surface, the crown or root can be divided by vertical lines into mesial, middle, and distal thirds. Vertical lines can divide the mesial or distal surface (proximal surfaces) of the crown or root into facial (labial or buccal), middle, and lingual thirds.

Line Angles and Point Angles

Imagine a grid of horizontal and vertical lines overlaying the facial, lingual, mesial, or distal surface of the tooth.

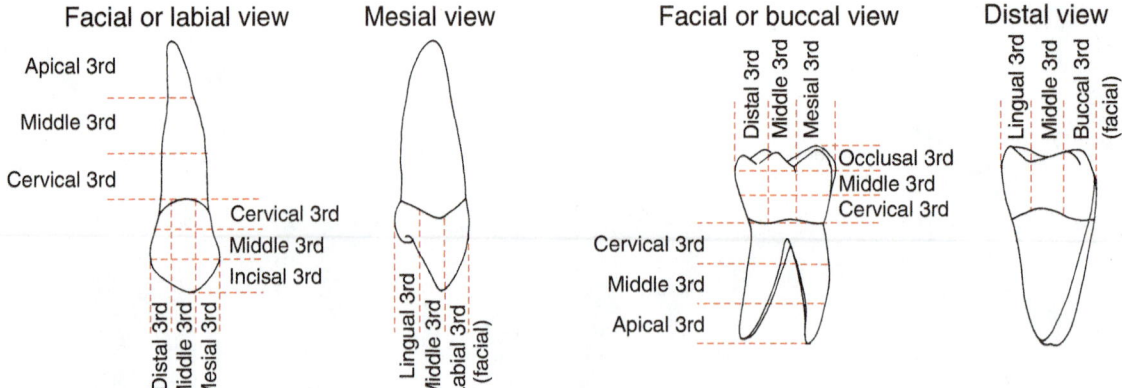

Figure 8–10 Arbitrary division of teeth into thirds.

Each of these lines represents a surface. You can describe a specific area of a tooth by referring to the intersection of the horizontal and vertical lines on that grid (Figure 8-11). The intersection of the two lines, called an external **line angle**, is named according to the two surfaces that those lines represent by changing the "al" ending of the first surface to an "o" and combining that word with the name of the second surface. For example, if you imagine a grid on the facial surface of a molar crown, you would refer to the line angle of the distal and cervical thirds as *distocervical*. Some other possible names of line angles from other surfaces are mesioincisal, linguo-occlusal, and buccocervical. Additionally, "middle third" is sometimes used as a reference point, but it is more common to hear "middle toward incisal edge" or "middle toward gingival margin" to specify a region. Those terms, along with "midline" or "long axis of the tooth," are useful when attempting to describe a particular location in space.

You can also refer to the intersection of three tooth surfaces at a point. This intersection is known as a **point angle** (see Figure 8-11). In this case, you would visualize a three-dimensional grid over the surface of a tooth (like a cube). For example, the point at which the mesial, lingual, and incisal surfaces meet would be called the "mesiolinguoincisal point angle."

Anatomical Structures and Landmarks

Tooth morphology is the study of a tooth's shape and structure. As you learned in Chapter 7, a tooth consists of a crown and a root. Although variations occur among the surface features of each tooth, and particularly among teeth of different individuals, every tooth has certain features of the crown and root in common.

Features of the Crown

The anatomic crown is the entire enamel-covered part of the tooth, some of which is below the gingiva, and the clinical crown is the portion of the crown that is visible in the oral cavity. For the purpose of this discussion, *crown* refers to the anatomic crown, although you will only be able to see these features on the clinical crown of a patient's tooth.

Cusps and Ridges

The peaks on the incisal surfaces of canines and the occlusal surfaces of premolars and molars are called **cusps.** Canine teeth may be referred to as *cuspids*, because they have only one cusp. Premolars are called **bicuspids**, although some have more than two cusps. Cusps are named for where they are located on the tooth. On a premolar with two cusps, the cusps are named for the tooth surface nearest each cusp: buccal and lingual. When a tooth has three or more cusps, the cusps are named according to the line angle of the closest corner: mesiobuccal, mesiolingual, distobuccal, and distolingual.

Four cusp ridges meet at the cusp tip—that is, the peak of the cusp—to form a rounded, four-sided pyramid (Figure 8-12). Three of these cusp ridges are named according to the tooth surface they extend toward: mesial,

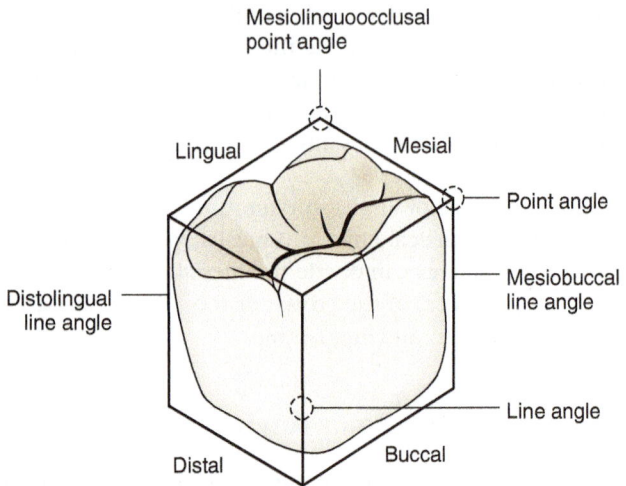

Figure 8–11 Line and point angles.

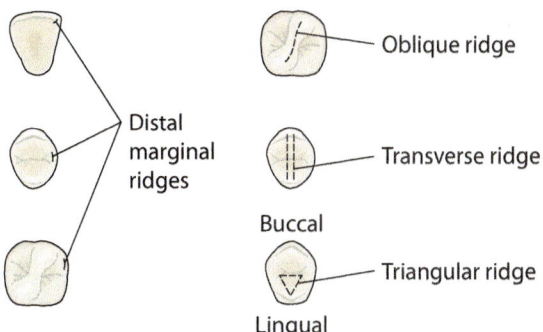

Figure 8–12 Examples of marginal, oblique, transverse, and triangular ridges.

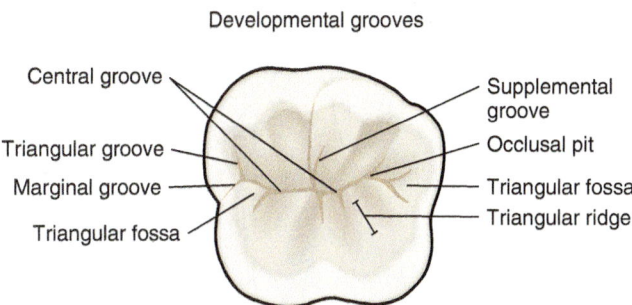

Figure 8–13 The labial and lingual view of cusp tips, slopes, ridges, fossae, and cingulum of a maxillary and mandibular canine.

distal, and facial (labial or buccal). The fourth cusp ridge is the triangular ridge. All major cusps of posterior teeth each have a **triangular ridge** that runs from the cusp tip to the center of the occlusal surface. The triangular ridges of cusps on opposite sides of the tooth join at the depression in the occlusal surface to form the **transverse ridge**. An **oblique ridge** consists of the meeting of the triangular ridges of the mesiolingual cusp and distobuccal cusp, which are diagonally across from each other. Oblique ridges are found only on maxillary molars.

Cusp ridges on the mesial and distal surfaces are also called *cusp slopes*. When cusps are viewed from the facial or lingual perspective, these slopes form an angle where they meet at the cusp tip. The sharpness or roundedness of the cusp angle can be used to distinguish between types of teeth. The areas where the cusp slopes meet the proximal surfaces are sometimes called the *shoulders* of the teeth, another feature that can be used in tooth identification.

Ridges of the facial surface of the teeth are less distinct than those of the lingual surface. The buccal ridge runs from the cervix to the occlusal surface (i.e., cervico-occlusally) along the vertical center of the premolar buccal (facial) surface. First premolars have a better-defined buccal ridge than second premolars. Canines have a similar ridge that runs cervicoincisally from the cusp tip along the labial (facial) surface—the labial ridge. A cervical ridge runs mesiodistally across the facial surface of all primary teeth as well as the permanent molars. This ridge is located in the cervical third of the buccal surface of the molar crown. The cervical ridge tends to be a pronounced bulge on primary molars but is fairly subtle on permanent molars.

A small bump called a **cingulum** (cingula is plural) is located on the lingual surface of the anterior teeth (i.e., canines and incisors), near the cervical area of the crown. **Marginal ridges** are the mesial and distal edges of the lingual surfaces of incisors and canines. These ridges angle toward the cingulum.

Incisors commonly have three small bumps called **mamelons** on their incisal surface when they first erupt. These mamelons form during the development of the facial surface. Mamelons usually wear down over time from contact between opposing incisors.

Grooves and Depressions

The occlusal surface of each posterior tooth has a valley, or **sulcus**, surrounded by the peaks of the cusps. Within the sulcus are multiple grooves in which the cusp ridges converge. These grooves allow food particles to be carried toward the tongue or cheeks when chewing.

Major features of the tooth or lobes on the occlusal surface are separated by distinct linear depressions formed while the tooth was developing, called **developmental grooves** (Figure 8-13). These grooves are named according to where they are located. The central developmental groove, or **central groove**, runs mesiodistally along the buccolingual center of the sulcus. Developmental grooves also run from the middle of the central groove to the buccal and lingual surfaces (called the *buccal* and *lingual grooves*, respectively), separating the mesial and distal cusps. Fossa developmental grooves branch off toward the corners of the tooth at the mesial and distal ends of the central groove and are identified according to which corner they point toward; for example, a fossa groove that points toward the distolingual corner of the tooth would be called the "distolingual fossa groove."

Supplemental grooves are smaller and less distinct than developmental grooves and are not located between lobes or other notable features of the tooth. When enamel fails to fuse along a groove during tooth development, a narrow slit called a **fissure** forms deep within the groove. Fissures are likely spots for dental caries to begin, and they can occur within any of the grooves.

Small depressions called **fossae** (fossa is singular) are located between the marginal ridges on the lingual surfaces of anterior teeth and on the occlusal surfaces of posterior teeth (see Figure 8-13). Faulty enamel calcification deep within a fossa leads to pit formation. **Pits** are pointed depressions in the enamel surface (see Figure 8-13).

Features of the Root

The cervix, or neck, of the tooth is the tapered area where the crown and root meet. The anatomic root is the entire cementum-covered part of the tooth. The tip of the root is called the **apex**, and the **apical foramen** is the small

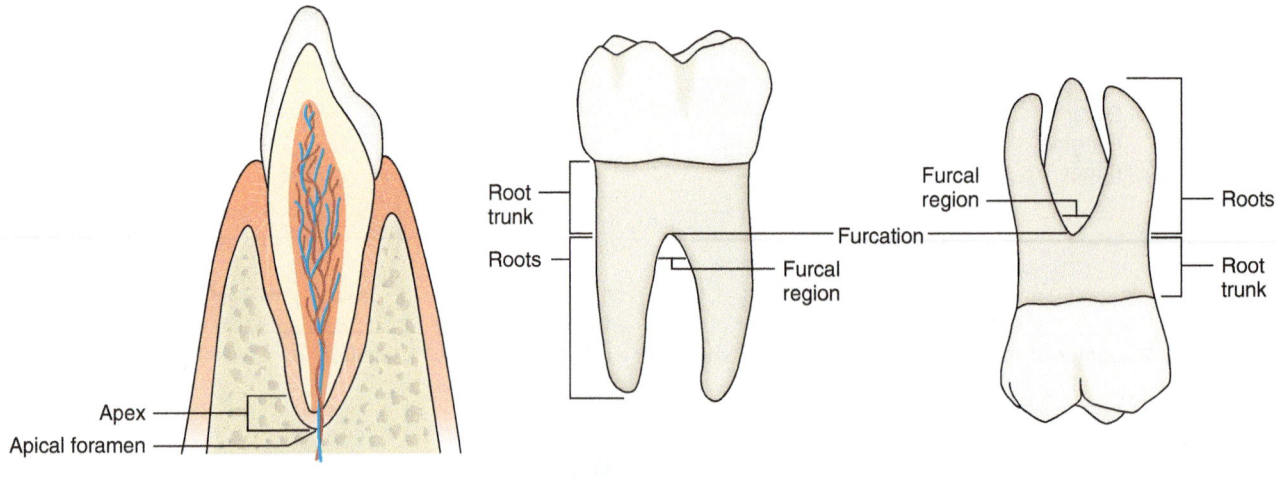

A. Apex and apical foramen **B.** Bifurcation **C.** Trifurcation

Figure 8-14 Teeth roots. **A.** The apex and apical foramen. **B.** Bifurcated roots. **C.** Trifurcated roots.

opening at the apex where nerves and blood vessels enter the root to connect with the tooth pulp (Figure 18-14A).

Teeth with two or more roots have a root trunk, or trunk base, near the cementoenamel junction before the root splits. The place where the root trunk branches off into separate roots is the **furcation**. If a tooth has two roots, the division is called a **bifurcation** (Figure 8-14B); the division into three roots is a **trifurcation** (Figure 8-14C). The **furcal region** is the area between two or more roots.

CHECKPOINTS

8-6 What four features are visible on the occlusal surface of a patient's tooth?

8-7 What is the difference between developmental and supplemental grooves?

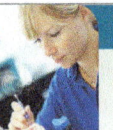

Voice of Experience

Knowing the anatomy and characteristics of each kind of tooth is very important for tooth identification, particularly when you are charting from radiographs or assisting with a dental exam. If an individual is missing teeth or if teeth have shifted, you will need to be familiar enough with what each tooth looks like to determine which teeth are present and which are missing. For example, the number of cusps and roots on a tooth can help you determine whether a tooth is a second premolar or a first molar.

The Primary Dentition

Twenty teeth make up the primary dentition: ten on each arch, five in each quadrant. Each quadrant consists of a central incisor, a lateral incisor, a canine, a first molar, and a second molar—there are no premolars in the primary dentition. Several characteristics differentiate primary dentition from permanent:

- Each primary tooth is smaller than its permanent counterpart (e.g., primary maxillary canines are smaller than permanent maxillary canines).
- Healthy primary teeth are whiter than healthy permanent teeth.
- Pulp cavities of primary teeth are larger in proportion to the size of the teeth than pulp cavities of permanent teeth.
- Primary teeth are more prone to wear (attrition) and decay because layers of enamel and dentin are thinner and the teeth are less mineralized.
- Roots of primary teeth are longer in proportion to the crown size than those of permanent teeth.
- Roots of primary molars are spread wider than their crowns to accommodate the permanent teeth as they move into position before eruption.

Maxillary Central Incisors

Primary maxillary central incisors (Figure 8-15) are the only incisor crowns of either dentition with a greater mesiodistal length than incisocervical length (i.e., the crown is wider than it is tall). The labial surfaces of maxillary central incisors are smooth, with no ridges. The incisal edges are also smooth and lack mamelons. From the labial perspective, distal surfaces are more convex than the mesial.

The lingual surfaces of the crowns narrow toward the gingiva. The cingula of primary maxillary central incisors tend to be larger relative to crown size than the cingula of other teeth. Because the cingula are fairly large, lingual fossae are found only in the incisal or middle thirds. Marginal ridges of a maxillary central incisor are usually well-defined, and in some cases are so prominent that the incisor resembles a shovel.

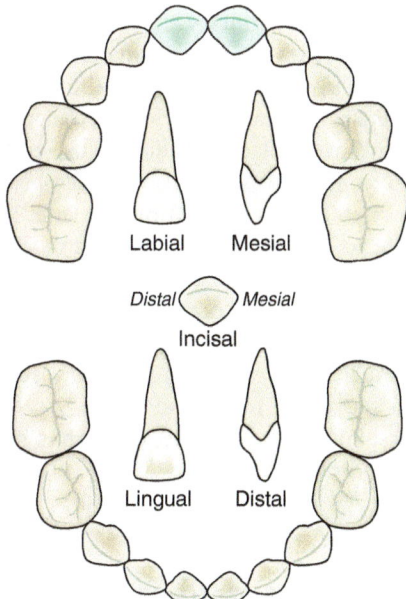

Primary maxillary central incisors

Figure 8–15 Primary/deciduous dentition with maxillary central incisors noted in blue.

Maxillary Lateral Incisors

The crown shape of a primary maxillary lateral incisor (Figure 8-16) is much like that of the maxillary central incisor, except that it is less symmetrical. The maxillary lateral incisor is proportionally narrower than the maxillary central incisor: The incisocervical distance is greater than the mesiodistal. Lateral incisors have a more rounded angle on the distoincisal edge than do central incisors. Like the max-

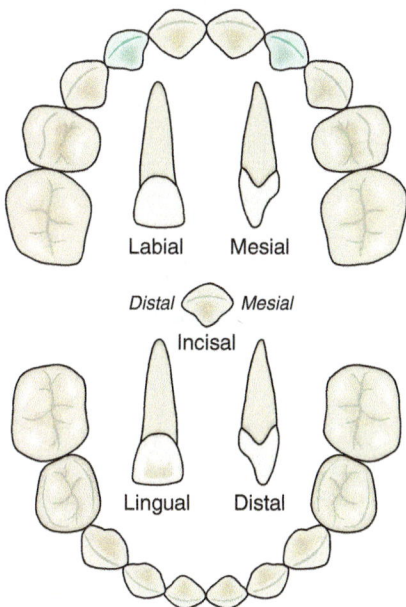

Primary maxillary lateral incisors

Figure 8–16 Primary/deciduous dentition with maxillary lateral incisors noted in blue.

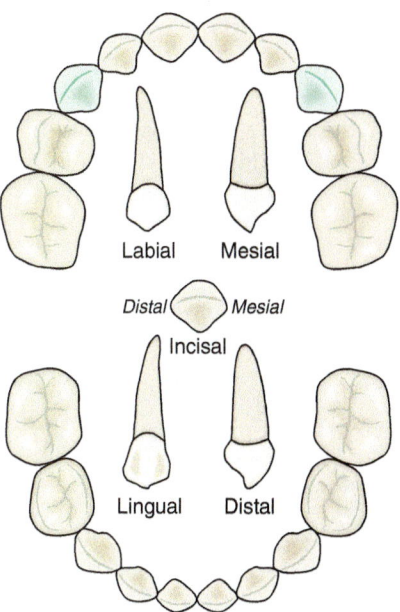

Primary maxillary canines

Figure 8–17 Primary/deciduous dentition with maxillary canines/cupids noted in blue.

illary central incisors, however, the distal surface of the maxillary lateral is more convex than the mesial surface.

Maxillary Canines

Maxillary canine (Figure 8-17) crowns are nearly as long as they are wide. The facial surface of the maxillary canine crown tapers at the cervix more so than on the mandibular canines. The mesial and distal surfaces are convex. Cusp ridges are often sharply angled with a distinctly pointed cusp tip, giving the facial surface of the maxillary canine a pentagon shape. Maxillary canines have longer mesial cusp ridges than distal cusp ridges, which is a unique characteristic. Another unique aspect of maxillary canines is that their mesial and distal contact areas are near the cervicoincisal center of the crowns. Primary canines are thicker than incisors in the cervical third of the crown. Roots of maxillary canines are the longest of the primary teeth.

Maxillary First Molars

Crowns of the first molars of both dental arches are wider mesiodistally than the permanent first premolars that replace them. Primary maxillary first molars (Figure 8-18) look somewhat like their replacement first premolars. The maxillary first molars generally have four cusps, two of which are more distinct: the mesiobuccal and mesiolingual cusps. The distobuccal and distolingual cusps tend to blend in with the marginal ridges along the distal surface. The three-cusp type of first molar lacks a distobuccal cusp. The mesiobuccal cusp of the maxillary first molar is the longest and the second sharpest; the mesiolingual cusp is

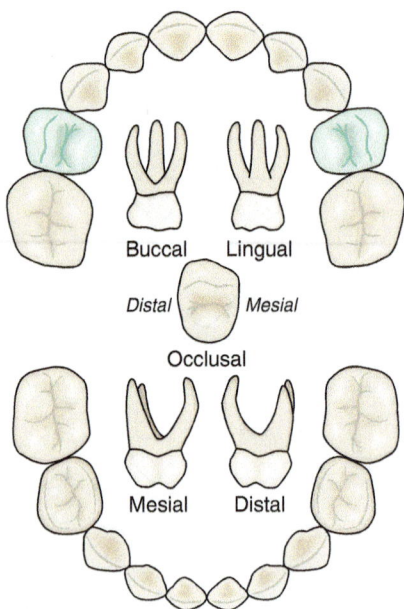

Primary maxillary first molars

Figure 8–18 Primary/deciduous dentition with maxillary first molars noted in blue.

the sharpest and the second longest. Maxillary first molars have thin, widely spread, trifurcated roots with mesiobuccal, distobuccal, and palatal portions. The root trunk is short because the trifurcation is near the cervix.

Maxillary Second Molars

There are three four-cusp and three three-cusp types of primary maxillary second molars (Figure 8-19). Maxillary

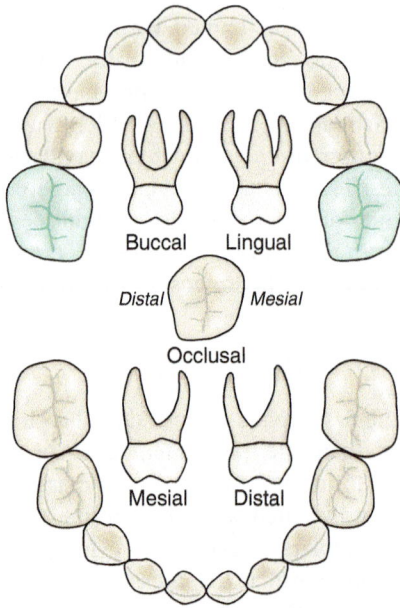

Primary maxillary second molars

Figure 8–19 Primary/deciduous dentition with maxillary second molars noted in blue.

second molars of the primary dentition look very much like a smaller version of the permanent maxillary first molars, which erupt just distally. Even the cusp ridges and fossae of primary second molars are similar to those of the permanent first molar, including a cusp of Carabelli in some instances. From a proximal view, the crowns of the maxillary second molars taper from the large bulge of the cervical ridge to the smaller occlusal surface. The crown also narrows from mesial to distal when viewed from an occlusal perspective. Both maxillary and mandibular second molars are wider mesiodistally than their permanent second premolar replacements. Maxillary second molar roots have a short root trunk and are trifurcated. Like the maxillary first molar, the second molar has mesiobuccal, distobuccal, and palatal roots.

Mandibular Central Incisors

Mandibular central incisors (Figure 8-20), like their maxillary counterparts, have a smooth labial surface. Their lingual surface has a cingulum and small fossae. Marginal ridges of the mandibular central incisors are less distinct than on the maxillary central incisors.

Mandibular Lateral Incisors

Crowns of primary mandibular lateral incisors (Figure 8-21) are slightly larger than those of mandibular central incisors, which is the opposite size order of the maxillary incisors. The shapes of the lateral incisors are less symmetrical overall than the central incisors. There are a cingulum and fossae on the lingual surface of the primary mandibular lateral incisor, but the marginal ridges are faint.

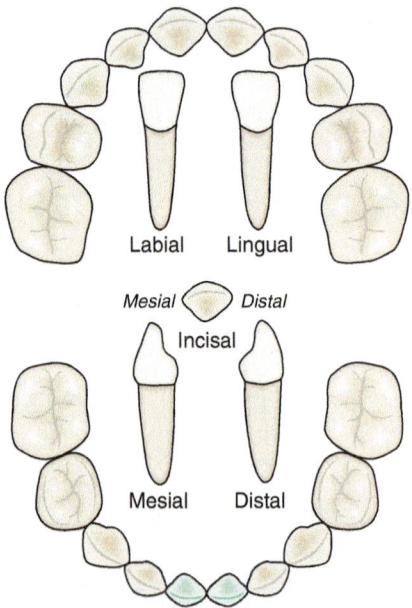

Primary mandibular central incisors

Figure 8–20 Primary/deciduous dentition with mandibular central incisors noted in blue.

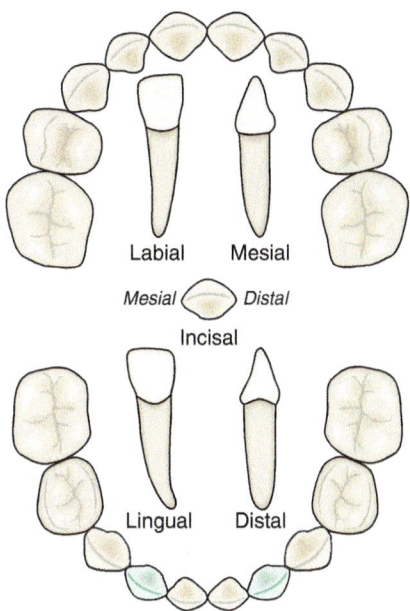

Primary mandibular lateral incisors

Figure 8–21 Primary/deciduous dentition with mandibular lateral incisors noted in blue.

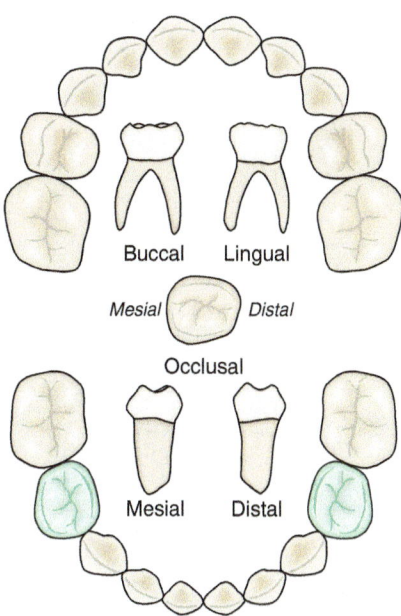

Primary mandibular first molars

Figure 8–23 Primary/deciduous dentition with mandibular first molars noted in blue.

Mandibular Canines

Primary mandibular canines (Figure 8-22) are longer than they are wide. Cusp tips of mandibular canines are pointed like maxillary canines, but the cusp ridges are less angled. Cusp slopes are longer on the distal side than on the mesial

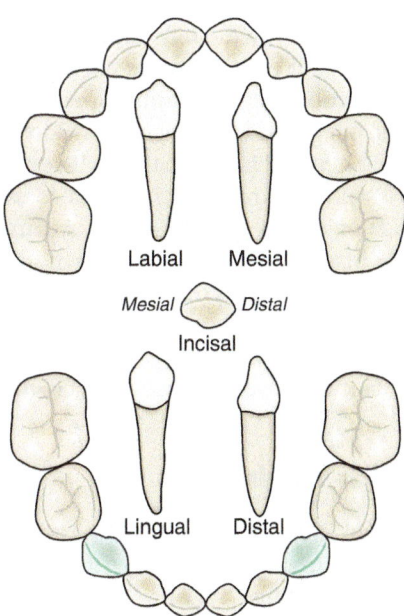

Primary mandibular canines

Figure 8–22 Primary/deciduous dentition with mandibular canines/cuspids noted in blue.

side. From an incisal view of mandibular canine crowns, the cingula tend to be either centered or slightly distal of center.

Mandibular First Molars

Mandibular first molars (Figure 8-23) of the primary dentition have a unique shape: They are unlike any of the primary or permanent molars or the premolars. The first molar has four cusps, but the cusps may be difficult to distinguish. The marginal ridge on the mesial surface may be the most unique aspect of the mandibular first molars. This mesial marginal ridge is overdeveloped to the point of resembling a cusp; it is positioned nearer to the occlusal surface than the smaller distal marginal ridge. The mesiobuccal cusp is the largest cusp overall, in both height and width. The occlusal outline of the crown is wider mesiodistally than buccolingually, giving it an oblong or rectangle shape. Unlike roots of the primary maxillary molars, the mandibular first molars are only bifurcated, with widely spread mesial and distal portions.

Mandibular Second Molars

Like maxillary second molars, mandibular second molars (Figure 8-24) resemble the permanent first molars of their respective arch. They share a similar shape as well as similar positioning of cusp ridges and fossae. Mandibular second molars have five cusps: mesiobuccal, distobuccal, distal, mesiolingual, and distolingual. The three buccal cusps are roughly the same size, and they are all slightly

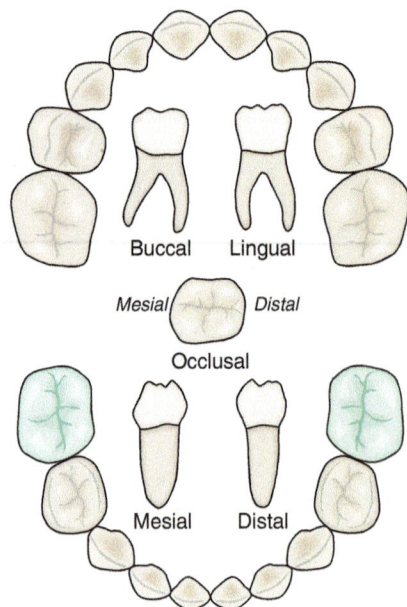

Buccal Lingual

Mesial Distal

Occlusal

Mesial Distal

Primary mandibular second molars

Figure 8–24 Primary/deciduous dentition with mandibular second molars noted in blue.

larger than the two lingual cusps. The cervical ridges of the mesial surface are more prominent on the second molars than on the first molars of the same arch. Primary mandibular second molars have bifurcated mesial and distal roots.

CHECKPOINTS

8-8 What are five characteristics of the primary dentition?

8-9 Which primary teeth typically have four cusps? Which have five cusps?

The Permanent Dentition

The permanent dentition has a total of 32 teeth: 16 teeth on each arch and 8 in each quadrant. Each quadrant consists of a central incisor, a lateral incisor, a canine, a first premolar, a second premolar, a first molar, a second molar, and a third molar.

Maxillary Central Incisors

Maxillary central incisors (Figure 8-25) have the longest crown of any of the teeth and the widest crown of all the incisors. The labial surface of the crown is fairly flat and symmetrical, and it is usually longer than it is wide. The cervical third is the narrowest part of the crown

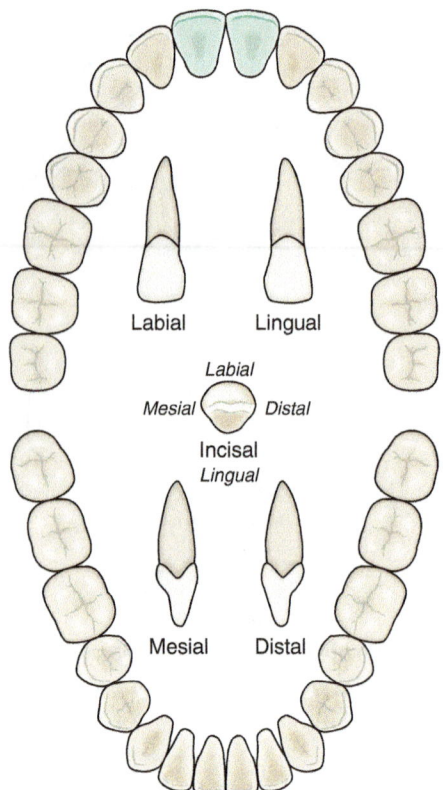

Labial Lingual

Labial

Mesial Distal

Incisal

Lingual

Mesial Distal

Maxillary central incisors

Figure 8–25 Permanent dentition with the maxillary central incisors noted in blue.

(mesiodistally), and the incisal third is the broadest. In most cases, the mesioincisal angle of the crown is almost a right angle. The root of a maxillary central incisor is nearly the same length as the crown (only slightly longer), making this the shortest root relative to the crown size. Maxillary central incisor roots resemble blunt-tipped cones: They are thick near the cervix and narrow quickly toward the tip.

The maxillary central incisor has a well-developed cingulum located distally off-center, and the lingual fossa is large. The marginal ridge on the mesial side is longer than the one on the distal side. Mamelons are frequently found on the incisal surfaces of newly erupted maxillary central incisors, but they usually wear away by adulthood. From the incisal view, the maxillary central incisor has a triangular shape because of its relatively flat face and its distinctly curved cingulum.

Maxillary Lateral Incisors

Maxillary lateral incisors (Figure 8-26) are much smaller than the central incisors, but they may be larger than either of the mandibular incisors. There is a great deal of variation in the shape of the maxillary lateral incisor from one individual to another: They may look somewhat like the maxillary central incisor; they may be asymmetrical; or they might have a peg shape. In some individuals,

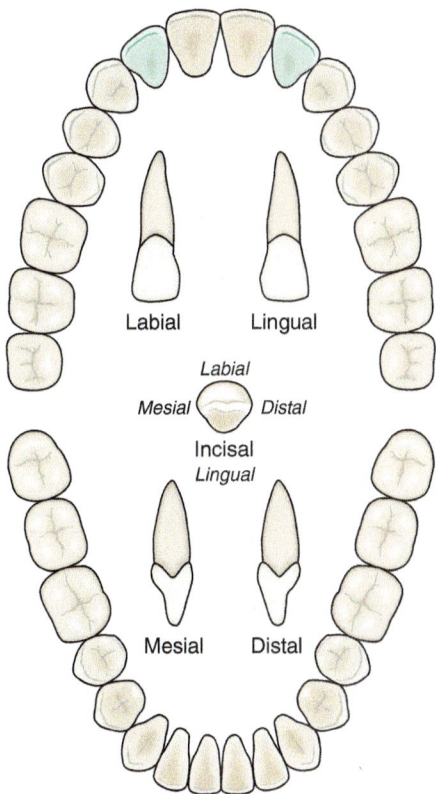

Maxillary lateral incisors

Figure 8–26 Permanent dentition with the maxillary lateral incisors noted in blue.

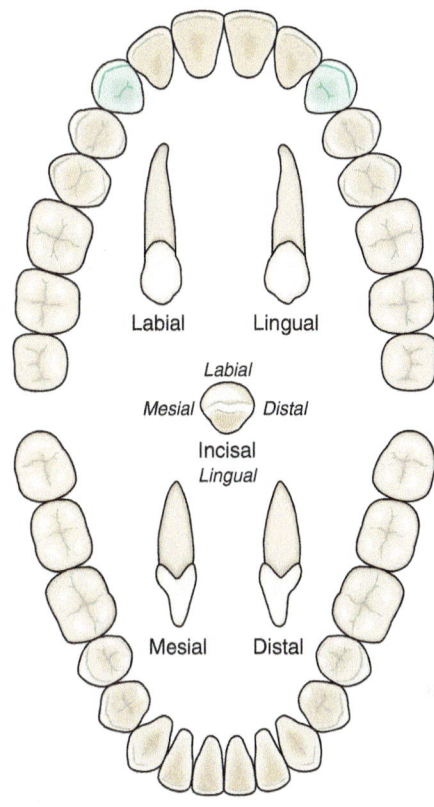

Maxillary canines

Figure 8–27 Permanent dentition with the maxillary canines/cuspids noted in blue.

the maxillary lateral incisors may not even develop. The labial surfaces of the maxillary lateral incisors tend to be more convex than the maxillary central incisors. The root of the maxillary lateral incisor is longer and thinner than that of the maxillary central, and the apical third of the root has a slight distal bend.

The incisal edge of the maxillary lateral incisor slopes toward the cervix from the mesial side to the distal side, giving it a longer mesial marginal ridge than distal (like the maxillary central incisor). The distal marginal ridge of the maxillary lateral incisor curves more so than the mesial marginal ridge, which is nearly straight.

Maxillary Canines/Cuspids

Maxillary canines (Figure 8-27) are the longest teeth in the oral cavity, although the *crowns* of the maxillary central incisor and mandibular canines are longer. Like the roots of their primary predecessors, roots of maxillary canines are the longest of any teeth and are relatively thick. Canines are cuspids, and so, unlike incisors, their incisal edges are divided by mesial and distal cusp ridges.

The labial surface of a canine is more convex than an incisor, with a vertical labial ridge that runs from the cervix to the cusp tip. Maxillary canines have more prominent

labial ridges than mandibular canines. On the lingual surface, the maxillary canine has a large cingulum that is centered with the cusp tip. The lingual ridge of the maxillary canine is usually larger than either the mesial or distal marginal ridge, although the lingual fossae are sometimes indistinct, particularly if the tooth surface is worn.

Maxillary First Premolars/Bicuspids

Maxillary first premolar (Figure 8-28) crowns are larger than those of the maxillary second premolars. Usually the root of the maxillary first premolar is slightly bifurcated, with a buccal and lingual portion. The shoulders (i.e., where the cusp slopes meet the proximal surfaces) are broad and distinctly angled on maxillary first premolars.

In contrast to all other premolars, the buccal cusp tip of the maxillary first premolar is located slightly distal, rather than being centered or slightly mesial. Another difference in the maxillary first premolar is that the mesial cusp ridge of the buccal cusp is longer than the distal cusp ridge. Maxillary first premolars have a buccal cusp that resembles a maxillary canine in that the cusp angle is sharply pointed, almost at a right angle, and the buccal ridge is prominent. The lingual cusp of the first premolar is much shorter than the buccal cusp, and it is located slightly toward the mesial.

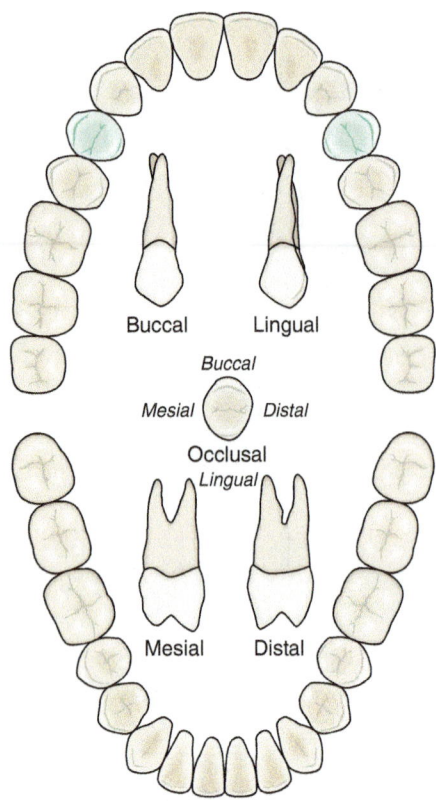

Maxillary first premolars

Figure 8–28 Permanent dentition with the maxillary first premolars/bicuspids noted in blue.

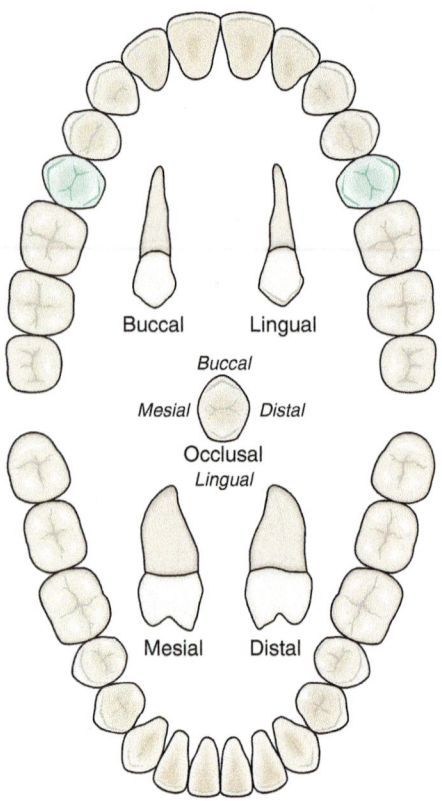

Maxillary second premolars

Figure 8–29 Permanent dentition with the maxillary second premolars/bicuspids noted in blue.

The positions of the buccal and lingual cusps give the maxillary first premolar a distinctly asymmetrical occlusal outline.

The central groove of the maxillary first premolar is over one-third the mesiodistal length of the occlusal surface. On most maxillary first premolars the mesial marginal ridge is crossed by a developmental groove called the *mesial marginal ridge groove*, which intersects with the central groove. Sometimes a distal marginal groove is also present on a maxillary first premolar.

Maxillary Second Premolars/Bicuspids

Although the crown of the maxillary second premolar (Figure 8-29) is smaller than that of the first premolar, it has a longer root. Unlike the maxillary first premolar, the second premolar typically has only a single root, which is about twice the length of the crown. The shoulders of the second premolar are rounded rather than angled. The buccal cusp of the maxillary second premolar is generally less sharply pointed than the first premolar, and the buccal ridge is less distinct. On maxillary second premolars the cusps are almost the same length, with the lingual cusp just slightly shorter. Both the buccal and lingual cusps are located slightly toward the mesial. A maxillary

second premolar has a shorter central groove than the first premolar, but it has more supplementary grooves. Mesial and distal marginal ridge grooves are much less common on maxillary second premolars.

Maxillary First Molars

Maxillary first molars (Figure 8-30) usually have the largest crowns overall of any teeth on the upper jaw. There are typically four major cusps on a maxillary first molar, with the following order of cusp heights: mesiolingual (tallest), mesiobuccal, distobuccal, and distolingual (shortest). A fifth cusp, the **cusp of Carabelli**, may be found on the lingual surface of the mesiolingual cusp. This fifth cusp is named for Georg von Carabelli, the Austrian dentist who first described it in the 1800s. The cusp of Carabelli, whether small or large, is essentially nonfunctional because it is considerably shorter than the mesiolingual cusp tip near which it is located. The distolingual cusp of a maxillary first molar is fairly wide, which makes the lingual half of the crown as wide (or wider) than the buccal half. Aside from a three-cusp mandibular second premolar, the maxillary first molar is the *only* posterior tooth that does not narrow toward the lingual surface.

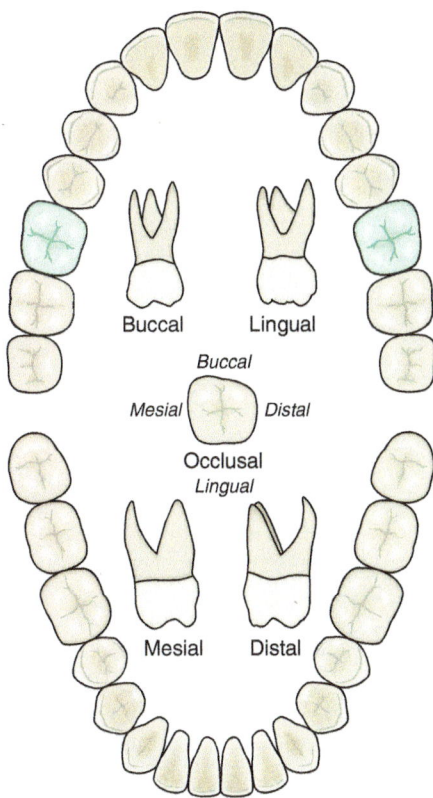

Maxillary first molars

Figure 8–30 Permanent dentition with the maxillary first molars noted in blue.

From an occlusal view, the maxillary first molar looks similar to a rhombus (a slanted square) with sharper angles at the mesiobuccal and distolingual edges. The crown is slightly larger buccolingually than mesiodistally. An oblique ridge crosses diagonally from the mesiolingual cusp to the distobuccal cusp. The crown of a maxillary first molar tapers toward the distal surface. On maxillary first molars each of the four major cusps (i.e., excluding a cusp of Carabelli) has a distinct triangular ridge. The mesiolingual cusp, which is the largest cusp, typically has two triangular ridges: the distal triangular ridge forms an oblique ridge with the distobuccal triangular ridge, and the mesial triangular ridge forms a transverse ridge with the mesiobuccal triangular ridge. The oblique ridge is prominent on the maxillary first molar.

Maxillary first molars have four fossae on their occlusal surface: the central fossa (largest), an elongated distal fossa, a mesial triangular fossa, and a distal triangular fossa (smallest). There are five distinct developmental grooves on a maxillary first molar: central, buccal, distal oblique, lingual, and transverse (a groove of the oblique ridge). The central groove of the maxillary first molar extends from the mesial fossa over the mesial transverse ridge and into the central fossa, where it ends. The buccal groove extends from the central fossa toward (and sometimes onto) the buccal surface. The distal oblique groove runs parallel to the oblique ridge along its distal side from the distal triangular fossa to

the lingual surface, where it becomes the lingual groove. The transverse groove of the oblique ridge is a distinct groove that crosses the oblique ridge and continues into the central groove.

Both maxillary first and second molars have trifurcated roots: mesiobuccal, distobuccal, and lingual roots. Although the three roots are close to the same length, usually the lingual root is longest and the distobuccal is shortest. Unlike roots of mandibular molars, which are furcated near the cervix, maxillary molars are furcated near the area where the cervical third of the roots meets the middle third. The mesiobuccal and distobuccal roots are spread wider on maxillary first molars than on second molars.

Maxillary Second Molars

Maxillary second molars (Figure 8-31) are generally the second largest crowns of the upper dentition, although a few individuals have larger second molars than first molars. Maxillary second molars can have either four cusps or three cusps, although the four-cusp type is more common. The three-cusp second molar has only one lingual cusp. The height order of the four-cusp maxillary second molar is the same as for the maxillary first molar: mesiolingual (tallest), mesiobuccal, distobuccal, and distolingual (shortest). There is no cusp of Carabelli on a maxillary second molar.

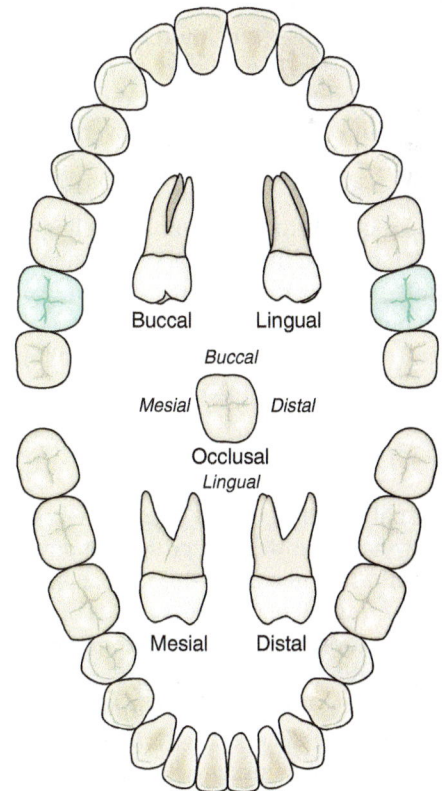

Maxillary second molars

Figure 8–31 Permanent dentition with the maxillary second molars noted in blue.

Four-cusp second molars are less square than first molars, and three-cusp molars are roughly heart shaped. The distolingual cusp of the maxillary second molar is relatively smaller than that of the first molar, so the maxillary second molar tapers lingually, like most posterior teeth. Maxillary second molars taper more noticeably than maxillary first molars both from buccal to lingual and from mesial to distal. The mesiobuccal cusp of a maxillary second molar gives the crown a distinctly slanted appearance from the occlusal view in part because the mesiobuccal cervical ridge is so prominent and in part because the distolingual cusp is so small. However, the mesiolingual cusp is the largest cusp overall.

The four-cusp maxillary second molar has similar ridge, fossa, and groove features as the maxillary first molar. Each of the four cusps has at least one distinct triangular ridge. The transverse ridge formed by the mesiobuccal and mesiolingual cusps is usually well developed on the maxillary second molar, but the oblique ridge is smaller than on the first molar. Like the maxillary first molar, the occlusal surface of the four-cusp maxillary second molar has central, distal elongated, mesial triangular, and distal triangular fossae. The four-cusp maxillary second molar typically has the same five distinct grooves as the maxillary first molar.

Three-cusp maxillary second molars, which have only one lingual cusp, do not have the elongated distal fossa of the four-cusp type. There are typically four triangular ridges on the three-cusp molar, which form one transverse ridge and one oblique ridge. The number of grooves is affected by the missing distolingual cusp and distal fossa: only the central groove, buccal groove, and transverse groove of the oblique ridge are present.

Roots of maxillary second molars are trifurcated into a mesiobuccal root, a distobuccal root, and a lingual root. The root trunk is longer on the maxillary second molar than on the first molar, but the roots follow the same height order: lingual (longest), mesiobuccal, distobuccal (shortest). Maxillary second molar roots are usually closer together and straighter than first molar roots.

Maxillary Third Molars

Although maxillary third molars (Figure 8-32) vary in size, they typically have the shortest crowns of any permanent maxillary teeth. The maxillary third molar has a particularly irregular crown: it may have as few as one cusp and as many as eight cusps. Compared to the maxillary first and second molars, the maxillary third molar generally has a small occlusal surface with a greater number of ridges and supplemental grooves. The relative size of the cusps on the maxillary third molar is usually the same as for the first and second maxillary molars, with the mesiolingual cusp usually being the tallest and largest overall, followed in order by the mesiobuccal cusp, the distobuccal cusp, and the distolingual cusp. Crowns of maxillary third molars

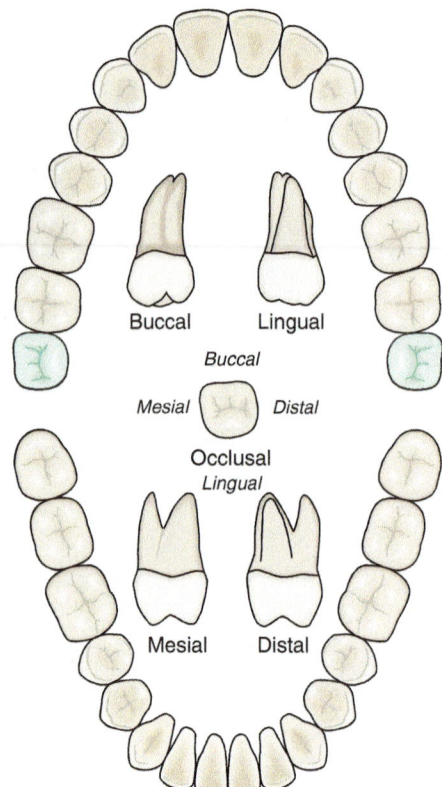

Maxillary third molars

Figure 8–32 Permanent dentition with the maxillary third molars noted in blue.

usually narrow from buccal to lingual and from mesial to distal. Maxillary third molars tend to have shorter roots but proportionally longer root trunks than maxillary first and second molars. They usually have three roots (mesiobuccal, distobuccal, and lingual), like the maxillary first and second molars, but the roots are often fused along most of their length.

Mandibular Central Incisors

Mandibular incisors (both central and lateral) (Figure 8-33) have the most consistent shape of any of the teeth when comparing teeth of different individuals. Mandibular central incisor crowns are generally the narrowest teeth in the oral cavity. Crowns of mandibular central incisors are symmetrical, such that it would be difficult to distinguish the left incisor from the right outside of the context of their placement on the mandibular arch. Even from the incisal perspective, they are very symmetrical mesiodistally. The roots of both central and lateral mandibular incisors are about the same size in proportion to their crowns, and both are proportionally longer than the roots of maxillary incisors.

From a facial view, mesial and distal outlines of mandibular central incisor crowns are mostly straight, but they

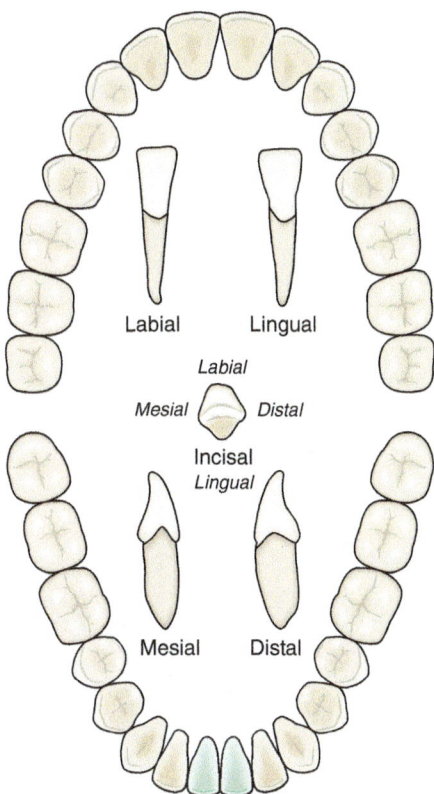

Mandibular central incisors

Figure 8–33 Permanent dentition with the mandibular central incisors noted in blue.

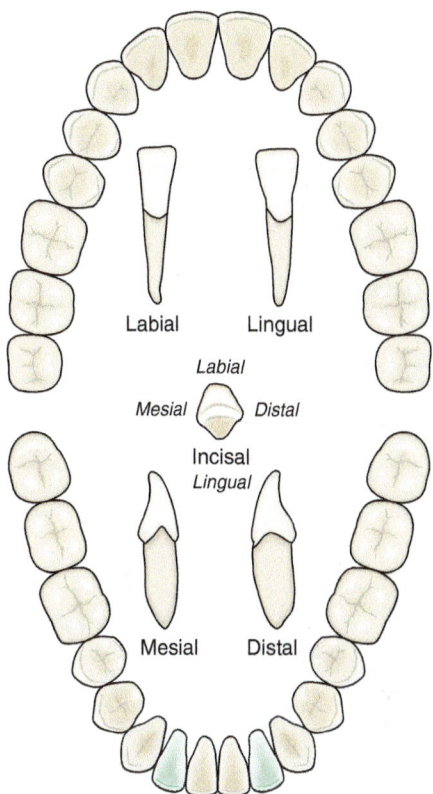

Mandibular lateral incisors

Figure 8–34 Permanent dentition with the mandibular lateral incisors noted in blue.

taper toward the cervix. The cingulum of a mandibular central incisor is small, the lingual fossa is fairly smooth, and the marginal ridges are faint. The cingulum is centered along the root axis line. On the incisal surface, newly erupted mandibular central incisors may have mamelons, but they are usually worn away over time.

Mandibular Lateral Incisors

Mandibular lateral incisors (Figure 8-34) are larger overall than the mandibular central incisors, unlike the size difference of the maxillary incisors. The mandibular lateral incisors look similar to the mandibular central incisors, except that they are less symmetrical. Crowns have a slight tilt toward the distal, making the distal outline shorter than the mesial. The mesioincisal angle of the mandibular lateral incisor is more nearly a right angle than the distoincisal angle, which is somewhat rounded.

On the lingual surface, the mesial marginal ridge is somewhat longer than the distal marginal ridge because the cingulum is just distal of the root axis line. The off-center cingulum makes the lateral incisor mesiodistally asymmetrical when viewing it from the incisal perspective, so right and left incisors are easy to differentiate from one another as well as from the mandibular central incisors. Mamelons may also be found on the incisal surface of lateral incisors early on.

Mandibular Canines/Cuspids

Mandibular canines (Figure 8-35) have a slightly longer crown and shorter root than maxillary canines, although they are the longest tooth overall on the mandibular arch. The mandibular canines have narrower crowns (mesiodistally) than the maxillary canines. Crowns of mandibular canines have a convex facial surface like maxillary canines, but the surface is smoother because the labial ridge is less distinct.

From the labial view, the mesial outline of the mandibular canine is nearly flat and lines up almost perfectly with the mesial side of the root, whereas the distal outline extends beyond the distal side of the root. The mandibular canine has a shorter, less prominent cingulum than the maxillary canine, and it is distally off-center. The distal marginal ridge on the lingual surface of a mandibular canine tends to be more noticeable than either the mesial marginal ridge or the lingual ridge.

Mandibular First Premolars/Bicuspids

Mandibular first premolars (Figure 8-36), like maxillary molars, have only two cusps. They are longer than mandibular second premolars. From the buccal view, a mandibular first premolar resembles a maxillary canine: the

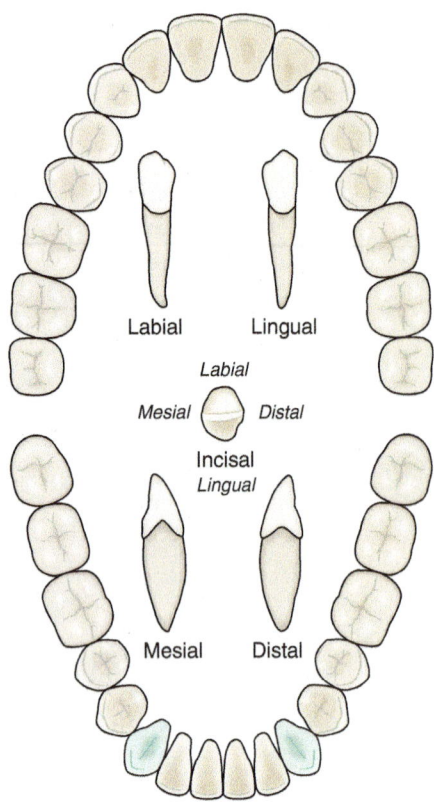

Mandibular canines

Figure 8–35 Permanent dentition with the mandibular canines/cupids noted in blue.

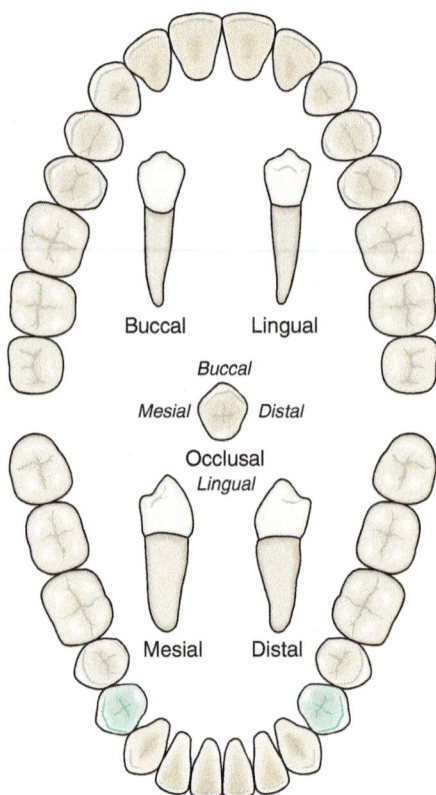

Mandibular first premolars

Figure 8–36 Permanent dentition with the mandibular first premolars/bicuspids noted in blue.

buccal cusp is long, centered over the root, and sharply angled. Crowns of mandibular first premolars are pentagon shaped from the buccal perspective. The lingual cusp of a mandibular first premolar is essentially a transition from the cingulum of a canine to the larger lingual cusp of a mandibular second premolar. Although the lingual cusp of the mandibular first premolar is pointed, it is usually too short to be functional. Mesiodistal width of the mandibular first premolar is narrower toward the lingual.

There is often a mesiolingual groove on the first premolar's occlusal surface that separates the mesial marginal ridge from the mesial slope of the lingual cusp, and rarely a similar distolingual groove is present. The transverse ridge is so prominent on the mandibular first premolar that it separates the grooves on the occlusal surface, so a central groove is rare. Rather than a single central groove, the occlusal surface of a mandibular first premolar typically has separate mesial and distal developmental grooves. When the mesiolingual groove is present, it connects to the mesial groove. Mesial and distal fossae of the mandibular first premolar have deep pits that are prone to decay.

Mandibular Second Premolars/Bicuspids

Mandibular second premolars (Figure 8-37) may have two or three cusps. Although the crown of the mandibular second

premolar is shorter than that of the mandibular first premolar, the second premolar has a longer root, which is about twice the length of the crown. As with the maxillary premolars, the buccal cusp of the second premolar is blunter than that of the first premolar. Because of its blunted buccal cusp tip, the crown of the mandibular second premolar looks more like a square than a pentagon from the buccal view. A mandibular second premolar with two cusps has a narrower lingual mesiodistal width, like the mandibular first premolar. In contrast, a three-cusp mandibular second premolar, which has two lingual cusps, is at least as wide (mesiodistally) on the lingual side as on the buccal side, and sometimes the lingual is wider. The lingual cusp of a two-cusp second premolar is smaller than its buccal cusp but larger overall than the first premolar's lingual cusp. Both lingual cusps on a three-cusp second molar are smaller than the buccal cusp, and the distolingual cusp is usually smaller than the mesiolingual cusp.

Like maxillary second premolars, two-cusp mandibular second premolars have many more supplemental grooves than first premolars. The two-cusp premolar has well-developed triangular ridges, but the transverse ridge that they form is not so prominent that it disrupts the central groove, which is distinctly curved around the buccal triangular ridge. Although a three-cusp second premolar has three triangular ridges, none of them connect to form a transverse ridge. A three-cusp premolar does not actually

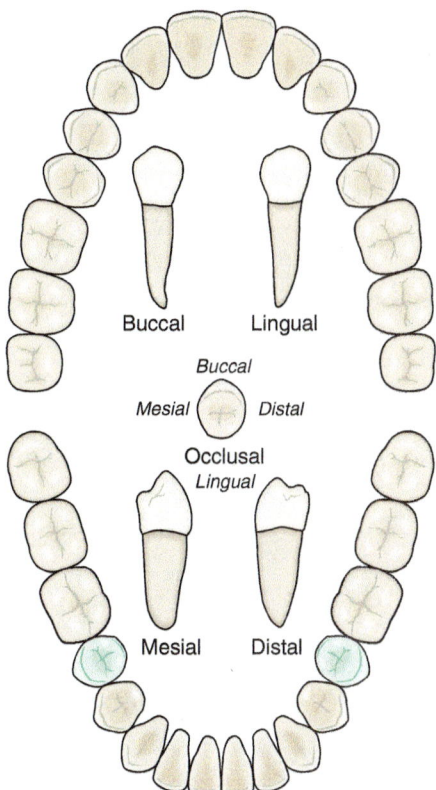

Mandibular second premolars

Figure 8–37 Permanent dentition with the mandibular second premolars/bicuspids noted in blue.

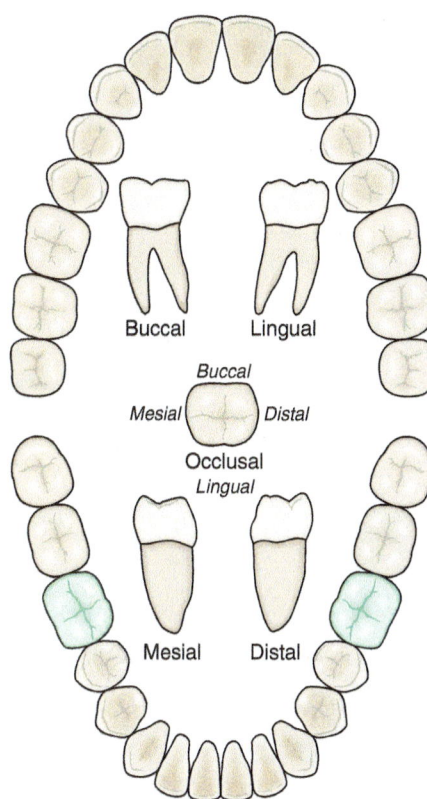

Mandibular first molars

Figure 8–38 Permanent dentition with the mandibular first molars noted in blue.

have a central groove, but instead it has three distinct fossae: mesial, central, and distal. These fossae are connected by supplemental grooves. The central fossa of the three-cusp premolar is distal to the center of the occlusal surface and is usually the largest of the three fossae. The lingual groove, which is unique to the three-cusp second premolar, extends from the central fossa to the lingual surface, separating the two lingual cusps.

Mandibular First Molars

Mandibular first molar (Figure 8-38) crowns tend to be larger than mandibular second molar crowns, and they have the greatest mesiodistal width of all the teeth. There are usually two lingual and three buccal cusps on the mandibular first molar, with the following height order: mesiolingual (tallest), distolingual, mesiobuccal, distobuccal, and distal (shortest). Notice that the height order of the cusps on mandibular molars differs from maxillary molars. Although the lingual cusps are longer than the buccal cusps, the root axis has a lingual tilt that puts the buccal cusps at a higher level. For mandibular first molars with three buccal cusps, there are two buccal grooves: a long mesiobuccal groove that divides the mesiobuccal and distobuccal cusps, and a short distobuccal groove that divides the distobuccal and distal cusps.

The mandibular first molar typically resembles a pentagon from the occlusal view, because of the five cusps. Mandibular first molars are wider mesiodistally than buccolingually. Although the mesial cusps of the first molar appear larger from the occlusal view than the distal cusps, the crown does not taper as noticeably toward the distal as the second molar crown. Mandibular first molars have two transverse ridges: one formed by the triangular ridges of the mesiobuccal and mesiolingual cusps, and one formed by the triangular ridges of the distobuccal and distolingual cusps. The triangular ridges of the buccal cusps are shorter than those of the lingual cusps because the lingual cusps are taller.

Both four- and five-cusp mandibular first molars have two roots. The mesial root is somewhat longer than the distal root, and both roots are roughly twice the length of the first molar crown. Roots of the mandibular first molar are bifurcated near the cervical line, making the root trunk fairly short. Mandibular first molar roots are more widely spread than those of the mandibular second molars.

Mandibular Second Molars

Mandibular second molars (Figure 8-39) have only four cusps: mesiolingual (tallest), distolingual, mesiobuccal, and distobuccal (shortest). The second molar has the same cusp

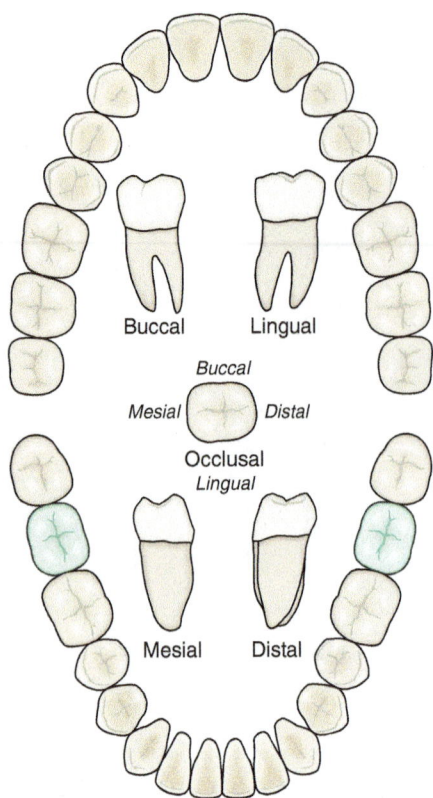

Mandibular second molars

Figure 8–39 Permanent dentition with the mandibular second molars noted in blue.

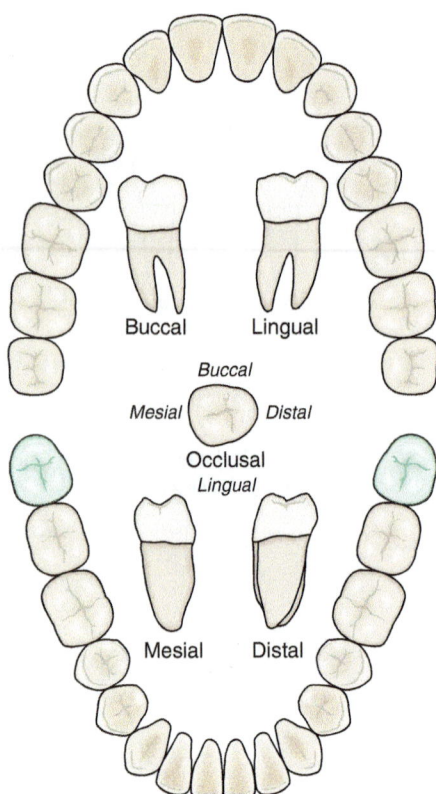

Mandibular third molars

Figure 8–40 Permanent dentition with the mandibular third molars noted in blue.

size order as the four-cusp first molar. Because the mandibular second molar has four cusps instead of five, it has only one buccal groove, which separates the mesiobuccal and distobuccal cusps. The mesiodistal width is greater than the buccolingual width on the mandibular second molar. From an occlusal view, the mandibular second molar looks rectangular but has a slight tapering toward the distal. Triangular ridges of the mesiobuccal and mesiolingual cusps and of the distobuccal and distolingual cusps form two transverse ridges on the mandibular second molar, like the mandibular first molar, with the longer triangular ridges on the lingual cusps.

Mandibular second molars, like the first molars, have two roots that are about twice as long as the second molar crown. Also like the first molars, the mesial root of the second molar is longer than the distal root. The roots of mandibular second molars tend to be more parallel than those of the first molars. The mandibular second molar roots taper toward the apex more so than the first molar roots, giving them a pointed appearance.

Mandibular Third Molars

Mandibular third molars (Figure 8-40) generally have the shortest crowns of all mandibular permanent teeth, which

is similar to their maxillary counterparts—the circumference is smaller, just as with the maxillary third molars. Also like the maxillary third molars, the mandibular third molars can vary considerably in shape and size. The mandibular third molar crown may have a similar appearance to either the mandibular first or second molar, or it may look entirely different. The lingual cusps are usually larger than the buccal cusps, and the mesiolingual cusp tends to be the largest overall. Of the buccal cusps, the mesiobuccal is typically the largest. From the occlusal view, the mandibular third molar looks oblong or rectangular and has a greater width mesiodistally than buccolingually. Mandibular third molars have mesial and distal roots, like mandibular first and second molars, but the roots are usually fused. When the roots are not fused, they have a proportionally long root trunk. Regardless of root orientation, mandibular third molars have much shorter roots than other mandibular molars.

✓CHECKPOINTS

8-10 Which permanent teeth are most likely to have an oblique ridge?

8-11 Which permanent tooth roots are typically bifurcated? Which are typically trifurcated?

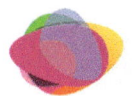

Chapter Highlights

✦ The three stages of dentition are primary, mixed, and permanent.

✦ The dentitions may be divided into two arches, four quadrants, or six sextants.

✦ Primary dentition is made up of 20 primary teeth, with two incisors, a canine, and two molars in each quadrant.

✦ Mixed dentition begins around age 6 years when the first permanent teeth begin to erupt and ends when the last primary tooth is exfoliated and replaced by a permanent tooth.

✦ Permanent dentition consists of 32 permanent teeth, with each quadrant containing two incisors, one canine, two premolars, and three molars.

✦ The five surfaces of the tooth are the incisal or occlusal, mesial, distal, lingual, and facial (labial or buccal). The surfaces of a tooth can be divided into horizontal and vertical thirds to more accurately describe where a feature of a tooth is located.

✦ Permanent teeth are larger overall than the primary teeth they replace. Primary teeth have longer roots than permanent teeth in proportion to their crown height.

✦ Incisors have a thin, flat biting surface for cutting food.

✦ Maxillary central incisors are larger than maxillary lateral incisors in both primary and permanent dentitions, whereas mandibular lateral incisors are larger than mandibular central incisors in both dentitions.

✦ Canines are cuspids with pointed incisal edges for cutting food. Canine teeth are usually the longest teeth overall in their respective dentition and arch.

✦ Premolars have an occlusal surface for grinding food as well as a sharp cusp tip for cutting food. Although there are no premolars in the primary dentition, the permanent premolars replace the primary molars.

✦ Molars tend to have shorter crown heights than other classes of teeth, but their crowns are larger overall than other classes of teeth because they are wider mesiodistally and buccolingually.

Review Questions

1. Which term does not apply to the surface of the teeth on the cheek side of the dental arches?

   a. Labial

   b. Facial

   c. Lingual

   d. Buccal

2. Which class of tooth has no cusp?

   a. Incisor

   b. Canine

   c. Premolar

   d. Molar

3. When two adjacent teeth of the same arch do not contact, the space between them is called

   a. Interproximal space.

   b. Embrasure space.

   c. A fissure.

   d. A diastema.

4. Which primary teeth are usually the first to erupt?

   a. Maxillary central incisors

   b. Maxillary lateral incisors

   c. Mandibular central incisors

   d. Mandibular lateral incisors

5. Which of these teeth has the longest root in the primary dentition?

   a. Maxillary central incisors

   b. Maxillary canines

   c. Mandibular first molars

   d. Mandibular canines

6. Which of the following teeth is most likely to have mamelons?

   a. Permanent maxillary central incisor

   b. Permanent mandibular first premolar

   c. Primary maxillary central incisor

   d. Primary mandibular canine

7. Mixed dentition typically begins around which age?

   a. 2 years

   b. 6 years

   c. 8 years

   d. 12 years

8. Which class of tooth is most likely to have a cusp of Carabelli?

   a. Maxillary first molar

   b. Maxillary second molar

   c. Mandibular first molar

   d. Mandibular second molar

9. How many cusps does a mandibular first molar have?

   a. Two

   b. Three

   c. Four

   d. Five

Active Learning Exercises

1. Draw a basic chart of the primary dentition. Use colored pencils to identify the ages at which the teeth will "fall out" (exfoliation). Now draw a basic chart of the permanent dentition and identify when they typically erupt.

2. Discuss the differences between line angles and point angles.

Application Activities

1. Use the terminology you have learned in this chapter to describe your own teeth. Select one of your teeth and write a clinical description using correct terminology to describe its class, surfaces, and location in the oral cavity.

PREPARING FOR CERTIFICATION EXAMS

Review the topics "Tooth Classifications and Functions" in this chapter to prepare for the Dental Assisting National Board (DANB) exam.

part III

Oral Health Preservation and the Prevention of Dental Disease

chapter 9

Dental Caries and Periodontal Disease

CHAPTER OUTLINE

CHAPTER CHECKLIST

On completion of this chapter, students will be able to:

- ☑ Explain how caries occurs, including the role of bacteria and dietary carbohydrates.
- ☑ Describe the important role saliva plays in neutralizing and preventing caries.
- ☑ Explain why young children and older adults are at special risk for caries.
- ☑ Describe early childhood caries.
- ☑ Explain how caries is classified by stage and location.
- ☑ Describe the various ways used to detect and treat caries.
- ☑ Describe how periodontal disease occurs, including the role of bacteria and an individual's immune system.
- ☑ Describe the conditions that can increase a person's risk for periodontal disease.
- ☑ Identify the stages of periodontal disease.
- ☑ Describe the clinical signs of gingivitis.
- ☑ Describe the clinical signs of periodontitis.
- ☑ Describe the diagnosis and treatment of periodontal disease.

KEY TERMS

calculus (KAL-kyoo-lus) – a mineralized bacterial plaque, covered on its external surface by nonmineralized, living bacterial plaque

caries (KARE-eez) – infectious disease of teeth caused by acidogenic bacteria with dissolution of enamel and dentin or cementum and dentin

cavitation – the formation of a cavity in the enamel of a tooth, the final stage in the caries process

demineralization (dee-mihn-uh-rih-lih-ZAY-shun) – major stage in the dental caries process in which minerals, primarily calcium and phosphorous, are dissolved from tooth structure by acids formed by acidogenic bacteria, primarily mutans streptococci and lactobacilli

early childhood caries (ECC) – the presence of one or more decayed, missing, or filled tooth surfaces in any primary tooth in a child before 6 years of age

gingivitis – a reversible condition; inflammation of the gingiva as a response to bacterial plaque on adjacent teeth; characterized by erythema, edema, and fibrous enlargement of the gingiva without resorption of the underlying alveolar bone

incipient lesion – beginning stage of caries, usually not visible upon examination

lactobacilli (lak-to-buh-SIL-lie) – bacteria that produce lactic acid when they encounter dietary carbohydrates

mutans streptococci (MYOO-tanz strep-toh-KOK-sigh) – infectious bacteria (*Streptococci mutans*) primarily responsible for caries

periodontitis – an irreversible condition; inflammatory disease of the periodontium occurring in response to bacterial plaque on adjacent teeth; characterized by gingivitis, destruction of alveolar bone and periodontal ligament, apical migration of the epithelial attachment resulting in formation of periodontal pockets, and possibly, if left untreated, eventual loosening and exfoliation of teeth

plaque – deposits on teeth, composed primarily of bacteria and acids

remineralization – healing process in which minerals are redeposited in the demineralized tooth structure; accomplished by the protective factors of the saliva and the action of fluoride to inhibit demineralization and interfere with the enzymatic requirements of bacteria

root caries – a soft, progressive lesion of cementum and dentin that involves bacterial infection and invasion

Introduction

Many processes are ongoing inside the human mouth, including constant demineralization and remineralization of teeth. When demineralization outpaces remineralization and certain bacteria are present, dental **caries** (also known as tooth decay) can occur and create cavities.

When bacteria spread to the tissues that surround the teeth (periodontium), periodontal disease can occur. An infection of these tissues is called **gingivitis**. If such an infection continues untreated, it may lead to a more serious condition, **periodontitis**, which involves not only the gingival tissue but also the supporting bone of the teeth. Tooth loosening and bone destruction follow unless periodontitis is halted by proper treatment and improved dental hygiene. Periodontal disease is the leading cause of tooth loss in adults over age 45 years.

Dental caries and periodontal diseases are preventable. As a dental assistant, you play a key role in helping to educate patients about how caries and periodontal disease occur as well as how to prevent them.

Dental Caries

Development of Caries

Teeth are composed of enamel, dentin, pulp, and cementum. Enamel and dentin, high in mineral content, are the surface materials. Enamel—the hardest substance in the body—is more than 95% mineral, and dentin is approximately two-thirds mineral in composition. If the outer enamel of the teeth is damaged or worn away, the risk of caries is increased.

Four factors are needed for a carious lesion to develop: a susceptible tooth, a source of energy (any type of carbohydrate), decay-inducing bacteria, and time. If one of these four required elements of the "decay formula" is missing (as when the first three factors coexist, but only for a short period, or when a baby's mouth is not yet host to decay-inducing bacteria), the chain of decay is broken, and decay cannot take place.

When a carbohydrate is introduced into the oral cavity, a 20-minute "acid attack" occurs. When any type of

carbohydrate is consumed, whether it is a sugar or a starch, the saliva becomes very acidic for approximately 20 minutes. During this time the teeth are assaulted by an acidic environment that contributes to the demineralization of the tooth structure.

To limit the frequency of acid attacks, individuals should limit the amount of carbohydrates eaten between meals and brush and floss (or chew sugarless gum) after eating. Rinsing the mouth out with water after a meal will also help reduce these attacks.

Too commonly, patients sip sugary drinks all day long. These drinks include not only sodas, but also sports drinks; natural juice drinks; and coffee or tea with added milk, creamer, and/or sugar. Patients tend to forget that the intake of some liquids may be contributing to the development of decay. As a dental professional, make sure your patients understand that every time a carbohydrate is introduced to the oral cavity, an acid attack takes place. Be sure to ask patients not only about their food intake, but also their liquid intake and the frequency of the liquid intake.

Voice of Experience

I see many people who drink a soda over a long period of time. They take a sip and then put the cap back on. They take another sip 20 minutes later, then another 15 minutes later, then another 10 minutes later, and so on. Unfortunately, this intermittent sipping puts the oral environment under a constant acid attack—before the 20 minutes required for the oral cavity to recover from acidity to a more neutral pH passes, another drink is taken. If you take sips of soda throughout the day, the pH of your mouth is never allowed time to recover from the acid attack that is constantly occurring.

Because of this, it's better to drink a soda or any other sugary drink (including coffee, if milk or creamer [which contain the natural sugar lactose] or sugar has been added) in one sitting. If you want to drink a sugary drink, drink it and get it over with, allowing your mouth to have to battle only one acid attack. The same is true for snacks: If you decide to snack, eat your snack all at once—do not graze on it throughout the day.

The oral cavity is also host to many bacteria. Among the types typically found in the mouth—and the bacteria primarily responsible for caries—are **mutans streptococci** (MS) (*Streptococcus mutans*) and **lactobacilli** (LB).

These bacteria convert carbohydrates (sugars and starches) into acids during the digestion process, lowering the pH at the tooth surface and increasing the rate of tooth demineralization beyond that of **remineralization**; thus, the tooth deteriorates. Without the presence of these specific bacteria, dental caries would not occur.

MS and LB are aerobic in nature, meaning that they require the presence of oxygen to survive. Unlike anaerobic bacteria (that is, bacteria that does not need oxygen to thrive in the oral environment), MS and LB do not play a significant role in periodontal disease because they must remain above the gumline in order to survive.

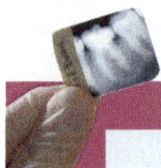

Dental Facts

The term *caries* is derived from Latin, meaning "rottenness."

Areas on teeth where bacteria accumulate as a biofilm—typically at the gingival margin and interproximally—are called **plaque** (Figure 9-1). MS, which are disease-producing bacteria, are commonly found in dental plaque. This sticky film helps to trap the bacteria and the acids they produce against the teeth.

These acids can be neutralized by saliva and products, such as toothpaste and mouthwash. Left untreated, however, plaque-trapped bacteria and acids can over time dissolve the mineral content of teeth (**demineralization**). Plaque, then, is a key factor in creating the environment in which caries occurs.

Saliva is a natural cleanser. If plentiful and thin enough, saliva helps to cleanse teeth by diluting acids from plaque. Saliva naturally contains enzymes and antibacterial components, which help to retain calcium, remineralize teeth, neutralize acids, and destroy bacteria. Therefore, good saliva flow is essential to help prevent caries. When saliva flow is impaired due to illness, medication, or other reasons, the risk for decay increases.

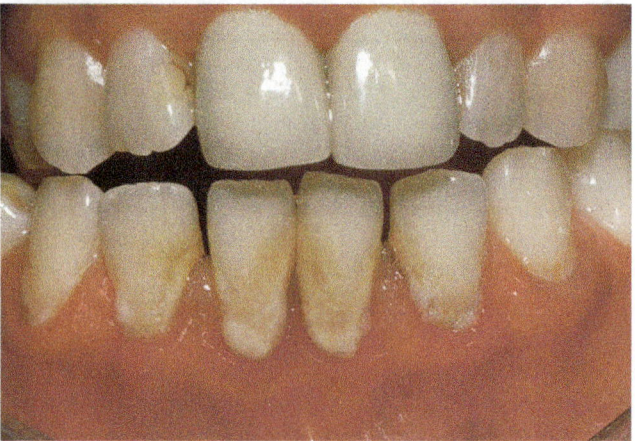

Figure 9–1 Severe accumulation of plaque along the gingival margins and interproximal surfaces.

The processes that naturally occur in the oral cavity cannot always handle the strains of modern life. The typical American diet features an abundance of carbohydrates eaten throughout the day, which increases the risk for caries. Many adults have a number of dental amalgams already, which also increases risk for additional caries, because these restored areas are more prone to bacteria.

Dental caries is so widespread that it is the most common chronic disease among U.S. children and possibly the most common disease among humans. Despite the fact that people have experienced caries throughout recorded history, it is a preventable disease. Frequent toothbrushing and flossing, especially after snacking on foods containing carbohydrates, can decrease the risk of caries or prevent its occurrence entirely.

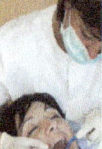

Voice of Experience

There's so much information we could share with patients that it can be overwhelming. I try to pick one or two things to emphasize with a patient during each visit—the take-away message I want them to remember. I mention it once or twice casually and then reiterate it at the end of the visit. I have found that they take my advice more to heart when I limit it to one or two key things at a time.

CHECKPOINTS

9-1 What are two bacteria responsible for causing caries?

9-2 What do these bacteria need to produce acid and cause caries to begin?

9-3 What helps to trap bacteria and acids on the teeth?

9-4 What naturally occurring substance helps to neutralize acid and remineralize teeth?

9-5 What is the most common chronic disease among children in the United States?

Particular Risk Groups—Young Children and Older Adults

In addition to diet, causes of dental caries include heredity, mechanical problems, and endocrine disorders. Diet begins to affect tooth health even before birth. Because tooth development begins *in utero*, a mother's diet during pregnancy—the nutrition the mother shares with her baby in the months before birth—is important to enable the formation of healthy teeth in the baby.

The bacteria that cause caries are transmissible and infectious. At birth, a baby's mouth does not contain MS. Typically, these bacteria are transmitted in short order through the saliva of a parent, sibling, or caregiver. This transmissibility highlights the importance of oral hygiene and dental care within a family.

A child's primary teeth are slightly more vulnerable to decay because they contain more water than their permanent replacements. The water in tooth enamel allows acids to flow into and minerals to flow out of the tooth. This vulnerability is very real—the most prevalent disease of childhood is **early childhood caries (ECC),** which is defined as the presence of one or more decayed, missing, or filled tooth surfaces in any primary tooth in a child between birth and 6 years of age.

ECC can affect any child but occurs most often in families with lower socioeconomic status and in others with limited access to dental care. Among certain populations, ECC is a significant public health problem, according to the American Dental Association.

ECC can be caused by routine use of a nursing bottle at bedtime or prolonged at-will breast-feeding. Other names for the condition are *nursing bottle mouth*, *baby bottle syndrome*, *baby bottle caries*, and *prolonged nursing habit*.

When the baby's sucking is active, the liquid passes beyond the teeth. However, as the baby falls asleep, pools of liquid (milk or a sweetened beverage) collect about the teeth. Maxillary anterior teeth and primary molars are the first to be affected. Mandibular anterior teeth are rarely affected because the nipple covers them.

ECC is an infectious and contagious disease. Dental professionals should educate parents that children's teeth are susceptible to caries as soon as they begin to erupt.

Older adults as well as young children are vulnerable to dental caries. With age, the gingiva can recede from the teeth on its own. The pockets created toward the base of the teeth by gingival recession begin to collect plaque (Figure 9-2) and over time plaque-released acids demineralize the tooth, creating dental caries. Moreover, because root surfaces are softer than enamel or dentin, they are especially vulnerable to decay.

Because older adults are more likely to have more dental amalgams, this population also is susceptible to caries around these restorations. When amalgams weaken, bacteria can penetrate and caries can occur. This is called *recurrent* or *secondary caries*.

CHECKPOINTS

9-6 Why is it important for pregnant women to practice good nutrition?

9-7 How are mutans streptococci bacteria usually transmitted to a newborn?

9-8 What are some causes of early childhood caries?

9-9 In what ways are older adults more vulnerable to dental caries?

Stages of Dental Caries

Dental caries occurs when more minerals are lost from enamel (an effect caused by the increased level of acid released by plaque) than are deposited and can take months or years to develop. The process has two distinct stages:

1. **Incipient lesion**—when decay begins to demineralize the enamel and penetrate the dentin; may be called a "white lesion or spot."
2. Untreated incipient lesion—when the affected area develops into an overt lesion and cavitation—the development of a cavity (carious lesion)—occurs.

Dental caries is also described by where in the mouth it occurs:

- Pit and fissure (Figure 9-3)—begins in a minute crevice in the enamel, where three or more lobes of a developing tooth join in an imperfect enamel plate (occlusal pits of molars and premolars), or at the endings of grooves of the teeth (buccal grooves of a mandibular molar).
- Smooth surface—begins in surfaces where there is no pit, groove, or other crevice or in areas where plaque is protected from removal (proximal tooth surfaces protected near a contact area, cervical thirds of teeth, and other difficult-to-clean areas).
- **Root caries**—a soft, progressive lesion of cementum and dentin. Gingival recession is necessary for root caries to occur. Because cementum is softer than enamel and dentin, root caries can occur more quickly than enamel caries.
- Secondary or recurrent caries—occurs in small spaces between a tooth and its restorative application, where bacteria can thrive in an area of a small leakage.

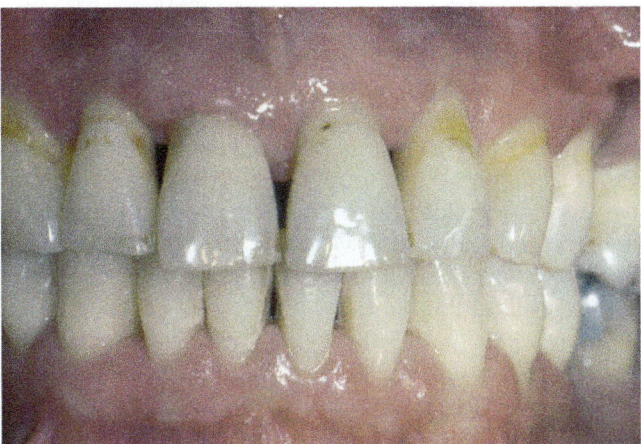

Figure 9–2 Generalized gingival recession and the exposed roots.

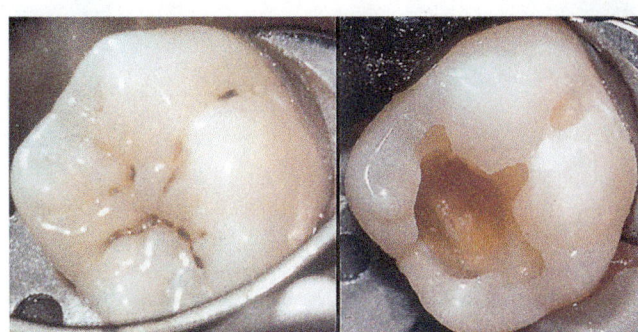

Figure 9–3 Occlusal pit and fissure and buccal groove caries.

✔ CHECKPOINTS

9-10 What are the two distinct stages of caries?

9-11 What are the types of caries, by location in the mouth?

Classification of Caries

The standard method for classifying and charting dental caries was developed by G. V. Black, a noted dental educator who divided the classes according to surfaces of the teeth. Each class is represented by a Roman numeral. The categories, which are standard throughout dentistry, are customarily used for carious lesions, cavity preparations, and finished restorations. For more information on how Black's classification system is used in patient treatment, see Chapter 20, Oral Diagnosis and Treatment Planning.

Caries Detection

Before the advent of current methods for detection of early-stage caries, detection involved treating end-stage caries, or *cavities*.

Incipient caries is not initially visible by clinical observation. Often, the first clinical sign of caries is the presence of a white area on the surface of the tooth, best visible under bright light, but with the enamel surface as yet unbroken by the ongoing acidic demineralization (Figure 9-4). Although you can use a blunt probe to lightly examine the surface of the tooth, you should not pick or scratch the affected tooth, which will require remineralization with saliva and increased levels of fluoride.

Untreated, a lesion breaks down the enamel over the demineralized area, which is visible to observation and irregular to the gentle application of the side of a blunt probe (Figure 9-5). A white area later in the process of caries may be characterized by slight surface roughness, showing initial breakdown of the surface. This tooth may respond to remineralization through the use of fluoride and good oral hygiene.

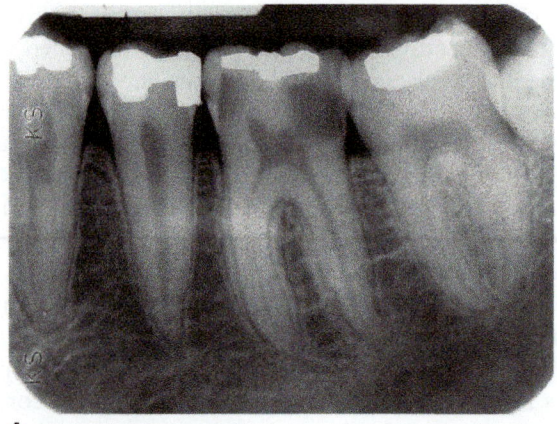

A

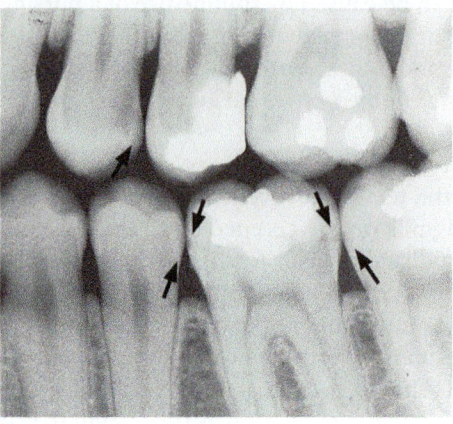

B

Figure 9–5 The process of caries. (**A**) Class V demineralization of the cervical and incisal edge of a maxillary lateral incisor. (**B**) Radiographic image of several class II lesions (*arrows*).

By the time caries has progressed to the point of **cavitation**, at which a cavity has developed in the enamel through the demineralization caused by plaque-released acids, this condition may be easily apparent to the dental professional. Radiographs are often used for confirmation or to check for interproximal and root caries.

Caries can also be detected using a dye that visually distinguishes between nondecayed and decayed tooth structures. The dye is applied to the suspected lesion and allowed to penetrate for a few seconds before being rinsed off. Areas of decay will retain the dye, thus indicating to the dentist that caries are present.

Another diagnostic instrument is the laser caries detector (Figure 9-6). This battery-powered device employs laser to reveal differences in tooth density, which are indicated by varying wavelengths (0–99) of fluorescent light. Little fluorescent light occurs when the laser is directed onto healthy teeth. The presence of caries, however, causes higher levels of this light.

Effective on both primary and permanent teeth, the laser detector is not effective for interproximal decay or that which is beneath sealants or restorations due to inaccessibility in these areas.

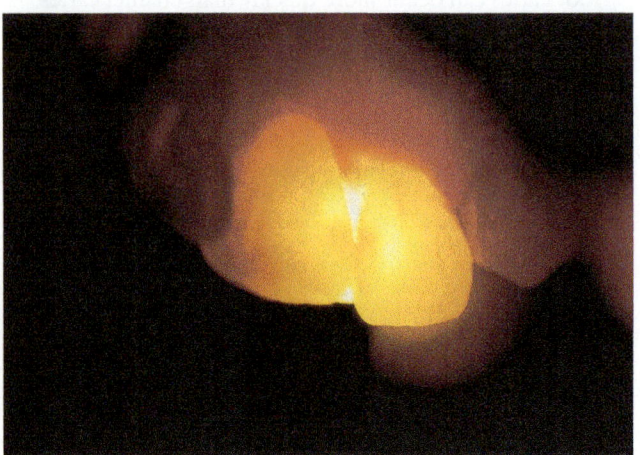

Figure 9–4 Class III incipient caries are visible under light.

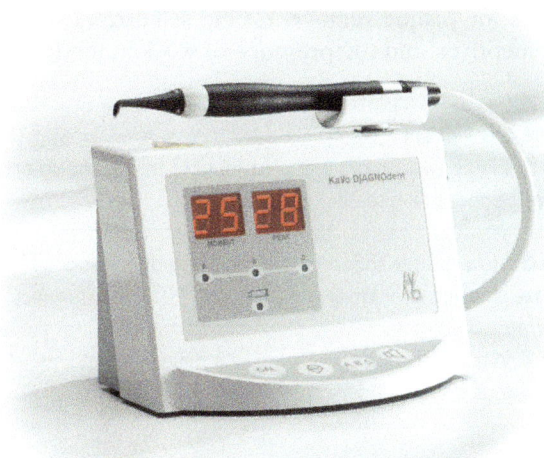

Figure 9–6 A battery-powered laser caries detector.

Caries Treatment

Today, the dental profession focuses on preventing caries in addition to repairing it. (See Chapter 10, Prevention of Caries and Periodontal Disease, for prevention information.)

Teeth that are determined to be in the process of demineralization and candidates for remineralization may be treated as follows. A significant step in this process is patient education. Steps to remineralize teeth in the early stages of caries include:

- Restore any true caries.
- Use sealants to close any pits and fissures.
- Encourage family members and close contacts to have necessary restorative dental care to eliminate transmissible caries-causing bacteria.
- Address any dry mouth conditions that limit saliva production.
- Increase personal fluoride use, including fluoridated water and use of dental products several times per day with no further eating or drinking after the last use of the day.
- Encourage good oral hygiene habits: brush after every meal when possible, or at least rinse with water after eating; brush at least twice daily and floss at least once daily.
- Avoid sugary drinks; water is the best fluid for the body and mouth.
- Reduce between-meal snacking.
- Chew sugar-free gum containing the sugar substitute xylitol after eating.
- Use a prescription dental rinse before bed or a brush-on dental product.

- Schedule frequent dental hygiene appointments for professional therapy, self-care instruction, and fluoride varnish applications.

Teeth with advanced caries will need restorative treatment. As a dental assistant, you will prepare and mix the materials used in this process. If you work in a state in which doing so is within the scope of practice, you also may place some materials in the patient's mouth. In either case, you need general knowledge of the materials used so you can prepare them, help educate the patient, and assist the dentist or hygienist.

In some instances, rapidly progressing caries called *rampant caries* may develop. This form of caries affects multiple teeth simultaneously, and, because of the aggressive nature of the disease, a swift treatment plan that includes preventive, therapeutic, and restorative elements is vital. Small children who routinely use a nursing bottle at bedtime or who breast-feed for prolonged periods may be at particular risk for this disease (see section on early childhood caries, earlier in this chapter). Other high-risk groups are individuals who have dry mouth (because of inadequate saliva output; these can include some patients with diabetes, habitual stimulant users, users of alcohol, and those under excessive stress, among others) and older adults (due to natural recession of the gingival margin with age).

Extra Patient Care

When a patient has a sudden increase in caries or cavities, it is important to discover why. A logical place to start this discussion is diet. When the patient is a child, try to hold the discussion when a parent is present. Inquire about the presence of carbohydrates in the diet, reminding the patient that this includes sugary or starchy food, candy (including gum), and drinks (including milk). Also ask about oral hygiene habits, including how often and how well the patient brushes and flosses. After pinpointing problematic areas and habits, advise the patient and, if applicable, parent what behaviors and changes in diet help reduce the risk for caries, describing proper brushing, flossing, and eating habits.

Periodontal Disease

Research shows that periodontal disease is one of the most widespread diseases among adolescent and adult Americans, affecting an estimated 67 million people. Many individuals who have it are unaware of its presence and its potential effects. Although females tend to practice better self-care than males, natural female hormonal variances often adversely affect gingival tissues. Environmental factors also put individuals who have lower levels of education and income at greater risk of developing periodontal disease.

The severity of periodontal disease increases with age. This may be due to risk factors associated with increased age—medication use, systemic illness, stress, and the impact of several years of smoking—or cumulative effects rather than age itself.

The Process of Periodontal Disease

Before 1960, clinicians believed that periodontal disease was caused solely by the presence of calculus (tartar) deposits acting as a mechanical irritant to the tissue. In later years, it was believed that bacteria in dental plaque caused periodontal disease. In recent years, research has fundamentally changed our understanding of periodontal disease—that the interaction of the patient with the bacteria, including how a person's immune system reacts to infection and inflammation, controls whether or not periodontal disease occurs. Some people are more at risk than others, for reasons both of habit and of heredity.

Oral conditions that increase the risk of periodontal infection include those that increase plaque retention, such as **calculus**. The surface of a calculus deposit is irregular and is always covered with disease-causing bacteria. As calculus deposits build up, they can lead to irregular surfaces and other alterations of the contours of the teeth that are difficult or impossible for patients to clean (Figure 9-7). Even slight buildups of calculus can lead to plaque retention. Because a living layer of bacterial plaque always covers a calculus deposit, dental calculus plays a significant role in contributing to periodontal disease. It is difficult to bring either gingivitis or periodontitis under control in the presence of dental calculus, and it is essential to remove these deposits.

Various oral conditions that increase the risk for periodontal infection include abnormal tooth structure, poorly contoured restorations (which limit access to tooth

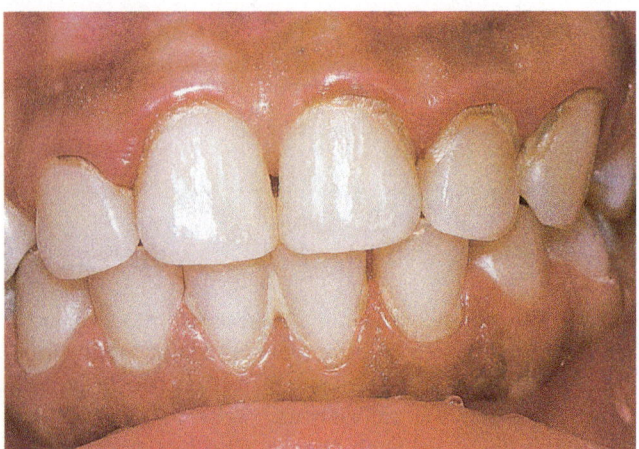

Figure 9–7 Calculus found interproximally and along the gingival margins contributes to periodontal disease.

surfaces for plaque removal during self-care), use of oral contraceptives, and the presence of wisdom teeth.

CHECKPOINTS

9-15 Name two factors that contribute to the likelihood of having periodontal disease.

9-16 How has the theory about the cause of periodontal disease changed over time?

9-17 What oral condition can make it difficult to get periodontal disease under control?

Risk Groups

Certain factors can increase a person's risk for periodontal disease, including tobacco use (including the use of smokeless tobacco), diabetes, osteoporosis, hormone alterations (particularly in females; these can include puberty, pregnancy, menopause, and postmenopause), psychological stress, and genetic influences (for about 30% of people).

Smoking is the most preventable risk factor for periodontal disease. Some studies suggest that smokers are as much as 11 times more likely than nonsmokers to have the bacteria that cause periodontal disease, 4 times more likely to have advanced forms of the disease, and twice as likely to become toothless after the age of 65 years. These risks increase with the number of cigarettes smoked each day. Recent studies have shown that tobacco and the chemicals in cigarettes inhibit or repress the body's immunity cells. These white blood cells, called *macrophages*, are often called "first responders" in the healing process. For this reason, most smokers suffer a more aggressive form of alveolar bone loss related to their body's inability to fight disease.

People who have diabetes may have difficulty combating infection, thus putting them at greater risk for periodontitis. The bacterial infection and inflammation that occur with periodontitis can also aggravate existing diabetes as well as make it more difficult to control when both conditions are present. Moreover, some research suggests that periodontitis may in fact increase the risk for developing diabetes.

Hormone-influenced periodontal disease affects some adolescents, pregnant women, and those who take birth control medication as a result of the body's exaggerated response to the presence of plaque when hormone levels are fluctuating.

In addition, increased age (gingival detachment intensifies with age), tooth abnormalities (such as poorly contoured restorations and abnormally shaped teeth), the presence of wisdom teeth (which may be home to increased populations of bacteria), and treatment for cancer in the bone (bone-strengthening drugs may cause decay in the jawbone) are all risk factors for periodontal disease.

From the Dentist's Perspective

The dental assistant has a wealth of knowledge to share with the patient in the mission of preventing periodontal disease. For example, the dental assistant can describe and demonstrate proper brushing and flossing techniques, explain the importance of oral care after eating and the role nutrition plays in caries, describe the importance of regular dental cleanings, and explain to parents how bacteria are transmissible and how their oral hygiene can affect their children. The more professionals who impart this information to patients, the better. I count on my dental assistants to play a significant role in patient education.

Dental Facts

Smoking may be responsible for more than half of the cases of periodontal disease among adults in the United States. Smokers are 2.6 to 6 times more likely to exhibit periodontal destruction than nonsmokers.

After smokers quit smoking, their periodontal health returns, over time and with adequate care, to a healthier state.

Undesirable Effects on Overall Health

In addition to conditions that increase the risk for periodontal disease, the disease itself may adversely affect a person's general health. The bacteria that cause periodontal disease can enter the bloodstream and spread to cause infections in other parts of the body. This infection can contribute to the development of heart disease; premature, low-birth-weight babies; poorly controlled diabetes; and respiratory diseases.

Research shows that patients who show evidence of bacteria associated with periodontitis may have an increased risk of developing cardiovascular disease, including atherosclerosis, myocardial infarction, and stroke. It is thought that the long-term effect of chronic periodontitis, such as extended bacterial exposure, may lead to cardiovascular disease. Research also shows that older adults who have higher levels of some bacteria that cause periodontal infection have thicker carotid arteries—a strong predictor of stroke and heart attack.

In addition to negatively affecting cardiovascular health, periodontitis affects respiratory conditions. Studies show that inhaling bacteria from the oral cavity into the lower respiratory tract can worsen chronic obstructive pulmonary disease, possibly causing infection in this area.

Some studies have demonstrated that pregnant women who have periodontitis may, as a result of inflammation subsequent to the spread of periodontal bacteria, be more likely to have preterm births with low-birth-weight babies. Moreover, periodontitis is a risk factor for halitosis; infection (as of a prosthetic joint subsequent to joint replacement surgery); bone decay in the jaw (and, thus, tooth loss); and, in older adults, cognitive impairment.

The best way to limit bacteria from the oral cavity from entering the bloodstream is by maintaining good periodontal health. Inflamed or ulcerated gingival tissue makes an individual vulnerable to bacteria spread.

CHECKPOINTS

9-18 List some of the conditions that increase the risk for developing periodontal disease.

9-19 Name the most preventable risk factor for periodontal disease.

9-20 What must occur for periodontal disease to adversely affect other areas of a person's health?

9-21 List some of the areas of health that periodontal disease can have a negative effect on.

Stages of Periodontal Disease

The changes that occur with periodontal disease can be divided into three distinct stages: subclinical gingivitis, gingivitis, and periodontitis.

Subclinical Gingivitis

In subclinical gingivitis, disease-causing bacteria have begun to accumulate near the gingival margin. This stage of periodontal disease has no visible clinical signs and can only be detected microscopically.

Development of Gingivitis

Gingivitis is a bacterial infection that is confined to the gingiva; its symptoms include inflammation, soreness, and bleeding. Unlike the damage caused by periodontitis, the damage that gingivitis causes to the tissues of the periodontium is reversible. Gingival diseases usually involve inflammation of the gingival tissues, most often in response to acids released by the bacterial plaque that forms through the interaction of oral flora with food. (However, a small percentage of gingivitis is not caused by bacterial plaque, but results from viral infections, fungal infections, skin diseases, hormonal changes, allergic reactions, or mechanical trauma.)

The tissues of the periodontium, including the gingiva, periodontal ligament, cementum, and alveolar bone (Figure 9-8), play a vital role in maintaining the health and function of the periodontium, and the body responds to bacterial invasion with marked changes in these tissues, including irritation, swelling, sores, and purulent discharge. However, by contrast to periodontitis, no permanent damage is sustained to tissues or bone.

Clinical gingivitis occurs when the bacterial infection is not resolved in the early accumulation phase, with bacteria then penetrating into the underlying connective tissue. This phase is characterized by changes that have

Figure 9–8 Tissues of the periodontium.

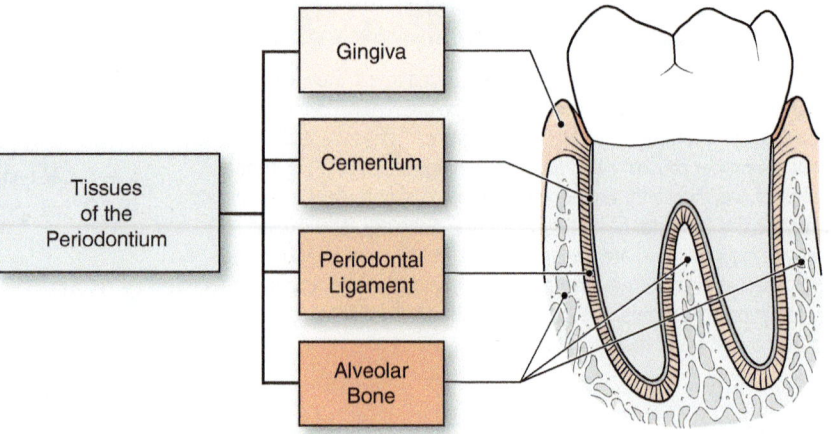

clinically visible signs (Figure 9-9). Bleeding and swelling may occur upon gentle probing, and probing depths may be greater than 3 millimeters due to swelling of the tissues. This phase may persist for years without ever leading to periodontitis. Gingivitis is characterized by changes in the "3 Cs" of gingival tissues: color, contour, and consistency. When gingivitis is present, the gingival tissue is usually red or reddish-blue, and the edges are swollen.

Cultural Diversity

The soft tissues (gingiva) of the mouth can vary according to patients' ethnic backgrounds and other factors without indicating gingivitis. We think of healthy gingiva as typically pink, firm, and stippled. However, it is also very common to see what is called *melanin pigmentation* on the soft tissue. Melanin pigmentation is seen in individuals with higher levels of melanocytes, which give rise to a darker skin color. Most commonly seen in those of African heritage, melanin pigmentation is a completely benign variation of normal tissues. Lifestyle and cultural practices may also contribute to gingival darkening. For example, smokers may be prone to staining, and studies are currently being conducted to determine whether parents who smoke have a direct effect on the gingival staining observed in their children. Some African and Middle Eastern cultures tattoo the buccal gingiva both for perceived beautification and clinical purposes.

CHECKPOINTS

9-22 Is the damage to the periodontium caused by gingivitis reversible?

9-23 List the clinical signs of gingivitis.

Development of Periodontitis

If plaque remains, gingivitis may proceed to **periodontitis**, a permanently destructive infection of the periodontium that can do serious harm to the soft tissues around the tooth root, resulting in irreversible destruction to the tissues and bones of the periodontium. As the inflamed gingiva pulls away from the tooth, bacteria (in particular, *Actinobacillus actinomycetemcomitans*, *Porphyromonas gingivalis*, *Bacteroides forsythus*, *Treponema denticola*, *Treponema socranskii*, and *Prevotella intermedia*) colonize the pockets thus formed, causing further inflammation and, ultimately, bone loss.

This deep-seated inflammation loosens tooth ligaments and allows deeper bacterial invasion in the soft tissue (possibly requiring drainage and antibiotic treatment) and in the pulp (only through an existing fissure), the soft central

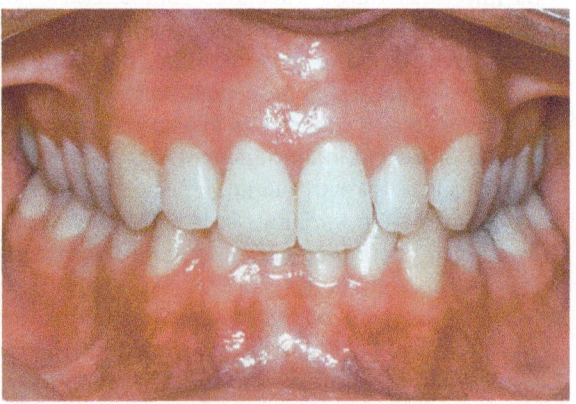

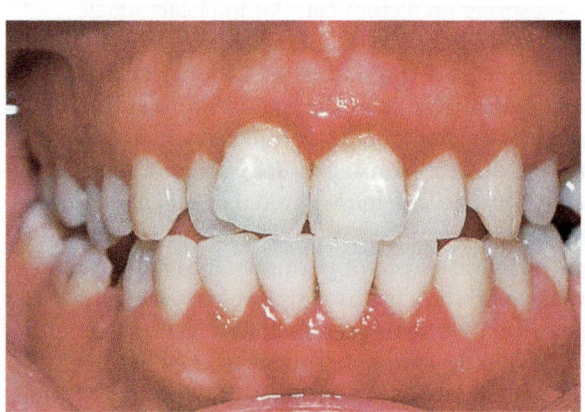

A　　　　　　　　　　　　　　　　　　　　B

Figure 9–9 **A.** Normal healthy gingiva. **B.** Gingivitis; red gingival margins with blunted interdental papillae.

tissue of the tooth that contains blood vessels and nerves. Periodontal disease causes far more tooth loss than does caries.

Periodontitis is characterized by visible alterations in the color, contour, and consistency of periodontal tissue. Some tissue may appear spongy, with a smooth, shiny, bright-red or purplish-red appearance; other tissue may appear light pink, with a firm, rigid consistency. The edges of the tissue are swollen or tough and may bleed upon probing or emit purulent material. Probing depths are 4 millimeters or greater.

There are three major categories of periodontitis:

■ Chronic—Signaled by red or swollen gingiva, bleeding during brushing, a bad taste in the mouth, persistent halitosis, sensitive teeth, loose teeth, and purulent material around teeth and gingiva; usually does not involve pain; clinical appearance is evident to dental professionals; bone loss may be evident on radiographs; most commonly detected in adults older than age 35 years.

■ Aggressive—Begins in childhood, adolescence, or early adulthood; affected tissue may have normal clinical appearance; probing reveals deep pockets around affected teeth; characterized by rapid destruction of periodontal ligament, rapid loss of supporting bone, poor response to periodontal therapy, and high risk for tooth loss.

■ Less common types—A manifestation of clinical disease (e.g., Down syndrome, poorly controlled diabetes, acquired immunodeficiency syndrome, juvenile periodontitis), necrotizing periodontal diseases, and abscesses of the periodontium; associated with endodontic lesions, developmental or acquired deformities and conditions, mucogingival deformities or conditions, and occlusal trauma.

CHECKPOINTS

9-24 Is the damage to the periodontium from periodontitis reversible?

9-25 Does gingivitis always proceed to periodontitis?

9-26 List some clinical characteristics of periodontitis.

Diagnosis of Periodontal Disease

Signs of periodontal disease can be observed or are measurable by the clinician. Examples include gingival redness, swelling, bleeding, detachment of periodontal tissue from tooth, tooth mobility, and loss of alveolar bone support. Symptoms the patient may experience include pain, itching of the gingiva, blood on the bed pillow, and a bad taste in the mouth. Some patients have no symptoms, which leads some clinicians to call periodontitis a "silent disease."

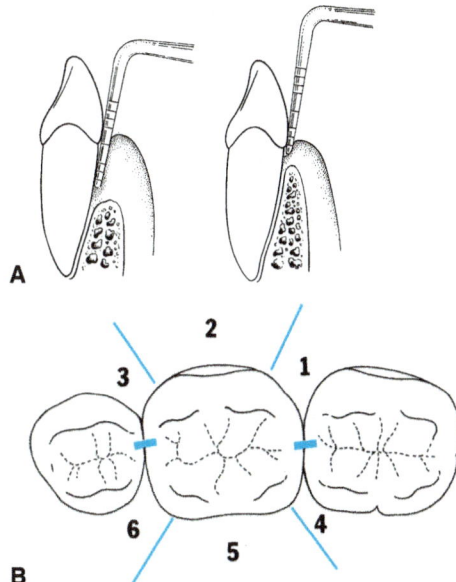

Figure 9–10 A. Probing the pocket depth from the gingival margin to the attachment of periodontal tissue. **B.** Probing depths for each of six areas around the tooth.

The clinical periodontal assessment is a fact-gathering process to provide a comprehensive picture of the patient's periodontal health status. The objectives are to look for clinical signs of inflammation and damage to the periodontium and to determine if it is healthy or diseased. Documentation of clinical findings serves as a baseline to measure periodontal disease activity and success of treatment.

One component of the assessment is probing depth measurements (Figure 9-10). These measurements are made from the free gingival margin to the base of the pocket and recorded to the nearest full millimeter. Measurements are recorded for six specific sites on each tooth—distofacial, facial, mesiofacial, distolingual, lingual, and mesiolingual.

Bleeding on gentle probing comes from ulcerations in the soft tissue wall of a periodontal pocket or from where portions of the epithelium have been destroyed. Penetrating the soft tissue with excessive probing force also could cause bleeding. Exudate, or purulent material, also may occur during probing.

The level of the free gingival margin in relationship to the cementoenamel and mucogingival junctions should be measured and charted (Figure 9-11), as should horizontal and vertical tooth mobility. This movement is assessed by trapping the tooth between two dental instrument handles (horizontal) and using the end of an instrument handle to put pressure against the occlusal or incisal surface of the tooth (vertical). Although the periodontal ligament normally allows some slight movement of the tooth in its socket, the amount of this natural tooth movement is so slight that usually it cannot be seen with the naked eye. The clinician should expect to find no visible movement in a periodontally healthy tooth.

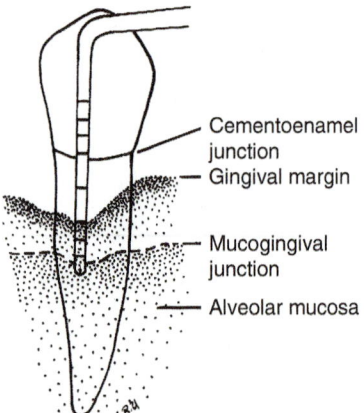

Figure 9–11 The relationship of the gingival margin to the cementoenamel and mucogingival junctions.

Teeth also should be checked for the presence of plaque and dental calculus. Both should be removed, and patients should be counseled in self-care measures such as proper brushing and flossing techniques and habits. Gingival inflammation also should be assessed. Alveolar bone loss should be determined through radiographic imaging (Figure 9-12).

A key component of the periodontal assessment is an accurate gingival description. To describe diseased periodontal tissues, it is important to know what healthy tissues look like (see Table 9-1). In the presence of bacterial plaque at the gingival margin, however, inflammation results in clinical changes in the tissue.

The stages of development of gingivitis and periodontitis are divided into four stages:

- Initial lesion—inflammatory response to bacterial accumulation occurs within two to four days of irritation; no clinical evidence of change appears in the earliest phases; slight marginal redness with enlargement occurs as the infection develops.

- Early lesion (Figure 9-13A)—increased inflammatory response is evident 7 to 14 days after bacterial accumulation; early signs of gingivitis become apparent, with slight gingival enlargement; healthy tissue may be restored and condition reversed.

- Established lesion (Figure 9-13B)—clear evidence of inflammation is present, with marginal redness, bleeding on probing, and spongy marginal gingiva.

- Advanced lesion—bacteria produce irritants and inflammation spreads through the loose connective tissue; pockets form and loss of bone and mobility occurs.

Check Your Ethics

An older adult patient, Mrs. Fisher, who is a regular patient at the office, arrives for a routine examination. As you are seating her, she mentions that she has been having financial problems and that her oral health is the least of her worries. When the dentist comes in, Mrs. Fisher exclaims, "At my age, I don't care if my teeth hurt. It's normal for my age. I'd just rather not know if anything is wrong!" Later the dentist notices some signs that indicate the early stages of periodontal disease, but he completes the examination without mentioning any long-term risks to Mrs. Fisher. What should you do? How should the examination be documented in the patient's chart?

CHECKPOINT

9-27 What are the clinical assessments that should be performed by the dentist or dental hygienist to assess periodontal health?

Treatment of Periodontal Disease

Today, the treatment of periodontal disease is directed at managing the bacteria and local and systemic conditions that increase the risk for periodontal disease.

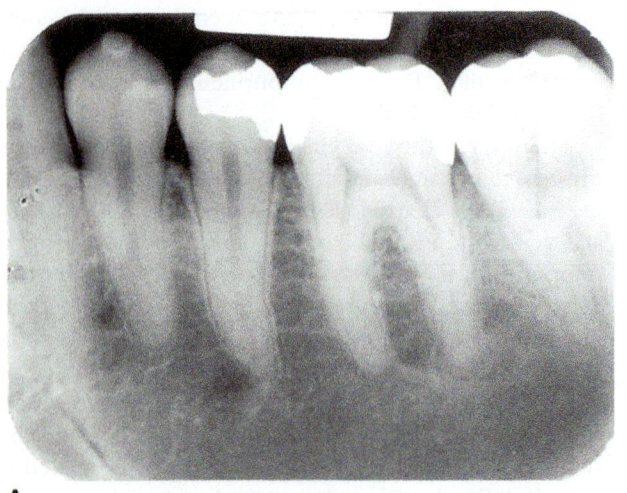

A

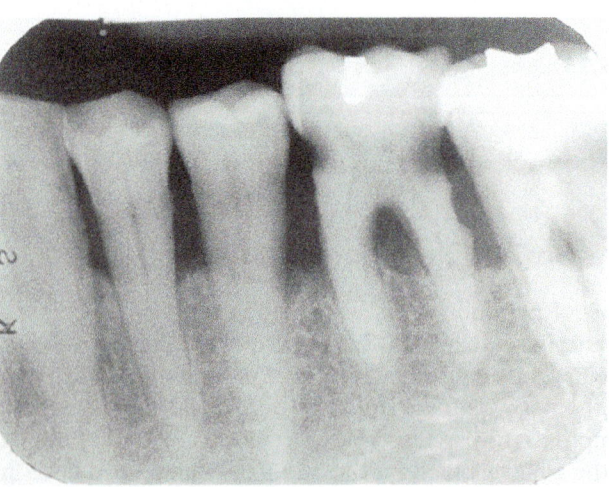

B

Figure 9–12 A. Normal bone level. **B.** Generalized bone loss.

TABLE 9-1	Clinical Appearance of Healthy Tissue versus Gingivitis	
	HEALTHY PERIODONTAL TISSUE	**GINGIVITIS**
Color	Uniform pink Possibly lighter shade in fair-complected blondes and darker in dark-complected brunettes	Bright red due to increased blood flow to the tissue in response to acute inflammation With chronic inflammation, color appears bluish red or purplish red
Size	Tissue lies snugly around tooth and firmly against alveolar bone	Enlargement of marginal and interproximal tissues, in a few areas or entire mouth
Shape	Gingival margin meets tooth with tapered, flat, or slightly rounded edge Follows curvature of tooth to create scalloped contours Papilla come to a point and fill space between teeth	Gingival margin meets tooth in a rolled, thickened edge Interdental papilla are bulbous, blunted, or cratered
Consistency	Attached gingival tissue firmly connected to underlying cementum and alveolar bone Tissue elastic and springs back when probed gently	Swollen, soft, spongy, and non-elastic Tissue easily compressed and retains imprint of probe when pressure is applied
Texture	Surface of attached gingival tissue is firm, may have dimpled appearance	Surface has increased fluid from inflammatory response, causing smooth, shiny appearance Tissue appears stretched
Margin	Gingival margin at or slightly above CEJ	Gingival margin may move further above CEJ
Bleeding	No bleeding upon probing	Spontaneous bleeding upon probing
Exudate	No discharge of purulent material	Purulent material may be visible upon pressure

CEJ, cementoenamel junction.

Professional care includes maintenance appointments as needed to assist patients in controlling disease. Self-care includes educating patients about plaque control techniques and the role bacterial plaque plays in periodontal disease.

Therapy for periodontal disease strives to control the bacterial challenge to the patient, minimize the impact of systemic factors, eliminate or control local risk factors, and stabilize the attachment level. This therapy includes:

- Treatment of emergency conditions
- Extraction of hopeless teeth
- Self-care education, including counseling for nutrition and smoking cessation

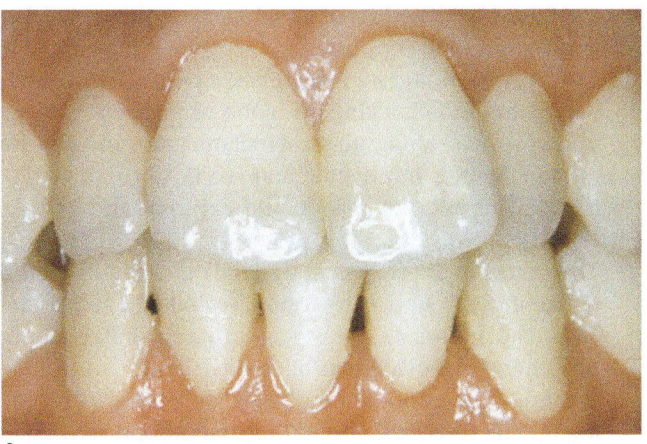
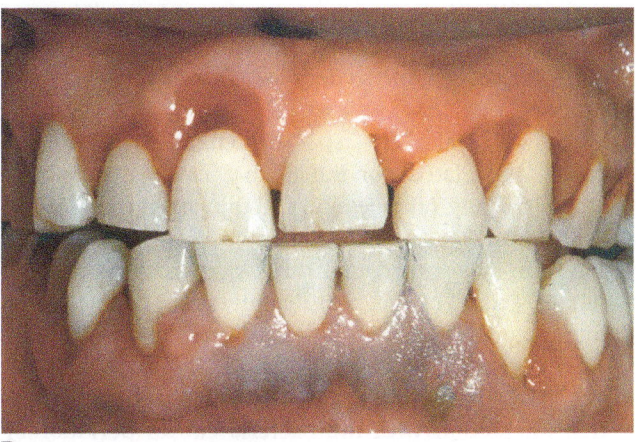

A   B

Figure 9–13 **A.** Early stage of gingivitis shows plaque and marginal inflammation. **B.** Chronic periodontitis shows pronounced changes in the appearance of the gingiva.

- Antimicrobial, fluoride, and occlusal therapy, which may include orthodontics
- Caries control and temporary restorations
- Placement of dental implants
- Root canal therapy
- Periodontal surgery
- Nonsurgical periodontal procedures, which may include root scaling, planing, and bite adjustment
- Replacement of missing teeth
- Dental restorations

Apply it

A pregnant patient has an appointment for a checkup. Most new mothers are eager to optimize their babies' health. What have you learned that you can share with this patient?

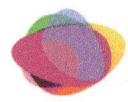

Chapter Highlights

- ✦ Demineralization and remineralization of teeth is an ongoing process. When demineralization outpaces remineralization, dental caries can occur.
- ✦ Among the types of bacteria in the mouth are mutans streptococci (MS) (*Streptococcus mutans*) and lactobacilli (LB). MS and LB convert dietary carbohydrates (sugars and starches) into acids during the digestion process.
- ✦ Areas on teeth where bacteria accumulate—typically at the gingival margin—are called *plaque*. Plaque helps to trap bacteria and acids against the teeth.
- ✦ Left untreated, bacteria and acids can dissolve the mineral content of teeth (demineralization).
- ✦ Good saliva flow is essential to prevent dental caries.
- ✦ The bacteria that cause caries are transmissible, including from parents, siblings, and caregivers to babies, which makes the practice of good oral hygiene within a family even more important.
- ✦ The most prevalent disease of childhood is early childhood caries, which is defined as the presence of one or more decayed, missing, or filled tooth surfaces in any primary tooth in a child between birth and 6 years of age.
- ✦ Early childhood caries can be caused by routine use of a nursing bottle at bedtime or prolonged at-will breastfeeding. Parents should be educated that children's teeth are susceptible to decay as soon as they begin to erupt.
- ✦ Older adults also are especially vulnerable to dental caries. Age-related conditions that cause this vulnerability are gingival recession and the presence of dental amalgams.
- ✦ The two stages of dental caries are incipient lesions, when decay begins to demineralize enamel, and untreated incipient lesions, when overt lesions develop and cavitation occurs.
- ✦ Bacterial plaque plus an individual's immune system interaction with the bacteria causes periodontal disease. Conditions that increase risk for periodontal disease include tobacco use, diabetes, osteoporosis, hormone alteration, psychological stress, and genetic influences.
- ✦ The bacteria that cause periodontal disease can enter the bloodstream and spread, leading to infections in other parts of the body and contributing to heart disease; premature, underweight babies; poorly controlled diabetes; and respiratory diseases.
- ✦ Gingivitis is a bacterial infection that is confined to the gingiva. The tissue damage that gingivitis causes is reversible.
- ✦ Gingivitis is characterized by bleeding upon gentle probing, probing depths that may be greater than 3 millimeters, red or reddish-blue tissue, and swollen edges.
- ✦ Periodontitis is a bacterial infection of all parts of the periodontium. The tissue damage is irreversible.
- ✦ Periodontitis is characterized by spongy tissue with a bright-red or purplish-red and smooth, shiny appearance; light pink tissue with a firm, rigid consistency; swollen or tough edges; bleeding or purulent material emission upon probing; and probing depths that may be greater than 4 millimeters.
- ✦ Signs of periodontal disease include gingival redness, swelling, bleeding, loss of attachment, mobility, and loss of alveolar bone support.
- ✦ Assessment should include checking probe depth measurements and checking for blood or purulent material upon gentle probing, gingival inflammation and gingival margin levels, horizontal and vertical tooth mobility, the presence of plaque and calculus, and alveolar bone loss.
- ✦ The stages of development of gingivitis and periodontitis are initial lesion, early lesion, established lesion, and advanced lesion. As the stages progress, inflammation becomes more evident as bacteria spread.
- ✦ Treatment of periodontal disease is directed at managing the bacteria, oral conditions, and other diseases and risk factors and stabilizing the attachment level.

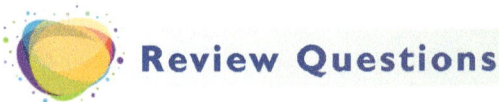 **Review Questions**

1. Dental caries is which of the following?

   a. Transmissible

   b. Infectious

   c. Preventable

   d. All of the above

2. What are the areas on teeth where bacteria accumulate?

   a. Dentin

   b. Cementum

   c. Pulp

   d. Plaque

3. What do bacteria interact with to produce acids in the mouth?

   a. Saliva

   b. Fluoride

   c. Carbohydrates

   d. Lactobacilli

4. Which of these does *not* increase a child's risk for dental caries?

   a. The presence of primary teeth, which contain more water than permanent teeth

   b. The child's reading habits

   c. The child's family's socioeconomic status

   d. The child's routine use of a bottle at bedtime

5. Which of these does *not* describe an area where dental caries occurs?

   a. Pits and fissures

   b. Small spaces between a tooth and its restorative appliance

   c. Gingiva

   d. Smooth surfaces

6. Which of these should you avoid doing to a tooth affected by demineralization?

   a. Scratching

   b. Examining

   c. Shining a bright light on

   d. Remineralizing

7. Which of these is *not* an effective way to remineralize teeth?

   a. Increasing personal use of products containing fluoride

   b. Decreasing snacking

   c. Seeing the patient at frequent dental hygiene appointments for fluoride varnish applications

   d. Increasing teeth's exposure to sunlight

8. Which of these is the current theory about the cause of periodontal disease?

   a. Bacteria cause periodontal disease.

   b. Bacterial plaque plus an individual's immune response reaction to infection and inflammation cause periodontal disease.

   c. Gingivitis always leads to periodontal disease.

   d. Calculus deposits are a mechanical irritant to tissue.

9. Which of these is the most preventable risk factor for periodontal disease?

   a. Menopause

   b. Psychological stress

   c. Diabetes

   d. Tobacco use

10. Which is not a sign of clinical gingivitis?

   a. Bleeding upon probing

   b. Red or reddish-blue tissue

   c. Swollen edges

   d. Horizontal and vertical tooth movement

Active Learning Exercises

1. List and discuss the stages of periodontal disease. Create a professional dialogue to discuss the various stages of the disease with your patient.

2. If a patient cannot afford to undergo periodontal surgery, what less costly alternatives might be suggested?

Application Activities

1. Why do you think diet and personal habits are important for maintaining good oral health? Write a paragraph or two describing how you, as a dental assistant, would explain to a patient the importance of personal factors in maintaining good oral health.

2. To help educate parents about early childhood caries, create a chart that outlines the causes and risk factors for the disease, including strategies for prevention.

PREPARING FOR CERTIFICATION EXAMS

Review the following topics in this chapter to prepare for the Dental Assisting National Board (DANB) exam:

- Introduction

- Development of Caries

- The Process of Periodontal Disease

- Stages of Periodontal Disease

Prevention of Caries and Periodontal Disease

CHAPTER OUTLINE

CHAPTER CHECKLIST

On completion of this chapter, students will be able to:

- ☑ Describe the oral hygiene products and strategies available for patient self-care.
- ☑ Compare and contrast manual and automatic toothbrushes.
- ☑ Explain the role of fluoride in preventive care.
- ☑ Identify the elements of an effective patient education program.
- ☑ Demonstrate the various toothbrushing techniques.
- ☑ Demonstrate proper flossing technique.
- ☑ Describe the methods and strategies for patient risk testing.

KEY TERMS

dental floss – twisted or untwisted thread made of fine, short silk or synthetic fibers, frequently waxed; used for cleaning the interproximal spaces and between the contact areas of the teeth

dental stimulator – device used to massage and increase blood flow in the gingival tissue, frequently made from rubber or wood

dental tape – a wide thread similar to dental floss, composed of fine, short silk or synthetic fibers; used for cleaning interproximal spaces and between contact areas of teeth

dentifrice (DEN-tuh-fris) – any preparation used to cleanse teeth, e.g., a tooth powder, toothpaste, or tooth wash

enamel hypoplasia (hi-poh-PLAY-zhuh) – developmental disturbance of teeth characterized by deficient or defective enamel matrix formation

floss threader – a flexible device resembling a large needle used to transport floss under fixed bridges or behind appliances such as orthodontic wires

fluorosis (fluh-ROH-sis) – a condition caused by an excessive intake of fluoride (2 ppm or more in drinking water), characterized mainly by mottling, staining, or hypoplasia of the tooth enamel

halitosis (hal-ih-TOH-sis) – malodorous breath caused chiefly by bacteria in the oral cavity, and exacerbated by various dietary choices or physical conditions; also called bad breath

interproximal (in-ter-PROK-sih-mul) brush – a brush with nylon bristles meant to penetrate the interproximal space to clean the tooth surface and stimulate the gingival tissue

mouth rinse – a liquid used to clean the oral cavity and treat disorders of oral mucosa; also known as mouthwash

systemic fluoride – fluoride that is ingested and absorbed through the bloodstream

topical fluoride – fluoride that is applied directly to the tooth surface and that penetrates the outermost layer of enamel

xerostomia (ze-roh-STOH-mee-uh) – an oral condition wherein the mouth is dry due to a lack of saliva

xylitol (ZYE-lih-tol) – a sugar substitute that has been shown to help prevent dental caries

Introduction

Modern dentistry is primarily concerned with treating and preventing oral disease. Patients who are motivated to develop and follow a comprehensive oral self-care regimen are much less likely to suffer from dental caries and periodontal disease.

A key part of the dental assistant's job is to help patients understand why self-care is so important and how to best take care of their teeth and gingiva between visits to the dentist's office. Thus, you should be thoroughly familiar with the most current oral hygiene products on the market, know their strengths and weaknesses, and be able to advise patients on which products will work best for them.

Clinical Experience

Patients often have more practical questions about the self-care products they are advised to use and turn to the dental assistant for information. Staying informed can help you guide patients about where to purchase self-care products and their approximate costs. You should also be familiar with generic brands so you can suggest cost-saving alternatives when necessary.

This chapter covers the products and methods patients can use to assist in their own dental care. Ultimately, successful dentistry is a partnership between the dental office and patients. As in any partnership, trust is essential, and in oral health care, this trust is based on the dental professionals' familiarity with and understanding of the various oral health products and resources available today.

Self-Care and Oral Hygiene Aids

Today's patients have a greater selection of oral hygiene products available to them than at any other time in history. Even toothbrushing can seem complicated by the array of toothbrush designs and dentifrices available.

But not all these products are appropriate for every patient. It is important to help patients understand their unique needs—given their diets, dental history, age and health status, and motivation level—and what will work best for them. With every patient, you should encourage open, honest communication so the most effective oral self-care plan can be developed.

At the same time, you should be an encouraging, motivational, and informed partner for your patients. With the right approach, dental assistants can make an enormous difference in their patients' lives.

Patient Motivation

Motivation levels vary widely among different patients—even patients within the same family. It is very important to listen closely to patients as they describe their oral hygiene habits. Ask specific questions regarding the frequency of oral hygiene practices. Sometimes a patient's idea of good oral hygiene may be different from the dental assistant's, so it is important to get as much information as possible. For example, many patients may not be fully aware of the danger that carbohydrates pose to the health of the oral cavity and teeth; even fewer will understand how wide an array of foods—such as milk—can be sources of carbohydrates.

This information will form the basis of future communication. Dental assistants can help patients develop better oral hygiene habits, and even patients with excellent oral hygiene will appreciate the occasional suggestion to refresh their skills or recommendations for new products that are suitable for them.

Developmental Stages

As patients move through their lives, their dental needs change according to their developmental stage. The following is a guide to help dental assistants better understand the unique needs of different developmental stages.

Dental Care for Infants and Children to 5 Years

Early dental care begins in infancy, before the baby's first teeth even come in. Parents and caregivers can gently wipe the baby's gingiva with a clean cloth. This can wipe away plaque and reduce the number of bacteria in the oral cavity. Perhaps equally important, it will begin to acclimate the baby to the concept of oral hygiene.

During infancy, parents and caregivers can begin to teach good oral habits. Infants should never be put to bed with a nursing bottle containing milk or any sweet or sugary drinks. This intensive exposure to sugar can result in a condition known as *early childhood caries* (Figure 10-1) (see Chapter 9, Dental Caries and Periodontal Disease).

As the primary teeth come in, caregivers can begin using a toothbrush and infant toothpaste. Many brands of toothpaste are designed for young children. These typically do not contain fluoride and are flavored in varieties more pleasing to young children. It is highly recommended not to use a fluoridated toothpaste for children under the age of 2 years, because young children cannot completely spit and rinse the mouth well after brushing, and are, thus, more apt to swallow toothpaste. At this age, the idea is both to care for the deciduous teeth and get the child used to toothbrushing and flossing. Over time, the child can take over some of the brushing, but young children should always be supervised, and it is often necessary for the parent or caregiver to finish brushing for them. Children do not have the dexterity to thoroughly brush and floss until about the age of 8 years. Caregivers or parents should also follow through with flossing for young children.

Dental visits in these early years are important. Dentists and dental hygienists can help clean the child's teeth and introduce the child to the idea of preventive dentistry. Office visits should always be a pleasant experience in which children are introduced to the instruments used in dentistry and the habits that comprise good oral hygiene. Good experiences at a young age can set the stage for a lifetime of good oral hygiene habits and comfort with the dentist's office.

Dental Care from Ages 5 to 19 Years

As children pass from young childhood into adolescence and their teen years, they go through profound transformations in their ability to learn new information, form habits, work with authority figures, and take proper care of their teeth. Their dentition also changes throughout these years as deciduous teeth gradually fall out and are replaced by permanent teeth. Orthodontic appliances are common among adolescents ages 10 to 15 years, and nutrition and oral hygiene habits can vary widely or be substandard.

The most important element of working with children and adolescents is to provide the right information, coupled with examples and motivation. Good habits developed in these years are likely to last a lifetime. Younger children are often motivated simply by praise, whereas appeals can be made to teenagers' desire to fit in with the crowd and attract interest from their peers. Dental offices can use poster boards of success stories, videos, and in-office demonstrations to show how plaque and caries form as well as how to properly brush and floss teeth.

Teaching about nutrition is also helpful. The consumption of sugary beverages has skyrocketed in recent decades, especially among children and adolescents. In addition, children often drink juice and sports drinks that may contain a great deal of hidden sugar. Dental assistants can help make children aware of how much sugar they are consuming, and the effect that doing so can have on their teeth. In addition to giving advice for immediate application, dental assistants can point out to children future lifestyle choices that can pose oral health risks, including drug use; tobacco use, whether smoking or smokeless; and snacking or sipping drinks throughout the day (which exposes the mouth to continuous acidic attack, demineralizing the teeth), instead of eating or drinking at a single sitting.

Dental Care for Adults Up to 60 Years of Age

By the time they reach adulthood, many patients have developed good oral hygiene habits and are active partners in their own dental health. However, this is not always the case. Just because a patient is an adult, you should not assume there is no need for continuing education. It sometimes helps to brush up on basic skills, and patients might appreciate a demonstration about proper brushing and flossing.

Gingivitis is common among adults, largely due to inadequate brushing and flossing. Gingivitis is characterized by red and swollen gingival tissue. This tissue often bleeds during brushing and, especially, flossing, and the

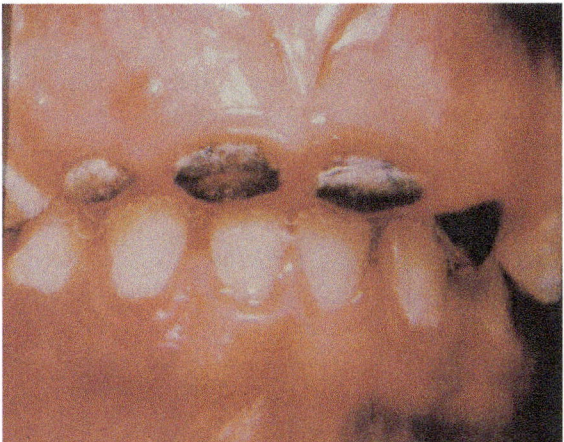

Figure 10-1 Early childhood caries. Also known as *baby bottle mouth*, this condition occurs when babies are allowed to bring a bottle or "sippy cup" to bed. Note the nearly complete loss of tooth structure of maxillary incisors, the abscess on the gingival tissues, and cervical plaque on the mandibular incisors.

patient might experience sensitivity to cold or transient pain. It is important to stress that gingival bleeding during toothbrushing does not mean the area should be avoided. To the contrary, patients should be encouraged to spend extra time in this area—removing plaque near the gingival margin is the best way to fight gingivitis.

If gingivitis is allowed to advance, it becomes periodontitis. This disease is characterized by the formation of pockets between the gingiva and the teeth. As pocket depth increases, the level of the bone holding the teeth may be affected, resulting in bone loss. As bone is lost around the teeth, the teeth will become loose, which, in turn, may result in tooth loss.

Adults suffering from any form of gingival disease should be encouraged to learn more about their condition and how to treat it themselves. Adults are commonly busy (which can discourage a good oral health regimen) and may also fail to grasp the long-term implications of inadequate oral hygiene. You can gently but firmly remind patients of the importance of tooth care and supplement areas where patient knowledge is lacking.

Dental Care for Adults Over Age 60 Years

At this age, the patient's focus might shift to keeping their natural teeth for the rest of their lives. Patients should be made aware that losing teeth is not a natural part of aging—there is certainly no reason patients should routinely lose teeth to oral disease.

At the same time, however, oral hygiene may become complicated by additional factors, such as other diseases and/or medications. Diseases, such as arthritis and stroke, can reduce mobility and make it harder to properly brush and floss. Diabetes can affect circulation in the gingival tissue. Dental assistants can recommend that patients in these situations use special products, such as toothbrushes designed for arthritic hands or dental floss holders that feature small strips of floss embedded in plastic handles.

Medications, too, can affect oral health. Dry mouth (**xerostomia**) is a relatively common side effect of some chronic medications. Patients suffering from dry mouth should know that saliva is an important part of oral health because it helps cleanse the mouth and reduce plaque. Patients suffering from dry mouth can suck on sugar-free hard candies, chew gum, and drink water to stimulate saliva production or, in extreme cases, use saliva replacement. Some chewing gum is designed specifically for patients who have xerostomia.

Nutrition is a persistent concern for some older adults, and numerous studies have shown a close link between oral health and nutrition at this age. Patients who are missing teeth may have a hard time chewing and, therefore, might avoid healthful but hard-to-chew foods like vegetables and fruits. This, in turn, can result in malnutrition that accelerates oral disease. It is very important with older adult patients to stress the connection between nutrition and oral health.

Finally, older adult patients might have appliances and even amalgams that are many decades old and may need to be replaced or fixed.

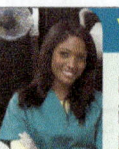

Voice of Experience

In our office, all new dental assistants practice giving patient demonstrations when they are first hired. It makes a big difference! Patients do not appreciate being reprimanded, which is actually counterproductive. We use phrases like, "That's good, but let's try modifying your technique a little bit and see how that feels" or "You're doing a good job. Maybe we can address such-and-such a little, just to refresh, and see if it works even better."

Brushing

Toothbrushing is one major part of a successful oral self-care health program (together with flossing). Ideally, patients should be thoroughly educated in proper brushing techniques from an early age and develop healthy habits they carry into adulthood. Proper toothbrushing is covered under the section Teaching Patients Effective Toothbrushing, later in this chapter. This section will deal with some of the products available and how they can be used to enhance oral hygiene.

The basic concept of a toothbrush is the same no matter what type is used. The brush invariably features a head that contains bristles of varying stiffness, size, and shape, which are used to cleanse tooth surfaces and massage gingival tissue to stimulate blood flow. The brush will also feature a shank and a handle (Figure 10-2). Within this basic design, however, there is wide variation. Moreover, even though they may brush their teeth once or twice (or sometimes more times) a day, many patients use toothbrushes incorrectly.

The two basic types of toothbrushes are manual and automatic. Manual toothbrushes are available in a range of styles, shapes, and sizes. There is no such thing as a perfect toothbrush that suits every patient. Rather, patients should choose their brush based on what works best for their own oral health regimen. The parts of a manual toothbrush include:

- *Head.* The head of the toothbrush is covered with bristles, usually arranged in rows. Bristles can be made

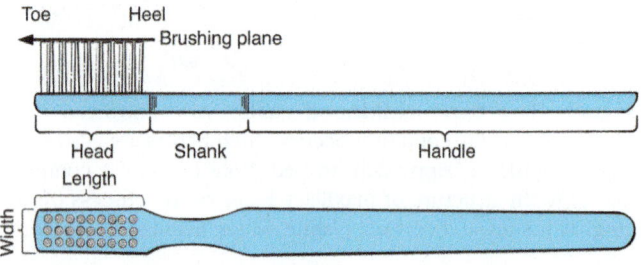

Figure 10–2 Parts of a toothbrush.

from nylon or natural fibers. Most dentists and dental hygienists prefer nylon bristles because they last longer and retain their shape better than natural fibers. The exact configuration of the bristles depends on the brush manufacturer. The head can be oval, rectangular, or some other geometrical shape. Bristles can be of uniform length or arranged in alternating rows of shorter and longer bristles to penetrate deeper into the interproximal area and the grooves on the tooth surface (Figure 10-3). Bristles are available in hard, medium, or soft textures. Most dentists recommend soft bristles because they are more flexible on tender oral tissue and do not abrade the enamel.

- *Shank*. The shank connects the head to the handle. Shanks vary in thickness and can be straight or angled to allow for easier access to posterior teeth. The choice of a shank depends on the patient's oral cavity and preference. The priority is making sure the patient is easily able to reach posterior teeth while brushing.
- *Handle*. Toothbrush handles range in style and shape from simple and unadorned handles to ergonomic and studded designs that are meant to increase grip. Some handles also include rubber tips for gingival stimulation, as well as tongue and cheek cleaners. The choice of a handle depends on the patient's preferences and unique needs.

Automatic toothbrushes have been around for more than 50 years, and their design has advanced considerably. Like manual toothbrushes, automatic toothbrushes have a head that is connected to a handle. However, in most designs, the toothbrush head is replaceable, and the handle is a larger unit that contains the motor. Some varieties have a timer built in that helps ensure patients pay attention to the proper brushing time (usually 30 seconds in each of four quadrants in the oral cavity: upper right, upper left, lower right, and lower left). The handle typically is designed to rest on a charger, which replenishes the built-in power supply.

An automatic toothbrush head may move in a variety of motions, depending on the brand and its design (Figure 10-4). The possible motions include elliptical, semicircular, vibrating, orbital, and reciprocating. Additionally, some models also use sound waves to enhance the brush's effectiveness. The motion of the head helps determine what kind of dentifrice and brushing motion should be used.

Any type of toothbrush can also be used to brush the tongue. Tongue brushing is recommended to help remove bacteria and decaying food from the rear of the tongue, thus creating an oral environment less damaging to tooth enamel. Brushing the tongue daily also often reduces **halitosis** (bad breath).

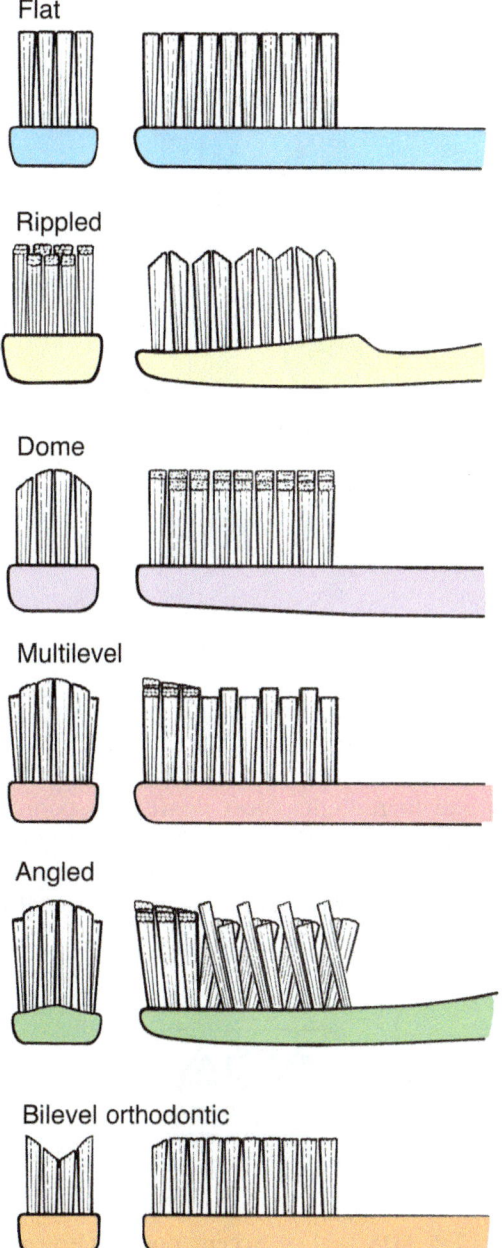

Figure 10–3 Manual brush trim profiles. A variety of filament profiles are available. In addition to the classic flat-planed brush, other trims include rippled, domed, bilevel, multilevel, and angled.

Flat

Rippled

Dome

Multilevel

Angled

Bilevel orthodontic

Cultural Diversity

Clean teeth are not always achieved with a Western-style toothbrush. A common practice among Muslims is cleaning the teeth with a miswak, or chewing stick, which is a twig from the arak tree. The inner bark of the common walnut tree, called dendasa, is also used to clean teeth in parts of Eastern Europe, the Middle East, and Northern Asia. Betel nuts, which are commonly found throughout the tropical Islands of the Pacific as well as some Asian countries, are chewed for their stimulant effects, but the constant chewing is also believed to preserve the tooth surface and clean the gingiva.

Figure 10–4 Power brush trim profiles. Power brushes are made in a variety of brush head shapes, such as oval, teardrop, rectangular, and round. Some power brushes have two different heads on the same brush or interchangeable brush heads.

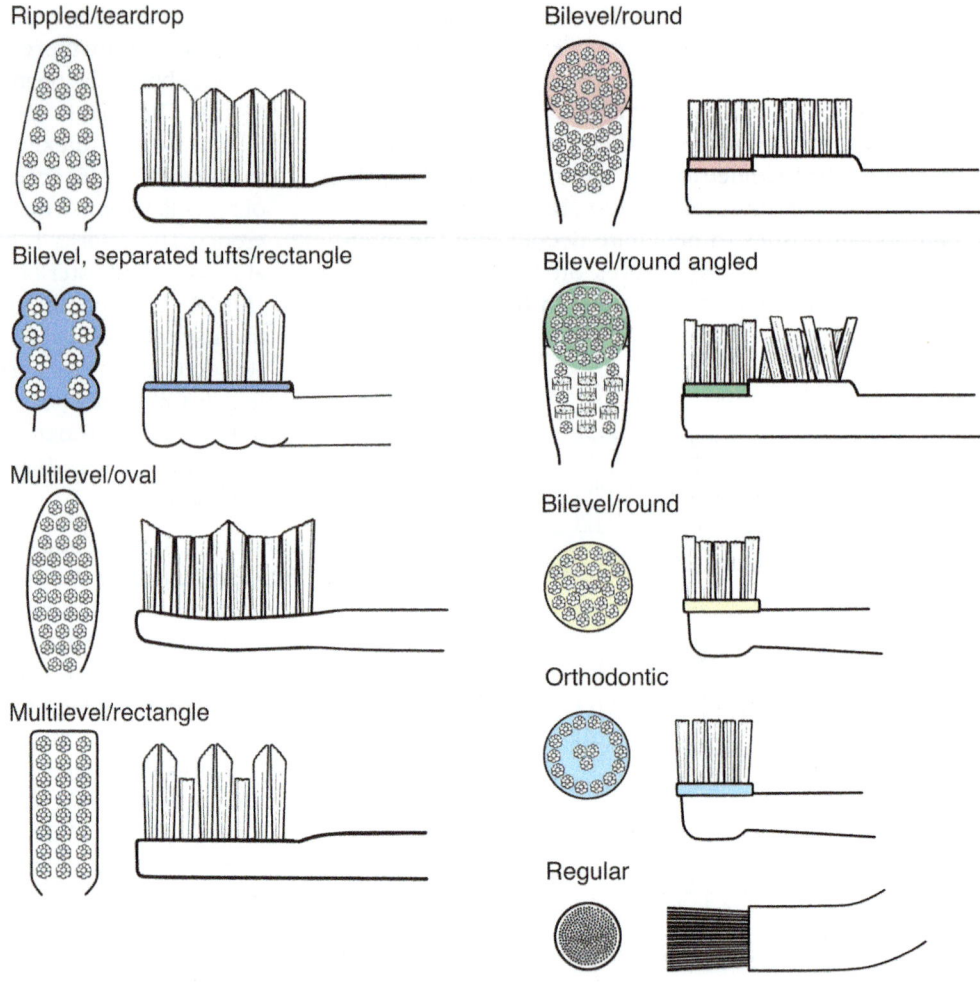

Rippled/teardrop

Bilevel, separated tufts/rectangle

Multilevel/oval

Multilevel/rectangle

Bilevel/round

Bilevel/round angled

Bilevel/round

Orthodontic

Regular

The ADA Seal of Acceptance

The American Dental Association (ADA) introduced its Seal of Acceptance (Figure 10-5) in 1931 to help consumers and dental professional distinguish between products that legitimately helped advance oral health and the various tinctures, potions, and powders that were being advertised as cure-alls for oral disease. The program is voluntary, meaning that manufacturers are not required to seek the ADA Seal of Acceptance as a condition for offering a dental product for sale. However, the ADA Seal of Acceptance means that a product has been examined by ADA expert consultants and the ADA Council on Scientific Affairs and been judged safe and effective. Certification under the ADA Seal of Acceptance program lasts for 5 years, after which time the manufacturer may reapply. As of 2009, more than 300 products carried the ADA Seal of Acceptance.

According to ADA requirements, a Seal Statement must be displayed as part of the product's information and advertising, along with the Seal itself. The Seal Statement explains why the ADA accepted the product into its program. Usually, the statement is one of efficacy, assuring patients that the product can be safely relied upon for oral care, and that the product's advertising and labeling accurately reflects the product's purpose and suitability. Patients can be directed to the ADA website, www.ada.org/sealprogramproducts.aspx, for a list of products that have earned the ADA Seal of Acceptance.

Dentifrice

Dentifrice is another word for *toothpaste*. As with toothbrushes, consumers literally have dozens of types of dentifrices to choose from, including different textures, flavors, and ingredients. Most dentifrices contain fluoride. Depending on their ingredients, dentifrices are also formulated with agents designed to increase whitening, reduce sensitivity, and control stains. Additionally, some

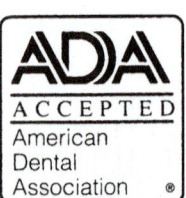

Figure 10–5 ADA Seal of Acceptance. The American Dental Association, Council on Scientific Affairs, awards the Seal to consumer products that meet ADA guidelines for safety and effectiveness. Printed with permission of the American Dental Association.

dentifrices are compounded from organic ingredients and are available as gels, pastes, and even powders and liquids.

Before a discussion of the various ingredients in dentifrices, there are a few generalities that can be applied to any toothpaste. First, patients should seek out a dentifrice that carries the American Dental Association (ADA) Seal of Acceptance (see box). Second, most dentists and hygienists recommend a fluoride-containing dentifrice, for both children and adults. The issue of fluoridation, however, can be controversial to some people. This is covered in greater depth in the Fluoridation section later in this chapter. Finally, most dentists advise against a highly abrasive dentifrice, because it can aggravate gingival tissue and wear away enamel.

Beyond these broad suggestions, a dentifrice should be chosen by each patient, with the assistance of a dental professional's recommendations, to fit the patient's needs and preferences. A dentifrice may include any of the following ingredients:

- *Whitening agents*. Dentifrices might contain a whitening agent, such as hydrogen peroxide or carbamide peroxide. Whether or not whitening dentifrices work is a subject of some controversy, with a lack of long-term, controlled studies. However, these dentifrices are safe for use, although they may aggravate some patients with oral sensitivities. If patients are very concerned about white teeth, they can be referred for an appointment to determine whether a bleaching or whitening office procedure may be appropriate.
- *Dentifrice for sensitive teeth*. Dentifrices designed for sensitive teeth contain ingredients that fill tiny openings in exposed dentin. These openings can expose tender nerve endings. One such ingredient is strontium chloride. Alternatively, dentifrices might include potassium nitrate, which reduces the transmission of pain. It is important to remind patients that it may take a week or two of use for sensitivity to diminish.
- *Calculus control*. Calculus-control toothpastes contain sodium pyrophosphate, which combines in the oral cavity with the chemicals that cause calculus and wash it away. These formulations do not actually remove existing calculus but can help prevent the build up of additional calculus. Note that this toothpaste is effective only on calculus that forms above the gumline; also note that some patients may be sensitive to sodium pyrophosphate and should not use this dentifrice.
- *Organic and herbal preparations*. Organic and herbal toothpastes are available in a wide variety of formulations, based on any number of natural and organic ingredients. The criteria for selecting an organic dentifrice are the same as selecting a conventional dentifrice: it should contain fluoride and, ideally, the ADA Seal of Acceptance.

✓ CHECKPOINTS

10-1 How long do most dentists recommend patients brush their teeth?

10-2 What can parents do for infant children before tooth eruption?

10-3 Is tooth loss a normal part of aging?

10-4 What is the American Dental Association Seal of Acceptance? What does it mean?

Dental Floss and Tape

Dental floss and **dental tape** are designed to clean the interproximal areas between teeth. Dental floss is round, whereas dental tape is flat. They are both equally effective if used correctly.

Even thorough toothbrushing can only clean three of the five surfaces on teeth. However, plaque and calculus also develop on the interproximal areas that a brush can't reach, just as on the larger surfaces.

Although many people maintain regular brushing habits, regular flossing is somewhat rarer. Thus, patients might need to be reminded of the benefits of using floss and dental tape, both for caries prevention and gingival health.

Adults often benefit from a simple demonstration of how to use dental floss and dental tape. Patients should be encouraged to practice in the office until they have mastered the technique. It also sometimes helps to remind patients that gingival bleeding is common at the outset of a flossing program. This is not a sign that they should stop flossing, but it is a sign that the flossing is working to condition the gingival tissue.

To correctly floss, the string or tape should be held taut and then gently massaged along the tooth surface and under the gingiva on both sides of the interproximal space (Figure 10-6). Like brushing, flossing should not be aggressive and painful. Dental floss or tape should be used before toothbrushing. This allows the fluoride in the dentifrice to penetrate into the newly cleaned interproximal space.

A variety of flosses and tapes are available on the market today, including flavored and fluoridated flosses, stretchy flosses, waxed and unwaxed flosses, and fabric flosses. The choice of a particular floss depends on the patient's preference and unique dentition. Research studies have not shown any particular type of floss to be superior.

However, some types of floss might be easier for certain patients to use. Patients should be encouraged to switch varieties until they find one that can easily penetrate the interproximal space and perform its job. Some patients dislike unwaxed floss because it is narrower and shreds more easily than waxed floss. These patients should be encouraged to use waxed floss.

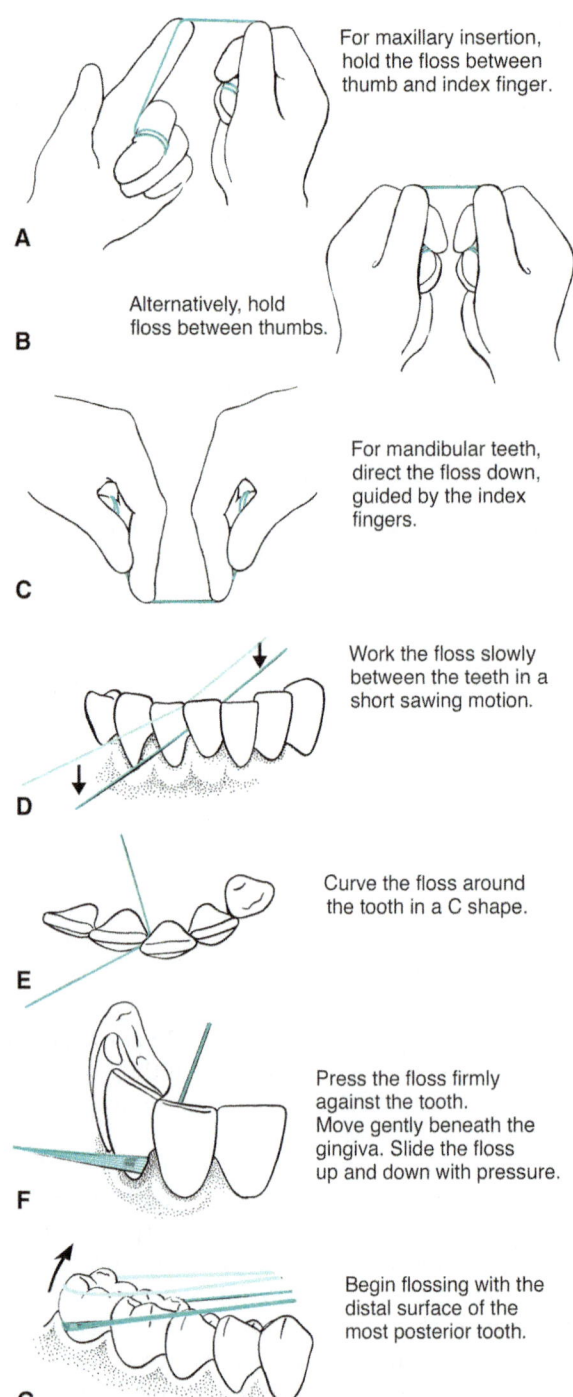

For maxillary insertion, hold the floss between thumb and index finger.

Alternatively, hold floss between thumbs.

For mandibular teeth, direct the floss down, guided by the index fingers.

Work the floss slowly between the teeth in a short sawing motion.

Curve the floss around the tooth in a C shape.

Press the floss firmly against the tooth. Move gently beneath the gingiva. Slide the floss up and down with pressure.

Begin flossing with the distal surface of the most posterior tooth.

Figure 10–6 Use of dental floss, shown in steps **A** through **G**.

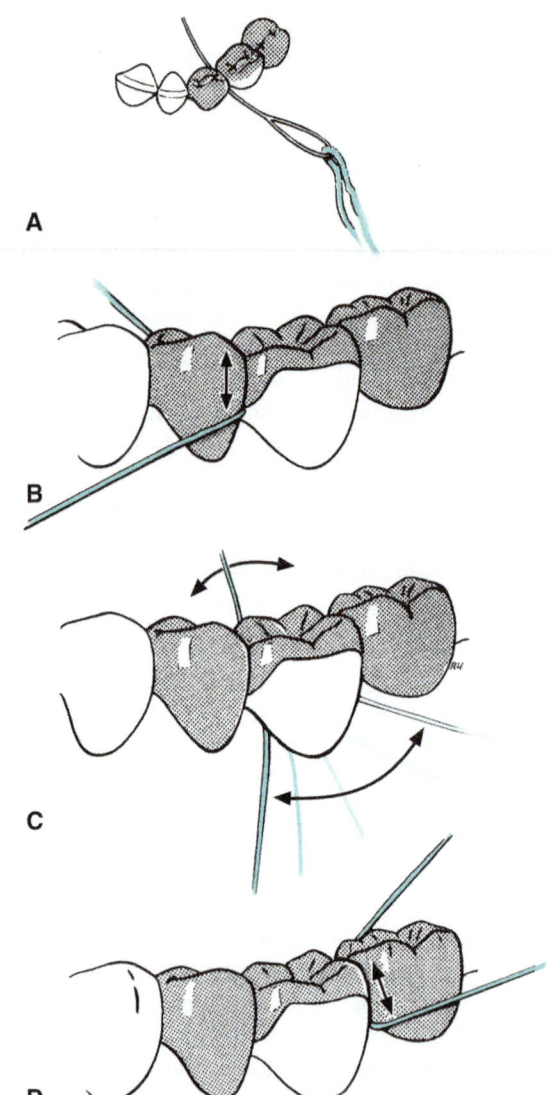

Figure 10–7 Use of floss threader. A. Use floss threader to draw the floss between the teeth of the dental appliance. **B.** Remove the threader, leaving the floss in place. **C.** and **D.** Move floss back and forth to remove dental biofilm.

For patients who cannot hold the floss or tape unaided, a variety of devices are available that hold floss or tape in a plastic handle, stretched between two arms, to allow for easier floss use or tooth access. A device called a **floss threader** is also available for dental appliances (Figure 10-7). This device resembles a large plastic needle with an oversized eye. It works just like a sewing needle: The floss is threaded through the eye, then the threader is pulled through the area to be flossed. Once through, the floss is removed from the threader and left in place to perform its function. This is somewhat more time consuming, and many patients with fixed bridges, orthodontic wires, and other appliances often skip flossing, despite its many benefits to oral health. These patients should be encouraged and shown how to use a threader.

Oral Irrigation

Oral irrigation involves devices that use a jet of water to forcefully expel particles from the interproximal area as well as massage the gingiva with the pulsing water jets. These devices are particularly helpful for patients who cannot or will not floss and those who have oral appliances that make adequate flossing difficult. This includes patients with orthodontic devices, implants, and other appliances.

Although oral irrigation devices help remove plaque and can be an aid to any patient, they are not a substitute for brushing and flossing.

Interdental and Periodontal Aids

Interdental and periodontal aids are designed to complement a brushing and flossing regimen (Figure 10-8).These products are often designed for patients with gingival or periodontal disease or conditions such as diabetes that make them more susceptible to oral disease. Interdental aids include:

■ **Interproximal brush.** This is a small wire device covered with short bristles on one end. It looks somewhat like a pipe cleaner, although the bristles are typically white nylon. Interproximal brushes are available in a variety of configurations, from inexpensive wire devices to devices that resemble a full-sized toothbrush (see Figure 10-8). The purpose of this device is to aid in cleaning interproximal areas or around hard-to-clean appliances such as orthodontic wires.To use the device, the patient inserts it into the area to be cleaned and gently rotates it. Like flossing, this should be done before brushing to allow fluoride to penetrate into the newly cleaned areas.

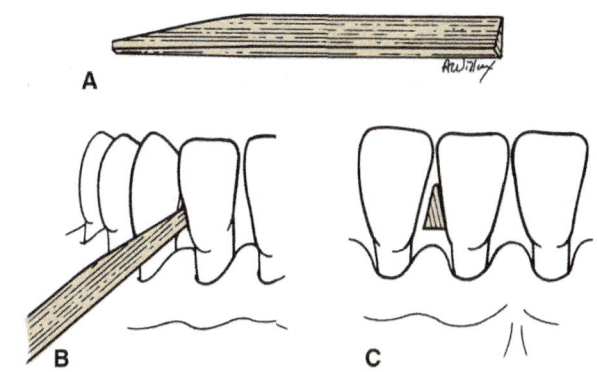

Figure 10–9 Wooden interdental cleaner. A. The 2-inch wooden triangular cleaner. **B.** Application on the proximal surface of a tooth. The base of the triangle is on the gingival side. **C.** The side of the triangle is rubbed in and out against the proximal surface to remove dental biofilm,

■ **Dental stimulator.** Dental stimulators are sometimes included on the handle of a toothbrush, or they can be sold as separate devices (Figure 10-9). These devices are designed to be inserted gently into the interproximal area and rotated lightly to massage the gingival tissue (something that may also be done, carefully, with the fingers), stimulating blood flow to the gingiva and conditioning the tissue—something of benefit to every patient. Wooden dental stimulators should be moistened before use to make them softer and easier on the tissue.

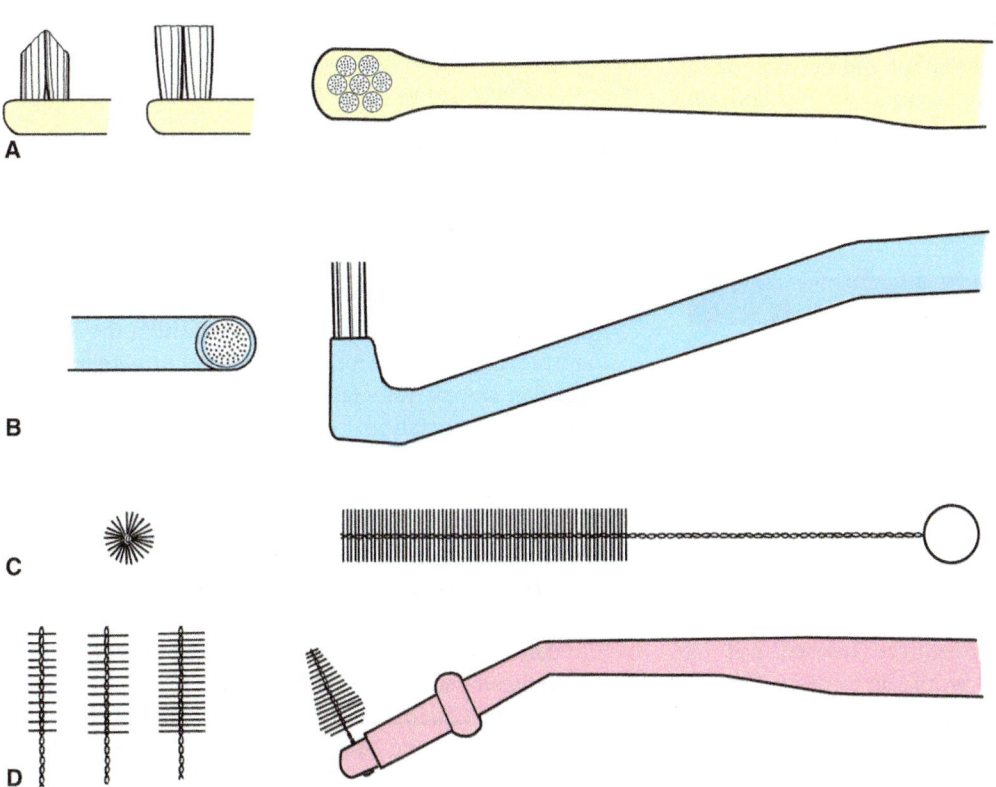

Figure 10–8 Single tuft and interproximal brushes. A. Single-tuft brush with tapered and flat groups of filaments. **B.** Single-tuft brush on handle with angulated shank. **C.** Interproximal brush with filaments twisted into a fine wire that ends in a handle. **D.** Insert brushes for a reusable handle with an angulated shank.

Mouth Rinses

Mouth rinses (or *mouthwash*) are used to flush debris from the oral cavity, freshen the breath, and in some cases, deliver fluoride. Some of the formulas also kill oral bacteria, which reduces the formation of oral calculus and helps fight against gingivitis. Mouth rinses, however, are not a substitution for a comprehensive program of brushing and flossing.

Some patients who are at high risk of caries might benefit from a fluoridated mouth rinse. Prescription mouth rinses generally contain 0.63% stannous fluoride or 0.2% sodium fluoride, whereas over-the-counter formulations contain 0.05% sodium fluoride.

These rinses should be used after brushing, and care should be taken not to swallow the rinse because it is inadvisable to consume excessive fluoride (see Fluoridation section later in this chapter). Fluoride rinses should be swished in the mouth for 1 minute, then spat out. Afterward, patients should refrain from eating or drinking for 30 minutes to allow the fluoride time to work. Some of the fluoridated rinses (e.g., those that contain stannous fluoride) can also help reduce tooth sensitivity.

Recently, a number of mouth rinses have also been developed to whiten teeth. These rinses usually contain the same whitening ingredients as whitening dentifrice. Patients should be advised that they are not dangerous to use, but that they can aggravate sensitive teeth. If patients develop tooth sensitivity after using a whitening mouth rinse, they should discontinue its use. The effectiveness of whitening rinses remains a subject of study, with a lack of long-term, high-quality studies showing their effectiveness.

Advise patients to read the list of ingredients on a mouthwash prior to using it. Some mouthwashes contain high amounts of alcohol and are not recommended for children or recovering alcoholics.

Dental Facts

Believe it or not, mouth rinses have been with us for thousands of years—although the ancients had a much different idea of what made a good rinse! In ancient Egypt, the first known mouthwash was made from the urine of preadolescent boys.

Chewing Gum

In eras past, children were routinely advised not to chew too much gum or they would get caries. This is still true for many sweetened gums, but new varieties of gum have been introduced that actually help *prevent* dental caries.

The act of chewing gum by itself can be beneficial for oral health. It exercises the jaw muscles, and, by stimulating saliva production, it helps to carry away debris in the oral cavity, including acidic plaque. Some patients with xerostomia, whether caused by illness, age, or medications, try to alleviate their condition by chewing gum. Some newer gums are formulated with **xylitol**, a nonfermentable sugar alcohol used as a sugar substitute similar to aspartame, sorbitol, and saccharine. However, among these, only xylitol has been shown to help prevent caries. It is thought to work by preventing bacteria from producing acid and inhibiting the growth of the *Streptococcus mutans* bacteria.

From the Dentist's Perspective

In my office, I rely on dental assistants to work closely with patients and show them how to use all the oral health products we recommend. This means I need dental assistants who stay current with the field and, especially, professionals who can really educate my patients and show them how to be the best partner possible in their own dental health.

Preventive Dentistry

Fluoridation

Derived from fluorine, fluoride is a mineral nutrient thought to prevent caries and support healthy teeth. Use of fluoride may slow tooth demineralization and enhance remineralization. Although use of fluoride may begin even before tooth eruption and continue throughout life, levels of use change as patients age.

However, the subject of fluoridation has become increasingly controversial over the past few decades. People who are opposed to fluoridation of drinking water cite, among other reasons, the following:

- Opposition to the use of fluoride by several prominent global health institutions, among them the Pasteur Institute, the U.S. Environmental Protection Agency, the Canadian Dental Association, and the International Chiropractors Association.
- The banning of fluoridation or the refusal to fluoridate in many nations, including Austria, Belgium, China, the Czech Republic, Denmark, Finland, France, Germany, Hungary, India, Israel, Japan, Luxembourg, the Netherlands, Northern Ireland, Norway, Scotland, Sweden, and Switzerland.
- Opposition to the use of fluoride by prominent dental health figures such as Dr. Hardy Limeback (former president of the Canadian Association for Dental Research; current head of the University of Toronto Department of Preventive Dentistry), and Brian A. Burt (professor

emeritus at the University of Michigan School of Public Health, Department of Epidemiology).

This section examines how fluoride works and some of its effects. When confronted with questions about fluoride, dental assistants should be able to address patients' concerns by presenting factual information.

Biology of Fluoride

Fluoride is a naturally occurring substance. It can be found in small amounts in plants and animals, although the majority of the fluoride to which modern humans are exposed is through fluoridation programs and commercial foods and beverages. Fluoride can be absorbed through the bloodstream, in the gastrointestinal tract, or directly by the outermost layer of tooth enamel during a topical application.

Use of fluoride may begin even before tooth eruption. Prior to eruption, the developing tooth is exposed to a small amount of maternal fluoride. Once it reaches the tooth, the fluoride replaces the hydroxyl ion on a structure called the *apatite crystal*, creating a new structure called the *fluoroapatite crystal*, which supplements tooth enamel and adds mass to the tooth. By this means, fluoride accumulates in bone and enamel, increasing their mass but also increasing their brittleness. Fluoride can also promote tooth remineralization to an extent and discourage some oral bacteria.

Just after tooth eruption, the absorption rate for fluoride reaches its peak level; at this time fluoridation is often begun through topical treatments.

As a person goes through life, fluoride use will change as well. In particular, medical authorities recommend that fluoride never be given to children, whether through treatments or toothpaste, and some advise against fluoride in drinking water. Similarly, patients with kidney disease or acquired immunodeficiency syndrome are at increased risk of fluoride poisoning, as are older adults. Adults with root exposure are encouraged to have in-office fluoride treatments out of concern that the roots of their teeth are not covered by enamel and are, thus, more prone to decay.

Fluoride Delivery

The various fluoride compounds are delivered to the teeth as either of two forms:

- **Systemic fluoride.** Fluoride that is ingested is systemic fluoride. This is absorbed through the bloodstream and delivered to teeth through the tiny blood vessels that supply the oral cavity. The kidneys are able to process and excrete only about half the body's fluoride intake; the remainder accumulates in the pineal gland, the bones, the teeth, and even the brain. Patients can obtain systemic fluoride from foods, beverages, and supplements. However, as stated by the U.S. Centers for Disease Control, "[fluoride's] actions primarily are topical for both adults and children"; systemic fluoride, thus, does not have its primary effect on teeth, but as a substance retained, in increasing amounts over time, within the body.

- **Topical fluoride.** Topical fluoride is applied directly to the surface of the tooth. Topical fluoride delivery systems include dentifrices, foams, rinses, gels, tablets, varnishes, and other methods. The main source of topical fluoride is toothpaste, which brings fluoride into direct contact with the enamel on a daily basis. Because fluoride should not be ingested, young children should be closely supervised during toothbrushing to make sure they do not swallow the toothpaste or the topical fluoride treatments that may also be given in the office (see Topical Fluoride Treatments section later in this chapter).

Systemic fluoride is available in some foods that naturally contain fluoride, and, in many cities, community water supplies contain supplemental fluoride. The fluoridation of community water began in 1945, when the city of Grand Rapids, Michigan, began adding small amounts of fluoride to the drinking water. Dental caries in the city dropped by about 60%, and other cities soon followed suit; however, modern research has failed to uphold a connection between ingestion of fluoride and reduction in caries. Some bottled water also contains fluoride.

Today, about 60% of cities and municipalities in the United States, and about 40% in Canada, fluoridate their water. However, fluoridation is not uniform, and in many countries, adding fluoride to drinking water is prohibited because of widespread concern about fluoride toxicity.

Topical Fluoride Treatments

Topical fluoride treatments are sometimes given to children who live in areas without fluoridated drinking water. They may also be given to other patients, including children who are at high risk of dental caries.

Topical fluoride is administered in a gel or foam that is applied directly to the teeth for a specified amount of time after they have been cleaned. The frequency of application depends on the type of fluoride used. Typically, topical fluoride is administered once or twice a year.

Topical fluoride treatments include:

- 2% sodium fluoride. Applied at 1-week intervals for 4 weeks (usually at ages 3, 7, 11, and 13 years), sodium fluoride is also used for patients with composite or porcelain restorations, because acidulated fluoride may cause pitting.
- 1.23% acidulated phosphate fluoride. This is the preferred option by most dentists and is applied once or twice a year in a gel or foam form, or as a varnish coated on the teeth using an applicator.

Procedure 10-1 Applying Topical Fluoride

In some states, dental assistants are allowed to apply topical fluoride as an expanded function after meeting additional training and licensing requirements.

Topical fluoride is available in gels and foams.

Materials needed (Fig. P10-1-1):

- Topical fluoride
- Disposable applicator trays
- Saliva ejector
- Air/water syringe
- Cotton rolls
- Timer
- Appropriate personal protective equipment (PPE)

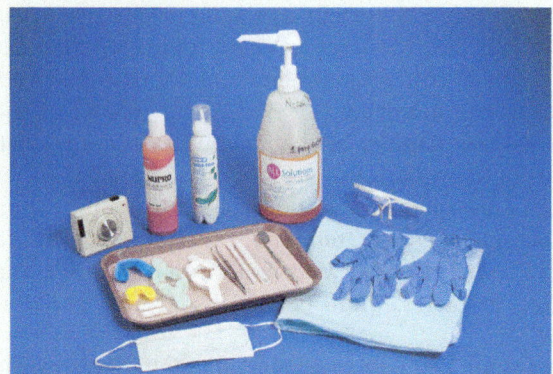

Figure P10-1-1

1. Put on appropriate PPE.
2. Begin by selecting the appropriate size disposable tray. Trays should adequately cover all teeth, but not extend beyond the distal surface of the most posterior tooth (Fig. P10-1-2). Trays are available as single- or double-arch trays, but not all patients can accommodate a double-arch tray.

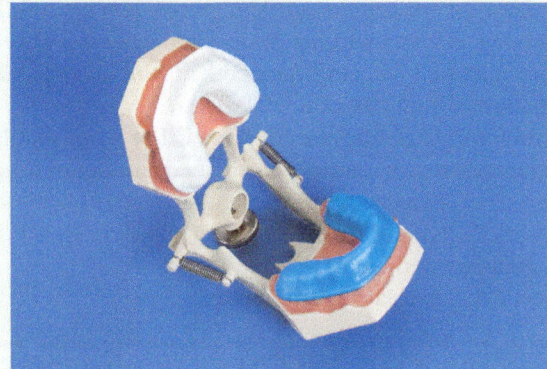

Figure P10-1-2

3. Make sure that no calculus is present. If it is, request that a hygienist or dentist remove it before beginning. Fluoride cannot penetrate through calculus, but it can penetrate through plaque.

4. Explain the procedure to the patient (Fig. P10-1-3). Ask if the patient would like water to drink before beginning the procedure, because it will be necessary for the patient to abstain from food or drink for 30 minutes following the treatment.

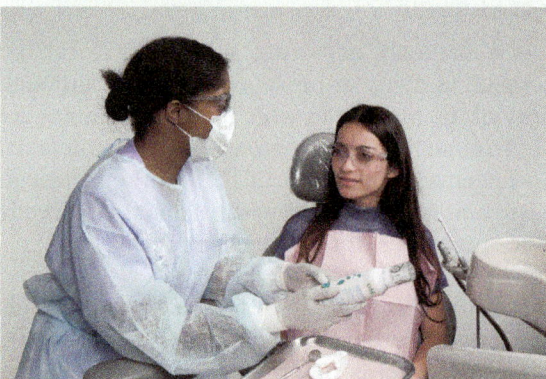

Figure P10-1-3

5. Seat the patient in an upright position to prevent accidental ingestion of the fluoride. Instruct him or her not to swallow any fluoride during the treatment.

6. Load the fluoride into the tray, using only as much as the manufacturer recommends for that type of fluoride and the patient's age (Fig. P10-1-4). Do not overload the tray.

7. Dry the teeth using the air/water syringe (Fig. P10-1-5).

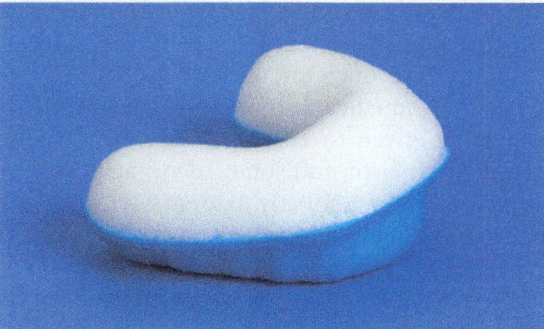

Figure P10-1-4

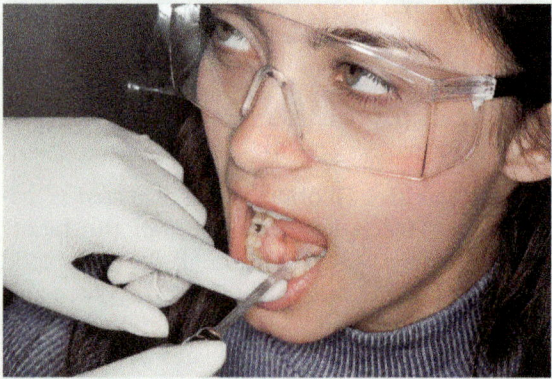

Figure P10-1-5

Procedure 10–1 Applying Topical Fluoride (Continued)

8. Insert the tray into the patient's oral cavity (Fig. P10-1-6A), placing cotton rolls between the arches. Instruct the patient to gently bite down on the cotton rolls, which will spread the fluoride throughout the teeth (Fig. P10-1-6B). After this initial step, remove the cotton rolls, quickly place the saliva ejector in the patient's mouth, and ask the patient to tilt his or her head forward to prevent accidental swallowing of fluoride during the treatment (Fig. P10-1-6C).

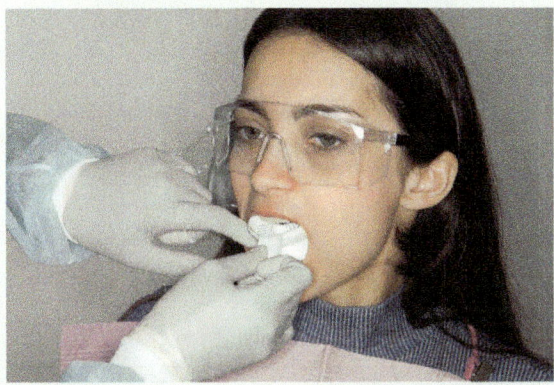

Figure P10-1-6A

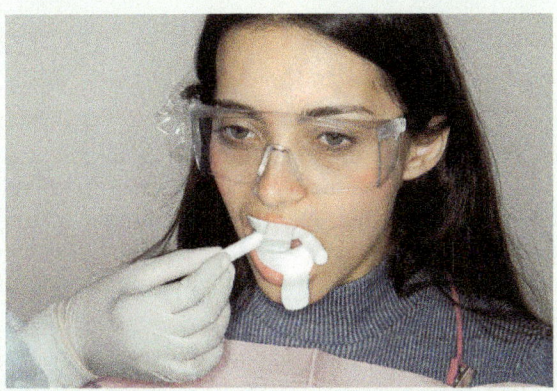

Figure P10-1-6B

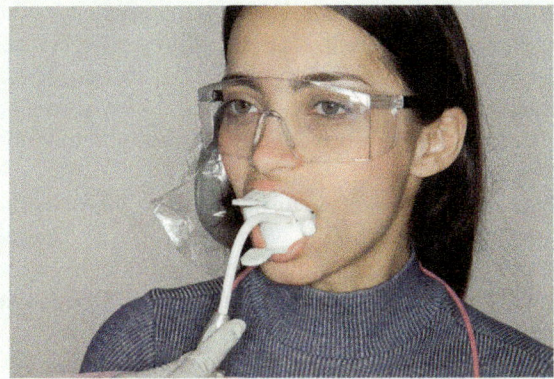

Figure P10-1-6C

9. Set the timer for the appropriate time, based on the form of fluoride (Fig. P10-1-7). Stay with the patient throughout the treatment.

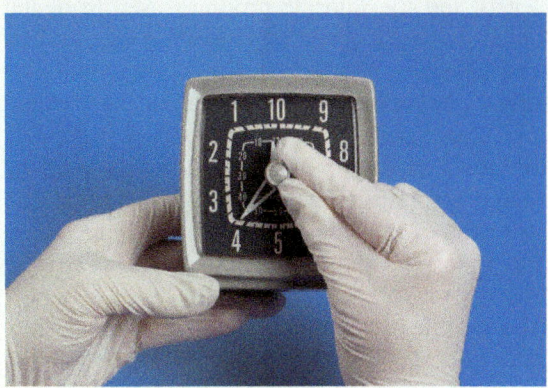

Figure P10-1-7

10. Remove the tray after the timer has ended. Tell the patient not to swallow any fluoride or rinse the oral cavity. Immediately use the saliva ejector or high-volume oral evacuator to remove excess saliva and fluoride from the oral cavity for the patient (Fig. P10-1-8).

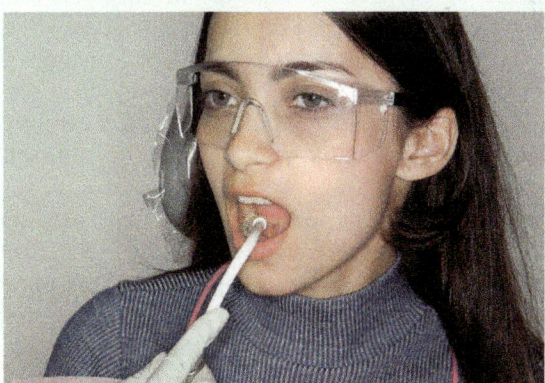

Figure P10-1-8

11. Make a note of the procedure in the patient's record. Instruct the patient not to eat, drink, rinse, or brush for at least 30 minutes. If some fluoride is accidentally swallowed and upsets the patient's stomach, advise the patient to drink milk or ingest milk of magnesia.

Fluoride Toxicity

A large body of research has been conducted into the ideal fluoride levels, and the fluoride products used in dental practices pose no health threat to patients, as long as they are used responsibly.

The normal level of fluoride found in fluoridated drinking water is 1 part per million (ppm), or 1 part fluoride per million parts of water. When fluoridation programs are considered, it is important to take into account all the potential sources of fluoride in a patient's life, including community water, oral health products, and any other sources.

It is important that patients not receive too much fluoride, because fluoride, like many nutrients, can be toxic at high levels. There are two forms of fluoride toxicity:

- *Acute.* This condition is very rare. Acute fluoride poisoning occurs when people ingest potentially fatal amounts of fluoride. A lethal dose of fluoride can be 2.5 mg/kg in an adult (for a 165-pound adult, less than 190 milligrams), 125 milligrams (less than a child-sized tube of flavored toothpaste) in an 8-year-old, and less than 60 milligrams in infants. If acute fluoride poisoning is suspected (e.g., a patient consumes a fluoride-containing product), emergency medical services should be contacted, and the person should be encouraged to drink milk, which calms the stomach and reduces nausea.
- *Chronic.* Chronic fluoride poisoning occurs when patients are exposed to high levels of fluoride over a longer period of time. This might occur, for example, if a patient regularly swallows fluoride rinses, drinks fluoridated water, and consumes multiple other streams of fluoride. Chronic fluoride poisoning can result in several conditions:
  - Skeletal hypermineralization. Sometimes called *crippling fluorosis*, this is a degenerative bone condition.
  - Mottled enamel. Mottled enamel is characterized by uneven coloration of the enamel (**enamel hypoplasia**) caused by exposure to excess fluoride levels during tooth development (Figure 10-10). This condition is known as **fluorosis.** It occurs after long-term exposure to fluoride levels ranging from 1.8 to 2.0 ppm, an exposure level possible because not only drinking water but also many commercial foods and beverages contain fluoride. (Moreover, fluoride collects in high levels in dried plants; some people have developed fluorosis merely by habitual consumption of tea.)

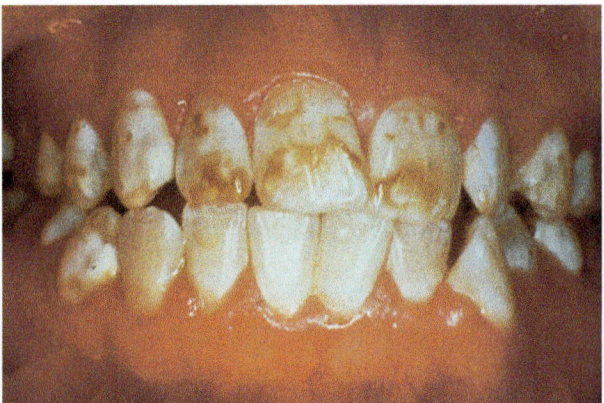

Figure 10–10 Mottled enamel. Moderate to severe staining due to fluorosis.

CHECKPOINTS

10-5 What's the difference between dental floss and tape? Which is better?

10-6 What is xylitol?

10-7 What is the usual level of fluoride in drinking water?

10-8 When is the absorption rate of fluoride the highest?

10-9 What is the condition called when children are exposed to too much fluoride?

Patient Education

An effective self-care oral health regimen depends on successful patient education. As the number of dental products on the consumer market proliferates, it is more important than ever to make sure that patients are armed with accurate information. The elements of an effective patient education program include:

- *Information.* Patients should be thoroughly briefed in the products that are beneficial to them, including universal products like toothbrushes and specialized products for unique needs. For example, patients who are at high risk for caries might benefit from oral rinses containing supplemental fluoride. Likewise, dental assistants can help patients understand how nutrition and lifestyle habits contribute to healthy teeth and gingiva.
- *Product demonstrations.* During in-office visits, dental assistants can help patients with the proper technique for brushing, flossing, and using other products, such as interdental stimulators and floss threaders. Occasional updates can be helpful.
- *Encouragement.* Oral health self-care is a habit, and good habits lead to good results. It is always a good idea to interact with patients in an encouraging way, offering them motivation and information as well as advice on how to obtain optimal results. It is important to strike the right balance between sharing the

consequences of poor oral health (but be careful not to frighten patients, which can be counterproductive) and offering encouragement that everyone, no matter their situation, can create solid oral health self-care habits that will benefit them for a lifetime. When you make recommendations to a patient, be sure to document them in the patient's chart for the office's records.

Teaching Patients Effective Toothbrushing

Like any tool, a toothbrush is only as effective as its operator. Effective toothbrushing means cleaning all the available surfaces of teeth. Most dentists and hygienists recommend that patients brush their teeth for 2 to 3 minutes, following the same pattern every time. Patients should brush twice a day ideally, in the morning and at night. Motivated patients can be encouraged to brush after every meal, including lunch. Patients should be advised that toothbrushing does not mean a vigorous attack on their teeth. Powerful scrubbing can actually damage teeth (by deteriorating tooth enamel) and gingival tissue (by detaching gingival tissue from the tooth surfaces) and may cause toothbrush abrasion.

When asked to demonstrate their toothbrushing, patients are often surprised by how long 2 to 3 minutes actually is—it turns out they have been brushing their teeth for only a fraction of the recommended time. Some patients correct this by using timers, others by counting the number of strokes in each area. Patients should

be encouraged to use whatever method works, as long as they adequately brush.

No matter how thoroughly a patient brushes, toothbrushes cannot reach into the interproximal areas. Ideally, brushing should follow flossing, thus cleaning all five surfaces of the teeth.

When it comes to actually brushing, dentists have developed several techniques to guide patients in the right motions to both clean teeth and stimulate the gingiva, including:

- Bass and Modified Bass Brushing Technique. This is the most frequently recommended technique. It was developed by Dr. C. Bass. Bass brushing removes plaque along the gingival margin.
- Modified Stillman Brushing Technique.
- Charters Brushing Technique

These techniques are distinguished by the placement of the bristles and the motion of the toothbrush head. They are covered more completely in Procedures 10-2, 10-3, and 10-4.

Check Your Ethics

Toothbrushing

You are working with a patient to demonstrate the proper brushing technique, but the patient is not getting it. After a minute or two, you realize that you are late for the next patient. What is the right thing to do?

Procedure 10-2 **Teaching the Bass Brushing Technique**

The Bass brushing technique is the easiest to learn and provides a thorough cleansing of the gingival margin, but it does not clean the remaining tooth surfaces as well as the other techniques. The following steps can be used to teach patients how to use this technique. Allow patients to practice in front of a hand mirror in the office so they can see the motions.

Materials needed:

- Toothbrush
- Hand mirror
- Appropriate PPE

1. Put on appropriate PPE.
2. Teach patients how to use the Bass brushing technique, outlined in steps 3–5.

3. Hold the brush with the bristles at a 45-degree angle to the gingival sulcus, placing the bristles directly against the tissue (Fig. P10-2-1).

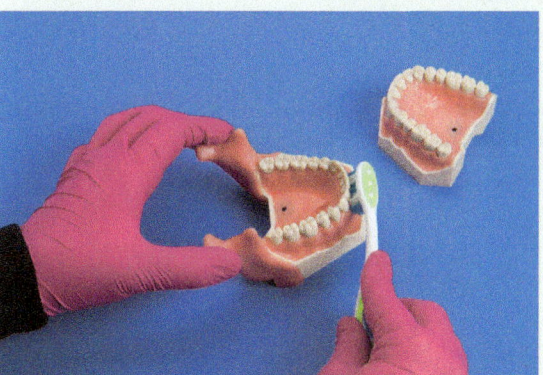

Figure P10-2-1

Procedure 10–2 Teaching the Bass Brushing Technique (Continued)

4. Use short, back-and-forth strokes to vibrate the brush head (without moving the tips of the bristles) against the sulcus for 10 seconds in each area until all areas have been cleaned (Fig. P10-2-2).

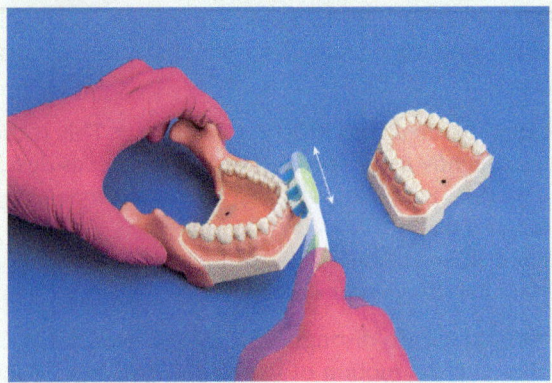

Figure P10-2-2

5. To use the modified Bass technique, after the vibration motion is completed at the sulcus in each area, sweep the

bristles along the tooth surface, toward the biting surface of the tooth (Fig. P10-2-3). This is sometimes called a "rolling stroke." It is designed to remove plaque and debris from the tooth surface.

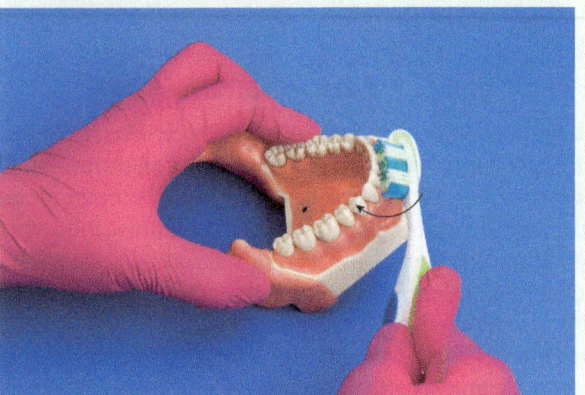

Figure P10-2-3

6. Have patients practice and correct their technique as necessary.

Procedure 10–3 Teaching the Modified Stillman Brushing Technique

The modified Stillman technique begins with the bristles held in a different orientation and helps stimulate the gingiva, increasing blood circulation. The following steps can be used to teach patients how to use this technique. Allow patients to practice in front of a hand mirror in the office so they can see the motions.

Materials needed:

- Toothbrush
- Hand mirror
- Appropriate PPE

1. Put on appropriate PPE.
2. Teach patients how to use the modified Stillman brushing technique, outlined in steps 3–6.

3. Begin by placing the brush next to the target teeth, with the flat surface of the toothbrush head on the same plane as the biting edge of the tooth (Fig. P10-3-1).

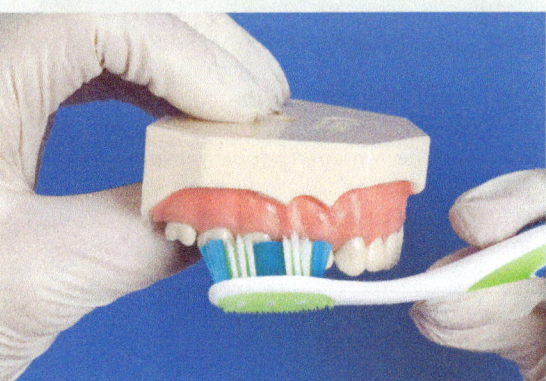

Figure P10-3-1

Procedure 10–3 Teaching the Modified Stillman Brushing Technique (Continued)

4. Rotate the bristles downward (a gingival stimulation technique), so they come into full contact with the gingival sulcus, and gently vibrate the toothbrush head, as in the Bass method, while counting to 10 (see Fig. P10-2-2).

5. Repeat the same motion at least 5 times in every area.

6. Optionally, add a rolling stroke, by sweeping the bristles along the tooth surface, toward the biting surface of the tooth, after the vibration is done (Fig. P10-3-2).

7. Have patients practice and correct their technique as necessary.

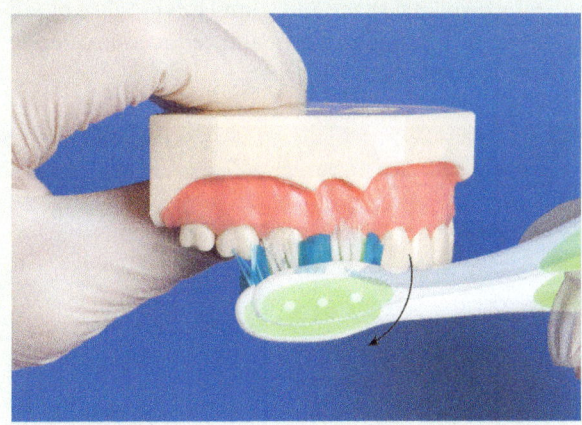

Figure P10-3-2

Procedure 10–4 Teaching the Charters Brushing Technique

The Charters brushing method is especially useful for patients with orthodontic appliances and those who need a little extra cleaning in the interproximal areas. It is less effective, however, at massaging the gingival sulcus. The following steps can be used to teach patients how to use this technique. Allow patients to practice in front of a hand mirror in the office so they can see the motions.

Materials needed:

- Toothbrush
- Hand mirror
- Appropriate PPE

1. Put on appropriate PPE.

2. Teach patients how to use the Charters brushing technique, outlined in steps 3–5.

3. Begin by placing the toothbrush near the target teeth with the bristles facing toward the biting surface of the tooth and the toothbrush head facing the apices. The bristles should be covering the gingival sulcus (Fig. P10-4-1).

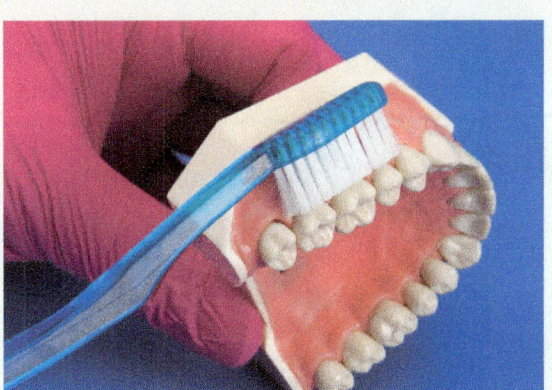

Figure P10-4-1

4. Press the bristles toward the teeth and vibrate the toothbrush head, as in the Bass method, for 10 seconds. (see Fig. p10-2-2) Repeat until all areas have been cleaned.

5. Because this technique does not clean the occlusal surface, a rolling stroke motion (see Procedure 10-2) should precede this method to effectively clean all the tooth surfaces (see Fig. P10-3-2).

6. Have patients practice and correct their technique as necessary.

Teaching Patients Effective Flossing

Properly used, dental floss (or dental tape) removes plaque from the interproximal space and stimulates gingival blood flow, resulting in healthier gingiva and reduced incidence of gingivitis and periodontal disease.

Once patients have made the choice of which floss works best for them, you can assist them in the correct technique to use it, as outlined in Procedure 10-5.

Procedure 10-5 Teaching Flossing Technique

Materials needed:

- Dental floss or tape
- Hand mirror
- Appropriate PPE

1. Put on appropriate PPE.

2. Provide patients with a length of floss or tape about 18 inches long (Fig. P10-5-1). You can either demonstrate this first, or invite them to wash their hands and then guide them through performing the procedure themselves. Either way, patients should have the opportunity to demonstrate flossing technique unaided after they have learned the proper technique. If demonstrating flossing technique for your patient, a hand mirror is necessary so that the patient can see what you are doing.

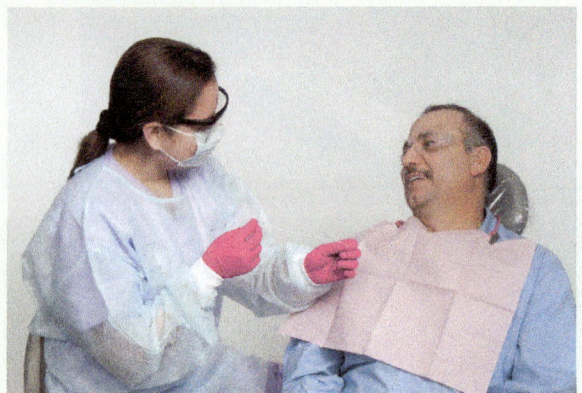

Figure P10-5-1

3. Wrap the floss around the middle or ring fingers on both hands, leaving about 3 inches of working floss between the hands (Fig. P10-5-2A).

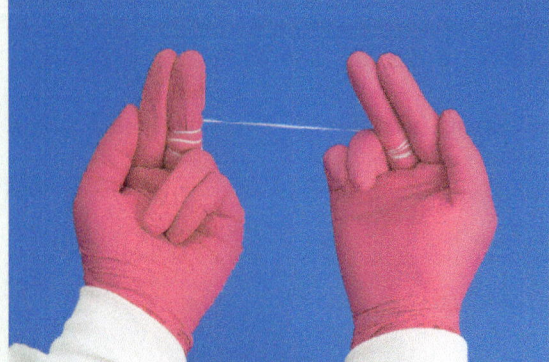

Figure P10-5-2A

4. Grip the working floss with the thumb and index finger, reducing the working space to less than 1 inch (Fig. P10-5-2B). This is the floss that will do the actual work.

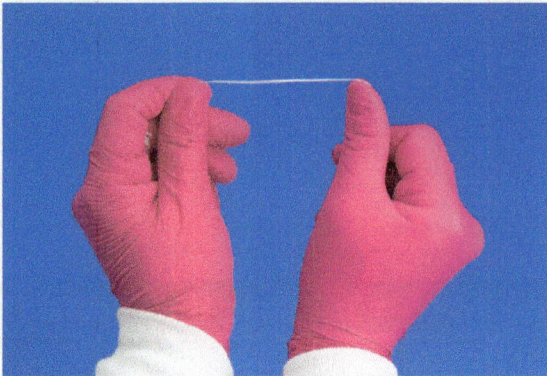

Figure P10-5-2B

5. Direct the floss to the target teeth, using thumbs and index fingers to position it between the teeth. Using a gentle sawing motion, guide the floss between the teeth. Do not snap it into place or violently saw it into the gingival tissue.

6. Do the side of one tooth first, followed by the adjacent surface of the proximal tooth. The correct motion involves bending the floss into a C-shape that conforms to the tooth surface, then gently moving the floss up and down. The floss should be pressed down gently into the gingival sulcus. When resistance is encountered, this means you've reached the bottom of the gingiva and should press no further (Fig. P10-5-3A).

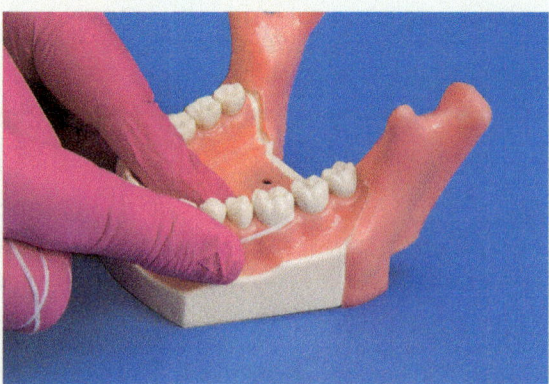

Figure P10-5-3A

Procedure 10–5 Teaching Flossing Technique (Continued)

7. Repeat this step for the adjacent surface of the proximal tooth, pressing down gently into the gingival sulcus (Fig. P10-5-3B).

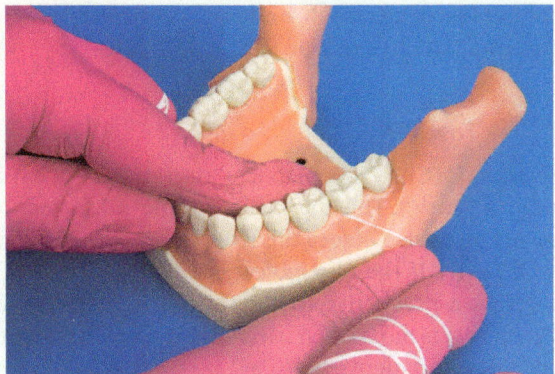

Figure P10-5-3B

8. Repeat steps 5–7 for all interproximal areas, alternately using the thumbs or index fingers to guide the floss, depending on whether you are doing maxillary or mandibular teeth. As you are flossing, slide the floss so you are using a fresh section rather than frayed or dirty floss.

9. Instruct the patient that, unlike brushing, flossing need be performed only once daily. Optimally, patients will floss before bed, thus removing the day's accumulation of plaque and food (Fig. P10-5-4).

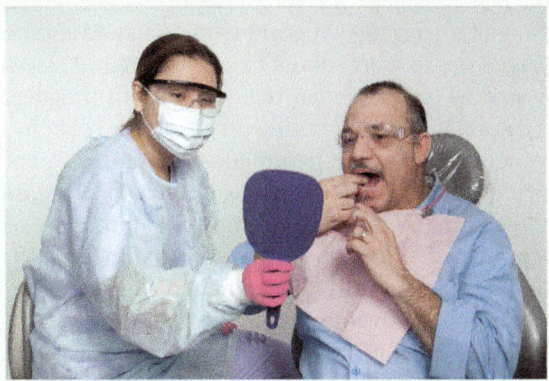

Figure P10-5-4

Nutrition

Comprehensive patient education involves a basic understanding of how nutrition affects the oral cavity. The connection between loss of teeth among older adults and malnutrition is well documented. Moreover, carbohydrates should also be eaten with care—not over prolonged periods, which causes the mouth to suffer a constant influx of acids. Likewise, there is a clear association between the consumption of sugary beverages, such as fruit juice and soda, and dental caries in infants and children. Prompt brushing after consuming carbohydrates is important. Similarly, care should be taken to brush soon after eating meat, lest fibers remain caught between teeth and release acids that will attack the tooth surfaces; likewise, acidic foods should be eaten in a single sitting (to minimize the duration of tooth exposure to acid), and the teeth should be brushed as soon after as is possible.

The role of nutrition in oral health goes far beyond prevention, however. Patients can benefit from nutrition counseling after oral surgery, after they have had oral appliances put in, and even during major life changes, such as having access to school cafeterias or moving into a first apartment. It should be noted that the rules of good nutrition are universal—they apply to dental assistants as well as patients.

A healthy diet consists of the right foods, eaten in the right proportions. Generally speaking, patients should strive to eat a diet that balances macronutrients (carbohydrates, fats, and proteins as well as water and fiber) in healthful proportions. A healthy diet is rich in vitamins and minerals, preferably derived from whole foods, and low in saturated fat, trans fat, and simple carbohydrates like processed sugar.

An excellent resource for dietary recommendations can be found at www.mypyramid.gov. This website is maintained by the United States Department of Agriculture and the United States Department of Health and Human Services. Based on the updated food pyramid, it offers personalized dietary advice.

These principles are discussed in greater detail in Chapter 11, Nutrition.

Patients with Special Conditions

Some patients may have special conditions that impact their oral health. Such patients include pregnant women and patients with oral cancer or other diseases, such as diabetes, that can complicate oral health. In this situation, the dental assistant has two primary functions:

1. Assist the dentist or hygienist as he or she develops a comprehensive oral health care plan for the patient. This might include instructing the patient in techniques used to clean teeth and gingiva.
2. Help the patient use the appropriate products for his or her condition. This can include anything from prescription rinses and oral irrigation devices to dental floss and methods of helping patients manipulate toothbrushes, including electric toothbrushes and customized toothbrush handles.

Note the following considerations for patients with special needs:

- Pregnant patients. The vomiting associated with morning sickness raises the acid level in the oral cavity, which can be harmful to teeth. Additionally, patients may be concerned about additional gingival bleeding caused by increased blood volume during pregnancy. The best approach to these patients is to find a time of day that women can best tolerate brushing (the toothbrush itself can sometimes stimulate gagging). Pregnant women should also be encouraged not to worry about excessive gingival bleeding, as long as they maintain their oral health program. This is a normal tendency during pregnancy.
- Oral cancer and cancer treatment. Cancer treatment can have profound effects on the oral cavity. Patients can suffer from dry mouth caused by chemotherapy or radiation, and they may be increasingly vulnerable to infection and dental caries. Some patients may elect to use home fluoride treatments, using custom-fitted fluoride trays, and nutritional counseling might be in order. Above all, be encouraging, positive, and empathetic.
- Older adult patients. Tooth loss is not a normal part of aging, but older adult patients might suffer from any number of diseases that complicate oral health care, including heart disease, diabetes, arthritis, and stroke. These conditions can limit mobility and directly affect oral health by reducing circulation. Dental assistants should be familiar with the patient's medical conditions and their implications for oral health. They should be able to recommend products for patients who have a hard time manipulating toothbrushes and floss. This might include large, soft handles for toothbrushes, interdental aids, and flossing sticks as opposed to string floss.

Patient Risk Testing

Risk testing involves assessing the patient's current risk level for developing oral diseases. This can include tools such as a food diary, which tracks a patient's intake of foods that might compromise oral health. It also requires that dental assistants listen closely to their patients, especially when they talk about their oral health care regimen. Many patients believe they are doing everything right, but are surprised to learn that they are brushing ineffectively, not brushing for long enough, or flossing improperly. All of these raise the patient's risk profile.

Caries Risk Test

A caries risk test (CRT) is available to assess a patient's risk of developing caries. This kit uses a simple saliva test to measure pH level and detect the level of bacteria present in the oral cavity. If the test indicates a patient is susceptible to caries, a preventive treatment plan can be implemented. This test is most often used with pediatric patients or other high-risk patients.

Plaque Identification

Plaque identification is a powerful visual aid that can be used to focus all patients on the state of their oral health by providing them a visual representation of their brushing and flossing habits. Plaque identification is possible through the use of a disclosing agent; these agents are available as tablets or liquids. When used correctly, they stain plaque red, allowing patients to actually see how much plaque is present on their teeth. Disclosing agents can be used in the dental office or at home.

The use of disclosing agents is simple. Patients chew the tablets or swish the liquid according to the package instructions. Any plaque on the teeth will be stained red. Before using the disclosing agent, patients should be warned that it will turn their oral cavity red. However, they can be reassured that this is not a permanent stain. Most disclosing agents fade after about 30 minutes.

Procedure 10-6 Applying Disclosing Agent for Plaque Identification

This procedure covers the in-office use of a disclosing agent. Patients can adapt this for use at home.

Materials needed:

- Disclosing agent (and applicator if needed)
- Hand mirror
- Appropriate PPE

1. Put on appropriate PPE.
2. Explain to the patient the function of disclosing agents and how they operate.
3. If using a liquid disclosing agent, apply the disclosing agent on all accessible tooth surfaces using a cotton tip applicator. If using a tablet disclosing agent, have the patient chew up the tablet, swish it around in the mouth for 15 seconds, then spit it out.
4. Supply the patient with a hand mirror so he or she can inspect the results. Use a dental mirror to draw attention to hard-to-see areas.
5. Afterward, instruct the patient in proper brushing and flossing techniques (see Procedures 10-2 through 10-5). The disclosing agent can be reapplied to demonstrate the results of effective techniques.

Pit and Fissure Sealants

Pit and fissure sealant, also called *dental sealant* or *enamel sealant*, is a clear composite that is applied to teeth to protect the occlusal surface and grooves. Often used for adolescents, pit and fissure sealants are an important and powerful tool in preventive dentistry. Many adolescent patients who have pit and fissure sealants have never experienced any dental caries. Depending on the scope of the practice act of the state in which they are employed, dental assistants are sometimes responsible for applying dental sealant. This technique is covered in more depth in Chapter 43, Pediatric Dentistry.

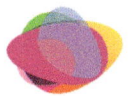

Chapter Highlights

- ✦ Dental assistants are a key part of patient education. During patient interactions, dental assistants should be encouraging, motivational, and ready with accurate information.
- ✦ Patients' needs change as they age, and it is important to know patients' state of understanding and their needs.
- ✦ Tooth loss is not a normal part of aging and can be prevented or minimized with adequate oral hygiene.
- ✦ Toothbrushes are available in many styles and shapes; no one toothbrush is the best, but different toothbrushes may suit different patients. Most dentists recommend soft bristles.
- ✦ Patients should brush their teeth at least twice a day, for 2 to 3 minutes each time.
- ✦ The American Dental Association (ADA) Seal of Acceptance is affixed to products that the ADA has judged as effective.
- ✦ Dentifrice, or toothpaste, is available in a wide variety of styles and flavors. Most dentists recommend a nonabrasive dentifrice.
- ✦ Flossing should be done before brushing.
- ✦ Interdental aids can be used to complement adequate brushing and flossing.
- ✦ Mouth rinses can include over-the-counter or prescription formulations. Some mouth rinses contain fluoride or whitening agents.
- ✦ Fluoridation has been shown to reduce dental caries and other oral health problems. At high levels, fluoride can be toxic and result in various medical problems. Topical fluoride treatments are recommended for patients at high risk of dental caries.
- ✦ There are several toothbrushing techniques often recommended, including the Bass technique, modified Stillman technique, and Charters technique.
- ✦ Nutrition affects the teeth and oral health.
- ✦ Patient risk testing using a disclosing agent can provide a powerful visual symbol of a patient's plaque status.

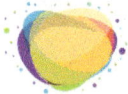

Review Questions

1. What is dentifrice?
   a. An oral appliance used to correct alignment
   b. Mouth rinse
   c. Toothpaste or other products used to cleanse teeth
   d. The practice of dentistry

2. Which artificial sweetener has been proven to prevent caries?
   a. Sorbitol
   b. Xylitol
   c. Aspartame
   d. Saccharine

3. How many tooth surfaces can a toothbrush reach?
   a. 1
   b. 2
   c. 3
   d. 4

4. The best toothbrush is:
   a. One that fits the patient's needs.
   b. A full-sized one.
   c. Automatic.
   d. Manual.

5. What is a dental stimulator?

   a. A bracing mouth rinse

   b. A device used to massage the gingival tissue

   c. A device used to clean the interproximal space

   d. An automatic device that measures plaque deposits

6. What is the usual level of fluoride in community water supplies?

   a. It varies by community

   b. None

   c. 1 ppm

   d. 10 ppm

7. Which form of fluoride is superior?

   a. Sodium fluoride

   b. Stannous fluoride

   c. Acidulated phosphate fluoride

   d. It depends on the application

8. Chronic exposure to high levels of fluoride can result in:

   a. Death.

   b. Mottled enamel and fluorosis.

   c. Neurological deficits.

   d. None of the above.

9. The best brushing technique for a patient with orthodontic appliances is:

   a. Modified Bass

   b. Modified Stillman

   c. Charters

   d. They are all equally effective

10. What does disclosing agent do?

   a. Stain plaque red

   b. Stain caries red

   c. Guarantee an accurate dental history

   d. Help diagnose periodontitis

Active Learning Exercises

1. Take a trip to the local supermarket. Make a list of all of the oral self-care aids they carry that you currently recommend to your patients. List them according to use and price. How could sugarless chewing gum be considered an oral self-care aid? Explain the role and benefits of chewing sugarless gum.

2. Identify and discuss the various types of fluoride. What are the modes of application and who benefits most from each type?

3. Role-play a scenario to discuss the prevention of periodontal disease. Be sure to address self-care and frequency of dental visits and use language appropriate for the particular patient.

Application Activities

1. At home, practice using each of the major brushing techniques discussed in the chapter and make a list of the pros and cons of using each method. Be prepared to share your list with the class.

2. Use the Internet to research current innovations in oral hygiene products. Write a paragraph or two about a new product that you feel would be especially useful.

3. Pick one method of oral health care (i.e., toothbrushing or flossing) discussed in the chapter and create a detailed plan to educate patients on properly performing the technique at home. Your plan should include a brief summary of the technique, the steps you would take to demonstrate the technique, and useful phrases you could use to encourage patients to regularly and correctly perform the technique at home.

PREPARING FOR CERTIFICATION EXAMS

Review the following topics in this chapter to prepare for the Dental Assisting National Board (DANB) exam:

- **Introduction**
- **Self-Care and Oral Hygiene Aids**
- **Patient Motivation**
- **Developmental Stages**
- **Brushing**
- **Dental Floss and Tape**
- **Oral Irrigation**
- **Interdental and Periodontal Aids**
- **Mouth Rinses**
- **Fluoridation**
- **Patient Education**
- **Patient Risk Testing**

chapter 11

Nutrition

CHAPTER OUTLINE

CHAPTER CHECKLIST

On completion of this chapter, students will be able to:

- ☑ Explain how nutrition affects oral health and the importance of patient education about nutrition
- ☑ List the macronutrients and micronutrients and how they impact overall health.
- ☑ Describe the role of macronutrients in the diet.
- ☑ Describe the difference between vitamins and minerals.
- ☑ Identify the ways in which nutrients specifically affect oral health.
- ☑ Identify ways to maintain healthy nutrition, including describing the new food guide pyramid and explaining food labels.
- ☑ Describe the two most common eating disorders, including their symptoms and risk factors.
- ☑ List the signs and symptoms of eating disorders likely to be seen by a dental professional.
- ☑ Give examples of inappropriate dieting methods.
- ☑ Explain how not having teeth impacts patient nutrition.

KEY TERMS

anorexia nervosa (an-oh-REK-see-uh ner-VOH-suh) – an eating disorder in which an individual refuses to eat and/or exercises excessively in order to maintain a very low body weight; often simply called *anorexia*

basal metabolism – the amount of energy (or calories) the body needs to maintain important functions while at rest, such as cellular function, body temperature, respiration, and heart beat

binging – eating an excessively large amount of food in a single sitting, usually more than one individual would normally eat; a behavior seen in individuals with bulimia nervosa

bulimia nervosa (buh-LEE-mee-uh ner-VOH-suh) – an eating disorder in which individuals binge and purge in order to control their weight; often simply called *bulimia*

calorie – scientifically, the amount of heat needed to raise the temperature of 1 kg of water 1 degree Celsius; also a measure of the amount of energy contained in a given food

carbohydrate – sugar and starch nutrient

eating disorders – psychological disorders in which people take extreme actions to control their weight or eating habits

enamel erosion – the wearing away of the outer enamel of the tooth; common in patients with bulimia nervosa who regularly make themselves vomit

fat – a nutrient that provides energy and helps the body use vitamins properly; includes both oils and solid fats

female athlete triad – three conditions that girls and young women who exercise vigorously or play sports intensely are at risk for; includes disordered eating, loss of menstrual period, and weakening of the bones

fiber – a type of complex carbohydrate that the body cannot digest; found in fruit, vegetables, beans, and whole grains

macronutrient – a nutrient that the body needs large amounts of in order to function and survive; includes carbohydrates, protein, fat, water, and fiber

metabolism – a measure of the rate at which energy is released from cells

micronutrient – a nutrient that the body needs small amounts of in order to function and survive; includes vitamins and minerals

mineral – a chemical element needed to maintain body structure and body functioning

nutrition – the study of what people eat and how the body uses food to function

nutrient – a food substance necessary for the body to live and function properly

organic food – food that has been grown and processed in nontraditional ways, usually to reduce pollution or environmental waste, to reduce the use of chemicals, or to feed and raise livestock differently

protein – a nutrient made up of amino acids responsible for building, maintaining, and repairing all of the body's muscles and tissues; includes mostly animal meat, eggs, and milk products, but also some vegetables, legumes, and nuts

purging – getting rid of food in the body; in bulimia nervosa, usually occurs after binging by forcing oneself to vomit by sticking a finger or object down the throat or using laxatives

Recommended Dietary Allowances (RDAs) – guidelines that tell how much of a nutrient is needed for nearly all people (about 98%) to stay healthy, depending on age and gender

saturated fat – a type of fat that generally comes from animals, such as in meat, eggs, and milk products, but also found in coconut, coconut oil, and palm oil

simple carbohydrate – a sugar carbohydrate that is quickly digested and used by the body for energy; includes table sugar, fruit and sugar from fruit, molasses, and sugar from milk

unsaturated fat – a type of fat that comes from plant sources; can be divided into monounsaturated fat, such as nuts, olives and olive oil, peanut oil, and avocados, and polyunsaturated fats, such as corn, flax seed, and canola oils

vitamin – a complex substance that aids digestion and allows cells to use food for fuel; may be fat soluble or water soluble

Introduction

One of a dental assistant's main responsibilities is educating patients about their oral health, including the role nutrition plays in maintaining oral health. To do this, you must understand how nutrients affect the development and health of the teeth and oral tissues, and you must be able to recognize deficiencies in a patient's diet by the effect they have on oral health. You may also play a vital role by recognizing the signs and symptoms of eating disorders and discussing these issues with the patient. A thorough understanding of proper nutrition makes the dental assistant a valuable asset to the dental office team.

Nutrition and Dental Caries

Nutrition is the study of what people eat and how the body uses food to function. Proper nutrition is one of the most important ways to prevent dental caries. When bacteria in the oral cavity encounter any type of carbohydrate, they produce acid that breaks down the surface of the tooth and eventually leads to caries. All types of carbohydrates increase the risk of dental caries. This includes table sugar that is added to food as well as naturally sweet food, such as fruit, molasses, and honey. Sweets that are sticky, like jelly beans or caramel, may

be especially likely to cause caries, because these foods have a tendency to adhere to the tooth surface, which encourages plaque build up and a proliferation of bacteria. In addition to sugar, starchy foods, such as beans and potatoes, become acidic when cooked. Although sugar substitutes do not contain sugar and, therefore, do not cause dental caries, they may be used in products that contain other cariogenic substances. For example, although diet soda contains no sugar, the acid in soda can erode the tooth enamel.

Each exposure of the tooth surface to carbohydrates or other cariogenic food in a meal or snack increases the amount of acid on the teeth. Therefore, in terms of oral health, the quantity of cariogenic food is not as significant as *how often* the teeth are exposed. For example, continuous snacking on potato chips over the course of an afternoon is more damaging to the teeth than eating the same portion of potato chips in one sitting. Frequent exposure to cariogenic substances does not allow time for a remineralization period to occur, thus exposing the teeth to acid for a prolonged period of time.

Nutrition and Health

Nutrition is important for more than just maintaining healthy teeth; it is essential for maintaining a healthy body. When people hear the word "nutrition," they often think about diet. Although food choices are certainly important, good nutrition includes many aspects of eating, such as:

- How you eat
  - Eat three balanced meals
  - Eat meals that include a variety of different types of foods
  - Eat reasonable portion sizes; there is no need to completely avoid sweets and other tasty treats as long as portion sizes aren't too large
- When you eat
  - Avoid food at least 2 hours before bed
  - Do not snack between meals
  - Do not skip meals—especially breakfast
- What you drink
  - Drink plenty of water—at least eight 8-ounce glasses per day
  - Keep intake of alcohol to a minimum
  - Skip sodas and other sugary drinks; remember that soda is basically liquid sugar!

From the Dentist's Perspective

The mouth is literally the gateway for a person's overall health. What goes into the oral cavity can affect the entire body. That's why my job is about more than just helping people have healthy teeth. By providing nutritional advice and giving patients important tips on how to improve their diet, I'm helping them lead healthier lives—and that includes oral health. I make sure my entire office has the same philosophy, too. I often share with staff research articles and news stories about diet and nutrition, and we discuss how these might impact our patients. I also make sure to ask my patients about their eating habits in front of the dental assistants so they can learn what questions to ask and see how to approach the topic.

Nutrients

Nutrients are food substances necessary for the body to live and function properly. **Macronutrients** are nutrients the body needs large doses of in order to function and survive. These typically include carbohydrates, protein, and fat as well as water and fiber. Virtually all food contains at least one macronutrient; all are needed to maintain a balanced diet. Table 11-1 lists the nutritional values for some common foods.

Carbohydrates

Sugar and starch nutrients are known as **carbohydrates**. Table sugar, honey, fruit and fruit sugar (called *fructose*), molasses, and sugar from milk (called *lactose*) are examples of **simple carbohydrates**. These are digested and used by the body for energy very quickly. However,

they cause the amount of sugar in the blood to rise and fall rapidly, which, over time, can damage the pancreas, heart, and blood vessels. Healthier forms of carbohydrates that do not cause such rapid changes in blood sugar are complex carbohydrates. These are digested and used by the body slowly and include whole grains, legumes (such as peas and beans), potatoes, and other vegetables. Once digested, all carbohydrates—whether grain, fruit, or vegetable—are converted to a simple sugar, and any sugar that isn't used for energy gets stored as fat. Each gram of carbohydrate contains 4 calories. It is recommended that approximately 50% of an average person's daily calorie intake be in the form of carbohydrates.

Sugar increases the risk of dental caries. Rather than trying to eliminate sugar completely, encourage patients to decrease the frequency of consumption of sugary foods and drinks. For example, sipping soda all day is much more damaging than enjoying a single soda with a meal. Patients may also want to look for satisfying foods that are lower in sugar.

Patients can defend against the effects of sugar by brushing their teeth right after eating sweet treats. Although complex carbohydrates are converted to sugar in the body, they do not promote bacteria growth as quickly as simple carbohydrates. Encourage patients to stick to complex carbohydrates as much as possible, which are healthier in general.

Fiber

Dietary **fiber** is a type of complex carbohydrate that comes from plants and cannot be digested by the body. Because fiber is only broken down in the colon, it slows the digestion process, which can create a feeling of fullness and satisfaction after eating. It also slows the rate at which sugar is absorbed into the bloodstream, which helps blood sugar levels remain even. Fiber keeps the large intestine, or *colon*, clean of bacteria and aids in keeping the bowels working properly. Many studies have shown a connection between eating fiber and a lower risk of cholesterol, heart disease, colon cancer, and diabetes. Fiber is found primarily in fruits, vegetables, beans, and in complex carbohydrates like whole grains. Fibrous foods usually require more chewing, which produces saliva and helps ward off dental caries. The recommended daily intake of fiber is 25 to 35 grams.

Proteins

Protein is made up of amino acids, which are considered the building blocks of the body. Protein is needed to build, repair, and maintain all of the body's muscles and tissues, including those of the heart, lungs, and other vital organs. Each gram of protein contains 4 calories. Protein also aids digestion and muscle movement and helps build fingernails and hair. Without the amino acids found in proteins, cells could not carry oxygen or function properly. Maintaining a good intake of protein

TABLE 11-1   Nutrition Values for Common Foods

FOOD/PORTION SIZE	PROTEIN (G)	TOTAL FAT (G)	TOTAL DIETARY FIBER (G)	CARBOHYDRATE (G)
Apple, raw, unpeeled	Trivial amount	Trivial amount	3.3	21
Carbonated beverage, cola, 12 fl oz	0	0	0	38
Carbonated beverage, cola, sweetened with aspartame, 12 fl oz	0	0	0	Trivial amount
Bagel, cinnamon-raisin, 4" bagel	9	2	2	49
Bologna, beef and pork, 2 slices	7	16	0	2
Cereal, Puffed Rice, 1 cup	Trivial amount	Trivial amount	0.2	13
Cheeseburger, regular size, with condiments	16	14	2.1	27
Chicken pot pie, frozen entrée, 1 small pie	13	29	1.7	43
Chocolate chip cookie, medium, commercially prepared, enriched, 1 cookie	1	2	0.3	7
Mashed potatoes, homemade, with whole milk and margarine, 1 cup	4	9	3.2	35
Milk, 2% milkfat, 1 cup	8	5	0	12
Pineapple, raw diced, 1 cup	1	1	2.2	19
Pizza, meat and vegetable topping, regular crust, 1 slice	13	5	1.7	21
Salad dressing, Thousand Island, 1 tbsp	6	0.9	0.1	2

is one of the simplest and most effective ways to stay healthy. There are eight essential amino acids. An essential amino acid is one that must come from food and is required by the body for normal growth and maintenance of body tissues.

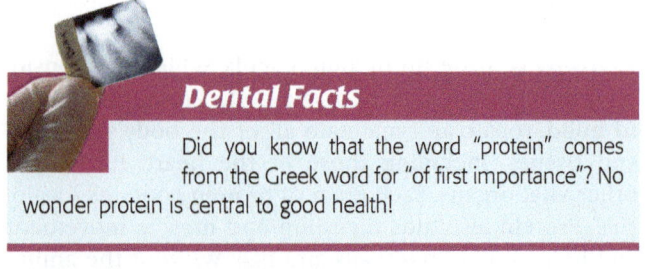

Dental Facts

Did you know that the word "protein" comes from the Greek word for "of first importance"? No wonder protein is central to good health!

There are two categories of proteins: complete and incomplete. Most animal foods, including meat, eggs, and milk products, supply the necessary amount of protein needed by the body. These types of foods are considered complete proteins because they provide all eight essential amino acids. Some nonanimal products, such as grains, legumes, and nuts, contain a fairly small amount of protein; these are incomplete proteins. Foods categorized as incomplete proteins are lacking or low in one or more of the essential amino acids. This means that this type of food should not be a person's only source of protein. However, these smaller-protein foods can be eaten together in order to achieve a healthy amount of protein. Proteins generally require more chewing, which produces saliva in the oral cavity and helps "wash" the teeth of sugars and food particles. Saliva also reduces acid in the oral cavity, making protein an important tool in fighting dental caries.

Fats

Fats are nutrients that provide energy and help the body properly use other nutrients such as vitamins; fats also provide heat insulation and protect body organs. Each gram of fat contains 9 calories. They include oils as well as fats that are solid at room temperature like butter. **Saturated fats** generally come from animal sources, such as meat, eggs, and milk products, but also include coconut, coconut oil, and palm oil. Saturated fats are solid at room temperature. **Unsaturated fats** come from plant sources and can be divided into two types: monounsaturated and polyunsaturated fats. Polyunsaturated fats include corn, flax seed, soybean, and canola oils. Monounsaturated fats include nuts, olives and olive oil, peanut oil, and avocados.

Saturated fat has been associated with higher rates of cancer, heart disease, and cardiovascular problems, though more research is needed to fully understand its effect on the body. Unsaturated fat, however, is considered "good fat" because of its association with lower levels of heart disease and cancer. It is important to note that some foods contain a type of unsaturated fat called *trans-fatty acids*, which research shows may be even more harmful than saturated fat. Trans-fatty acids are found in shortening and margarine. Patients should avoid trans-fatty acids as much as possible.

Water

Water is needed for every function in the body to work properly. Without water, cells cannot access and use nutrients, and waste cannot be eliminated. About 60% of human body weight is water. However, the body cannot store water, which is why it is so important to drink an adequate amount of water every day. Most doctors recommend drinking at least eight 8-ounce glasses of water daily. Water may be treated with fluoride, which is essential to building strong teeth and fighting dental caries. Like saliva, water also helps "wash" teeth of sugars and food particles, which can build up in the gingival tissue and between teeth. Rinsing the oral cavity with water after eating can help remove cariogenic substances before they cause damage.

Vitamins and Minerals

Although the body needs relatively large amounts of macronutrients to survive, it needs only small amounts of vitamins and minerals, which are called **micronutrients**. Some studies suggest that vitamins and minerals can prevent diseases such as cancer or heart disease. Other studies, though, have found unclear results. Recommendations on whether individuals should take supplemental vitamins and minerals to prevent these diseases have not yet been established. However, eating a balanced diet composed of all of the macronutrients can help the body get the micronutrients it needs.

Vitamins are complex substances that aid digestion and allow cells to use food for fuel. All vitamins are organic compounds that are produced by either plants or animals. Some vitamins, called *fat-soluble vitamins*, dissolve in fat and, therefore, are easily stored in the body. Fat-soluble vitamins are vitamins A, D, E, and K. Other vitamins rapidly dissolve in water; these *water-soluble vitamins* are not easily stored, which means the body needs a new supply each day. The B vitamins and vitamin C are water-soluble vitamins. Deficiencies of vitamins B or C can result in a variety of conditions that affect oral health, including angular cheilitis, a condition characterized by cracks at the corners of the lips; glossitis, a condition in which the filiform papillae of the tongue are missing; and scurvy, a disease characterized by gingival bleeding. For more information about these conditions, see Chapter 12, Oral Pathology.

Minerals are chemical elements needed to maintain body structure and body functioning. Minerals perform many jobs, such as helping blood clot properly, keeping muscles healthy and able to contract, and allowing nerves and cells to communicate with one another. Unlike vitamins, minerals are inorganic substances. They are not made by animals or plants directly, but rather are in dirt and water and are eaten and absorbed by animals and plants. The body needs larger amounts of some minerals, called *major minerals*, and only tiny amounts of others.

Although all minerals are needed for good oral health, some play an especially large role in keeping teeth strong and healthy. These include calcium, phosphorus, and fluoride. (For a detailed look at fluoride, see Chapter 10, Prevention of Caries and Periodontal Disease.) Further, calcium and phosphorus require vitamin D and magnesium in order to carry out their functions, so these are important for dental health as well. The major vitamins and minerals needed to maintain body functioning are outlined in Table 11-2.

It is important to remember that vitamins and minerals do not supply energy; only carbohydrates, proteins, and fats supply energy. Vitamins and minerals help the body function properly, promoting good health and increasing energy. Taking a multivitamin does not supply the body with energy; this is a myth. Encourage patients to supply their body with all necessary nutrients by eating healthy foods on a daily basis rather than making poor food choices and attempting to supplement with a daily vitamin.

CHECKPOINTS

11-1 What nutrients make up the macronutrients and micronutrients?

11-2 How do carbohydrates increase the risk of dental caries?

11-3 What is the difference between saturated and unsaturated fats?

11-4 Which micronutrients play a strong role in keeping teeth healthy?

TABLE 11-2 Major Minerals and Vitamins

MAJOR MINERAL	SOURCE	WHAT DOES IT DO?
Calcium (most abundant mineral in the body)	Milk products (including cheese and yogurt), eggs, green vegetables, legumes (including peas and beans)	Bone and teeth formation Blood clotting Nerve and muscle activity
Iodine	Seafood, iodized salt	Component of thyroid hormones; necessary for normal reproduction and growth
Fluoride (considered a trace element since only a small amount is needed)	Fluoridated water, seafood, tea	Helps prevent dental caries
Magnesium	Leafy green vegetables, nuts, soybeans, bananas, seafood	Helps calcium and phosphorus carry out their functions
Phosphorus	Meat, fish, poultry (chicken and turkey), egg yolks, milk products	Bone and teeth formation
Potassium (electrolyte)	Fruit (bananas), meat, seafood, milk products, vegetables, grains	Regulates fluids in the body Nerve and muscle activity
Sodium (electrolyte)	Nearly all foods, table salt	Regulates fluids in the body Nerve and muscle activity
Iron	Liver, red meats, egg yolks, dried fruits (raisins), leafy green vegetables	Aids in formation of hemoglobin, which supplies oxygen to the cells

VITAMIN	SOURCE	WHAT DOES IT DO?
Vitamin A (retinol)	Orange fruits and vegetables, dark green vegetables, liver, eggs, milk products	Reproduction Boosts immune system Keeps skin and eyes healthy
Vitamin B1 (thiamin)	Pork, cereal, grains, legumes, nuts, meats	Nerve activity
Vitamin B2 (riboflavin)	Meat, eggs, liver, leafy green vegetables, grains	Helps other minerals carry out their functions
Vitamin B12 (cyanocobalamin)	Meat, eggs, and milk products	Cell production Nerve activity
Vitamin C (ascorbic acid)	Citrus fruits, green vegetables, potatoes, orange fruits	Maintains skin and eye health Protects cells against breakdown
Vitamin D (calciferol)	Fatty fish (including salmon and tuna), liver, eggs, milk	Helps calcium and phosphorus carry out their functions
Vitamin E (tocopherol)	Seeds, green vegetables, nuts, grains, oils	Protects cells against breakdown
Vitamin K	Liver, cabbage, leafy green vegetables	Bone formation Blood clotting
Folate B9 (folic acid)	Vegetables, liver, legumes, seeds	Development of red blood cells Prevention of birth defects such as spina bifida

Dietary Recommendations

The United States Department of Agriculture (USDA) and the United States Department of Health and Human Services have teamed up to provide the public with tools and recommendations to maintain good health. They suggest eating a variety of foods and balancing a nutritious diet with regular physical activity. Fruits, vegetables, and grains are encouraged, whereas saturated fats and trans-fatty acids are highly discouraged. Salt and sugar certainly make food taste better, but for ideal health, encourage patients to skip these seasonings and enjoy their food's natural flavors. Spices, such as pepper, garlic, and salt-free spice mixes, also provide a boost of flavor without harming health.

Energy Balance

All food contains energy, which is measured as a food's **calories**. The nutrients release energy from the cells, which the body uses for fuel. The measure of the rate at which energy is released from cells is called **metabolism**. Cells release energy when the body is in motion, but they also release energy while the body is at rest. Energy is needed in order for the body to perform the necessary functions to stay alive, including maintaining temperature, respiration, and heartbeat. The amount of energy the body needs to maintain these important functions while at rest is called **basal metabolism**. The balance between energy taken

in (by eating food) and energy burned (through activity and/or through basal metabolism) impacts whether an individual maintains, gains, or loses weight. Studies indicate that obesity may play a role in periodontal disease, because obese patients are shown to have a higher frequency of periodontal disease. Promotion of healthy nutrition, adequate physical exercise, and weight control may be factors in preventing periodontal disease or slowing its progress.

How many calories should be consumed each day? Men and women have different energy balance needs, as do individuals who engage in physical activity and individuals who get no exercise at all. Table 11-3 gives two simple formulas for determining an individual's basal metabolic rate, which helps determine how many calories are needed each day.

To keep the right balance of calories, make sure to eat the right amount of each macronutrient. The number of carbohydrates, protein, and fat each person needs may be somewhat

---

TABLE 11-3 Basal Metabolism and Calorie Needs

DETERMINE YOUR BMR

Step 1	Find weight in kilograms ■ Do this by dividing weight in pounds by 2.2
Step 2	Multiple weight in kilograms by: ■ 0.9 if you are a woman ■ 1.0 if you are a man
Step 3	Multiple this number by 24 = This is your BMR!

DETERMINE YOUR DAILY ENERGY NEEDS

Step 1	Find your BMR
Step 2	Find your physical activity level range numbers (see below)
Step 3	Multiple your BMR by each physical activity level number
Step 4	Add to each total your BMR; these two numbers give the range of calories you need to eat each day to maintain weight

ACTIVITY LEVEL	IF YOU ARE MALE, MULTIPLE BY...	IF YOU ARE FEMALE, MULTIPLY BY...
Little = "couch potato"	0.25 and 0.40	0.25 and 0.35
Light = walking throughout the day but no planned exercise	0.50 and 0.75	0.40 and 0.60
Moderate = aerobic activity, such as running or swimming, several times per week	0.65 and 0.80	0.50 and 0.70
Heavy = daily intense exercise or athletics	0.90 and 1.20	0.80 and 1.00

BMR, basal metabolic rate.

TABLE 11-4 Energy Guidelines Based on a 2,000-Calorie Diet

NUTRIENT	PERCENT OF TOTAL CALORIES	AMOUNT
Carbohydrate	55 to 60%	■ No more than 300 grams ■ At least 25 grams should come from fiber
Fat	30% or less	■ No more than 65 grams ■ Less than 20 should come from saturated fat
Protein	15 to 20%	■ Between 75 and 100 grams

different based on gender, age, weight, physical activity level, and whether he or she has a medical diagnosis, such as diabetes or high cholesterol. The average American adult eats a 2,000-calorie diet. The exact amount of each macronutrient needed is based on the total calories eaten (Table 11-4).

A caloric intake that balances the body's needs for energy leads to maintaining the same weight. That does not mean, however, that the person's weight is in the best range for optimal health. A common way to determine whether one is in a normal weight range or under- or overweight uses the body mass index (BMI) scale, which assigns a value based on the person's height and weight. Although other individual factors must also be considered, BMI provides a general evaluation of a person's body weight (Figure 11-1).

Food Guide Pyramid

The USDA has published dietary guidelines for nearly 100 years. The most recent guidelines, published in 2005, are called *MyPyramid* and can be found online at the website www.mypyramid.gov (Figure 11-2). This food guide pyramid shows five colored bands representing five different categories of foods; the width of each band shows the relative amount of that category that should be eaten.

BMI	19	20	21	22	23	24	25	26	27	28	29	30	31	32	33	34	35
Height	Weight in pounds																
4'10"	91	96	100	105	110	115	119	124	129	134	138	143	148	153	158	162	167
4'11"	94	99	104	109	114	119	124	128	133	138	143	148	153	158	163	168	173
5'	97	102	107	112	118	123	128	133	138	143	148	153	158	163	168	174	179
5'1"	100	106	111	116	122	127	132	137	143	148	153	158	164	169	174	180	185
5'2"	104	109	115	120	126	131	136	142	147	153	158	164	169	175	180	186	191
5'3"	107	113	118	124	130	135	141	146	152	158	163	169	175	180	186	191	197
5'4"	110	116	122	128	134	140	145	151	157	163	169	174	180	186	192	197	204
5'5"	114	120	126	132	138	144	150	156	162	168	174	180	186	192	198	204	210
5'6"	118	124	130	136	142	148	155	161	167	173	179	186	192	198	104	210	216
5'7"	121	127	134	140	146	153	159	166	172	178	185	191	198	204	211	217	223
5'8"	125	131	138	144	151	158	164	171	177	184	190	197	203	210	216	223	230
5'9"	128	135	142	149	155	162	169	176	182	189	196	203	209	216	223	230	236
5'10"	132	139	146	153	160	167	174	181	188	195	202	209	216	222	229	236	243
5'11"	136	143	150	157	165	172	179	186	193	200	208	215	222	229	236	243	250
6'	140	147	154	162	169	177	184	191	199	206	213	221	228	235	242	250	258
6'1"	144	151	159	166	174	182	189	197	204	212	219	227	235	242	250	257	265
6'2"	148	155	163	171	179	186	194	202	210	218	225	233	241	249	256	264	272
6'3"	152	160	168	176	184	192	200	208	216	224	232	240	248	256	264	272	279
	Healthy weight						Overweight					Obese					

Figure 11-1 Adult body mass index (BMI) chart. Locate the height in the left-most column and read across the row for that height to the weight of interest. Follow the column of the weight up to the top row that lists the BMI. BMI of 18.5–24.9 is the healthy weight range, BMI of 25–29.9 is the overweight range, and BMI of 30 and above is in the obese range.

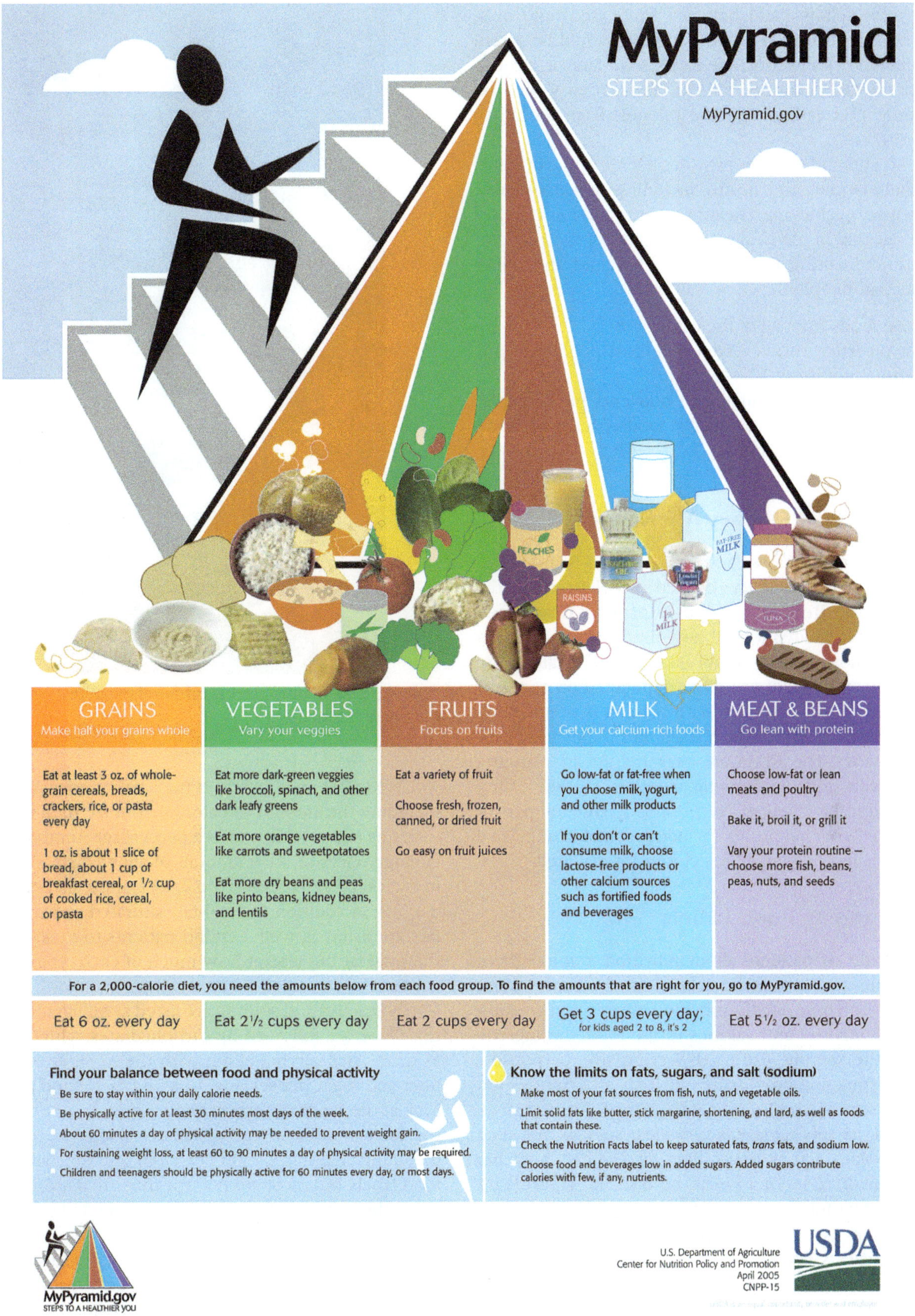

MyPyramid
STEPS TO A HEALTHIER YOU
MyPyramid.gov

GRAINS	VEGETABLES	FRUITS	MILK	MEAT & BEANS
Make half your grains whole	Vary your veggies	Focus on fruits	Get your calcium-rich foods	Go lean with protein
Eat at least 3 oz. of whole-grain cereals, breads, crackers, rice, or pasta every day 1 oz. is about 1 slice of bread, about 1 cup of breakfast cereal, or ½ cup of cooked rice, cereal, or pasta	Eat more dark-green veggies like broccoli, spinach, and other dark leafy greens Eat more orange vegetables like carrots and sweetpotatoes Eat more dry beans and peas like pinto beans, kidney beans, and lentils	Eat a variety of fruit Choose fresh, frozen, canned, or dried fruit Go easy on fruit juices	Go low-fat or fat-free when you choose milk, yogurt, and other milk products If you don't or can't consume milk, choose lactose-free products or other calcium sources such as fortified foods and beverages	Choose low-fat or lean meats and poultry Bake it, broil it, or grill it Vary your protein routine — choose more fish, beans, peas, nuts, and seeds

For a 2,000-calorie diet, you need the amounts below from each food group. To find the amounts that are right for you, go to MyPyramid.gov.

Eat 6 oz. every day	Eat 2½ cups every day	Eat 2 cups every day	Get 3 cups every day; for kids aged 2 to 8, it's 2	Eat 5½ oz. every day

Find your balance between food and physical activity
- Be sure to stay within your daily calorie needs.
- Be physically active for at least 30 minutes most days of the week.
- About 60 minutes a day of physical activity may be needed to prevent weight gain.
- For sustaining weight loss, at least 60 to 90 minutes a day of physical activity may be required.
- Children and teenagers should be physically active for 60 minutes every day, or most days.

Know the limits on fats, sugars, and salt (sodium)
- Make most of your fat sources from fish, nuts, and vegetable oils.
- Limit solid fats like butter, stick margarine, shortening, and lard, as well as foods that contain these.
- Check the Nutrition Facts label to keep saturated fats, *trans* fats, and sodium low.
- Choose food and beverages low in added sugars. Added sugars contribute calories with few, if any, nutrients.

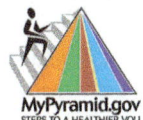

MyPyramid.gov
STEPS TO A HEALTHIER YOU

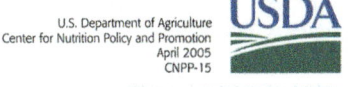

U.S. Department of Agriculture
Center for Nutrition Policy and Promotion
April 2005
CNPP-15

USDA

Figure 11–2 MyPyramid Food Guidance System. U.S. Department of Agriculture, Center for Nutrition Policy and Promotion, April 2005. Available at http://www.mypyramid.gov.

The narrow yellow band between fruits (red) and milk (blue) represents oils; very little of these should be eaten. The pyramid does not include sugar, solid fats, or alcohol because the USDA considers these "extras" that should be eaten only after eating adequate amounts from the other categories.

The MyPyramid website provides a wide range of information about diet and health, including how to plan a healthy menu, achieving a healthy weight, and information about engaging in physical activity. As part of their recommendations in using the food guide pyramid, the USDA suggests that people:

■ choose foods from all of the categories
■ focus on fruits and vegetables, as most people do not eat enough of these
■ select foods that are higher in nutrients but lower in calories; this means avoiding fast foods, packaged foods, and simple carbohydrates

Recommended Dietary Allowances

In 1941, the United States Food and Nutrition Board of the National Academy of Sciences created a set of dietary guidelines called the **Recommended Dietary Allowances (RDAs)**. These guidelines tell how much of a nutrient is needed for most people (about 98%) to stay healthy. The RDA of a given nutrient can differ depending on age, gender, and factors such as whether a woman is pregnant or breastfeeding. The RDAs are revised and published every 10 to 15 years. The RDAs are very helpful in planning healthy meals and determining whether current eating habits need to be changed. Nutrition is an integral part of an individual's overall health, including dental health. Total body health and oral health are closely intertwined.

Understanding Food Labels

When talking to patients about nutrition, remind them to read the nutrition food labels on food packaging (Figure 11-3). These labels provide valuable information about the nutrients and calories in the food, the ingredients, and the serving size used. Serving size, or portion, is key in estimating how many nutrients and calories are eaten. The serving size is listed at the top of the food label. Sometimes the serving size is very clear, such as one slice or two cookies. Other times, figuring out just how big (or how small) a serving is can be difficult. Figure 11-4 provides a helpful guide for estimating common serving sizes of many foods. Also keep in mind that some nutrition content may change when the food is prepared. For example, the nutritional information for popped popcorn is quite different than the information for unpopped kernels. Labels often list information as both prepared and unprepared, so tell patients to pay close attention to the right numbers.

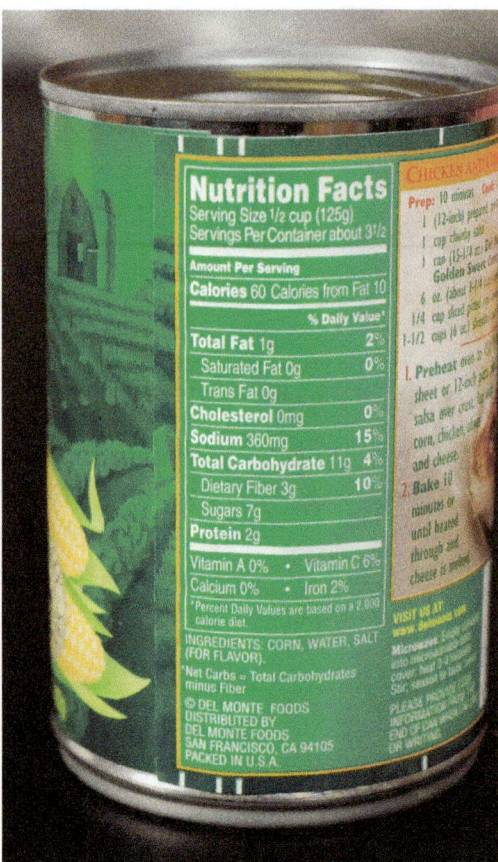

Figure 11-3 A nutrition food label. Note the serving size at the top of the label.

Listed after serving size is the total calories per serving, including the amount of calories from fat. Total fat is listed in grams per serving and as a percentage number. The percentage refers to what amount of allowed fat is contained in each serving, based on the 2,000-calorie diet recommendations. In addition to total fat, saturated and unsaturated fats are listed as well. Remind patients to look not just at the total fat but also at how much of each type of fat is in the food.

Cholesterol and sodium are listed as milligrams per serving. These are followed by carbohydrates, which are listed as grams per serving along with the number of grams of fiber and sugar per serving. As with fats, remind patients to look at the types of carbohydrates in each serving, not just the total number of carbohydrates. Some micronutrients, including vitamins A and C, calcium, and iron, are listed on food labels, but most are not. For those that are, food labels show the percent of the daily recommended value in each serving.

Food labels can also show whether a product is organic. **Organic food** is food that has been grown and processed in different ways, usually to reduce pollution or environmental waste, to reduce the use of chemicals, or to feed and raise livestock differently. For example, organic farmers may use animal manure for fertilizer rather than chemical

What's in a Serving?

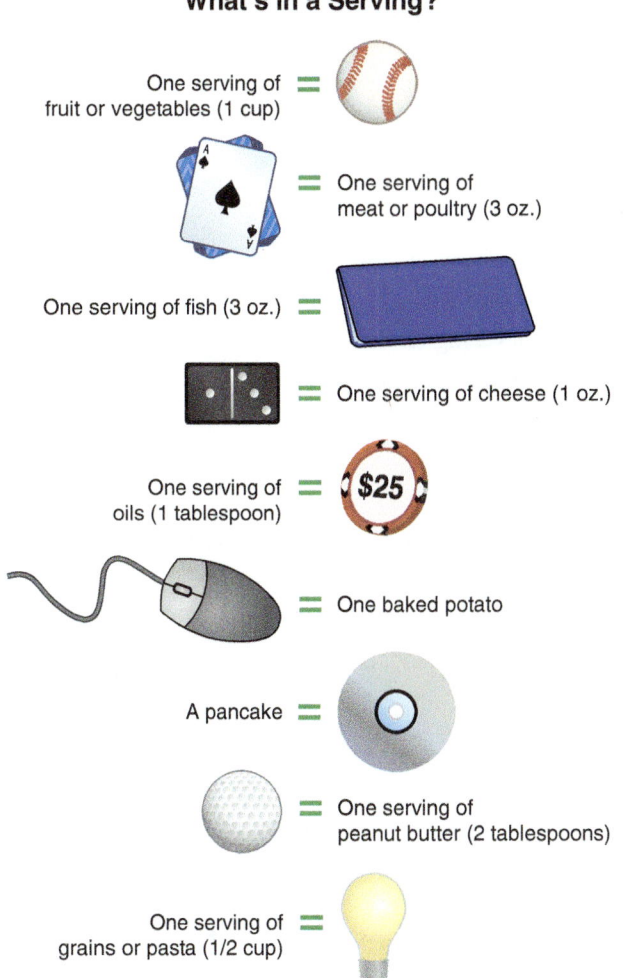

One serving of
fruit or vegetables (1 cup) **=**

= One serving of
meat or poultry (3 oz.)

One serving of fish (3 oz.) **=**

= One serving of cheese (1 oz.)

One serving of
oils (1 tablespoon) **=** $25

= One baked potato

A pancake **=**

= One serving of
peanut butter (2 tablespoons)

One serving of
grains or pasta (1/2 cup) **=**

Figure 11–4 Serving size guide. Use these common items to help remember serving sizes.

fertilizers, or may avoid putting hormones or medicines in their animal feed. The USDA certifies that foods labeled as "organic" must meet strict standards and that at least 95% of the ingredients are organically produced. The USDA seal confirms that the food is organically produced, although foods are not required to display the seal (Figure 11-5). Sometimes food labels contain terms such as "all-natural" or "free-range," which may mean the food is healthier or that the animals were raised in a more humane environment, but does not necessarily mean that the product is

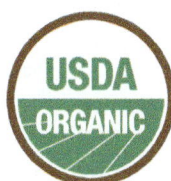

Figure 11–5 United States Department of Agriculture organic seal. This seal certifies that the food has been organically produced.

TABLE 11-5 Meaning of Health Claims	
HEALTH CLAIM	**MEANING**
Healthy	Low in fat, saturated fat, cholesterol, and sodium and has at least 10% daily value of protein, iron, calcium, fiber, and vitamins A and C
Good source of, more added	10% more daily value of given nutrient than original recipe
High, rich in, excellent source of	20% or more of the given nutrient per serving
Less, fewer, reduced	25% less of given nutrient than original recipe
Low, little, few, low source of	Frequent consumption of food will not exceed daily value

organic. Only the USDA seal indicates that the food is certified as organic.

The U.S. Food and Drug Administration (FDA) website (www.fda.gov) is frequently updated with the latest food labeling guidelines. Table 11-5 explains the meaning of some common health claims found on food labels. Table 11-6 provides an overview of the FDA requirements that must be met in order to make particular health claims.

Diet Analysis and Modification

When is it time to make dietary changes? For some patients, having a medical condition may result in needing to make dietary changes. Patients with diabetes may need to control carbohydrates, for instance. Other diet-related problems, such as food allergies, may require patients to avoid certain foods. One of the most common reasons for making diet changes is to control weight. This may mean eating fewer calories overall, or perhaps focusing on eating less of a particular nutrient, usually fat. A nutritional counselor is a professional, often a registered dietician, who can help patients learn what changes are needed and how to make them. If patients have serious concerns or questions about diet, advise them to ask their doctor for a referral to see a nutritional counselor.

Patients can do several things on their own to improve their diet. Keeping a food diary helps track what is eaten throughout the day. People often eat snacks or take extra helpings without noticing, which makes a food diary a very useful and eye-opening tool. Physical activity not only helps burn calories, but also provides multiple benefits, such as:

- Maintaining healthy weight
- Increasing circulation

TABLE 11-6 FDA Requirements to Meet Health Claims

CLAIM	REQUIREMENT
Fat free	0.5 g of fat per serving or less
0 g trans fat	<0.5 g of trans fat per serving
Low fat	3 g of fat per serving or less
Less fat	25% less fat than original recipe
Light (fat)	50% less fat than original recipe
Saturated fat free	0.5 g of saturated or trans fat per serving or less
Cholesterol free	2 g or less saturated fat per serving and <2 mg cholesterol per serving
Low cholesterol	2 g or less saturated fat per serving and <20 mg cholesterol per serving
Reduced calorie	25% fewer calories than original recipe
Low calorie	40 calories or less per serving
Light (calories)	One-third fewer calories than original recipe
Extra lean	5 g fat or less, 2 g saturated fat or less, 95 mg cholesterol/100 g serving of meat, poultry, or seafood
Lean	10 g fat or less, 4.5 g saturated fat or less, 95 mg cholesterol/100 g serving of meat, poultry, or seafood
High fiber	5 g or more per serving
Sugar-free	0.5 g or less per serving
Sodium-free (salt-free)	0.5 g or less per serving
Low sodium	140 mg or less per serving
Very low sodium	35 mg or less per serving
Heart Healthy	Low in saturated fat, cholesterol, and sodium

FDA, U.S. Food and Drug Administration.

- Strengthening the heart and lungs
- Building muscles
- Keeping bones strong
- Improving sleep
- Decreasing stress

All patients should get some form of physical activity on a regular basis. Patients who are under age 35 years and are in good health can usually start an exercise program on their own. However, patients over age 35 years and those who may have health problems need to speak with a doctor before starting regular exercise. It is especially important for patients with certain medical disorders, such as high blood pressure and heart disease, to seek doctor approval before beginning an exercise program.

Patient Education

When educating patients about diet, it is important to consider several factors before giving recommendations. These include the patient's age, geographic background, medical conditions, and social and financial situation. Some cultures and religions have guidelines that include or exclude certain foods. For example, some cultures eat lots of grains and vegetables; others do not eat animal products. Be sensitive to these differences before recommending that a patient change his or her diet. Remind patients that nutritional information is available at most restaurants and encourage patients to make sensible choices. Many restaurants also have nutritional information available online. Table 11-7 has some tips you can share with your patients about simple changes they can make in food preparation to make their meals healthier.

CHECKPOINTS

11-5 What do the color bands on the MyPyramid stand for?

11-6 How many grams of carbohydrates, protein, and fat are recommended for the average adult, based on a 2,000-calorie diet?

11-7 Name at least five items listed on a food label.

TABLE 11-7 Tips for Healthy Food Preparation

INSTEAD OF...	TRY...
Frying meats and vegetables	▪ Grilling ▪ Baking ▪ Broiling ▪ Roasting
Cooking with butter or vegetable oil	▪ Using non-stick spray ▪ Sautéing in broth ▪ Cooking with healthier oils, such as olive and canola oils
Buying packaged soups	▪ Preparing homemade soups with natural spices, herbs, and fresh vegetables
Using fatty cuts of meat	▪ Buying lean cuts of poultry and meat ▪ Sticking to white meat rather than dark meat ▪ Trimming the excess fat before cooking
Eating chocolate or pastry desserts	▪ Eating desserts that are naturally sweet, like fresh fruit
Selecting white, starchy breads	▪ Choosing whole grain breads that are rich in fiber and full of complex carbohydrates

Eating Disorders

Eating disorders are psychological disorders in which people take extreme actions to control their weight or eating habits. The two most common eating disorders are anorexia nervosa and bulimia nervosa. Eating disorders are very serious and can even result in death. Individuals with eating disorders usually have significant dental problems, which means that dental professionals are likely to see these patients in their office at some point.

Anorexia Nervosa

Anorexia nervosa, often referred to simply as *anorexia*, is a disorder in which a person has a strong desire to be excessively thin. As a result, patients purposely starve themselves by refusing to eat, exercising excessively, or misusing diet pills. Most individuals with anorexia are female, although about 10% are male. Signs and symptoms of anorexia include:

- Having an extremely low body weight or BMI
- Refusing to eat or starving oneself
- Expressing unusually strong fears of gaining weight
- Being overly concerned with weight and body shape in general

Anorexia nervosa carries very serious health consequences, including death. The lack of nutrition forces the body to break down its own muscles and organs, including the heart. Bones may become weak and stop growing altogether. Severe malnutrition can negatively impact all systems in the body, including the teeth and periodontal tissues. There is often a lack of important micronutrients, such as potassium, sodium, and calcium, which are needed to maintain heart and brain functioning. As a result of significantly poor nutrition, women with anorexia may have a reduction in the hormone estrogen, which can cause them to stop menstruating.

Emotionally, patients with anorexia may have low self-esteem and feel depressed. Often patients feel they need to be thin in order to achieve perfection or to be considered attractive or beautiful. People with anorexia may have extremely negative feelings about their body, believing that they are overweight or refusing to believe that they are underweight. They may also feel that they have little control over their own lives and that managing diet and weight is a way to get this control back. Table 11-8 outlines common risk factors for anorexia nervosa.

Patients with anorexia often need to be treated by a psychiatrist or psychologist, who are health care professionals trained to treat mental illnesses. Treatment often involves taking medications and talking to a mental health professional through a technique called *psychotherapy*. Because patients may refuse to eat, treatment can also include hospitalization at a special facility designed to help people overcome anorexia.

Bulimia Nervosa

Bulimia nervosa, often called *bulimia*, differs from anorexia in two important ways. First, unlike anorexia in which patients deliberately starve themselves, patients with bulimia engage in **binging**, in which they eat unusually large amounts of food in a single sitting—typically

TABLE 11-8 Risk Factors for Anorexia Nervosa

BIOLOGICAL	EMOTIONAL	SOCIAL
■ Female gender ■ Caucasian race ■ Possible genetic factors such as a family history of depression	■ Wanting to be "perfect" ■ Having very low self-esteem ■ Feeling a need to get control over one's life ■ Perceiving oneself as excessively overweight or unattractive ■ A history of childhood sexual abuse ■ Coming from a family that is over-controlling, high-achieving, and/or over-protective	■ Movies, television, and magazines that send the message that being beautiful means being thin ■ Western culture in general, which promotes thinness as an ideal state among women ■ Certain professions, such as modeling, dancing, and acting, that require extremely low body weight ■ Commercials and advertisements that encourage dieting and concern with shape, weight, and eating

much more food than an individual would normally eat. Often, binges consist of high-calorie foods like sweets and fried foods. Second, after binging, patients engage in **purging**, or behaviors to rid their body of food. Usually this involves causing oneself to vomit by sticking a finger or an object down the throat. However, patients may also purge by taking high doses of laxatives. Other patients avoid food for long periods of time (also called *fasting*) or exercise excessively. This is why bulimia is known as a "binge-and-purge" disorder. In addition to the binging and purging behaviors, symptoms of bulimia include:

■ Feeling as though one is "out of control" while binging
■ Having an especially negative view of one's body or shape

As with anorexia, serious health complications can occur from bulimia. The effects of the stomach acid from vomiting can cause dehydration, acid reflux in the stomach after eating, abnormal heart rhythms, inflammation of the throat, ulcers, and constipation. Frequent vomiting may seriously jeopardize oral health, as contact with corrosive stomach acid can severely erode tooth enamel. As a result of causing oneself to vomit, patients may have calluses or scars on the back of their hands from their teeth. The loss of important micronutrients, such as potassium and sodium, can cause the heart to stop. Although death in bulimia is less common than in anorexia, it does occur.

Many of the risk factors for bulimia are the same as for anorexia, shown in Table 11-8. Bulimia nervosa is more common in females than males and often begins between the ages of 13 and 20 years, though many patients continue to struggle with the disorder throughout their lives, even after treatment. Treatment for bulimia can include medications as well as psychotherapy. The disorder can be difficult to diagnose because, unlike patients with anorexia who are noticeably thin and underweight, patients with bulimia are often of average or slightly higher than average weight. Patients with bulimia may be very good at hiding their binging and purging behaviors, which can also make diagnosis difficult.

Check Your Ethics

You see a patient with bruising on her palate. You're not sure of the cause, but you suspect that she could be forcing herself to vomit. It also occurs to you the bruises could be signs of forced sexual activity. You are a little worried that you might be "jumping to conclusions," but you don't want to overlook what could be signs of a serious problem. What do you do?

Eating Disorders and Oral Health

Dental professionals are often among the first to notice when someone has an eating disorder. Knowing what oral signs and symptoms to look for in patients with anorexia or bulimia may not only help improve patients' oral health, it may lead to treatment that can save their lives. Bulimia nervosa is particularly harmful to the teeth and oral cavity due to the strong effects of stomach acid. The extreme under-nutrition in anorexia also causes dental problems. Nutrients that promote oral health, such as calcium, iron, and vitamin B, may be lacking, which can increase the risk of dental caries and periodontal disease. Learn to recognize these common dental signs and symptoms of eating disorders:

■ Worn away tooth enamel (called **enamel erosion**), especially on the lingual surfaces of the anterior maxillary teeth (Figure 11-6)
■ Fillings that appear raised or dark, due to erosion
■ Yellowing of the teeth
■ Sore throat
■ Cracks in the corners of the mouth from opening wide to purge
■ Bleeding on the roof of the mouth caused by trauma from the finger or object used to induce vomiting
■ Swollen salivary glands, which give the jaw a wide, square-like appearance
■ Decreased saliva, dry mouth, or thick saliva
■ Inflamed and bleeding gingival tissue
■ A burning feeling on the tongue

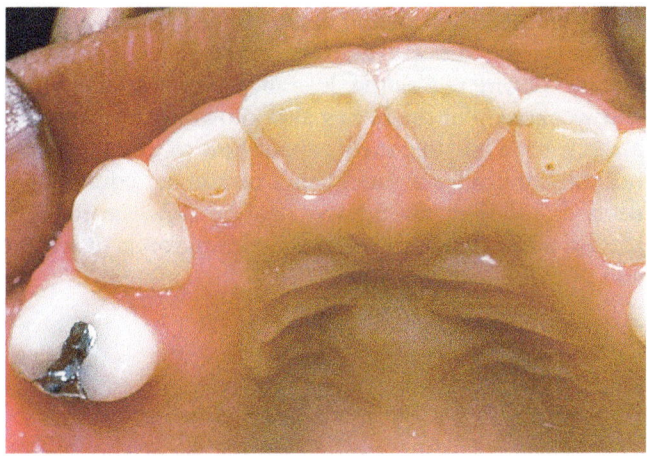

Figure 11–6 Erosion caused by chronic vomiting in bulimia.

- Tooth, tongue, and mouth sensitivity, especially to temperature and pain
- Possible tooth loss
- Halitosis, especially in anorexia due to the body burning its own body tissue for energy

Apply it

Jane has been a patient at your office for several years. You notice that her teeth seem to be getting yellower. On this visit, you also notice that the enamel seems to be wearing down. You remember that during her last visit, her throat and mouth appeared unusually red. During this visit, the redness is even brighter. When you lightly press against her gingival tissue, you notice bleeding. When you question Jane about possibly having bulimia nervosa, she tells you that managing her weight has nothing to do with her teeth. How would you respond to Jane? What information is important for her to know to help her understand how this behavior is impacting her teeth?

Damage to the teeth and oral cavity can be permanent without treatment. Home treatments can be effective in helping eating disorder patients begin the process of repairing their teeth. The dental team can provide tools for sensitive teeth, such as toothbrushes with soft bristles and toothpaste that is nonabrasive. Oral irrigating devices can be helpful for cleaning without irritating the gingiva, which may bleed easily. Sodium fluoride increases a tooth's resistance to acid erosion and strengthens the root of the tooth. Daily fluoride can be prescribed as a mouthwash or as a gel for a custom-made dental tray. Dental professionals can also prescribe saliva replacements. It is important to provide patients with oral hygiene instructions specific to their condition. Remind a patient with bulimia not to brush immediately after purging because the environment of the mouth is very acidic after vomiting. Brushing immediately after vomiting tends to push the acids back onto the teeth. Instruct the patient to rinse first with water or a mixture of baking soda and water. This action helps reduce the acidic environment of the oral cavity.

Dental professionals are on the front lines of helping to diagnose eating disorders, yet it is not uncommon for clinical staff to feel uncomfortable asking patients about whether they might have an eating disorder. For adult patients, ask them directly if they are having problems with their eating (see Table 11-9) and provide a referral to a physician for further evaluation. For patients under the age of 18 years, speak with the parents. In both cases, make it clear that dental treatment will take place alongside any medical treatment the patient receives. As a health professional, you have a responsibility to act if you believe a patient's health is in danger. Remember that eating disorders can be deadly. No matter how uncomfortable it may be, take the time to talk to a patient any time there are signs that an eating disorder may be present.

TABLE 11-9 If You Suspect an Eating Disorder

KEYS TO REMEMBER	WHAT YOU CAN DO
Respect patient privacy	Talk to the patient one on one; if other assistants are in the room, ask them to step out so that the patient has as much privacy as possible.
Open up	It is okay to be honest and admit that the topic is uneasy. Try something like, "This is a little uncomfortable, but I need to ask you something important about your health."
Be direct	Be professional, but ask the patient directly if you suspect an eating disorder may be present. Try something like, "I notice some problems with your teeth that are very similar to what we see in people with eating disorders. Do you have an eating disorder?"
Show that you care	Remind the patient that his or her health is your biggest concern. Try not to make the patient feel embarrassed, ashamed, or guilty. Use statements that show care and concern, such as: ■ "I know this might be difficult to talk about." ■ "Your health is what is most important." ■ "I am here to help you however I can." ■ "What can I do to help you with this?"

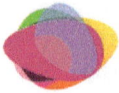

Voice of Experience

Ever hear the phrase, "less is more"? I have found that when approaching patients about personal, sensitive topics, sometimes you can do more by actually doing a little bit less. When I saw a patient whom I suspected might have bulimia nervosa, rather than being angry or asking lots of questions, I found it helpful to take a quieter approach. I gently asked whether she had any struggles with eating, and she gradually began opening up and sharing her concerns. Eventually, she admitted that she had been binging and purging, and then we were able to talk about resources available to help her. It is not unusual for patients to feel afraid to share personal information with the dentist—it may feel too much like sharing with a parent or teacher! As a dental assistant, I feel lucky that I can put my patients at ease and be an important resource for them.

Inappropriate Dieting

Most people at some point in their lives will go on a diet to lose weight. Dieting can be either healthy or unhealthy depending on the methods used. Appropriate dieting includes following the guidelines suggested by the USDA, such as eating balanced meals made up of large amounts of fruits and vegetables, maintaining an adequate number of calories, drinking at least eight 8-ounce glasses of water each day, and getting regular exercise.

Unfortunately, there are also unsafe methods of dieting. Repeatedly going "on" and "off" diets is known as "yo-yo dieting," and it can damage the body's metabolism. This can make losing weight in the future very difficult. "Fad" diets are ones that only allow one or two types of foods, or that eliminate all foods of a certain color or nutrient. These diets deny the body of important vitamins and minerals. Also, once a "fad" diet is stopped, the person is likely to not only gain back the weight lost but additional pounds as well (called *rebound weight gain*). Rebound weight gain is also a problem for yo-yo dieters. Diets that are extremely low in calories are dangerous and can lead to serious health problems, such as brain and heart damage. Individuals who exercise vigorously or play sports intensely may be at risk for using inappropriate diets to keep weight down and enhance their athletic performance. In girls and young women, this can lead to a combination of conditions known as the **female athlete triad**. These conditions include disordered eating, loss of the menstrual period, and weakening of the bones, also known as *osteoporosis*. Make sure to talk to patients about how to diet safely and healthily, and refer a patient to a nutritional counselor if needed. Although weight loss may be slow, appropriate dieting means long-term success, both in terms of weight and overall health.

Lack of Teeth

When the bone and gingival tissue of the oral cavity become infected, tooth loss can occur. People who are lacking teeth, especially in the back of the mouth, may develop nutritional and bowel problems due to their choice of foods. Patients lacking teeth often avoid foods that require more chewing, such as meat, raw vegetables, fresh fruits, and even some types of bread. In turn, they may eat softer foods, such as those containing high amounts of fat or simple carbohydrates. This can lead to a decrease in important vitamins, minerals, and fiber and an increase in cholesterol and sugar. Patients who are missing teeth also often cannot chew their food properly, which makes food more difficult to swallow and digest. Digestive problems are not uncommon in individuals who are missing teeth.

Many older adult patients have some or all of their teeth missing. Be especially mindful of how missing teeth can impact nutrition and health among these patients. For any patients with missing teeth, it is not unusual for a dentist to give a referral to a nutritional counselor for recommendations on how to eat safely and properly.

CHECKPOINTS

11-8 In what ways does anorexia nervosa differ from bulimia nervosa?

11-9 What are some common oral signs and symptoms that a patient may have an eating disorder?

11-10 What health problems can come from lacking teeth

Chapter Highlights

+ Proper nutrition is an important part of preventing dental caries, especially when it comes to eating carbohydrates.
+ Macronutrients include carbohydrates, protein, fat, water, and fiber.
+ Carbohydrates include sugars, called *simple carbohydrates*, as well as starches and vegetables, called *complex* *carbohydrates*. Complex carbohydrates are considered healthier than simple carbohydrates because they keep blood sugar levels even and are generally higher in fiber.
+ Protein helps build, repair, and maintain the body's muscles, tissues, and organs. Proteins usually come from animal products, such as meat, eggs, and milk products,

but smaller amounts of protein can be found in some vegetables and grains.

✦ Fat is needed to help the body use nutrients properly and includes saturated and unsaturated types of fat. Saturated fats are considered unhealthy and generally come from animals, whereas unsaturated fats, or "good fats," come from plants and seeds.

✦ Micronutrients are vitamins and minerals. Vitamins come from plants and animals and are needed for cells to use food for fuel. Minerals are chemical elements found in the soil and water that are needed to maintain body structure and functioning.

✦ All food contains energy, called *calories*; too few calories can damage organs and cells, but too many calories can cause weight gain.

✦ People need different amounts of calories based on age, gender, and other factors, but the average adult should consume no more than 300 grams of carbohydrates, between 75 and 100 grams of protein, and no more than 65 grams of fat (and less than 20 grams of saturated fat) daily.

✦ The Recommended Dietary Allowances are guidelines that tell how much of a nutrient is needed to keep nearly all people (about 98%) healthy, depending on age and gender.

✦ Food labels are on all packaged foods and provide valuable information about a food's calories, serving size, and nutrients.

✦ Some patients may need to make changes to their diet, such as people with certain medical conditions (like diabetes), food allergies, and excessive weight. A dietician or nutritional counselor is a professional who can help figure out what changes in diet need to be made.

✦ Anorexia nervosa is an eating disorder in which individuals starve themselves in order to keep their weight very low. It can lead to serious problems with the heart, brain, and other organs. It can even lead to death.

✦ Bulimia nervosa is an eating disorder in which individuals eat excessive amounts of food, called *binging*, and then rid the body of food, called *purging*.

✦ Eating disorders are very harmful to oral health and can cause problems such as wearing away of tooth enamel (enamel erosion), bleeding or bruising of the roof of the mouth, lack of saliva, swollen salivary glands, and possible tooth loss.

✦ Patients who are missing teeth, such as older adult patients, may suffer from poor nutrition due to difficulty chewing food properly. They may avoid foods that require a lot of chewing, such as meat, raw vegetables, and fresh fruits.

 **Review Questions**

1. Which macronutrient carries the greatest risk for developing dental caries?

   a. Sugar

   b. Protein

   c. Carbohydrates

   d. Fat

2. Which of the following statements about simple and complex carbohydrates is true?

   a. Simple carbohydrates are considered healthier because the body uses them for energy quickly.

   b. Complex carbohydrates are considered healthier because they keep the blood sugar stable and are higher in fiber.

   c. Simple carbohydrates are considered healthier because they are higher in fiber and easier to digest.

   d. Complex carbohydrates cause more oral problems than simple carbohydrates because they require more chewing.

3. Unsaturated fats come from what sources?

   a. Polyunsaturated fats include corn, flax, and canola oils, whereas monounsaturated fats include olive oil, avocados, and nuts.

   b. Polyunsaturated fats include animal products, such as meat and eggs, whereas monounsaturated fats include olive oil, avocados, and nuts.

   c. Polyunsaturated fats include corn, flax, and canola oils, whereas monounsaturated fats include animal products, such as meat and eggs.

   d. Polyunsaturated fats come from animal sources, whereas monounsaturated fats come from plant sources.

4. Which are needed along with calcium and phosphorus to help build strong teeth and bones?

   a. Vitamins D and K

   b. Fluoride and magnesium

   c. Vitamin E and fluoride

   d. Vitamin D and magnesium

5. The Recommended Dietary Allowances:

    a. State that 98% of people should follow the MyPyramid food guide.

    b. State how much of a nutrient is needed for most people (about 98%) to stay healthy.

    c. State how many calories are needed for most people (about 98%) to stay healthy.

    d. State how many vitamins and minerals are needed to stay healthy about 98% of the time.

6. Food labels do not include which of the following?

    a. Amount of saturated and unsaturated fat per serving

    b. Amount of cholesterol per serving

    c. Complete amount of vitamins and minerals per serving

    d. Amount of fiber per serving

7. Healthy nutrition includes which of the following?

    a. Reducing exercise to avoid bodily injuries

    b. Limiting water to no more than eight 8-ounce glasses of water per day

    c. Eating three balanced meals consisting of a variety of foods

    d. Avoiding all fats and sugars

8. Which of the following statements about patient education and nutrition is true?

    a. Tell all patients to eat from all categories of food, regardless of their background.

    b. Do not discuss nutrition with patients; instead, tell patients to see a dietician or nutritionist for information.

    c. Ask patients what foods they like to eat and encourage them to eat only those.

    d. Provide general guidelines about eating healthy meals, such as those consistent with United States Department of Agriculture recommendations.

9. Anorexia nervosa is defined by which symptoms?

    a. Binging and purging

    b. Refusing to eat and purging

    c. Exercising excessively and having an average body weight

    d. Refusing to eat and having a very low body weight

10. All of the following may be risk factors for anorexia nervosa except:

    a. Female gender.

    b. A desire for perfection.

    c. Average or high self-esteem.

    d. Involvement in jobs such as dancing, modeling, and acting.

11. Unlike in anorexia nervosa, patients with bulimia nervosa:

    a. Are not at risk for death.

    b. Can develop dental problems.

    c. Do not go out of their way to hide their disorder.

    d. Are usually average or slightly above average in weight.

12. Which of the following is NOT a common dental problem associated with repeated vomiting?

    a. Swollen salivary glands, giving the jaw a square-like appearance

    b. Excessive saliva

    c. Loss of tooth enamel

    d. Sensitivity to temperature and pain

13. When oral signs and symptoms of an eating disorder are present:

    a. Make the patient an appointment to see a physician, but do not ask the patient any questions.

    b. Only ask the patient questions about his or her teeth.

    c. Ask the patient gently but directly whether he or she is struggling with an eating disorder.

    d. Make a note in the chart and follow the patient for 6 months before questioning.

14. "Yo-yo" and "fad" diets:

    a. Can damage the metabolism and make future weight loss much harder.

    b. Only occur in women.

    c. Are not important for dental care.

    d. Are safe as long as the patient is taking vitamins.

15. Patients who are missing teeth, such as older adult patients:

    a. Do not usually go to the dentist.

    b. May need a referral to a nutritional professional.

    c. Should not have problems eating fruit and bread.

    d. May have digestive problems due to eating too many raw vegetables.

Active Learning Exercises

1. Make a journal of the daily food you consume for one week. Evaluate the journal and identify those foods with the potential to facilitate dental caries. What replacements or substitutions could you make? What other modifications could you make to limit your intake of such foods?

2. Imagine treating a patient with severe lingual erosion. You suspect the patient may be bulimic, or may have been at one time. Create a dialogue to open a non-threatening discussion regarding this condition. Be sure to establish an atmosphere of comfort and trust in your discussion.

3. Discuss quantity versus frequency of cariogenic foods. Which is more cariogenic in nature: Consuming a large chocolate bar at one sitting, or eating the chocolate bar over the course of the day?

Application Activities

1. Spend 3 days keeping a food diary. At the end of the third day, calculate the average amount of calories, carbohydrates, protein, and fat you have eaten. Were your amounts higher or lower than you thought they would be? How do they compare with United States Department of Agriculture recommendations?

2. What are some easy ways you can make healthy diet changes over the next week? Can you replace your favorite fried food with something baked? Can you add more fruits and vegetables to your plate? Make a list of five changes you can make over the next week to improve your diet.

3. What might you do if you thought a friend had an eating disorder? Would you talk to him or her? Consider what things you could say as well as how your friend might react. If your friend gets angry, how might you respond? What would you say if your friend denied having a problem?

4. Visit your favorite fast food restaurant and obtain the nutritional information for your favorite fast food meal. (You can also usually find this information on the restaurant's website.) Gather all the nutritional information for the meal, including total calories, sodium content, fat content, total carbohydrates, total protein content, and any vitamins or minerals. Be sure to include all foods and any liquids you consume along with the meal, such as soda, iced tea, coffee, alcohol, etc. Bring this information to class to share. How did you feel once you compiled the nutritional information? Were you surprised by the amount of calories, sodium, fat, and sugar? After reviewing the information, will you continue to eat these foods or will you attempt to make healthier choices? Or do you feel your food choices are already pretty healthy?

PREPARING FOR CERTIFICATION EXAMS

Review the topic "Nutrition and Dental Caries" in this chapter to prepare for the Dental Assisting National Board (DANB) exam.

Oral Pathology

CHAPTER OUTLINE

CHAPTER CHECKLIST

On completion of this chapter, students will be able to:

- ☑ Describe the tools used to diagnose oral pathologies.
- ☑ Identify the classifications of oral lesions.
- ☑ Describe the various types of oral lesions.
- ☑ Identify oral conditions associated with human immunodeficiency virus/acquired immune deficiency syndrome infection.
- ☑ Describe the origin and treatment of various pathologies affecting the hard and soft tissues.
- ☑ Describe the two kinds of oral carcinomas.
- ☑ Describe abnormalities that may occur during tooth development.

KEY TERMS

abscess – a sac filled with purulent material and surrounded by inflamed tissue that forms as a result of localized infection

aphthous (AF-thus) ulcer – stomatitis characterized by intermittent episodes of painful oral ulcers that are covered by gray exudate, are surrounded by a halo, and range from several mm to 2 cm in diameter; they are limited to oral mucosa membranes; sometimes called a *canker sore*

biopsy – the process of removing tissue from a patient for diagnostic examination

blister – a fluid-filled, thin-walled structure under the epidermis or within the epidermis

bulla (BUL-uh) – a fluid-filled blister greater than 1 cm in diameter appearing as a circumscribed area of separation of the epidermis from the subepidermal structure or as a circumscribed area of separation of epidermal cells caused by the presence of serum; plural is *bullae*

carcinoma – any of the various types of malignant neoplasm derived from epithelial cells, chiefly glandular (adenocarcinoma) or squamous cell carcinoma

cellulitis – inflammation of subcutaneous, loose connective tissue

congenital condition – existing at birth, referring to certain mental or physical traits, anomalies, malformations, diseases, and like findings, which may be either hereditary or due to an environmental influence

cyst – an abnormal sac containing gas, fluid, or a semisolid material, with a membranous lining

ecchymosis (eh-kuh-MOH-sis) – a discoloration of the skin caused by extravasation of blood into the skin, differing from petechiae only in size (i.e., larger than 3 mm in diameter)

erosion – tooth loss due to chemical or unknown factors; also a shallow ulcer in the mucosa, with no penetration of the mucosa

erythroplakia (ih-rith-roh-PLAY-kee-uh) – a red, velvety, plaquelike lesion of mucous membrane that often represents a malignant change

etiology (ee-tee-OL-uh-jee) – the science and study of causes of disease and their mode of operation

fistula (fis-CHOO-luh) – an abnormal passage from one epithelial surface to another

glossitis – inflammation of the tongue

granuloma – term applied to nodular inflammatory lesions, usually small or granular, firm, persistent, and containing compactly grouped modified phagocytes

hematoma – localized mass of extravasated blood relatively or completely confined within an organ or tissue; blood is usually clotted or partly clotted; for example, a bruised area

idiopathic – denoting a disease of unknown cause

lesion – wound or injury; any abnormal tissue

leukoplakia (loo-kuh-PLAY-kee-uh) – white patch of oral mucous membrane that cannot be wiped off and cannot be diagnosed clinically as any specific disease entity

macule – a flat area, up to 1 cm in diameter, differing perceptibly in color from surrounding tissue; small discolored patch or spot on skin, neither elevated above nor depressed below skin's surface; for example, freckles

metastasize – the shifting of disease or its local manifestations from one part of the body to another; spread of a disease process from one part of the body to another, as in appearance of distant neoplasms in an area removed from the locale of the original neoplasm

neoplasm – abnormal tissue that grows by cellular proliferation more rapidly than normal and continues to grow after the stimuli that initiated the new growth cease

nodule – a small node; in skin, a node up to 1 cm in diameter, solid, with palpable depth

palpate – to examine by feeling and pressing with the palms of hands and fingers

papule – a circumscribed, solid elevation up to 1 cm in diameter on the skin

petechiae (pih-TEE-kee-ee) – minute (1–2 millimeter) hemorrhagic spots on mucosa or skin that do not blanch even when pressed

plaque – patch or small differentiated area on body surface

purpura (PUR-pyur-uh) – a large area of skin discoloration caused by underlying bleeding

pustule – a circumscribed, superficial elevation of the skin, up to 1 cm in diameter, containing purulent material

sarcoma – connective tissue neoplasm, usually highly malignant, formed by proliferation of mesodermal cells

stomatitis – inflammation of the mucous membrane of the mouth

teratogen (TARE-uh-toh-jen) – any agent or factor that induces or increases the incidence of abnormal prenatal development

ulcer – a lesion through skin or mucous membrane resulting from loss of tissue, usually with inflammation

vesicle – a small bladder or bladder-like structure; a small, less than 1 cm, circumscribed skin elevation containing fluid; for example, a blister

Introduction

Oral pathology is the study of diseases of the oral cavity. Dental assistants cannot diagnose diseases. Only a dentist can do that. If you notice something unusual in the oral cavity during a dental procedure, legal and ethical considerations prevent you from speculating about a diagnosis with a patient. Instead, quietly point it out to the dentist. This should be done in a way that does not alarm the patient. Dental assistants serve a valuable role by observing patients and bringing anything unusual to the attention of the dentist. In many cases, dental assistants have a unique perspective on the patient's oral cavity. They see it from a different angle than the dentist and may also see a pathology when taking oral radiographs.

It is important to be able to recognize normal anatomy and structures and also possible abnormalities. With a basic understanding of the signs and symptoms associated with diseases affecting the oral cavity, you can play a vital role in detecting oral pathologies.

The Language of Pathology

When dentists or other physicians discuss pathologies, they use a number of terms that dental assistants should be familiar with:

- **Etiology**: the cause of the disease
- **Idiopathic**: a disease of unknown origin
- **Biopsy**: a tissue sample analyzed to diagnose certain conditions
- **Palpate**: to feel or rub something to get an understanding of its size, tenderness, and texture
- **Inflammation**: a specific immune system response that includes swelling, redness, and tenderness

✓ CHECKPOINT

12-1 What is an idiopathic condition?

Diagnosing Oral Pathologies

The steps to diagnosing an oral pathology depend on the condition itself. Dental assistants cannot legally diagnose oral pathologies, and they should never relate their suspicions to a patient. It is important not to express alarm to a patient, through words or through body language. If a dental assistant sees something unusual, he or she should remain calm and objective and discreetly bring it to the dentist's attention. The dentist will follow certain steps and rely on certain tools to arrive at a diagnosis. These tools include the dental history, clinical diagnosis, microscopic findings, dental radiographs, surgical findings, and laboratory findings. Each of these will be described in greater detail below.

Dental History

The dental history is often the first place a dentist turns for information. This important record should include the patient's history of oral health, including any previously diagnosed conditions, as well as a general medical history, family history, and information, such as smoking status and lifestyle habits, all of which might help the dentist make a decision.

The family history is especially important because many diseases are genetic in nature. They are passed from parent to child. For example, a family history of cancer is an important diagnostic element because, for certain cancers, there is a greater chance of offspring developing cancer, and additional screening may be warranted.

The dental history, however, is not usually enough to make a diagnosis by itself. The dentist will need more information from the patient's unique circumstances to complete the investigation. Often, the dentist uses information or results from a variety of tests or examinations to make a diagnosis.

Clinical Diagnosis

Many conditions are diagnosed based on their clinical appearance and feel. This is where the dentist's expertise comes into play. Lesions and pathologies will be evaluated based on their size, texture, appearance, color, location, and any other observable traits. Some conditions, such as fungal infections in the mouth and fissured tongue, can be more easily diagnosed by clinical diagnosis alone. During a clinical examination, the dentist might palpate the lesion, observe it closely, or compare it to similar lesions to help arrive at a diagnosis.

Microscopic Findings

Microscopic findings include biopsy findings. In a biopsy, a small sample of tissue is removed from a suspicious

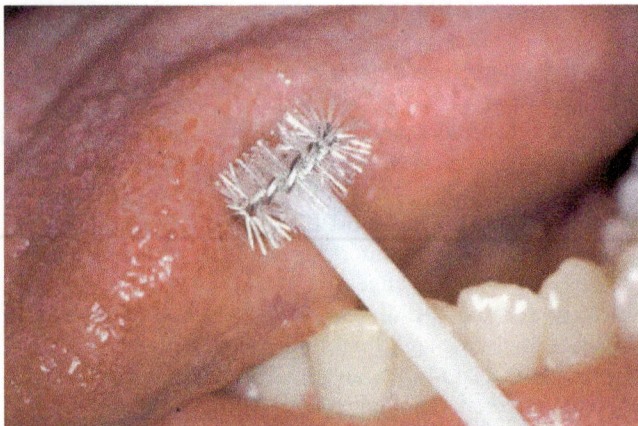

Figure 12–1 An example of using the brush biopsy technique to obtain cells from a lesion on the lateral border of the tongue. (Photo provided by CDx Laboratories, Inc., Suffern, NY.)

area and examined under a microscope. Biopsies can be performed by the dentist or hygienist in the office. Many cancers can only be definitively diagnosed by microscopic findings, and biopsy samples are often sent to off-site labs for examination. Some dentists may refer the patient to an oral surgeon or specialist for the biopsy. Different types of biopsies may be performed depending on the suspicious lesion (Figure 12-1).

Dental Radiographs

Radiographs are an invaluable tool for diagnosis. In general, patients should always have an updated set of radiographs in their dental record. If the dentist is suspicious of a lesion, or if the records need updating, a patient might be asked to have radiographs taken. These can be used to diagnose impacted teeth, dental caries, cysts, abscesses, and various bone lesions (Figure 12-2). For more information on dental radiography, please see Part VII: Dental Radiography.

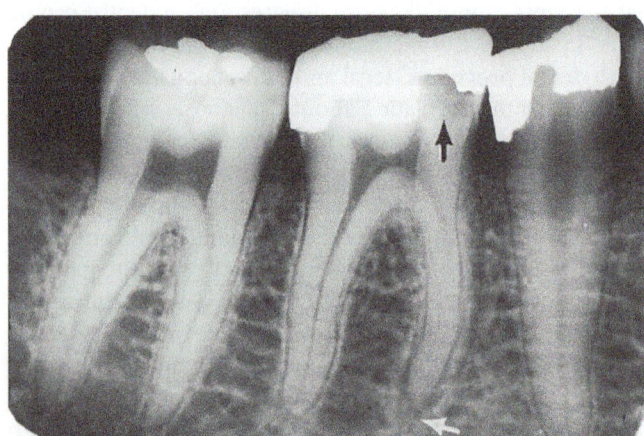

Figure 12–2 A radiograph of acute apical abscess. Note the abscess at the white arrow. The black arrow shows a carious lesion under the restoration.

Surgical Findings

Surgical findings are discovered during the course of a surgery and can help make a diagnosis. Surgeries can be exploratory or conducted for another condition. An example of a situation that might require surgery is unusual findings on a dental radiograph. A dentist might not be able to distinguish, for example, between certain types of bone cysts on a radiograph and will perform a surgery to tell if further treatment is needed or not.

Laboratory Results

Lab results typically include blood tests, urine tests, and culturing of microorganisms to determine their type. A wide variety of conditions can be diagnosed based on lab tests, although, in some cases, dentists have to combine lab tests with other diagnostic tools to make a diagnosis.

CHECKPOINTS

12-2 Which dental office employees are legally able to diagnose oral pathologies?

12-3 What key traits are evaluated during a clinical examination of a lesion?

Oral Lesions

Lesions are any type of abnormal tissue. A wound, a cyst, or a tumor might all be described as oral lesions. Any type of lesion is worth investigating, even if only to make sure a simple cut is healing well.

Oral lesions are classified by their position in relation to the mucosa and whether they are flat or raised. Lesions can be characterized by the following descriptions:

- Below the mucosal surface
- Above the mucosal surface
- Even with the mucosal surface
- Flat or raised

Lesions Below the Mucosal Surface

Some lesions may begin at the mucosal surface and extend down into the tissue or be located entirely under the mucosal surface (Figure 12-3). These types of lesions include the following:

- **Ulcers** are small craters in the mucosal surface. They are normally inflamed and painful, and they range in size from a few millimeters to several centimeters in diameter. Ulcers can be caused by other diseases, such as oral cancer, or by aggravation of the mucosa by

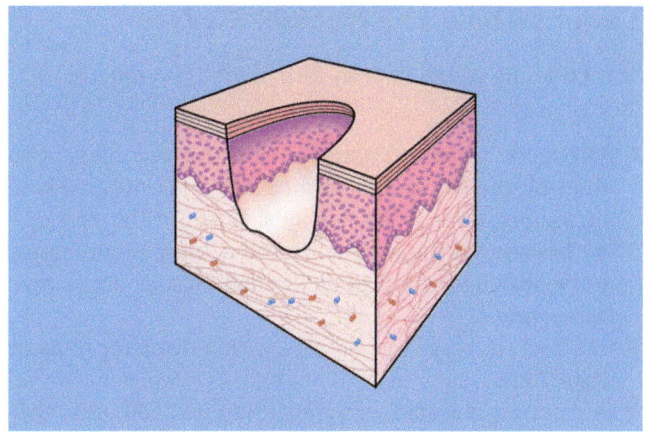

A

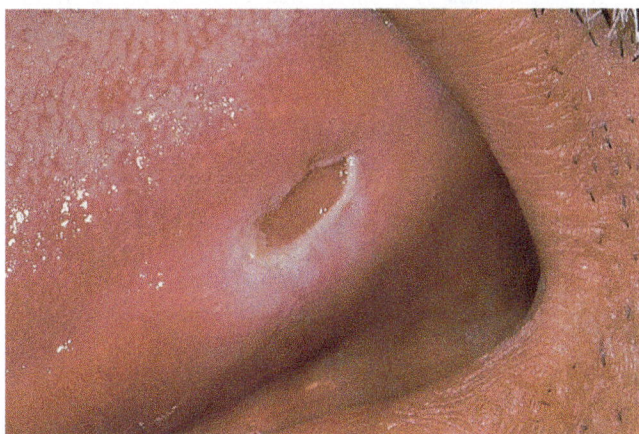

B

Figure 12–3 Ulcers. A. Illustration and **B.** photograph of an ulcer, a lesion below the mucosal surface.

trauma or foreign substances such as tobacco products. Food, chemicals, and autoimmune responses can also lead to ulcers. The location of the lesion affects the type of treatment needed.

- **Erosions** are caused by mechanical activity, such as chewing or the friction of an orthodontic appliance. These shallow wounds are often inflamed and have ragged, ill-defined margins. They are located wherever there is contact between whatever caused the injury and the mucosa.
- An **abscess** is a small sac filled with purulent material caused by infection with bacteria or other microorganisms. They can either be sealed off or connected to the surface of the mucosa by a **fistula**. Abscesses may be located at the apex of the tooth or within the periodontal membrane. The location of the abscess affects the type of treatment needed.
- **Cysts** are small sacs. They can be solid tissue or partly or completely filled with fluid. There are many causes of cysts, some benign and some requiring treatment. Many dentists suggest the removal of impacted wisdom teeth because, over time, cysts can form around the crown of an unerupted tooth.

Lesions Above the Mucosal Surface

Several kinds of lesions can form above the mucosal surface (Figure 12-4):

- **Blisters** are raised areas of skin that are filled with fluid. Blisters are usually formed as a result of some kind of trauma, such as friction or a burn. In the oral cavity, because of the constant motion, blisters commonly burst, leaving behind an ulcer. Small blisters are known as **vesicles**.
- **Bullae** are very large blisters, with a diameter of more than 1 cm.
- A **pustule** is a small, elevated lesion that contains purulent material (pus).
- A **hematoma** is a blister that contains blood. Hematomas are caused by a ruptured blood vessel near the surface of the mucosa. They are sometimes caused during injection of an oral anesthetic. If a hematoma occurs during injection, the dentist can treat it with gentle pressure, which causes the blood to be redistributed beneath the tissue.
- **Papules** are small, elevated areas of skin. They can vary in pigmentation and texture.

- **Plaques** are any abnormal patches of skin. They are slightly raised, and they may be off-color compared to the rest of the mucosa. Oral skin plaques are not related to dental plaque.

Lesions Even with the Mucosal Surface

Lesions that form even with the mucosal surface are usually clearly marked by pigmentation or discoloration (Figure 12-5). They include:

- **Ecchymosis** is a discoloration of the skin that results from pinpoint hemorrhages that cause blood to pool in subcutaneous tissue. Commonly called *bruising*, ecchymosis is typically the result of trauma.
- **Macules** and patches are areas of different texture or color. This is a descriptive term, not a diagnosable condition.
- **Petechiae** are tiny spots of red or purple caused by localized hemorrhaging. These tiny bruises are often caused by hemorrhage or strain.

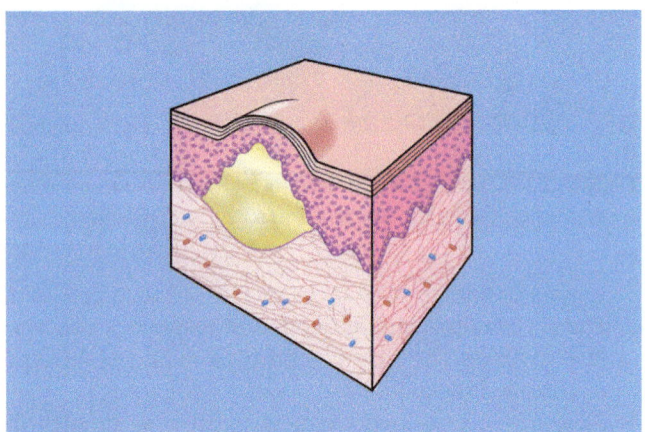

A

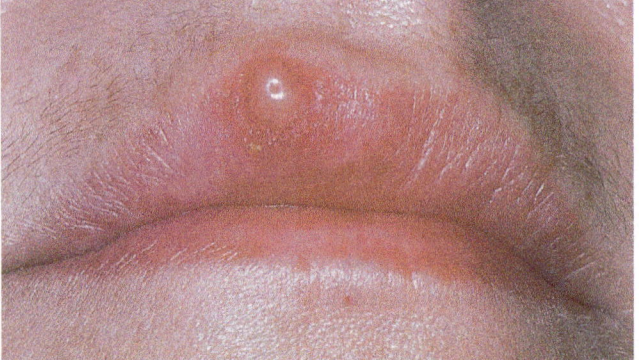

B

Figure 12–4 Vesicles. A. Illustration and **B.** photograph of a vesicle, a small blister above the mucosal surface.

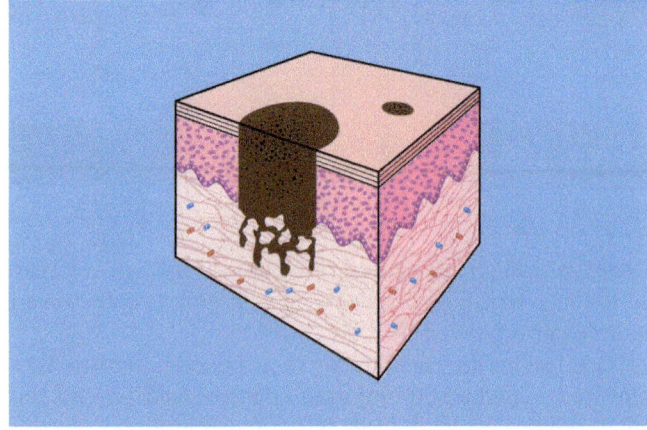

A

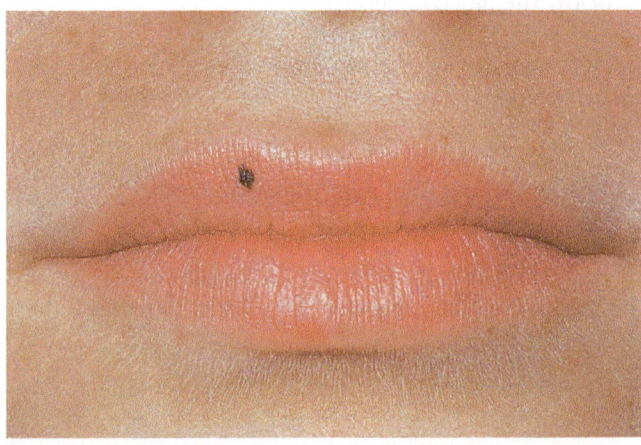

B

Figure 12–5 Macules. A. Illustration and **B.** photograph of a macule, a lesion even with the mucosal surface.

■ **Purpura** is a term used to describe a large area of skin discoloration caused by underlying bleeding. Both petechiae and ecchymosis are forms of purpura.

Flat or Raised Lesions

Three types of lesions may lie flat with the mucosal surface or be raised above it (Figure 12-6):

■ **Nodules** are small, round lumps that are located beneath the mucosa but protrude outward. When palpated, they usually feel like frozen corn kernels.

■ **Neoplasms** are tumors. Medically speaking, a neoplasm is made from new tissue that serves no obvious purpose. Neoplasms can either be malignant (cancerous) or benign (harmless). A biopsy is usually required to definitively diagnose oral cancer.

■ A **granuloma** is a neoplasm that contains granulated tissue. The suffix *-oma* is used to describe a tumor. Not all granulomas are located above the mucosal surface; they can also be located within the bone.

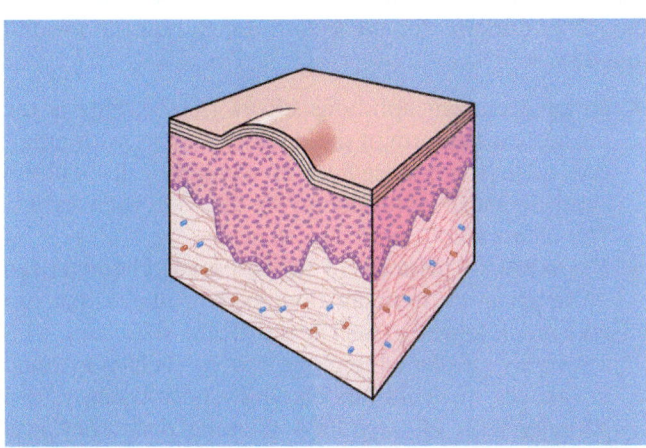

A

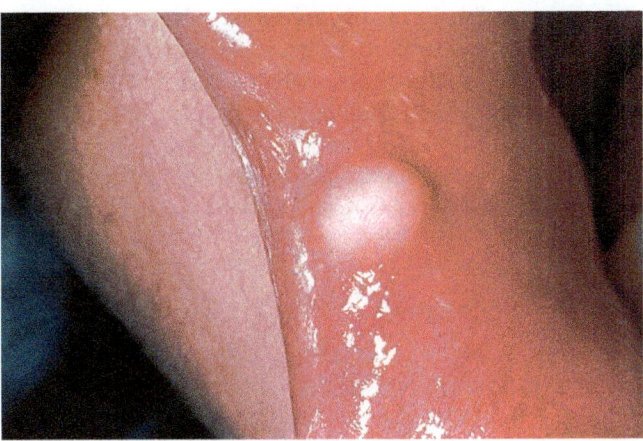

B

Figure 12–6 Nodules. A. Illustration and **B.** photograph of a nodule, a lesion that is located below the mucosal surface but protrudes outward.

CHECKPOINTS

12-4 How is an ulcer different from an abscess?

12-5 What is a bulla?

12-6 What is an ecchymosis?

Hard and Soft Tissue Diseases and Associated Lesions

Many diseases and conditions can affect the oral cavity. Although a dental assistant cannot diagnose conditions, it is still important for dental assistants to recognize the most common lesions. The dentist should be alerted to the presence of any unusual lesion.

Lesions of Uncertain Cause

Leukoplakia

Leukoplakias are white patches that occur anywhere in the oral cavity (Figure 12-7). Leukoplakias normally are not pathologic but should not be ignored. Leukoplakias often occur before malignant lesions develop, and they are frequently caused by high-risk activities, such as tobacco use (including smokeless tobacco) and excessive alcohol consumption. Leukoplakias can also be caused by vitamin A deficiency, cheek biting, and any form of oral aggravation such as poorly fitting dental appliances.

Leukoplakia lesions can vary in appearance and size from very small, white, almost transparent, bumps to a heavy, warty plaque. They may appear leathery. The lesions are firmly fixed to the underlying tissue and cannot be

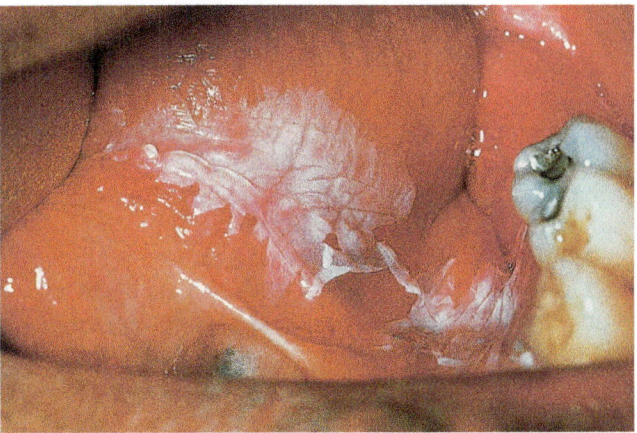

Figure 12–7 Leukoplakia. Note the white patches on the floor of the mouth and the ventral tongue.

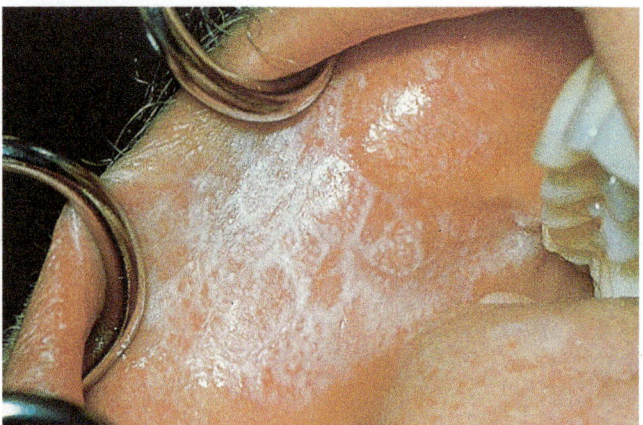

Figure 12–8 Lichen planus is white papules that form webbing.

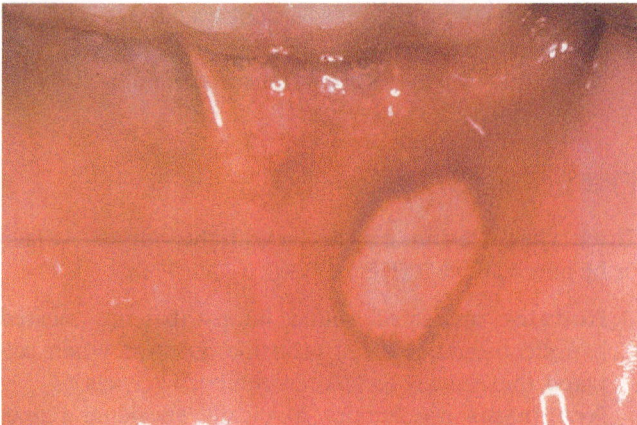

Figure 12–9 Aphthous ulcer is also known as *canker sore.* Note the red border.

scraped away or wiped away, which distinguishes them from thrush.

Leukoplakias should be distinguished from hairy leukoplakias, which are associated with human immunodeficiency virus (HIV) infection. These are covered further in the Oral Complications of HIV/AIDS Infection section later in the chapter.

Lichen Planus

Lichen planus can affect both the oral mucosa and the skin (Figure 12-8). On the skin, these lesions appear as flat, red papules. In the oral cavity, they are tiny white papules that form characteristic circles and webbing. This pattern is known as *Wickham striae.*

There are two forms of lichen planus, and both are relatively common. The regular form is chronic and benign and without symptoms. There is also an erosive form that, over time, causes degeneration of the outer layer of skin in the oral cavity. This can result in swelling and tenderness, and the patient may be sensitive to certain foods.

Lichen planus is treated with topical steroids.

Aphthous Ulcer

Aphthous ulcers are commonly known as *canker sores* (Figure 12-9). They are common lesions, and little is understood about their underlying cause. Outbreaks are sometimes associated with trauma and stress, food allergies, highly acidic foods, and hormonal changes, and they are often found in patients with weakened immune systems. Aphthous ulcers tend to run in families.

Aphthous ulcers should not be confused with herpes lesions, which are caused by a virus and are highly contagious. In contrast, aphthous ulcers cannot be transmitted to others. Herpes lesions occur on attached tissue, such as the lips or the gingiva, whereas aphthous ulcers occur on movable tissue, such as mucous membranes.

A typical aphthous ulcer begins with a burning or stinging sensation in the oral cavity, usually on the mucosa

lining the inside of the cheek or on the tongue, the floor of the mouth, or the inner lip. A papule forms soon afterward, which bursts and leaves behind a painful ulcer. Round or oval in shape, the shallow ulcer typically has a white-gray or yellowish center surrounded by a red border. The ulcers can be infected with bacteria, which causes further discomfort and swelling. The number and length of duration for the lesions depend on the form of the disease:

- Minor recurrent aphthous ulcers (RAUs). This is the most common form of the disease. Patients with minor RAU might experience five or fewer outbreaks of ulcers annually, usually with one to six ulcers in their mouth. The ulcers take 7 to 10 days to heal.
- Major RAUs. This form of the disease is characterized by much more frequent outbreaks of ulcers that can take much longer to heal. It is typically associated with a severely weakened immune system, such as is found in cancer patients undergoing chemotherapy and patients with HIV/acquired immune deficiency syndrome (AIDS).

Even the mild form of aphthous ulcers can cause considerable discomfort for patients, depending on the individual lesions themselves. Dental care may have to be rescheduled to avoid pulling or stretching the sensitive tissue.

Aphthous ulcers are usually treated with a topical painkiller. Over-the-counter products are available for patients to use.

Geographic Tongue

Geographic tongue is a condition that affects about 2% of the population. People with geographic tongue have red, smooth patches on the dorsal and lateral surfaces of the tongue. The patches are often surrounded by a whitish or pale border. The condition takes its name from the shifting pattern of patches, which resemble a map. The condition has no symptoms and treatment is not necessary.

Pathologies of Infectious Origin

Infectious agents can affect the oral cavity in one of two ways: microorganisms can directly cause lesions, such as an oral herpes infection, or an infectious agent such as HIV/AIDS can weaken the immune system and make a patient more vulnerable to lesions. An accurate, current medical history is vital when it comes to diagnosing oral lesions caused by infectious agents.

When treating patients with potentially infectious agents, it is vital to practice effective infection control to prevent the spread of the microorganism. According to current standards, all patients and all body fluids should be treated as potentially infectious. Infection control is covered in greater depth in Chapter 14, Disease and Infection Control.

Cellulitis

Cellulitis is an inflammatory condition that is caused by bacterial infection, usually a streptococcus bacterium (Figure 12-10). Cellulitis occurs when the bacterial infection spreads in the skin and tissues immediately beneath the skin. It can occur anywhere in the body and is sometimes seen in the legs of patients with poorly controlled diabetes. However, cellulitis can occur anywhere bacteria gain entry to the body, including through cuts, scrapes, bites, and other lesions. Patients may experience cellulitis as a result of an untreated dental abscess.

Symptoms of cellulitis include swelling, redness, heat, fever, and pain. The symptoms are related to the severity of the infection. A rapidly spreading, severe infection can be accompanied by a high fever and intense, throbbing pain. Infections can stay localized, or they can spread to nearby lymph nodes, the brain, or even the bloodstream, causing potentially serious damage.

Cellulitis is typically diagnosed by its appearance and symptoms. Treatment is with antibiotics. Symptoms will usually resolve within a few days of antibiotic treatment.

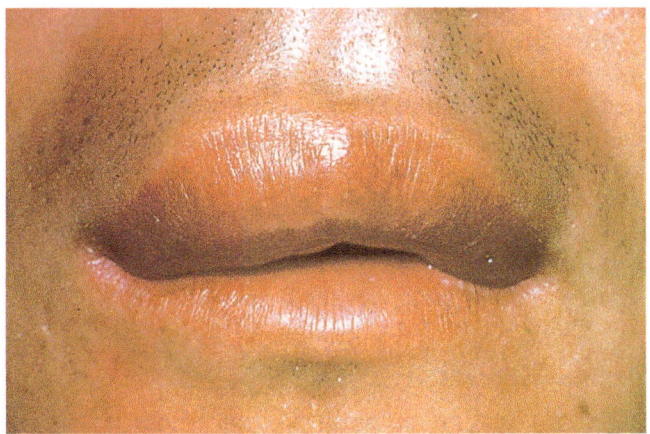

Figure 12–10 Cellulitis. This patient's swelling of the lip is caused by an abscessed incisor.

Herpes Simplex Lesions

The herpes virus is typically spread through direct contact with a herpes lesion. Once the virus has successfully colonized a host, it causes periodic outbreaks resulting in painful lesions and blisters, often referred to as a *cold sore* or a *fever blister* (Figure 12-11A). Herpes lesions can affect the eyes, nose, and lips. Oral herpes lesions may appear singly or in clusters. The initial infection usually occurs in children and may be mild, with isolated ulcers, or characterized by widespread oral ulcers, which is called *herpetic gingivostomatitis* (Figure 12-11B). Children can become infected by adults who are carrying the virus but do not have symptoms.

During the initial infection, an individual experiences a fever and body aches. This stage might be mistaken for the flu or another viral infection. Afterward, the lesion appears, typically located on the lips (*herpes labialis*) or on the inside of the cheeks and lips. The lesions can range in size from very small, pinhead blisters to blisters up to 1/4-inch in diameter.

Topical treatments such as Abreva® are available to reduce the duration and severity of the outbreak, and oral antiviral drugs are sometimes taken to reduce the frequency

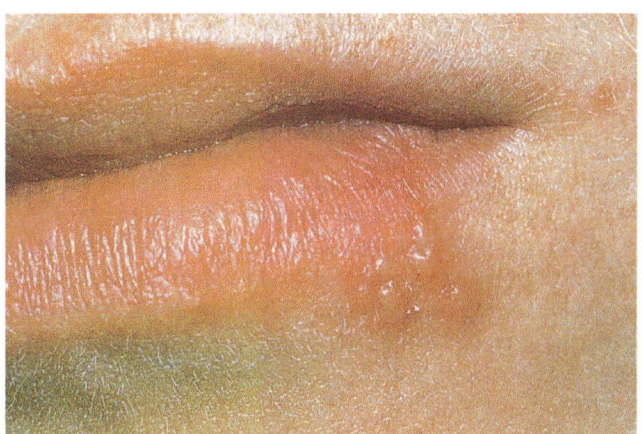

A

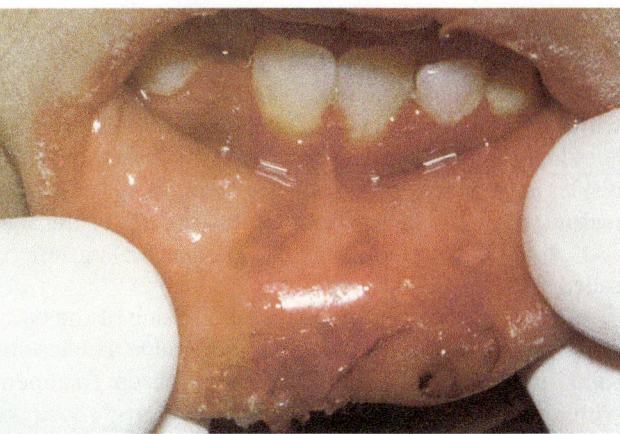

B

Figure 12–11 Herpes simplex. A. Clustered vesicles seen in recurrent *herpes labialis*. The lesions are also known as *cold sores* or *fever blisters*. **B.** Herpetic gingivostomatitis in a child.

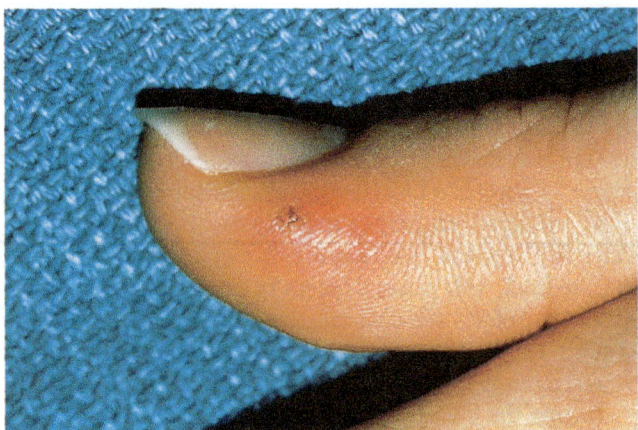

Figure 12–12 A herpetic whitlow caused by autoinoculation of the herpes virus.

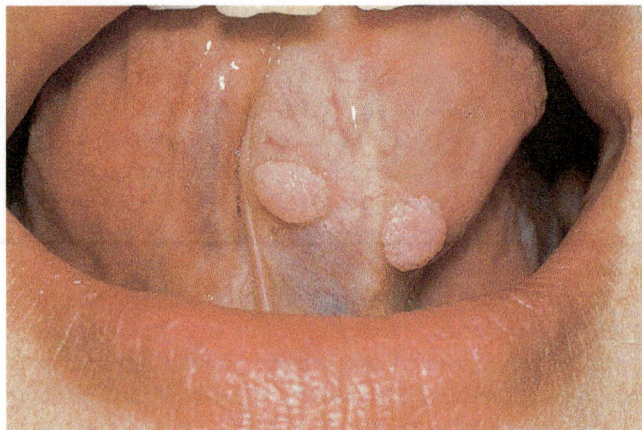

Figure 12–13 Human papillomavirus (HPV). Condyloma acuminate, also known as *venereal warts*, is caused by HPV types 6 and 11.

of outbreaks. A typical herpes episode lasts 10 to 14 days. Any patients with herpes lesions that last longer than 1 month should be screened for HIV/AIDS status, because there is a connection between long-lasting outbreaks and HIV infection.

Herpes blisters can be extremely painful, and it may be impossible to treat a patient with active herpes lesions. Stretching the skin can cause patient discomfort. In addition, the lesions may break and spread to the patient's eyes or other areas. Herpes is an infectious disease, and dental assistants should be aware that there is a risk of transmission. Careful attention should be paid to infection control. Wearing gloves is not an absolute barrier against infection. Some dental practices request that patients suffering from an active herpes infection reschedule their appointment.

If the herpes virus penetrates a break in the skin, a *herpetic whitlow* might result. This is a crusted sore on the skin that can be extremely painful (Figure 12-12).

For more information about the herpes simplex virus, see Chapter 13, Understanding Microbiology.

Herpes Zoster

Herpes zoster is the virus that causes chickenpox in children and shingles in adults. Typically, a child is infected with herpes zoster and has chickenpox, and then the virus goes into remission. During the person's lifetime, the virus resides in the nerve cells. Then, at a later age, for unknown reasons, the virus travels from the nerve cells to the skin and causes outbreaks of painful, red and scaling lesions called *shingles*.

Shingles are typically confined to one side of the body. They can be very painful and uncomfortable. The lesions can last for several weeks before they clear up. Treatment with an antiviral medication, such as acyclovir (Zovirax), valacyclovir (Valtrex), or famciclovir (Famvir), may speed healing and lessen discomfort.

There is a connection between shingles outbreak and immune system health. Patients who are infected with HIV,

as well as those who are undergoing treatment for cancer, are more likely to experience an outbreak of herpes zoster lesions.

Human Papillomavirus

Human papillomavirus (HPV) is a common virus responsible for a variety of warts and lesions that can occur throughout the body (Figure 12-13). More than 100 forms of HPV exist. Most types produce only minor skin ailments; some forms, however, can cause a variety of cancers, including cervical cancer and oral cancers. An HPV vaccine is available that is recommended for girls and young women. HPV infection is more common among adolescents and adults than children. Together with herpes, HPV is the most common viral infection of the oral cavity. Infection with HPV is a risk factor for oral squamous cell carcinoma, which is covered more completely in the Carcinomas section.

HPV causes small white warts in the oral cavity. They typically occur on the hard palate, lips, tongue, or gingiva. The warts are white in appearance, with tiny whitish spikes or a slightly hairy appearance. They may also have a cauliflower-like appearance. Warts associated with HPV have well-defined margins.

Treatment for oral HPV consists of removing the lesions, usually with a laser or surgically. However, they often return. Patients with HPV should be closely monitored for oral cancers. HPV is highly contagious. Infected patients can unknowingly transmit the disease by putting their hands in the mouth and then touching other objects. Warn patients of the risk of transmitting the disease to others and carefully follow proper infection control procedures when working with a patient who has HPV.

Actinomycosis

Actinomycosis is a bacterial infection of the oral cavity that can involve the jaw bones (Figure 12-14). The main symptoms are pain, localized swelling, tenderness, and

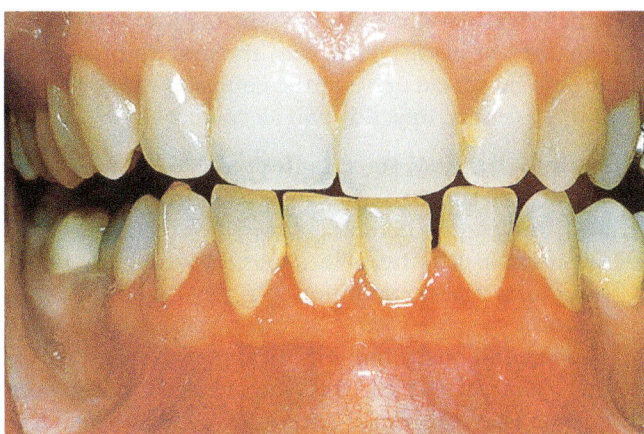

Figure 12–14 Actinomycotic gingivitis affecting the marginal gingiva.

discharge of purulent material. Before the age of antibiotics, actinomycosis was relatively common and sometimes resulted in death. Today, with available antibiotics, it is easily treated. The greatest risk factors for developing an actinomycosis infection are poor oral hygiene and dental caries.

Candidiasis

Candidiasis is an infection with the *Candida albicans* fungus (Figure 12-15). The infection is common, especially among newborns (when it is called *thrush*). It does not typically appear among healthy adults, but infection with *Candida* is an important symptom for other diseases. It often occurs in HIV patients, whose compromised immune systems are not capable of fighting off infection. Other risk factors for candidiasis include diabetes, antibiotic treatment, xerostomia, and chemotherapy.

Three forms of candidiasis are commonly seen. Signs and symptoms vary, depending on the infection:

- *Thrush (Pseudomembranous Candidiasis)*. This infection appears as a thick white covering, or plaque, over the oral mucosa. It is a relatively common infection among newborn children and rarely seen in adults. If symptoms are present, they usually include halitosis (bad breath) and a bitter taste in the mouth.

  Treatment consists of wiping away the plaques with sterile gauze, then applying antifungal drugs or using an antifungal mouthrinse. Once the plaques are removed, they do not reappear, and the infection is resolved.

- *Hyperplastic Candidiasis*. This infection resembles thrush, but it cannot be removed by scraping or wiping away. It is a common complication of infection with HIV/AIDS. It is typically treated with antifungal medication, which should resolve the plaques within 14 days. If a patient has this infection, and the plaques cannot be healed, the patient should be tested for HIV status.

- *Atrophic Candidiasis*. Atrophic candidiasis is usually a complication of antibiotic treatment. The plaques are reddish and appear on the tongue and palate. The most common symptom is burning upon swallowing. Atrophic candidiasis is treated with antifungal medications, which typically resolve the plaques within 14 days. If the lesions do not disappear, the patient should be tested for the type of candida infection, HIV status, and other conditions.

Acute Necrotizing Ulcerative Gingivitis

Formerly known as *trench mouth*, acute necrotizing ulcerative gingivitis (ANUG) is a serious disease affecting the gingival tissue (Figure 12-16). Symptoms include pain, redness, bleeding, spreading infection, and a strong, foul odor from the oral cavity. It is typically caused by high stress, coupled with poor oral hygiene, lack of sleep, and poor general health. Smoking and nutritional deficiencies are risk factors for the disease. It was first called trench mouth because it was common among soldiers who lived in trenches. Today, it is more often seem among adolescents and college students around exam time.

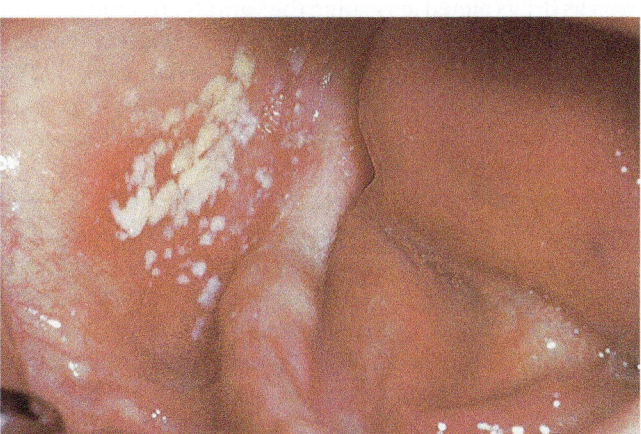

Figure 12–15 Acute pseudomembranous candidiasis in a patient with diabetes.

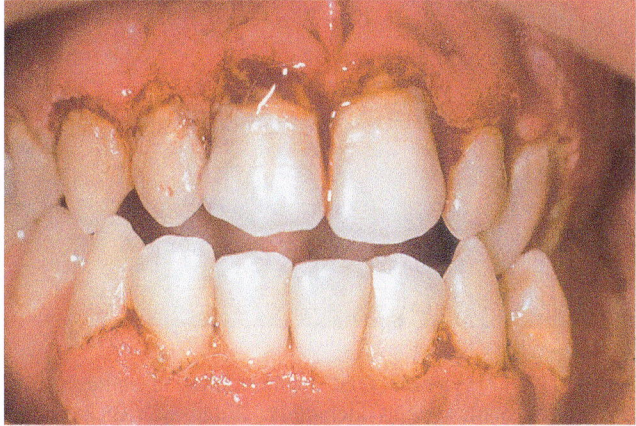

Figure 12–16 Acute necrotizing ulcerative gingivitis. Formerly known as *trench mouth*, this disease is seen today among adolescents and college students.

Treatment for ANUG involves a complete dental cleaning, thorough debridement, and, if infection is present, treatment with oral antibiotics to kill any bacteria. After treatment is complete, the patient will remain at a heightened risk for gingival diseases and recurrences, so special care must be paid to oral hygiene and overall health. Patient instruction and motivation for self-care are needed. Chapter 10, Prevention of Caries and Periodontal Disease, outlines self-care techniques patients can use to improve oral hygiene, and Chapter 11, Nutrition, presents a detailed look at the nutritional requirements for maintaining good health.

Syphilis

Syphilis is a venereal disease of bacterial origin. It used to be a significant source of mortality before antibiotic treatment was developed to cure the disease. Syphilis has three stages of involvement with the oral mucosa. These stages can be spread out over the course of years, depending on the general infection and its course:

- During the first stage, a lesion called a *chancre* appears on the lip. The chancre can be up to 1/2 inch in diameter. It is hard and raised. Over time, it crusts over and usually heals in about a month. The lesion resembles a herpetic lesion and may be mistaken for herpes.
- The second stage typically occurs within a year of the chancre. During this stage, more oral lesions appear. They are one of two types: a mucous patch or a split papule. During this stage, the disease is highly infectious.
- In the third stage, the final lesion appears. This lesion is known as a *gumma*. The gumma is a dangerous lesion that can destroy bone and cartilage and result in permanent deformity.

Syphilis can also affect fetuses during development. Children born to mothers with syphilis may suffer from a condition known as *Hutchinson incisors* (Figure 12-17A). This condition is characterized by notched or serrated edges on the anterior incisors of the secondary dentition. It is caused by abnormal prenatal development of these teeth. Syphilis may also affect the molars, which may appear rounded or stubbled, somewhat like raspberries or mulberries. This condition is sometimes referred to as *mulberry molars* (Figure 12-17B).

Oral Complications of HIV/AIDS Infection

HIV is a virus that does not directly physically affect the oral cavity. Instead, the virus attacks the immune system, eventually progressing to AIDS. At that stage, the immune system is seriously compromised, and the body is vulnerable to opportunistic infections. There is no cure for AIDS. Instead, physicians treat the disease with powerful antiviral drugs meant to bolster the patient's immune system as well as drugs aimed at treating the various complications of AIDS, which include pneumonia, tuberculosis, herpes, hepatitis, and hyperplastic candidiasis. Death among AIDS patients is caused by an opportunistic infection. For more information about the HIV virus and AIDS, see Chapter 13, Understanding Microbiology.

Pathologies of the oral cavity often precede the progression from infection with HIV to the development of full-blown AIDS, or they are used as indicators of viral status. Oral lesions are frequently among the earliest signs to appear. The fungal infection candidiasis is strongly associated with HIV infection. Viral infections, such as herpes lesions and hairy leukoplakia, are also common.

Bacterial infections may also be present. Periodontal infections associated with HIV infection tend to show more severe symptoms and to progress more rapidly

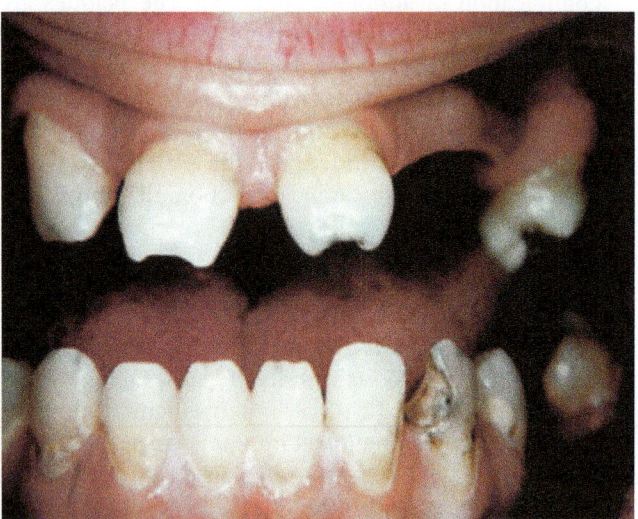

A

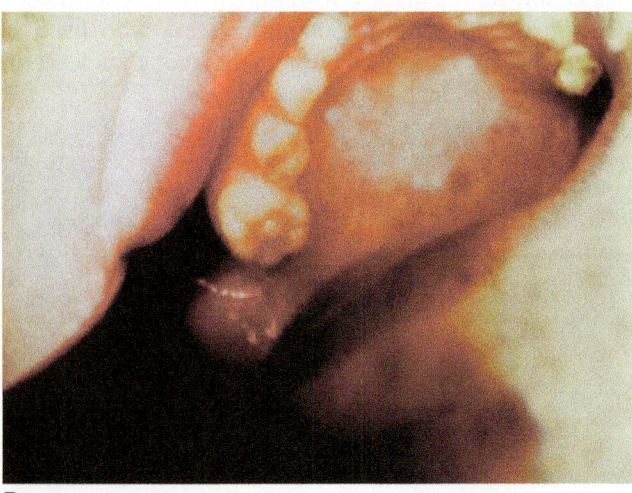

B

Figure 12–17 Syphilis. Oral manifestations in children born to mothers with syphilis include **A.** Hutchinson incisors and **B.** mulberry molars. (From Sweet RL, Gibbs RS. *Atlas of Infectious Diseases of the Female Genital Tract*. Philadelphia: Lippincott Williams & Wilkins, 2005.)

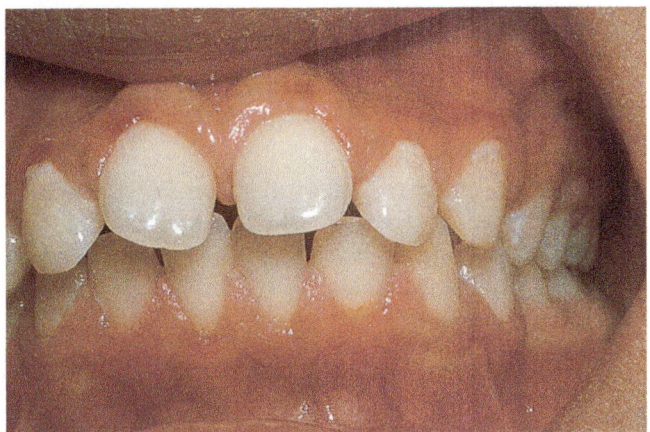

Figure 12–18 Linear gingival erythema. A severe form of gingivitis is often seen in patients with human immunodeficiency virus.

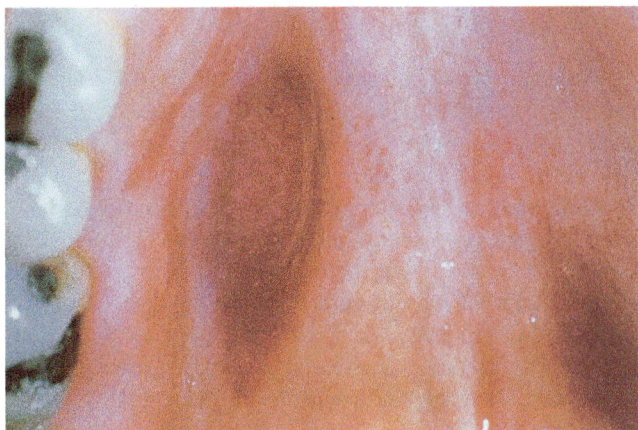

Figure 12–20 Kaposi sarcoma is a tumor that appears almost exclusively in patients with acquired immune deficiency syndrome.

than periodontal conditions in individuals who are not immunosuppressed. A severe form of gingivitis called *linear gingival erythema* is often seen in patients who are HIV positive (Figure 12-18). This condition is characterized by a 2- to 3-mm red band that appears along the gingival margin. Spontaneous bleeding and bleeding on gentle probing can occur.

An increased incidence of ANUG has been observed in patients with HIV, and a weakened immune system makes individuals vulnerable to various periodontal infections, including rapidly progressing periodontitis.

Oral complications known to affect patients who have HIV/AIDS include:

■ *Hairy Leukoplakia.* Hairy leukoplakia resembles candidiasis (Figure 12-19). It appears as a white covering along the sides of the tongue that cannot be wiped away. Over time, it can spread to cover the entire dorsal surface of the tongue. Caused by the Epstein-Barr virus, there is no cure for hairy leukoplakia. It is one of the first clinical manifestations of HIV infection and is considered an indicator of viral status. If a patient is diagnosed with hairy leukoplakia and has never been tested for HIV

status, the dentist will likely recommend testing. Most patients with this condition will test positive for HIV.

■ *Kaposi Sarcoma.* Kaposi sarcoma is a tumor that appears almost exclusively in patients with AIDS; before the advent of AIDS, Kaposi tumors were very rare in the United States. The vascular tumor appears as a bluish or purple flat nodule on the palate (Figure 12-20). Kaposi sarcomas can also appear elsewhere on the body. Over time, as the tumor enlarges, it may bleed and hurt. There is no cure for Kaposi sarcoma. At present, surgery is sometimes used to excise (remove) part or all of the tumor, and radiation and low-dose chemotherapy might be recommended. Nevertheless, Kaposi sarcomas are aggressive and invasive, and the prognosis is generally poor once the tumor is advanced. This is a relatively common cause of death among patients with AIDS.

■ *Lymphoma.* Lymphoma is the term used to describe a malignancy of the lymph nodes. There are lymph nodes throughout the body, including in the region near the oral cavity. The first symptom of lymphoma is often swelling and tenderness in the affected nodes, or ulceration of the affected nodes. Dentists can often detect swollen and tender lymph nodes in the head and neck region by palpating these areas. A biopsy of the lesion is usually required for diagnosis.

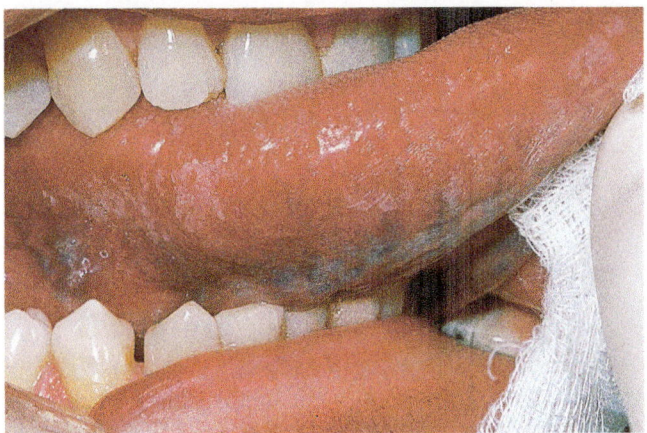

Figure 12–19 Hairy leukoplakia is one of the first manifestations of human immunodeficiency virus infection.

CHECKPOINTS

12-7 What is a leukoplakia and how is it caused?

12-8 What is an aphthous ulcer and how is it treated?

12-9 Which kind of herpes simplex virus causes oral herpes?

12-10 Describe thrush and identify the organism that causes it.

12-11 Hairy leukoplakia and Kaposi sarcoma are often complications of what disease?

Pathologies of Physical Origin

Many of the physical lesions seen in the dental office are self-inflicted. Patients bite their cheeks; devices and appliances cause abrasions; or utensils or other objects held in the mouth may cause injuries to the soft tissue.

Additionally, the dental team can cause injury to the oral cavity. Dental instruments must be handled with extreme caution to avoid tearing the oral mucosa or aggravating an existing injury. Even sponges or gauze squares can cause injury if they are left in place too long. If one of these items dries to the mucosa, it can adhere, so when it is removed, it will take a layer of skin with it and leave behind a tiny ulceration.

Hyperplasia

Hyperplasia is the medical term used to describe the formation of new, noncancerous cells or tissue (Figure 12-21). In the oral cavity, hyperplasia can be caused by aggravation and friction against the sensitive tissues, like that found with dentures. At first, small ulcerations appear that eventually evolve into folds of excess tissue. The best treatment for hyperplasia is to remove the aggravating factor. For example, a patient might forgo wearing dentures for a few days, until the swelling is reduced. In the meantime, the dentures can be remade or outfitted with a soft lining that does not aggravate the oral tissue.

Mucocele

A mucocele is a small, raised bump caused by a blocked salivary gland or duct. These usually occur at the back of the lower lip, as a result of patients accidentally biting their lips. The resulting trauma to the salivary gland seals the salivary duct, causing fluid to build up under the skin. The mucocele appears as a small, pebble-like protrusion. In some cases, a mucocele is caused by small particles that block the salivary duct. Treatment for a mucocele involves draining the blocked duct and gland. If the lesion recurs, the duct and gland may need to be removed.

Radiation Injury

Radiation is sometimes used to treat cancers of the head and neck; however, the patient might experience a number of radiation-induced side effects that specifically affect the oral cavity. These include:

- Deformity of developing teeth. Developing teeth subjected to excess radiation may be undersized, deformed, or without roots.
- Ulceration. Swelling and ulceration can occur immediately after the radiation therapy. This soft tissue injury should heal on its own, although the length of time to heal depends on the patient's overall health. After it heals, the tissue may be pigmented.
- Xerostomia. *Xerostomia* is the medical word for dry mouth. Radiation therapy to the oral area can sometimes destroy the salivary glands, meaning the patient will stop producing saliva. The resulting extreme dry mouth raises the risk of dental caries, oral infection, and gingival disease. Saliva replacements can be used to bring some relief.
- Death of bone. Known medically as *osteonecrosis*, this condition can occur when the jaw bone is directly exposed to high levels of radiation. Patients with this condition are at increased risk of jaw fractures and should avoid tooth extractions, if at all possible. In some cases, complete tooth extraction might be recommended before radiation therapy to prevent necrosis (death) of the jawbone and ensuing complications.

Amalgam Tattoo

An amalgam tattoo occurs when small particles of amalgam are trapped under the surface of the oral mucosa during a dental procedure (Figure 12-22). This can occur

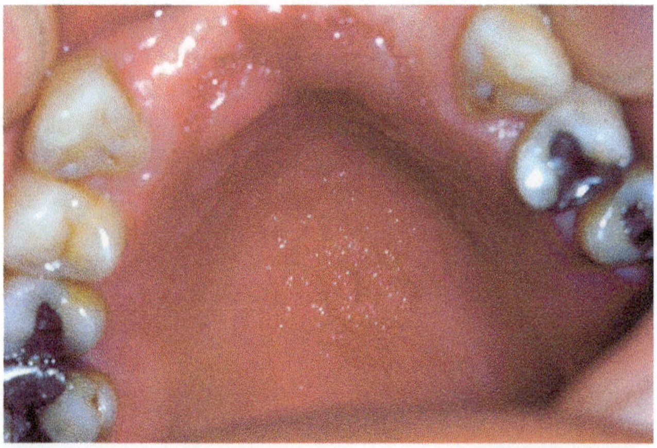

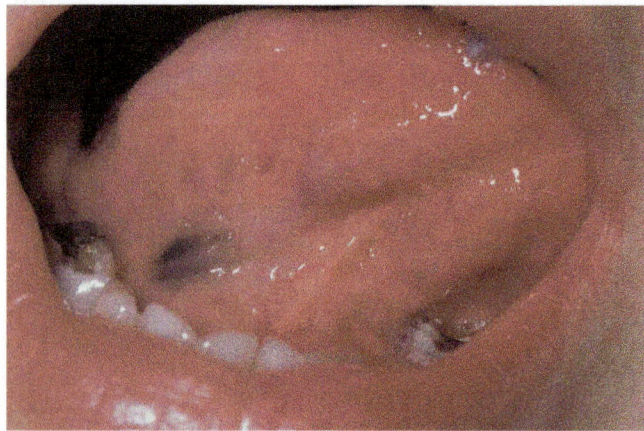

Figure 12–21 Hyperplasia. This patient had been wearing a temporary partial prosthesis to replace the maxillary incisors for several years. The poor fit of the prosthesis was related to the papillary hyperplasia seen here.

Figure 12–22 This amalgam tattoo was caused when amalgam was accidentally introduced into the soft tissues when an amalgam restoration was being placed. (Courtesy of Dr. Peter Jacobsen.)

during oral surgery or during preparation for a crown procedure. The risk is higher in tissue with more severe abrasion.

Amalgam tattoos appear as bluish or purple spots on the tissue. They are harmless, however, and no treatment is necessary. To prevent amalgam tattoos, the area should be flushed thoroughly during procedures that use amalgam. Dental dams can also help prevent amalgam tattoos by reducing the risk of loose amalgam in the oral cavity.

Cosmetic Piercing

Oral piercing is increasingly common, and more and more areas of the oral cavity are being pierced. Used as a form of artistic and self-expression, patients might pierce their lips, tongues (both horizontally and vertically), both the maxillary and mandibular frenums, and their uvulas. Multiple piercings are also seen, and some patients pierce their tongue multiple times.

During piercing, a needle is rapidly inserted through the tissue, and then a temporary object is inserted to hold open the hole while the tissue heals. Swelling at this stage is common, and bleeding can range from minor to severe, depending if blood vessels were involved. In extreme cases, during tongue piercing, swelling can actually threaten to close the airway, and the patient may be hospitalized on an emergency basis. Infection is also a risk during this phase because oral injuries can take several weeks to heal.

Once the original wound has healed, the temporary object is removed from the hole and the permanent ornament is placed. In tongue piercings, this is usually a small barbell-like piece of jewelry that is screwed into place. Other ornaments include hoops and studs.

Despite the popularity of oral piercing, the practice involves a lengthy list of possible side effects, including:

- Chipped and cracked teeth
- Recession of gingival tissue
- Abscess
- Aggravation and ulceration of soft tissues in contact with the piercing
- Increased salivation
- Increased risk of infection
- Sensitivity to cold and heat
- Sensitivity to metal
- Scarring
- Problems with chewing
- Speech impairment
- Increased risk of hepatitis C transmission

Patients who are considering oral piercing should be made aware of these risks and advised to practice scrupulous care of their piercing wound to prevent complications.

Extra Patient Care

If patients tell you they want an oral piercing, you can help them prepare by giving them information on how to treat the wound after the piercing and how to avoid long-term problems. The following online resources offer some handy tips:

Oral Piercing Risks and Safety Measures:
www.safepiercing.org/piercing/oral-piercing-risks

Oral Piercing: An Overview
ijahsp.nova.edu/articles/vol6num3/pdf/cooper.pdf

Check Your Ethics

A minor comes into the office, and during her exam, mentions that she wants to get her tongue pierced and asks about the risks. When you follow up, you find out that her parents do not know of her plans. She begs you not to tell them because they "would kill [her]. Anyway, it's not like it's their mouth." How should you react?

Split Tongue (Tongue Forking)

Tongue splitting is a cosmetic procedure in which the tip of the tongue is slit down the middle to give the person a reptilian, forked tongue. It can be surgically reversed. Tongue splitting carries fewer risks to the teeth than oral piercing, in part because there are no metal ornaments left in the mouth. However, patients with split tongues may have trouble swallowing and making certain sounds. Additionally, the surgical wound is susceptible to infection.

Abrasion

An abrasion is an injury caused by excessive friction against a tooth or oral structure. The most common cause of abrasive injuries is improper toothbrushing, with too much pressure on the brush. Abrasions can also be caused by nervous oral habits (such as chewing on a pen cap) and appliances in the mouth. Treatment of the wound depends on its severity and location, and, if necessary, patients should be educated on the proper way to brush and use other oral appliances.

Pathologies of Chemical Origin

The most common chemicals to cause oral pathologies include tobacco and drugs, such as aspirin and antibiotics. These agents can affect the tongue as well as tissue in the oral cavity. The medical term for a condition that affects the tongue is **glossitis**, which means swelling and inflammation of the tongue.

Nicotine Stomatitis

Nicotine stomatitis is caused by repeated exposure to tobacco smoke. **Stomatitis** is inflammation of the oral mucosa. It is characterized by small ulcers covered with a grey exudate and surrounded by a small red halo (Figure 12-23).

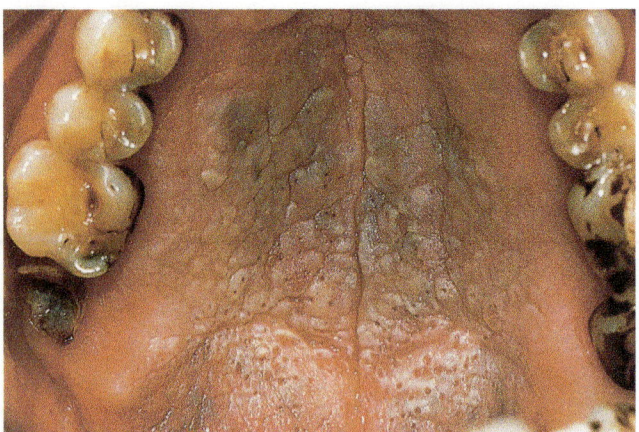

Figure 12–23 Nicotine stomatitis. Inflammation of the oral mucosa characterized by small ulcers covered with a gray exudate.

Although all smokers are susceptible to nicotine stomatitis, the condition is somewhat more common among pipe smokers. Pipe smokers are more likely to hold their pipe in the same place in the mouth every time they smoke, and because pipe tobacco is wetter and unfiltered, it can be hotter and harsher than cigarette smoke.

Patients with nicotine stomatitis will initially develop a red blister. Over time, the red area will be covered by a white layer of fibrous (corrugated-looking) tissue. Additionally, nearby salivary glands will be hyperkeratinized, or swollen.

This condition is benign, but smokers should be made aware of it. Additionally, the risk of oral cancer is higher among people who use tobacco products, and they should be encouraged to quit. See Chapter 16, Pharmacology, for information about smoking cessation programs.

This condition can also appear among frequent marijuana users, in which it is typically located in the middle anterior sections of both the maxillary and mandibular lips. In this case, the lesion is caused by exposure to the unfiltered, very hot ends of rolled marijuana cigarettes.

Aspirin Burn

As aspirin burn occurs when patients hold aspirin against the gingiva, tucked between the lip and the sensitive gum tissue. This is sometimes used as a home remedy for pain. Aspirin contains acetylsalicylic acid. The direct exposure of sensitive tissue to aspirin causes a white lesion that can extend from the gingival tissue to the lining of the mucosa. These lesions typically hurt after the aspirin is removed. They will heal on their own but may be sensitive.

Snuff and Chewing Tobacco

Snuff and chewing tobacco are smokeless tobacco. Snuff is a finely ground powder that can be inhaled through the nostrils or packed into a wad or pellet for chewing. Chewing tobacco is available in leaf form or plug form. Both are tucked into a space between the lip and the gingiva. All forms of smokeless tobacco contain nicotine and are addictive. These are not safe substitutes for smoking tobacco products.

People who use smokeless tobacco are vulnerable to a number of oral conditions, including oral cancers and cancer of the esophagus and larynx as well as periodontal disease and the eventual loss of teeth. In the early stages, lesions caused by smokeless tobacco are whitish, hardened, and vary in size, depending on how often tobacco is used and how much is typically used. Patients with early lesions from smokeless tobacco should be educated about the risks of using smokeless tobacco.

Gingival Hyperplasia

Overgrowth of the gingival tissues may occur due to the effects of certain medications, including some medications used to treat heart disease, as well as phenytoin and other anticonvulsive drugs commonly used by patients with epilepsy. When related to phenytoin use, gingival enlargement may also be called *Dilantin hyperplasia*. The severity of the hyperplasia depends on the dosage and length of time the patient has taken the medication. Meticulous oral hygiene may reduce the occurrence and severity of gingival overgrowth. In severe cases, the excess gingival tissue may be surgically removed.

Hairy Tongue

Hairy tongue is caused when the tiny filiform papillae on the tongue grow too long, eventually resembling tiny hairs. In some extreme cases, the papillae grow so long as to interfere with breathing and swallowing. Over time, the papillae are stained yellow, brown, or black by food and liquid, sometimes earning the nickname "black hairy tongue" (Figure 12-24). Hairy tongue may also cause halitosis.

This condition may occur for unknown reasons, as a result of poor dental hygiene, or by antibiotic use upsetting the natural flora balance in the mouth. Other drugs that might cause black hairy tongue include chemotherapy and the use of hydrogen peroxide–based mouthwash. To treat the condition, patients should be advised to discontinue what-

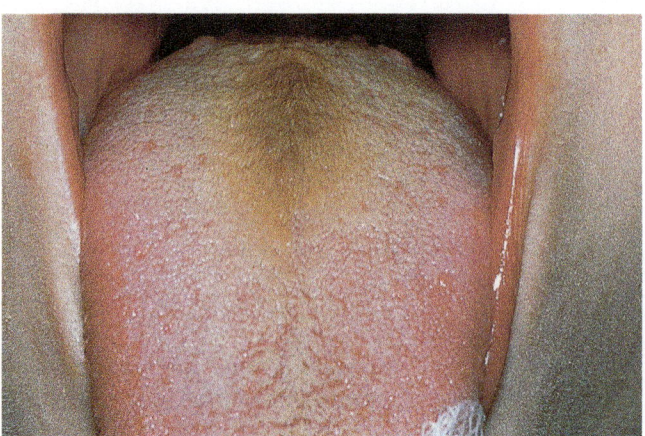

Figure 12–24 Black hairy tongue.

ever is causing it, if possible. Good oral hygiene, including tongue brushing, should prevent it from returning. If the papillae are so long that they interfere with the patient's swallowing or breathing, they may need to be trimmed.

Voice of Experience

It might be hard to believe, but black hairy tongue can be caused by mouthwash or even poor brushing. In our office, one of the dental assistants recently started using an off-brand of whitening mouthwash and soon began experiencing symptoms of hairy tongue. Within a few weeks, her tongue had turned completely black! Fortunately, after she stopped using the mouthwash, her symptoms disappeared completely.

From the Dentist's Perspective

Dental students are often fascinated by black hairy tongue. It seems hard to believe that the tongue can be trimmed like hair! But it's true. Hairy tongue (white or black) is caused by overgrowth of filiform papillae on the surface of the tongue. When these are stained by food and liquid, the condition is nicknamed "black hairy tongue." In most cases, simply discontinuing the cause of the overgrowth, combined with brushing and scraping the tongue, will resolve the condition and discourage the growth of new papillae. However, if the tiny, thread-like papillae are long enough to cause aggravation, they can be trimmed using a carbon dioxide laser or even scissors.

Oral Cancers

Oral cancers are relatively common, and, if not treated, they can be deadly. Tobacco and alcohol use are strong risk factors for oral cancer. Other cancers can involve the jaw bones, the palate, the tongue, and the floor of the mouth. A **carcinoma** is a malignant neoplasm that arises from epithelial tissue. A **sarcoma** is a malignant neoplasm that arises from connective tissue or bone. A biopsy should be performed on any oral lesion that does not heal within 2 weeks.

Oral cancers can **metastasize**, or spread, to lymph nodes, surrounding tissue, or nearby organs in the head and neck. Treatment of oral cancer depends on its location, the type of cancer, and its stage of development. Available treatment options include surgery to remove tumors, chemotherapy, and radiation therapy. One or more of these approaches might be used.

Erythroplakia

Erythroplakias are red patches in the oral cavity that are not connected to any obvious source of inflammation (Figure 12-25). They are smooth and somewhat velvety in appearance and typically occur in the soft palate or on the floor of the mouth. These are most often seen in patients who have smoked or used excessive amounts of alcohol for many years.

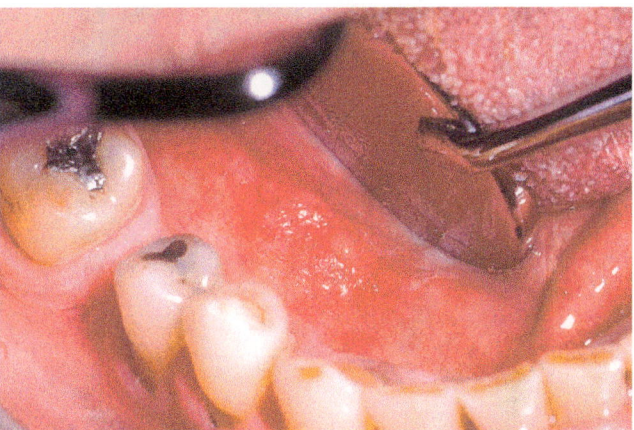

Figure 12–25 Erythroplakias. Red patches on the floor of the mouth that are not connected to any obvious source of inflammation.

Erythroplakias are serious. In the vast majority of cases, a biopsy will reveal that the plaque is malignant. Early diagnosis and treatment is critical. In the early stages, the plaques can be removed surgically without further intervention. In later stages, however, after the malignancy has penetrated deeper into the mucosal tissue, chemotherapy and radiation may be necessary.

Leukemia

Leukemia is cancer of the white blood cells and organs that produce white blood cells. Leukemia affects the bone marrow, where white blood cells are produced from stem cells, although leukemia cells can also invade other organs. Among patients with leukemia, great numbers of immature white blood cells are produced. There are several types of leukemia. They are classified by which type of white blood cells are affected and which organs in the immune system are invaded by cancerous cells.

From a dental point of view, early indications of leukemia often can be noticed by examining the oral cavity. Signs and symptoms might include ulceration, bleeding and hemorrhage, a red-colored gingiva, and a spongy feeling to the gingiva.

Carcinoma

Carcinomas are cancers that invade the epithelial tissue. From there, they can rapidly metastasize to other organs. There are two kinds of carcinomas that affect the oral cavity.

- *Squamous Cell Carcinoma.* About 90% of oral cancers are squamous cell (Figure 12-26A). These cancers originally affect the epithelial layers of the soft tissues in the oral cavity. They often appear as small ulcers, especially under the tongue, on the sides of the tongue itself, and on the soft palate. Risk factors for squamous cell carcinoma include tobacco use and long-term alcohol use.

In the early stages, squamous cell carcinomas may appear as whitish plaques that spread. As the disease

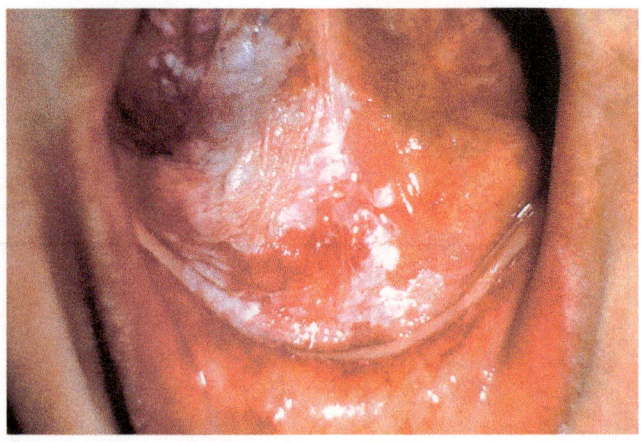
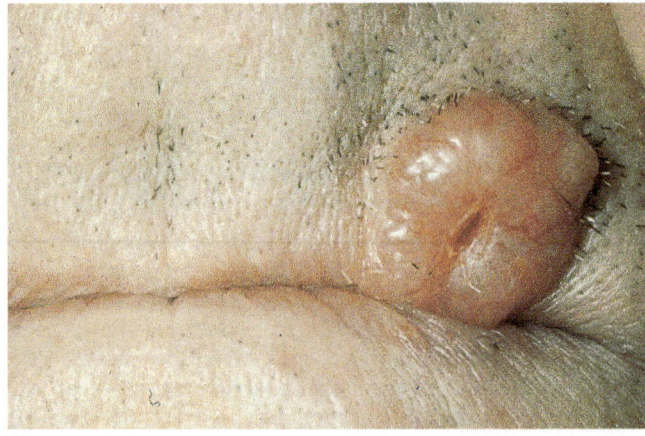

A   **B**

Figure 12–26 Carcinoma. **A.** Squamous cell carcinoma on the floor of the mouth. **B.** Basal cell carcinoma on the edge of the lip.

progresses, it forms an ulcer that grows into surrounding tissues. Over time, the ulcer develops a margin.

Early detection and treatment is critical. In the early stages, these cancers can often be successfully treated with surgery. However, if the cancer has metastasized, treatment might involve radiation and chemotherapy, and the mortality rate rises.

■ *Basal Cell Carcinoma.* Basal cell carcinomas are the most common skin cancers, although squamous cell is more common in the oral cavity (Figure 12-26B). These cancers typically form in the skin cells of the lips, head, and neck, the areas where sun exposure is the greatest. Patients with occupations that require high levels of sun exposure are at an increased risk for basal cell carcinoma. These occupations may include farmers, carpenters, and landscapers. Always advise patients to use sun block on the face and lips.

Surgery is the typical treatment for a basal cell carcinoma. Because these cancers only rarely metastasize to surrounding tissues, the treatment rate is very good. Once a person has had one basal cell carcinoma, the risk of recurrence is high, so it is important to maintain regular checkups.

Benign Tumors

In addition to malignant tumors, several forms of benign neoplasms can occur in the oral cavity.

■ *Papilloma.* A papilloma is a small, cauliflower-shaped tumor caused by a virus. These range in size up to 3 cm and vary in color from white to red. Treatment is through surgery.

■ *Fibroma.* A fibroma is a tumor of the connective tissue. They are typically found in areas such as the inside of the cheek, where chewing motion aggravates the epithelial layer and causes growth of the connective tissue cells. The tumors are typically dome shaped, pink, and smooth. Treatment is surgical removal of the fibroma. They rarely return once removed.

Hormonal Disturbances

Oral lesions can sometimes be caused by changes in hormone status, such as those that occur with pregnancy or during puberty. In most cases, the conditions resolve as soon as the hormonal situation is resolved (e.g., the patient passes through puberty or is no longer pregnant). However, hormonally mediated changes in the gingival tissue can lead to further problems if the patient is careless about oral hygiene. It is important to practice good oral hygiene to reduce bleeding and the risk of further problems.

Gingival Changes

Gingival changes can occur during puberty or pregnancy, when hormone levels are much higher than normal. It is important to practice conscientious self-care during these times in addition to getting regular professional dental hygiene care. This is especially crucial for pregnant patients, because recent studies indicate a link between periodontal disease and preterm birth and low-birth-weight babies.

■ *Pubertal gingival enlargement.* This condition occurs during puberty and is characterized by enlarged,

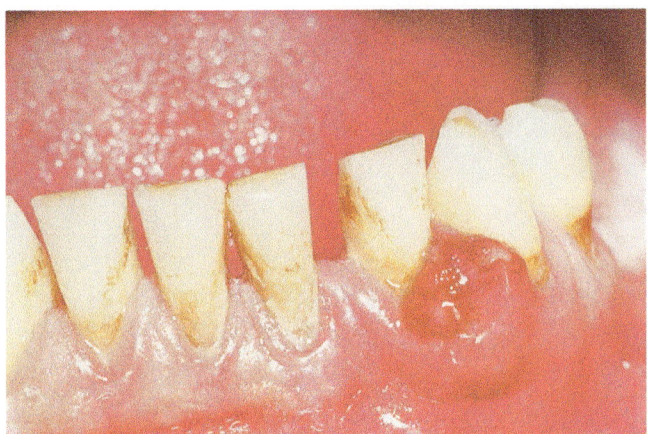

Figure 12-27 Pyogenic granuloma. Benign, nonpainful tumor also known as a "pregnancy tumor."

swollen gingival tissue. The tissue may bleed more easily, and it may be spongy and red. It is more common among girls than boys. There is no treatment, other than good oral hygiene to reduce the risk of further gingival conditions. After puberty, the gingiva should return to normal with proper self-care and professional therapy. The consensus, however, is that adult periodontal disease gets its start from unresolved pubertal gingivitis.

- *Gestational gingivitis.* Much like gestational diabetes, gestational gingivitis occurs only during pregnancy. It resembles pubertal gingival enlargement in appearance, with swollen, sensitive gingival tissue that bleeds more easily. Good oral hygiene should be practiced.

Pyogenic Granuloma

Pyogenic granulomas are sometimes referred to as "pregnancy tumors," although they can also appear in nonpregnant women and in men. Pyogenic granulations occur when granulated tissue grows rapidly due to local irritation, resulting in a red mass ranging in size from a few millimeters to several centimeters across, located near the gingival margin (Figure 12-27). These benign tumors are not painful. Pyogenic granulomas can be removed surgically, but they often reappear. These tumors are caused by hormonal disturbances; as soon as hormone levels return to normal, they disappear.

Developmental Disorders

Developmental disturbances fall into two categories: environmental and genetic. Both can affect the way teeth and oral structures grow in a developing fetus. An abnormality that is present at birth is called a **congenital condition**. This term is used interchangeably to describe both environmental and genetic disorders. In many cases, the exact cause of a congenital abnormality will never be known. For some disorders, it is possible that a complex interplay of genetics and environmental conditions affected the developing fetus. For other conditions, the exact cause will be known.

Not all congenital abnormalities require treatment. In other cases, such as cleft palate, correction will be necessary to help the child eat and speak.

Environmental disorders are caused by outside influences that act on the developing fetus. Anything that can harm a developing fetus is known as a **teratogen**. Teratogens include many types of drugs (e.g., prescription, illicit, and over the counter), chemicals, radiation, and even fever and nutritional deficiencies.

Genetic disorders are caused by defects in the chromosomes that direct oral development. Genetic factors are passed down from one or both parents, although the parents might not have the disorder themselves. Genetic factors influence everything about a developing fetus, including jaw size, tooth size, and possible abnormal development.

Disturbances in Hard and Soft Tissues

A number of conditions can affect the hard and soft tissues, including:

- *Cleft lip and cleft palate.* Cleft lips occur when the nasal processes fail to join during development, resulting in an abnormal opening between the maxillary process and the intermaxillary segment (Figure 12-28A).

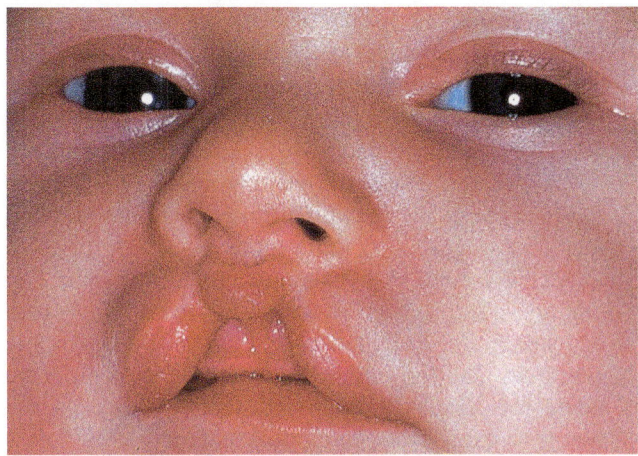

A

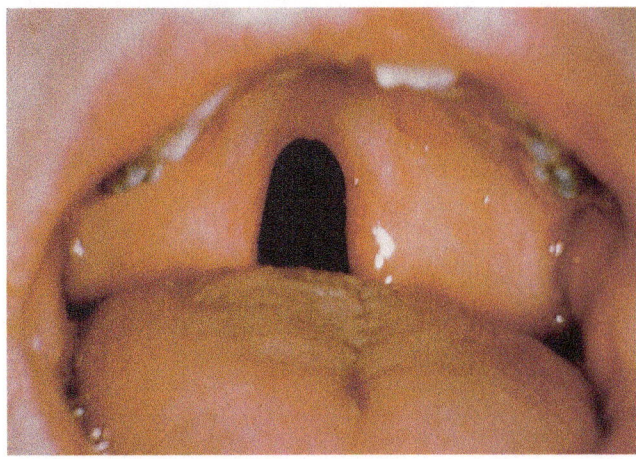

B

Figure 12-28 A. Cleft lip. **B.** Cleft palate.

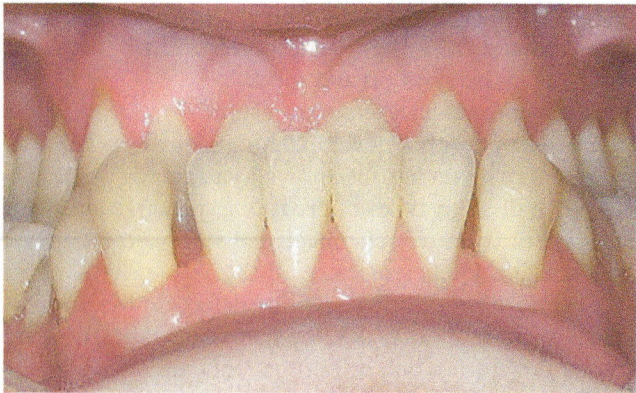

Figure 12–29 Class III malocclusion. Caused by macrognathia.

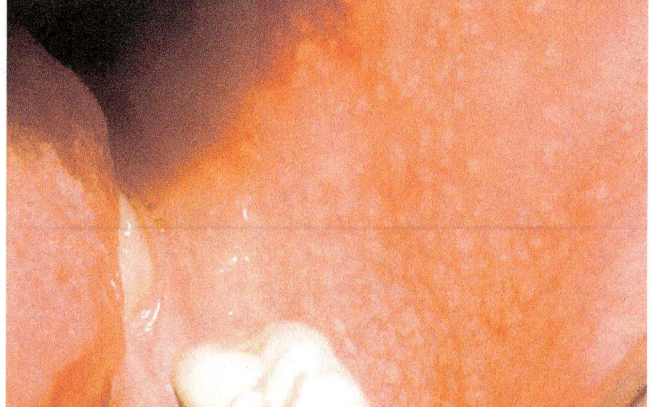

Figure 12–31 Fordyce spots. Sebaceous oil glands near the surface of the epithelium that appear as light yellow spots.

Cleft palates occur when the maxillae fail to join with the primary palate during development, resulting in an abnormal opening in the palate (Figure 12-28B). Surgery is usually required to close the openings and correct speech and swallowing problems.

- *Macrognathia.* Macrognathia is abnormally large jaws, especially in the mandibles, resulting in a class III malocclusion (Figure 12-29).
- *Micrognathia.* Micrognathia is abnormally small jaws, especially in the mandibles, resulting in a class II malocclusion (Figure 12-30).
- *Exostoses.* Exostoses are bony outgrowths that typically occur on the mandibular or maxillary palate; they are also called *tori* (see below).
- *Tori.* Tori are bony outgrowths that can occur in the midline of the palate (torus palatinus) or on the lingual surface of the mandible (torus mandibularis) that may lead to several complications. Food may become impacted around tori, making it difficult to clean certain areas. The tissues covering tori are extremely thin and susceptible to irritation or scratches by food while eating. In addition, these outgrowths may complicate dental radiographs, so dental assistants should place the film with care. Treatment is usually unnecessary unless tori obstruct a dental appliance such as dentures. Then

they can be removed surgically in order to create a foundation for the prosthesis.

- *Fordyce spots.* These appear as light yellow spots in the oral cavity (Figure 12-31). In actuality, they are sebaceous oil glands near the surface of the epithelium. They are a normal occurrence in up to 80% of the population. No treatment is necessary.
- *Ankyloglossia.* Commonly called "tongue tied," this condition occurs when the lingual frenum is attached near the tip of the tongue, thus limiting its movement in the oral cavity (Figure 12-32). Speech and sounds are often affected because of the tongue's reduced range of motion. Dental assistants should watch for signs of this in children, and, if ankyloglossia is suspected, bring it to the attention of the dentist. A simple test can be performed by asking the child to stick the tip of the tongue out and move it from side to side to see if restriction is present. Treatment is a simple surgical procedure to sever the lingual frenum.
- *Fissured tongue.* About 5% of the population has deep wrinkles on the tongue surface known as *fissures.* The cause of fissured tongue is unknown, but it is theorized to be caused by long-term vitamin deficiencies or chronic trauma. No treatment is necessary,

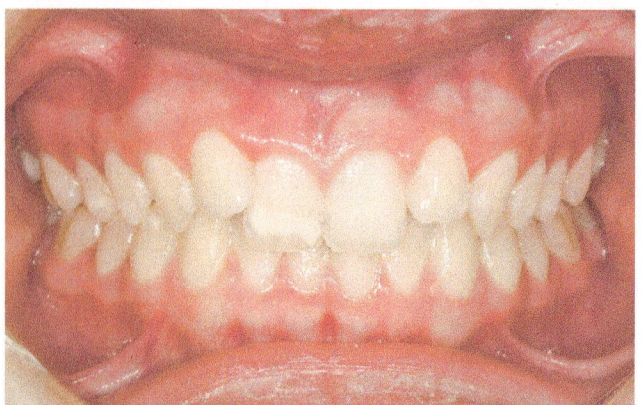

Figure 12–30 Class II malocclusion. Caused by micrognathia.

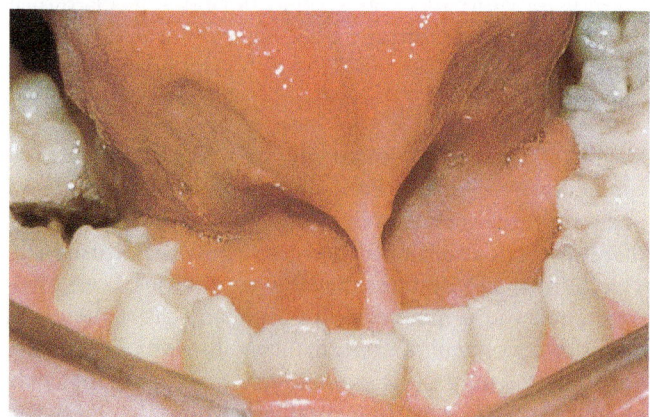

Figure 12–32 Ankyloglossia. Also known as "tongue tied."

although patients might choose to irrigate the fissures occasionally to reduce the likelihood of debris getting stuck in the fissures and causing aggravation.

■ *Bifid tongue.* A bifid tongue occurs when the lateral halves of the anterior tongue do not fuse together during development. Patients will have an extra flap or tag of muscle at the back of their tongue. No treatment is necessary unless the patient complains of irritation or discomfort.

Disturbances in Tooth Development and Eruption

The following abnormalities can occur while the teeth are developing or during eruption:

■ *Ameloblastoma.* This is a tumor caused when the remnants of tooth lamina fail to disintegrate after tooth buds are formed (Figure 12-33).

■ *Amelogenesis imperfecta.* This inherited condition occurs when the tooth enamel is discolored, partly missing, or very thin. Because these teeth can be extremely susceptible to dental carries, they are sometimes covered with composite or crowns.

■ *Ankylosis.* This occurs when the tooth fuses with the alveolar bone. This restricts the tooth's ability to erupt normally, so it may appear below the occlusal plane of adjacent teeth. Also, the deciduous tooth cannot be shed normally because it is fused to the bone. It typically affects deciduous molars. Removal can be complicated and the dentist might have to use a bur and handpiece to dislodge the tooth from the bone.

■ *Anodontia.* This is the congenital absence of teeth. It most often affects the third molars, or "wisdom teeth," although it also sometimes affects maxillary lateral incisors and mandibular second premolars. Anodontia can also affect primary teeth.

■ *Dens in dente.* This Latin phrase translates as "tooth within a tooth." In this condition, a small, tooth-like enamel lump is present at the base of a normal tooth. This kind of tooth is visible on radiographs as "tooth within a tooth" (Figure 12-34).

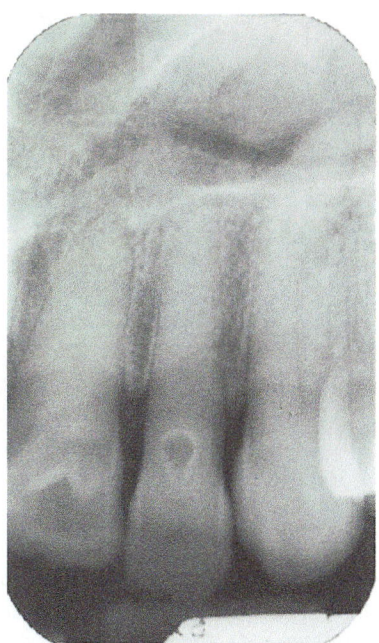

Figure 12–34 Dens in dente. Radiograph showing tear-shaped tooth within a tooth.

■ *Dentinogenesis imperfecta.* This condition occurs when the tooth enamel is very thin, and the tooth is off-color (Figure 12-35). Enamel on teeth affected with this condition chips away soon after eruption. The teeth are also lacking pulp chambers and root canals. It normally affects both primary and permanent teeth. People with this condition typically experience very fast tooth wear because they are lacking protective enamel.

■ *Fusion.* Fusion occurs when the enamel and dentin of two adjacent teeth become fused together, resulting in one continuous oversized tooth. There may be a slight indentation between the two original teeth. This condition typically affects anterior mandibular primary teeth.

■ *Gemination.* Gemination is the opposite of fusion: instead of two teeth fusing, one tooth bud attempts to divide, leaving an indentation on the incisal or occlusal surface.

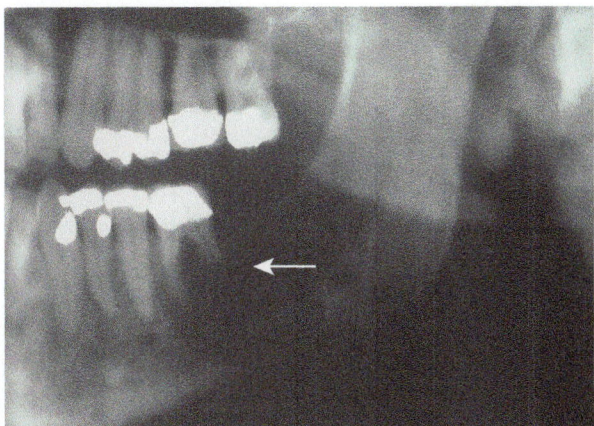

Figure 12–33 Ameloblastoma. Radiograph showing a tumor (arrow) caused by remnants of tooth lamina. (Courtesy of Dr. Harvey Kessler.)

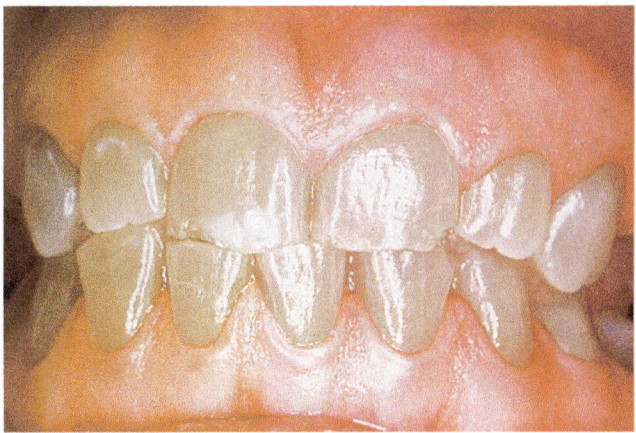

Figure 12–35 Dentinogenesis imperfecta. Amber colored teeth with excessive wear.

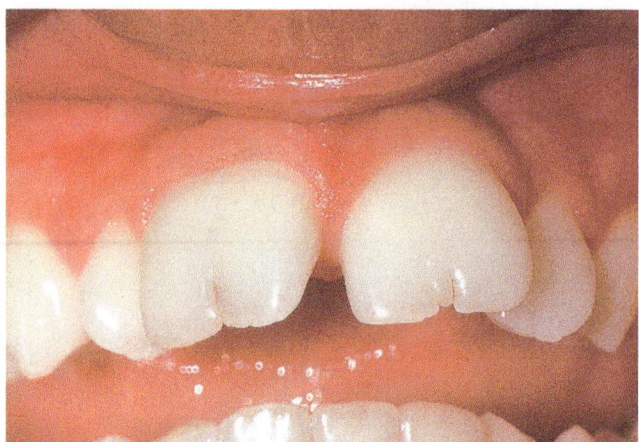

Figure 12–36 Macrodontia. Abnormally large teeth.

- *Macrodontia*. Teeth affected with this condition are abnormally large (Figure 12-36). It can affect all teeth, or just one or two.
- *Microdontia*. Teeth affected with this condition are abnormally small (Figure 12-37). It can affect all teeth, or just one or two. This condition is sometimes associated with genetic syndromes, such as Down syndrome.
- *Neonatal teeth*. Neonatal teeth are present at birth or erupt within the first month. The most common neonatal teeth are mandibular incisors. These teeth lack roots and are usually shed very quickly. They are often removed to prevent the infant from swallowing them as they are shed. Normal primary tooth development follows.
- *Supernumerary teeth*. Supernumerary teeth are any teeth in excess of the normal 32. Supernumerary teeth are typically dwarfed, but they can be normal in size and appearance. They usually appear in the maxillary anterior or third molar region.
- *Twinning*. This occurs when the tooth bud successfully divides, resulting in the creation of two mirror-image teeth from one tooth bud.

Nutritional Disturbances

Nutritional disturbances are the result of inadequate nutrition. They can result from a poor diet, from psychological disorders such as bulimia, or from absorption or systemic problems.

Vitamin Deficiencies

Like all organs, the teeth and oral cavity need adequate vitamins and nutrients to thrive. (See Chapter 11, Nutrition, for a detailed examination of how nutrition affects dental health.) The most common vitamin deficiency to affect the oral cavity is a lack of the B-complex vitamins. Lack of essential vitamins can result in the following conditions:

- *Angular cheilitis*. Angular cheilitis is a lesion that forms in the juncture of the upper and lower lips, in the corner of the mouth (Figure 12-38). The lesion usually extends from the interior to the exterior, thus involving both oral mucosa and skin where the lips meet. Besides a lack of vitamin B, this condition can also be caused by patients who compulsively lick their lips and among patients with ill-fitting dentures that result in the corners of the mouth collapsing inward. Because the area is constantly wet, it is prone to the *Candida albicans* fungus. Treatment for this condition depends on its cause. If the cause is lack of B vitamins, the patient will be advised to get adequate B vitamins. If it is caused by ill-fitting dentures or an anatomical problem, new dentures or crowns might be recommended to restore the normal aspect of the mouth.
- *Glossitis*. Inflammation and changes to the tongue can be caused by lack of vitamin B. In glossitis, the filiform papillae are missing, resulting in smooth spots on the tongue itself, thus the condition is sometimes referred to as "bald tongue." Patients may be sore and will sometimes avoid food. Treatment consists of making sure the patient obtains all the necessary vitamins and nutrients.

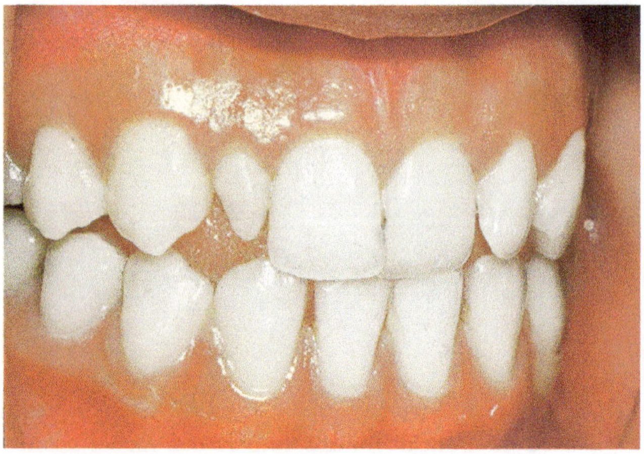

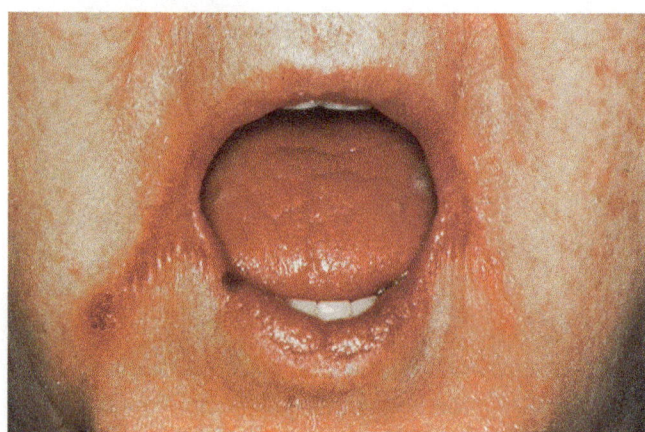

Figure 12–37 Microdontia. Abnormally small teeth.

Figure 12–38 Angular cheilitis, shown in an older adult.

- *Scurvy.* Scurvy is a condition resulting from a vitamin C deficiency. Once associated with sailors who lacked a source of vitamin C during long sea voyages, the disease is rare in modern times. Individuals whose diet is lacking in fresh fruit and vegetables, such as older adults, patients with alcoholism, and infants and children, may develop the disease. A patient with scurvy exhibits gingival bleeding, general weakness, anemia, and skin hemorrhages. Patients suffering from scurvy are given vitamin C treatment.

Anorexia Nervosa and Bulimia Nervosa

Anorexia nervosa (anorexia) and bulimia nervosa (bulimia) are psychological conditions that can result in malnutrition and significant oral complications. Anorexia is a condition in which the desire to be excessively thin leads to a refusal to eat. Bulimia is characterized by cycles of binging and purging.

People with anorexia are often significantly underweight and may be severely malnourished, which can cause oral complications. In contrast, patients with bulimia are often of average or slightly above average weight and may effectively hide their condition. In fact, by recognizing the oral symptoms of bulimia, dental professionals may be among the first people to recognize bulimia in a patient.

The vomiting associated with bulimia can cause extensive damage to the teeth. Frequent exposure to corrosive stomach acid causes the lingual surface of the anterior teeth to become decalcified and gradually lose their enamel. The posterior teeth may also be affected as their occlusal surfaces are eroded and existing dental work is compromised. The patient may also suffer from an above average number of dental caries and swelling of the parotid glands.

See Chapter 11, Nutrition, for a detailed discussion of anorexia and bulimia.

Other Disorders

Varix

Varix is the oral equivalent of varicose veins elsewhere in the body (Figure 12-39). This condition is seen primarily in older adults. It is characterized by the extension and weakening of veins in the oral cavity, especially beneath the tongue or in the buccal mucosa. These veins are visible as purplish lines, just like varicose veins. No treatment is necessary.

Bell Palsy

Bell palsy is a condition that causes temporary paralysis on one side of the face. The cause is unknown, but it may be due to an immune system reaction or a viral infection. Several viruses have been linked to Bell palsy, including

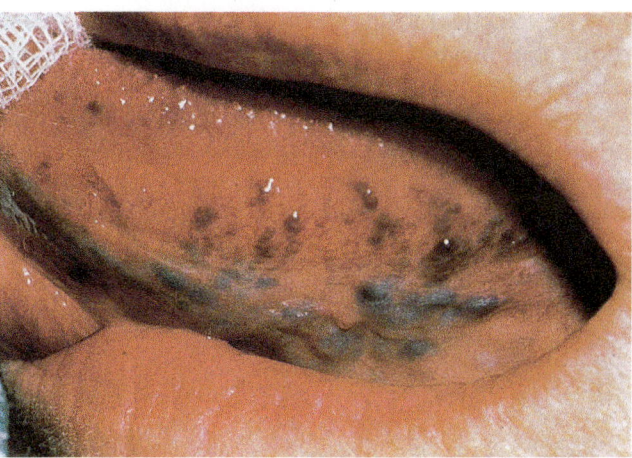

Figure 12–39 **Lingual varices** shown on the ventral tongue.

the Epstein-Barr virus and the herpes simplex virus. The first symptom is typically pain that begins behind one ear, followed by a progressive and sudden weakening of the facial muscles.

The severity of the condition ranges from mild weakness to complete paralysis. Patients with Bell palsy may be unable to close the eye on the affected side of the face, and their saliva production may be affected. Treatment usually consists of antiviral drugs, along with corticosteroids to reduce swelling of the affected nerves. Eye drops may be prescribed to moisten the affected eye.

Bell palsy usually heals on its own, depending on the severity of the paralysis. Partial paralysis can resolve within 1 to 2 months, whereas full paralysis may take up to 6 to 12 months. In some cases, lingering weakness may remain for life.

Fibromyalgia

Fibromyalgia is a chronic disorder of the muscles and tendons that causes widespread pain and tenderness. It is much more common in women than men, and the cause of fibromyalgia is typically unknown. There are several forms of fibromyalgia, including a variety that affects the temporomandibular joint.

In the temporomandibular form, the muscles used in chewing may become very sensitive and painful, sometimes prohibiting patients from opening the mouth fully. This condition can be caused by clenching the jaw or grinding the teeth during sleep. Treatment for this form of fibromyalgia relies on mouth guards to stop patients from grinding their teeth at night, along with pain relief and sometimes antidepressants, which have been shown to reduce the nighttime symptoms.

Trigeminal Neuralgia

Trigeminal neuralgia is a pain condition that affects the trigeminal nerve, which carries sensory information from the face to the brain. The cause may be unknown, or there may be structural abnormalities that cause compression of the trigeminal nerve. It can also be caused by tumors compressing the nerve or by multiple sclerosis.

Among patients with trigeminal neuralgia, specific spots on the face are sensitized, resulting in extreme pain if pressure is applied. This may include the cheeks, lips, or tongue. Even toothbrushing can cause jolts of excruciating pain.

Trigeminal neuralgia can complicate dental treatment. Pain relief should be provided. Treatment usually involves anticonvulsants, which help stabilize nerves, and in some cases, surgery may be necessary.

CHECKPOINTS

12-17 What causes pyogenic granulomas?

12-18 What is a congenital condition?

12-19 Angular cheilitis can be linked to a deficiency of which vitamin?

12-20 What congenital condition affecting tooth development is linked to Down syndrome?

Chapter Highlights

- ◆ Oral pathology is the study of diseases and lesions in the oral cavity. Although dental assistants cannot diagnose oral conditions, they can play a crucial role by alerting the dentist to any unusual oral conditions.
- ◆ Tools involved in diagnosing oral pathologies include the dental history, clinical diagnosis, microscopic findings, radiographs, surgical findings, and lab results.
- ◆ The term *lesion* refers to a type of abnormal tissue. Lesions are classified by their relation to the mucosal surface: below, above, even with, or flat or raised.
- ◆ Lesions below the mucosal surface include ulcers, erosions, abscesses, and cysts. Lesions above the mucosal surface include blisters, bullae, pustules, hematomas, papules, and plaques. Lesions even with the mucosal surface include ecchymosis, macules, petechiae, and purpura. Flat or raised lesions include nodules, neoplasms, and granulomas.
- ◆ Lesions of infectious origin include herpes, cellulitis secondary to infection with the streptococcus bacteria, herpes zoster (shingles), human papillomavirus, actinomycosis, syphilis, human immunodeficiency virus/acquired immune deficiency syndrome, and candidiasis.
- ◆ Oral complications of acquired immune deficiency syndrome include hairy leukoplakias and Kaposi sarcoma.
- ◆ *Hyperplasia* means growth of new, noncancerous tissue; it frequently results from friction with a dental appliance.

- ◆ Radiation treatment can cause a number of oral problems, including deformity of developing teeth, ulcers, xerostomia, and death of bone.
- ◆ Cosmetic piercing, especially tongue piercing, has a number of oral complications that patients should be aware of before committing to the procedure.
- ◆ Smoking and smokeless tobacco use is a major risk factor for several oral pathologies, including oral cancers.
- ◆ Hairy tongue is a condition caused by overgrowth of the filiform papillae on the tongue, which are then stained by food and drink.
- ◆ Oral cancers include squamous cell carcinoma and basal cell carcinoma. Squamous cell is more common, and is usually caused by tobacco use or excessive, long-term alcohol consumption.
- ◆ Papillomas and fibromas are noncancerous oral tumors.
- ◆ Pregnancy-related oral conditions include gingival enlargement and pyogenic enlargement, or noncancerous tumors.
- ◆ Congenital conditions are present at birth. These include various deformities of the teeth and other oral structures. Not all congenital conditions require treatment.
- ◆ Angular cheilitis is a lesion that forms where the lips meet. It can be caused by a lack of B vitamins and by excessive licking of the lips or ill-fitting dentures that allow saliva to pool in the corner of the mouth.
- ◆ Bulimia can cause significant oral damage as the teeth are exposed to corrosive stomach acid.

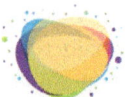

Review Questions

1. What does etiology mean?
   a. A disease of unknown origin
   b. A small, hard, raised plaque in the oral cavity
   c. The cause of a disease or pathology
   d. Swelling and tenderness

2. What is a biopsy?
   a. A sample of a tissue used for diagnosis
   b. Findings arrived at during oral surgery
   c. A compilation of all previous oral pathologies
   d. A biological agent that causes disease

3. What is an erosion?

    a. An inflamed crater in the oral cavity with well-defined margins

    b. Deep grooves or fissures in the tongue

    c. A congenital condition in which the baby is born with teeth that rapidly fall out

    d. A shallow wound with ragged margins that is often caused by friction

4. What is the difference between a pustule and a blister?

    a. Blisters are larger, whereas pustules are very small

    b. Blisters are filled with fluid, whereas pustules are filled with purulent material

    c. Blisters are benign, whereas pustules are usually malignant

    d. Blisters are very painful, whereas pustules are not painful

5. What is a macule?

    a. A blood-filled sac under the oral mucosa

    b. A small, elevated area of skin that varies in pigmentation and texture

    c. An area or patch that is colored differently than surrounding tissue

    d. A blister that contains blood

6. A neoplasm is

    a. A newly erupted tooth.

    b. A plasma-based growth from a bony organ.

    c. A painful ulceration.

    d. Newly formed tissue that serves no obvious purpose.

7. What condition is associated with Wickham striae?

    a. Nodules

    b. Oral cancers

    c. Lichen planus

    d. Candidiasis

8. How long will most minor canker sores last?

    a. 1 day

    b. 1 to 5 days

    c. 7 to 10 days

    d. Longer than a month

9. A patient arrives in the office with swelling caused by a local infection of the streptococcus bacteria. What is the most likely diagnosis?

    a. Cellulitis secondary to bacterial infection

    b. Sepsis

    c. Flesh-eating viral infection

    d. Swelling, pain, and inflammation

10. Oral human papilloma virus infection causes

    a. Intensely painful, bleeding blisters

    b. Small plaques on the mucosa

    c. Early tooth loss

    d. Small warts in the oral cavity

11. Acute necrotizing ulcerative gingivitis affects which oral structures?

    a. Tongue and palate

    b. Gingiva and teeth

    c. Lips and gingiva

    d. Tongue only

12. Kaposi sarcoma usually appears as what?

    a. Whitish, raised bumps on the tongue and cheeks

    b. Ulcerative holes in the gingiva

    c. Bluish or purple flat nodules on the palate

    d. Reddish plaques on the tongue

13. What are erythroplakias?

    a. White, furry growths on the gingiva and tongue

    b. Red patches in the oral cavity that are commonly malignant

    c. Grooves worn into the tooth enamel

    d. Fissures in the gingiva

14. Define tori.

    a. Bony outgrowths in the oral cavity

    b. Soft tissue flaps in the gingiva

    c. Hard, muscular lumps on the anterior of the tongue

    d. None of the above

15. What is the common term for ankyloglossia?

    a. Tongue tied

    b. Trench mouth

    c. Cleft palate

    d. Cleft lip

16. Ankylosis is what?

    a. Extra teeth in the oral cavity

    b. A lack of teeth in the oral cavity

    c. When the dentin of deciduous teeth fuses with the alveolar bone

    d. A tooth within a tooth

17. What are neonatal teeth?

   a. The first set of teeth, which arrive around 12 months of age

   b. Teeth that are present at birth or shortly after

   c. Extra teeth

   d. Teeth that fail to erupt

18. What are varix?

   a. Red, weakened, and extended veins in the oral cavity

   b. Malignant lesions

   c. A varied pattern of lesions

   d. A shifting network of smooth patches on the tongue

Active Learning Exercises

1. List some potential problems a patient with exostoses may encounter. What are the possible treatments for a patient with exostoses who may require a maxillary or mandibular prosthesis?

2. A patient experiencing sores in the junctures of the mouth has what condition? Which vitamin deficiency is responsible for the condition, and what medications are typically prescribed for it? Discuss any alternatives to taking medications.

3. Create a dialogue to discuss the manifestations of nicotine stomatitis. Be sure to include the associated visual cues, such as the corrugated-looking tissue and the hyperkeratinized palatal nodules (glands) that may look red or white in circumference. Which areas of the mouth are more prone to nicotine stomatitis?

Application Activities

1. Collect images of a variety of oral lesions and attempt to correctly identify them based on photographic evidence alone.

2. Practice patient education. Select one of the oral pathologies described in the chapter and write a paragraph or two describing some oral hygiene tips you would share with a patient suffering from the condition.

part IV

Basic Skills

chapter 13

Understanding Microbiology

CHAPTER OUTLINE

Introduction
The History of Microbiology
Types of Microorganisms
    Bacteria
    Protozoa
    Fungi

Algae
Viruses
Prions and Other Infectious Microorganisms
Bacterial Diseases
    Antibiotics: Issues in Treatment
    Important Bacterial Diseases

Viral Diseases
    Important Viral Diseases
The Immune System
    Natural Immunity and Acquired Immunity

CHAPTER CHECKLIST

On completion of this chapter, students will be able to:

☑ Discuss the history of microbiology.
☑ Identify the major microorganisms that pose a threat to human health.
☑ Describe important bacteria and their diseases.
☑ Describe important viruses and their diseases.
☑ Describe how the immune system helps prevent disease.

KEY TERMS

acute hepatitis – the initial stage of infection with the hepatitis virus; acute hepatitis may or may not convert into chronic hepatitis, depending on the strain of the virus and other, unknown factors; acute hepatitis ranges in severity from a mild, cold-like illness to a severe illness requiring hospitalization

aerobic – living in air; requiring oxygen to live

anaerobic – living without oxygen

bacilli (bah-SIL-lie) – a genus of aerobic or facultatively anaerobic, spore-forming, ordinarily motile bacteria containing gram-positive rods

chronic hepatitis – infection with the hepatitis virus that causes long-term and sustained live inflammation; chronic hepatitis ranges in severity from mild inflammation with no symptoms to severe inflammation that leads to cirrhosis of the liver

cocci (KOK-sigh) – a bacterium of round, spheroid, or ovoid form

diplococci (dih-ploh-KOK-sigh) – spheric or ovoid bacteria linked together in pairs

encephalitis (en-sef-uh-LIE-tis) – inflammation of the membrane surrounding the brain

etiologic (ee-tee-uh-LOJ-ik) agent – the specific cause of a disease, such as a bacteria or virus

facultative anaerobe (FAK-ul-tay-tiv AN-uh-robe) – an anaerobe that grows in the presence of air or under conditions of reduced oxygen tension

fever – a complex physiological response to disease that is characterized by a rise in core temperature, generation of acute phase reactants, and activation of immunologic systems

gram-negative bacteria – refers to the inability to resist decolorization with alcohol after being treated with Gram crystal violet stain; however, following decolorization, these bacteria can be readily counterstained with safranin, imparting a pink or red color to the bacteria when viewed by light microscopy

gram-positive bacteria – refers to the ability of a bacterium to resist decolorization with alcohol after being treated with Gram crystal violet stain, imparting a violet color to the bacterium when viewed by light microscopy

infection – invasion of the body by organisms that have the potential to cause disease

infection control – measures taken to prevent infection

inflammation – a fundamental, stereotyped complex of reactions that occur in affected blood vessels and adjacent tissues in response to an injury or abnormal stimulation caused by a physical, chemical, or biologic agent

interferons – a class of small proteins produced in response to viral infection and other biological and synthetic stimuli; interferons bind to specific receptors on cell membranes; their effects include inducing enzymes, suppressing cell proliferation, inhibiting viral proliferation, and enhancing the immune system

local infections – infections that are confined to a specific region of the body

microbiology – the science concerned with microorganisms, including fungi, protozoa, bacteria, and viruses

microorganisms – microscopic organisms

mold – a filamentous fungus, generally a circular colony that may be cottony, wooly, or glabrous, but with filaments not organized into large fruiting bodies, such as mushrooms

natural killer cells – large granular lymphocytes that kill targeted cells using antibody-dependent cell-mediated cytotoxicity

nosocomial (nose-oh-KOH-mee-uhl) infection – an infection acquired in a hospital

pathogenic (path-oh-JEN-ik) – causing disease or abnormality

pathogen (PATH-uh-jen) – any virus, microorganism, or other substance that causes disease

phagocytosis (fayg-oh-sigh-TOE-sis) – the process of ingestion and digestion by cells of solid substances

prion (PRY-on) – small, infectious proteinaceous particle

seroconversion (sir-oh-kun-VER-zhun) – the process by which, after exposure to an etiologic agent of a disease, the blood changes from a negative to a positive serum market for that specific disease

streptococci (strep-toe-KOK-sigh) – a genus of nonmotile, non–spore-forming, aerobic to facultatively anaerobic bacteria containing gram-positive, spheric, or ovoid cells that occur in pairs or short or long chains

systemic infection – an infection that occurs throughout the body

tinea (TIN-ee-uh) – a fungus infection

viroid – a fragment of RNA that is an infectious organism

yeast – a general term denoting true fungi of the family *Saccharomycetaceae* that are widely distributed

Introduction

Microbiology is the study of organisms that are too small to be seen with the naked human eye. These tiny organisms are called **microorganisms**. There are many kinds of microorganisms, including many that are beneficial to human health. In fact, the human intestine is colonized with beneficial microorganisms that aid in digestion and nutrient absorption.

However, some of the more familiar microorganisms are responsible for illnesses, many of which can be very serious. These include bacteria, viruses, fungi, and others. People who work in medical settings, including dental assistants (DAs), must take great care to protect both their patients and themselves from transmitting microorganisms and causing illness.

Any disease that is acquired in a medical setting is known as a **nosocomial infection**. The practice of antiseptic and protective measures to prevent infection is known as **infection control**. It is an extremely important element of a successful dental practice.

After a disease has been transmitted, it is up to medical professionals to identify the microorganism responsible and, if possible, treat the condition. Tools used in the diagnosis of microbial illnesses include a microscope, culture dishes for growing bacterial samples, and rapid test kits that can identify certain viral and bacterial illnesses. These kinds of diagnostic tests are not performed in dental offices.

This chapter will introduce and describe the most important microorganisms that DAs are likely to come into contact with, including bacteria and viruses, as well as introduce the immune system. For a more detailed discussion on preventing illness and aseptic techniques in the dental office, see Chapter 14, Disease and Infection Control.

The History of Microbiology

Before microbes were identified and studied, the medical profession had a number of implausible theories for what caused disease. In warmer regions, where mosquito-borne illnesses, such as yellow fever and malaria were common, the illnesses were blamed on swamp vapors, or *miasma*, which was thought to creep into the lungs and cause sickness.

In the 1840s, two doctors, Dr. Oliver Wendell Holmes in the United States and Dr. Ignaz Semmelweis in Vienna, speculated that poor infection control might be contributing to a very high mortality rate among new mothers. At the time, it was not uncommon for up to 25% of women to die immediately after childbirth from a fever. In Vienna, Dr. Semmelweis speculated that the new mothers might be catching a microbial disease from medical students, who frequently traveled straight from the morgue to the birthing rooms without washing their hands. Dr. Semmelweis ordered that all students and physicians had to wash their hands from then on, and the mortality rate in the birthing ward dropped to less than 1%.

It is not an understatement to say that the discovery of infectious microbes and, eventually, the development of methods for guarding against them and treating infections, has been one of the single greatest advances in human health.

Although most of the major advances in microbiology have taken place in the 20th and 21st centuries, the first microorganisms were actually observed by Anton Van Leeuwenhoek (1632–1723) in Holland. Van Leeuwenhoek ground lenses to make an early magnifying glass and used it to observe a drop of rainwater. He saw that the water was swarming with tiny moving organisms. Later, he observed microorganisms in a scraping from his own tooth. Today, Van Leeuwenhoek is considered the Father of Microscopy, and several of his basic designs are still used today (Figure 13-1).

Other pioneers in microbiology include:

■ *Ferdinand Julius Cohn* (1828–1898). Cohn was the first to classify bacteria as plants, and he later classified bacteria into four groups, depending on their characteristics. Cohn's work is important because he demonstrated that not all bacteria can be killed by boiling. Some kinds of bacteria transform into endospores when exposed to

high-stress environments. This information is critical to an understanding of modern antiseptic techniques.

■ *Louis Pasteur* (1822–1895). Pasteur's work was crucial to our understanding of bacteria. He demonstrated that both bacteria and endospores can be destroyed by high heat, and he proved that bacteria cause disease. Perhaps his most famous contribution was his discovery that broth did not spoil if it was exposed to very high heat, destroying the bacteria in the broth, and then kept in a sealed container so it could not be contaminated. This process took on his name and is today known as *pasteurization*. Finally, Pasteur worked with vaccines later in his career, showing that when patients are given a highly weakened form of some diseases, they become immune to the disease in the future. Pasteur is widely known as the Father of Microbiology.

■ *Robert Koch* (1843–1910). German biologist Koch was the first to link specific types of bacteria to specific diseases. He identified the specific bacteria strain that causes tuberculosis. He is also known for the Koch postulates, which are a set of conditions used to determine if a strain of bacteria is responsible for a specific disease. They are:
1. The bacteria must be present in all cases of the disease.
2. The bacteria must be isolated in a pure culture environment.
3. The bacteria must be able to cause the same disease in another person or animal.
4. The bacteria must be recovered and isolated again in a pure culture environment.

■ *Richard Julius Petri* (1852–1921). Petri worked as a lab assistant to Koch after he earned his doctorate in medicine. Petri developed the wide, shallow dish (i.e., *petri dish*) that is still used to culture bacteria. He also developed a method to introduce the bacteria to the dish. Today, bacteria are grown in petri dishes on a medium of agar, which provides a substrate for bacterial growth.

CHECKPOINT
13-1 Who is considered the Father of Microscopy? The Father of Microbiology?

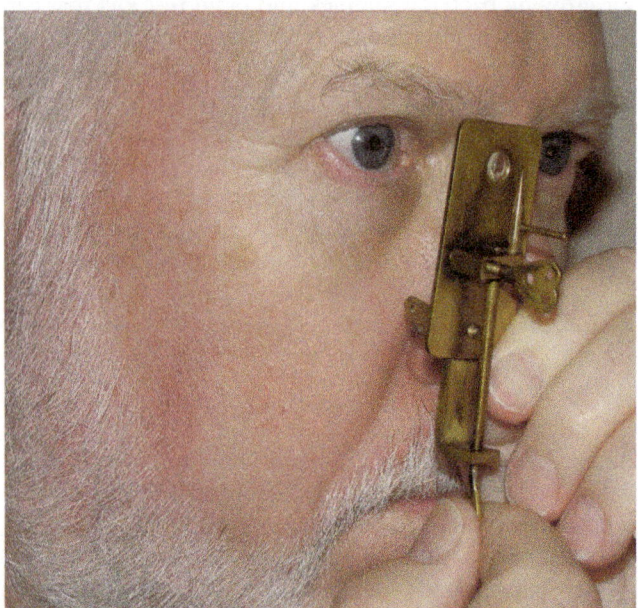

Figure 13-1 Leeuwenhoek's microscopes. Leeuwenhoek's microscopes were very simple devices. Each had a tiny glass lens, mounted in a brass plate. The specimen was placed on the sharp point of a brass pin. The entire instrument was 3 to 4 inches long and was held very close to the eye.

Types of Microorganisms

Researchers have identified many thousands of different microorganisms. Some of them are beneficial, whereas some cause disease. Microorganisms that cause disease are known as **pathogens** or are described as **pathogenic**. An invasion by pathogens is known as an **infection**. Infections, in turn, can be systemic or local.

■ **Systemic infections** are present throughout the body. They are usually spread by the bloodstream and might affect multiple organ systems. Most communicable diseases, such as influenza, are systemic diseases.

- **Local infections** are confined to a particular region or area of the body. The most common local infections are relatively harmless skin infections that occur when a scrape or cut becomes infected with a bacterial agent. The skin around the cut becomes red and puffy, and there may be a slight oozing, but the infection is limited to that immediate area and is relatively easy to treat. If a local infection seeps into the bloodstream, it becomes systemic and, consequently, much more dangerous.

If a microorganism, such as a bacteria or virus, causes a disease, it is known as the **etiologic agent**, or causative agent. Thus, when physicians and researchers talk about the *etiology* of a disease, they are talking about the underlying cause of a particular disease.

Certain conditions must be met for a microorganism to travel from one host to another and spread disease. This is known as the *chain of infection*. The chain of infection and disease prevention is covered in greater detail in Chapter 14, Disease and Infection Control.

Bacteria

Bacteria are among the most important microorganisms in a modern dental practice. They are the most common microorganisms and are prevalent everywhere.

Bacteria are among the simplest organisms on earth, although they are more complex than viruses (Figure 13-2).

Bacteria have a cell wall, but they lack a cell nucleus and many other structures that characterize higher-order cells. They do have DNA, but they do not have chromosomes. Unlike viruses, bacteria can replicate their own DNA and reproduce outside of a host cell.

Bacteria can live in an incredibly wide range of environments, from inside the human digestive tract to polar ice or hot springs to the immense cold and high pressure of the deepest ocean rift. Bacteria that require oxygen to live are called **aerobic**, whereas those that can live without oxygen are **anaerobic**. Bacteria that are able to thrive without oxygen, but will use it if it is available, are known as **facultative anaerobes**.

Some, but not all, bacteria produce resistant forms called *endospores* when exposed to a high-stress environment, such as increased temperature or lack of moisture. Endospores are easily transmitted through the air and are very difficult to kill, even with modern antiseptic techniques. Thus, bacteria that form endospores are particularly dangerous. Bacteria that form endospores include the anthrax species.

Bacteria are present in most environments in staggering numbers. It is estimated that one person's skin is permanently colonized by 1 billion bacteria. Most of them are *Staphylococcus* species, but there are others present as well, including *Propionibacterium* (which causes acne).

Under the right conditions, bacteria can reproduce with incredible swiftness. Some bacterial cells are able to reproduce through simple cell division every 20 minutes. This means a colony of just 10 bacteria can grow to a colony of more than 40,000 bacteria within 4 hours.

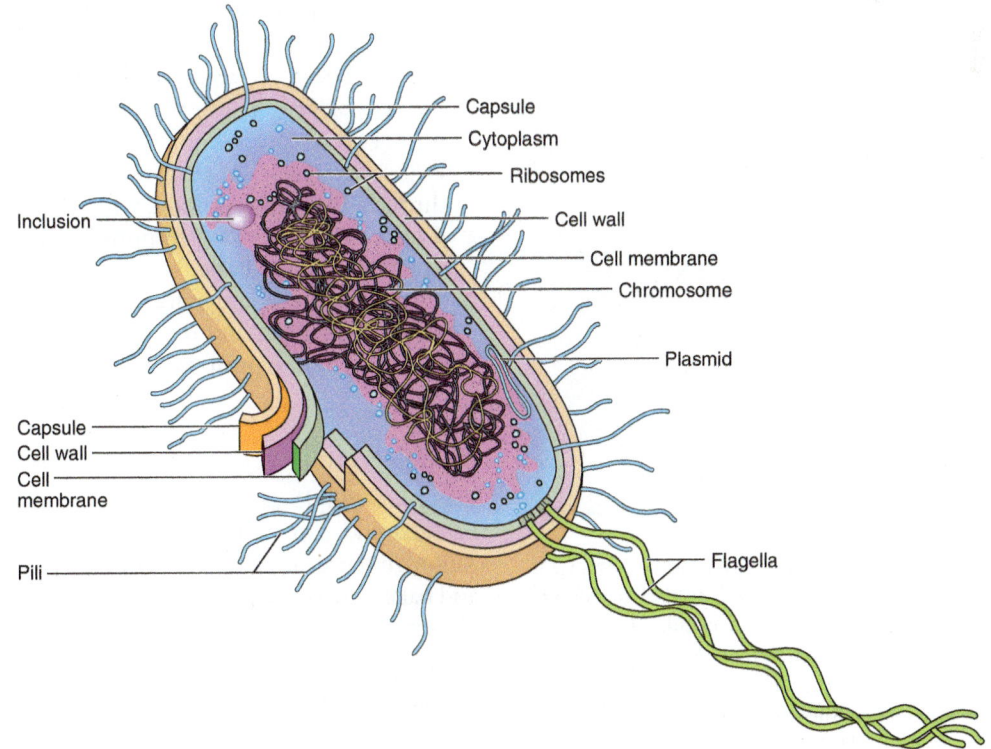

Figure 13-2 A typical bacteria cell is shown.

Identifying and Classifying Bacteria

Bacteria are present in many shapes and forms. Like other organisms, they are often identified by their genus and their species names. The genus name is written first, with a capital letter, followed by the species name in lowercase. Both genus and species are typically italicized when they appear in text. For example, the common *Escherichia coli* bacteria belong to the *Escherichia* genus and the *coli* species.

Bacteria are typically classified by their shape and color when stained by dyes (Figure 13-3). The following forms are recognized:

- **Gram-positive bacteria**. Gram-positive are thick-walled organisms. When exposed to a purple dye, followed by a decolorization with an acid wash and then restaining with a red dye, these bacteria remain purple.

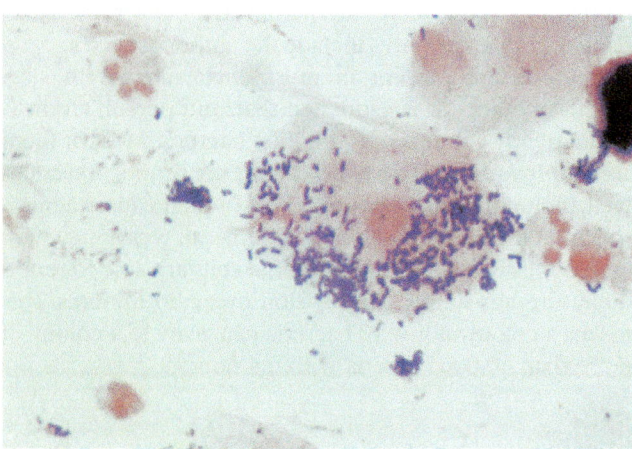

A

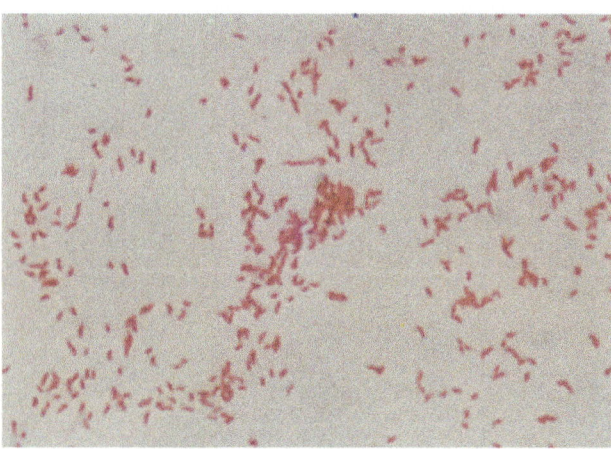

B

Figure 13–3 Gram staining. (A) Gram-positive bacteria (purple stain) can be seen on this pink-stained epithelial cell. **(B)** Gram-negative bacilli (red stain) can be seen as individuals and as short chains. (**A.** From Winn WC Jr, et al. *Koneman's Color Atlas and Textbook of Diagnostic Microbiology*, 6th ed. Philadelphia: Lippincott Williams & Wilkins, 2006. **B.** From Koneman E, et al. *Color Atlas and Textbook of Diagnostic Microbiology*, 5th ed. Philadelphia: Lippincott Williams & Wilkins, 1997.)

- **Gram-negative bacteria**. Gram-negative bacteria are thin-walled organisms. When exposed to the same dye procedure (known as the *Gram stain*), these bacteria emerge pink or red because the initial purple dye is washed from their thin cell walls.

Bacteria are also classified by their shape. These include:

- Round, or **cocci**. Cocci bacteria are round in shape. Those in pairs are called **diplococci**. Those arranged in chains are **streptococci**. Finally, those in large clusters are known as **staphylococci**. Round bacteria are responsible for many dangerous diseases, including pneumonia and scarlet fever.
- Elongated, or **bacilli**. These bacteria are shaped somewhat like cigars. All bacteria that form endospores are bacilli. These include tuberculosis, tetanus, and others.
- Curved. This group includes vibrios (e.g., cholera), spirilla, and spirochetes (e.g., syphilis).

For more information on specific diseases, see the Bacterial Diseases section later in the chapter.

Protozoa

Protozoa are single-celled organisms, but they are much larger and more complicated than bacteria. There are four main types of protozoa, which cause a number of diseases including amebic dysentery, African sleeping sickness, giardiasis, and malaria. Types of protozoa include:

- Amoebas. These are masses of cytoplasm that move by extending a part of their cytoplasm (known as a *pseudopod*) and filling in the extension. Amoebas cause amebic dysentery.
- Ciliates. These are small organisms that move through the use of tiny hairs called *cilia* that wave and, thus, propel the creature.
- Flagellates. These are small organisms that are propelled through the use of a long, whiplike structure called a *flagella*. Flagellates are responsible for African sleeping sickness and giardiasis.
- Sporozoa. These are parasitic organisms that cannot move themselves and rely on their host to live. Malaria is caused by the protozoa *Plasmodium*.

Fungi

Fungi are simple plant-like organisms that are larger than bacteria and can grow either outside or inside the body. Although there are many types of fungi, such as mushrooms and baker's yeast, only a few types are dangerous to humans.

Generally, dangerous fungi occur in two forms:

- **Molds**. These are fuzzy, branching, and multicellular organisms.
- **Yeasts**. These are single-cell organisms that form clumps.

Like some other microbes, fungi naturally occur on and in the human body. The human mouth, intestinal tract, and skin are colonized by *Candida* and *Aspergillus* fungi. These are not typically harmful but might represent a threat to a person with a compromised immune system, such as a patient with acquired immune deficiency syndrome (AIDS) or human immunodeficiency virus (HIV). *Candida* is also responsible for the condition known as *thrush*, which occurs on the oral mucosa and the tongue. Infections of the skin and mucosal membranes caused by fungus are known as **tinea**.

Diseases caused by fungi are known as *mycotic infections*, and they are treated with drugs called *antifungals*. Some infections are important and potentially very dangerous conditions, whereas others are less dangerous. Both athlete's foot and *tinea capitis*, or ringworm, are common and relatively harmless fungal diseases.

Dangerous fungal infections include *Pneumocystis jiroveci*, which causes a rare but very serious pneumonia among people with AIDS, and *Histoplasma capsulatum*, which causes infections deep in the lungs.

Algae

Algae are simple aquatic plants. They are very rarely responsible for disease and are generally not considered a threat in the dental practice.

Viruses

Viruses are extremely small microorganisms; in fact, as small as bacteria are, they are still very large compared to viruses. A typical virus is not visible under a normal light microscope but can only be viewed with a powerful electron microscope.

Viruses do not have independent metabolism and are not technically considered living organisms, even though they have RNA and DNA and can replicate. Except in special laboratory conditions, viruses can grow and divide only inside a host organism. Outside of a host, viruses are inert and inactive.

Viruses do not contain a cell wall but do have a core of RNA or DNA surrounded by a protein coating. Because they can only replicate inside a host organism, they are immune to the antimicrobial drugs, such as antibiotics, that are effective against bacteria. In recent years, antiviral drugs have been introduced that interfere with the virus's ability to replicate, but these drugs are not as effective as antibiotics and may cause much stronger side effects.

Viruses are very important infectious agents. Diseases caused by viruses include AIDS, hepatitis, influenza, herpes and chickenpox, and the common cold.

Viruses are classified in several different ways. They are sometimes classified by whether they have an RNA or DNA core, and whether their nucleic acid is single stranded or double stranded. In human cells, all cells except reproductive cells contain double-stranded DNA. Viruses might also be classified by their symptoms (e.g., yellow fever), the diseases they cause (e.g., measles, HIV, common cold), or by where they were first isolated and identified (e.g., West Nile, Ebola, Hanta).

For a more thorough discussion of the specific diseases caused by viruses, see the Viral Diseases section later in the chapter.

Prions and Other Infectious Microorganisms

Until recently, viruses were considered the smallest infectious agent. Now, however, researchers have uncovered even smaller disease-causing microorganisms—prions and viroids.

Prions are very small organisms that are not considered living organisms. A prion is made up solely of protein. The word "prion" is derived from the phrase proteinaceous infectious agents. Like viruses, prions can only duplicate themselves in cells, but they do not have RNA or DNA. In structure, a prion is more like a crystal or a snowflake, and it duplicates through very slow growth in brain tissue. Diseases caused by prions include Creutzfeldt-Jakob disease, a rare degenerative brain disorder characterized by impaired coordination and rapidly progressing dementia, and its bovine equivalent, bovine spongiform encephalopathy (BSE), often called *mad cow disease*. BSE has been linked to a variant form of Creutzfeldt-Jakob disease in humans.

Viroids are also tiny infectious organisms, but, so far, they do not appear to pose a threat to humans. Viroids are fragments of RNA with no protein coating. Researchers have identified them only in plants.

✓ CHECKPOINTS

13-2 A infection that occurs throughout the body is known as what?

13-3 What term is used to describe bacteria that require oxygen to live?

13-4 How fast can some bacteria reproduce?

13-5 What three shapes are used to classify bacteria?

13-6 What are the smallest microorganisms known to threaten human health?

Bacterial Diseases

Bacterial diseases are a significant threat to human health. To prevent the spread of bacterial and viral diseases, dental and medical offices practice strict infection control. Bacteria thrive in damp and dark environments, especially warm ones.

Under normal conditions, people are exposed to bacteria on a daily basis. However, a healthy immune system is capable of preventing most serious threats to health posed by bacteria. In more serious infections, treatment might be required. The standard treatment for a bacterial illness is antibiotics. For a more thorough discussion of the immune system and the role it plays in preventing bacterial infection, see the section titled, The Immune System, later in the chapter.

Antibiotics: Issues in Treatment

Antibiotics are agents produced by living cells that can destroy bacteria. Sir Alexander Fleming discovered the first commercially produced antibiotics in 1928, when he observed that colonies of *Staphylococcus aureus* were destroyed by the *Penicillium notatum* mold. He speculated that the mold contained a natural antimicrobial agent that killed bacteria.

The significance of his discovery, however, was not fully appreciated until the 1940s, when other researchers isolated, identified, and began to produce the active agent, called *penicillin*. When it was introduced, penicillin was considered a miracle drug—it achieved total remission in diseases and infections that were, until that point, considered incurable. Throughout World War II, penicillin was produced in staggering quantities through a partnership of private companies and the government, and it saved thousands upon thousands of lives from battlefield wounds and infections.

Since then, research into antibiotics has yielded a steady stream of stronger and more effective antibiotic agents. Even though penicillin itself is still in use, patients today are much more likely to be treated with a newer, stronger antibiotic.

However, as antibiotics became more and more common, researchers began to notice that some bacterial infections no longer responded to antibiotics as they once had. Because bacteria are rapidly dividing organisms, strains began to emerge that are resistant to common antibiotics. Known as *antibiotic-resistant bacteria*, these pose a serious threat to the effectiveness of antibiotics.

The most important of these newer, more dangerous bacteria is the methicillin-resistant *Staphylococcus aureus*, or MRSA. MRSA is an aggressive bacterium that cannot be killed with standard antibiotics and can result in a fast-moving, rapidly degenerating infection. MRSA is sometimes called the "flesh-eating bacteria" because of its ability to quickly destroy large areas of tissue.

MRSA is most commonly spread in areas of close contact, such as schools, military barracks, and medical settings. MRSA that occurs in a health care setting is known as *health care–associated MRSA*, or HA-MRSA. MRSA that occurs in the broader community is known as *community-associated MRSA*, or CA-MRSA. The bacteria can survive outside the human body, and it can be transmitted through the air, as opposed to only through direct contact.

Because of the threat of antibiotic-resistant bacteria, overuse of antibiotics is strongly discouraged. This affects the dental practice because many patients are prescribed antibiotics as a preventive measure during dental procedures. For example, patients with certain heart conditions, such as artificial heart valves, are often prescribed antibiotics because an infection could be potentially fatal, as are patients who have had any joint replacements. In recent years, however, researchers have begun to reconsider many of these recommendations and, in some cases, reverse them. If a patient demands antibiotics or is worried that antibiotics might be necessary, dental office employees should refer the patient to his or her regular physician. Note, however, that antibiotics are not effective in treating viral infections.

Important Bacterial Diseases

Bacterial diseases are among the most common and important of human illnesses (see Table 13-1). In a dental practice, assistants might be exposed to any number of bacterial diseases, including:

- *Gonorrhea.* Gonorrhea is a sexually transmitted disease that causes painful discharge, local lesions, and swelling and redness in the infected areas. Gonorrhea is usually a local infection, but can travel through the bloodstream to infect joints, cause fever and pain, and result in pus-filled spots on the skin.
- *Meningitis.* Meningitis is inflammation of the *meninges*, or the tissue covering the brain and spinal cord. Meningitis can be caused by viral or bacterial agents, and several different kinds of bacteria have been linked to meningitis, including *Neisseria meningitidis* and *Streptococcus pneumoniae*. Acute bacterial meningitis occurs most often in patients with compromised immune systems, such as those who have recently suffered from another illness. Symptoms include a stiff neck, fever, headache, sore throat, and vomiting. Acute bacterial meningitis is a very dangerous condition that can result in death in hours or days and needs to be treated immediately with antibiotics.
- *Tuberculosis.* Tuberculosis (TB) is a bacterial infection of the lungs caused by the *Mycobacterium tuberculosis* bacterium. TB bacterium can reside in the body for many years before causing an active infection. Once the disease becomes active, a person can spread the disease through coughing, sneezing, or talking. Symptoms of TB include fever, night sweats, cough, fatigue, and unintentional weight loss. On occasion, pulmonary tuberculosis spreads to other organs in the body. Other symptoms of TB include enlarged or tender lymph nodes in the neck or elsewhere, a crackling-like breath sound, wheezing, breathing difficulty, or chest pain. As the disease progresses, air or fluid may collect in the chest cavity, causing shortness of breath. Antibiotic treatment for TB may last 6 months because the bacteria are very slow growing.

TABLE 13-1 Important Bacterial Diseases

DISEASE	ORGANISM	TRANSMISSION
Gonorrhea	*Neisseria gonorrhoeae*	Sexually transmitted
		Mother to child
Meningitis	*Neisseria meningitis*	Airborne
		Close contact
Tuberculosis	*Mycobacterium tuberculosis*	Airborne
Typhoid fever	*Salmonella enterica*	Fecal contamination
Staph infections	*Staphylococcus aureus*	Airborne
		Close contact
		Compromised immune system
Strep throat	*Streptococcus*	Airborne
		Contaminated surfaces
E. coli	*Escherichia coli*	Contaminated food
Tetanus	*Clostridium tetani*	Blood-borne
		Lack of immunization
Pneumonia	Various bacteria	Airborne
		Close contact
		Opportunistic infections
Chlamydia	*Chlamydia trachomatis*	Sexually transmitted
Anthrax	*Bacillus anthracis*	Airborne
		Close contact
		Contaminated meat
Diphtheria	*Corynebacterium diphtheriae*	Close contact
		Lack of immunization
Whooping cough	*Bordetella pertussis*	Close contact
		Lack of immunization

- *Typhoid fever.* Typhoid fever is caused by the *Salmonella typhi* bacterium. Symptoms include high fever, abdominal pain, and rash. Typhoid fever is transmitted through fecal matter and urine, so inadequate handwashing is a risk factor for transmission. More than 99% of patients who are treated promptly with antibiotics recover.

- *Staph infections.* Staphylococci bacteria normally colonize the nose and skin in 20% to 30% of healthy adults. Staph infections become dangerous, however, when the bacteria penetrate the skin and cause infection. Staph infections range from local, pus-filled skin infections to life-threatening internal infections of the heart, lungs, and other organs. MRSA is considered the most dangerous kind of staph infection. Staph infections are also responsible for gangrene, toxic shock syndrome, and pneumonia. Symptoms of staph infections vary widely, depending on the site and scope of the infection.

- *Strep throat.* Strep throat is the most common infection caused by streptococci bacterium, although there are many disease-causing forms, and infection can occur in other areas besides the throat. Symptoms of strep throat include sore throat, fever, headache, and vomiting. Scarlet fever can result if the bacteria release a toxin that causes a widespread, pink-red rash on the abdomen, chest, and folds of the skin.

- *E. coli.* *Escherischia coli* is one of the microorganisms that causes gastroenteritis. The main symptoms of gastroenteritis are loss of appetite, nausea, vomiting, and stomach cramps. It is usually a food-borne illness, caused by ingestion of undercooked meats. It can also be transmitted through swimming in infected water or contact with infected fecal matter. Antibiotics are usually not used because the infection is typically mild in healthy adults. Among more vulnerable patients, however, the dehydration can be life threatening, and aggressive treatment may be required.

- *Tetanus.* Tetanus is caused by the *Clostridium tetani* bacterium. The bacteria can live in spores in the soil or animal feces and is sometimes transmitted through cuts with rusty objects or puncture wounds. Tetanus causes lockjaw and muscular spasms in the face and neck. Treatment usually involves an antibiotic to kill the bacteria and drugs designed to neutralize the toxins that have already been released by the bacteria.

- *Pneumonia*. Pneumonia is an infection of the lungs that can have many causes, including bacterial infection. Pneumonia is an important cause of death in the United States, killing up to 70,000 people annually. Successful prevention and treatment of pneumonia depends on identifying risk factors for pneumonia, such as a compromised immune system, and identifying the causative agent among existing patients. Vaccines are available to reduce the risk of viral pneumonia.

- *Chlamydia*. *Chlamydia trachomatis* is a sexually transmitted bacterium that can cause a disease that resembles gonorrhea. Chlamydia can often exist without symptoms in both men and women. The most common symptoms include painful urination and yellowish discharge.

- *Anthrax*. Anthrax is caused by infection with *Bacillus anthracis*. It typically affects the skin, lungs, or digestive tract. Anthrax is a spore-forming bacterium that can live in the soil and animal products for decades. Anthrax is highly lethal when inhaled and is one of the agents used in biological warfare. Anthrax can also cause potentially fatal skin infections. Vaccines exist against anthrax infection.

- *Diphtheria*. Diphtheria is a potentially fatal infection of the upper respiratory tract caused by *Corynebacterium diphtheriae*. Vaccination programs have largely wiped out diphtheria as a cause of illness in the developed world. Transmission of diphtheria is usually caused by coughing or sneezing infected droplets into the air. Treatment of diphtheria is accomplished with antibiotics and drugs used to neutralize the potent toxins released by the bacteria.

- *Whooping cough*. Also known as *pertussis*, whooping cough is caused by infection with the highly contagious *Bordetella pertussis* bacterium. Symptoms typically include a cough followed by a long, high-pitched indrawn breath. As with diphtheria, whooping cough has largely been eliminated in the developed world through the widespread use of vaccines.

CHECKPOINTS

13-7 Where do bacteria thrive?

13-8 Antibiotics are often recommended before dental surgeries to prevent infection of vulnerable patients. However, what recent development has caused doctors to reconsider the widespread use of preventative antibiotics?

13-9 Staph infections can infect which parts of the body?

13-10 Are vaccines effective against bacteria?

Viral Diseases

Viral illnesses are very common and range in seriousness from mild annoyances to life-threatening diseases that require aggressive treatment. Unlike bacteria, viruses cannot reproduce outside a living host cell, except in special laboratory conditions. Thus, infection control with viruses is easier because they are considerably easier to kill in the environment.

However, viral infections are harder to treat once they have gained entry to a host and begun to multiply. Viruses are not affected by antibiotics, and there are few effective antiviral agents. Those that do exist are expensive, have side effects, and do not destroy all the viruses. Some forms of viruses can lie dormant in the host organism for years or decades before being activated and causing infection. Treatment against viruses is often aimed at reducing symptoms to make the individual more comfortable for the duration of the disease.

Highly effective vaccines have been developed against several common and dangerous viruses, including influenza, measles, mumps, rubella, and hepatitis. However, there are challenges associated with vaccine development with some viruses. With influenza, for example, there are many different strains of the virus, and it tends to mutate quickly. For a vaccine to be effective, researchers have to first calculate which strain of influenza is expected to be prevalent and manufacture a specific vaccine against that strain. Some viruses, such as HIV/AIDS, do not have vaccines.

Important Viral Diseases

HIV/AIDS

HIV is a virus that causes AIDS. It can be transmitted by blood, semen, vaginal discharge, and purulent material.

HIV was not discovered in the United States until the early 1980s, although researchers believe it was active overseas for a long time before it came to the United States. It was first noticed in the United States in young, homosexual men, although now the disease rate is rising fastest in African American women. HIV can be transmitted through sexual contact, blood transfusions, exposure to cuts and scrapes on infected patients, during childbirth, and from needlesticks with infected needles.

Once HIV has gained access to the body, it launches an attack on the immune system. Specifically, the virus targets the T lymphocytes. These cells coordinate and activate the activities of other immune system cells. At first, the HIV cell uses T lymphocytes to replicate itself, destroying the cells in the process. At this stage, the person is often unaware that he or she has contracted HIV and is not contagious. However, within a few weeks of infection, the viral count may have increased to the point that transmission is possible.

Early in the disease, infection with HIV rarely causes any problems. Although the virus targets the body's immune system, an immune response is still mounted, and

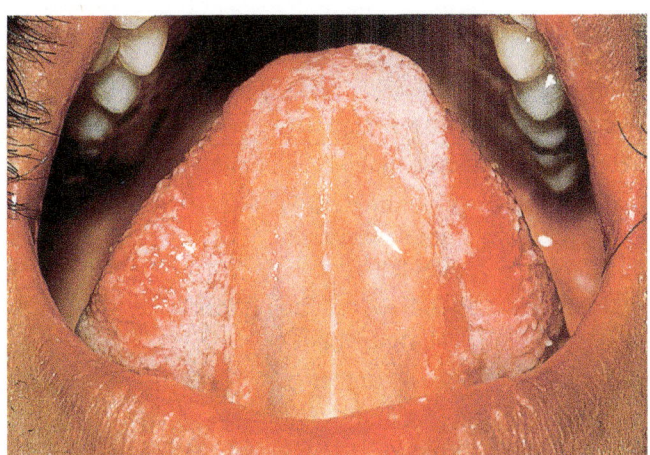

Figure 13–4 Colonies of yeast, *C. albicans.* The footlike extensions from the margins of the colonies are typical of this species. (From Winn WC Jr, et al. *Koneman's Color Atlas and Textbook of Diagnostic Microbiology*, 6*th* ed. Philadelphia: Lippincott Williams & Wilkins, 2006.)

the number of viral cells in the body is kept under control. During this stage, only mild symptoms might be present, including fever, swollen lymph nodes, and fatigue. This condition is sometimes called an *AIDS-related complex*. These symptoms might disappear after a few weeks as the body attempts to fight the virus.

An individual might have HIV for years before the infection worsens. HIV progresses to AIDS when the viral count in the bloodstream (i.e., the viral load) progresses to the point at which the body can no longer mount an effective immune response. At this stage, the patient becomes vulnerable to opportunistic infections, including pathologies of the oral cavity, such as lesions or fungal infections (Figure 13-4). Patients with AIDS often suffer from diseases that are relatively rare in people with healthy immune systems, including a cancer known as *Kaposi sarcoma*. Still other cancers of the immune system might develop. AIDS can also directly affect the brain, causing dementia, and patients with AIDS often suffer from *wasting*, a condition of significant weight loss and muscle degeneration with no apparent cause.

HIV/AIDS cannot be cured. However, in recent years, researchers have made significant progress in battling the disease. A multidrug regimen can reduce the viral load. This regimen includes drugs that interfere with the way HIV replicates itself and grows inside cells. However, to be effective, these drugs must be taken exactly as prescribed, and they have significant and unpleasant side effects. Intense work is continuing for a cure.

Hepatitis

Hepatitis is an inflammation of the liver. Although there are many causes of hepatitis, the most important to health care providers is viral hepatitis. Viral hepatitis is a contagious disease for which there is no cure. It is transmitted by direct contact with infected blood, or it can be transmitted through infected surfaces. Hepatitis is caused by one

of the five hepatitis viruses. The infection is usually broken down into two phases: acute and chronic.

Acute hepatitis occurs shortly after infection. Symptoms, which range from a mild flu-like illness to fatal liver inflammation, flare up suddenly and persist for a few weeks before fading. Many people who have acute hepatitis are unaware of their condition, depending on the strain of hepatitis (e.g., A and C often have very mild symptoms, whereas B and E often produce severe symptoms) and their particular response. For people with mild infection, acute hepatitis rarely requires treatment. People with more serious infection may require hospitalization.

Chronic hepatitis often occurs in people who have been infected with hepatitis C and, less commonly, hepatitis B. After recovery from acute hepatitis, these patients become carriers of the disease, and months or years later, develop chronic liver inflammation. In about two-thirds of cases, however, patients develop the disease without any known previous acute infection, even though they do have the virus. Chronic hepatitis can last for months or even years. Symptoms range from mild inflammation without significant liver damage to very serious inflammation that progresses to *cirrhosis* (scarring of the liver) and liver failure or liver cancer.

The five hepatitis viruses are:

- *Hepatitis A.* Typically transmitted by contact with infected feces, usually as a result of unsanitary hygiene. It can also be transmitted through infected food (e.g., shellfish harvested from infected water) or sexual contact. Hepatitis A is usually a mild infection with no symptoms. Recovery is typically complete, and it does not cause chronic hepatitis. A vaccine is available for hepatitis A.

- *Hepatitis B.* Hepatitis B is more difficult to transmit than hepatitis A but more important to the DA. It can be transmitted through infected blood by needlesticks and through contact with saliva, tears, milk, and other bodily fluids. Hepatitis B typically causes a short-lived acute phase, with symptoms including digestive upset, abdominal pain, fever, weakness, muscle pain, and jaundice. About 5% to 10% of acute patients will go on to develop chronic hepatitis. A significant number of people will also become asymptomatic carriers of the disease.

People who have been exposed to hepatitis B can be given an immune globulin drug within 14 days of exposure. This drug yields a weak protection to the virus and may prevent infection.

Vaccines are an important element in the prevention of hepatitis B and are recommended for all health care providers who might be exposed to the virus. A hepatitis B vaccine, Heptavax-B, was introduced in 1982, and additional vaccines have since been developed and introduced. Hepatitis B vaccines are given in a series of three shots into the arm. Studies have shown that administration in the arm is more effective than injection in the buttocks. The initial shot is followed by a second shot about 1 month later, with a third shot 6 months after the first shot. After the vaccine is administered, a blood test, called a *titer*, can detect the seroconversion rate, indicating that immunity has been achieved.

According to the Occupational Safety and Health Administration (commonly called *OSHA*), employers are responsible for offering the hepatitis B vaccine within 10 days of employment to new employees whose work may include tasks that involve potential exposure to blood, body tissues, or body fluids. Employees are free to decline the vaccine but must sign an informed refusal form that is kept on file. Employers, however, are not obligated to pay for the blood test to confirm seroconversion. This blood test is an important part of vaccination—if immunity was not conferred, the physician can adjust the vaccine and administer another dose. All DAs should make sure they receive this blood test.

Boosters for the hepatitis B vaccine are not recommended unless the employee has been directly exposed to hepatitis B or a patient has tested negative for seroconversion.

- *Hepatitis C*. Hepatitis C is similar in its symptoms to hepatitis B. However, there is no vaccine currently available, and about 75% of people infected with acute hepatitis C become carriers of the disease. Hepatitis C is most often spread through sharing needles.
- *Hepatitis D*. Hepatitis D can replicate only in the presence of hepatitis B and can only occur as a co-infection with hepatitis B. The hepatitis B vaccine also eliminates the risk of hepatitis D.
- *Hepatitis E*. Hepatitis E is spread through infected feces, which contaminates the food and water supply. Symptoms of acute viral hepatitis E may be severe, and epidemics sometimes occur in developing countries when the virus is spread through the water supply. No vaccine is available.

Table 13-2 summarizes the mode of transmission and availability of vaccines for each of the five hepatitis viruses.

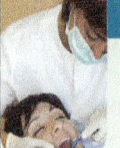

Voice of Experience

Even though we do not have to by law, my office makes sure that all employees who have been vaccinated against hepatitis B have the titer afterward to make sure the vaccination was effective. You would be surprised how many vaccinated people have a low titer count and need to redo their hepatitis B series. But of course, it's much better to know you are protected than to worry after a needlestick or other injury occurs, when people are more concerned about actually contracting hepatitis B. Better safe than sorry!

Herpes Simplex Viruses

Herpes simplex viruses (HSVs) cause recurring outbreaks of small, painful blisters in the infected region (Figure 13-5). There are two varieties of herpes: HSV-1 and HSV-2. HSV-1 typically infects the mouth and causes lesions on the lips, whereas HSV-2 is more commonly known as *genital herpes*. It is important to note, however, that this distinction is not

TABLE 13-2 Viral Hepatitis: Transmission and Vaccines

VIRUS	TRANSMISSION	VACCINE
Hepatitis A	Fecal–oral Contaminated food, water, shellfish	Yes
Hepatitis B	Blood, saliva, and all body fluids Sexual contact	Yes
Hepatitis C	Percutaneous blood Needles	No
Hepatitis D	Blood, saliva, and all body fluids	Hepatitis B vaccine also protects against hepatitis D because hepatitis B must be present in order for hepatitis D to develop
Hepatitis E	Fecal–oral Contaminated water	No

absolute: oral lesions can be caused by either type of the virus. There is no cure for herpes, although there are topical treatments to reduce the severity of the outbreak, and oral antiviral drugs are sometimes used.

Herpes viruses have two states: dormant and active. *Dormant herpes* resides in the nerve cells that supply the infected area. Every so often, the virus becomes active, traveling along the nerve cells to the skin, where it causes an eruption. The virus causes an eruption at different times when it travels along the nerve cells to the skin. The reason for activation is often unknown, although it can be triggered by stress, fever, menstruation, or, in the case of lesions on the lips, physical trauma such as dental work.

Herpes transmission can occur most easily when the virus is active, and cankerous sores are visible. During these times, the virus is present on the skin surface and in discharge in greater numbers. However, transmission is also possible when there are no sores evident. Studies have shown that the herpes virus can still be present even on skin that looks healthy.

The outbreaks caused by herpes can cause severe discomfort. Herpes-related lesions typically last 10 to 14 days and make eating and drinking extremely uncomfortable. If open sores are visible, dental work might be rescheduled, both for the patient's comfort and the dental care providers' safety. Herpes can be transmitted through breaks in the skin (e.g., herpetic whitlow) and can also affect the eyes (e.g., herpes simplex keratitis).

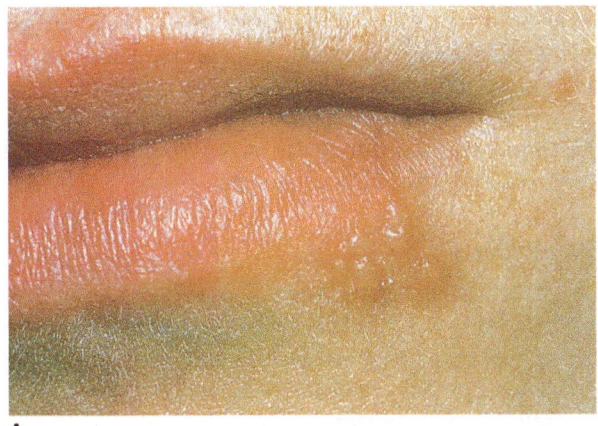

A

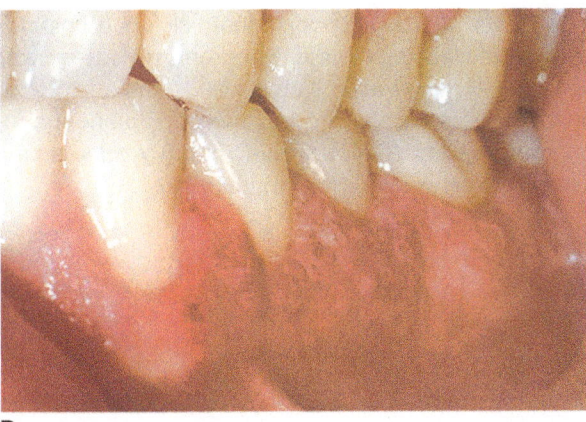

B

Figure 13–5 Herpes simplex viruses. (A) Recurrent herpes labialis showing clustered vesicles. **(B)** Recurrent herpes simplex showing multiple gingival ulcers.

From the Dentist's Perspective

Many people who enter my office do not appreciate that cold sores are actually caused by the herpes virus. Naturally, people are sensitive about herpes, and people are often hesitant to discuss the disease at all, even its oral form. It can be ever more difficult if the patient divulges a history of genital herpes. Yet as uncomfortable as it is, it's very important that patients feel they can talk about their herpes status in a safe, confidential, and professional environment. The fact is, we can only give the best patient care when we have all the information we need.

Common Cold

The common cold is one of the most common illnesses in the world. It is a viral infection of the nose, sinuses, throat, and large airways. Symptoms include runny nose and scratchy throat, fatigue, and, sometimes, a mild fever. Although there are many viruses than can cause the common cold, the most common are the rhinoviruses. There are more than 100 subtypes of rhinovirus.

Colds are easily spread through droplets and direct physical contact with an infected person's nasal secretions. In the dental office, treatment gloves and strict handwashing

protocols can greatly reduce the risk of contracting a cold from an infected patient. People are most contagious in the first 2 days after symptoms become apparent. The virus typically has a 1- to 3-day incubation period between infection and symptoms appearing.

There is no cure for the common cold, and, because there are so many viral agents that cause colds, there is no vaccine. The best prevention is excellent hygiene and infection control practices. Once a cold has been contracted, treatment is aimed at reducing the symptoms with a variety of over-the-counter medications. Symptoms typically last from 4 to 10 days, depending on the virus and the severity of the infection.

Influenza

Influenza is a very common viral illness that peaks every fall and winter. Influenza typically occurs in epidemics, in which large numbers of people get sick at once. The virus is easily transmitted through airborne droplets caused by sneezing and coughing, and many strains of influenza have been discovered. Symptoms of influenza include fatigue, muscle aches, runny nose, high fever, and headache. The onset of the flu usually causes a high fever before it moves into the respiratory tract later in the illness.

The virus has an incubation period of 24 to 48 hours after infection before symptoms begin to appear, and the symptoms generally last for up to 10 days. In many cases, the first few days of symptoms are so severe that patients are unable to work, go to school, or visit any doctors' offices. After the illness is over, a flu-related cough may persist for several weeks.

Infection from many common flu viruses can be prevented with annual vaccination. Every year, researchers try to identify the three most likely strains of flu to cause a worldwide epidemic and formulate a vaccine with these three strains. Vaccination is widely recommended, especially for children, older adults, people with compromised immune systems, and health care providers. DAs should make sure they receive a flu shot every fall to protect themselves against infection that season.

There is no cure for the flu, and treatment tends to focus on symptom relief with over-the-counter medications. Antiviral drugs, such as amantadine and rimantadine, might be used in someone who has just been exposed to flu or in the event of an epidemic.

Chickenpox

Usually thought of as a childhood disease, chickenpox is actually caused by the varicella-zoster virus, which is a member of the herpes family. In childhood, the disease causes characteristic red lumps on the skin and a slight fever. After the disease resolves, the virus goes into a dormant state in the nerve cells. It may reemerge years later, when the patient is an adult, as *shingles*. Shingles appears as clusters of small blisters, typically isolated to one side of the body. Adult shingles are painful and much more severe than the childhood version.

A vaccine against varicella-zoster is available, although the length of immunity is unknown.

Measles

Measles is a highly contagious viral infection that is transmitted through exposure to droplets or contact with contaminated surfaces. Symptoms include fever, runny nose, and a characteristic rash that appears 10 to 15 days after infection. The rash begins on the neck and spreads across the trunk. During the peak of the illness, the child's fever might exceed 104°F, and, in some very rare cases, the virus might infect the brain.

In most cases of childhood measles, the sickness resolves within a week or so after symptoms appear with no lasting side effects. However, secondary bacterial infections pose a threat, especially pneumonia. Antibiotics may be administered in this case.

At one time, measles was a very common and dangerous childhood infection. Measles has largely been eradicated in the United States and other developed countries through aggressive childhood vaccination. In recent years, however, many parents have opted against vaccination after a 1998 research report raised concern over a suspected link between the common MMR (measles, mumps, and rubella) vaccine and autism. Although most medical experts dispute the link, the ensuing controversy led to fewer vaccinations, which has resulted in an increase in measles cases in the United States.

Mumps

Mumps is a contagious viral infection that causes enlargement of the salivary glands, although it can also affect the testes, brain, and pancreas. Like measles, mumps is spread through inhalation of infected droplets coughed or sneezed out by an infected person or by direct contact with contaminated surfaces. Mumps is less contagious than chickenpox or measles but can still cause epidemics in nonvaccinated populations. It is most common in children but usually more severe in adults.

Mumps has an incubation period of 14 to 24 days after infection. The disease usually begins with chills, headache, and mild fever. Within 24 hours after symptoms begin, the salivary glands start to swell, peaking 48 hours later. As a result, eating is painful, and the fever can rise to 104°F. Most children recover without incident, but in some rare cases, symptoms reappear in about 2 weeks. In a small percentage of people, mumps can also infect the testes or lead to inflammation in the brain.

Mumps vaccination is routine in the United States and most developed countries.

West Nile Virus

West Nile virus is the common name for infection with a particular strain of the arbovirus. There are actually several types of arbovirus active in the United States, and all of them are spread by mosquitoes. Arboviruses cause severe inflammation of the brain (**encephalitis**). The first symptoms of infection

with an arbovirus are headache, drowsiness, and fever. This is followed by confusion, seizures, and coma. The disease often occurs as an epidemic as infected animals spread the disease.

There is no treatment for arbovirus. The best approach is prevention by controlling the mosquito populations that spread it during the summer months.

Mononucleosis

Mononucleosis, or "mono," is a common viral infection caused by the Epstein-Barr virus. Mononucleosis occurs most frequently in adolescents and young adults, although individuals of all ages can develop the infection. The infection is transmitted orally by direct contact with saliva; symptoms usually start 4 to 6 weeks after exposure to the virus. Because of the means of transmission, mononucleosis is commonly known as the "kissing disease." Symptoms include weakness and fatigue, fever, swollen lymph glands, and a severe sore throat. There is no specific treatment for mononucleosis. Symptoms usually resolve within several weeks, although more severe cases may last a month or two.

CHECKPOINTS

13-11 Are antibiotics an effective treatment against viral diseases?

13-12 What oral conditions are characteristic of the early stages of acquired immune deficiency syndrome?

13-13 The Occupational Safety and Health Administration requires employers to offer hepatitis B vaccines to employees whose jobs involve what kind of potential exposure?

13-14 What are some circumstances that can trigger a herpes outbreak?

The Immune System

The body has developed a number of defenses against the broad array of microorganisms that assault it on a daily basis. The most obvious defenses are mechanical, such as the skin. Healthy skin is a very effective barrier to illness, preventing bacteria, viruses, and other microorganisms from accessing the body. Other mechanical defenses include sneezing, coughing, vomiting, and diarrhea, which all expel microorganisms.

However, once a microorganism has gained access, the body's immune system kicks in to fight off infection and destroy invading organisms. The immune system is a complex series of defenses that act on different levels to identify invading organisms and waste and remove it. Elements of the immune system include fever, phagocytosis, inflammation, interferon, and natural killer cells.

■ **Phagocytosis**. Phagocytosis is the process in which white blood cells travel quickly to the site of an infection to remove waste and destroy foreign material.

- **Inflammation.** Inflammation is a local reaction designed to isolate and expel any foreign or irritating material in the body. Inflammation can be triggered by any foreign material, not just microorganisms. Splinters, cuts, burns, chemicals, and even excessive sun exposure can all cause inflammation. During the inflammatory reaction, blood flow to the area increases, and the region is flooded with white blood cells. The byproduct of inflammation is known as *purulent material* (or pus). It is a combination of dead white blood cells, pathogens, and destroyed cells. Inflammation results in local redness, swelling, pain, and warmth.
- **Natural killer cells.** Natural killer cells are a type of white blood cell that destroys abnormal body cells such as cancer cells.
- **Fever.** Fever is an increase in normal body temperature that stimulates the body's immune system and interferes with the ability of some microorganisms to multiply.
- **Interferon.** Interferon is produced within cells that have been invaded by viruses. It prevents nearby cells from producing more viruses.

Natural Immunity and Acquired Immunity

The above defenses are nonspecific, meaning that they are activated against an invader. The body also has specific defenses against particular invaders. This is the final line of defense against invading organisms. It is referred to generally as *immunity*.

There are two kinds of immunity: natural immunity and acquired immunity.

Natural Immunity

As the name suggests, natural immunity is inborn and inherited. Nonspecific defenses are part of the natural immune system. So is species immunity. Humans are born immune to certain illnesses that affect other animals, and vice versa. Natural immunity varies from individual to individual— some people seem never to get sick, while others catch every cold that crosses their paths. Natural immunity cannot be significantly manipulated, although adequate rest and a healthy diet will bolster natural immunity.

Acquired Immunity

Acquired immunity is immunity that is gained as a result of exposure to a specific virus or other pathogens. Acquired immunity is gained throughout life as a person is exposed to more and more pathogens. Acquired immunity depends on the manufacture of antibodies. These cells are produced in response to a specific pathogen once the body has identified it as dangerous. Forever afterward, they patrol the body, looking for that pathogen. If they encounter it, antibodies trigger an intense immune reaction that targets and destroys the pathogen before a dangerous infection can occur.

There are several types of acquired immunity:

- **Passive acquired immunity.** This occurs when antibodies from one person are transferred to another, conferring a short-lived immunity. The best example of this is the transfer of antibodies from a mother to her baby during breastfeeding. This kind of passive immunity lasts for about 6 months.
- **Naturally acquired immunity.** This occurs when a person contracts a disease; the body then identifies the invading organism and manufactures antibodies against it for future defense. From then on, the person is normally immune to the disease.
- **Artificial acquired immunity.** This occurs when a person is vaccinated against a disease, including both bacteria and viruses. Vaccines consist of tiny amounts of the antigen, which stimulate the body to produce antibodies. Some viral vaccines are live virus vaccines, meaning the person is injected with a tiny amount of the virus. These viruses have been treated to reduce their danger. Other vaccines are dead virus vaccines, meaning the vaccine contains only dead viruses.

CHECKPOINTS

13-15 Name the elements of the immune system.

13-16 How does fever act as a defense against microorganisms?

13-17 What are the two kinds of immunity?

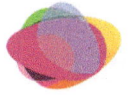

Chapter Highlights

- Microbiology is the study of microorganisms, including bacteria and viruses. Not all microorganisms are harmful to human health.
- The history of microbiology includes the development of microscopes, methods to achieve sterilization, linking bacteria to disease, and development of techniques to culture and kill microorganisms.
- Systemic infections occur throughout the body. Local infections are confined to a particular region of the body.

- Bacteria are rapidly dividing organisms that exist in staggering numbers, both inside and outside the body. Bacteria that require oxygen to thrive are aerobic. Bacteria that do not require oxygen are anaerobic.
- Bacteria are classified by their shape and arrangement as well as by their color when stained with dyes.
- Protozoa are single-celled organisms including amoebas, ciliates, flagellates, and sporozoa. Malaria is caused by a sporozoa.

◆ Fungi are plant-like organisms. Of the many kinds of fungi known, only a few are dangerous to humans.

◆ Viruses are very tiny organisms that consist of RNA or DNA wrapped in a protein coating. They cannot replicate themselves outside of a host cell. Viruses cannot be treated with antibiotics.

◆ Prions are smaller than even viruses; they are crystalline structures that grow in brain tissue and cause illness such as Creutzfeldt-Jakob disease.

◆ Antibiotic-resistant bacteria, such as methicillin-resistant *Staphylococcus aureus,* are posing a greater health threat as they become more common. Because of this, overuse of antibiotics is strongly discouraged.

◆ Infection control is essential to prevent bacterial and viral illnesses from spreading to dental care providers.

◆ Human immunodeficiency virus/acquired immune deficiency syndrome, hepatitis, and herpes are all viruses of concern to dental workers, who should be familiar with their symptoms and know how to prevent transmission.

◆ Vaccines consist of pieces of a live virus or dead virus that are administered to give immunity to a particular disease. Dental workers should be vaccinated against hepatitis B and receive annual flu vaccinations.

◆ The immune system involves a number of mechanical and natural barriers and processes designed to prevent illness.

◆ Acquired immunity is the result of being exposed to an illness after birth, or receiving antibodies from another person. Vaccines are a form of acquired immunity, as is the body's natural immunity to many diseases after recovering from them once. Natural immunity is inherited immunity against certain diseases.

 **Review Questions**

1. A disease acquired in a medical setting is known as a/an
   a. Health care professional infection.
   b. Nosocomial infection.
   c. Etiological infection.
   d. Health care–related illness.

2. Anton Van Leeuwenhoek is best known for what?
   a. Linking bacteria to specific diseases
   b. Discovering the human immunodeficiency virus
   c. Inventing the sterilization process
   d. Observing microorganisms in a drop of rainwater

3. The Koch postulates help determine if
   a. A bacteria is responsible for a particular disease.
   b. A bacteria is anaerobic or aerobic.
   c. A virus is responsible for a particular disease.
   d. None of the above.

4. What are pathogens?
   a. Another word for microorganisms
   b. Simple aquatic plants
   c. Microorganisms that cause disease
   d. Dead white blood cells

5. An etiologic agent does what?
   a. Prevents disease
   b. Identifies a disease-causing organism
   c. Causes disease
   d. Divides rapidly when exposed to heat

6. What is the function of an endospore?
   a. To multiply fungi
   b. To protect certain bacteria when exposed to stress
   c. To destroy viral material
   d. To spread protozoan illnesses

7. Acquired immunity can be obtained through
   a. Vaccination.
   b. Diet and exercise.
   c. Inheritance from mother's side of family.
   d. Hard work.

8. Gram-positive bacteria
   a. Are thin-walled organisms.
   b. Have no cell wall.
   c. Live underground.
   d. Are thick-walled organisms.

9. Staphylococci bacteria are what?
   a. Cigar-shaped clusters
   b. Round clusters
   c. Round chains
   d. Pairs of round bacteria

10. Which of the following diseases is caused by protozoa?
    a. Acquired immune deficiency syndrome
    b. Mumps
    c. Malaria
    d. Dysentery

11. What is a yeast?

    a. Clumping fungi

    b. Cluster of fuzzy bacteria

    c. Plant

    d. Fuzzy, multibranching fungi

12. Dental health care providers should be vaccinated against

    a. Influenza.

    b. Hepatitis B.

    c. Human immunodeficiency virus/acquired immune deficiency syndrome.

    d. A and B.

13. What is a viroid?

    a. Crystalline structure that grows in brain cells

    b. Superlarge virus

    c. Fragment of RNA with no protein coating

    d. Genetically engineered virus

14. Methicillin-resistant *Staphylococcus aureus* is dangerous because it

    a. Is fast replicating.

    b. Survives for long periods outside the human body.

    c. Is transmitted through mosquitoes.

    d. Is resistant to most common antibiotics.

Active Learning Exercises

1. Identify the three major shapes of bacteria and draw a picture of them. List two types of illness or disease associated with each of the three shapes and their corresponding treatments, if any. What precautions should the dental team take to avoid transmission?

2. List five diseases caused by viruses. Research the Center for Disease Control and Prevention (www.cdc.gov) website and identify any available vaccinations for the diseases. Do these diseases require boosters or is revaccination necessary after a certain period of time?

3. Which fungus manifests on the oral mucosa and often the tongue? What two names are given to the condition associated with this fungus? What classification of drugs may be used to treat this condition?

Application Activities

1. Visit the Centers for Disease Control and Prevention (CDC) website (www.cdc.gov) and do additional research on one of the viruses discussed in the chapter. Review the material available from the CDC, focusing on methods for preventing transmission of the disease. Make a list of five things you could do in the dental office to minimize the risk of transmission. Be prepared to discuss your findings in class.

PREPARING FOR CERTIFICATION EXAMS

Review the following topics in this chapter to prepare for the Dental Assisting National Board (DANB) exam:

- **Protozoa**

- **Fungi**

- **Viruses**

- **Prions and Other Infectious Microorganisms**

- **Important Bacterial Diseases**

chapter 14

Disease and Infection Control

CHAPTER OUTLINE

CHAPTER CHECKLIST

On completion of this chapter, students will be able to:

- ☑ Explain the steps in the chain of infection and the points at which the chain of infection can be broken.
- ☑ Identify the types of infections that can occur and the agents that cause infection.
- ☑ Describe the various infection control techniques used in a dental office.
- ☑ Describe the steps involved in proper handwashing.
- ☑ Describe the various types of personal protective equipment commonly used in a dental office and when they should be used.
- ☑ Identify the disinfectants commonly used in a dental office.
- ☑ Explain the purpose and use of the ultrasonic cleaner.
- ☑ Identify the various dental instruments that require sterilization.
- ☑ Describe the procedures involved in maintaining the dental waterline.

KEY TERMS

anaphylaxis (an-uh-fih-LAK-sis) – an immediate, transient immunologic (allergic) reaction characterized by contraction of smooth muscle and dilation of capillaries due to release of pharmacologically active substances (histamine, bradykinin, serotonin), classically induced by the combination of antigen (allergen) and antibody

biofilm – thin coating of microorganisms that forms on a body surface, especially the surface of a tooth

Bloodborne Pathogen Standard – Occupational Safety and Health Administration regulation for reducing the risk of transfer of disease-producing microorganisms transmitted by means of blood, tissue, and body fluids

cavitation (ka-vih-TAY-shun) – the production by ultrasound of small, vapor-containing bubbles in a liquid

chain of infection – the required set of conditions for an infectious microorganism to transfer from one host to another host

colony-forming unit (CFU) – the measure of unit used to gauge water safety; colony-forming units are made up of coliform bacteria, which at high enough concentrations can cause illness

contact dermatitis (der-muh-TIE-tis) – inflammatory rash marked by itching and redness resulting from cutaneous contact with a specific allergen (allergic-contact dermatitis) or irritant (irritant-contact dermatitis)

disinfectant – an agent capable of destroying pathogenic microorganisms or inhibiting their growth

disinfection – destruction of pathogenic microorganisms or their toxins or vectors by direct exposure to chemical or physical agents

fomites (FOH-mie-teez) – objects such as clothing, towels, and utensils that may harbor a disease agent and are capable of transmitting it

fungicide (FUN-juh-side) – agent that destroys fungus

Hazard Communication Standard – Occupational Safety and Health Administration regulation concerned with alerting workers about exposure to possibly dangerous chemicals in the workplace

portal of entry – the point at which a pathogen enters the body and gains access to susceptible tissues, where it may cause disease or infection

portal of exit – the means by which a pathogen exits the reservoir and may gain access to a new host

reservoir – living or nonliving material in or on which an infectious agent multiplies and develops and is dependent on for its survival in nature

sharp – any medical/dental instrument or any disposable material that is sharp or may produce sharp pieces; should be disposed of in a biohazard container

sporicide (SPOR-uh-side) – any agent that kills bacterial spores

standard precautions – current guidelines for prevention of infectious diseases and nosocomial infections as established by the Centers for Disease Control and Prevention; these precautions state that health care workers should avoid contact with all bodily fluids, including saliva and blood, regardless of a patient's diagnosis or possible infectious status

sterile – the condition of being aseptic, or free from all living microorganisms and their spores

sterilization – the destruction of all microorganisms in or about an object

universal precautions – a set of procedural directives and guidelines to prevent parenteral, mucous membranes, and nonintact skin exposures of health care workers to bloodborne pathogens; this term has generally been replaced by the term *standard precautions*

virucide (VIE-ruh-side) – an agent active against virus infections

virulence (VIR-yuh-lunz) – the disease-evoking power of a pathogen

Introduction

Infection control is a vital part of a successful dental practice. Every member of the dental team is required to use infection control procedures—a single break in the defense against infection can result in the transmission of disease.

Infection control procedures are designed for both the safety of the patient as well as the safety of the people who work with patients, including dental assistants (DAs), dental hygienists, and dentists. Infections can be transmitted a number of ways, including by direct and indirect contact with pathogens. Some types of microbes can survive on surfaces, and some are resistant to simple cleaning solutions.

Infection control begins before the patient enters the office, by maintaining a hygienic work environment, and ends after the patient leaves, with the safe disposal of medical waste.

From Classroom to Clinic

Highly contagious matter, such as bacteria and viruses, can spread very easily. The dental assistant can help prevent cross-contamination in the office with safe hygiene practices and careful disinfecting. Your knowledge of infection control will ensure your safety and that of the rest of your team.

This chapter also covers the requirements of government agencies and industry groups that regulate infection control, including the Occupational Safety and Health Administration (OSHA), the Centers for Disease Control and Prevention (CDC), and the American Dental Association (ADA).

Transmission of Disease

Effective infection control is aimed at preventing the transmission of disease. Unlike past ages, when diseases were thought to ride on vapors and fogs, the transmission of disease is well understood today. The method by which a disease moves from one host to another is referred to as the **chain of infection.**

The Chain of Infection

The chain of infection describes the steps that a microbe takes as it travels from one host to another spreading infection (Figure 14-1). People are not infected with every microbe they are exposed to—if that was the case, humans would likely be extinct. Instead, a number of conditions must be present for a microbe to successfully move from one host to another. The idea behind infection control is to break this chain somewhere along the path, so even if dangerous microbes are present,

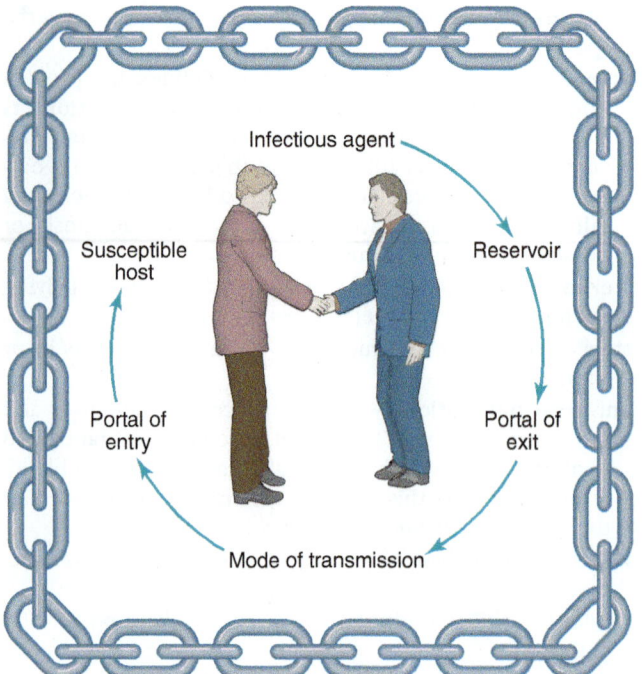

Figure 14–1 Chain of infection. The six components of the infectious disease process are shown.

they cannot infect anybody. The elements of the chain of infection include:

- Infectious agent
- Reservoir
- Portal of exit
- Mode of transmission
- Portal of entry
- Susceptible host

Infectious Agent

An infectious agent must be present for infection to occur. In addition to the microbes covered in Chapter 13, Understanding Microbiology, infectious agents can also include chemical or physical agents. Chemical agents include pesticides, cleaning agents, and industrial chemicals. Physical agents include heat, radiation, noise, and light. In a dental practice, however, the term *infection control* is always associated with control of biological agents such as bacteria and viruses.

Infectious agents must be present in sufficient numbers to accomplish infection. A single virus or a few dozen bacteria are unlikely to successfully infect a new host (although it is certainly possible). Infection can only be accomplished when the infectious agent overwhelms the target host's defense mechanisms.

Reservoir

A **reservoir** is best described as a hospitable environment for an infectious agent to thrive and multiply. The most common reservoirs for biological infectious agents are other people. An example would be a patient infected with an influenza virus: The patient provides a hospitable reservoir where the influenza virus can replicate itself and thrive between transmissions. It is important to note that people can carry infectious agents with no symptoms or visible signs of infection. Some people can even carry the human immunodeficiency virus (HIV) virus with no signs of infection or symptoms of illness. These people can still transmit the disease.

Different biological infectious agents have different reservoir requirements. For example, many bacteria can thrive outside the human body. Some viruses can survive outside a host organism, whereas others will quickly die once exposed to the environment. Similarly, some viruses can be transmitted by animal reservoirs, whether or not they actually infect those animals.

An object that is contaminated with an infectious agent is called a **fomite**. An example of a fomite is an x-ray positioning device that is contaminated with virus-containing saliva. In this case, the fomite is a less-than-ideal environment, but as long as the virus can survive long enough for transmission, it is an effective reservoir.

Portal of Exit

The **portal of exit** is how the infectious agent leaves the reservoir and travels to a new host. A portal of exit is not necessarily a literal exit such as a nostril. A portal of exit might be the sputum or mucus in which the viral agent travels after the patient sneezes. Portals of exit include sputum, mucus, blood, saliva, vaginal or penile discharges, urine, purulent material and secretions, feces, or any other means of transportation for an infectious agent. In some cases, eye fluids and breast milk may also be portals of exit.

Mode of Transmission

The mode of transmission is the actual method by which the infectious agent moves from the portal of exit to the new host (through the portal of entry; see the next section). Depending on the agent, infectious agents can be transmitted by one, or several, of the following modes of transmission in the dental office:

- *Direct transmission*. Direct transmission occurs through person-to-person contact. An example would be transmission of a virus through touching a person's infected blood, saliva, or mucus. Sexually transmitted diseases are transmitted through direct means, as are colds and influenza.
- *Indirect transmission*. Indirect transmission, or cross-contamination, occurs when the infectious agent is transferred to a second surface and then transmitted from there to a new host. An example is

contaminated saliva droplets moving from a patient's oral cavity to a dental film and from the dental film to a DA. Handwashing is an excellent prevention method for indirect transmission, because infectious agents are often transmitted on objects that are physically handled.

- *Airborne transmission.* Airborne transmission describes the transmission of an infectious agent that is airborne in droplet, spray, spatter, or aerosol form. Many kinds of infectious organisms are present in the saliva and mucous secretions of an infected person. When such a person sneezes or coughs, the infectious agent may be forcefully ejected into the air in a fine spray (which has prompted CDC recommendations of sneezing into the crook of the arm). Aerosols can also be created by the handpiece and the ultrasonic scaler as well as the air and water syringe. Depending on the size of the droplets, the agent might remain suspended in the air; smaller droplets can remain suspended for an indefinite period of time. The most common organisms transmitted by aerosol include bacteria. The best defense against airborne transmission is an intact physical barrier, such as a face mask or intact, healthy skin.
- *Parenteral transmission.* Parenteral transmission occurs when an infectious agent is spread through breaks in the skin. These are typically caused by needle-stick injuries, cuts, abrasions, bites, and scrapes. Blood-borne agents, such as hepatitis and HIV, can be spread in this way.

There are additional modes of transmission, such as food or water transmission or transmission through third-party vectors such as mosquitoes, but these are rarely an issue in a dental practice.

Portal of Entry

The **portal of entry** is the means of entry into the body. The body is equipped with a number of barriers to keep infectious pathogens out. The skin is the largest of these. Healthy, intact skin is an excellent physical barrier. Other defense mechanisms include sneezing and coughing, vomiting, and diarrhea, all of which are designed to expel organisms before they can cause an infection.

The most common portals of entry include:

- Oral and nasal cavities, which lead to the respiratory tract and gastrointestinal system;
- Genitourinary tract, which is a common portal of entry for sexually transmitted diseases;
- Circulatory system, which can be accessed through cuts, scrapes, and needlesticks; and
- Placental system, which allows mothers to pass infectious organisms to their fetuses.

Susceptible Host

The final step in the chain of infection is the presence of a susceptible host. A susceptible host is any organism that can provide a suitable environment for an infectious agent to thrive. In this case, the term is used to describe people, both patients and employees, who might become infected and ill.

Not all infectious organisms have the same capacity for infection. The measure of an infectious agent's power to infect is known as **virulence**. Some organisms, such as the common cold, are very easily transmitted from host to host. They readily overcome barriers and easily colonize new hosts. They can be spread through a number of modes of transmission. Other infectious agents are less virulent and cannot infect a host as easily.

Just as not all infectious organisms are equal, not all hosts are equally vulnerable to infection. A number of factors affect the potential for infection. A host who is easily infected is called a *compromised host.* An example of a compromised host is someone whose immune system has been reduced by chemotherapy treatments for cancer.

Other factors that affect susceptibility include:

- Immunization/vaccination status—full immunization protects against many diseases.
- Disease status—the presence of additional diseases can weaken one's immunity; acquired immune deficiency syndrome (AIDS)/HIV specifically targets the immune system and increases chances of opportunistic infection.
- Age—older and younger patients may have reduced immune function.
- Lifestyle factors—factors such as extreme stress, exhaustion, malnourishment, drug and alcohol addiction, and risk practices such as sharing needles all increase susceptibility.
- Occupation—people who work in occupations with high exposure to infectious agents, such as hospital workers, or those who work in industrial settings with a high burden of toxic exposure, may have decreased immunity.
- Heredity—susceptibility is inherited to some degree, with some people seemingly more vulnerable to infection.

Breaking the Chain of Infection

For a pathogen or infectious agent to successfully move from one host to another, each link in the chain of infection must be intact. A disruption at any point impedes the process of causing a new infection. Thus, the purpose of infection control is to erect barriers that cause disruptions in the transfer of infectious agents. This can occur at any of the following points:

1. *Infectious agent and reservoir reduction.* The key to infection is often the number of infectious agents that are present. As stated earlier, it is unlikely that a few dozen bacteria or a single virus can successfully colonize a new host. Although it is impossible to eliminate infectious organisms outside of a completely sterile environment, infection control techniques aim to dramatically reduce the number of organisms present in the environment, thus reducing the odds of indirect transmission. Methods to accomplish this include disinfection, sterilization, and thorough cleaning of surfaces that have come into contact with potentially infectious agents. Specific techniques for each of these methods will be covered later in this chapter.

   Another obvious method is to remove the reservoir from the area. In the dental office, this means canceling appointments for patients who are obviously ill or a DA who is ill staying home from work. In medical terms, this is known as *isolation*. In practical terms, it is common courtesy not to potentially infect patients or other employees.

2. *Portal of exit and mode of transmission.* To successfully cause an infection, an infectious agent must leave the reservoir and travel to a new host. This process can be disrupted by many of the same techniques used to reduce the number of infectious agents and prevent the formation of reservoirs. Sterilization, cleansing, and disinfection of all possible surfaces that might carry infectious agents will reduce the ease of transportation. Additionally, open wounds should be dressed and clean, and DAs and employees should be protected from aerosol droplets with face masks. All surfaces that have come into contact with potentially infectious organisms should be carefully cleaned.

3. *Portal of entry and host.* Once again, many of the same methods used to deny an infectious agent a mode of transmission can be used to deny the agent a portal of entry. Exposed skin should be intact and healthy, and DAs and employees should always wear face masks and gloves when they are working directly with patients. Aerosol droplets are often invisible and can linger, so the mere absence of visible splatter should not be taken as reassurance that no infectious organisms are present. Similarly, DAs should follow a diligent handwashing protocol, washing their hands before and after contact with patients or any device or item that has come into direct contact with the patient. Some means of denying a portal of entry include wearing examination gloves, masks, gowns, and safety glasses.

   Finally, the chain of infection can be broken between the infectious agent and the host. Proper nutrition, adequate rest and exercise, and current immunizations can all help to prevent infection, even if an infectious agent does gain entry.

Types of Infection

An infection occurs when disease-causing organisms, known as *pathogens*, cause illness. Infections can be local infections, meaning they are confined to a single area or region of the body, or they can be systemic infections, meaning they are present throughout the body. Skin infections are common local infections. Systemic infections include most viruses and some dangerous bacterial infections.

A number of organisms can cause infection:

- Bacteria
- Viruses
- Protozoa
- Fungi
- Prions

These infectious agents are covered in greater detail in Chapter 13, Understanding Microbiology.

CHECKPOINTS

14-1 What are the steps in the chain of infection?

14-2 What is a fomite?

14-3 What are the modes of transmission?

14-4 Give examples of a portal of entry?

14-5 What's the difference between a systemic infection and a local infection?

Prevention of Disease Transmission

Disease prevention is a major focus in modern dentistry. Infection control techniques have advanced rapidly over the past few decades, and, today, all DAs must be thoroughly acquainted with the regulatory and professional bodies that govern infection control as well as the regulations and recommendations that constitute effective infection control.

Regulations are created by government agencies and carry the weight of law. They must be followed, and there is usually an inspection and enforcement mechanism in place to make sure dental offices are compliant. When new regulations are introduced, there is usually an adoption period so offices can bring themselves in line with the new code.

Recommendations are made by industry organizations or government agencies and are not mandatory.

The main organizations that are active in infection control in dental offices include:

- ADA
- CDC
- OSHA
- U.S. Food and Drug Administration (FDA)
- Environmental Protection Agency (EPA)

Each of these is discussed at greater length in the following sections.

Infection Control Practices

Infection control is a routine part of all modern dental practices. According to the principle of **universal precautions**, all patients are treated as if they are potentially infectious. This means that all blood is treated as if it is harboring HIV, hepatitis, or other infectious organisms. Universal precautions are valuable for two reasons. The first is that it is often impossible to tell by sight alone if a patient is potentially infected—and not all patients always give accurate information in their medical histories. The second is it prevents legal complications that might occur if dental offices were to discriminate between one class of patients as potentially infectious and another as "safer."

The universal precautions standard has been expanded to an approach known as **standard precautions**. According to standard precautions, all bodily fluids, including saliva and blood, should be treated as reservoirs for infectious agents. In practical terms, there is no difference in the dental office between universal and standard precautions because dental offices have always treated saliva and other bodily excretions as if they harbored infectious organisms.

CDC Guidelines for Dental Practices

The CDC is a federal public health agency that falls under the umbrella of the Public Health Service, within the U.S. Department of Health and Human Services. The CDC is responsible for many of the recommendations and guidelines that govern modern infection control, including the standard precautions that are used by every dental practice.

In 2003, the CDC released the *CDC Guidelines for Infection Control in Dental Healthcare Settings—2003*. The document is available from the CDC and can be accessed at www.cdc.gov/mmwr/PDF/rr/rr5217.pdf, or by calling 770-488-6054. The CDC updated the standard precautions in 2007, and the following year they updated disinfection and sterilization procedures in health care facilities. These comprehensive guidelines cover a wide range of infection control practices at dental offices.

CDC Guidelines for Infection Control in Dental Healthcare Settings

- Use of standard precautions rather than universal precautions
- Work restrictions for healthcare personnel infected with or occupationally exposed to infectious diseases
- Management of occupational exposures to blood-borne pathogens, including postexposure protection for work exposures to hepatitis B virus, hepatitis C virus, and human immunodeficiency virus
- Selection and use of devices with features designed to prevent sharps injury
- Use of hand-hygiene products and surgical hand antisepsis
- Prevention of contact dermatitis and latex hypersensitivity
- Sterilization of unwrapped instruments
- Ensuring quality of dental water
- Infection control during dental radiology
- Aseptic techniques for parenteral medications
- Preprocedural mouth rinsing for patients
- Infection control during oral surgical procedures
- Infection control when using laser/electrosurgery plumes
- Prevention of transmission of tuberculosis
- Prevention of transmission of Creutzfeldt-Jakob disease and other prion-related diseases
- Infection control program evaluation
- Research considerations

Source: *CDC Guidelines for Infection Control in Dental Healthcare Settings—2003*

The CDC guidelines represent the standard of care of dental practice infection control. The following sections are based on CDC recommendations. The CDC divides its recommendations into categories based on the scientific evidence supporting the recommendation. Categories include:

- *Category IA*: Strongly recommended for implementation and strongly supported by well-designed experimental, clinical, or epidemiological studies.
- *Category IB*: Strongly recommended for implementation and supported by experimental, clinical, or epidemiologic studies and a strong theoretical rationale.
- *Category IC*: Required for implementation as mandated by federal or state regulation or standard. When IC is used, a second rating can be included to provide the basis of existing scientific data, theoretical rationale, and applicability. Because of state differences, an absence of an IC rating does not necessarily mean state regulations do not exist.
- *Category II*: Suggested for implementation and supported by suggestive clinical or epidemiologic studies or a theoretical rationale.

Handwashing and Hand Hygiene

Handwashing is one of the most basic, yet most effective, forms of infection control. The hands provide an excellent mode of transportation for infectious agents, representing a danger for both patients and dental professionals. See the box on this page for the CDC's general considerations on hand hygiene.

There is good reason for continual handwashing. Hands should be washed before gloves are put on because the gloves can have tiny rips or tears. They should then be washed after gloves are removed in case the skin was contaminated, either through a torn glove or during the act of glove removal itself.

Handwashing should also be performed after any bare-handed contact with a potentially contaminated surface, including fixed surfaces, such as tables or x-ray units, and mobile surfaces, such as trays, cups, handpieces, and instruments.

Handwashing should include liquid soap. Bar soaps, which are frequently kept wet or in small pools of water, may be contaminated with bacteria, which tend to multiply rapidly in wet, warm, and dark environments.

As a final note, frequent handwashing can lead to dry skin and other problems. To prevent this, DAs should use moisturizing lotions (that are free from petroleum products if latex gloves are worn) to keep their skin moistened, and their hands should always be thoroughly dried after handwashing and before insertion into treatment gloves.

For a description of the best handwashing technique, see Procedure 14-1, Handwashing.

Alcohol-Based Hand Rubs

Alcohol-based hand rubs are a relatively new product (Figure 14-2). These products are typically dispensed as gels. They are waterless and do not require access to water. To use them, a small amount is squirted on the skin, and then rubbed thoroughly over the hands. The hands should be air dried, not dried with a paper towel. The alcohol in the product kills infectious organisms and then quickly evaporates.

Alcohol-based rubs have become popular in the medical professions because they are effective. Some of the products also contain moisturizers that help protect against dry skin.

It is important to note, however, that alcohol-based rubs are dose dependent, meaning they must be used according to the manufacturer's instructions to be effective. Additionally, they are not a substitute for proper handwashing. Alcohol-based rubs are best used in conjunction with a comprehensive handwashing program.

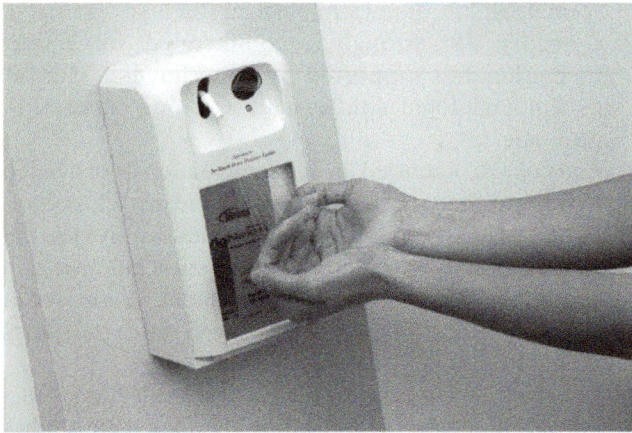

Figure 14–2 Alcohol-based hand rubs. This waterless gel kills infectious organisms and then quickly evaporates.

CDC Guidelines on Hand Hygiene

General Considerations

1. Hands should be washed with either a nonantimicrobial or antimicrobial soap and water when hands are visibly dirty or contaminated with blood or other potentially infectious material. If hands are not visibly soiled, an alcohol-based hand rub can also be used. Follow the manufacturer's instructions with both soaps and alcohol-based hand rubs, including washing the hands for the appropriate time, usually 2 to 6 minutes for most soaps. (Recommendation level: IA)
2. Hands should be washed:
   a. When they are visibly soiled. (Recommendation level: IA, IC)
   b. After barehanded touching of inanimate objects likely to be contaminated by blood, saliva, or respiratory secretions. (Recommendation level: IA, IC)
   c. Before and after treating each patient. (Recommendation level: IB)
   d. Immediately after removing gloves. (Recommendation level: IB, IC)
3. Surgical hand cleaning should be performed before donning sterile surgical gloves for oral surgical procedures. (Recommendation level: IB)
4. Liquid hand-care products should be stored in either disposable closed containers or closed containers that can be washed and dried before refilling. (Recommendation level: IA).

Special Considerations

1. Hand lotions can be used to prevent skin dryness associated with frequent handwashing. (Recommendation level: IA)
2. Avoid products that might damage latex gloves, including ingredients in lotions and other antiseptic products, as well as petroleum-based or other oil moisturizers. (Recommendation level: IB)
3. Keep fingernails short, with smooth, filed edges to make cleaning easier and prevent tears to gloves. (Recommendation level: II)
4. Do not wear artificial nails or extenders. (Recommendation level: IB)
5. Do not wear hand or nail jewelry if it makes wearing gloves more difficult or threatens to damage the gloves. (Recommendation level: II)

Procedure 14–1 Handwashing

Materials needed:

- Sink with running water
- Liquid soap
- Disposable paper towels

1. Remove jewelry, rings, watches, and any other adornments. Ideally, nails should be neatly trimmed, and acrylics should not be worn. These accessories provide a place for bacteria to harbor (i.e., a reservoir).

2. Turn on water, either using a foot control, an automatic, motion-activated valve, or by holding a paper towel or using an elbow to touch the faucet (Figure P14-1-1). It is best to avoid skin-to-metal contact with the faucet, because it may be contaminated.

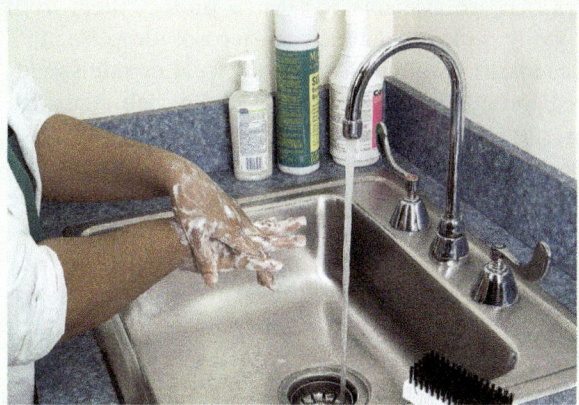

Figure P14-1-3

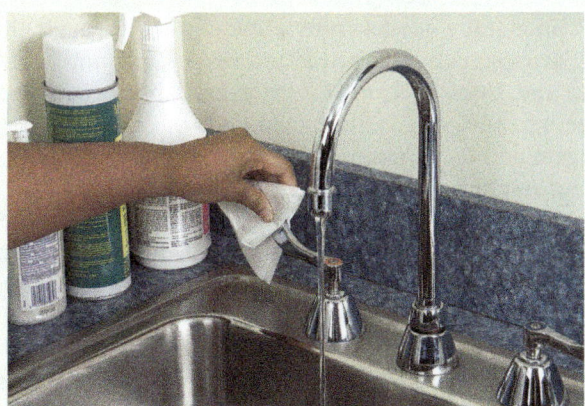

Figure P14-1-1

3. Apply soap and lather. Use a generous amount of soap and lather the hands completely (Figure P14-1-2). Make sure to wash in a downward motion, washing between fingers and thumb as well as upper and lower sides of each hand (Figure P14-1-3). When washing, make a cup with one hand to scrub under the nails, then repeat on the other hand, making sure to clean under every fingernail.

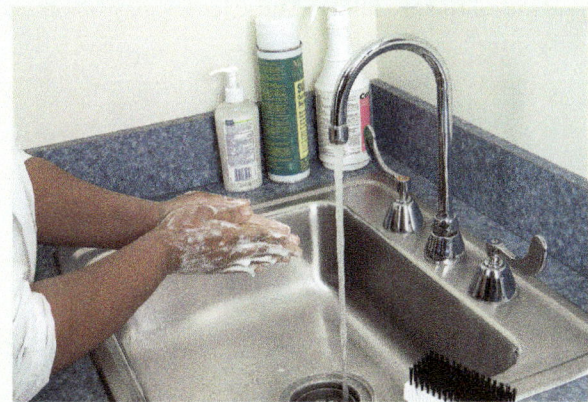

Figure P14-1-2

4. Rinse under running water (Figure P14-1-4). Rub hands vigorously under water to make sure all soap and debris are removed.

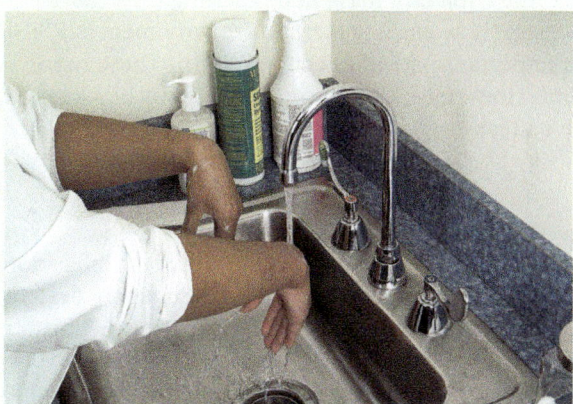

Figure P14-1-4

5. Repeat steps 3 and 4. The first washing serves to remove the surface debris, whereas the second removes tenacious microorganisms. Rinse with cool water to close the pores.

6. Dry hands with a paper towel (Figure P14-1-5). Do not use a linen towel or any other reusable cloth. These cloths can stay moist and warm and provide a perfect breeding ground for bacteria. When drying, dry the hands first, followed by the wrists.

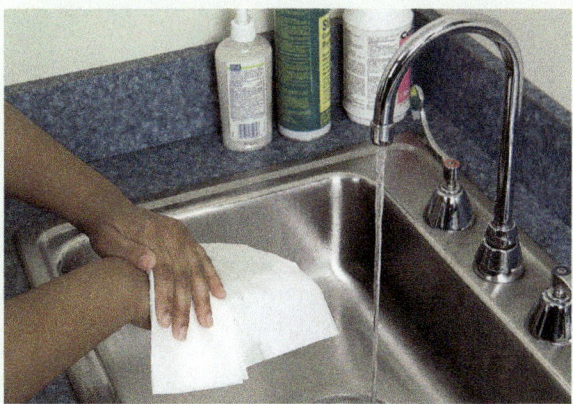

Figure P14-1-5

7. Use a paper towel to turn off the faucet and another clean paper towel to clean the sink and counter.

Personal Protective Equipment

Personal protective equipment (PPE) includes the many barriers that are available to DAs to protect them from saliva, body fluids, splatter, and aerosol droplets. PPE includes masks, respirators, safety eyewear or side shields on eyeglasses, face masks, surgical gowns, lab coats, lab aprons, surgical hats, gloves, and closed shoes (to protect against dropped sharp or hot instruments or objects).

According to OSHA regulations, employers must provide a basic level of PPE to protect health care providers. However, the exact combinations of protective barriers used depend on the situation. Use of high-speed handpieces, for example, creates a potentially contaminated aerosol that can linger in the air. In this case, DAs would want to make sure their faces are totally covered. By contrast, taking a medical history is a much less risky situation, and it may be safe to forgo a full face mask in this setting.

No matter how clean or sterile an environment is, PPE is still an important part of infection control. These barriers deny infectious organisms a portal to entry by blocking off sensitive areas such as the nasal passages, eyes, and oral cavity.

Masks

Masks cover the nose and oral cavity to prevent inhalation of droplets and splatter (Figure 14-3). Common devices that create potentially contaminated aerosol or splatter include the dental handpiece, ultrasonic scaler, and air-water syringe. Even with proper use of the high-volume evacuator, splatter can still occur.

Masks should *never* be reused from patient to patient. A new mask should be used with *every* patient. Masks should be put into place before the DA's final handwashing and donning safety eyewear and gloves.

Masks are available in two basic styles: flat and domed. Both are held in place with elastic loops or cloth ties that go around the ears or head and secure the mask to the face. The mask should be a snug fit—there should be no room

for any tiny drops to slide between the mask and the skin. Some masks might have a thin, flexible piece of metal over the bridge of the nose that, when pinched, causes the mask to fit tightly into place.

After a procedure, the mask should be removed by hooking fingers into the tie or elastic bands and removing the mask. Avoid touching the front of a potentially contaminated mask. Masks should never be worn dangling around the neck or ear. Used masks should be discarded immediately after the procedure is over and must never be placed on countertops or anywhere else except for trash receptacles.

Protective Eyewear

Protective eyewear includes goggles and glasses or side shields on eyeglasses (Figure 14-4A) that are designed to block infectious agents from gaining entry through the eyes. Viruses, such as hepatitis and herpes, can potentially infect the eyes, as can *Staphylococcus* bacteria. Other dangers to the eyes include flying bits of debris, such as amalgam and tooth fragments, and caustic chemicals. Eye damage might be irreversible.

Protective eyewear is not the same as corrective lenses or contact lenses. Dental care providers who wear corrective lenses or contact lenses should still wear protective eyewear when appropriate. According to the CDC, protective eyewear should include side, top, and bottom protection. Larger eye protection devices are available to fit over corrective lenses.

Dental offices also need to provide eye protection to patients during procedures that might cause splatter. This eyewear should be treated the same as eyewear provided to the dental staff. According to the CDC, eyewear should be cleaned with soap and water, or if visibly soiled, it should be cleaned and disinfected between patients.

An additional kind of eyewear is available to protect the eyes from potentially damaging light sources such as the lasers used to cure fillings. These lenses may be orange

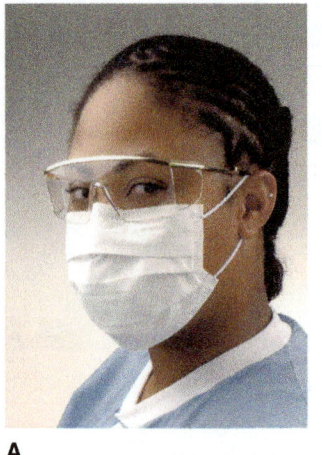
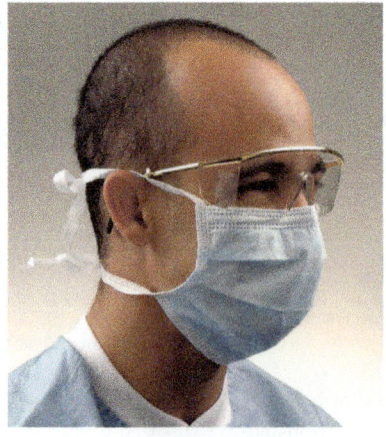
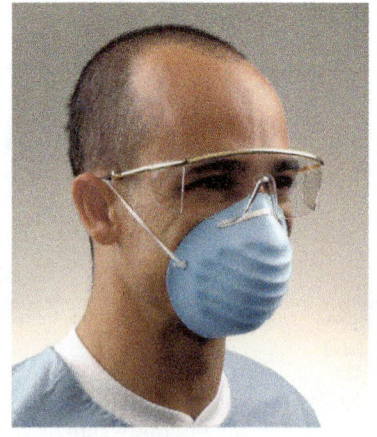

| A | B | C |

Figure 14-3 **Masks.** **(A)** Earloop style. **(B)** Surgical tie-on style. **(C)** Molded cup style.

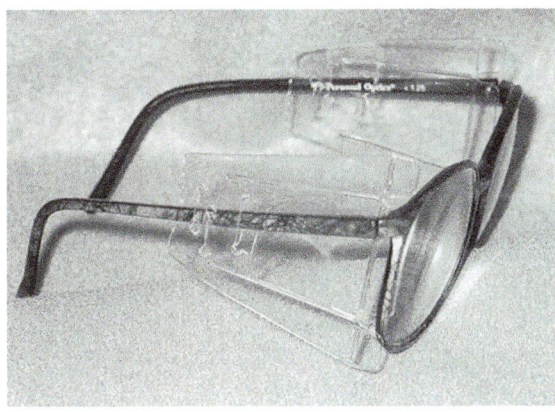

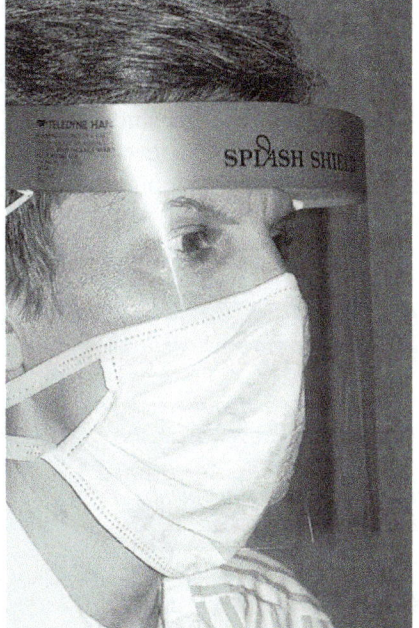

Figure 14–4 Protective eyewear. (A) Glasses with side shields. **(B)** Face shield worn over separate mask.

A   B

colored and will protect against damage to sensitive eye tissues during curing and bonding.

Protective eyewear should be put on after masks but before handwashing and donning examination gloves.

Face Shields

A face shield is a device that looks somewhat like a tennis visor with a clear plastic shield extending from the top down to the chin or neck (see Figure 14-4B). These physical barriers are designed to keep splatter and debris away from the entire face.

Face shields can be highly effective at blocking debris but, by themselves, do not protect from inhalation or aerosol. Thus, face shields often work in conjunction with face masks (in fact, some face shields are attached to masks) in situations in which aerosol is a concern.

Face shields should be put on before the final handwashing and gloving.

Protective Clothing

Protective clothing includes the many forms of clothing that are worn to protect dental workers from splatter, blood, saliva, sharps, and other hazards they might come into contact with. Items of protective clothing include gowns, uniforms, lab coats, jackets, pants, scrubs, surgical hats, and surgical shoe covers (Figure 14-5). According to OSHA, an employer has to provide protective clothing to employees.

The particular items of protective clothing to be worn with each patient depend on the nature of the visit. Oral surgery, for example, requires more protective clothing than does taking a routine radiograph series because of the increased likelihood of coming into contact with blood, saliva, and other body fluids. Protective clothing should:

- Be resistant to fluids. This includes most modern fabrics, such as cotton, polyester blends, and other fabrics.
- Provide full coverage. This means long sleeves, full pant legs, and high necks.

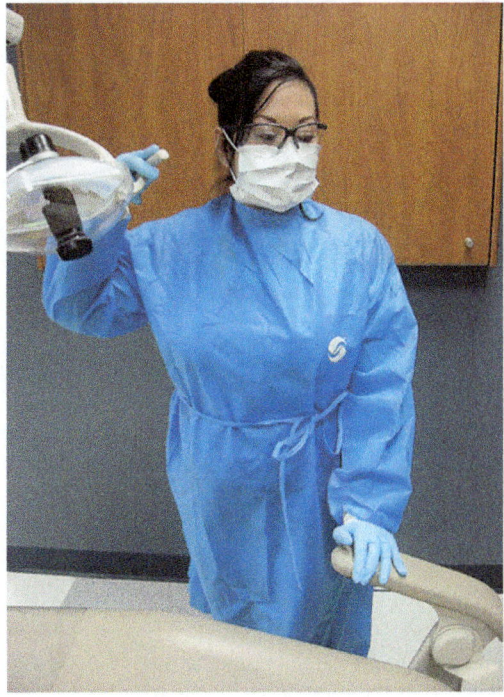

Figure 14–5 Protective clothing, including gown, gloves, mask, and eyewear.

- Be free from potential points of entry or reservoirs, such as zippers, buttons, pockets, and other adornments.
- Be tucked under protective gloves.

Protective clothing should be worn only in the office and not worn between patient appointments. DAs should never wear their lab coats or treatment gowns when stepping outside the office, going to lunch, or running errands.

Finally, a note on laundering PPE: Employees are prohibited from taking designated PPE home to launder. These items must be laundered by the employer. Most dental offices have a service that specializes in medical laundry that will pick up the items to be laundered, or they must be washed in the office using proper protocol.

Procedure 14-2 **Putting On Personal Protective Equipment**

Protective clothing should be put on before handwashing and gloving. The exact items to be worn depend on the procedure, but it is always better to be overprotected rather than underprotected. The following procedure covers putting on protective clothing, face and eye protection, and gloves.

Materials needed:

- Appropriate protective clothing
- Surgical mask
- Protective eyewear
- Handwashing station
- Gloves

1. Put on appropriate protective clothing (lab coat, treatment gown, lab gown, lab apron, or clinical jacket). Protective clothing should be worn over street clothes (Figure P14-2-1).

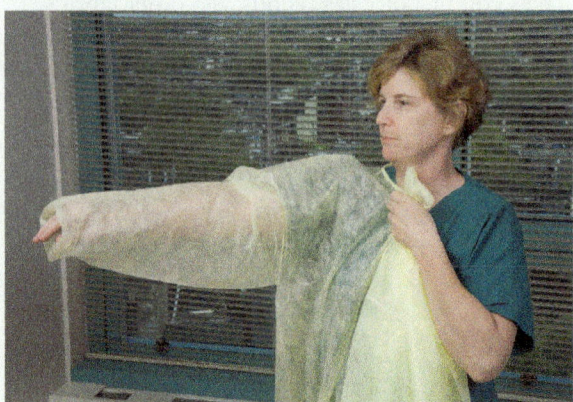

Figure P14-2-1

2. Put on mask by looping both elastic bands over your ears or tying the cloth ties behind your head and fitting the mask snugly to your face. If the mask includes a piece of metal at the nose, lightly pinch the bridge of your nose so the mask conforms to your nose. The mask should not be loose or hanging (Figure P14-2-2).

3. Put on protective eyewear (Figure P14-2-3).

4. Wash hands. Remember to thoroughly rinse and dry hands to reduce contact dermatitis.

5. Pull on gloves one at a time. Hold gloves at the cuff to pull them on. Be careful not to compromise the integrity of the glove by breaking or tearing the material. Gloves should always be put on last in the sequence of applying PPE (Figure P14-2-4).

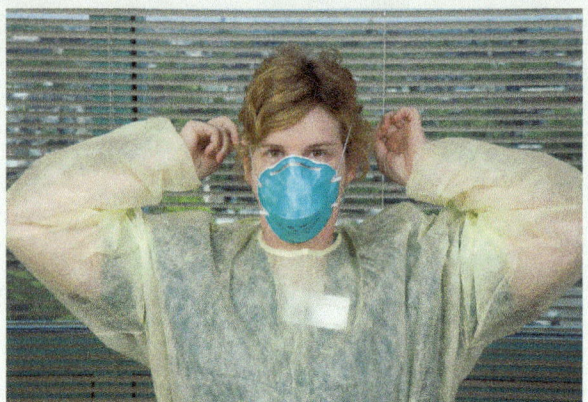

Figure P14-2-2

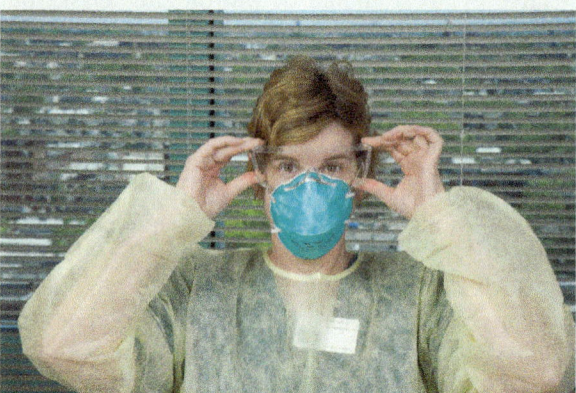

Figure P14-2-3

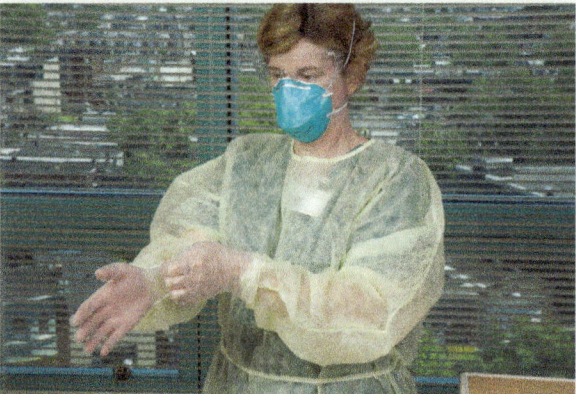

Figure P14-2-4

Gloves

Gloves are a basic and critical part of infection control (Figure 14-6). They provide an effective barrier against infectious agents and prevent the indirect spread of infectious agents when used properly. Gloves should be worn any time there is a chance of contact with a potentially infected surface or substance, including blood; saliva; tools; surfaces; and supplies, such as paper cups and trays.

A variety of gloves are used in dental offices, including *examination gloves* (nonsterile) and *surgical gloves* (sterile). These two types of gloves are regulated by the FDA and must meet certain standards for use. Other types of gloves include overgloves, utility gloves, cotton gloves for sensitive skin protection under gloves, heat-resistant gloves, and others.

Examination gloves are the most common gloves worn by DAs. These gloves are typically available in a range of sizes from small to extra large, and they are designed to fit either hand. Examination gloves are not sterile; they are designed as a protective physical barrier between the patient and the DA. Because of the issue of latex allergies, examination gloves are available in both latex and nonlatex (vinyl). For more information on latex allergies, see the box, Latex Allergies.

Among people who are not latex sensitive, latex gloves are generally favored. Many dental office employees feel they fit better, and they provide better tactile sensation

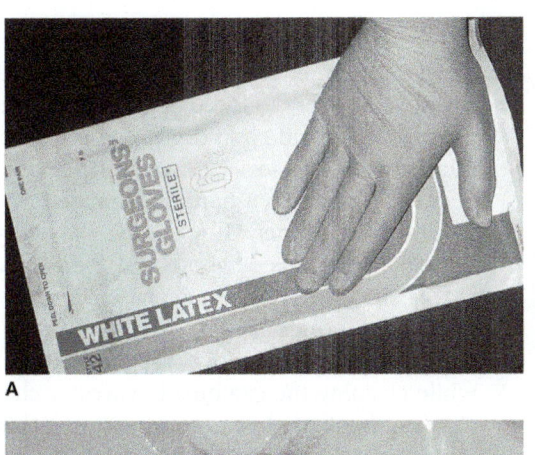

A

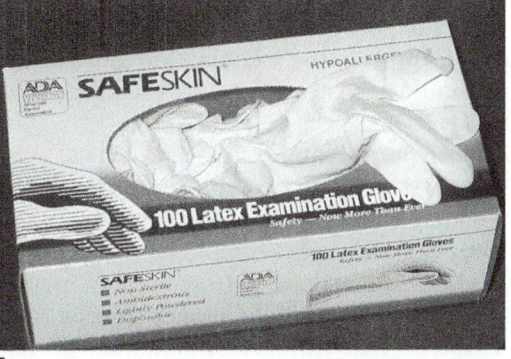

B

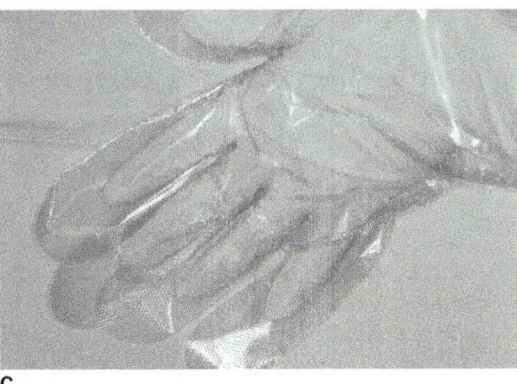

C

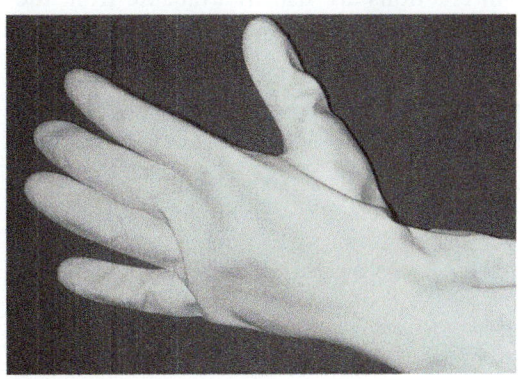

D

Figure 14–6 **Types of gloves.** **(A)** Sterile surgeon's glove. **(B)** Nonsterile exam glove. **(C)** Overglove. **(D)** Utility glove.

than vinyl gloves. In the past, vinyl gloves were more rigid and tore more easily.

Sterile surgical gloves are the same ones worn by surgeons in hospital operating rooms. These gloves are sold in pairs with a right and a left hand. Also regulated by the FDA, these gloves are worn during oral surgery that involves contact with larger amounts of blood and/or cutting through tissue and bone. Sterile surgical gloves made from latex, vinyl, styrene, and synthetic copolymer are available.

Infection Control and Gloves

Proper use of gloves will ensure that infection control is maintained. The following principles should always be followed regarding gloves:

1. Gloves must be changed between patients. Disposable gloves should not be washed between patients but should be removed and discarded. Before new gloves are donned, the hands should be washed according to proper handwashing protocol.
2. If a glove is damaged (e.g., torn, punctured, ripped, etc.), it is no longer effective as a barrier mechanism. The DA should immediately excuse himself or herself from the procedure, remove the gloves and discard them, then wash the hands. The procedure can continue after regloving.
3. To avoid cross-contamination, examination gloves should never come into contact with any other surface in the dental office while worn. If the DA has to leave chairside, overgloves should be worn or a barrier used to protect the examination gloves. The overgloves should be discarded before the procedure continues.
4. Many chemicals in a dental office can damage synthetic gloves. Dental office employees should be aware of which chemicals are present that might interact with their gloves. Examples of potentially dangerous chemicals include petroleum jelly, hydrogen peroxide, alcohol, acrylic monomer, solvent, acid etch, and others. Descriptions of potential glove/chemical interactions are usually available from the glove manufacturer.

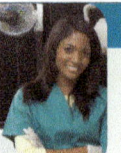

Voice of Experience

Watch Out for Cross Contamination!
It is easy to forget sometimes, but anything you touch with your examination gloves can become contaminated. This means pens, clipboards, cups, and charts. I always remind my staff to be aware of their exam gloves and to pay special attention to anything they touch before degloving. The less you touch, the less chance there is of a problem!

CDC Guidelines for Gloves

1. Wear medical gloves when a potential exists for contacting blood, saliva, spatter, or mucous membranes. (Recommendation level: IB, IC)
2. Wear a new pair of medical gloves for each patient, remove them promptly after use, and wash hands immediately to avoid transfer of microorganisms to other patients or environments. (Recommendation level: IB)
3. Remove gloves that are torn, cut, or punctured as soon as feasible and wash hands before regloving. (Recommendation level: IB, IC)
4. Do not wash surgical or patient examination gloves before use or wash, disinfect, or sterilize gloves for reuse. (Recommendation level: IB, IC)
5. Ensure that appropriate gloves in the correct size are readily accessible. (Recommendation level: IC)
6. Use appropriate gloves (e.g., puncture resistant and chemical resistant utility gloves) when cleaning instruments and performing housekeeping tasks involving contact with blood or spatter or chemicals. (Recommendation level: IB, IC)
7. Consult with the glove manufacturer regarding the chemical compatibility of glove material and dental materials used. (Recommendation level: II)

Source: *CDC Guidelines for Infection Control in Dental Healthcare Settings—2003*

Additional Kinds of Gloves

Besides examination gloves and surgical gloves, the following gloves are used in dental offices. These are not regulated by the FDA.

- *Overgloves.* Also known as "food-handling gloves," overgloves are large, clear, lightweight plastic gloves that easily slide over a gloved hand. These are not examination gloves and should not come into contact with the patient. Overgloves are worn whenever it becomes necessary to touch a noncontaminated object, such as a drawer or cabinet. They can be slid on quickly, used to perform the needed task, and then discarded. Overgloves should never be reworn or cleaned and should be used only once.
- *Utility gloves.* Utility gloves are heavy, thick gloves used while cleaning the examination area or cleaning potentially contaminated trays and instruments. These gloves are designed to provide a protective physical barrier. They are not examination gloves and should never come into contact with a patient. Utility gloves are not disposed of after every use—they can be washed, sterilized, and reused. However, utility gloves should be disposed of when a pair becomes cracked and worn. It is best if every employee who cleans examination areas or instruments has his or her own designated pair of utility gloves.
- *Autoclavable utility gloves.* Autoclavable utility gloves are utility gloves that can be sterilized in the autoclave sterilization unit after use.

Latex Allergies

Latex gloves are very common in medical settings, but their heavy use has coincided with a rise in latex sensitivities. As latex, a natural product made from the milky sap of the *Hevea brasiliensis* tree, has become more common in treatment settings, latex sensitivities and allergies have become more common in both medical professionals and patients. Such allergies may be accompanied by partner food allergies, including allergies to avocados, bananas, chestnuts, kiwifruits, and other latex and rubber products, including prophylactic cups, nitrous oxide masks, and dental dams.

The CDC has set guidelines for handling latex in the dental office, including:

1. Educate dental health professionals regarding the signs, symptoms, and diagnoses of skin reactions associated with frequent hand hygiene and glove use. (Recommendation level: IB).
2. Screen all patients for latex allergy, including a medical history, and refer patients for a medical consultation if a latex allergy is present or suspected. (Recommendation level: IB).
3. Ensure a latex-free environment for patients and dental health professionals with a known latex allergy.
4. Have emergency treatment kits with latex-free products available at all times. (Recommendation level: II).

Latex problems fall into two categories: sensitivities and allergies. Latex sensitivities are common among people who have frequent contact with latex.

Contact Dermatitis

Contact dermatitis is a surface reaction to latex that is limited to the first few layers of skin. It is not a true allergy, meaning that it does not involve an immune system response. Instead, contact dermatitis is caused by contact with substances that contain chemicals that irritate the skin. Reactions typically include red, dry, cracked, and irritated skin. A reaction will occur almost immediately.

Contact dermatitis is worsened by frequent handwashing and the use of antimicrobial agents. Incomplete rinsing and drying and using a scrub brush during handwashing also contribute. The cornstarch powder in gloves can also worsen contact dermatitis. The cornstarch itself is not an irritant, but it transmits the latex chemicals more efficiently to the skin.

To reduce contact dermatitis, hands should be thoroughly rinsed after washing and then completely dried. Gloves should be changed often to prevent perspiration inside the gloves, which also worsens the condition. Finally, the use of lotions and emollients to keep skin moisturized and protected will reduce dermatitis.

Type IV Allergic Reaction

A type IV allergic reaction is a local allergic reaction to the proteins in the chemicals used to process latex, as opposed to the latex proteins themselves. It involves the immune system, and symptoms appear in 24 to 72 hours. Symptoms are similar to those of contact dermatitis but are more severe and may include oozing blisters. The allergic reaction begins where the latex had contact to the skin, but it can spread.

Once this type of allergic reaction has occurred, it's very important to eliminate latex exposure in that person. Nonlatex gloves or hypoallergenic gloves should be provided, and the allergic person should be aware of all possible sources of latex in the dental office.

Type I Allergic Reaction

A type I allergic reaction occurs within minutes of contact with latex. It is an immune-mediated allergic reaction in which the body identifies the latex proteins as pathogens and mounts an aggressive, systemic immune response. Type I allergic reactions can be extremely dangerous—people who are highly sensitive to latex proteins are at risk of death from **anaphylaxis**.

Symptoms of anaphylaxis or anaphylactic shock include coughing, wheezing, shortness of breath, and runny eyes and nose. These symptoms are caused by rapid swelling of the respiratory tract, which makes it difficult to breathe.

People who have latex allergies should avoid all contact with latex and be treated in latex-free environments. Even the cornstarch used to coat the insides of gloves, which may contain latex proteins, poses a threat to these people. During degloving, cornstarch can become airborne and then inhaled, triggering an allergic reaction.

Anaphylactic shock is a medical emergency. If a dental professional or patient exhibits signs of anaphylactic shock after exposure to latex, emergency medical care should be sought.

Procedure 14–3 Removing Contaminated Gloves

Once treatment gloves have been used, they are considered contaminated. The following degloving procedure can help reduce the risk of spreading infectious agents.

Materials needed:

- Gloves
- Biohazard receptacle

1. Hook a gloved finger under the outside cuff of one glove and peel the glove from your hand, inverting the glove as it comes off. The idea is to turn the glove inside out, thus trapping all potentially contaminated material inside the inverted gloves (Figure P14-3-1).

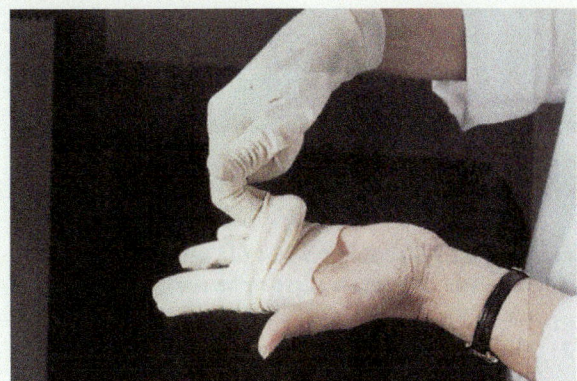

Figure P14-3-1

Procedure 14–3 **Removing Contaminated Gloves (Continued)**

2. Hold the inverted, removed glove in the palm of your still-gloved hand (Figure P14-3-2).

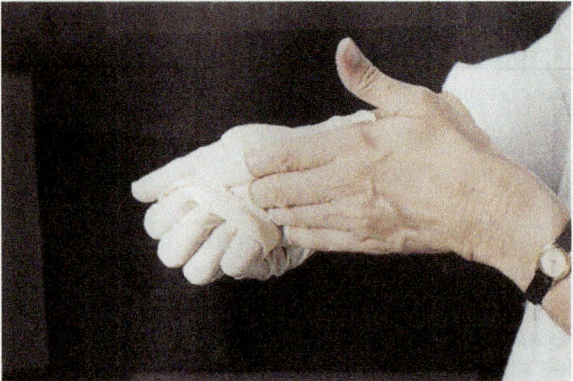

Figure P14-3-2

3. Slip your ungloved fingers under the cuff of the glove you are still wearing, next to the skin, and pull it outward and off.

This glove will also invert, trapping the first glove inside and presenting the skin-side of the glove to the outside (Figure P14-3-3).

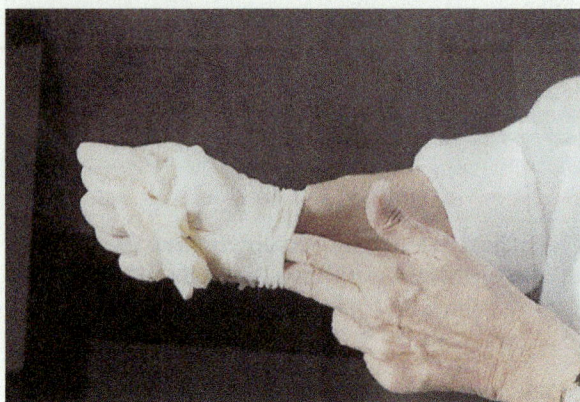

Figure P14-3-3

4. Dispose of used gloves in a waste receptacle.

Protective Barriers

Protective barriers are physical barriers that contain and control contamination (Figure 14-7). Anything that can become potentially contaminated should be covered by a protective barrier. This includes handles, knobs, counter surfaces, faucets, handpieces, air-water syringes, high-volume evacuators, saliva ejectors, pens and pencils, and tubing. Protective barriers are often made of disposable plastic,

Figure 14–7 Protective barriers. Barriers on **(A)** air and water syringe handle and **(B)** the saliva ejector and high-speed air evacuator handles should be changed between patients.

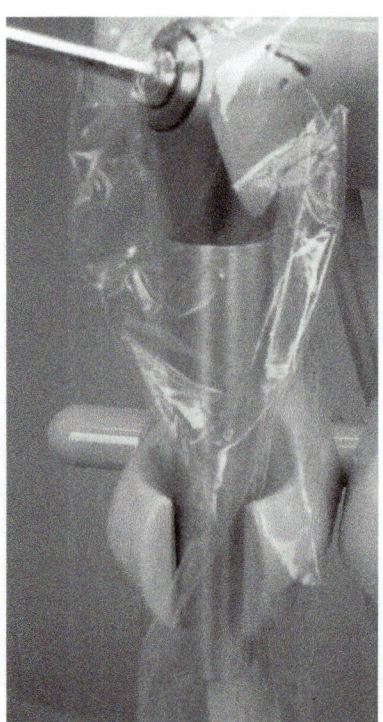

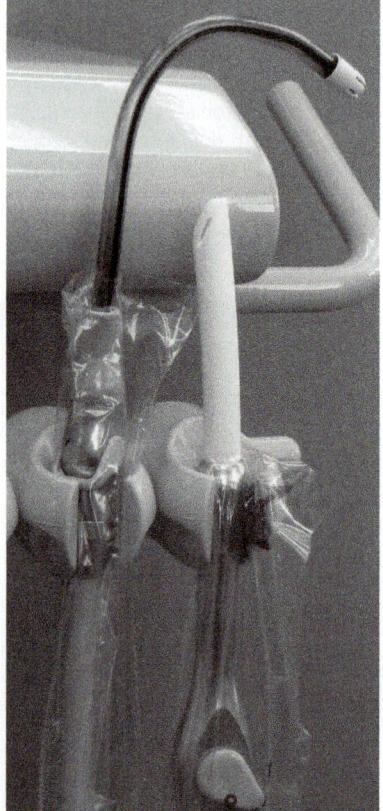

A   **B**

and special products have been introduced that conform to hard-to-cover areas, such as the tubing that connects the air-water syringe. Protective barriers should be changed between every patient and disposed of in a safe manner. When handling protective barriers, always wear PPE and utility gloves. These surfaces should be treated as potentially contaminated.

OSHA's Bloodborne Pathogen Standard

Along with the CDC and other government agencies, OSHA helps regulate workplace safety. The disposal of medical waste, including sharps and potentially contaminated material, is covered in greater depth in Chapter 15, Safety Regulations. However, OSHA is also active in infection control through the **Bloodborne Pathogen Standard**, or BBP. The BBP is officially supported in the CDC's guidelines.

The BBP was issued in 1991 in response to the high number of needlesticks and other injuries that could cause transmission of bloodborne diseases such as hepatitis and HIV/AIDS. It was revised in 2001 at the mandate of the Needlestick Safety and Prevention Act, which was passed by Congress.

The BBP is a comprehensive protocol designed to protect employees from bloodborne illness. Among its provisions are:

- All potentially infectious materials such as blood, saliva, cerebrospinal fluid, and visibly contaminated body fluids should be considered infectious.
- Employees should wash hands immediately following glove removal.
- No eating, drinking, or smoking should be permitted in work areas.
- Food and drink should not be stored in work areas.
- Needles should never be recapped (but if recapping is unavoidable, only use a one-handed technique), bent, or broken.
- Efforts should be made to minimize splashing of blood and potentially infectious materials.
- Employees should wear personal protective equipment including eye protection, gloves, and protective clothing.

The BBP also covers **sharps**. Sharps are defined as any object that can easily pierce protective barriers and skin. This includes the following:

- Needles
- Scalpels
- Blades of all sorts
- Disposable air-water syringe tips
- Burs
- Orthodontic brackets and wires
- Endodontic reamers, files, barbed broaches, and burs
- Broken glass
- Pieces of metal or metal instruments that are broken and sharp

According to the BBP, sharps containers should be readily accessible and close to the work area. Sharps containers should be puncture resistant and clearly labeled or color-coded to reduce confusion. They should be leak-proof and have a cover to close them. Finally, sharps containers should be routinely replaced so there is no risk of overflow.

For more information on handling exposure incidents under the BBP, see sidebar, Reporting an Exposure Incident: OSHA Rights and Responsibilities.

> ### Reporting an Exposure Incident: OSHA Rights and Responsibilities
>
> Despite the best precautions to protect employees from bloodborne pathogens, exposure incidents are still relatively common. Once an exposure incident has occurred, immediate action should be taken by both the employee and the dentist.
>
> 1. Any employee who has had an exposure incident must immediately report it to the employer.
> 2. The employer directs the employee to a qualified health care professional for a medical evaluation and follow-up. OSHA regulations do not cover the exact nature of the evaluation and follow-up, but they say that the dentist must refer the employee to a licensed health care professional to receive the most current evaluation. The evaluation is paid for by the employer.
> 3. The dentist has to document the incident, including the nature of the incident and the circumstances surrounding it, as well as vaccination status. This report is included in the employee's file, and a copy is provided to the health care professional who performs the evaluation. The dentist must also contact the source patient (if known) and ask for his or her consent for testing for hepatitis B and HIV and then disclose the results of these tests to the exposed employee. Denial of permission by the source patient has to be noted in the incident report.
> 4. After the examination, the health care professional will provide the results to the dentist. In turn, the employer must provide counseling to the exposed employee and prophylaxis and evaluation of any reported illness. Vaccination for hepatitis B will be provided if the employee was not vaccinated previously, or in high-risk cases, post-exposure drugs must be administered to reduce the risk of transmission.
> 5. The dentist will provide a copy of this health care professional's report to the employee.
> 6. Exposed employees have the right to refuse testing or delay testing up to 90 days. They may choose to opt for a simple blood test to determine hepatitis and human immunodeficiency virus (HIV) status, or only hepatitis and decline HIV testing. Blood samples have to be saved for 90 days. All tests must be performed by an outside accredited laboratory at no cost to the exposed employee.

Along with the BBP, OSHA has developed a **Hazard Communication Standard**. The hazard communication was developed to educate employees about the potentially toxic chemicals in their workplace and how to use, handle, and dispose of those chemicals. This is covered in greater depth in Chapter 15, Safety Regulations.

Additional Regulations

The CDC and OSHA are the main regulatory agencies that govern infection control, but a number of additional professional, state, and federal agencies exert control and influence over the operation of a dental office, including the following:

- Professional Associations:
  - ADA. The ADA is the main professional body for the dental industry. It recommends infection control best practices to supplement and support CDC guidelines.
  - American Dental Assistants Association (ADAA). Just as the ADA represents the interest of dentists, the ADAA represents the interests of professional DAs. Membership is open to DAs as well as office personnel, such as receptionists and office managers.
  - ADHA. This group represents dental hygienists.
  - Organization for Safety and Asepsis Procedures (OSAP). OSAP is a not-for-profit organization dedicated to infection control in dentistry. Membership includes dentists, dental hygienists, DAs, researchers, consultants, and members from government and academia. OSAP provides recommendations to the dental profession on such issues as disinfection, sterilization, water line management, and any other infection-control related issues.
- Government Agencies:
  - CDC. A federal agency devoted to public health, the CDC published the *Guidelines for Infection Control in Dental Healthcare Settings—2003*, which is the clinical standard for infection control. In 2007, the CDC updated the standard precautions. In 2008, the CDC published an update for disinfection and sterilization procedures in health care facilities, which includes dental offices.
  - FDA. As regards dentistry, the FDA is concerned with the safety, manufacture, and sale of medical devices. The FDA regulates devices such as sterilizers, ultrasonic cleaners, gloves, masks, protective eyewear, dental handpieces and instruments, dental chairs, and other equipment that comes into contact with patients. The FDA must approve all dental and medical devices approved for sale in the United States and can remove potentially dangerous products from the market.
  - EPA. The EPA is concerned with the effectiveness of disinfectants. All EPA-approved disinfectants are tested by the agency to ensure they are effective and meet manufacturers' claims. The EPA also regulates the disposal of chemicals and waste materials used in the dental office.
  - OSHA. OSHA is a division of the Department of Labor. This regulatory agency is tasked with protecting American workers in all settings, including medical and dental offices. The OSHA Bloodborne Pathogen Standard and Hazard Communication Standard are used in all dental offices to protect employees from infectious agents and alert them to potentially toxic chemicals in their workplace.

Immunizations

Immunizations are a standard part of infection control. Most Americans receive a course of vaccinations as children against diseases such as mumps, measles, and rubella. As a result, these diseases have become much less common.

In the dental office, only hepatitis B vaccination is covered by OSHA regulation. According to OSHA, all employees must be offered the hepatitis B vaccination within 10 days of starting employment. A blood titer taken after vaccination can determine how effective the vaccine is. This test is not mandated by law, but it is highly recommended to ensure that the vaccination was effective.

Medical professionals are also recommended to receive vaccination against influenza. The flu vaccines are given annually; they target the three most likely strains of flu that researchers predict will be prevalent that year. Flu vaccines are not mandated by OSHA, but many employers require them.

For more on vaccination, see Chapter 13, Understanding Microbiology.

CHECKPOINTS

14-6 Define standard precautions.

14-7 Which type of soap is best for handwashing?

14-8 Is it acceptable to let a mask dangle during a patient visit?

14-9 What is the most common type of gloves used in the dental office?

14-10 What are the three most common reactions to latex?

14-11 What is the Bloodborne Pathogen Standard?

14-12 What happens after a possible exposure to a bloodborne pathogen?

Disinfection

Disinfection is the process of removing most microbes from surfaces. This is different from **sterilization**, which is the process of removing all microbes from surfaces, thereby rendering them **sterile**.

Areas that should be disinfected include any areas in the office that are likely to be contaminated by saliva, blood, bodily fluids, or contaminated aerosol. This especially includes areas that cannot be protected by disposable plastic barriers or sterilized. These areas provide potential reservoirs for microorganisms, some of which can live exposed to the environment for a long time. *Mycobacterium tuberculosis*, for example, can live on surfaces for weeks.

Chemicals used to disinfect are known as **disinfectants**. Disinfectants are regulated by the EPA, which subjects them to rigorous tests to determine which microorganisms they destroy and how effective they are. All disinfectants must carry the EPA approval on their label, along with instructions on how to use the product and other valuable information, such as shelf life, precautionary statements, and storage and disposal instructions.

It is important to use the product exactly according to label instructions. For example, if a product must sit on a surface for 10 to 15 seconds to be effective, users should make sure to include this time in their cleaning regimen.

All offices should have a posted schedule for cleaning, assigning responsibilities among the staff clearly. It is best to keep initialized and dated records of who cleaned which area so nothing is left to chance. Treatment rooms should be cleaned and disinfected between every patient. For more on cleaning the treatment rooms, see Procedure 14-5: Cleaning and Disinfecting the Treatment Room.

Classes of Disinfectants

Disinfectants are classified according to their ability to kill the *M. tuberculosis* organism. Tuberculosis was chosen because it is an especially hardy organism. The assumption is that if a disinfectant can kill *M. tuberculosis*, it can kill any other organisms on surfaces.

Disinfectants are also sometimes labeled according to which type of organism they are most effective against. **Sporicides** are most effective against spores. **Virucides** are most effective against viruses. **Fungicides** are most effective against fungal organisms.

The EPA recognizes the following classes of disinfectants:

- *High-level disinfectant.* Defined as a disinfectant that kills most, but not all, of *M. tuberculosis* spores. Extremely strong agents are sometimes labeled as sporicidal.
- *Intermediate-level disinfectant.* Defined as a disinfectant that does not normally kill all *M. tuberculosis* spores.
- *Low-level disinfectant.* Defined as a disinfectant that kills viruses (which are generally easy to kill outside the body), fungi, and most bacterial organisms, but does not kill bacterial spores, which are typically much more difficult to kill.

Chemical Disinfectants

Common disinfectants used in dental offices are listed in Table 14-1 and include:

- *Chlorine dioxide.* Chlorine dioxide is a high-level disinfectant and sterilant. It can be used as a rapid-acting

TABLE 14-1 Disinfectants				
DISINFECTANT	**LEVEL**	**ADVANTAGES**	**DISADVANTAGES**	**CONTACT TIME**
Chlorine dioxide	High	■ Rapid-acting surface disinfectant ■ Sterilant (6 hours contact)	■ Must be used with cleaning solution ■ Corrosive to metals ■ Irritating to skin and eyes	3 minutes to disinfect
Glutaraldehyde	High	■ Used as immersion disinfectant ■ Long effective period	■ High toxicity ■ Corrosive to metal	10–90 minutes to disinfect
Iodophor	Intermediate	■ Nontoxic	■ May stain surfaces ■ Short effective period	5–10 minutes
Sodium hypochlorite	Intermediate	■ Rapid disinfection ■ Economical	■ Corrosive to metal, plastic, and fabric ■ Irritating to skin and eyes ■ Unstable solution	10 minutes
Synthetic phenols	Intermediate	■ Noncorrosive and can be used on metal, glass, and rubber	■ May degrade plastics over time ■ Must be prepared daily to be effective	10 minutes
Alcohol	Not EPA registered	N/A	N/A	N/A

EPA, Environmental Protection Agency; N/A, not applicable.

surface disinfectant (3 minutes of contact) or a slower-acting sterilant (6 hours of contact). Chlorine dioxide has two main drawbacks: It is a poor cleaning solution that does not penetrate organic material, and it is corrosive. Chlorine dioxide should not be used on any products made from steel, as well as aluminum, copper, or brass. It must be prepared daily.

- *Glutaraldehyde*. Glutaraldehyde is a high-level disinfectant and sterilant. Slower acting than chlorine dioxide, it needs 10 to 90 minutes to disinfect, and 6 to 10 hours to sterilize. However, glutaraldehyde is often used for overnight sterilization of plastic utensils that cannot withstand the heat of the sterilization unit. The main drawbacks to glutaraldehyde include its high toxicity and its corrosive abilities. Glutaraldehyde should only be used in a very well-ventilated area, and utensils that will have direct patient contact must be very well rinsed with water before coming into contact with patients. Some glutaraldehyde solutions can be reused for up to 28 days.

- *Iodophor*. Iodophor is classified as an intermediate-level hospital disinfectant. It requires 5 to 10 minutes of contact time to work, and care must be taken to dilute iodophor according to the label instructions. Iodophor contains iodine, so repeated use on white surfaces, such as countertops, can result in staining. Iodophor has a relatively short effective period, so solutions should be changed every 3 days at the minimum.

- *Sodium hypochlorite*. Sodium hypochlorite, or household bleach, is an intermediate-level disinfectant. The most common product on the market is the 5.25% cleaning solution widely available in grocery stores, although sodium hypochlorite is also an ingredient in some labeled disinfectants. Sodium hypochlorite is not an EPA-registered disinfectant, and as a result, is no longer recommended as a disinfectant in dental settings under the latest CDC guidelines; however, it is still widely used. Typically, it is diluted in a 1:10 ratio with water, meaning that 1 cup of 5.25% bleach is added to 10 cups of water before cleaning. Disinfection is achieved in 10 minutes of surface contact. Sodium hypochlorite has a number of drawbacks, including:
  - It is highly unstable and must be prepared daily.
  - It is highly corrosive to metals, plastics, and fabrics.
  - The fumes can be highly irritating to the eyes and nose.
  - It is potentially dangerous when combined with other cleaning products.

- *Synthetic phenols*. Synthetic phenols are intermediate-level disinfectants that are EPA registered. These broad-spectrum disinfectants kill a majority of microorganisms with 10 minutes of surface contact. Synthetic phenols are available as sprays and can be used safely on metal, glass, and rubber. They are also sometimes used as holding solutions for instruments, although they leave a residue that must be carefully rinsed off before patient use. Synthetic phenol solutions must be prepared daily.

- *Alcohol*. Ethyl and isopropyl alcohol were once widely used as disinfectants. However, because of their rapid evaporation rate and their poor action against microorganisms in blood and saliva, alcohols are no longer recommended for use in dental offices, according to the ADA, CDC, and OSAP.

> Many disinfectants and cleaning solutions require mixing before they are effective. When placing a prepared disinfectant solution into another bottle, such as a spray bottle or immersion bottle, it is very important to label the new container along with any cautions. Anyone in the office should be able to tell at a glance what the contents of a bottle are and if they are flammable, corrosive, or toxic.

Immersion Solutions

Many of the common disinfectants are used as immersion solutions for both disinfecting and sterilizing. It is important to note that the contact times might be different when comparing surface disinfection and immersion sterilization. Additionally, the clock may have to be reset every time a new instrument is added to the immersion solution, thus potentially introducing new infectious agents. Sterilization times can range up to 30 hours, depending on the product. Always follow label instructions.

When using immersion solutions, PPE should always be worn. Many of these chemicals are toxic and should never be used at their immersion concentrations as surface disinfectants.

Ultrasonic Cleaning

An ultrasonic cleaner uses sound waves to prepare objects for sterilization. After all visible matter has been removed from the items to be cleaned, the ultrasonic cleaner then removes any remaining debris, including calculus, scale, saliva, blood, and other material. While using an ultrasonic cleaner, heavy utility gloves and PPE should be worn. Instruments placed into an ultrasonic cleaner are contaminated and may include sharps. Special plastic or metal holding trays can reduce the risk of a puncture but not eliminate it.

Before instruments are moved to an ultrasonic cleaner, they are frequently stored in an immersion precleaning bath consisting of an approved disinfectant. This bath begins to loosen the hardened debris and starts the cleaning process. Instruments can remain in the bath until the DA is ready to remove them and begin the cleaning.

When the DA is ready, the immersion bath full of instruments should be carried to the sterilization area, the instruments carefully removed (with tongs or puncture-resistant utility gloves) and then placed into the baskets for cleaning.

During operation, the ultrasonic cleaner produces sound waves that cause bubbles in the special ultrasonic cleaner cleaning solution. This process is called **cavitation**. The bubbles then implode, or burst inward. These bubbles "scrub" the instruments free in preparation for sterilization. However, ultrasonic cleaning *does not* sterilize instruments. Instruments in the ultrasonic bath should remain immersed until they are visibly clean, about 5 to 15 minutes.

Ultrasonic cleaning solution is a special solution designed for use in ultrasonic cleaners. Never use a nonapproved disinfectant in an ultrasonic cleaner. This may actually "set" the debris and make it harder to remove. Ultrasonic cleaning solutions should be clearly labeled.

After the cleaning cycle, the instruments can be removed from the ultrasonic bath. They are then thoroughly rinsed and dried and prepared for sterilization.

Care for the Ultrasonic Cleaner

Ultrasonic cleaners should be considered contaminated. The ultrasonic cleaning solution must be cleaned at least every day, or whenever the solution becomes cloudy. When the solution is changed, the tray should be rinsed with water, disinfected, rinsed again, and dried. To prevent the risk of aerosol and airborne contaminants, face masks, eyewear, and gloves should be worn while cleaning an ultrasonic unit.

To test the ultrasonic unit, submerge the lower half of a sheet of lightweight aluminum foil vertically in a fresh liquid bath for 20 to 30 seconds. Afterward, the surface of the aluminum foil should be finely textured as a result of the cavitation action. If any section greater than a 1/2-inch square is free from the pebbling, the machine is not working to full capacity and needs to be repaired.

Procedure 14-4 Cleaning and Disinfecting Surfaces

The following steps should be taken to clean and disinfect a surface. Remember that the procedure varies depending on the disinfecting solution used. Always use a disinfectant according to its label directions.

Materials needed:

- PPE, including eyewear, utility gloves, and face mask
- Disinfectant solution and disposable towels

or

- Premoistened disinfecting wipes

1. Put on PPE, including eye protection, clean utility gloves, and face mask.

2. If not using premoistened wipes, spray the disposable towel with a disinfectant solution (Figure P14-4-1).

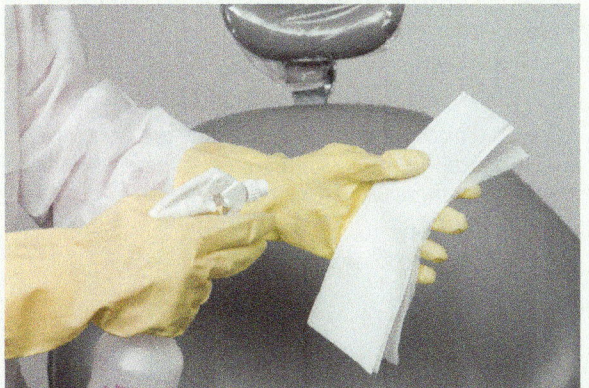

Figure P14-4-1

3. Wipe all surfaces free of debris, tissue, saliva, etc. (Figure P14-4-2).

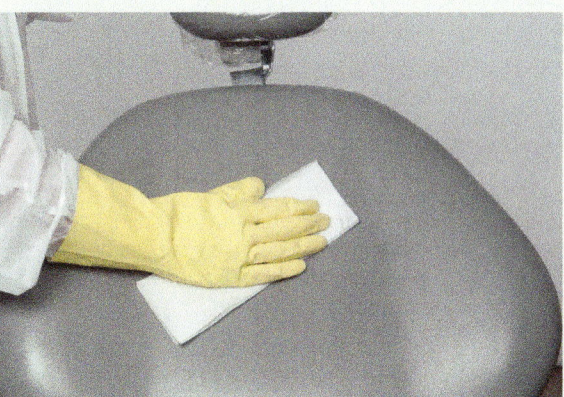

Figure P14-4-2

4. Once surface debris has been removed, wipe all surfaces again with a new disinfectant-sprayed paper towel or premoistened wipe.

5. Allow the disinfectant to remain on all surfaces for the required time, according to the type of disinfectant.

6. Wipe all surfaces clean.

7. Allow all surfaces to thoroughly dry before applying protective barriers or showing new patients into the treatment area.

Environmental Infection Control

The CDC recognizes two classes of environmental surfaces in the dental office: *clinical contact surfaces* and *housekeeping surfaces*.

■ Clinical contact surfaces are surfaces that are at risk of coming into direct contact with spray or spatter generated during dental procedures. These surfaces should be protected with surface barriers and cleaned with a low- or intermediate-level disinfectant. High-level disinfectants or chemical sterilants should not be used to clean them.

■ Housekeeping surfaces are surfaces such as floors, walls, and sinks. These should be cleaned with a detergent and water or an EPA-registered low-level disinfectant on a routine basis.

The vast majority of cleaning energy is expended on clinical contact surfaces. The OSAP has further classified clinical contact surfaces into three groups:

■ *Touch surfaces* are directly touched during procedures. These include handles, knobs, switches, computers, writing implements, telephones, etc.

■ *Transfer surfaces* are not directly touched but may come into contact with contaminated instruments. These include trays and handpiece holders.

■ *Splash, spatter, and droplet surfaces* are not touched by members of the dental team or instruments but may come into direct contact with splash or spatter. These include countertops and the dental chair.

Wherever possible, clinical contact surfaces should be protected by physical barriers, such as disposable plastic wrap that is changed between patients. Touch surfaces and transfer surfaces should be disinfected between patients. Splash, spatter, and droplet surfaces should be cleaned and disinfected at least every day.

Procedure 14–5 Cleaning and Disinfecting the Treatment Room

The treatment room should be cleaned and disinfected between patients. The following procedure outlines the basic steps in cleaning treatment areas.

Materials needed:

■ PPE, including utility gloves and eyewear

■ Disinfectant solution and disposable towels

or

■ Premoistened disinfecting wipes

1. Remove treatment gloves.

2. Put on protective gear, including utility gloves, protective eyewear, and other PPE. Do not use examination gloves to clean because the latex in these gloves may disintegrate with the chemicals used while cleaning.

3. Prepare the disinfectant solution if it is not already prepared. Make sure you are using correctly formulated disinfectant solution that is within its effective date.

4. Make sure that any instrument trays and immersion baths with instruments have been removed to the sterilization area.

5. Remove all disposable physical barriers such as plastic wrap (Figure P14-5-1).

6. Wipe down all clinical contact areas with a premoistened wipe or a disposable towel sprayed with disinfectant (see Figures P14-4-1 and P14-4-2).

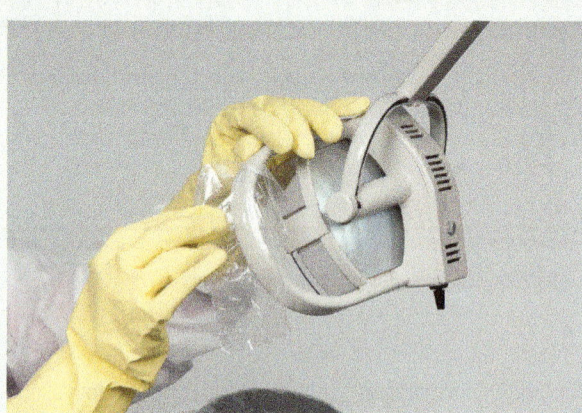

Figure P14-5-1

7. Wipe down all clinical contact areas again with a new disinfectant-sprayed paper towel or premoistened wipe and leave it on for the appropriate kill time, according to the label instructions.

8. Wipe all clinical contact areas clean with paper towels.

9. Allow all clinical contact areas to dry before new patients are introduced to the treatment area. If there is not time, manually dry them with a clean cloth.

10. Dispose of all paper towels, wipes, and disposable physical barriers in an appropriate receptacle.

Sterilization

Sterilization is the removal of all microorganisms from a surface or object. A variety of forms of sterilization are used in the dental office, including heat, chemical, and steam. Which one is best depends on the item to be sterilized.

All objects that penetrate or come into direct contact with the patient's skin or mucosa must be sterilized after use. Sterilization is typically the responsibility of the DA, so it is essential that all DAs learn the proper technique for each type of sterilization.

Objects Needing Sterilization

The CDC classifies all patient care objects into three groups: critical, semi-critical, and noncritical. The level of cleaning varies among the three groups, depending on their use.

- *Critical instruments* are used to penetrate soft tissue or bone. Examples include needles, scalpels, scalers, forceps, and other surgical instruments. All critical instruments require sterilization.
- *Semi-critical instruments* are used to touch mucous membranes or used in the intraoral cavity. However, they do not break the soft tissue barrier. Examples include amalgam condensers and dental mirrors. Semi-critical instruments require sterilization or high-level disinfection.
- *Noncritical instruments* only come into contact with intact skin; they do not touch mucosal membranes and are not used in the intraoral cavity. Examples include the radiograph head. They require intermediate to low-level disinfection or basic cleaning.

Precleaning and Packaging Before Sterilization

After a procedure is done, contaminated instruments should be transported to a designated sterilization area. This area should be easy to access from all patient care areas but should not be in a high-traffic area. Contaminated instruments should be carried in a covered, solid container to reduce the potential for dropping or exposing these materials anywhere in the facility. The sterilization area should be equipped with the necessary PPE, such as utility gloves, masks, and protective eyewear.

Typically, the DA or hygienist will carry trays of contaminated instruments and disposable items to a receiving area in the sterilization area. There, the disposable items are discarded along with medical waste, and the contaminated instruments are either processed immediately or placed into a holding solution until they can be processed. Holding solutions are typically noncorrosive solutions that help loosen organic debris and begin the cleaning process. These are not disinfectants or sterilization solutions. Holding solutions might include enzymatic solutions or even common dishwasher detergent. All holding solutions should be considered highly contaminated and changed frequently.

The first step in the sterilization procedure is to preclean the instruments. This typically includes ultrasonic cleaning (see previous section on ultrasonic cleaning) or cleaning in an approved automatic washer (much like a common dishwasher). Some of these devices operate at a high heat level and are capable of killing most microorganisms and, thus, disinfecting instruments.

Once the precleaning is done, the instruments are ready for packaging. Packaging is often done to reduce the risk of contamination immediately after sterilization. If newly sterilized instruments are exposed to the environment after sterilization, they might pick up airborne bacteria or other microorganisms. To reduce the risk of contamination, sterilized items should never be carried around in the sterilization area. Sterilization packaging materials are regulated by the FDA as medical devices. It is essential to use only FDA-approved sterilization packaging with the appropriate type of sterilization. Using the wrong material might damage the instruments or compromise the sterilization procedure.

Many types of sterilization units work with both packaged and unpackaged instruments.

Sterilization Methods

Several different sterilization methods are used in dental offices. Each has its advantages and disadvantages and may be used in different situations. The individual approaches are covered below. They include:

- Liquid chemical sterilization
- Ethylene oxide sterilization
- Dry heat sterilization
- Chemical vapor sterilization
- Steam autoclave sterilization

Liquid Chemical Sterilization

Liquid chemical sterilization is used for objects that cannot withstand heat sterilization. This includes anything made from rubber and many plastics. Items such as rubber dam guides and radiograph film-holding devices are typically liquid sterilized.

The items to be sterilized are completely immersed in the liquid solution and left there for the required length of time. This is typically between 6 and 10 hours, depending on the solution used. The main drawbacks to liquid sterilization are the length of time required to complete the process, the toxicity of the chemicals (good ventilation is needed), and the fact that once items are removed from the liquid bath, they might be contaminated again as they are rinsed and packaged for use.

Ethylene Oxide Sterilization

Low-temperature sterilization can also be accomplished in an ethylene oxide sterilization unit. Items are placed in the unit, which is activated and bathes the instruments inside in ethylene oxide gas. A high-temperature unit (although still safe for most plastics) can complete sterilization in 2 to 3 hours, whereas a room-temperature unit needs 12 hours to achieve sterilization. Also, after sterilization, porous instruments require at least 16 additional hours to let the toxic ethylene oxide gas fully dissipate from the material. Ethylene oxide sterilization units are infrequently used in dental offices.

Dry Heat

Dry heat sterilization accomplishes sterilization by exposing instruments to temperatures of at least 320°F to 375°F (160°C–190°C) for 1 hour. The advantage to this unit is that it does not cause corrosion or dulling of cutting edges. It is also very reliable and can be used with loose or packaged instruments. However, plastics, fabrics, and rubber items cannot be placed in this machine because they will melt. One type of dry heat sterilization, called *forced air sterilization*, works in as little as 6 minutes. This device circulates the heated air inside the device rapidly, causing more rapid transfer of heat.

Chemical Vapor Sterilization

Chemical vapor sterilizers create a sterilizing fog from chemicals including alcohol or formaldehyde. The units typically operate at 270°F (132°C), and they are very reliable and easy to monitor. The main advantage to this form of sterilization is the lack of water vapor inside the unit. Thus, metals and other materials do not corrode as rapidly. The unit also works relatively quickly, and it can sterilize both loose and packaged instruments. The main disadvantage is the toxicity of the chemicals used in the unit. When the door is opened after sterilization, toxic chemicals are released into the environment, potentially causing irritation. Good ventilation is essential, and any dental personnel exposed to these devices should wear monitoring badges that measure exposure to airborne chemicals.

Steam Autoclave Sterilization

Steam sterilization is the most common form of sterilization found in dental offices. Most offices have an autoclave sterilization unit (Figure 14-8). These units use pressurized steam to rapidly sterilize both wrapped and unwrapped instruments. Autoclave sterilizers typically have four cycles:

- Heat up
- Sterilizing
- Depressurization cycle/venting
- Drying

During the heat-up cycle, the unit produces steam between 250°F (121°C) and 270°F (132°C) at 15 lbs. of steam pressure. It operates for a set amount of time, depending on the need. Items usually require 3 to 30 minutes for sterilization, depending on whether and how they are packaged. Different autoclave units operate along slightly different lines. Some produce a vacuum before sterilization to help force heated steam through the unit, whereas others produce several surges of heated steam. Autoclaves are available in different sizes and configurations. Many units require distilled water to be used in the machine.

Autoclave packaging is very important. Follow the manufacturer's instructions exactly to package instruments for the autoclave unit. Steam must be allowed to penetrate the package to reach the instrument inside.

Steam autoclave sterilization is very efficient and fast. Flash sterilization of loose instruments can be accomplished in some cases in as little as 3 minutes. The main drawback to steam autoclave sterilization is wear and tear on instruments. After repeated sterilization, cutting edges will dull, and instruments will rust and corrode.

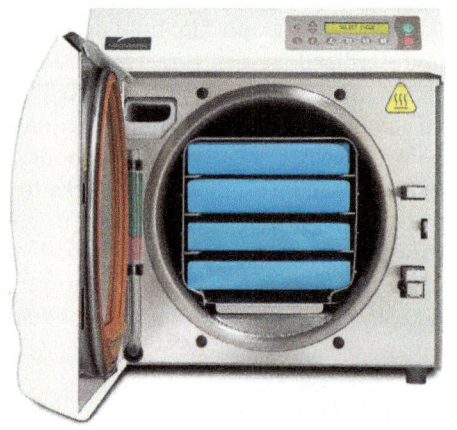 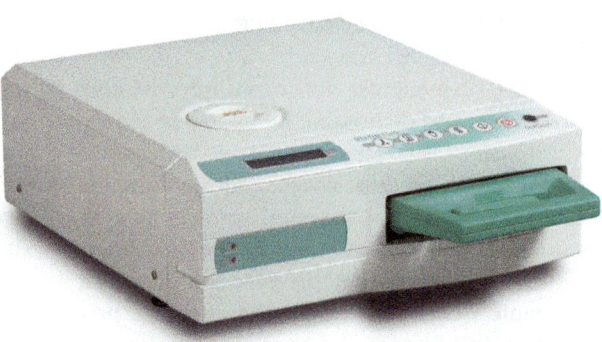

Figure 14–8 Steam autoclave sterilizers. Units produce steam from distilled water for 3 to 30 minutes to sterilize instruments.

Procedure 14-6 Packaging Instruments and Loading an Autoclave Sterilization Unit

Multiple kinds of autoclave sterilization units are available, and each unit has its own specific techniques. It is best when using a new autoclave machine to read the manufacturer's instructions for using that machine and thoroughly familiarize yourself with methods of sterilizing both packaged and unpackaged instruments. The procedure below is representative of an autoclave unit, but differences may exist between various units. (Note, too, that the Statim sterilizers are able to quick-sterilize items.)

Materials needed:

- PPE, including utility gloves, vinyl examination gloves or overgloves, and eyewear
- Cleaning solution
- Autoclave unit
- Corrosion inhibitor
- Packaging materials appropriate for the autoclave unit being used
- Distilled water, if needed

1. Put on appropriate PPE, including utility gloves and eyewear.

2. Clean instruments using an ultrasonic cleaner before they are sterilized (Figure P14-6-1). Pat objects dry with a paper towel.

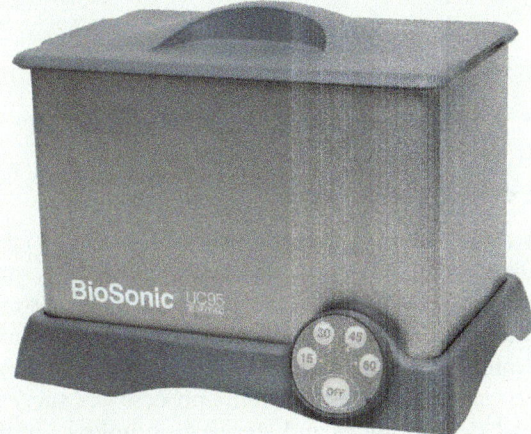

Figure P14-6-1

3. Use a corrosion inhibitor on nonstainless tools and burs to extend lifespan. A corrosion inhibitor is typically a 1% sodium nitrate solution.

4. Package, seal, and label instruments, including the date of sterilization, according to the manufacturer's instructions for that package type. Packages are typically made from film or paper pouches, nylon wrap, or paper-wrapped cassettes (Figure P14-6-2).

5. Place the sealed items in the autoclave. Allow a reasonable distance between packages—do not pile packages atop one another. There must be room for steam to circulate. Put the larger packages at the bottom of the unit (Figure 14-6-3).

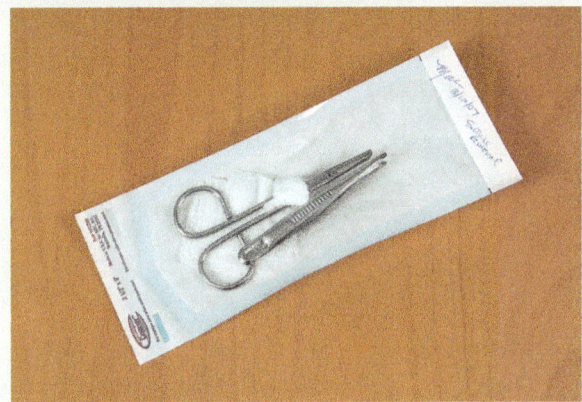

Figure P14-6-2

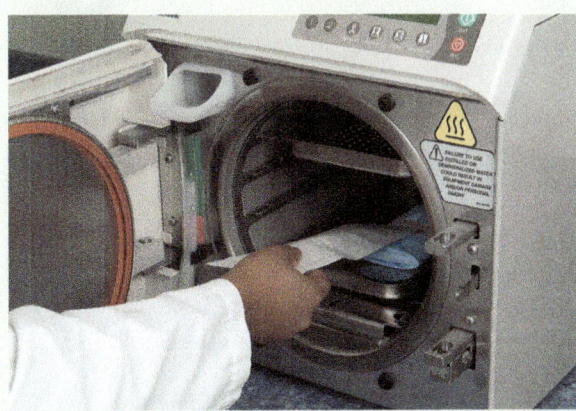

Figure P14-6-3

6. Insert the sterilization indicator.

7. Make sure the autoclave has enough water. Most units require distilled water because tap water contains minerals that can damage or clog the machine. If additional water is needed, add water (Figure P14-6-4).

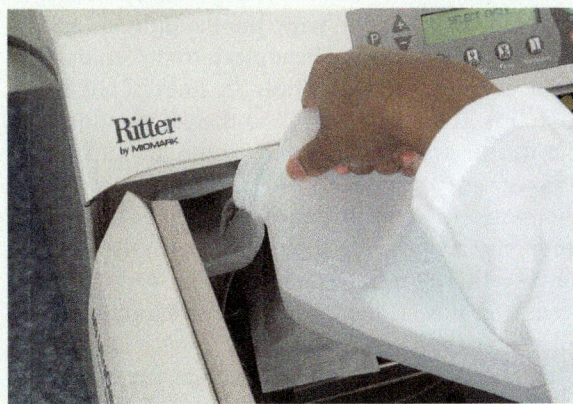

Figure P14-6-4

Procedure 14–6 Packaging Instruments and Loading an Autoclave Sterilization Unit (Continued)

8. Set the autoclave controls, including the time, temperature, and pressure (Figure P14-6-5). Unwrapped instruments can be sterilized at 270°F (132°F) at 15 lbs. of pressure for 3 minutes. Refer to the manufacturer's instructions for requirements for specifics.

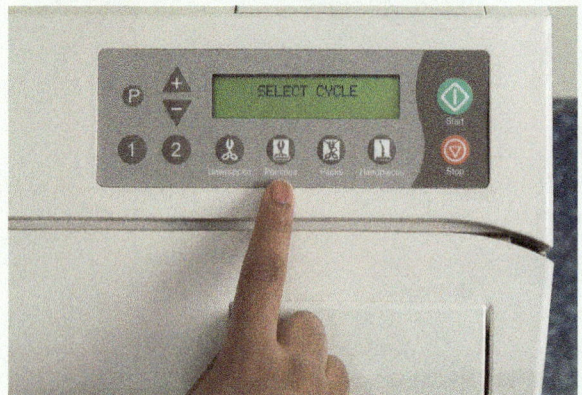

Figure P14-6-5

9. Close the door and activate the unit (Figure P14-6-6).

10. At the end of the cycle, vent the steam into the room if the machine does not automatically vent (most do). Allow the unit's drying cycle to dry the instruments and cool them.

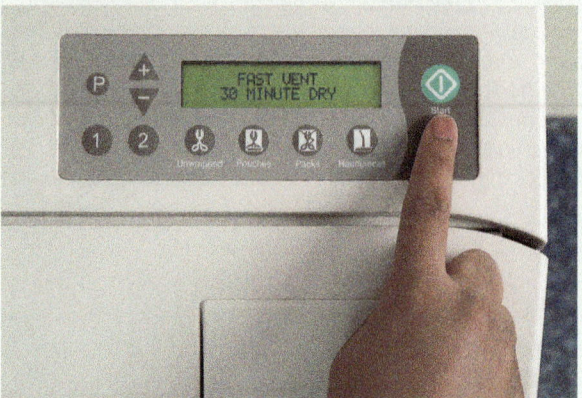

Figure P14-6-6

11. Wash hands and wear vinyl examination gloves or overgloves (avoid latex gloves due to allergen issues) before handling sterile equipment packages. Remove sterile packages from the unit and place into the clean area. Do not carry sterilized instruments through the processing area for contaminated instruments.

12. Store sterilized instruments properly until required.

Handpiece Sterilization

Handpieces are expensive and heavily used pieces of dental equipment. Therefore, they have to be sterilized, but it is important to use a system that will not damage the handpiece during frequent sterilizations and shorten its life.

After use with a patient, wipe the handpiece clean of visible debris and attach the handpiece to the unit with a bur in place. Run it briefly to flush the lines of any water, air, and debris. Then, take it back to the sterilization area, where it can be washed according to the manufacturer's instructions. Use only the soap recommended by the manufacturer, and scrub it under water with a brush. If the handpiece is approved for use in an ultrasonic unit, you can use the ultrasonic unit for those parts that are approved. After it is cleaned, lubricate the handpiece with a manufacturer-approved lubricant (or none at all, depending on the make). After it is lubricated, place the handpiece back on the unit with a bur and run it briefly again to flush out any extra lubricant. The fiber optics on the handpiece can be cleaned with a cotton swab and isopropyl alcohol.

To sterilize a handpiece, closely follow the manufacturer's instructions. Handpieces can be sterilized in steam units in the appropriate packaging. Most handpieces cannot tolerate heat above 275°F (135°C).

Sterilization Monitoring

No matter what kind of sterilization unit is used, successful sterilization depends on the completion of several steps. Any break in the process can result in failed sterilization and instruments that still harbor microorganisms. Because microorganisms cannot be seen by the naked eye, there's no way to intuitively tell if the process was successful. Instead, dental offices and sterilization units carefully monitor the process to make sure that all the steps are followed and the process was successful.

In addition to keeping careful records of the machine's dials and knobs, there are two basic forms of sterilization monitoring: chemical and biologic.

Biologic monitoring is the only way to guarantee a sterilization unit is running as it is supposed to. In this form of monitoring, three specially prepared paper strips are used. One is placed loose in the machine, one is placed within sterilization packaging, and one is used as a control strip (Figure 14-9A). These strips contain bacterial endospores that are resistant to disinfection. The spores in the test strips do not pose a threat to human health. Once the strips are in place, the machine is used as normal, with a full load. Then the strips are cultured to see if any of the bacteria survived. The culturing process is performed either in an in-office

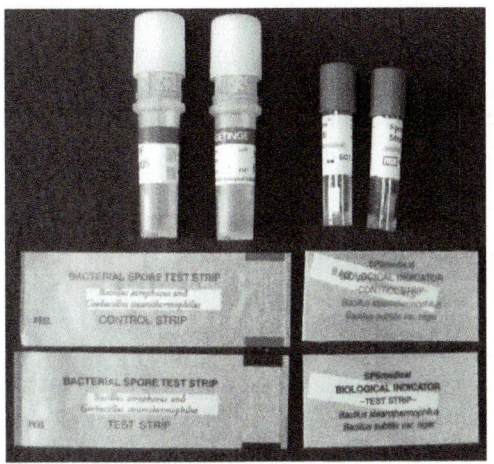
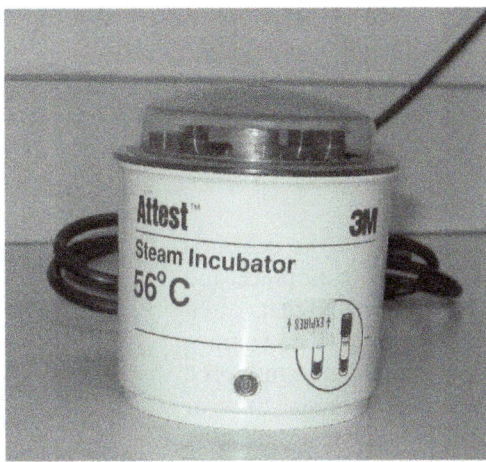

A   B

Figure 14–9 Biologic monitoring. (A) Examples of biologic indicators. **(B)** In-office incubator.

incubator (Figure 14-9B) or at an outside laboratory by a company that specializes in sterilization monitoring. The culturing process takes several days to complete, so the test is not immediate. However, a positive test indicates that the sterilization unit is not working as it should. The CDC, ADA, and OSAP recommend at least weekly biologic monitoring.

It is important to use the correct type of spore strips. Spore strips vary depending on the type of sterilization unit. Some spore strips contain more than one kind of spore and can be used in several different types of units. Check the product labeling to make sure that the spore strips are compatible with the sterilization unit.

The second form of monitoring is *chemical monitoring*. Chemical monitoring uses special chemical labels or inks that react with the sterilization environment. There are two basic types:

- Process indicators are used on the outside of sterilization packages. Examples of process indicators include autoclave tape and color-change labels. These indicators use special ink that change color based upon their exposure to heat. In other words, when the unit hits 270°F (132°C), for example, the tape will change color.
- Dosage indicators are used in sterilization units that rely on chemical vapors at certain concentrations, dry heat, or steam.

Chemical monitoring is useful on a day-to-day basis to confirm that the *conditions* required for sterilization were present. However, neither form of chemical monitoring actually measures the *effectiveness* of sterilization. Neither can confirm that sterilization has actually taken place. As a result, chemical monitoring has to be used in conjunction with biologic monitoring.

Handling and Storage of Sterilized Instruments

The final step in sterilization is handling and storing sterilized instruments. Instruments wrapped in sterilization packages should remain in their packages until they are opened to be used. If a sterilization package is damaged in any way—is ripped, becomes wet, or is punctured—the instruments inside need to be resterilized. The intact packages of sterilized instruments should be stored in a clean, dry, and cool place. There is no limit to how long sterilized instruments can be stored in packages as long as the packaging remains intact.

As a final note, sterilized instruments and packages should never be stored in the same place as precleaned instruments or instruments awaiting sterilization. Sterilization areas should be clearly divided into "clean" areas and "contaminated" areas. Once an object has been sterilized, it should never be taken into the contaminated area.

Procedural Practices and Other Considerations

In addition to the procedures outlined earlier in this chapter, several other practices are commonly used to reduce the risk of infection. The key to any infection control program is consistency and predictability—it makes sense to take any measures that will reduce the risk of microorganisms.

Antiseptic Mouth Rinses

Antiseptic mouth rinses are available to patients for use before procedures. These are not required by OSHA or any other agency, but they are an excellent precaution. An antiseptic mouth rinse will reduce the number of microorganisms in the patient's mouth, minimizing the opportunity

From the Dentist's Perspective

Sterilization is so important to my practice that we make sure to have a posted protocol of monitoring and checking the autoclave machine. But I still encourage my assistants to pay close attention with their ears and eyes. If anything sounds wrong, or the machine just does not appear to be operating correctly, I want them to bring it to my attention so we can check the machine. It's good for our patients, and it's good for the practice.

Voice of Experience

If I have doubts about whether something in the dental office is clean enough, I just ask myself, "Would I let a family member use it?"

for exposure by aeration or spatter. The most common antiseptic mouth rinse is 0.12% chlorhexidine gluconate.

Other Techniques for Infection Control

The following tools are also commonly used for infection control:

- *High-volume evacuator* (HVE). The HVE is designed to reduce spray from the high-speed handpiece and air-water syringe. HVE units have traps that catch items evacuated from the patient's mouth. These traps must be cleaned regularly. Traps should be considered highly contaminated areas, and it is essential to wear proper protective clothing while cleaning and flushing the HVE.
- *Dental dams.* Dental dams are used to reduce saliva and spray during procedures. They are made from rubber and provide a shield over the open oral cavity. Dental dams, however, are not perfect seals, so they provide only partial protection. Masks, gloves, and protective eyewear must still be worn.
- *Disposable supplies.* One-time use, disposable supplies are an excellent way to prevent cross-contamination. These supplies are frequently made from paper, plastic, or light metal. They are designed for a single use and then should be discarded. (To prevent accidental reuse, adopt the habit of crumpling or breaking each supply item—such as snapping a cotton tip applicator—immediately after use.) Never reuse disposable supplies, even in the same patient. Also, such supplies cannot tolerate sterilization or disinfection. They should be disposed of as medical waste. Their major drawback is expense: Disposable supplies are often more expensive than reusable supplies.

> ## Check Your Ethics
>
> As a dental assistant, you observe the dentist "double-dipping" a cotton swab back into the local anesthetic, potentially contaminating the anesthetic. You are not sure if the dentist was aware of doing it—he did not seem to be paying attention—but he is sitting chairside at the moment. What is the appropriate course of action?

Dental Waterlines

Dental waterlines are the small plastic tubes that connect the water supply to the handpiece, air-water syringe, and scaler. These lines are typically 1/8 to 1/16 of an inch in diameter and made from pliable plastic. Like any water-carrying tube or pipe, they can become infected with colonies of bacteria (not viruses, which cannot multiply in waterlines) and pose an infection risk.

Community water is not sterile. All water coming into office buildings, homes, and dental offices carries microorganisms. In the United States, water quality is measured by detecting the levels of coliform bacteria. According to the EPA, community water should contain no more than 500 **colony-forming units** (CFUs) per milliliter (ml). In dental offices, the ADA recommends a lower maximum level of 200 CFUs.

How Waterlines Become Contaminated

Dental waterlines are often more contaminated than regular waterlines because they are potentially contaminated by two sources: community water and backflow.

As water travels through any line, the bacteria, fungi, and other organisms in the water eventually adhere to the line. Once adhered, they are coated with a protective layer of slime. This is known as **biofilm** (Figure 14-10). Biofilm forms anywhere that water is in contact with an appropriate surface. The green film inside a poorly maintained aquarium is an example of biofilm.

However, in addition to the natural organisms carried in community water, dental lines are also exposed to organisms from the patient's oral cavity. When a patient closes his or her mouth around the low-volume saliva ejector and then releases, a vacuum is formed that causes a small amount of saliva to travel backward into the saliva ejector. Additionally, there is a very small risk of backflow into the handpiece or air-water syringe.

Backflow prevention devices are available to reduce the risk of backflow and cross-contamination with the handpiece and air-water syringe. Also, all waterlines and handpieces should be flushed for 20 to 30 seconds between patients to reduce the number of microorganisms in the line.

Maintaining Clean Water

Water quality is a concern with dental waterlines. Several methods are used to obtain the best quality water. According to the CDC, waterlines should be flushed at the beginning of each day.

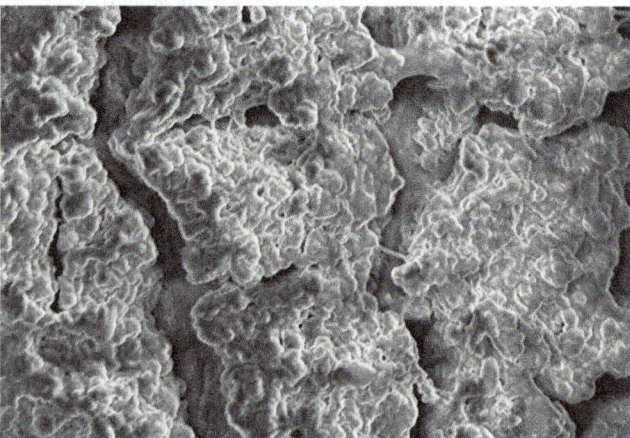

Figure 14-10 **Biofilm.** Scanning electron micrograph of biofilm buildup in a dental waterline, ×2,500.

Microfiltration cartridges can also be installed in the waterlines to help filter out organisms. These disposable cartridges should be inserted as close as possible to the handpiece or air-water syringe, and they must be changed daily.

Newer systems are also equipped with self-contained water reservoirs. These systems have an external water source that usually provides sterile, distilled water to the waterlines. The pressure is supplied by an air pump that pushes the water through the lines. Because the air is a potential source of microbes, the water cannot be considered sterile, but it is much cleaner than community water. These systems must be maintained according to the manufacturer's instructions, including cleaning the water reservoirs and flushing/disinfecting the waterlines. Although the water is higher quality than community water, the lines still need to be cleaned periodically.

Cleaning waterlines is accomplished with chemicals that attack and remove biofilm. Biofilm is very resistant to chemicals, so it's important to follow instructions and regularly maintain the lines. Inadequately maintained lines can result in water with much higher CFUs than even community water.

Two kinds of chemicals are available to reduce biofilm:

- *Continuous-use chemicals*. These are added to the water supply on a constant basis. They can be used with self-contained water systems to even further reduce the level of CFUs. At the concentration they are used, these biocides are not harmful to humans.
- *Shock treatments*. These are strong chemicals that are used specifically to attack biofilm and disinfect waterlines. Household bleach can be used as well as commercial disinfectants. To disinfect the lines, purge them with air, then fill with disinfectant and allow the disinfectant to remain in-line for the appropriate length of time (per the manufacturer's instructions). After disinfecting, purge the chemical from the lines and flush with water before use. Be careful because many of these chemicals can damage the waterlines, so always follow the manufacturer's instructions. This should be done on a weekly basis.

Monitoring Water Quality

The only way to guarantee that water falls within acceptable ranges for CFUs is to test the water coming from the lines. Commercial services are available that will take water samples and test them. Alternatively, water quality indicators (WQIs) are available for in-office use. Follow the manufacturer's instructions for use with a WQI.

Radiography and Laboratory Equipment

Infection control techniques should also extend to the radiography room, darkroom, and anywhere else where potentially contaminated objects are taken. Infection control during radiographic procedures is covered in Chapter 30, Producing Intraoral Dental Radiographs. Infection control during radiograph processing is covered in Chapter 32, Film Processing, Mounting, and Evaluation.

CHECKPOINTS

14-13 What is the difference between disinfection and sterilization?

14-14 What are the two classes of environmental surfaces recognized by the Centers for Disease Control and Prevention?

14-15 What is the purpose of an antiseptic mouth rinse?

14-16 How do dental waterlines become contaminated?

 **Chapter Highlights**

- The chain of infection describes the steps that a microbe takes as it travels from one host to another. Steps include the reservoir, portal of exit, mode of transmission, portal of entry, and susceptible host.
- A reservoir is a hospitable environment where a microbe can thrive and multiply. Humans are excellent reservoirs.
- Modes of transmission include direct, indirect, airborne, and parenteral.
- People with lowered immune function, such as older adults and those suffering from an illness, are more vulnerable to infection.
- Universal precautions were developed to help health care providers deal with infection risk. According to universal precautions, all blood should be treated as if it is potentially infectious.

- Universal precautions were expanded into standard precautions, which recommend that all bodily fluids and patients be treated as potentially infectious.
- The Centers for Disease Control and Prevention's *Guidelines for Infectious Control in Dental Healthcare Settings—2003* are the standard for infection control in the dental industry. In 2007, the CDC updated the standard precautions, and, in 2008, they published an update for disinfection and sterilization procedures in health care facilities, including dental offices.
- According to the Centers for Disease Control and Prevention, hands should be washed when they are visibly dirty, after touching possibly contaminated objects or patients, and immediately after removing examination gloves.
- Protective masks, eyewear, and clothing should be worn to prevent the spread of infection.

+ Types of gloves include examination gloves, surgical gloves, utility gloves, over-gloves, and autoclavable utility gloves.
+ Latex allergies are on the rise. Employees and patients who are sensitive to latex should be provided a latex-free environment.
+ The Occupational Safety and Health Administration's Bloodborne Pathogen Standard regulates the use of sharps and exposure incidents to possibly contaminated blood.
+ Disinfection is the removal of most microorganisms from an object or surface. Disinfection guidelines are issued by the Centers for Disease Control and Prevention.
+ Sterilization is the complete removal of microorganisms from an object or surface. Sterilization guidelines are issued by the Centers for Disease Control and Prevention. Different types of sterilization include steam pressure (autoclave), chemicals, and heat.
+ Each dental office should have a clearly defined protocol for disinfection and sterilization.
+ Dental waterlines can become contaminated with bacteria and fungi. Waterlines should be flushed daily and chemically cleaned weekly to remove biofilm.

 **Review Questions**

1. A reservoir of infection is
   a. A hospitable environment where a microbe can multiply.
   b. A large group of microbes.
   c. A liquid that contains living organisms.
   d. A method of treating infection.

2. Infectious organisms can gain access into the body in which of the following ways?
   a. Breaks in the skin
   b. Mucous membranes
   c. Inhalation
   d. All of the above

3. According to standard precautions
   a. All blood should be tested for human immunodeficiency virus/acquired immune deficiency syndrome and hepatitis.
   b. Dental assistants should take extra precaution with sick patients.
   c. All bodily fluids should be treated as contaminated.
   d. Patients should be asked for their infection status before all procedures.

4. Masks
   a. Do not need to be worn with face shields.
   b. Should be replaced after every patient.
   c. Should be replaced at the end of every day.
   d. Can be worn around the neck when not in use.

5. Examination gloves
   a. Should be washed thoroughly between patients.
   b. Should never come into contact with many common chemicals.
   c. Should never come into contact with anything outside the exam area.
   d. b and c.

6. Latex allergies
   a. Are becoming less common.
   b. Are not dangerous.
   c. Result from infrequent contact with poorly washed latex.
   d. Range in severity from mild to life threatening.

7. According to the Bloodborne Pathogen Standard
   a. Only blood should be considered contaminated.
   b. Only visibly infected fluids are dangerous.
   c. All bodily fluids should be considered infectious.
   d. All blood should be tested for infectious organisms after exposure.

8. After an exposure to potentially contaminated blood
   a. Employees must report it immediately.
   b. Employers have to refer employees to a qualified health care professional for an examination.
   c. The incident has to be documented.
   d. All of the above.

9. A sterile object
   a. Has no living organisms on it.
   b. Has fewer living organisms on it.
   c. Is freshly cleaned.
   d. Cannot be contaminated.

10. A high-level disinfectant is one that
    a. Sterilizes objects after short exposure.
    b. Is commonly used to disinfect surfaces.
    c. Kills most organisms.
    d. Kills viruses.

11. Which two disinfectants are also used as sterilants?

　a. Chlorine dioxide and iodophor

　b. Glutaraldehyde and chlorine dioxide

　c. Sodium hypochlorite and glutaraldehyde

　d. Synthetic phenols and iodophor

12. What is the purpose of ultrasonic cleaners?

　a. To sterilize instruments

　b. To remove unsightly abrasions and stains

　c. To prepare items for sterilization

　d. To reduce the risk of puncture during dental procedures

13. According to the Centers for Disease Control and Prevention, which instruments should be sterilized?

　a. Noncritical instruments

　b. Semicritical instruments

　c. Critical instruments

　d. Semicritical and critical instruments

14. What is the main drawback to liquid chemical sterilization?

　a. Length of processing time

　b. Cannot sterilize plastics

　c. High heat

　d. Dangerous to operators

15. Biologic monitoring

　a. Tests to see if the conditions are appropriate for sterilization.

　b. Is the only true test of a sterilization unit.

　c. Is not dependable.

　d. Can only be conducted by outside labs.

16. To combat biofilm, dental waterlines should be disinfected

　a. Daily.

　b. Weekly.

　c. Monthly.

　d. Annually.

Active Learning Exercises

1.　List the Environmental Protection Agency's three disinfection levels. List corresponding disinfectants that fall under each category. Create a chart that could be used in the office for all employees listing the efficacy and advantages and disadvantages of each.

2.　What are the differences between biological monitors and process indicators? How and when are they used? Why is autoclave tape not an indication that sterilization has been attained?

3.　What three factors must be achieved in order to ensure sterilization has taken place in a steam autoclave? List them and the appropriate recommendations for use.

Application Activities

1.　Visit the Occupational Safety and Health Administration (OSHA) website (www.osha.gov) and locate the Bloodborne Pathogens Standard. Take some time to read through the provisions outlined in the document and think about how these standards apply in a dental office. Write down three scenarios involving potential exposure to bloodborne pathogens in a dental office and describe what you could do to maintain compliance with the OSHA standards.

2.　Think about the last time you had an infection. Review the chain of infection described at the beginning of the chapter and write down how each step in the chain applied to your own infection.

3.　Practice following the handwashing techniques described in Procedure 14-1.

PREPARING FOR CERTIFICATION EXAMS

Review the following topics in this chapter to prepare for the Dental Assisting National Board (DANB) exam:

- **The Chain of Infection**
- **Types of Infections**
- **Infection Control Practices**
- **Disinfection**
- **Environmental Infection Control**
- **Sterilization**
- **Procedural Practices and Other Considerations**

chapter 15

Safety Regulations

CHAPTER OUTLINE

Introduction

Government and Professional Agencies

Waste Management

    Classification of Waste

Dental Office Waste

Hazardous Materials

    Chemical Exposure

    Physical Hazards and Spills

Biological Hazards

CHAPTER CHECKLIST

On completion of this chapter, students will be able to:

- ☑ Define *recommendations* and *regulations*.
- ☑ Identify types of waste commonly encountered in a dental setting, the two categories of waste, and the proper procedures for disposal.
- ☑ Identify hazardous materials commonly used in a dental office and understand their labels.
- ☑ Identify three common means of chemical exposure.
- ☑ Describe the main components of the Hazard Communication Standard.
- ☑ Describe safety measures available for handling physical hazards and spills.
- ☑ Describe the procedures for correctly handling biological hazards.

KEY TERMS

acute toxicity – a medical condition caused by exposure to high levels of a toxic substance such as a chemical; acute toxic reactions typically occur within minutes of exposure and can include a range of symptoms from minor to life threatening

chronic toxicity – a medical condition caused by exposure to lower levels of a toxic substance over time; chronic toxic reactions often take years to become apparent and are often characterized by diffuse symptoms and organ damage, such as cancer, or kidney or liver failure

nonregulated waste – waste that is not regulated by any government agency, including normal office waste and used barrier material

regulated waste – hazardous waste that falls under the jurisdiction of a government agency, such as the Occupational Safety and Health Administration and the Environmental Protection Agency, or a local agency; regulated waste includes hazardous chemicals and potentially contaminated materials

Introduction

Infectious organisms are not the only potential dangers in dental offices. This chapter examines some of the chemicals and other hazardous materials that are commonly used in dentistry. It is important that dental assistants (DAs) are aware of the possible dangers in the office and the rules and regulations surrounding the use of hazardous materials.

Every dental office should have a written plan for handling hazardous materials. This plan should include descriptions of the materials used in the office, describe the handling and disposal requirements, and identify the person in charge of making sure that chemicals are stored safely and disposed of properly.

Government and Professional Agencies

The dental office is governed by a number of agencies, both professional and governmental. The most important of these include the American Dental Association (ADA), the Centers for Disease Control and Prevention (CDC), the Occupational Safety and Health Administration (OSHA), and the Environmental Protection Agency (EPA). Each of these organizations issues recommendations or regulations to help guide office practices.

- *Recommendations* are advisory standards issued by either professional associations or government entities. A recommendation does not carry the full weight of law, and, in the case of the CDC, recommendations are often ranked according to the weight of scientific evidence backing them up.
- *Regulations* are laws that must be followed. They are issued by governmental entities such as OSHA. New regulations are introduced relatively frequently. Typically, a regulation is proposed, and then there is a public comment period during which the affected groups can attempt to influence the regulation. After this period is over, the regulation is issued in its final form. There is usually an adoption period allowed so dental offices will have time to adapt to the new regulations. Regulations also have enforcement mechanisms, such as licenses, inspections, and fines for breaking the rules. Regulations can either be issued by regulatory agencies, or they can be passed as laws by state or federal governments.

A full list of professional associations and agencies that are active in dentistry can be found in Chapter 14, Disease and Infection Control.

CHECKPOINT
15-1 What is the difference between a recommendation and a regulation?

Waste Management

During the course of a normal day, DAs may be exposed to a number of potentially dangerous substances, objects, and chemicals. To keep the dental team safe, regulations have been designed to help manage the use and disposal of these items. The exact regulatory body that controls a given hazardous material depends on the nature of the material and where it is used.

For example, OSHA regulates the use of hazardous chemicals and potentially infectious items while they are being used in the office. Once these items are disposed of, however, many of them come under the jurisdiction of the EPA, which regulates items for their environmental impact.

Classification of Waste

Dental office waste falls into one of two categories:

- **Regulated waste**. This category includes sharps (e.g., used needles, scalpels, burs, orthodontic brackets and wires, and endodontic files and reamers). Other items of regulated waste include blood and objects that are soaked, caked, or drenched with blood or saliva; human tissue; and pathological waste. Special and very specific regulations govern the disposal of regulated waste. However, it is important to note that states and cities might have additional rules of their own. Dental offices should inquire with their local government agency, at the city and state levels, to make sure that all of the applicable laws are being followed.
- **Nonregulated waste**. Nonregulated waste includes used disposable barriers, nonbloody gauze, and other nonblood-related items that were used in the treatment room.

From Classroom to Clinic

In the clinical setting, not all items can be disposed of with "regular" trash, and it is essential that the dental assistant carefully follows waste management guidelines. It may even be up to you to educate the team members in your office about *nonregulated* versus *regulated* waste.

Figure 15–1 Biohazard symbol.

Regardless of the category of waste, any container of potentially infectious material must be clearly marked with a biohazard warning sign (Figure 15-1). This is for the safety of both the public and employees.

From the Dentist's Perspective

I cannot stress enough how important it is to have dental assistants who know how to handle waste properly. In our busy practice, we generate many kinds of waste, and we live in a town with strict environmental regulations. All it takes is one mistake to incur a hefty fine, so experienced, knowledgeable assistants can really save the practice!

Dental Office Waste

Like any medical office, dental offices generate a wide range of waste products that need to be disposed of safely and with as little environmental impact as possible. As previously mentioned, any disposal container that holds potentially infectious material must be labeled with a biohazard warning label. Guidelines for specific types of waste are outlined in the next sections.

Extracted Teeth

Extracted teeth are regulated waste because they are potentially infectious. The only exception is if the teeth are sterilized and returned to the patients. Before disposal, teeth should be sterilized, either in a chemical immersion bath or with a steam autoclave sterilization unit. Teeth that contain amalgam should never be sterilized in a steam or dry heat unit, however, because the heat can cause the amalgam to release toxic mercury vapors, which, when heated, become eight times more toxic. These teeth should be sterilized in an immersion chemical bath. After teeth are sterilized, they can be disposed of according to state or local regulations.

Sharps

Sharps are defined as any object that is capable of slicing, cutting, or puncturing the skin and potentially transmitting infectious diseases. These objects must be placed in

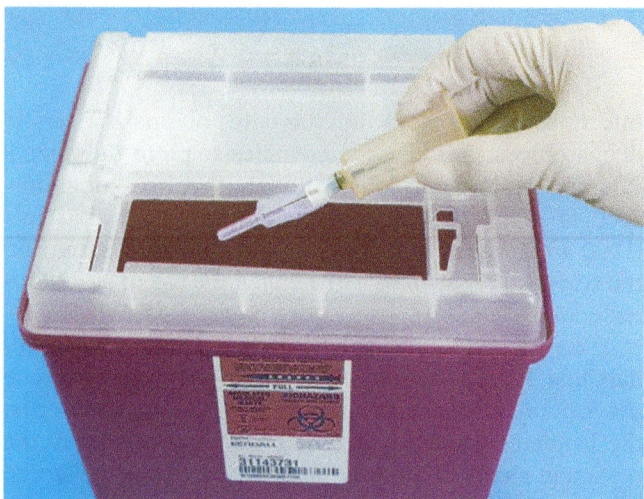

Figure 15–2 Sharps container. Note the biohazard symbol on the container.

special sharps containers (Figure 15-2). A sharps container is usually red, for identification purposes, and should be:

- Leak proof
- Clearly labeled for sharps
- Puncture resistant
- Equipped with a lid or cap

Once the sharps container is full, it should be sealed; sterilized, if possible, in the autoclave; and sent to an agency that specializes in sharps disposal. For more information on sharps disposal and what goes into sharps containers, please see Chapter 14, Disease and Infection Control.

Radiographic Supplies

Radiographic procedures generate several kinds of waste, including nonregulated barriers; potentially contaminated biohazardous and disposable waste, such as saliva-soaked cotton rolls; and chemicals used during processing. Each of these must be handled in accordance with its type of waste.

Any regulated, potentially infectious waste, such as saliva-soaked cotton rolls, should be disposed of by placing these items in containers labeled as biohazardous and sent to the appropriate waste facility. This kind of waste is regulated by the EPA and sometimes also by local and state laws.

Chemicals used during radiographic processing include:

- *Fixer*. Fixer is high in silver nitrate, which is a toxic metal. This kind of waste is either treated on-site in the dental office, or sent off-site for treatment. An on-site treatment program uses a special silver recovery unit that removes toxic silver from the solution. If the solution will be processed off-site, it should be safely stored in sealed containers until the disposal company can pick it up. Disposal companies should be able to offer advice and guidelines on how to package and store silver solution.

- *Developer*. Developer is considered a hazardous waste because of its high pH (it is a strong base). Liquids with pH levels outside of acceptable ranges might damage the local water treatment facilities or plumbing if they are poured down drains. Contact local governmental agencies for guidelines on how to dispose of these chemicals.

Objects Containing Lead

Lead is an environmental contaminant, and the EPA regulates its disposal. High lead levels in water and the environment are related to damage to wildlife and humans. Dental offices generate several forms of lead-containing waste:

- *Lead foil*. Radiograph film packets contain lead foil to protect the unexposed film. These can be recycled through a licensed recovery facility. Lead-based foil should not be thrown in the regular garbage or it will contaminate landfills and potentially contaminate groundwater.
- *Lead-lined boxes*. At one time, dental film was commonly stored in lead-lined boxes to protect it from scatter radiation and ruin. These boxes were typically covered on the inside with unpainted lead, and it was not uncommon that the film inside would become covered with a fine powder of lead oxide. The U.S. Food and Drug Administration recommends that these boxes no longer be used, and they are no longer on the market. Film should be stored according to the manufacturer's instructions. If a dental office has one of these boxes, it should be sent to an appropriate recovery and recycling facility in the community. Lead-lined boxes should *never* be disposed of in the garbage.

Amalgam

Scrap dental amalgam contains mercury, which is regulated as a hazardous material. Mercury vapor is highly toxic, and mercury contamination in groundwater supplies is dangerous to wildlife and humans. Numerous studies have shown that mercury contamination is common among open-ocean and freshwater fish.

Mercury amalgam waste should be stored in a designated, clearly labeled container. The label should contain the date the container was designated for use as an amalgam waste container, along with the name, address, and phone number of the dental practice. If the amalgam is stored in liquid, the liquid should be considered highly contaminated with mercury traces and never poured down the drain, where it would eventually reach the community water supply. Amalgam containers should be handled by a mercury disposal company according to local and EPA regulations.

Disinfectants and Cleaners

A number of cleaners and disinfectants are commonly used in the dental office. Disinfectants that are used as immersion sterilants should be considered contaminated with infectious organisms and disposed of as biohazardous material. Solutions containing more than 2% glutaraldehyde are usually regulated as hazardous waste, while solutions containing less than 2% glutaraldehyde can sometimes be poured into the drain. Disposal of these solutions also depends on the flashpoint. Call the local waste management agency for specific guidelines for handling used disinfectants and cleaners.

Additionally, the containers used to hold disinfectants, cleaners, and other chemicals should be considered hazardous. Never use empty chemical containers to hold another chemical because there is a risk of a chemical reaction. Guidelines for disposing of empty containers are found on the product label or the material safety data sheet (discussed later in the chapter). Local waste management companies can also advise on how to dispose of used containers.

CHECKPOINTS

15-2 What are the two categories of dental waste?

15-3 What is a sharp?

15-4 What component of amalgam requires regulation as a hazardous material?

Hazardous Materials

Like blood, hazardous chemicals in the dental office fall under the jurisdiction of OSHA. Hazardous chemicals are defined as any chemical that can cause injury or a health hazard. This class includes cleaners, disinfectants, and sterilants as well as the numerous chemicals used to process radiograph film, create amalgam, and for other functions. Chemicals are considered hazardous if they are toxic, flammable, corrosive, or can form toxic compounds when mixed with other chemicals.

Chemical Exposure

There are numerous ways DAs might come into contact with hazardous chemicals in the office:

- *Skin contact*. Skin contact occurs when the chemical comes into contact with unprotected skin. Some chemicals are reactive with the materials found in examination gloves and other items of personal protective equipment. It is important to take the necessary precautions, including wearing the right forms of protection, when working with chemicals that can damage on contact. Not all chemicals will cause immediate injury upon contact. In some cases, repeated contact will slowly develop into a nonallergic condition called *contact dermatitis*. This is a skin condition characterized by rashes, redness, and irritation.

- *Inhalation*. Inhalation occurs when a person breathes in vapors, fumes, dust, or gases of hazardous chemicals. This can cause direct damage to the lungs, either immediately or over time. Alternatively, the chemicals can be absorbed through the tiny blood vessels in the lungs and enter the blood stream.
- *Ingestion*. Ingestion occurs when a person inadvertently swallows or eats a hazardous chemical. This is relatively uncommon in dental offices, but can happen if hands are not washed properly before lunch or if food is eaten in areas where chemicals are handled.

Chemical exposure, and the damage it causes, is usually *dose dependent*. In other words, the danger is related to how much of the chemical was present and how long it remained in contact. Damage that occurs very quickly, after a very short exposure, is known as **acute toxicity**. An example of acute toxicity is a chemical burn after spilling a strong acid or base on bare skin. Symptoms of acute toxicity depend on the chemical, but they are often strong and might include nausea, burning eyes and blurring vision, vomiting, burning lungs and throat, headache, and fainting.

An acute chemical exposure should be treated as a medical emergency. However, be aware that treatment varies for different types of chemical exposure, and it is never safe to guess at the appropriate course of action after an exposure. Follow the treatment guidelines listed in the material safety data sheet for the chemical, described below.

In contrast, **chronic toxicity** occurs over time, usually after exposure to much smaller amounts on a consistent basis. Chronic toxicity often has no immediate symptoms or only minor symptoms that are easily dismissed. An example might be breathing vapors from an exposed chemical over months or even years. Depending on the chemical, chronic toxicity raises the risk of developing internal diseases, including certain cancers, liver and kidney diseases, nerve disorders, and fertility problems.

Acute and chronic exposure events can occur with the same chemicals. The difference is usually the amount and length of exposure. Acute events are characterized by greater exposure to more chemicals.

Check Your Ethics

You see an employee dumping large amounts of chemical fixer down the drain. The employee sees you, and knows you saw him dumping the fixer. He asks you not to say anything so he will not get in trouble. What should you do?

OSHA's Hazard Communication Standard

OSHA's Hazard Communication Standard is designed to protect employees from exposure to hazardous chemicals, and, if exposure does occur, protect them from future injury and provide a guide on how to handle an exposure incident. It is the companion guideline to the Bloodborne Pathogen Standard.

Under the Hazard Communication Standard, employers must alert employees about hazardous chemicals used in the workplace and develop a *hazard communication program*. The aim of a hazard communication program has several elements, each of which must be completed. According to the Hazard Communication Standard, new employees must be trained in the use and handling of hazardous chemicals within 30 days of beginning employment and annually thereafter. A certificate of training must be kept within the employee's personnel file.

Elements of the Hazard Communication Standard include:

- A chemical inventory form
- A material safety data sheet
- Labeling of all chemicals with quantity, physical state, and hazard class, among other elements

Chemical Inventory Form

The chemical inventory is a complete list of all the hazardous chemicals used in the office. This list should include cleaners, sterilants, composites and bonding materials, amalgam, impression agents, and anything that might pose a threat. The list must be updated every time a new hazardous material enters the office. The chemical inventory should also include a material safety data sheet for every chemical present (see below).

Material Safety Data Sheets

The material safety data sheet (MSDS) is provided by the manufacturer. Even though the dental practice may receive the MSDS from the dental vendor, the law requires the manufacturer to generate this document. This all-encompassing document includes critical information about the chemical's toxicity as well as information on how to handle exposure events. Each chemical in the office must have an MSDS on file in the chemical inventory. If no MSDS is provided by the manufacturer, whoever coordinates the Hazard Communication Standard program from the dental office should call and obtain it as soon as possible. This is a legal requirement.

The MSDS provides a wealth of data about a chemical, including its ingredients, properties and uses, and detailed hazard data. See Table 15-1 for descriptions of the information provided on the MSDS.

TABLE 15-1 **Sections of a Material Safety Data Sheet**

SECTION	TITLE	DESCRIPTION
I	Product Identification	Provides manufacturer, including address and contact information. Also provides product name and number and emergency contact information.
II	Hazardous Ingredients of Mixtures	Contains a list of all hazardous ingredients, sorted by percentage of product weight and permissible exposure limit. This information must match the product label.
III	Physical Data	Describes the material and gives some of its physical properties, such as evaporation rate, freezing point, boiling point, and others.
IV	Fire and Explosion	Describes the material's flashpoint and firefighting procedures to put out a fire. Also describes any potential toxins released as a result of a fire.
V	Reactivity Data	Describes the material's stability and lists any other materials with which the product might be incompatible.
VI	Health Hazard Data	Describes the health hazards associated with the material, including symptoms of overexposure, routes of exposure, and chronic and subchronic effects.
VII	Emergency and First Aid Procedures	Describes how to treat exposure incidents (e.g., in case of contact with eyes or skin).
VIII	Spill and Leak Procedures	Describes how to handle leaks and disposal.
IX	Protection Measures	Lists all the protection measures that should be taken when using and handling the material, including personal protective measures, such as gloves, eye protection, and inhalation protection.
X	Special Precautions	Describes any special or unique precautions that should be taken when handling, storing, or transporting the product.

Voice of Experience

Every employee in our office is trained on how to read material safety data sheets (MSDSs) and use the MSDS log, but only one dental assistant is put in charge of the log. Although it might seem like just paperwork, this is an important responsibility. The MSDS log has an alphabetized list of every chemical we use, and, in an emergency, it is an invaluable resource because it tells us exactly how to locate the MSDS.

Product Labeling

Much of the information on the MSDS is duplicated on the product's label. If a manufacturer's label is not on the container, the dental office should label the container and make information on its contents available to employees. All containers in the office should be clearly labeled with their contents. This includes containers in which disinfectants or cleaners are mixed prior to use such as placing materials in separate spray bottles.

The only exceptions to this labeling requirement are certain consumer products, such as food products, drugs, cosmetics, alcoholic beverages, and tobacco products. Over-the-counter drugs are also exempt from labeling standards if they are intended to be used by employees within the office.

National Fire Protection Association Labels

The National Fire Protection Association (NFPA) has devised a widely used labeling system that alerts people to the contents of any container (Figure 15-3). A simple diagram on the container is easy to understand and quickly communicates hazards associated with the chemicals inside the container.

The NFPA symbol is a color-coded diamond with four sections (blue, red, yellow, and white). Each section is associated with a different property, and each is assigned a number from 0 to 4 to describe the danger of the material within. The higher the number is, the greater the danger. The only exception is the white diamond, which is assigned either a ₩ or OX symbol to describe its reactivity. The breakdown of the label is:

RED: Flammability
   0 = Nonflammable
   1 = Combustible if heated
   2 = Combustible liquid flashpoint of 100°F to 200°F
   3 = Flammable liquid flashpoint below 100°F
   4 = Highly flammable gas or liquid

BLUE: Health Hazard
   0 = No hazard
   1 = Possibly irritating
   2 = Harmful if inhaled or absorbed

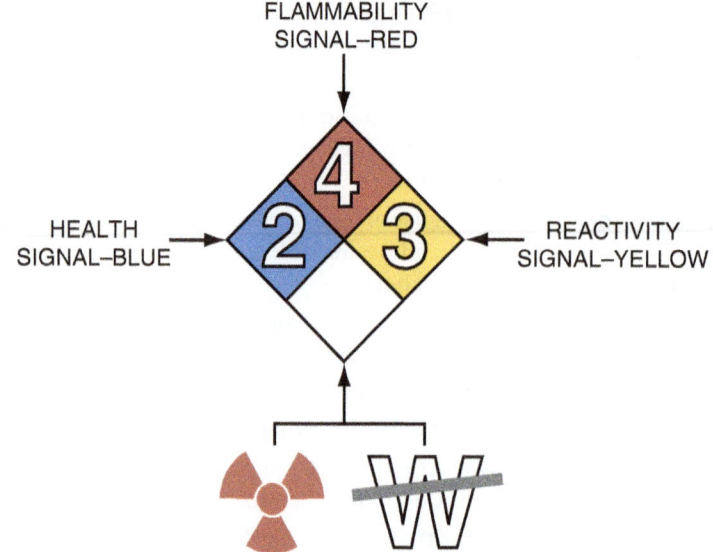

FLAMMABILITY
SIGNAL–RED

HEALTH
SIGNAL–BLUE

REACTIVITY
SIGNAL–YELLOW

RADIOACTIVE OR WATER REACTIVE

Identification of Health Hazard Color Code: **BLUE**		Identification of Flammability Color Code: **RED**		Identification of Reactivity (Stability) Color Code: **YELLOW**	
	Type of possible injury		Susceptibility of materials to burning		Susceptibility to release of energy
SIGNAL		SIGNAL		SIGNAL	
4	Materials that on very short exposure could cause death or major residual injury even though prompt medical treatment was given.	4	Materials that will rapidly or completely vaporize at atmospheric pressure and normal ambient temperature, or that are readily dispersed in air and that will burn readily.	4	Materials that in themselves are readily capable of detonation or of explosive decomposition or reaction at normal temperatures and pressures.
3	Materials that on short exposure could cause serious temporary or residual injury even though prompt medical treatment was given.	3	Liquids and solids that can be ignited under almost all ambient temperature conditions.	3	Materials that in themselves are capable of detonation or explosive reaction but require a strong initiating source or that must be heated under confinement before initiation or that react explosively with water.
2	Materials that on intense or continued exposure could cause temporary incapacitation or possible residual injury unless prompt medical treatment is given.	2	Materials that must be moderately heated or exposed to relatively high ambient temperatures before ignition can occur.	2	Materials that in themselves are normally unstable and readily undergo violent chemical change but do not detonate. Also materials that may react violently with water or that may form potentially explosive mixtures with water.
1	Materials that on exposure would cause irritation but only minor residual injury even if no treatment is given.	1	Materials that must be preheated before ignition can occur.	1	Materials that in themselves are normally stable, but that can become unstable at elevated temperatures and pressures or that may react with water with some release of energy, but not violently.
0	Materials that on exposure under fire conditions would offer no hazard beyond that of ordinary combustible material.	0	Materials that will not burn.	0	Materials that in themselves are normally stable, even under fire exposure conditions, and that are not reactive with water.

Figure 15–3 National Fire Protection Association 704 marking system.

3 = Corrosive or toxic; avoid contact or inhalation

4 = Potentially fatal with short exposure

YELLOW: Instability

    0 = Not reactive when mixed with water

    1 = May mildly react if heated or mixed with water

    2 = Unstable and may violently react if mixed with water

    3 = Potentially explosive if shocked, heated under confinement, or mixed with water

    4 = Explosive at room temperature

WHITE: Special Notice

    W̶ = Reactive with water

    OX = Oxidizing agent

With regard to the white section, these are the only two symbols approved by the NFPA. However, some companies add symbols identifying what personal protective equipment (PPE) should be used when handling the chemicals or other symbols describing if the chemical inside is corrosive. The NFPA designed its symbol to be simple and easily understood, however, and does not condone the use of extra symbols within any of its quadrants.

Physical Hazards and Spills

Despite the best precautions, spills and exposure incidents still occur. It is essential that every dental office have a hazardous material plan, which is maintained and updated by one of the office employees. As part of the Hazard Communication Standard, every employee must be trained in this plan as well as handling and storing the chemicals in the office.

Safety measures are described below.

Hand Protection

Hand protection is essential while working with chemicals. Even chemicals that may not cause immediate damage can result in chronic injury through long-term exposure. Gloves should always be used with hazardous chemicals, but it's important to note that latex and nonlatex examination gloves are not protective against hazardous chemicals. In fact, some chemicals can react with latex.

Instead, chemical-resistant utility gloves should be worn when handling toxic material (refer back to Chapter 14, Figure 14-6D). These gloves are made from a variety of materials, including neoprene or industrial-grade nitrile. If there is any question about which form of hand protection to use, consult the MSDS or the product label, which should contain information about safety precautions for handling the material.

Eyewash Units and Eye Protection

The eyes are particularly vulnerable to certain chemicals. Splashes, droplets, vapors, and sprays all pose a potentially serious threat to eye health, including potential blindness.

Accidents can occur when carrying containers full of chemicals, pouring chemicals, or using them. Protective eyewear should always be used. Similar to the eyewear used in infection control, the eyewear should have side panels to protect the eyes from the side. Eyewear should conform to the face, leaving little room for droplets to run down under the lenses.

Although curing lights or lasers are not chemicals, eyewear should nevertheless be worn when working with them. These devices can cause damage to the eyes. Check with the manufacturer of the device to see what form of eyewear is recommended.

In case a chemical accidentally gets into the eye, OSHA requires that all workplaces that use chemicals have eyewash stations (Figure 15-4). A variety of eyewash stations are commercially available. Some units hook up to normal faucets and produce a wide, gentle jet of water that can be used to irrigate and flush out the eye. Alternatively, wall-mounted units used solely for eyewashing are available.

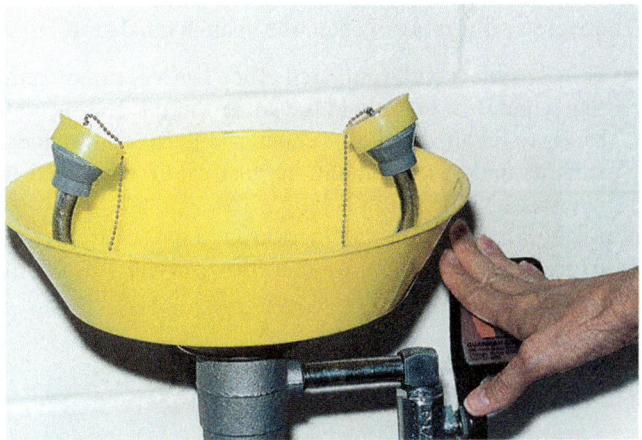

A

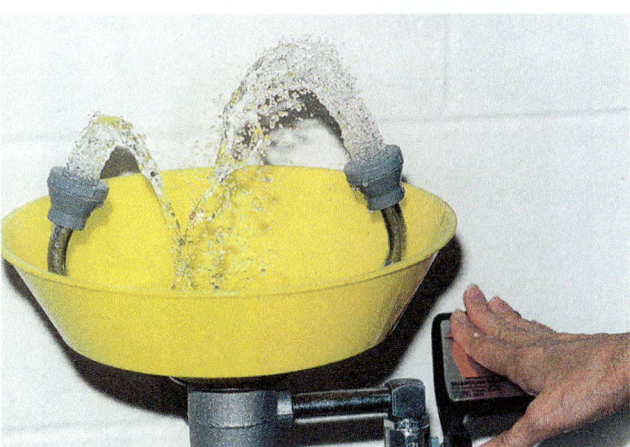

B

Figure 15–4 Eyewash station. (A) Press the lever at the right of the basin. **(B)** The stream of water forces the caps from the nozzles. Lower your face and eyes into the stream and continue to wash the area until eyes are clear.

According to OSHA, all eyewash stations should be inspected monthly, and a record must be kept of the inspections. Additionally, many dental offices run wall-mounted eyewash stations for 3 minutes every week to flush the waterlines of microbial buildup.

All employees must be trained in the proper use of an eyewash station.

Protective Clothing

Items of protective clothing include gowns, jackets, and rubber and neoprene aprons. The aprons are recommended when mixing corrosive chemicals or working in the darkroom. For further information on protective measures, the chemical's MSDS sheet or label should have handling precautions and recommendations for what PPE to wear. See Chapter 14, Disease and Infection Control, for more information on protective clothing and equipment.

Inhalation Protection

There are two forms of protection against inhalation:

- *Ventilation.* A well-ventilated office has less fumes, particles, and dust floating in the air, so there is less opportunity to inhale dangerous chemicals. Even small spaces, such as darkrooms, should be adequately ventilated if chemicals are in use.
- *Face masks.* Most examination face masks are made from paper and may or may not provide the level of protection necessary for chemicals. People who are particularly sensitive to any chemicals, or who have allergies or asthma, might want to use a mist respirator face mask. Any face mask should both be fluid repellant and protect from particle inhalation (Figure 15-5).

Cleaning Broken Glass

Broken glass is considered a sharp, and, depending on what was in the glass container, it may be potentially contaminated. DAs should never handle broken glass because of the risk of tear or puncture wound. Instead, glass should be swept into a dustpan or onto a sheet of cardboard and then disposed of in a sharps container.

Laundry Procedures

Laundry items, such as gowns, aprons, coats, and scrubs, should be considered potentially contaminated and, if they were worn during cleaning or handling chemicals, a possible chemical hazard. Laundry should be removed carefully to prevent contamination of the clothes underneath and any direct contact between exposed skin and potentially dangerous substances on the laundry. Gloves should always be worn when working with laundry. Laundry should be placed into a container that is clearly labeled with the biohazard label. Laundry is typically sent off-site for cleaning by companies that specialize in medical laundry. Consult with the laundry company to get their list of precautions and packing instructions.

Handling Chemical Spills

Despite the best precautions, chemical spills will sometimes happen. In the event of a chemical spill, the MSDS or product label should be consulted immediately to learn the best way to clean it up. During the clean-up, DAs should wear appropriate PPE and take every precaution. Water should never be automatically thrown onto a chemical spill unless the MSDS indicates that water is safe, and the chemical will not react with the water.

Special care should be taken with mercury, which is used in amalgam. Mercury is highly toxic even in small doses. It can be absorbed through the skin and the vapors can be inhaled. Mercury has been shown to cause genetic mutations in animals and humans after exposure. All dental offices should be equipped with a mercury spill kit. The mercury spill kit will include the tools used to clean mercury spills—mercury-absorbing powder, mercury-absorbing sponges, and disposal equipment—and thorough instructions on their use. Appropriate PPE includes utility gloves, masks, and eye protection. Mercury should always be disposed of according to local ordinances. If the office does not have a mercury spill kit, a turkey baster or eye dropper may be used to draw up the spilled

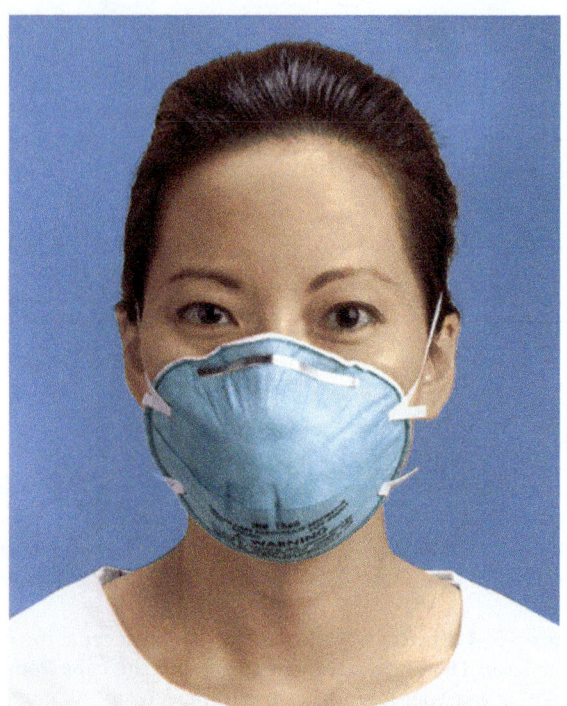

Figure 15–5 N95 respirator face mask. (Courtesy Brevis Corp. Salt Lake City, UT.)

mercury. Never use a vacuum because the heat generated from the vacuum will make the spill vapors eight times more toxic.

Biological Hazards

Biological hazards in the dental office include infectious organisms such as bacteria and viruses. These topics are covered in depth in Chapters 13, Understanding Microbiology, and 14, Disease and Infection Control.

Control of biological hazards includes:

- *Handwashing and PPE.* Both handwashing and PPE are also used in the handling of hazardous chemicals. It's important to note the differences, however. Some chemicals react with water and should not be washed off with water immediately. Also, the gloves used to protect DAs from infectious organisms are not protective against corrosive chemicals. Special chemical-resistant gloves should be used when handling chemicals. Eye protection, aprons, masks, and other items of PPE are often the same, but remember that any PPE that was potentially exposed to contaminated bodily fluids should be treated as contaminated and removed as soon as possible.
- *OSHA's Bloodborne Pathogen Standard.* The Bloodborne Pathogen Standard is the companion policy to the Hazard Communication Standard. This standard is designed to educate workers about the risks of infectious diseases carried by objects and fluids that are potentially contaminated with blood. According to the Bloodborne Pathogen Standard, all potentially infectious materials, such as blood, saliva, cerebrospinal fluid, and other body fluids should be treated as potentially contaminated. The standard also clearly spells out the rights and responsibilities of employers and employees after a possible exposure to a bloodborne disease.
- *Sharps management.* Sharps include needles, scalpels, burs, broken glass, and any other object that can easily pierce protective barriers and skin. According to the Bloodborne Pathogen Standard, sharps containers should be readily accessible and close to the work area. They must be clearly labeled as sharps containers, puncture resistant, leak proof, and covered.
- *Disinfection and sterilization.* Disinfectants and sterilants are considered hazardous chemicals. Their use in the office is regulated by OSHA, and their disposal is often regulated by the EPA or by local ordinance.

Following OSHA Regulations

As a final note on OSHA's Bloodborne Pathogen Standard and Hazard Communication Standard, copies of the regulations are provided through OSHA at no cost (www.osha.gov). Dental offices are required by law to provide training in OSHA regulations and to keep records of steps taken to comply with the regulations. Exposure events are also required to be documented. To effectively manage OSHA programs, one employee should be given overall responsibility for the Bloodborne Pathogen Standard and Hazard Communication Standard programs, including record keeping and making sure the regulations are followed. This person is often a DA.

CHECKPOINTS

15-5 Which government agency regulates hazardous chemicals?

15-6 What are some of the means by which members of the dental office team might come into contact with hazardous chemicals at work?

15-7 Which chemicals in a dental office must include a MSDS on file?

15-8 Can examination gloves be used as protection when handling hazardous chemicals?

15-9 How often should eyewash stations be inspected?

15-10 What are the two forms of protection against inhalation of hazardous materials?

Chapter Highlights

- ✦ Hazardous materials in the dental office include chemicals and materials, such as amalgam, bonding agents, bleaches, and acid etch.
- ✦ A regulation is a law that must be followed. Regulations are issued by government agencies, such as the Occupational Safety and Health Administration and the Environmental Protection Agency as well as local governmental bodies.
- ✦ Regulated waste is waste whose handling and disposal falls under the jurisdiction of a governmental body. This includes potentially contaminated waste, biological waste, and many chemicals.
- ✦ Extracted teeth must be sterilized before they are disposed of or given to patients.
- ✦ Sharps are regulated waste; they should be stored in clearly marked sharps containers and disposed of by an agency that specializes in sharps disposal.
- ✦ Radiographic supplies are regulated waste and should be disposed of according to federal and local guidelines.

◆ Dental amalgam contains mercury, which is highly toxic. Amalgam waste must be stored in a clearly marked container in the dental office and disposed of by a mercury disposal company.

◆ The handling of chemicals in the dental office is governed by the Occupational Safety and Health Administration's Hazard Communication Standard. Every dental office needs to have a written plan for dealing with the use and disposal of hazardous waste.

◆ Every chemical in the dental office must have a material safety data sheet (MSDS) on file. This document details the properties of the chemical and first aid and safety precautions associated with it. MSDSs are typically provided by the manufacturer.

◆ The National Fire Protection Association's diamond label is used to easily identify hazardous chemicals. The color-coded label helps identify if the chemical is flammable, reactive with water, stable, and a health hazard.

◆ When handling chemicals, dental assistants must take all the necessary precautions, including wearing masks, gloves, and eye protection where necessary.

◆ Broken glass is considered a sharp and should always be cleaned up with a broom and dustpan and stored in a sharps container.

 **Review Questions**

1. An environmental *recommendation* is
   a. Subject to fines if broken.
   b. Not a law but a suggested practice.
   c. Only authorized by the Occupational Safety and Health Administration.
   d. None of the above.

2. An example of unregulated waste is
   a. Used needles.
   b. Amalgam waste.
   c. Bloody gauze and pads used in an examination.
   d. Disposable barriers.

3. Sharps include
   a. Used needles.
   b. Broken glass.
   c. Burs.
   d. All of the above.

4. Which agency regulates waste once it leaves the dental office?
   a. Occupational Safety and Health Administration
   b. Centers for Disease Control and Prevention
   c. Environmental Protection Agency
   d. American Dental Association

5. Which is an example of chronic toxicity?
   a. Exposure to fumes over time that cause lung cancer
   b. Spilling fixer on your hand and burning your skin
   c. Mercury spills that release clouds of mercury vapor
   d. Fainting after exposure to a chemical spill

6. What does the material safety data sheet describe?
   a. Federal regulations for handling materials
   b. A chemical's properties and safety data
   c. Local regulations for handling materials
   d. None of the above

7. Material safety data sheets should be on file for
   a. Only chemicals with high toxicity.
   b. Only chemicals with a pH above 9 or below 5.
   c. Only chemicals that are federally regulated.
   d. All chemicals used in the office.

8. The blue diamond on the National Fire Protection Association label indicates what?
   a. Flammability
   b. Health hazard
   c. Instability
   d. Reactivity

Active Learning Exercises

1. What are engineering and work practice controls? Go to the Occupational Safety and Health Administration (OSHA) and the Centers for Disease Control and Prevention (CDC) websites and research how these practices can be incorporated into the dental office. Who is responsible for ensuring these practices and why?

2. Imagine that you start working in an office and realize that there is no Material Safety Manual or labeling system. How could you explain the importance of this system to the office? How could you help incorporate such a system?

3. Identify the differences between regulated and nonregulated waste. Make a chart of five chairside procedures and their associated materials. Identify each material as regulated or nonregulated waste.

Application Activities

1. Draw a diagram of the National Fire Protection Association label and fill in what each of the quadrants stands for, with numerical ratings.

2. Develop a sample hazardous materials handling plan for a dental office.

PREPARING FOR CERTIFICATION EXAMS

Review the following topics in this chapter to prepare for the Dental Assisting National Board (DANB) exam:

- **Dental Office Waste**

- **Occupational Safety and Health Administration's Hazard Communication Standard**

- **Physical Hazards and Spills**

- **Biologic Hazards**

chapter 16

Pharmacology

CHAPTER OUTLINE

CHAPTER CHECKLIST

Upon completion of this chapter, students will be able to:

- ☑ Explain how a drug's chemical, generic, and brand or trade names differ.
- ☑ Describe the purpose behind each section of a written prescription.
- ☑ Describe the routes of drug administration.
- ☑ Describe the drug classifications outlined in the Comprehensive Drug Abuse Prevention and Control Act.
- ☑ Describe the most common used and abused drugs and how they may affect dental care.
- ☑ Describe the most common prescription drugs and what they are used to treat.
- ☑ Differentiate between *synergistic effects* and *side effects.*
- ☑ Describe the importance of the *Physician's Desk Reference*, including the type of information it contains on each drug.
- ☑ Describe the role of the dental assistant in handling and dispensing medications.

KEY TERMS

amphetamine – stimulant; some are used to treat narcolepsy and attention deficit disorder

analgesic – a drug used to relieve pain

anaphylaxis – rare, potentially life threatening allergic reaction to a drug

anesthetic – a drug used to prevent or control the perception of pain

antibiotic – a drug used to treat infections

anticholinergic (an-tee-koh-lih-NUR-jik) – a drug that inhibits secretions; used in dentistry to inhibit saliva production

antihistamine – a drug used to relieve allergy symptoms, such as a runny nose or watery eyes

antihypertensive – a drug that reduces blood pressure

barbiturate – a sedative derived from barbituric acid

brand name – the name assigned to a drug by its manufacturer

contraindication – a condition or instance in which a particular drug should not be used

DEA number – the identifying number assigned to medical professionals who prescribe controlled substances

depressant – a drug or agent that slows the speed of bodily processes and physical reactions

Drug Enforcement Agency (DEA) – federal agency within the Department of Justice; enforces controlled substance laws

drug interaction – occurs when one drug alters the effect of another

efficacy (EF-ih-kuh-see) – the effectiveness of a drug in accomplishing its intended purpose

generic – a drug identified by its nonproprietary name rather than by brand name

infective endocarditis (en-doh-kahr-DIE-tis) – infection of the valves and lining of the heart

inhalation – administering drugs or medications by inhaling them through the mouth or nose

intradermal administration – injecting drugs and medications beneath the epidermis

intramuscular administration – injecting drugs or medications into a muscle

intravenous administration – administering drugs directly into a vein

local-action drug – a drug applied to the skin or mucosa as an ointment, lotion, or gel; affects only the area of the body where it is directly applied.

narcotic – any of a variety of opioid drugs, including opium and cocaine

nitrous oxide – an inhaled anesthetic used in dentistry

NSAIDs – nonsteroidal anti-inflammatory drugs; includes commonly used over-the-counter analgesics

oral administration – administering drugs orally

oral thrush – candidiasis of the mouth

overdose – a lethal or toxic amount of a drug

pharmacokinetics (far-muh-koh-kih-NET-iks) – how a drug is absorbed, distributed, and metabolized within the body

pharmacology – the study of drugs and their effect on living organisms

Physician's Desk Reference **(PDR) –** comprehensive reference work on drugs in current use

prophylactic – a preventive measure; as when giving a drug to prevent rather than treat infection

rectal administration – administering drugs and medications through the rectum

sedative – a drug that reduces excitement, including anxiety

side effect – an unintended result of drug use

stimulant – a drug or agent that increases the speed and efficiency of bodily processes

subcutaneous administration – injecting drugs or medications just below the skin

sublingual administration – placing drugs beneath the tongue until they dissolve

synergistic effect – a drug interaction that occurs when drugs produce an effect that is greater than the sum of their separate actions

therapeutic – relating to the use of drugs to treat illness and disease

topical administration – administering drugs through lotions or gels applied to the skin

toxicology – the scientific study of poisons and their effects

trade name – the brand name of a drug

tranquilizer – a drug that relieves anxiety and promotes relaxation

transdermal administration – delivering medications through a skin patch

Introduction

Pharmacology refers to the study of drugs and their actions on living organisms:

- How drugs originate (organic or synthetic)
- What they are composed of (chemical formulation)
- How they are used to treat patients (therapeutic use)
- What happens in the body as a result of taking the drug (pharmacodynamics)
- They mechanics of how drugs accomplish their work within the body (**pharmacokinetics**)
- The potential for poisoning and other adverse effects (**toxicology**).

Drugs are increasingly used to treat a wide variety of diseases and conditions. Their potential misuse, intentional or otherwise, is also increasing. It is important for dental assistants (DAs) to understand how various classes and types of drugs affect bodily functions, and how these effects might influence dental care. Knowledge of pharmacology—especially of drugs used in dental care or those potentially abused by patients—helps professional DAs provide better quality patient care.

Patient Medical History

A DA's responsibilities include obtaining an accurate medical history from patients and carefully documenting both prescription drugs and those purchased over the counter (OTC). As you obtain this history, you will usually be concerned with prescription and OTC drugs that are legally obtained. Drugs that are legally obtained, however, may still be abused by patients. DAs should be able to recognize signs of drug abuse and should remain aware of which specific types of prescription or OTC drugs patients are more likely to abuse.

DAs should also make note of any possible abuse of illegal drugs. Illegal drugs, or street drugs, carry many health risks and can also interact adversely with drugs used in dentistry. You also should be able to recognize when a patient in your care may be under the influence of drugs or alcohol. If you notice a possible problem, you have an ethical obligation to let the dentist know. Just remember to discuss any concerns in private. As a health care professional it is your duty to maintain patient confidentiality at all times.

Classification of Drugs

Drugs originate from a variety of sources. Throughout medical history, plants have been the source of many different drugs. Some drugs originate from animal products. Drugs originating from these living sources are referred to as *organic drugs*. Drugs synthesized in a laboratory or made from inorganic materials are referred to as *synthetic* or *inorganic drugs*.

Not every drug is a medicine. Drugs are substances that alter processes within the body. Medicines are drugs specifically used to treat diseases and conditions. Legal drugs are classified according to their availability to the public and their potential for abuse. They are identified by a brand name, generic name, or chemical formulation.

- A **brand name**, sometimes referred to as a **trade name**, is assigned to a drug by its manufacturer when the drug finally comes onto the market. A brand name is always capitalized and may be followed by a registered trademark. An example of a brand name drug is Valium.
- The **generic** name of a drug is not capitalized, and a generic drug does not have patent protection. It may be used by any drug company. Names of generic drugs are drawn from their chemical compounds and are chosen during the drug's research and development stage. The generic name of Valium is diazepam.
- A drug's chemical formulation is the first name given to it. It identifies the chemical make-up of the drug. The chemical name of Valium is 7-chloro-1,3-dihydro-1-methyl-5-phenyl-2H-1,4-benzodiazepin-2-one.

✓ CHECKPOINTS

16-1 What type of drugs originate from living sources such as plants or animals?

16-2 What type of drug name is Sudafed?

Drug Prescriptions

A dentist may sometimes direct a DA to complete a prescription and leave it for the dentist to sign. Only physicians, dentists, physician assistants, and nurse practitioners, however, may legally write prescriptions. Each of these medical professionals is assigned an identifying number by the **Drug Enforcement Agency (DEA)**, the federal agency within the Department of Justice that enforces controlled substance laws. This number is known as the medical professional's **DEA number** and must appear on each sheet of the prescription pad they use to write prescriptions. The DEA number is assigned to individual dentists, not to the dental offices in which they practice. When a dentist or other prescribing medical professional retires from practice, his or her assigned DEA number retires with him or her.

A prescription is a highly structured document. It is written in several parts and must be complete to ensure that patients will receive the correct drug in the manner the dentist intended.

All prescriptions should be written clearly and legibly. The DA should make sure a copy is kept for future reference in the patient's chart. Some prescription pads are printed in triplicate and numbered sequentially to make this easier. A prescription has four main parts (Figure 16-1):

- *Heading.* This appears at the top of the prescription pad and notes the dentist's full name, degrees earned, office address, and office phone number. In many dental practices this identifying information is often preprinted on the pad. The appropriate DEA number appears here or at the close of the prescription near the signature line. Some law enforcement agencies advocate not preprinting the dentist's DEA number on prescription forms.
- *Superscription.* Appearing directly below the heading, the superscription contains blank lines where the dentist can enter the patient's name and address as well as the date the prescription was written. The patient's age, gender, and home phone number may also be written here. This information may prove helpful to the pharmacist in filling the prescription. Age and gender are among the factors that can affect drug dosage.

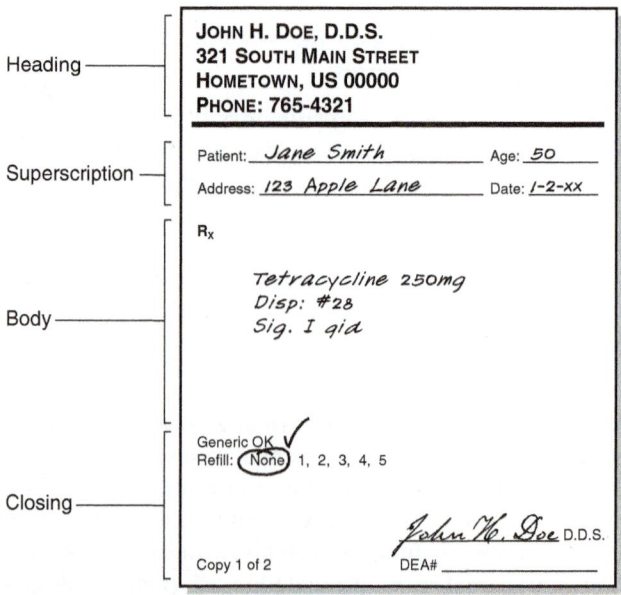

Figure 16-1 A prescription form.

TABLE 16-1 **Traditional Latin Phrases Used When Prescribing**

LATIN ABBREVIATION	CORRESPONDING LATIN PHRASE	MEANING IN ENGLISH
aa	*ana*	of each
ac	*ante cibum*	before meals
bid	*bis in die*	twice a day
q2h	*quaque 2 hora*	every 2 hours
q4h	*quaque 4 hora*	every 4 hours
q6h	*quaque 6 hora*	every 6 hours
sig	*signa*	take
stat	*statim*	immediately
tid	*ter in die*	three times a day
qid	*quater in die*	four times a day
qh	*quaque hora*	every hour
pc	*post cibos*	after meals
hs	*hora somni*	at bedtime
prn	*pro re nata*	as needed

- *Body of the prescription.* This part of the prescription is labeled with an Rx symbol. This longstanding symbol for a medical prescription is thought to be an abbreviation for the Latin term "recipe," meaning "to take." The body of a prescription is further divided into two other parts. The first is an *inscription* where the dentist "inscribes" or writes the name of the drug to be dispensed, the form in which it should be dispensed, its strength, and the dose to be given at one time. The second portion of the body of the prescription is the *subscription*. Here, the dentist subscribes, or specifies, the number of doses, and how the drug should be taken. The dentist also includes any special instructions to the pharmacist here.
- *Closing of the prescription.* The dentist closes the prescription with a personal signature and instructions on whether and how many times the prescription may be refilled. The dentist also notes whether a generic drug may be substituted for the brand name drug prescribed. If a generic drug is not acceptable, the dentist writes the abbreviation DAW, meaning "dispense as written," at the close of the prescription.

Certain abbreviations of Latin phrases are traditionally used when a dentist inscribes or subscribes how a drug should be taken. Table 16-1 contains some examples.

Security Measures

In any dental office, prescription pads must be kept in a secure location to prevent theft or misuse. They must never be used as a substitute for note paper or used for anything other than their intended purpose.

CHECKPOINTS

16-3 Whether a generic drug may be substituted for the brand name prescribed is indicated where on a prescription?

16-4 What does the abbreviation *prn* stand for when used on a prescription?

Routes of Drug Administration

Drugs and medications may be administered in a number of ways depending on the drug (Figure 16-2). The dentist will determine which of these routes is most beneficial for the patient. Not all of the 10 routes of drug administration possible are used in dentistry.

- **Oral administration** is the most common method of drug administration. The drug is swallowed, usually with a glass of water. Tablets, pills, capsules, and liquid medications are all administered orally.
- **Sublingual administration** is placing a drug under the tongue until it is absorbed. Small pills and sprays may be administered in this fashion.
- **Inhalation** is inhaling a drug through the nose or mouth. This method offers the quickest route for medications to reach the lungs. For example, patients with asthma may carry an inhaler to administer medication quickly in emergencies. In dentistry, the anesthetic **nitrous oxide**, sometimes called "laughing gas" for the feeling of euphoria it may briefly produce, is administered through inhalation.

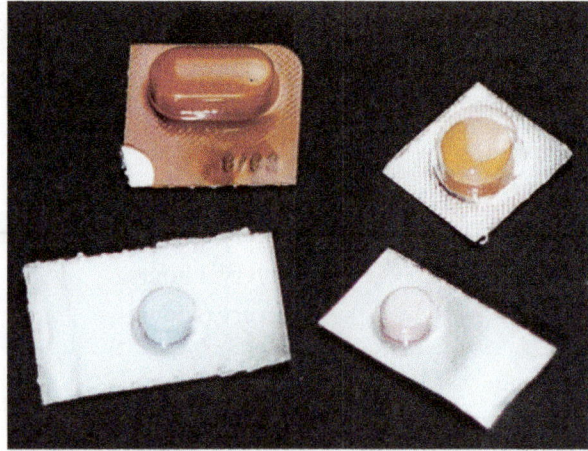

A

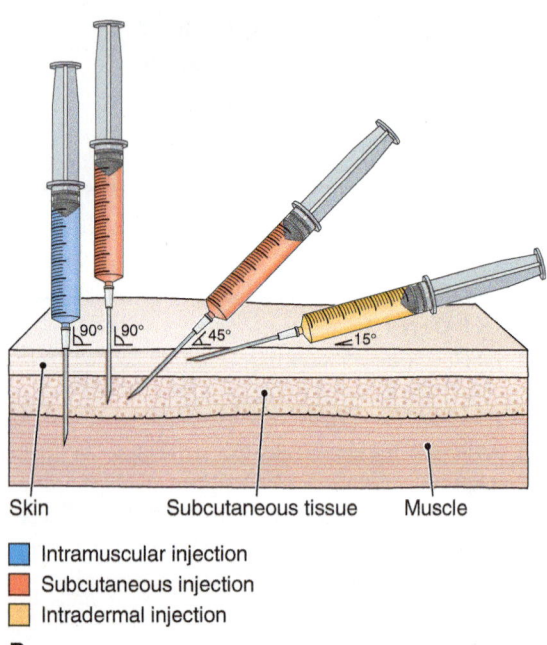

Skin   Subcutaneous tissue   Muscle

■ Intramuscular injection
■ Subcutaneous injection
■ Intradermal injection

B

Figure 16–2 Routes of medication administration. (A) Unit dose packages for oral medications. **(B)** Comparison of angles of insertion for intramuscular, subcutaneous, and intradermal injections. (Reprinted with permission from Cohen BJ. *Medical Terminology: An Illustrated Guide*. Philadelphia: Lippincott Williams & Wilkins, 2003.)

■ In **topical administration**, drugs are applied to the skin surface or mucosa in the form of creams, lotions, gels, or ointments. In dentistry, topically applied drugs are used to numb an area of the oral cavity prior to injection with an anesthetic. Topical application drugs are **local-action drugs** or local drugs. They deliver their effects at the site of application and do not enter the bloodstream to travel throughout the body.

■ **Transdermal administration** delivers medication through a patch applied to the surface of the skin. Medication from the patch is released into the body at an appropriate and consistent pace. Nicotine skin patches, for example, lessen the symptoms of withdrawal for smokers who are quitting.

■ **Intravenous (IV) administration** involves injecting medications or therapeutic substances directly into a vein. This method hastens the body's response to medication.

■ In some cases, drugs may be absorbed through the rectum as enemas or suppositories. This is referred to as **rectal administration**.

Drugs are injected into the body through a variety of routes of administration. So-called "shots" actually take a variety of forms depending on the drug that is being injected:

■ **Intramuscular administration** injects drugs into the muscle tissue. This results in a slower, but longer-lasting response to the medication.

■ **Subcutaneous administration** injects drugs directly *under* the skin.

■ **Intradermal administration** injects drugs directly *into* the skin.

✔ CHECKPOINT

16-5 A skin patch administers drugs through which route of administration?

Drug Laws

Five federal laws protect consumers by regulating the manufacture, distribution, and sale of drugs in the United States. Before the enactment of the Pure Food and Drug Act in 1906, drugs were not regulated, and their composition and purity varied widely. This act established the first federal regulations for the composition, distribution, and sale of drugs.

The 1938 Pure Food, Drug, and Cosmetic Act specifies that the federal agency known as the *U.S. Food and Drug Administration (FDA)* will control all food, drug, and cosmetic advertising and sales in the country. It also mandates that a drug's safety must be determined before it can be sold to consumers. Amendments to the act in 1951 and 1965 establish the use of labels to warn consumers of potential side effects such as drowsiness, set additional regulations against tampering, and require manufacturers to show the effectiveness as well as safety of drugs they introduce to the market.

The Comprehensive Drug Abuse Prevention and Control Act of 1970 classifies drugs according to their abuse potential. A related law, the Controlled Substances Act, assigns enforcement of laws regarding controlled substances to the DEA. The DEA concerns itself with controlled substances only. Medications that are not subject to abuse are not regulated by the DEA.

✔ CHECKPOINT

16-6 Which law established the first federal regulations for the composition, distribution, and sale of drugs?

Controlled Substances

Controlled substances are specific drugs whose use may result in abuse or physical and psychological dependency. Physical dependency results in mild to severe physiological symptoms, called *withdrawal symptoms*, such as vomiting, sweating, or trembling, if the drug is abruptly stopped. Psychological dependency refers to an acquired need or craving for the feeling brought on by the drug.

The possession and use of controlled substances is governed by the Controlled Substances Act. Controlled substances are classified according to the likelihood and potential severity of their abuse by consumers. The following Drug Schedule is part of the Comprehensive Drug Abuse Prevention and Control Act of 1970.

I. Schedule I drugs are considered to have a high potential for abuse, to currently have no accepted medical use, or to lack a consensus of safety even under medical supervision. Schedule I drugs include both highly addictive drugs, such as heroin, as well as the much less addictive drug marijuana (which, its schedule notwithstanding, is in medical use in 14 states) and the nonaddictive hallucinogenic drugs mescaline and lysergic acid diethylamide (commonly known as *LSD*).

II. Schedule II drugs have a high potential for abuse, but also have accepted medical uses. Use and abuse of these drugs can lead to psychological and physical dependence. Schedule II drugs include codeine, morphine, certain tranquilizers, and stimulants. Prescriptions for these drugs must be made in writing and cannot be refilled.

III. Schedule III drugs have a lower potential for abuse than Schedule II drugs and also have recognized medical uses. Compounds made from Schedule III drugs are routinely prescribed in dental practice and used in the dental office. Schedule III drugs include stimulants and tranquilizers as well as compounds such as Tylenol no. 3 (acetaminophen with codeine). Prescriptions for Schedule III drugs may be refilled.

IV. Schedule IV drugs have less potential for abuse than Schedule III drugs and also have established medical uses. Schedule IV drugs include anti-anxiety drugs, antidepressants, and sedatives not included in Schedules I through III. Prescriptions for Schedule IV drugs may be refilled five times within a 6-month period.

V. Schedule V drugs have the least potential for abuse. They are often compounds made from small amounts of drugs included in Schedules I through IV. Schedule V drugs may include antidiarrheal medications and cough medications. Some Schedule V drugs are available without a prescription.

CHECKPOINT

16-7 In which category of the schedule of controlled substances do medically useful drugs with a high potential for abuse, such as codeine and morphine, appear?

Extra Patient Care

As you gather medical and dental histories from patients, you may encounter individuals who are not sure of the exact name of a medication they regularly take. You may be able to obtain a more accurate and complete medical history if you ask these individuals to bring their prescriptions with them the next time they visit the office. Information on the labels should help answer your questions and may even open up an opportunity for further discussion.

Over-the-Counter Drugs and Herbal and Other Supplements

Over-the-Counter Drugs

OTC drugs are sometimes referred to as *patent medicines* and may be obtained at pharmacies, grocery stores, and other retail establishments without a prescription. Some medical and dental offices may also dispense OTC medications. The FDA evaluates OTC drugs for safety and **efficacy** (effectiveness). OTC drugs commonly used by consumers include analgesics for pain relief, antacids for an upset stomach, and expectorants and cough suppressants for relief of cold symptoms. Some OTC analgesics are known as *nonsteroidal anti-inflammatory drugs*, abbreviated as **NSAIDs**. Aspirin and ibuprofen are examples of NSAIDs. Dentists and DAs who discuss the use of OTC drugs with their patients must remember that, although OTC drugs may be available without a prescription, their use may still involve side effects, adverse effects, and drug interactions.

Herbal and Other Dietary Supplements

Use of herbal and other dietary supplements is widespread. If a patient is a regular user of a dietary or herbal supplement, this information should be noted in his or her health history. DAs may encounter patients who have questions regarding supplements they are using. Some supplements have the potential to interact with prescription and other drugs. Refer any patient questions regarding side effects or synergistic effects of herbal supplements to the dentist.

Herbal and other dietary supplements may prove helpful to some patients. Patients should be cautioned, however, regarding the use of these or any other substances not approved by the FDA or the American Dental Association (ADA). Current law requires supplement manufacturers themselves to determine the safety of their product before they place it on the market; the FDA will, however, monitor safety once the supplement is being sold, and investigate and take action against any unsafe supplement on the market. The FDA also regulates product claims, labeling, package inserts, and any accompanying literature. The Federal Trade Commission regulates advertising of dietary supplements.

Commonly Used and Abused Drugs

Alcohol

Ethyl alcohol, found in wine, beer, and other alcoholic beverages, is one of the oldest drugs known to humanity. Alcohol, like other **depressant** drugs, slows bodily processes and reactions. Its effects are felt rapidly because it is absorbed directly into the bloodstream and carried throughout the body. People experiencing the effects of alcohol are said to be "intoxicated," "inebriated," or "drunk." The legal definition of intoxication in most states in the United States is a blood alcohol level of 0.8%–0.10%. Symptoms of inebriation include a marked loss in judgment, impaired physical coordination, slowed reactions to stimuli or events, and slurred speech.

Alcohol and Public Health

Alcohol abuse is a serious public health issue. According to the National Institutes of Health, more than half of all motor vehicle accidents are caused by impaired driving, which includes driving under the influence of alcohol or other drugs. More than 40% of traffic deaths nationwide are specifically alcohol related.

Expectant mothers who drink large amounts of alcohol put their developing babies at increased risk of developing numerous serious birth defects. These defects are sometimes referred to as *fetal alcohol syndrome*.

Alcoholism

Most adults can consume moderate amounts of alcohol safely. Some people, however, acquire a psychological and physical dependence on alcohol. Some of these individuals may have been born with a specific gene (a genetic disposition) that makes it more likely they will develop a dependence on alcohol. Dependence on alcohol is known as *alcoholism*, and the disease affects between 17 and 18 million adult Americans. Features of alcoholism include:

- Persistent cravings for alcohol
- The need to drink progressively larger amounts of it to feel any effect
- Inability to stop drinking
- Physical dependence characterized by withdrawal symptoms such as nausea, sweating, or trembling if drinking stops

If alcoholism goes untreated it can contribute to cardiovascular disease and to some cancers. Alcoholism can also lead to brain damage and cause dementia, a condition characterized by memory loss, confusion, agitation, and an inability to carry out normal activities of living. Untreated alcoholism can also result in liver scarring and damage, causing cirrhosis. The scarred liver tissue associated with cirrhosis cannot perform the work of a healthy liver, such as cleansing the blood of impurities, helping digest food, fighting infection, and storing energy. If the underlying causes of scarring are not addressed, cirrhosis eventually results in death.

CHECKPOINT

16-8 Untreated alcoholism can result in liver damage and scarring known as what?

Alcohol and Dental Care

Some patients may use alcohol in an attempt to ease their fears of dental examination and treatment. DAs should make note of any signs of inebriation or recent alcohol consumption, such as an odor on the breath, and call them to the attention of the dentist. Few medicines can be taken safely while a person is drinking alcohol. Many prescription medications and OTC products have special warnings on the label that caution patients not to use them while using alcohol. Certain drugs used in dentistry can interact adversely with alcohol. For example, diazepam (Valium) may cause severe drowsiness when used with alcohol.

Alcohol can depress the appetite, causing individuals who abuse alcohol to neglect their diet. An improper diet can adversely affect oral health. In these and other cases, DAs should call the dentist's attention to any deterioration in a patient's dental health they believe may be caused by malnutrition.

Tobacco

Tobacco contains the drug nicotine. Smokers and others who are addicted to tobacco use are actually addicted to nicotine. Unlike alcohol, which is a depressant, nicotine is a stimulant. **Stimulants** temporarily increase the speed and efficiency of bodily processes but may also cause health problems as well as anxiety and depression when their effects wear off. Tobacco is smoked in cigarettes, pipes, or cigars or chewed as smokeless tobacco.

Tobacco has no medicinal use and is, therefore, never used in medicine. Smoking is a known health hazard, both to smokers themselves and those in their vicinity who must breathe the smoke secondhand. Cancer—especially lung cancer—and heart disease are more prevalent in smokers than nonsmokers. The carbon monoxide in tobacco smoke interferes with the body's ability to properly oxygenate the blood and supply oxygen to the bodily organs. This shortage of oxygenated blood forces the heart to work harder over all the years that an individual continues to smoke tobacco and is responsible for much of the heart disease caused by smoking. In addition, as a *vasoconstrictor*, nicotine increases blood pressure.

Smokeless Tobacco

Despite the fact that it is not smoked, smokeless tobacco, sometimes called *chewing tobacco*, also causes serious health issues. Risks associated with chewing tobacco include:

- Oral cancers
- Pulling away of gingiva from the teeth
- Decay of exposed tooth roots
- White patches and red sores within the oral cavity that can turn into cancer (Figure 16-3)

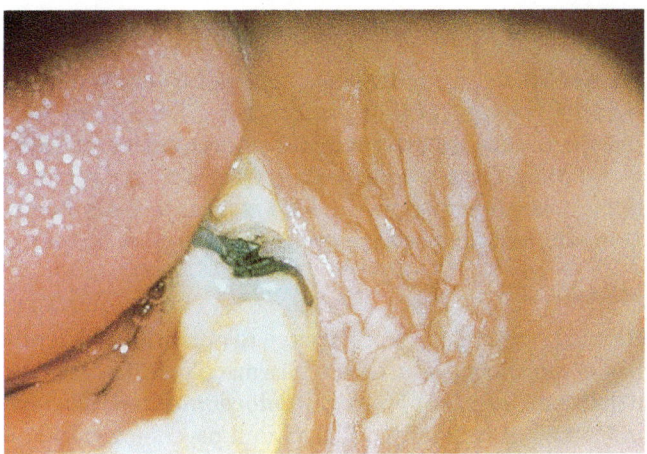

Figure 16–3 Snuff dipper's patch on the mucobuccal fold.

Tobacco and Dental Care

Tobacco, whether smoked or chewed, increases the risk of a number of dental and oral health problems, including:

- Halitosis
- Stained teeth
- Periodontal disease

Patients may complain to DAs that they find it impossible to stop smoking or using tobacco. Products are available to assist patients in gradually reducing their craving for nicotine. These products provide a substitute source of nicotine that is gradually reduced over time to alleviate symptoms of withdrawal. Individuals should follow precisely any instructions for use of the product, and should be encouraged to discuss its use in detail with their doctor or pharmacist. Available products include:

- *Nicotine gum.* Chewing this gum also acts as a substitute oral activity to take the place of smoking or chewing tobacco.
- *Nicotine skin patches.* These are applied directly to the skin at the same time each day.
- *Prescription drugs.* Available medications include bupropion (Zyban), an antidepressant drug that decreases nicotine cravings and reduces nicotine withdrawal symptoms, and varenicline tartrate (Chantix), a drug that blocks the effect that nicotine has on the brain and reduces nicotine withdrawal symptoms.
- Community health departments and other health care facilities, such as hospitals, may offer *smoking cessation programs and workshops.* DAs may want to familiarize themselves with these offerings and mention appropriate ones to patients anxious to quit smoking.

Professional DAs are expected to model good health habits. A dental practice may be reluctant to hire or retain a DA who smokes. Prospective assistants may wish to consider enrolling in smoking cessation programs available in their area, or may wish to ask their personal physicians or local health clinics about available and effective products.

Caffeine

Caffeine is a stimulant found in coffee, tea, soft drinks, chocolate, and cocoa. Like all stimulants, it increases the speed and efficiency of bodily processes. Because of this, it also increases heart rate and nervous system activity. Caffeine is habit forming, but, under normal circumstances, these common beverages and foods are safe to eat and drink. Caffeinated beverages may, however, stain the teeth of patients who ingest them frequently.

Dental Facts

Tea is second only to water as the world's most common beverage. So familiar is it that most of us do not think of it as an herbal medicine. Yet Indian, Chinese, Japanese, and Korean traditional medicine is believed to have made use of it for thousands of years. All three of the main types of tea—black, oolong, and green tea—are derived from the same plant, Camellia sinensis, which grows best in subtropical climates where it receives plenty of sun and moisture. Tea's qualities as a stimulant and diuretic are well known in the West, and clinical and scientific studies continue to examine the possible use of its chemical compounds in preventing or addressing a wide assortment of medical conditions and illnesses, including asthma, cancer, osteoporosis, and even oral leukoplakia. Brought to Western cultures in the 6th century by Turkish traders and again in the 18th century by Dutch traders, tea may offer far more to dental patients than those stubborn stains familiar to hygienists and dental assistants.

Marijuana

Marijuana consists of a dry, shredded mix of stems, flowers, seeds, and leaves of the hemp plant, *Cannabis sativa*. It is most commonly smoked in cigarettes, called "joints," or in pipes. Marijuana itself is known by various street names, including "pot," "grass," and "weed." Research continues into possible medicinal uses of marijuana, including treating eye diseases such as glaucoma, lessening nausea and vomiting in cancer patients undergoing chemotherapy, and lessening severe pain, if taken in moderate doses. Some states have legalized its use for medical purposes, but it remains illegal under federal law, although the use of medical marijuana that complies with state law is increasingly less frequently prosecuted at the federal level. Marijuana is the mostly commonly abused illegal drug in the United States.

Side effects of marijuana abuse include increased heart rate, lung tissue damage associated with smoking the drug, abnormal hormone levels, and abnormal sperm production. Use of marijuana does not result in a physical dependency, as with alcohol, but may result in psychological dependence. Noticeable side effects vary among individuals, but may include memory problems as well as effects on speech, social behavior, and learning ability.

Check Your Ethics

Although dental assistants (DAs) must advocate for their patients, they must also remain vigilant about possible drug abuse among their patients and be knowledgeable about it in the community at large. A DA who encounters a patient under the influence of marijuana, for example, is faced with a dilemma. It may be possible to treat such a patient successfully, and dental professionals may even disagree on how advisable it might be. The side effects of marijuana, however, include some that could potentially obstruct quality dental care. An increased heart rate is one of the most noticeable side effects of marijuana abuse, but problems with memory, as well as effects on speech and social behavior, could diminish accurate and thorough communication between dentist, patient, and DA. Diminished or impaired communication could frustrate treatment efforts and even jeopardize the safety of dental procedures.

Cocaine

Cocaine is a highly addictive illegal drug whose long-term use is known to cause pronounced anxiety, restlessness, and irritability. Other known side effects include heart problems that can prove fatal, breathing problems that can result in respiratory distress and death, strokes, mental illness, violent behavior, and digestive problems. Purified cocaine that resembles a crystalline rock is known commonly as "crack" and usually smoked in pipes. Symptoms of withdrawal from cocaine include intense craving, anxiety, and depression. Cocaine abuse is often accompanied by alcohol consumption; this combination is one of the most common causes of drug-related deaths.

Cocaine and Dental Care

The powder form of cocaine is inhaled into the nose or rubbed over the gingiva. Because cocaine is abrasive, signs of its abuse may appear on the teeth and gingiva. These abrasions may appear similar to toothbrush abrasions, but will occur over a wider area. Long-term use of inhaled cocaine damages nasal mucosa.

CHECKPOINT

16-9 Abuse of which illegal drug can cause signs of abrasion on the teeth and gingiva?

Ecstasy

Ecstasy (MDMA) is an illegal synthetic drug that gained popularity during the 1980s among teens and young adults associated with the electronic music scene. Because of its prevalence at dance clubs and raves, ecstasy is known as a "club drug." Typically used in pill or tablet form, the drug produces enhanced self-confidence and feelings of empathy and emotional warmth. The effects of ecstasy typically last 4 to 6 hours. Side effects include increased energy and higher heart rate, blood pressure, and body temperature. Research indicates that the drug may cause depression, sleep problems, and anxiety for days to weeks after a dose.

Narcotics

Narcotics are highly addictive depressants that have been used for thousands of years to relieve pain. Opium is an example of a narcotic that has been in use for centuries around the world. Morphine and codeine are medicinally used narcotics derived, like opium, from the seed pod of the Asian poppy. Drugs derived from opium poppies are known as *opiates*.

Heroin

Heroin is an illegal narcotic related to opium and currently has no medicinal use. Other pharmacological names for heroin are *diamorphine*, *acetomorphine*, and *diacetylmorphine*. It is highly addictive both psychologically and physically. An individual who abuses heroin does not take long to develop a tolerance to the drug. Progressively larger quantities of the drug are needed to produce the same feelings of euphoria, drowsiness, and loss of pain previously experienced. Use of progressively larger quantities of heroin puts the individual at risk for an **overdose**, ingestion of a potentially fatal amount of the drug.

An overdose of heroin is characterized by vomiting, diarrhea, decreased respiration, and decreased heart rate. Symptoms of shock may set in and the individual may fall into a coma. Any individual suspected of having overdosed on heroin should be immediately taken to a hospital for treatment.

Individuals who abuse heroin may inject the drug intravenously or subcutaneously, or may inhale it. Heroin users who inject the drug, and share needles with others while doing so, run a serious risk of contracting bloodborne diseases such as hepatitis and human immunodeficiency virus (HIV).

A person who is dependent on heroin will begin to exhibit symptoms of withdrawal within 12 hours after stopping the drug. Symptoms of heroin withdrawal include an intense craving for the drug, hot and cold flashes, stomach cramps, vomiting, diarrhea, trembling, muscle pain, and bone pain.

Morphine

Unlike heroin, morphine is a legal prescription narcotic used for the relief of severe pain. It may be used to treat postsurgical pain, pain from myocardial infarction or heart attack, and pain from terminal cancer. Because it is also highly addictive, its medicinal use is limited to cases in which its strength and potency as a painkiller are truly necessary. Side effects of morphine include constipation, nausea, vomiting, and confusion.

Prescription morphine may take the form of time-release capsules or tablets, rectal suppositories, intramuscular injections, or IV drips. Treatment with morphine is closely monitored to prevent withdrawal symptoms when the drug is discontinued. Withdrawal symptoms include flu-like symptoms such as stomach and body cramps.

OxyContin

OxyContin is a controlled-release form of oxycodone prescribed for moderate to severe pain when a continuous, around-the-clock analgesic is needed for an extended period of time. A patient may experience fewer adverse reactions with oxycodone than morphine, and the drug is effective and generally considered safe for older adults when used as prescribed. The tablets are to be swallowed whole and should not be broken, chewed, or crushed. Oxy-Contin is increasingly being abused in the United States.

Codeine

Codeine is a legal prescription narcotic used, often in combination with other less potent drugs, to relieve pain, control coughing, or control severe diarrhea. Dentists may prescribe small amounts of codeine in combination with other medications to relieve mild to moderate pain. Like other opiates, codeine causes drowsiness and, if used over a long period of time, can prove physically and psychologically addictive, although less so than other opiates.

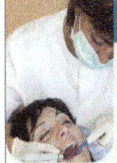

Voice of Experience

You never know when you will see it. Drugs can be abused by the most unlikely people. At least they seem unlikely. One day I was updating a medical history from a patient who had been with us since he was a child. He had moved out of town, and we had not seen him in quite a while. I noticed he was quieter than I remembered. I was about to ask him if he was feeling okay when he lifted his arm and rolled it slightly to the side to take hold of a cup of water he had asked for. I glanced down to start the history again and was shocked to see needle track marks on his arm. After a moment, I told him it was important to get his medical history as accurate and up to date as possible. I asked him if he was having any problems with medications, or if he had any questions for the dentist. Most of all, I just wanted to get him to talk, if I could. Maybe, just maybe, he would say something about his history and what was going on now. I asked him if he had been traveling. Living somewhere new? Was he back living at home now? He answered all my questions, but said nothing about drug use and reported no recent treatment for abuse.

Bloodborne illnesses surface often among drug abusers who share needles, but we exercise the same precautions with all patients. After I finished the history, I prepared myself to work with the patient and assist the dentist. I waited an extra moment, then excused myself to go and find the dentist. I needed to alert him about the unspoken part of our patient's history.

Hallucinogens

Hallucinogenic drugs cause hallucinations in the people who ingest or use them. Drug-induced hallucinations may take the form of sounds, visions, sensations, or emotional reactions that do not have a basis in reality. Some hallucinogenic drugs derived from plant and mushroom extracts have been used during traditional religious ceremonies for centuries. A person under the influence of a hallucinogen may see unusual colors, hear voices, or experience powerful shifts in emotions and perceptions. The perception of time and self may change. Some individuals experience profound personality changes. These powerful effects are what have led to the abuse of hallucinogenic drugs.

Many hallucinogens have a chemical structure similar to that of *neurotransmitters*, chemicals found naturally in the brain. Research suggests that hallucinogens work by temporarily attaching themselves to sites important to the natural functioning of neurotransmitters (receptor sites) and interfering with normal brain activity.

LSD

LSD is a synthetic drug first manufactured in a laboratory. It is one of the most notorious hallucinogens. First synthesized and discovered in 1938, it originates from a fungus that grows on wheat and rye. LSD has been illegal for many years and has no medicinal use. The hallucinogenic effects induced by LSD are referred to as a "trip" and may last as long as 12 hours. Flashbacks from "bad trips" can recur spontaneously for several years afterward. A habitual user may become psychologically dependent on the drug.

Psilocybin

Psilocybin is a hallucinogenic drug found in certain mushrooms that grow in tropical and subtropical regions of the United States, Mexico, and South America. Sometimes known informally as "magic mushrooms," these may be ingested in fresh or dried form, brewed into teas, or mixed with other foods. Hallucinogenic effects of psilocybin take about 20 minutes to appear and last approximately 6 hours. Side effects are psychological as opposed to physical and include changes in motor function and perception, panic reactions, and an inability to distinguish fantasy from reality.

Peyote

Peyote is a spineless cactus plant that contains the hallucinogenic drug mescaline. Native populations in parts of northern Mexico and the southwestern United States traditionally used the drug in religious ceremonies. Button-shaped discs are cut from the cap of the cactus and chewed, or boiled and brewed into tea. Side effects may include elevated body temperature, flushing, excessive sweating, increased heart rate, and lack of coordination. Psychological effects are similar to those of LSD. Effects of peyote use last about 12 hours. Repeated use of peyote can prove addictive and cause persistent cravings for the drug.

Phencyclidine

Phencyclidine, also known as *PCP*, is a particularly dangerous hallucinogen. It was originally developed as an anesthetic for use during surgery, but is no longer used for that purpose in humans. Phencyclidine is sometimes called "angel dust." It may be smoked, eaten, or inhaled. Psychological side effects include significant anxiety, paranoia, violent behavior, agitation, and memory loss. Physical effects include depressed respiration, nausea, vomiting, and convulsions.

Despite its serious adverse effects, PCP proves addictive in habitual users, who crave the drug and compulsively seek it out despite these adverse consequences.

CHECKPOINT

16-10 Hallucinogens are thought to interfere with which naturally occurring brain chemicals?

Commonly Prescribed Drugs

A DA may administer drugs, such as anesthetics, under the direction of the dentist, or may dispense drugs, such as analgesics, to the patient for later use at home.

Dentists, physicians, physician assistants, and nurse practitioners are the only professionals allowed to prescribe drugs. All these medical professionals exercise caution when prescribing. They explain drugs administered or prescriptions written and answer any patient questions. Dentists are more likely to prescribe or use anesthetics for pain prevention, analgesics for pain relief, antibiotics to fight infection, and tranquilizers for relief of anxiety. The DA records in the patient's dental history all drugs administered or prescribed as well as any OTC drugs discussed.

Package Inserts

Patients, dentists, and DAs may obtain additional information regarding a particular drug from the package insert accompanying it. A package insert typically describes the following:

- How the drug will affect the body—what kind of relief or effect it will offer
- For what condition(s) the drug is prescribed
- Any adverse effects experienced by users (e.g., drowsiness, nausea, sleeplessness)
- Any long-term adverse effects possible (e.g., liver or kidney damage)
- Special precautions to take while on the drug (e.g., do not drink alcohol or drive)
- **Contraindications**, or situations in which the drug should not be used.
- Dosage to be taken and route of administration.

CHECKPOINT

16-11 Situations or conditions in which a particular drug should not be used are known as what?

Barbiturates

Barbiturates are **sedatives** derived from *barbituric acid*. They may be used in dentistry to treat severe anxiety associated with dental treatment. The drug *phenobarbital* may be given in a liquid form to adult or pediatric dental patients. Barbiturates may also be used to treat conditions such as epilepsy, in which potential seizures may be averted by the depressed brain activity brought on by drugs such as phenobarbital.

Barbiturates prove highly addictive if abused, whether obtained through legitimate medical channels or sold illegally on the street. Symptoms of withdrawal from barbiturate addiction include stomach cramps, nausea, vomiting, and twitching.

Amphetamines

Amphetamines are stimulants. They increase heart rate, respiratory rate, and blood pressure. Amphetamines have few medical uses. They are not normally used in dentistry. In general medicine and psychiatry they may be used to treat narcolepsy, a condition in which individuals suddenly and unexpectedly fall asleep. Paradoxically, amphetamines are also used to treat attention deficit disorder in children, in whom they have a calming rather than stimulating effect. Amphetamines were once used as appetite suppressants but no longer are; today they are sold on the street under a variety of names, including "meth," "speed," and "crank."

CHECKPOINT

16-12 Which barbiturate is sometimes used in dentistry to treat severe anxiety associated with dental procedures?

Analgesics

Analgesics relieve pain. In dentistry, analgesics may be used to relieve the pain of toothache or postoperative pain. Analgesics may also be used to address chronic orofacial pain such as that caused by inflammation of the temporomandibular joint. OTC analgesics include aspirin, ibuprofen, and acetaminophen. Prescription analgesics include morphine and codeine. Aspirin normally is not recommended as a pain reliever following dental surgery or extraction because it thins the blood and increases bleeding. Possible side effects of some analgesics include nausea and stomach irritation.

Tranquilizers

Tranquilizers relieve anxiety and promote relaxation. They may be used in dentistry to relieve patient anxiety regarding upcoming procedures. Patients whose overpowering fear of dental pain previously caused them to avoid necessary dental work may be helped by judicious use of tranquilizers. Diazepam, also known as Valium, may be administered a half hour prior to a procedure to alleviate patient anxiety. Possible side effects of tranquilizers include dizziness and drowsiness.

Antihypertensive Drugs

Antihypertensive drugs reduce blood pressure and are, therefore, used to treat hypertension (high blood pressure). Hypertension affects approximately one in three Americans and causes stroke, heart attack, and heart failure if left untreated.

Drugs used to treat hypertension include:

- Diuretics
- Vasodilating drugs

- Adrenergic-blocking drugs
- Antiadrenergic-blocking drugs
- Calcium channel-blocking drugs
- Angiotensin converting–enzyme inhibitors
- Angiotensin II–receptor antagonists

Although these drugs work in different ways, the goal—to reduce blood pressure—is the same. Often, combinations of two drugs from different classes are used to improve the drugs' effectiveness. In addition, treatment with antihypertensive drugs is often combined with diet and exercise.

Antibiotics

Antibiotics are used to treat infection. Some antibiotics, such as penicillin, are derived from molds and fungi; others are manufactured synthetically. Broad spectrum antibiotics are effective against a wide variety of infections; other antibiotics target only specific infections. Bacteriocidal antibiotics, including penicillin, treat infection by directly killing all infecting organisms. Bacteriostatic antibiotics, such as tetracycline, treat infection by slowing and interfering with the metabolic processes of the infecting bacteria. Eventually, the individual's immune system disposes of the decreasing and weakened infecting organisms. No antibiotic is effective against viruses.

Chlorhexidine is an antibiotic dispensed as an oral rinse or topical gel treatment. It is used in dentistry to control the buildup of plaque and to treat gingivitis.

Other antibiotics are used in dentistry for a variety of purposes including eliminating infections, reducing bacteria associated with periodontal disease, and treating canker sores in the oral cavity.

Treatment with antibiotics may be **therapeutic** in response to an already active infection or it may be a **prophylactic** measure taken to prevent the development of infection. Table 16-2 outlines prophylactic regimens for some common antibiotics. In dentistry, prophylactic use of antibiotics is intended to prevent the development of **infective endocarditis** in patients whose medical history may make them unusually susceptible. Infective endocarditis is an infection of the heart's inner lining or of the heart valves. It develops when bacteria enter the bloodstream and travel to damaged or abnormal parts of the heart where they lodge and inflict further damage. Complications of infective endocarditis include destroyed heart valves and strokes resulting from the infection, both of which can prove fatal. Early treatment of endocarditis improves the chances of a good outcome. Endocarditis is treated with specific antibiotics depending on the bacteria causing it.

CHECKPOINT

16-13 Treatment with antibiotics that is intended to prevent the development of an infection is known as what?

Endocarditis is of concern in dentistry because bacteria can enter the bloodstream briefly following certain dental procedures. This is known as *transient bacteremia*. When a patient is undergoing an invasive procedure, the ADA guidelines call for administering prophylactic antibiotics to patients whose medical history may predispose them to developing infective endocarditis. These include:

- Patients with a history of heart valve replacement
- Patients previously infected with endocarditis
- Heart transplant recipients who develop heart valve problems
- Persons who have undergone certain procedures to correct specific heart problems they have had from birth
- Patients who have undergone a total joint replacement are also administered prophylactic antibiotics. Bacteria from the bloodstream may lodge in artificial hips, knees, or other artificial joints and cause infections that are difficult to treat.

Patients with these conditions should have antibiotic prophylaxis when undergoing procedures that involve manipulation of the gingival or periapical tissue or procedures in which the oral mucosa is cut or perforated. The ADA limits the prophylactic use of antibiotics to patients who would have the worst outcomes should infective endocarditis develop. These limitations reflect recent concerns in medicine and dentistry regarding the overuse of antibiotics.

Apply it

A new patient arrives for an extensive procedure. On his medical history he reports the replacement of a defective heart valve. American Dental Association guidelines call for using prophylactic antibiotic treatment to ward off any possibility of infective endocarditis. The patient insists he does not need premedication, saying that his doctor told him he does not require it. Overuse of antibiotics is the patient's primary concern.

What would you do first? Are there resources you could consult to confirm guidelines or check for updates?

If a need for premedication is confirmed, how would you again approach the patient? Would his attending cardiologist or other physician be available for consultation with your dentist? Could written medical clearance be obtained?

Resistance to Antibiotics

Concerns over the unnecessary use of antibiotics center on the resistance dangerous bacteria may develop to antibiotics that previously destroyed them effectively. This resistance can develop for a variety of reasons. Individuals prescribed an antibiotic may not continue taking the medication after they start feeling better. Prematurely stopping the drug leaves some disease-causing bacteria alive to multiply all over again. This time, however, they will have acquired a resistance to the antibiotic previously

TABLE 16-2 Prophylactic Regimens for Common Antibiotics

PATIENT TOLERANCE	DRUG AND DOSAGE	ROUTE OF ADMINISTRATION	WHEN TO ADMINISTER
Able to take standard general prophylaxis	Amoxicillin *Adults:* 2 g *Children:* 50 mg/kg	Oral	30 to 60 minutes before procedure
Unable to take oral medications	Ampicillin *Adults:* 2 g *Children:* 50 mg/kg or Cefazolin or ceftriaxone* *Adults:* 1 g *Children:* 50 mg/kg	Intramuscular or intravenous	30 to 60 minutes before procedure
Allergic to penicillin or ampicillin	Cephalexin* *Adults:* 2 g *Children:* 50 mg/kg or Clindamycin *Adults:* 600 mg *Children:* 20 mg/kg or Azithromycin or clarithromycin *Adults:* 500 mg *Children:* 15 mg/kg	Oral	30 to 60 minutes before procedure
Allergic to penicillin or ampicillin and unable to take oral medications	Cefazolin or ceftriaxone* *Adults:* 1 g *Children:* 50 mg/kg or Clindamycin *Adults:* 600 mg *Children:* 20 mg/kg	Intramuscular or intravenous	30 to 60 minutes before procedure

*Should not be used for patients with a history of anaphylaxis, angioedema, or urticaria with penicillin or ampicillin.
Adapted from Wilkins. *Clinical Practice of the Dental Hygienist,* 10th edition. Lippincott, Williams & Wilkins, 2008. Table 7-4; and http://www.americanheart.org/presenter.jhtml?identifier=11086.

used to destroy them. Resistance to previously effective antibiotics has become a serious public health issue.

Antibiotics can cause side effects in some people. These include nausea, diarrhea, and stomach pain. In severe cases, these can lead to dehydration. Some people develop skin irritations, such as itching and rash. Even breathing difficulty may develop in some cases. These potential developments illustrate the importance of accurate dental and medical health histories that include any previous drug allergies.

Some antibiotic side effects result from the destruction of naturally occurring and health-promoting bacteria. Destruction of these bacteria in the oral cavity, intestines, or vagina can prompt troublesome yeast infections, a condition called *candidiasis*. Candidiasis that develops in the oral cavity is known as **oral thrush** (see Chapter 12, Figure 12-15). Thrush and other yeast infections are treated with antifungal drugs.

Nystatin and Antifungal Agents

Nystatin is an antifungal agent used in dentistry to treat candidiasis of the mouth, also known as *oral thrush*. Thrush is normally caused by a weakened immune system, poorly fitted dentures, or by recent use of antibiotics. Nystatin is administered as a suspension or liquid that is held in the mouth and rinsed throughout it prior to swallowing. Patients should be advised to continue with nystatin treatment for 48 hours after symptoms of thrush have disappeared. Possible side effects of nystatin include stomach pain, nausea, vomiting, and diarrhea.

Nystatin ointment is used in dentistry to treat **angular cheilitis** (see Chapter 12, Figure 12-38) or candidiasis that develops at the corners of the mouth.

Antiviral Agents

Viruses, such as hepatitis, hand-foot-mouth disease, herpes simplex, recurrent herpes infection, herpes zoster, and HIV, can all cause viral infections within the oral cavity. Many times the infection appears as one or more oral lesions, often small and frequently located on or near the lips, or on the tongue. Antiviral agents to treat viral infections of the mouth may be administered in capsule, tablet, liquid, or ointment form. Acyclovir (Zovirax) is the most commonly used antiviral agent in dentistry.

Antihistamines

Antihistamines are used most commonly to relieve allergy symptoms, such as a runny nose or watery eyes. Side effects of antihistamines include drowsiness and abnormal dryness of mucous membranes. Antihistamines may interact with other drugs, including muscle relaxants, sleeping pills, drugs to treat hypertension, and alcohol.

Cholinergic Blocking Agents

Cholinergic blocking agents (**anticholinergics**), specifically atropine sulfate, are used in dentistry to inhibit the flow of saliva. Excessive saliva can make some dental procedures more difficult, including obtaining a proper impression for a crown or bridgework. Atropine may be administered approximately 2 hours prior to any procedure that would be adversely affected by excess saliva. Effects of atropine wear off some 4 to 6 hours following treatment. Side effects of anticholinergics include excessively dry mouth and blurred vision.

✓ CHECKPOINT

16-14 What are cholinergic blocking agents used for in dentistry?

Drug Side Effects, Adverse Effects, and Interactions

DAs must obtain as accurate a medical and dental history as possible from patients and carefully document both drugs prescribed and those purchased OTC. This careful history is essential for two reasons:

- **Side effects** are unintended results of drug use. These range from headaches, nausea, and diarrhea to more serious adverse effects, such as hypertension, fainting, or an irregular heartbeat (cardiac arrhythmia). Side effects of one drug can potentially interfere with the administration and effectiveness of other drugs, including drugs used during dental care.

- **Synergistic effects** occur when one drug interacts with another in a process known as **drug interaction**. Drug interactions can occur with OTC medications, prescription drugs, herbal supplements, alcohol, and even certain foods. Any of these interactions can alter the effects of drugs by making them less effective or by dangerously increasing their effect. Unforeseen synergistic effects can cause potentially dangerous or unsettling situations in the dental office.

Drug Allergies

An allergic reaction to a drug is not the same thing as a side effect. An allergic reaction to a drug may show up as a rash, hives, shortness of breath (dyspnea), or wheezing. Allergic reactions may appear within minutes or hours of exposure, depending on the route of administration for the drug.

A rare, but very serious allergic reaction, **anaphylaxis**, can prove life threatening. Anaphylaxis typically occurs upon second exposure to a drug that initially caused a milder allergic reaction such as hives. An anaphylactic reaction occurs throughout the body. Among its most dangerous effects is a tightening of the airways that can result in difficulty breathing (respiratory distress).

When obtaining a medical and dental history from a patient, DAs should list drug allergies prominently and repeat the information on each page of the dental record. Annoying, but commonly experienced side effects, such as dizziness, nausea, and diarrhea, are not allergic reactions to a drug and should *not* be indicated as such on the patient's record.

For information about treating a patient suffering from an allergic reaction, see Chapter 18, Responding to Medical Emergencies.

Physician's Desk Reference

The *Physician's Desk Reference* (PDR) is a valuable and widely used source of information on drugs currently in use. Its intended audience is physicians, dentists, nurse practitioners, and physician assistants, but it is a valuable resource for anyone. A professional DA must often understand particular medications or a class of medications better before administering or dispensing them to patients. The PDR lists drugs according to brand name, generic name, and chemical composition as well as by therapeutic classification

TABLE 16-3 Classification of Drugs

THERAPEUTIC CLASSIFICATION	USES	COMMON EXAMPLES
Analgesic	Relieve and control pain	Aspirin; acetaminophen; codeine
Antacids	Neutralize or reduce stomach acidity	Magnesia (Milk of Magnesia); calcium (Tums)
Antibiotic	Destroy or interfere with the growth of microorganisms	Penicillin; amoxicillin; tetracycline
Anticoagulants and thrombolytics	Prevent and dissolve blood clots	Coumadin; heparin; aspirin
Anticonvulsants	Control frequency and severity of seizures	Phenobarbital; phenytoin (Dilantin)
Antidepressants	Stabilize moods; treat depression	Fluoxetine (Prozac); amitriptyline hydrochloride (Elavil)
Antifungals	Destroy or retard the growth of fungi	Nystatin (Mycostatin)
Antihistamines	Relieve allergy symptoms	Chlorpheniramine maleate (Chlor-Trimeton); diphenhydramine hydrochloride (Benadryl)
Antihypertensives	Treat elevated blood pressure	Methyldopa; atenolol (Tenormin)
Anti-inflammatories	Reduce inflammation	Aspirin; ibuprofen (Motrin); naproxen (Naprosyn)
Antiviral agents	Inhibit viral replication	Acyclovir (Zovirax); azidothymidine
Bronchodilator	Dilate bronchi and relax smooth muscles of bronchial tree	Albuterol sulfate (Ventolin)
Cholinergic blocking agents	Inhibit secretions	Atropine sulfate; propantheline bromide
Contraceptive	Prevent ovulation	Provera; progestin
Decongestant	Reduce swelling of nasal passages	Pseudoephedrine hydrochloride (Sudafed)
Diuretic	Increase the secretion of urine by kidneys	Furosemide (Lasix); chlorothiazide (Diuril)
Emetics	Promote vomiting	Ipecac syrup
Hormones, female	Prevent symptoms of menopause	Estradiol (Estraderm); medroxyprogesterone acetate (Provera)
Hormones, male	Androgen therapy to treat testosterone deficiency	Fluoxymesterone (Halotestin)
Insulin and oral hypoglycemics	Control diabetes	Neutral protamine Hagedorn and Ultralente insulins; glipizide (Glucotrol); tolbutamide
Nitrates	Prevent and treat chest pain (angina)	Nitroglycerin (Nitrostat)
Thyroid and antithyroid agents	Increase or decrease amount of thyroid hormone produced	Levothyroxine sodium (T4) (Levothroid, Synthroid)
Tranquilizers	Promote relaxation; reduce anxiety	Alprazolam (Xanax); diazepam (Valium)

Adapted from Kronenberger, et al. *Comprehensive Medical Assisting*, 3rd edition. Lippincott, Williams & Wilkins, 2008. Table 23-1: Classification of Drugs.

(Table 16-3). The PDR offers the following information and more on each drug it lists:

- Chemical composition
- Generic name
- Brand name or names
- Properties

- Indications for its use, or the particular diseases and conditions for which it would be prescribed
- Contraindications against its use, or those conditions or instances in which it should *not* be used
- Dosages
- Side effects

The PDR is present in most medical and dental practices and is also available in libraries and bookstores. The website www.pdr.net offers free access to the PDR for physicians, dentists, nurse practitioners, physician assistants, and their practices.

The Role of the Dental Assistant

The professional DA is expected to maintain accurate records of drugs prescribed or dispensed to patients. If the drug was discussed in detail with the patient, important points of this discussion should be recorded. DAs may phone, fax, or send e-mail to pharmacies to confirm patient prescriptions issued by the dentist. These communications and prescriptions should be recorded in the patient record.

Although questions from pharmacists regarding patient prescriptions should always be referred to the dentist, many DAs come to know the local pharmacist well. They build and sustain a relationship with them that proves beneficial to both patients and dentists. Among other benefits, cases of patient drug abuse may come to light more quickly, and dental practices may benefit from the pharmacist's first-hand knowledge of newly introduced and available drugs.

Within the dental practice, DAs may be responsible for:

- Ordering prescription pads and ensuring that they are kept in a secure place
- Keeping the dentist's DEA number confidential
- Ensuring that necessary medications are kept in stock
- Placing controlled substances in locked cabinets and keeping them secure
- Choosing and maintaining a designated spot for drug samples left by pharmaceutical company representatives.

DAs also play a role in ensuring that a dental practice maintains all necessary records regarding controlled substances. The DEA requires that dental practices record the following and keep records on hand for at least 2 years:

- What controlled substances they received and when
- How and to whom the substance was dispensed
- The destruction of any controlled substances.

Officials at regional DEA offices throughout the country will answer questions regarding any of the drugs under their control. A DA can keep a dental practice updated on any changes regarding controlled substances by making sure the practice is on the list to receive periodic DEA informational mailings.

One of the most important professional obligations of the DA is facilitating communication with the patient regarding any use of prescription or OTC drugs. In addition, obtaining a full and accurate medical and dental history from the patient and consistently updating the histories of long-time patients helps dental practices prescribe and use only those drugs that will prove safe and most effective for their intended purposes. DAs should communicate all pertinent information to the dentist, who can make a final decision as to the appropriateness of any medication used prior to, during, or following a dental procedure.

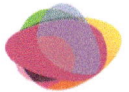

Chapter Highlights

- *Pharmacology* refers to the study of drugs and their actions on living organisms, including what drugs are composed of, how they are used, the effects they cause, and any potential for poisoning, overdoses, and other adverse effects.
- Knowledge of pharmacology helps dental assistants obtain a more accurate and complete medical history, assist in certain dental procedures, and dispense medications as needed under the supervision and direction of the dentist.
- Because drugs are increasingly used to treat a wide variety of diseases and conditions, it is important for dental assistants to understand how various classes and types of drugs affect bodily functions and influence dental care.
- Dental assistants should be able to recognize signs of drug abuse and should know which specific types of prescription and over-the-counter drugs patients are most likely to abuse.
- Legal drugs are classified according to their availability to the public and their potential for abuse. They are identified by brand name, generic name, or chemical formulation.
- Drugs and medications may be administered in a number of ways depending on the drug. Drugs may be

administered orally, sublingually, or rectally; inhaled; applied topically to the skin or mucosa; absorbed through a skin patch; or injected intravenously, intramuscularly, subcutaneously, or intradermally.

◆ The Controlled Substances Act assigns enforcement of laws governing controlled substances to the Drug Enforcement Agency. An official Drug Schedule assigns these drugs to one of five categories according to their potential for abuse, potential for medicinal use, and proven safety.

◆ Over-the-counter (OTC) drugs are sometimes referred to as *patent medicines* and may be obtained at retail establishments without a prescription. OTC drugs commonly used by consumers include analgesics for pain relief, antacids for upset stomach, and expectorants and cough suppressants for relief of cold symptoms.

◆ Three legal and habit-forming substances of concern to dental assistants are alcohol, tobacco, and caffeine. Use of each affects dental and oral health to some degree. Excessive use of alcohol and tobacco present a public health concern.

◆ Illegal drugs of concern include marijuana, cocaine, heroin, and hallucinogens such as lysergic acid diethylamide.

◆ Dental assistants must remain aware of potential side effects, synergistic effects, and adverse effects that may interfere with the administration and effectiveness of drugs used during dental care.

◆ An allergic reaction to a drug is not the same thing as a side effect. An allergic reaction to a drug may show up as a rash, hives, shortness of breath (dyspnea), or wheezing. A rare, but very serious allergic reaction, anaphylaxis, can prove life threatening.

◆ Dentists are most likely to prescribe anesthetics, analgesics, antibiotics, and tranquilizers.

◆ Some duties related to prescription drugs that a dental assistant may be expected to perform include maintaining accurate records of drugs prescribed or dispensed to patients, ordering prescription pads and keeping them secure, ensuring that necessary medications are kept in stock, placing controlled substances in locked cabinets and keeping them secure, choosing and maintaining a proper storage space for drug samples left by company representatives, and ensuring that the dental practice maintains all necessary records regarding controlled substances.

◆ A primary role of the dental assistant is to obtain and consistently update the medical and dental history from each patient, including the patient's use of prescription and over-the-counter drugs.

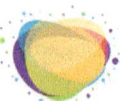 **Review Questions**

1. The recommended route of administration for the drug nitrous oxide is

    a. Oral.

    b. Transdermal.

    c. Inhalation.

    d. Intramuscular.

2. Codeine is sometimes dispensed combined with any of several other drugs to produce a greater pain-reducing effect than can be obtained by taking either in isolation. This is an example of which of the following?

    a. Synergistic effect

    b. Side effect

    c. Sublingual administration

    d. Anaphylactic reaction

3. Which medical professionals are allowed to *prescribe* medication to patients?

    a. Physicians, dentists, nurse practitioners, and physician assistants

    b. Physicians, dentists, dental hygienists, and dental assistants

    c. Physicians, dentists, and dental hygienists

    d. Physicians and dentists

4. Which of the following is *not* a route of drug administration?

    a. Oral

    b. Transdermal

    c. Sublingual

    d. Gastrointestinal

5. Smoking causes many cases of heart disease by

    a. Interfering with the body's ability to properly oxygenate the blood.

    b. Allowing nicotine to collect in the tissues of the heart.

    c. Causing shortness of breath (dyspnea) that results in lack of exercise.

    d. All of the above.

6. To which of the following categories does the commonly prescribed drug codeine belong?

    a. Narcotic

    b. Opiate

c. Analgesic

d. All of the above

7. Anaphylaxis, a systemic allergic reaction, is dangerous because

a. Its effects are not detectable.

b. It appears in a patient the first time a drug is used.

c. It causes airways to constrict, restricting breathing.

d. It causes hepatic hemorrhage.

8. Of the common types of drugs, dentists are most likely to use or prescribe

a. Anticonvulsants, painkillers, and cholinergic-blocking agents.

b. Antifungal agents, nitrates, and antihypertensives.

c. Antiviral agents, sedatives, and nonsteroidal anti-inflammatory drugs.

d. Anesthetics, analgesics, antibiotics, and tranquilizers.

9. Which antibiotic is dispensed as a mouth rinse and used in dentistry to treat plaque and gingivitis?

a. Lysergic acid diethylamide

b. Diazepam

c. Chlorhexidine

d. Acyclovir

10. Infective endocarditis, an inflammation of the lining of the heart, is of concern in dentistry because

a. It may interfere with the administration of nitrous oxide and other anesthetics.

b. Certain patients may be predisposed to developing it following dental procedures.

c. It can cause airways to constrict and cause respiratory distress.

d. It is complicated by the synergistic effects of drugs.

Active Learning Exercises

1. List three routes of administration for drugs, then identify two types of drugs that may be administered via each route. For example:
   Inhalation: Asthma medication, such as albuterol, and oxygen can be administered by inhalation.

2. Discuss the differences between tranquilizers and analgesics. What are some reasons a patient may need them for a dental visit?

3. Choose three of the most commonly prescribed drugs in the dental office. Look them up in the *Physician's Desk Reference* and make a chart including common use, possible side effects, adverse drug reactions, contraindications, and any dental considerations.

Application Activities

1. Create a simple double-column list summarizing antibiotic prophylaxis recommendations for dental procedures performed on high-risk patients. In the first column, list the procedures that require preventive antibiotics, and in the second column list those that do not.

2. Understanding how the abuse of drugs or alcohol can affect an individual's oral health will help you better communicate with patients who may be struggling with addiction. Select five of the commonly abused drugs discussed in the text. Using the library or the Internet for research, write a paragraph or two for each one describing possible oral health problems associated with abuse of the substance.

PREPARING FOR CERTIFICATION EXAMS

Review the following topics in this chapter to prepare for the Dental Assisting National Board (DANB) exam:

- **Introduction**

- **Commonly Prescribed Drugs**

- **Drug Side Effect, Adverse Effects, and Interactions**

- **Drug Allergies**

- **The Role of the Dental Assistant**

chapter 17

Vital Signs

CHAPTER CHECKLIST

On completion of this chapter, students will be able to:

☑   Identify the major vital signs.

☑   Describe factors that can affect each of the vital signs.

☑   Identify the different kinds of thermometers.

☑   Identity the common sites and methods for taking temperature.

☑   Describe how to measure respiration.

☑   Name the common body sites for measuring pulse.

☑   Describe the numbers that compose blood pressure readings, and explain what each means.

☑   Describe the correct technique for taking each of the major vital signs.

☑   Describe the purpose of electrocardiography.

KEY TERMS

antecubital (an-tee-KYOO-bih-tul) space – the inside fold of the arm, opposite the elbow

axillary thermometer – an instrument that is placed inside the armpit to measure temperature

blood pressure – the pressure of blood against the walls of the arteries as the heart pumps and relaxes

brachial (BRAY-kee-ul) artery – a blood vessel located in the upper arm that can be felt at the antecubital space

carotid (kuh-ROT-id) artery – a major blood vessel located in the neck, where the pulse can be felt under the jaw bone about halfway between the chin and the ear

diastolic (die-uh-STOL-ik) pressure – the pressure of blood on the walls of the arteries as the heart relaxes and fills up with blood

electrocardiogram – a test that measures the patterns of electrical activity and determines whether the heart is beating regularly or irregularly

femoral artery – a major blood vessel in the thigh, where the pulse can be felt inside the crease between the groin and the inner thigh

oral thermometer – an instrument that is placed under the tongue to measure temperature

palpate (PAL-pate) – to examine by feeling with the fingers or hands

pulse – the expansion and relaxation of an artery; also called a *pulsation*

pulse oximeter (ok-SIM-ih-ter) – a device that attaches to the finger and measures the amount of oxygen in the blood; used for patients under anesthesia to monitor vital signs

pulse rate – the number of pulsations measured per minute

pulse rhythm – the pattern of pulsations (e.g., steady, skipping)

pulse volume – the force of pulsations (e.g., strong, weak)

radial artery – a blood vessel in the lower arm and hand, where the pulse can be felt on the inside of the wrist, below the bone by the thumb

rectal thermometer – an instrument that is placed inside the rectum to measure temperature

respiration – the movement of oxygen into and carbon dioxide out of the lungs

respiratory depth – amount of oxygen inhaled and carbon dioxide exhaled

respiratory rate – number of breaths per minute

respiratory rhythm – pattern of breaths

sphygmomanometer (sfig-moh-muh-NOM-ih-ter) – a device for measuring blood pressure that includes an arm cuff, inflation bulb, and pressure gauge

stethoscope – an instrument used to listen to sounds in the heart, lungs, and other body organs; includes ear pieces that fit into the ear and a flat metal disc that is placed on the body and picks up sounds

systolic pressure – the pressure of blood on the walls of the arteries as the heart pumps and sends blood out to the rest of the body

temperature – the measure of heat in the body

tympanic thermometer – an instrument placed inside the ear's outer canal to measure body temperature

vital signs – physical measures of body functioning that provide important information about the basic systems that keep a person alive, such as breathing and heart functioning

Introduction

Monitoring the patient's physical health is one of your most important responsibilities. The well-being and safety of the patient may depend on knowing his or her **vital signs**. Vital signs are physical measures of basic body functioning. They provide important information about the basic body systems that keep a person alive, such as breathing and heart functioning. Vital signs commonly include temperature, respiration, pulse, and blood pressure. Electrocardiography may also be used to monitor some patients' heart function. By checking and understanding a patient's vital signs, you can detect indications of unsafe physical conditions and assist the patient accordingly, helping make the patient's appointment as safe and productive as possible.

Factors Affecting Vital Signs

Vital signs reveal much about how the patient's body is functioning, and high or low readings can occur for many reasons. For example, nervous or upset feelings can increase pulse rate and body temperature. Older adults often have lower respiration or blood pressure than other adults. Even beverages can impact vital signs. Ever notice how a hot cup of coffee can get your heart pumping?

If a patient's vital signs are higher or lower than normal, consider whether any of these factors may be present. If the patient seems upset or nervous, provide gentle reassurance. Has the patient just come in from cold or hot weather outdoors? If so, allow a few minutes for the patient to relax before proceeding. You may need to take the vital signs again but, in the end, having an accurate recording of the patient's vital signs is what is most important.

Temperature

The body's **temperature** is the measure of the balance between heat produced and lost by the body. The body produces heat two ways: *metabolism* (the normal physical and chemical processes that occur inside the body) and *muscle movement*. Heat can be lost by breathing, sweating, or elimination of bodily waste.

Temperature is measured using a thermometer, which can be placed at different sites on or inside the body (Figure 17-1). **Oral thermometers**, the most common type used, are placed directly under the tongue. **Axillary thermometers** are placed just inside the armpit. **Tympanic thermometers** are inserted inside the ear. For infants, **rectal thermometers** are gently inserted inside the rectum. Temperature can also be taken by placing a strip thermometer across the forehead.

Types of Thermometers

When taking an oral temperature, use a glass thermometer or a digital thermometer (see Figure 17-1). Glass thermometers have a glass tube that contains a silver bulb filled with a non-hazardous liquid that acts as a temperature sensor. Glass thermometers once contained the chemical mercury, which can be harmful to humans. Today's glass thermometers no longer contain mercury and are safe when used with care.

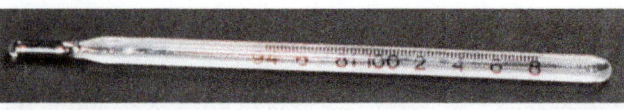

A

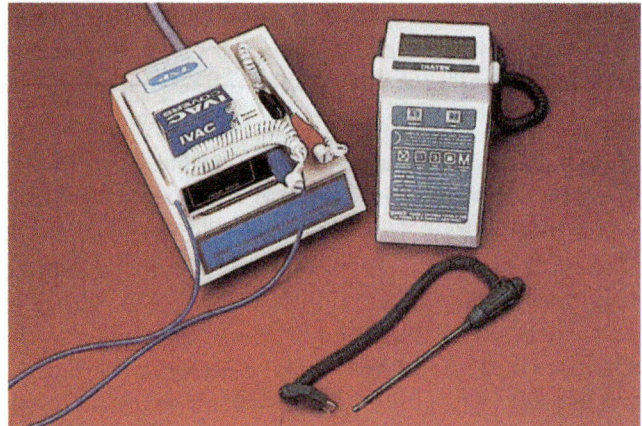

B

Figure 17–1 Thermometers. (A) Glass. **(B)** Two types of digital models with probes.

The patient's body heat causes the liquid inside the bulb to expand and slowly rise. Numbers written along the side of the thermometer show the temperature reading. After 3 minutes, the liquid will reach its highest point, and you can determine the patient's temperature by reading the number.

Digital thermometers are more common today than glass thermometers. Although they are used in the same way, digital thermometers have an electronic display that shows a patient's temperature in numerical digits. This makes them much easier to read. Digital thermometers contain a metal probe. Before using the digital thermometer, cover the probe with a plastic tube that can be thrown away afterward. This will prevent the spread of germs from patient to patient.

Digital thermometers use batteries and are kept in a base that is plugged into the wall. When the thermometer is not being used, keep it in its base in order to prevent the batteries from running low. Low batteries in a digital thermometer can cause it to show an incorrect reading.

Tympanic thermometers are usually used for children and infants over 3 months of age. A tympanic thermometer contains a short metal probe which is placed gently inside the ear. Like the digital thermometer, a plastic cover is placed over the tube and thrown away afterwards. Within about 2 seconds, a digital reading of the patient's temperature is displayed.

Axillary thermometers can be either glass or digital and are tucked gently inside the armpit. Forehead thermometers have an infrared light that measures heat from the body. They can be digital or may come in the form of disposable strips, which are placed directly on the forehead.

TABLE 17-1 Types of Thermometers and Normal Temperature Range

BODY SITE	TYPE OF THERMOMETER	NORMAL ADULT TEMPERATURE
Oral	Glass or digital	98.6°F
Axillary	Glass or digital	97.6°F
Tympanic	Digital	99.6°F
Rectal	Glass or digital	99.6°F

Temperature Scales

Two scales are used to read temperature. The Fahrenheit (F) scale is more commonly used in the United States, whereas in Canada and Europe the Celsius (C) scale is used. A normal body temperature is 98.6°F (37.0°C) but may be slightly higher or lower depending on where on the body it is taken (Table 17-1). Infants and young children usually have higher temperatures than teenagers and adults. Older adults often have slightly lower temperatures.

Table 17-2 describes some factors that can raise or lower body temperature. Make sure you are aware of these factors when you take the patient's temperature.

TABLE 17-2 Factors that Affect Temperature

Gender	Women tend to have higher temperatures than men.
Exercise	Burning calories raises your body temperature.
Time of day	People usually have a lower body temperature at the start of the day.
Emotions	If you're feeling stressed, nervous, or upset, your temperature can rise. If you're feeling blue or depressed, your temperature can fall.
Health	When you're feeling ill, you may have a slightly higher or lower temperature.
Environment	If the air around you is especially hot or cold, this can make your body temperature higher or lower as well.

Procedure 17-1 **Taking an Oral Temperature**

Digital Thermometer

Materials needed (Figure P17-1-1):

- Digital thermometer with base
- Disposable plastic probe cover
- Gloves

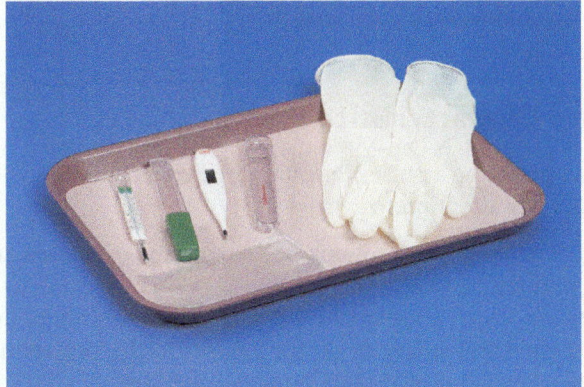

Figure P17-1-1

1. Wash your hands and put on a pair of gloves. Ask your patient if he or she has had anything to eat or drink, chewed gum, or smoked tobacco within the past 15 minutes. If so, wait 15 minutes until taking your patient's temperature. Failing to do so can cause an incorrect reading!

2. Place a new, clean plastic cover on the probe. Turn the thermometer on and wait for the "ready" reading on the display. Using the thermometer before it is "ready" can result in incorrect readings.

3. Gently place the probe under the patient's tongue and ask the patient to close his or her lips around the probe. Do not talk to the patient. If the patient's lips do not stay closed, the temperature reading may be incorrect.

4. The thermometer will beep when the reading is complete. Read the temperature on the display and remove the probe from the patient's mouth.

5. Throw away the disposable probe cover, turn the thermometer off, and return the thermometer to its base. You must keep the thermometer in the base so that the batteries do not run low.

6. Record the patient's temperature in the dental chart, including the date, time, and your signature.

Glass Thermometer

Materials needed (see Figure P17-1-1):

- Glass thermometer
- Sheath cover for protection
- Gloves

1. Wash your hands and put on a pair of gloves. Ask your patient if he or she has had anything to eat or drink, chewed gum, or smoked tobacco within the past 15 minutes. If so, wait 15 minutes until taking your patient's temperature. These can cause incorrect readings if you do not!

2. Make sure the thermometer is dry, clean, and free of cracks or breaks. Place a disposable plastic sheath over the thermometer to keep from spreading germs.

3. Hold the thermometer at eye level and turn it slowly on its side. If the reading is above 94.0°F, shake the thermometer until the reading falls below that level. The thermometer must be below 94.0° F before you can accurately take a temperature.

4. Gently place the probe under the patient's tongue and ask the patient to close his or her lips around the probe (Figure P17- 1-2). Do not talk to the patient. If the patient's lips do not stay closed, the temperature reading may be incorrect.

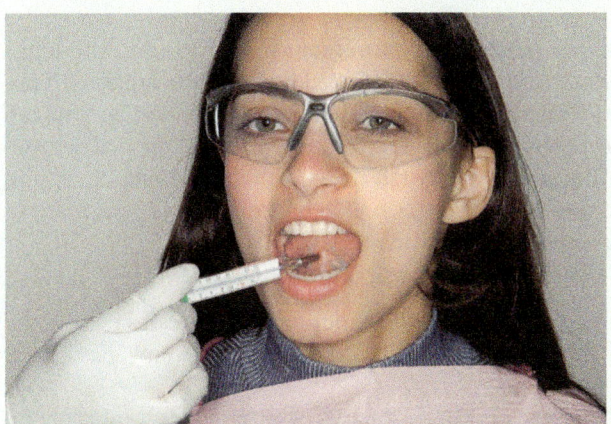

Figure P17-1-2

5. Leave the thermometer in place for 3 to 5 minutes before removing.

6. Hold the thermometer at eye level, keeping it on its side, and read the level to which the liquid has risen (Figure P17-1-3).

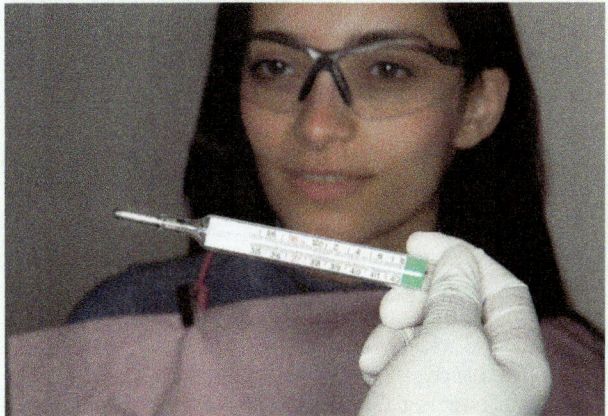

Figure P17-1-3

7. Clean and disinfect the thermometer according to the manufacturer's instructions.

8. Record the patient's temperature in the dental chart, including the date, time, and your signature.

CHECKPOINTS

17-1 What are the four most common vital signs?

17-2 Why are vital signs important to monitor?

17-3 What is the normal temperature for an adult?

17-4 What are four types of thermometers used to measure temperature?

Respiration

Respiration is the movement of oxygen into the lungs (*inhalation*) and carbon dioxide out of the lungs (*exhalation*). The brain generally controls respiration so you can breathe without having to think about it. Special sensors in the carotid artery tell the brain when too much carbon dioxide is in the lungs, which tells the lungs to respirate so carbon dioxide can be released.

Characteristics of respiration include:

- The **respiratory rate**, or number of breaths per minute
- The **respiratory rhythm**, or the overall pattern of breathing
- The **respiratory depth**, or amount of air inhaled and exhaled

In addition to these characteristics, respiration should be checked for any unusual sounds, such as wet or dry sounds (crackles) or high-pitched sounds (wheezing).

The normal respiration rate for a relaxed adult is 10 to 20 breaths per minute. Children and teen-agers may have as many as 30 breaths per minute. Respiration rate can be affected by a lack of oxygen resulting from an illness or other medical condition, by exercise, by strong emotions (such as being very upset), and by the use of tobacco or drugs.

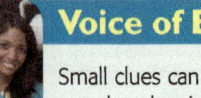

Voice of Experience

Small clues can lead to big discoveries. I have learned as a dental assistant that vital signs give me very important information about my patients' overall health. While measuring respirations, I discovered that an older patient had rapid breathing. After asking some questions, I realized that she had a larger, more serious health issue. By recognizing her abnormal breathing, I was able to ask the right questions and determine that she needed to go to the hospital. It turned out that she had pneumonia. Because I took her vital signs, she got the treatment she needed. On another occasion, taking the vital signs of a patient who felt unwell led to my discovery that he had missed his morning blood pressure medication. Even though they may seem routine and simple, vital signs carry important messages that I do not want to miss!

Pulse

Every time the heart beats, it pushes blood through the arteries. When the heart beats, the arteries expand. Between beats, the arteries relax. This expanding and relaxing motion is called a **pulse**, or *pulsation*. Arteries that are close to the skin are good for measuring pulsations because you can feel the pulse simply by touching, or **palpating**, with your fingers.

Pulse Characteristics

When palpating a pulse, there are three characteristics you should pay attention to.

- **Pulse rate** is the number of pulsations counted in 1 minute.
- **Pulse rhythm** refers to the pattern of the pulsations. Do they feel steady or do they skip? Do the pulsations occasionally slow down? Do they speed up?
- **Pulse volume** is the force of the pulsations. Does the pulse feel strong? Weak?

Take a pulse by gently palpating an artery with your fingers. Never use your thumb because it has a pulse of its own, which could be confused with the patient's.

Pulse Locations

There are several arteries where you can palpate a pulse (Figure 17-2). Most often, you will use the **radial artery**, located on the inside of the wrist below the thumb. Take a radial pulse by placing your index and middle fingertips just below the bone on the thumb side. The **brachial artery** in the upper arm can be felt on the inner fold of the arm, opposite the elbow. This space is called the **antecubital space**. The **carotid artery** is a major blood vessel felt on the side of the neck, near the Adam's apple (also called the *larynx* or *voice box*). It can be found by palpating just under the jaw bone, about halfway between the chin and the ear. The **femoral artery** is one of the largest blood vessels in the body, and its pulse can be felt inside the crease between the groin and the inner thigh.

Taking a Pulse

When taking a pulse, you need a watch or clock. While watching the second hand, count the number of beats for 1 minute. You can also count the number of beats for 30 seconds and double the number. Do not count for less than 30 seconds, though, because it is hard to detect any problems with the heartbeat in so short a time.

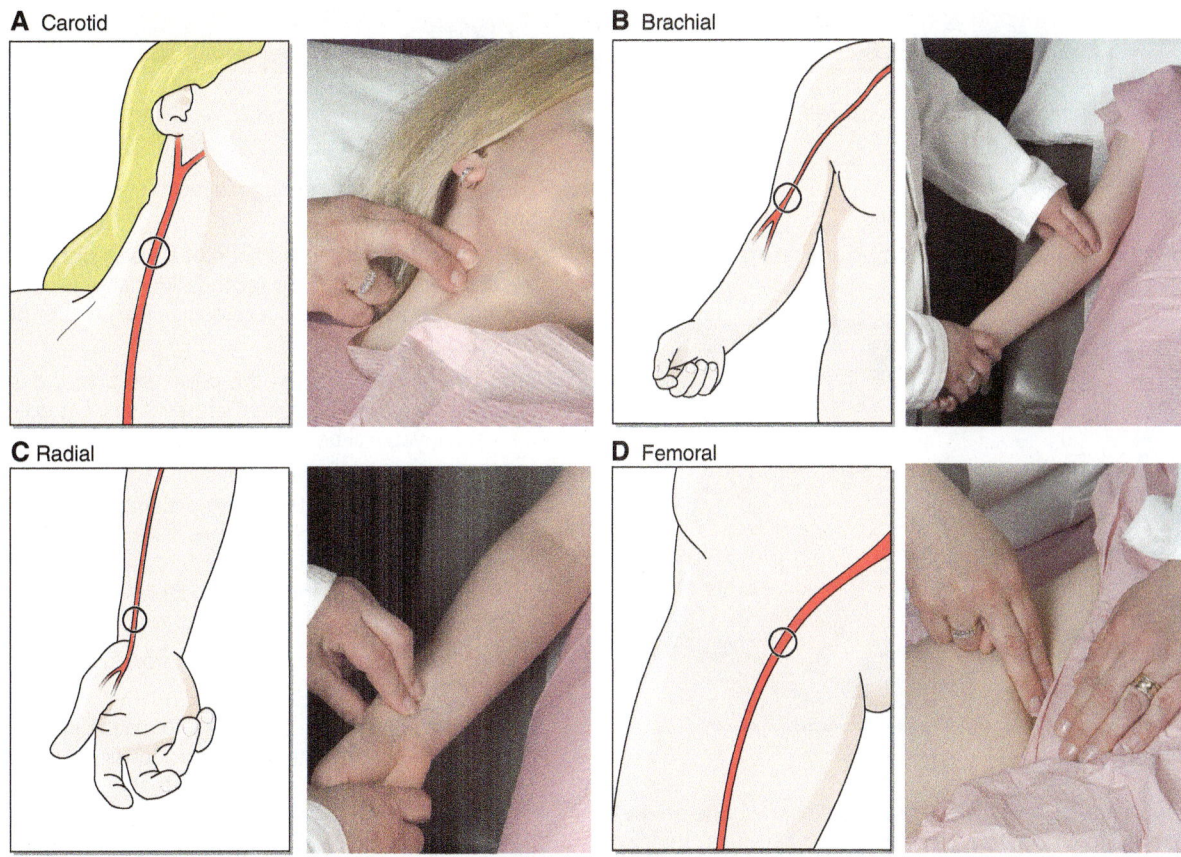

Figure 17–2 **Sites for palpation of pulses.** **(A)** Carotid. **(B)** Brachial. **(C)** Radial. **(D)** Femoral.

A **pulse oximeter** is a medical device that measures the amount of oxygen in the blood (Figure 17-3). It is used to monitor pulse and blood oxygen levels in patients who are under anesthesia. It attaches to the finger by a small plastic clip that is connected to a monitor. If blood oxygen falls too low, an alarm will sound. When a patient is intravenously sedated, a pulse oximeter is a helpful way of monitoring these vital signs.

For adults, a normal pulse ranges between 60 and 80 beats per minute. For children under the age of 10 years, it is slightly higher at 90 to 110 beats per minute. Infants under the age of 1 year have an even faster pulse at 110 to 170 beats per minute. Older adults typically have a lower pulse, ranging from 55 to 70 beats per minute.

Factors Affecting Pulse

The pulse's rate, rhythm, and volume are affected by many different factors. For instance:

- The pulse rate is lower early in the morning than at night.
- Women generally have a slightly higher pulse rate than men.
- People with smaller body sizes usually have a lower pulse rate than people with larger bodies.
- Exercise increases the pulse rate, as do strong emotions such as anger, fear, or excitement. On the other hand, feeling very down or blue can make the pulse rate lower.
- With a fever, the pulse rate is often higher.
- Medications can both raise or lower the pulse rate.
- A dramatic loss of blood (hemorrhage) or a lack of fluids (dehydration) can initially increase the pulse rate.

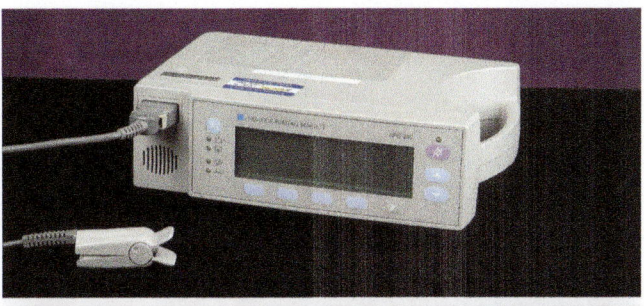

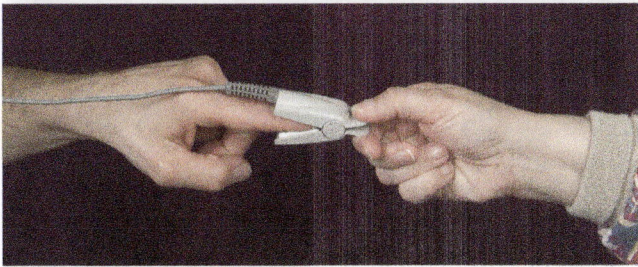

Figure 17–3 Pulse oximeter.

Procedure 17-2 Taking a Radial Pulse and Assessing Respiration

Pulse and respiration should be measured together, starting with the pulse.

Materials needed:

- A watch or clock with a second hand

1. Make sure the patient's arm is relaxed and resting comfortably in his or her lap.

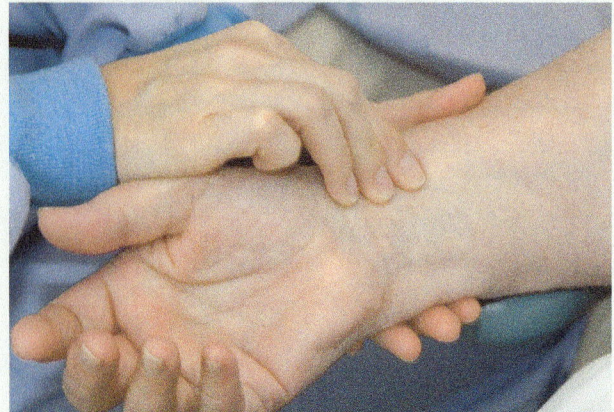

Figure P17-2-1

2. Gently palpate the radial artery just below the bone on the thumb side of the inner wrist with your index and middle

fingertips. Remember to use your fingers and not your thumb, which has a pulse of its own (Figure P17-2-1).

3. Press lightly but firmly enough to feel the pulse of the artery against your fingers.

4. While watching the second hand of a watch or clock, count the number of beats for 30 seconds. Multiply this number by 2 because pulse is always recorded as the number of beats per minute.

5. After you have completed the pulse, keep your fingers in place as you count the patient's respirations, but do not tell the patient you will be doing so. This may cause the patient to breathe abnormally slow or fast.

6. Count the number of times the patient's chest rises and falls for 30 seconds. Each complete rise and fall of the chest counts as 1. Multiply this number by 2 because respiration is always recorded as the number of breaths per minute.

7. Note the characteristics of the patient's respiration. Was the patient breathing unusually fast or slow? Did the patient seem to be struggling to breathe?

8. Record the pulse and respiration information in the dental chart, along with the date, time, and your signature.

Blood Pressure

With each beat of the heart, blood is forced through the arteries. The amount of pressure on the walls of the arteries is known as **blood pressure**. Blood pressure measurements include two numbers. The **systolic pressure** is the force on the arteries as the heart pushes blood into the blood vessels. **Diastolic pressure** is the force on the arteries when the heart relaxes and fills back up with blood. The systolic pressure should be higher than the diastolic pressure.

Measuring Blood Pressure

Blood pressure is measured in millimeters of mercury (mm Hg). The systolic number is written first, followed by the diastolic, and it is pronounced as systolic "over" diastolic. For example, 120/80, or "120 over 80," means that the systolic pressure is 120 mm Hg, and the diastolic pressure is 80 mm Hg.

Blood pressure is measured by placing a **sphygmomanometer**, or blood pressure cuff and gauge (Figure 17-4), around the arm, over the brachial artery. The cuff is inflatable and wraps around the upper arm. It is connected to a rubber ball by a short tube. When the ball is squeezed, the cuff inflates and tightens around the arm. As the cuff continues

to tighten, blood stops flowing through the brachial artery. A screw valve on the gauge allows the cuff to deflate so blood can flow through the artery again. Using a **stethoscope**, sounds of the systolic and diastolic pressure can be heard. A stethoscope is an instrument used to listen to sounds in the body. It has earpieces that fit into the ears and a flat metal disc

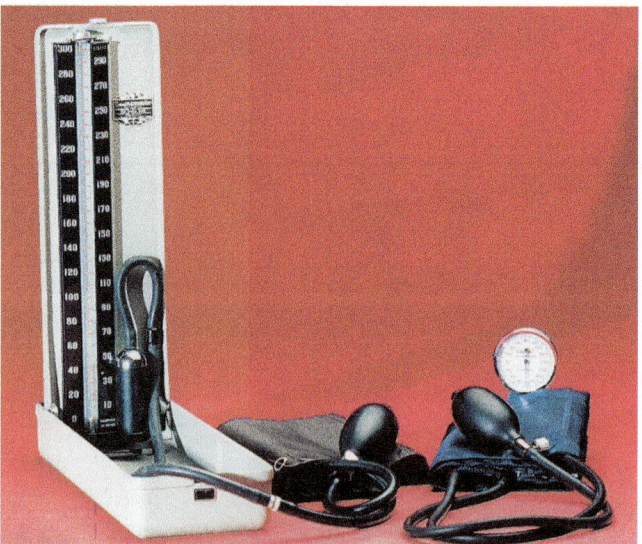

Figure 17-4 Sphygmomanometers. Mercury column (left) and aneroid (right).

TABLE 17-3 Five Phases of Korotkoff Sounds with Cuff Deflation

PHASE	DESCRIPTION	SOUND
Phase I	Blood flows back into the brachial artery; this is the systolic pressure.	This makes a sharp tapping sound.
Phase II	More blood continues to flow.	This makes a soft swishing sound.
Phase III	A large volume of blood now flows through the artery.	This makes a rhythmic, sharp, distinct tapping sound.
Phase IV	Blood flows through the artery easily.	This makes a soft tapping that becomes faint.
Phase V	The artery returns to its original state; this is the diastolic pressure.	The last sound disappears.

that is placed on the body to pick up sounds. These sounds of the heart as the pressure cuff deflates are called *Korotkoff sounds*, named after the Russian doctor who first described them. The five phases are described in Table 17-3.

Blood pressure readings can be influenced by many factors, such as too small or too large cuff size for the arm, exercise, strong emotions, medications, alcohol use, and heat or cold. Some patients experience a slight temporary increase in blood pressure due to anxiety while in a medical setting, called "white coat hypertension." Table 17-4 describes the standard blood pressure categories.

From the Dentist's Perspective

Ensuring the health and safety of my patients is my most important job. Having a dental assistant who knows how to correctly take a blood pressure reading is very valuable. If the patient has unusually high or low blood pressure, it can make procedures risky and can cause unnecessary harm to the patient. When I can trust that my dental assistant knows how to accurately take a blood pressure reading, that is one less thing for me to have to worry about—which means more time and energy can be devoted to the patient.

There are several types of blood pressure measuring equipment, and each has its own advantages and disadvantages (Table 17-5).

Electrocardiography

Electrocardiography refers to the electrical activity in the heart that allows it to beat. An **electrocardiogram** (ECG, or EKG) is a test that measures the patterns of electrical activity to determine whether the heart is beating regularly. When the patient is undergoing a dental procedure that requires anesthesia, an ECG can monitor the heartbeat during the procedure. An ECG uses electrodes on the chest to gather information about the heartbeat for the ECG. The machine prints out a strip of paper that shows patterns of electrical activity as the heart beats and relaxes. The printout can show whether or not the patient has an arrhythmia, or abnormal heart rhythm.

CHECKPOINTS

17-5 Why must you always palpate a pulse with your fingers but not your thumb?

17-6 What arteries are commonly used to take a pulse?

17-7 What are the two types of blood pressure readings and what does each mean?

TABLE 17-4 Blood Pressure Categories

BLOOD PRESSURE CATEGORY	SYSTOLIC PRESSURE mm Hg		DIASTOLIC PRESSURE mm Hg
Normal	less than 120	and	less than 80
Prehypertension	120–139	or	80–89
High (stage 1)	140–159	or	90–99
High (stage 2)	160 or higher	or	100 or higher
Hypertensive crisis	180 or higher	or	110 or higher

TABLE 17-5 Types of Instruments Used to Take Blood Pressure

INSTRUMENT	STRENGTHS	WEAKNESSES
Automatic (finger)	Finger equipment is easy to carry and easy to use.	Not as accurate as other blood pressure instruments.
Manual, mercury	This is the most common and most accurate type of blood pressure equipment used in health care.	Bulky and heavier than electronic equipment. Also, the mercury in the monitor can be harmful to humans if it breaks and the liquid spills. Manual equipment also requires a stethoscope.
Manual, aneroid	Just like the mercury equipment, the aneroid gauge is very common and highly accurate. However, it uses a spring rather than liquid mercury, so it poses fewer risks to patients.	Because they are lighter, these tend to break more easily. Requires a stethoscope.
Automatic (wrist, arm)	This style is easy to carry, easy to use, and is accurate. Also, no stethoscope is needed.	Automatic monitors are newer and have more parts, which can make them expensive to replace or repair. They also require batteries, which, if low, can lead to incorrect readings.

Procedure 17-3 Taking Manual Blood Pressure

Taking blood pressure should only take 5 to 10 minutes.
Materials needed (Figure P17-3-1):

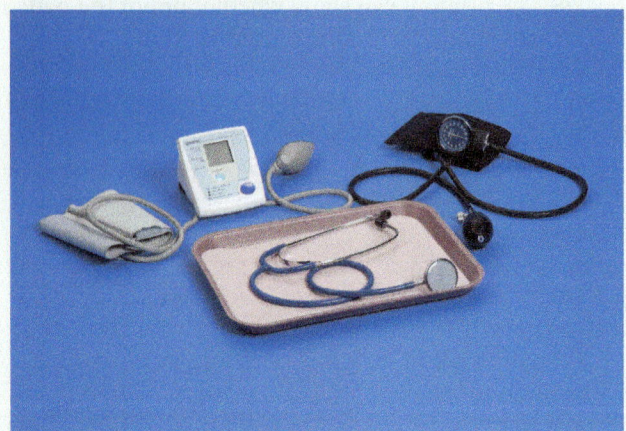

Figure P17-3-1

- Sphygmomanometer (pediatric and adult sizes)
- Stethoscope

OR

- Digital blood pressure machine

1. Usually the patient's right arm is used. Make sure the patient's arm is resting comfortably, either on his or her leg or on an object (such as a tabletop). The arm should be bent slightly with the palm facing up; legs should be uncrossed. (If the patient's arm is not relaxed and level with the heart, your reading can be incorrect. Crossed legs can increase blood pressure.) Keep the upper arm level with the patient's heart.

2. If needed, roll or push up the sleeve, but be sure it is not too tight. A tight sleeve can increase blood pressure. Choose the correct size cuff for the patient's arm size.

3. If you need to determine the maximum inflation level, strap the cuff onto the patient above the antecubital fossa, then locate the radial pulse pressure point, and close the sphygmomanometer valve. Palpate the radial pulse, watching the center of the manometer's mercury column. Quickly inflate the cuff to 80 mm Hg, then continue to inflate in increments of 10 mm Hg until the radial pulse disappears (note the reading of the mercury column at this point). Double-check to ensure the pulse is absent; if not, inflate the cuff another 10 mm Hg, repeating as necessary. After the pulse is confirmed as being absent, inflate the cuff another 30 mm Hg to ensure that the radial pulse has disappeared. This is the maximum inflation level.

Procedure 17-3 **Taking Manual Blood Pressure (Continued)**

4. Slide the deflated cuff over the arm and place it directly over the brachial artery—this should be about 2 inches (5 cm) above the antecubital space (Figure P17-3-2).

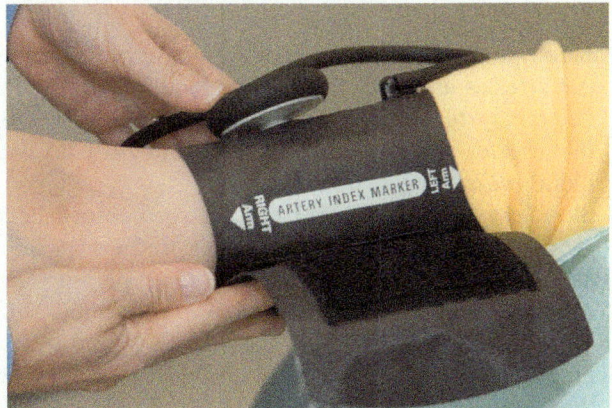

Figure P17-3-2

5. Tightly secure the cuff over the arm using the Velcro. The cuff should be tight enough to be able to barely slide one finger underneath it. A cuff that is too tight or too loose will give an incorrect reading.

6. Place the earpieces of the stethoscope in your ears with the earpieces facing forward and press the stethoscope disc (also known as the *chestpiece* or *head*) flat against the brachial artery with your nondominant hand (Figure P17-3-3).

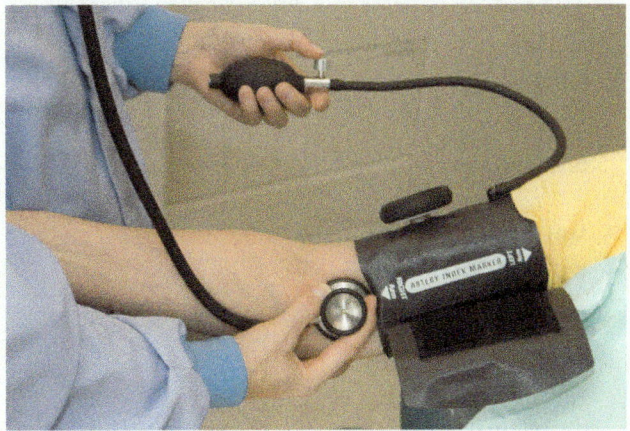

Figure P17-3-3

7. Turn the sphygmomanometer valve clockwise to lock it in place. An unlocked valve will prevent the cuff from inflating.

8. With your dominant hand, squeeze the ball and inflate the cuff quickly.

9. Watch the gauge on the cuff and stop pumping once it reaches the maximum inflation level you noted earlier. The sound of the pulse should have ceased. Overinflating can cause discomfort to the patient. However, if you underinflate, you will not get a correct systolic reading.

10. Once the cuff is fully inflated to the maximum level, turn the valve counterclockwise to begin releasing the air. You must do this slowly, at about 2 to 4 mm Hg per second. Deflating too quickly means you may miss the systolic reading. Deflating too slowly can cause incorrect readings.

11. Watching the gauge, note the number at which you hear the first clear thumping sound. This is the systolic pressure, or *Korotkoff Phase I*.

12. Slowly continue releasing air from the cuff and listen to the changes in sounds. Note the number on the gauge at which you hear the last sound—this is the diastolic pressure, or *Korotkoff Phase V*.

13. Record the two numbers and be sure to note the date, the time, and which arm was used, along with the date, the time, and your signature (Figure P17-3-4).

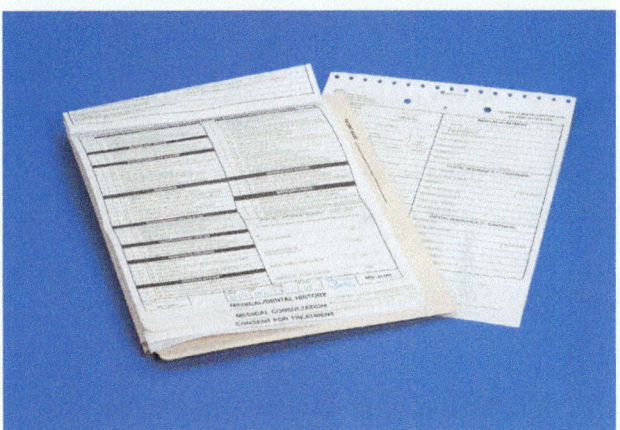

Figure P17-3-4

14. Remove the cuff from the patient.

15. Remove the stethoscope and disinfect the earpieces and metal disc.

Chapter Highlights

✦ Vital signs are important measures of basic body functions that keep a person alive, such as temperature, pulse, respiration, and blood pressure.

✦ Temperature is measured with a thermometer, which can be glass or digital.

✦ Different thermometers are placed at different body sites, such as oral, axillary, tympanic, rectal, and forehead thermometers.

✦ *Pulse* refers to the expanding and relaxing of the arteries as the heart beats. Characteristics of pulse include the *rate*, or number of beats per minute; the *rhythm*, or pattern of beats; and the *volume*, or force of the beats.

✦ Take a pulse by palpating an artery with your fingers, but never your thumb. The radial artery is the most common artery for palpating a pulse, but you can also use the brachial, carotid, and femoral arteries.

✦ Respiration is the process of breathing in oxygen and breathing out carbon dioxide.

✦ Characteristics of respiration include *rate*, or number of breaths; *rhythm*, or pattern of breaths; and *depth*, or amount of oxygen inhaled and carbon dioxide exhaled.

✦ Blood pressure is measured as the amount of force on the arteries as the heart pumps blood into the blood vessels (*systolic pressure*) and the amount of force on the arteries as the heart relaxes and fills back up with blood (*diastolic pressure*).

✦ Blood pressure is measured using an instrument called a *sphygmomanometer* (blood pressure cuff and gauge).

✦ Sounds heard when measuring blood pressure are called *Korotkoff sounds*. You listen to the sounds with a stethoscope.

✦ *Electrocardiography* refers to the electrical patterns in the heart as it beats.

✦ An electrocardiogram is a test that follows the pattern of the heart's electrical activity to determine whether the heart rhythm is normal or abnormal.

Review Questions

1. Which of these is not considered a vital sign?

   a. Temperature

   b. Weight

   c. Blood Pressure

   d. Respiration

2. What is the average normal oral temperature for an adult?

   a. 97.0°F

   b. 98.6°F

   c. 96.8°F

   d. 96.7°F

3. Which of these could cause a person's body temperature to be lower than the average normal?

   a. Female gender

   b. Exercise

   c. Older age

   d. Using a tympanic thermometer

4. The pattern of beats in a pulse is called what?

   a. Rate

   b. Rhythm

   c. Volume

   d. Palpation

5. What is the most common body location for taking a pulse?

   a. Antecubital space

   b. Carotid artery

   c. Radial artery

   d. Brachial artery

6. What is a normal resting pulse for adults?

   a. 40 to 60 beats per minute

   b. 60 to 110 beats per minute

   c. 80 to 120 beats per minute

   d. 60 to 80 beats per minute

7. Characteristics of respiration include
   a. Rate, rhythm, and depth.
   b. Rate, depth, and volume.
   c. Rate, rhythm, and volume.
   d. Depth, rhythm, and volume.

8. The systolic pressure
   a. Is written first and is usually larger than the diastolic.
   b. Is written second and is usually smaller than the diastolic.
   c. Is written first and is usually smaller than the diastolic.
   d. Is written second and is usually larger than the diastolic.

9. What is a normal blood pressure for an adult?
   a. 80/150
   b. 50/120
   c. 80/20
   d. 110/80

10. When taking a blood pressure, be sure the patient's arm is
    a. Hanging by his or her side.
    b. Raised above his or her chest.
    c. Resting comfortably at chest level.
    d. Extended straight in front of the body.

Active Learning Exercises

1. What is the importance of taking baseline vitals on every patient? What changes in vital signs may delay or alter dental treatment?

2. List the physiologic process by which blood pressure is taken. What happens at each stage (where does blood flow to and from)? Be sure to include an explanation of the systolic and diastolic readings.

3. Make a chart of acceptable readings for a healthy resting adult, including: pulse, blood pressure, respirations, and temperature.

Application Activities

1. Practice taking the vital signs of your classmates. If blood pressure instruments and thermometers are not available, just practice taking pulse and respiration. Compare measurements and see whether your readings of one another are nearly the same or very different.

2. Explore the different body sites for taking pulse by palpating the radial, brachial, and carotid arteries of three people. Compare their different pulse values. What factors might account for why some people have faster or slower pulses?

3. Make a two-column list. On one side, list all the factors that you can think of that might make a person's body temperature high. On the other side, list all the factors that might make a temperature low. Do the same for pulse, respiration, and blood pressure.

4. Select one of the four vital signs and write a paragraph or two about what to do if a patient has an unusually high or low reading in that area. What follow-up questions might you ask the patient? Do you need to wait and measure the vital sign again? If readings are still very high or very low, what should you do next?

PREPARING FOR CERTIFICATION EXAMS

Review the following topics in this chapter to prepare for the Dental Assisting National Board (DANB) exam:

- **Temperature**
- **Respiration**
- **Pulse**
- **Blood Pressure**

chapter 18

Responding to Medical Emergencies

CHAPTER OUTLINE

Introduction
Preventing Emergencies
    Emergency Preparedness
    Emergency Equipment and Supplies
Immediate Life Support
    The C-A-Bs of Life Support
    Cardiopulmonary Resuscitation

Airway Obstruction (Choking)
    Use of Oxygen
Responding to Common Medical Emergencies
    Nondental Emergencies
    Dental Emergencies
After the Emergency

Procedures
  18-1 Adult CPR
  18-2 Infant and Child CPR
  18-3 Using an AED
  18-4 Choking and Airway Obstruction
  18-5 Delivering Oxygen

CHAPTER CHECKLIST

On completion of this chapter, students will be able to:

- ☑ Describe the steps that can be taken to prevent medical emergencies.
- ☑ Describe the elements in an emergency preparedness plan.
- ☑ Identify the emergency equipment and supplies that are available in the event of a medical emergency.
- ☑ Describe how to provide immediate life support during a medical emergency.
- ☑ Describe the various nondental and dental medical emergencies, including how to respond appropriately to each one.
- ☑ Describe the appropriate steps to take after a medical emergency.

KEY TERMS

avulsed (uh-VULST) tooth – a tooth that has been forcibly removed from its socket; such a tooth can often be resituated and retained if given prompt medical attention

cardiopulmonary resuscitation (CPR) – restoration of cardiac output and pulmonary ventilation following cardiac arrest and apnea using artificial respiration and manual or mechanical closed chest compression

diabetes – a metabolic disease in which the body does not produce sufficient insulin or use it adequately to process the glucose in the blood, leaving high levels of glucose in the blood, resulting in symptoms ranging from chronic hyperglycemia and infection to water and electrolyte loss, ketoacidosis, and coma; may also cause low blood glucose levels in some situations

epilepsy – see *seizure disorder*

hemorrhage (HEM-er-ij) – an escape of blood through ruptured or unruptured vessel walls; internal or external bleeding

hyperglycemia (hi-per-glie-SEE-mee-uh) – an elevated level of glucose in blood plasma, with symptoms and signs that include hunger and thirst, fatigue, weight loss, depressed wound healing function, impotence, or coma; when prolonged, damage to various systems of the body may result

hyperventilating – greatly increased breathing rate that can cause carbon dioxide levels in the blood to drop below normal; may result in dizziness and confusion

322

hypoglycemia (hi-poh-glie-SEE-mee-uh) – a reduced level of glucose in blood plasma, with symptoms and signs that include anxiety, shakiness, double vision, headache, numbness, paralysis, and coma

myocardial infarction – sudden insufficiency of blood supply to an area of the heart muscle, usually as a result of blockage of a coronary artery; commonly called a *heart attack*

orthostatic (or-thuh-STAT-ik) hypotension – a form of low blood pressure that occurs when a seated patient quickly stands or suddenly changes position; accompanied by symptoms that may include lightheadedness, dizziness, obscured vision, and numbness; also called *postural hypotension*

seizure disorder – a chronic disorder characterized by some alteration of consciousness; clinical manifestations of the attack may vary from complex abnormalities or behavior, including generalized or focal convulsions, to momentary spells of impaired consciousness

sign – any abnormality indicative of a disease, discoverable on examination of a patient; an objective indicator of disease

stroke – any acute clinical event that impairs blood flow to a part of the brain for longer than 24 hours

symptom – any adverse phenomenon or undesirable departure from structural, functional, or sensational norm experienced by a patient; a subjective indicator of disease

transient ischemic attack – any acute clinical event that impairs blood flow to the brain for shorter than 24 hours, producing a sudden focal loss of neurologic function with complete recovery

traumatic intrusion – a condition in which newly erupted primary teeth are pushed back into their sockets as a result of trauma to the teeth

universal distress signal – a posture assumed by patients who are choking; patients stand with their hands at their throats

ventricular fibrillation – an abnormal heart rhythm in which the main pumping chambers of the heart, the ventricles, quiver and beat far too fast, thus reducing the supply of freshly oxygenated blood to the body

Introduction

A medical emergency is a situation in which a person requires immediate medical attention due to an illness or injury. Medical emergencies can happen to anybody, anywhere, at any time, including to patients in a dental office. Medical emergencies include injuries, heart attacks and strokes, and rapidly spreading infections as well as dental emergencies, such as lost teeth or other injuries to the oral cavity. All dental offices should have an emergency preparedness plan in place and be equipped with standard emergency medical supplies.

During a medical emergency, there is usually no time to consult a textbook or online resource on the condition and develop a treatment plan. Rather, a rapid, informed response is essential. Therefore, you should know how to recognize different conditions, provide basic treatment, and obtain comprehensive care as quickly as possible.

Although dental assistants (DAs) play a crucial role in emergencies, it is important to note that they do not play a lead role in treating or advising patients. Rather, they help the dentist recognize and treat conditions, or in an emergency, provide basic medical care until paramedics arrive.

The exception, of course, is if the DA is the only person present when the emergency occurs. In this situation, it is vital to soothe and calm the patient, call for the necessary help, and provide basic lifesaving emergency care. In this situation, your quick thinking, training, and skills can mean the difference between life and death.

Cultural Diversity

Gently touching a patient in American society out of caring or understanding is not uncommon. In the dental office, for example, an assistant may comfort a patient during an emergency situation with a pat on the shoulder or a squeeze of the hand. However, in other cultures, such as in the Orthodox Jewish faith, it is prohibited for touching to occur unless it is strictly for treatment.

Preventing Emergencies

Medical emergencies cannot always be prevented or anticipated. Dental examinations are stressful events for many patients—they may have elevated blood pressure and a rapid pulse and be sweating nervously when they are seated in the chair. This may or may not mean anything. In some cases, this stress can exacerbate an existing condition and result in a true emergency; in other cases, it is just nervousness.

The best way to prepare for and, hopefully, prevent a medical emergency is to be alert and gather as much information as possible. A thorough medical history is essential. Patients with medical conditions and patients who are taking drugs (both pharmaceutical and illicit drugs) should be monitored more closely. DAs who see any unusual signs in patients should quietly alert the dentist about their concerns—once a patient is under anesthesia, it is no longer possible to see how a patient is acting.

Emergency Preparedness

All dental offices should have an emergency preparedness plan, and all employees need to be trained in the plan. Training should include basic lifesaving procedures, such as how to administer cardiopulmonary resuscitation (CPR) or use an automatic external defibrillator (AED), as well as steps for calling for additional medical assistance. These will be covered in greater depth later in this chapter.

Elements of an emergency preparedness plan include:

- *Assigned roles.* During an emergency, coordination between office staff is essential. Specific roles for each member of the dental office team should be identified before an emergency occurs, so there is no confusion over who does what. Assigned roles should include:
  - Calling for emergency help, such as dialing 911 or the local emergency number
  - Retrieving any emergency medical equipment, such as oxygen or AED units
  - Performing basic life support, if needed
  - Rapidly reviewing the patient's medical history
  - Handling other people in the office
  - Serving as a "lookout" by standing outside and awaiting emergency medical services (EMS) personnel or flagging them down so they know where to go immediately upon arrival
- *Training and drills.* Training and drills should be conducted during non-emergency situations. Any employee who is expected to administer basic lifesaving skills, such as CPR or AED, should be trained and certified in the procedure, taking refresher courses as needed. Additionally, in-office drills should be conducted monthly to keep everyone's reflexes and training sharp. During a mock emergency, every member of the staff should participate, each in his or her assigned roles, and "extras" can even be brought in to play the role of worried patients.
- *Emergency numbers.* Emergency numbers should be posted next to every phone in the office, in an easy-to-locate spot. The emergency card should minimally include police, fire, ambulance, and poison control contact numbers (note that all may share the emergency number 911), and the numbers must be kept current (they should be checked at regular intervals). Additionally, numbers to the nearest hospital and local

oral surgeons should also be available—during dental emergencies, the skills of an oral surgeon might be more appropriate than paramedics. Staff members should also know who they are supposed to call. For most nondental emergencies, 911 is the best number to call unless a local number is used. It accesses all emergency services through a central dispatch that can organize the appropriate response. However, there might be exceptions to this: 911 services vary in urban and rural areas, and response times vary. It is best to have a plan in place for the best way to reach the appropriate help.

Emergency Equipment and Supplies

Like all medical offices, dental offices should be equipped with certain standard emergency medical supplies. These items will be covered in greater detail throughout this chapter, but the basic list should include an emergency medical kit (Figure 18-1). Employees should know how to use the supplies inside. Although the exact contents of the kit might vary, a basic emergency kit may include:

- Bandages and sterile gauze
- Adhesive tape and alcohol
- Sterile syringes, tracheotomy needle, and oral airway devices
- Blood pressure cuff (sphygmomanometer)
- Stethoscope
- Oxygen masks and emergency oxygen source (even if oxygen is available in the office)
- CPR barrier devices
- Emergency medications (see Table 18-1)
  - Epinephrine
  - Ammonia inhalant
  - Nitroglycerin

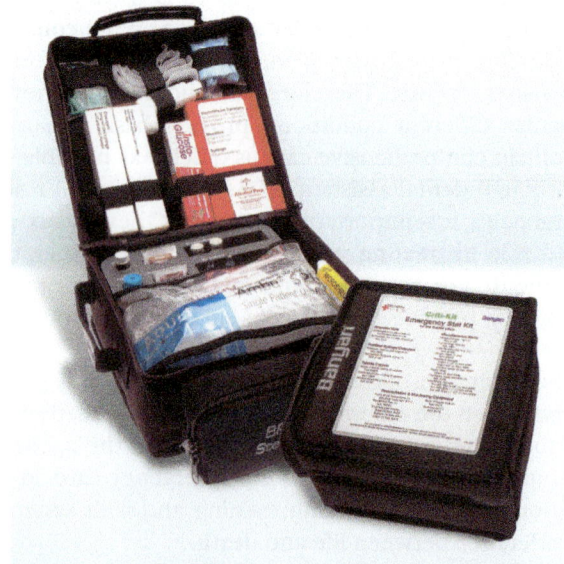

Figure 18-1 Emergency medical kit for the dental office.

TABLE 18-1   Emergency Medications

PURPOSE	DRUG NAME (BRAND)
Respiratory relief	Oxygen
Stimulant/fainting	Ammonia inhalants
Allergic reactions	Epinephrine (EpiPen)
	Diphenhydramine (Benadryl)
	Chlorpheniramine (Chlor-Trimeton)
Angina	Nitroglycerin
Bronchodilator	Albuterol (Ventolin)
Antiseizure	Diazepam (Valium)
Painkiller	Morphine, codeine
Antihypertensive	Methoxamine (Vasoxyl)
Heart stimulants for bradycardia	Atropine (Atropair)
Relief of mild-to-moderate pain	Ibuprofen (Advil, Motrin, Nuprin)
Treatment and prevention of infection in minor cuts and abrasions	Triple antibiotic ointment (Medi-Quik, Neosporin, Triple Antibiotic)

The items included in an emergency kit should be based on the dentist's training and capabilities; not all commercial kits are suitable for all dentists. The kit should be updated on a regular basis and the drugs checked weekly to make sure they have not expired. Everything in the kit should be clearly labeled and color-coded for easy access during an emergency.

Table 18-1 outlines common medications kept in a typical emergency medical kit. Check the kit weekly to make sure none of the drugs have expired, and promptly replace any expired drugs.

Additional Emergency Equipment

In addition, two other pieces of equipment are vital to keep in case of an emergency:

- *AED*. An AED is a specially designed tool used in case of fibrillation caused by cardiac arrest. The AED delivers an electrical shock to the heart to restart or normalize an erratic heartbeat. Modern AEDs are very simple to use. The machine will assess the patient's condition, program itself for the right amount of electricity delivered at the right time, and then deliver the shock. Because of their ease of use and effectiveness, these units are appearing in medical offices, airlines, arenas, and even gyms. Operators should be trained in its use. AEDs are covered more completely under the heading, Using an Automated External Defibrillator, later in this chapter.

- *Oxygen source*. Some dental offices have oxygen available in every treatment room. In case this system fails, all offices should also have emergency oxygen tanks. Emergency oxygen cylinders are always green and contain 100% oxygen. Oxygen is used to revive patients who are still breathing but not alert. A typical emergency oxygen unit contains tanks and back-up tanks as well as masks. The use of supplemental oxygen (the most commonly used drug in the dental office) is covered in greater detail in the section, Use of Oxygen, later in the chapter.

CHECKPOINTS

18-1 How often should the expiration dates of the drugs in the emergency kit be checked?

18-2 What does AED stand for? What is an AED used for?

Immediate Life Support

All employees in the dental office should be trained in lifesaving techniques, and each should know his or her role in an emergency. Regular mock drills help make sure that everyone can respond calmly and rapidly should an emergency arise.

During a medical emergency, it is important to stay alert and quickly and correctly assess the situation. Patients might present a wide variety of signs and symptoms during an emergency. **Symptoms** include anything the patient must personally identify, such as dizziness or pain. **Signs** are observable by a third party, such as a dentist or DA. Signs include fever, pallor, increased pulse or respiratory rate, or dilated pupils.

If a patient complains of unusual symptoms, or if worrisome signs are apparent to the DA, this information should be recorded. This information might be vital in the rescue effort.

The C-A-Bs of Life Support

Medical emergencies can be very stressful, but it is important to keep calm and stick to the plan. To help organize the relief effort, rescuers follow the acronym "C-A-B" to provide life support. This stands for:

- **Circulation**. Use chest compressions to stimulate circulation.
- **Airway**. Make sure the airway is open.
- **Breathing**. Restore normal breathing if possible, or initiate rescue breathing.

If the patient is in cardiac arrest, a "D" is also added for **Defibrillation**. For victims of cardiac arrest, use an AED to shock the heart into normal rhythm as soon as it is available.

These procedures are addressed in detail in the next section.

Cardiopulmonary Resuscitation

CPR is used for nonresponsive patients. All workers in a dental office should be trained in current CPR methods. The standards have changed over the years, most recently in 2010, when the AHA Guidelines for CPR changed the sequence of steps from A-B-C (Airway, Breathing, Chest compressions) to C-A-B (Chest compressions, Airway, Breathing) for adults, children, and infants.

The updated guidelines stress the importance of beginning chest compressions immediately. Studies have shown that chest compressions are the most important part of CPR. If two medical professionals are present, chest compressions should be constant.

During CPR, it helps if the patient is on a firm surface that allows for better compressions. However, in the dental office, patients may be in a dental chair, which may provide too soft of a surface. If compressions cannot be effectively performed in the chair, then the patient should be moved to the floor or other hard surface.

A key step in any CPR routine is to call for help, or direct someone else to call for help. Although CPR is helpful, it is not a substitute for advanced medical help and is only a temporary measure to keep the patient alive until medical help arrives.

See Procedures 18-1 and 18-2 for instructions for adult and infant CPR, respectively.

Procedure 18-1 Adult CPR

This procedure is described for one rescuer. If two trained rescuers are available, chest compressions should be administered constantly, with each rescuer performing 5 cycles of chest compressions before the other rescuer takes over. While these are the most current recommendations as of 2010, it is important that all staff members receive annual training to ensure that they are following the most current recommendations.

Materials needed (Figure P18-1-1):

- CPR mouth barrier

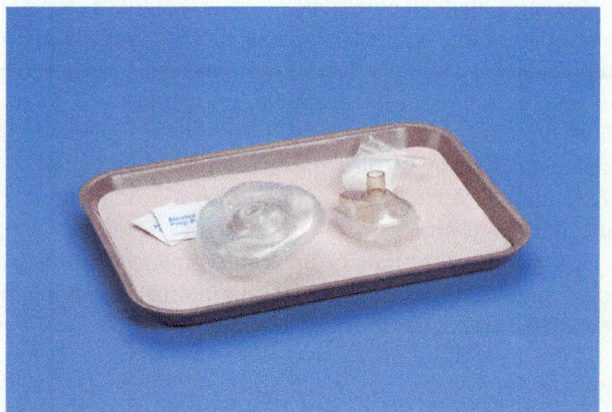

Figure P18-1-1

1. See if the patient is responsive by asking, "Are you okay?" Touch or tap the patient to see if he or she responds while simultaneously looking to see if the patient is breathing.

2. If the patient is unresponsive and is not breathing or is gasping, have someone call for help. If it is not possible for someone else to call, call for help immediately yourself and quickly return to the patient.

3. Check for the patient's pulse by pressing your fingers lightly against the patient's carotid artery for no more than 10 seconds (Figure P18-1-2). If you do not feel a pulse within 10 seconds, place the patient in the supine position and start chest compressions immediately.

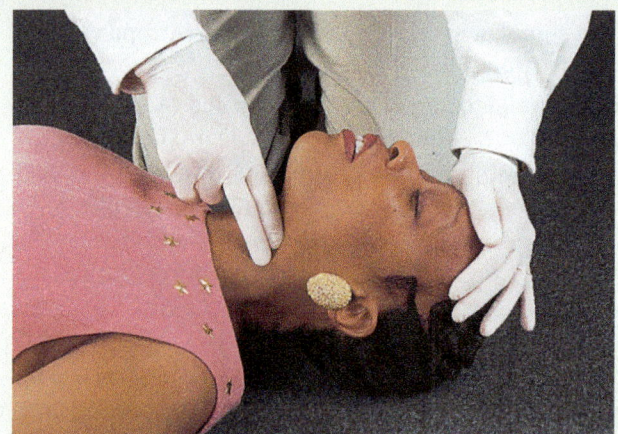

Figure P18-1-2

4. Place your hands on top of each other on the lower half of the patient's sternum. Center your shoulders over your hands. Compress the sternum at least 2 inches down at a rate of at least 100 compressions per minute (at least 3 compressions every 2 seconds)—"push hard and fast" (Figure P18-1-3).

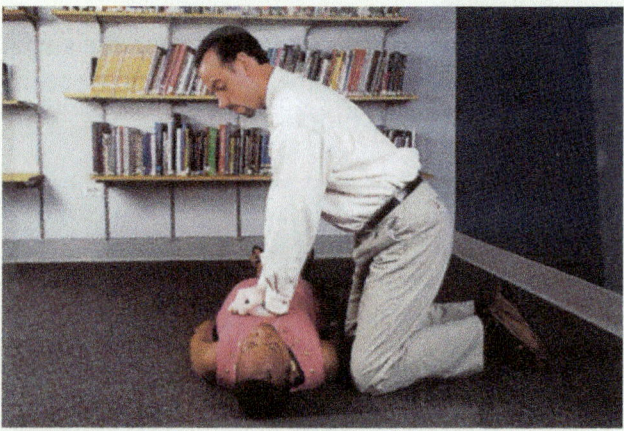

Figure P18-1-3

Procedure 18–1 Adult CPR (Continued)

5. Administer 30 compressions.

6. Once the compressions are completed, make sure the patient's airway is clear then use the head tilt-chin lift maneuver (Figure P18-1-4) to tilt the head back.

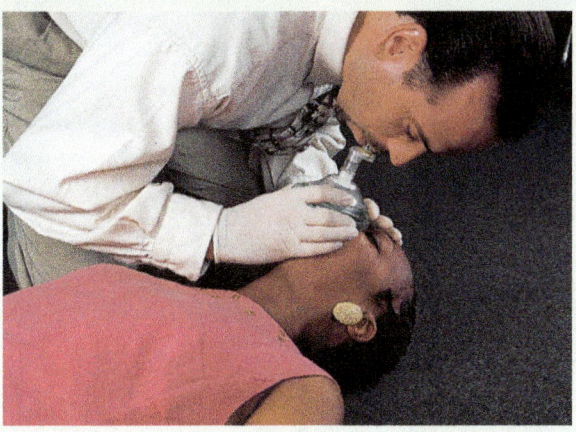

Figure P18-1-5

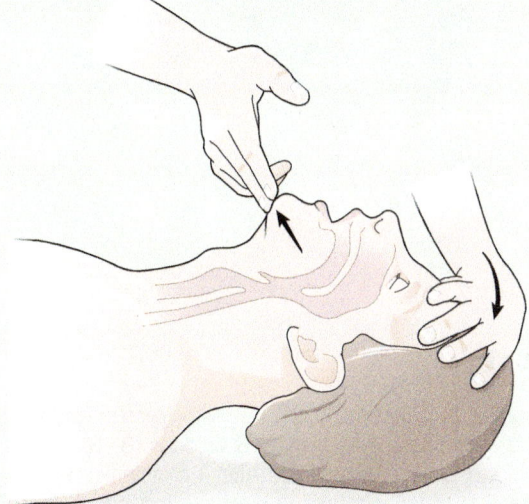

Figure P18-1-4

7. Position the CPR mouth barrier over the patient's mouth and nose.

8. Administer two rescue breaths by breathing slowly into the CPR mouth barrier (Figure P18-1-5). During rescue breaths, do not exhale sharply and do not force air into the patient's lungs. The patient's chest should gently rise. After the breaths, turn your head sideways to feel for the exhalation and watch the chest fall.

9. Check for a pulse with your fingers on the patient's carotid artery.

10. If a pulse is present, continue with rescue breaths, administering one breath every 6–8 seconds (8–10 breaths per minute). Do this for 1 minute. After 1 minute, recheck the pulse and continue with rescue breathing for as long as the pulse remains or until the patient is breathing unassisted.

11. If the patient does not have a pulse, administer 30 chest compressions.

12. Continue for five cycles of compressions and breaths, then stop to check for a pulse. If there is no pulse, continue with compressions and breaths at the same 30:2 ratio, stopping to check for a pulse every five cycles, until help arrives.

Procedure 18–2 Infant and Child CPR

This procedure is described for one rescuer. If two trained rescuers are available, chest compressions should be administered constantly, with each rescuer performing 5 cycles of chest compressions before the other rescuer takes over. While these are the most current recommendations as of 2010, it is important that all staff members receive annual training to ensure that they are following the most current recommendations.

Materials needed (see Figure P18-1-1):

■ CPR mouth barrier

1. See if the patient is responsive by asking, "Are you okay?" Touch or tap the patient to see if he or she responds while simultaneously looking to see if the patient is breathing.

2. If the patient is unresponsive and is not breathing or is gasping, have someone call for help. If it is not possible for someone else to call, perform CPR for 2 minutes then call for help yourself and quickly return to the patient. Infants and children have very little reserve oxygen, so it is

important to get some supply of oxygen to their systems before taking the time to call for help.

3. Check for the patient's pulse for no more than 10 seconds. In children older than 1 year old, press your fingers lightly against the patient's carotid artery; in infants 1 year and younger, check for pulse at the brachial artery. If you do not feel a pulse within 10 seconds, place the patient in the supine position and start chest compressions immediately.

4. For children (ages 1–8 years), use one or two hands, as needed, on the lower half of the sternum. For infants, use two fingers on the lower sternum (Figure P18-2-1). Center your shoulders over your hands. Compress the sternum at least one-third the depth of the chest (approximately 1.5 inches in infants and 2 inches in children) at a rate of at least 100 compressions per minute (at least 3 compressions every 2 seconds)—"push hard and fast".

Procedure 18-2 Infant and Child CPR (Continued)

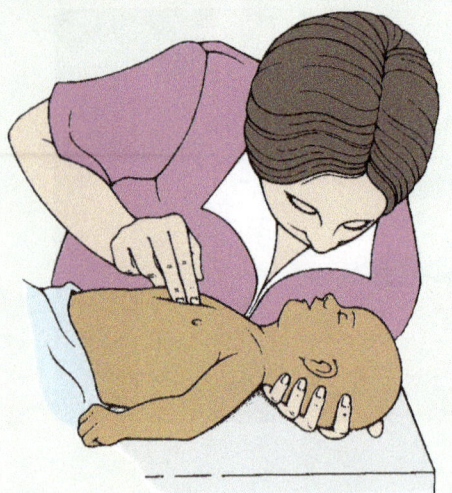

Figure P18-2-1

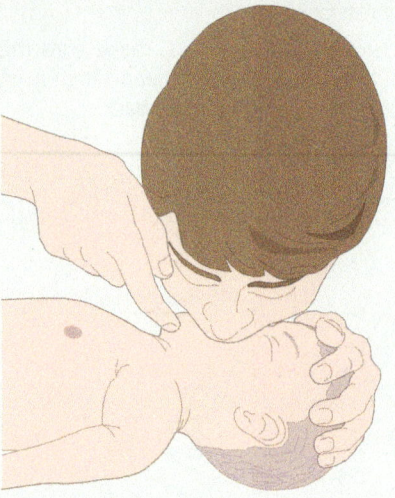

Figure P18-2-2

5. Administer 30 compressions.

6. Once the compressions are completed, make sure the patient's airway is clear then use the head tilt-chin lift maneuver to tilt the head back.

7. Position the CPR mouth barrier over the patient's mouth and nose.

8. Administer two rescue breaths by breathing slowly into the CPR mouth barrier (Figure P18-2-2). During rescue breaths, do not exhale sharply and do not force air into the patient's lungs. The patient's chest should gently rise. After the breaths, turn your head sideways to feel for the exhalation and watch the chest fall.

9. Check for a pulse with your fingers on the patient's carotid artery.

10. If a pulse is present, continue with rescue breaths, administering one breath every 6–8 seconds (8–10 breaths per minute). Do this for 1 minute. After 1 minute, recheck the pulse and continue with rescue breathing for as long as the pulse remains or until the patient is breathing unassisted.

11. If the patient does not have a pulse, administer 30 chest compressions.

12. Continue for five cycles of compressions and breaths, then stop to check for a pulse. If there is no pulse, continue with compressions and breaths at the same 30:2 ratio, stopping to check for a pulse every five cycles, until help arrives. NOTE: When two rescuers are present, compressions and breaths should be performed at a 15:2 ratio (2 rescue breaths given for every 15 compressions).

Using an Automated External Defibrillator

An AED delivers electrical shocks that are designed to "shock" the heart back into a normal rhythm (Figure 18-2). There are many reasons a patient might be unresponsive, including *cardiac arrest*. Cardiac arrest occurs when the heart has gone into an irregular rhythm that does not sustain blood flow and life. A variety of conditions can cause cardiac arrest, including heart attack and ventricular fibrillation. Because of advances in technology, AEDs have become increasingly easy to use—they are now located in any number of public locations and people are easily trained in their use.

AEDs should be used only on nonresponsive patients with no pulse. The sooner defibrillation is performed on a patient in cardiac arrest, the better the chances of survival without serious, debilitating injury. If defibrillation is performed within the first 5 minutes, the odds of survival are 50%. By 10 minutes, the odds of survival are very small.

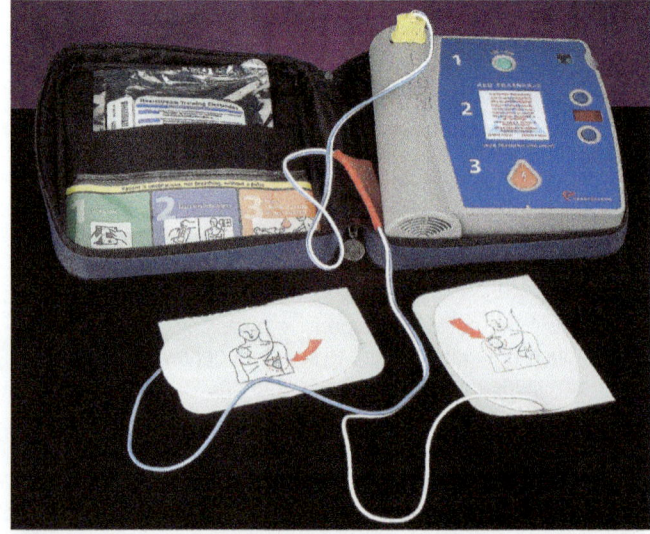

Figure 18-2 Automatic external defibrillators (AEDs). These may be used to defibrillate a life-threatening heart rhythm.

Procedure 18-3 **Using an AED**

Materials needed:

- AED machine
- CPR mouth barrier

1. Check for patient responsiveness and breathing as described in Step 1 of Procedure 18-1. If the patient is unresponsive and is not breathing or is gasping, begin CPR until the defibrillator is attached. Have someone call for help and retrieve the AED machine.

2. If you are the only rescuer, and no one is available to retrieve the AED, perform 30 chest compressions, then get the machine and call for help. If patient is an infant or child, perform 2 minutes of CPR before retrieving the AED and calling for help.

3. Follow the instructions on the unit to place the electrodes (Figure P18-3-1).

4. Press the analyze button on the AED.

5. If no shock is needed, continue with CPR until help arrives.

6. If a shock is advised, loudly instruct anyone in the area to stand clear of the patient, then deliver the shock or allow the machine to automatically deliver the shock.

7. After delivering the shock, the AED will again analyze the patient's heart rhythm. The patient must not be touched during this process.

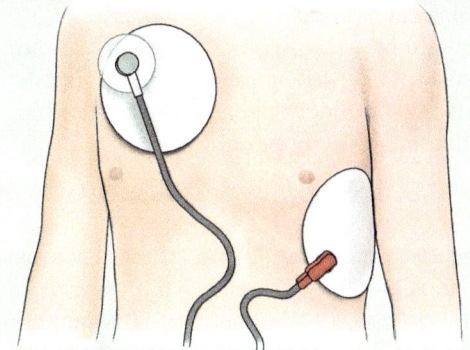

Figure P18-3-1

8. Continue to follow the instructions given by the AED, which will include either reshocking the patient or resuming CPR. Always assess the patient's breathing and pulse before resuming CPR.

9. Continue with attempts to defibrillate until the patient is revived and the machine indicates "no shock needed" or until help arrives.

When used correctly, the AED device will monitor the heart rhythm, determine which kind of abnormal rhythm is present, program itself to deliver the right form of defibrillation, and when the operator executes the command, deliver the electricity.

Airway Obstruction (Choking)

Choking, or airway obstruction, is a fairly common medical emergency encountered in a dental office. During dental treatment, patients are positioned with their heads back and their mouths open—in even the most controlled settings, it is possible for items to fall into the back of the throat and block the airway. Potential choking hazards include extracted teeth, crowns, amalgam, gauze and cotton rolls, instruments, and impression material.

The symptoms of an airway obstruction are usually immediate and obvious. Conscious patients who are choking frequently make the **universal distress signal**. This means the patient holds his or her hands to the throat in a position of distress. When patients exhibit this signal, ask, "Are you choking? Can you breathe?" They may or may not be able to answer, depending on how securely the item is lodged in the throat.

If a patient is indeed choking, the first step is to sit the patient up and have him or her attempt to cough or spit the object out. Oftentimes, the shift in gravity, combined with a forceful exhalation of air, will be enough to dislodge the object and end the emergency.

If this is not successful, however, the rescuer should attempt the *Heimlich maneuver* (Figure 18-3). To execute the Heimlich maneuver, get behind the patient, removing the patient from the chair if necessary, and wrap your hands around the waist. The rescuer's

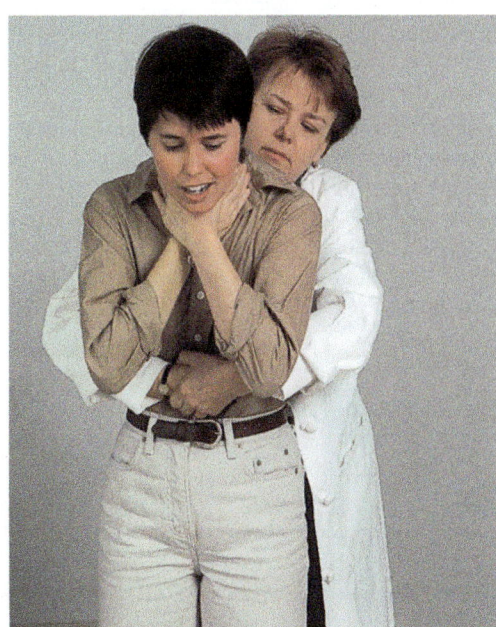

Figure 18-3 Heimlich maneuver being performed on a victim making the universal choking sign.

hands should be tightly wrapped into a double fist, which is then driven upward and back, into the patient's abdomen, above the navel. This motion should expel the object from the patient's throat.

If the rescuer cannot wrap his or her hands around the patient because of obesity or pregnancy, the hands can instead be positioned under the patient's armpits and quick thrusts delivered to the upper chest area.

Unconscious Choking

The Heimlich maneuver is used only on conscious patients who can stand under their own power. Airway obstruction, however, can become rapidly dangerous—the brain cannot be deprived of oxygen for more than a few minutes without the risk of serious injury or death.

If a patient becomes unconscious during attempts to dislodge the object or is found unconscious and not breathing, emergency services should be called immediately. Following that, the rescuer should open the victim's mouth wide and look for the object, except in case of seizure. If an object is visible in the patient's mouth, remove it with your fingers. If you do not see an object in the patient's mouth, begin administering CPR (see Procedure 18-1), then attempt to expel the object by straddling the patient and following the instructions in Procedure 18-4.

Use of Oxygen

Oxygen is commonly used during medical emergencies in the dental office. In many dental offices, oxygen is readily available in every room, piped through the wall for administration with nitrous oxide during routine dental procedures. In other offices, oxygen and nitrous are available on a cart that is wheeled in when needed. In addition to these two sources of oxygen, dental offices should also be equipped with a backup emergency oxygen kit. DAs should be trained on all forms of oxygen administration.

Procedure 18-4 Choking and Airway Obstruction

Materials needed:

- Gloves
- CPR mouth barrier

1. If symptoms of choking are apparent (e.g., the universal distress signal), ask the patient, "Are you okay? Can you breathe?"

2. If the answer is no (by shaking the head), sit the patient up in the treatment chair and have him or her attempt to cough out or forcefully expel the object. Sometimes a strong cough is enough to dislodge an object.

3. If the object cannot be expelled, get the patient into a standing position and stand behind the patient in order to perform the Heimlich maneuver.

4. To perform the Heimlich, loop your hands around the waist and grab one fist in your other hand. Position your hands just under the solar plexus and give repeated, sharp upward jabs into the abdomen to dislodge the object (see Figure 18-3). For pregnant and obese patients, stand behind and place your arms under their armpits and apply the same sharp, upward jabs to the upper chest.

5. Repeat until the object is dislodged, help arrives, or the patient becomes unconscious.

6. With an unconscious patient, call for help, then lay the patient on his or her back and perform the tongue-jaw lift to lift and move the tongue out of the way.

7. Put on gloves and perform a finger sweep to see if you can locate and dislodge the object.

8. If this fails, straddle the patient's thighs to perform a chest thrust. To perform a chest thrust, position your hands under the solar plexus and push upward to dislodge the object (Figure P18-4-1).

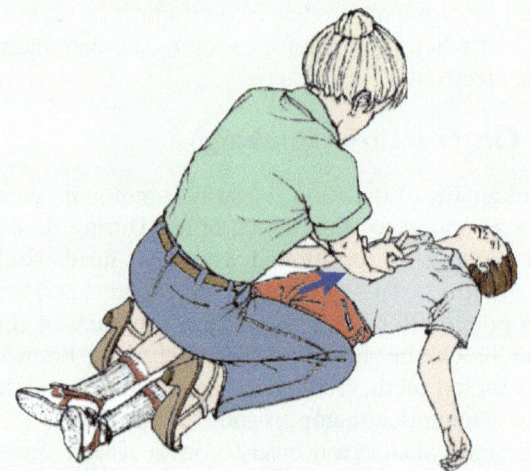

Figure P18-4-1

9. Continue until the object is dislodged or help arrives.

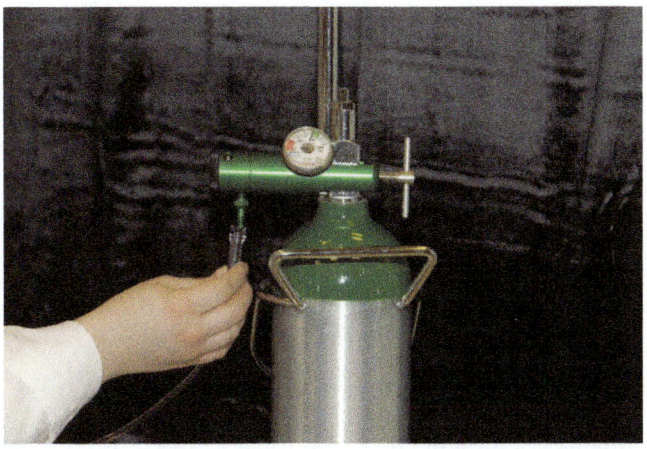
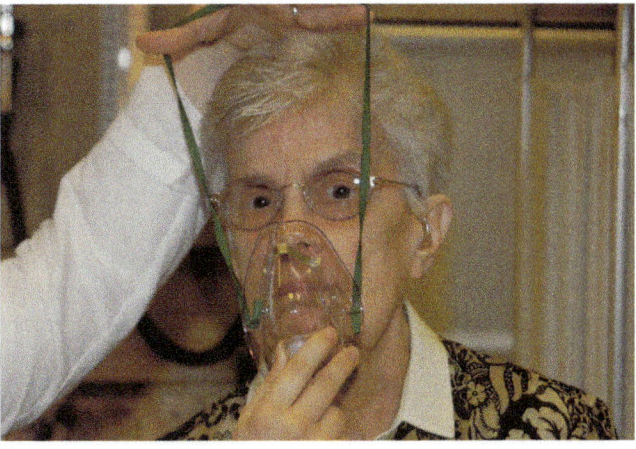

A   **B**

Figure 18–4 Administering oxygen. (**A**) Oxygen tank. (**B**) Secure the oxygen mask over the nose and mouth.

Oxygen Equipment

No matter how the oxygen is delivered, some equipment is common to all oxygen units (Figure 18-4). There will be a tank or oxygen source. Oxygen tanks are colored green to make them easier to identify. Tanks are fitted with a valve on the top so the DA can control the flow of oxygen and a pressure gauge showing how much oxygen is in the tank.

A tube runs between the tank and the face mask. Oxygen face masks are designed to fit securely against the patient's face, covering both the nose and mouth. To deliver oxygen, place the mask in position on the patient's face, looping the elastic around the back of his or her head. Slowly turn on the valve to start the flow of oxygen.

✔ CHECKPOINTS

18-3 What does the life support acronym "C-A-B" stand for?

18-4 What is the chest compression/breathing ratio for adult CPR?

Procedure 18-5 Delivering Oxygen

Materials needed:

- Oxygen tank
- Face mask

1. If the oxygen tank is not assembled, assemble following the manufacturer's instructions.
2. Place the patient in the *Trendelenburg position* if possible. In this position, the patient should be lying down, face up, with the feet above the heart level.
3. If the patient is conscious and lucid, explain what you are doing and why while you are doing it.
4. If using a nonrebreather mask, start the flow of oxygen prior to placing the mask on the patient. The reservoir bag should be filled half way with oxygen before the mask is placed on patient's face.
5. Loop the mask over the patient's face, making sure it fits snugly against the patient's nose and the oxygen tube is not obstructing the patient's breathing (Figure P18-5-1).
6. Start the flow of oxygen, if it wasn't already started in Step 4.

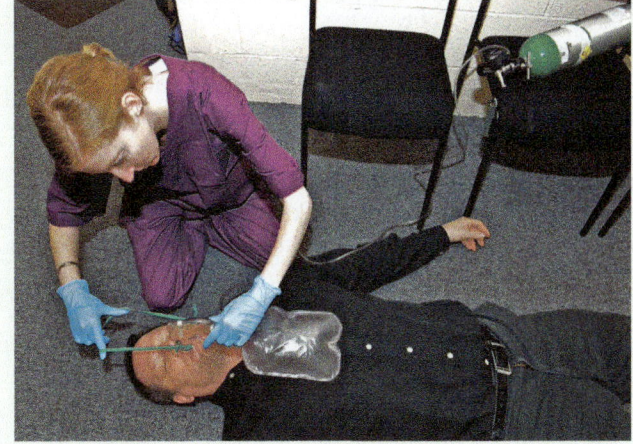

Figure P18-5-1

7. Have the patient breathe through his or her nose if possible.
8. Keep the oxygen flowing until the patient recovers or help arrives. Keep the patient calm and relaxed if possible.

Responding to Common Medical Emergencies

Dental visits are a time of high stress for many patients, which can exacerbate an existing medical condition. Medical emergencies in the dental office might be either dental or nondental in nature. It is important to quickly and correctly identify the symptoms and signs of an emergency and respond appropriately. In this section, common emergencies are described along with their symptoms and the correct course of action.

Nondental Emergencies

Nondental emergencies can include anything from heart problems to issues with pregnant patients.

Heart Attack (Myocardial Infarction)

A heart attack occurs when the blood supply to the heart muscle is disrupted, thus starving the heart muscle of oxygen. The most common cause of a heart attack is a blood clot that obstructs the coronary arteries, which feed the muscle with freshly oxygenated blood. This is most often the result of coronary artery disease, a condition in which the coronary arteries become narrowed and stiffened as a result of plaque deposits inside the narrow arteries. Risk factors for heart attack include diabetes, obesity, smoking, and a family history of heart attacks.

Heart attacks range in severity, depending on how severe the restriction of blood flow to the heart muscle is. Severe heart attacks can come on suddenly and result in very rapid deterioration and death. Less severe heart attacks are experienced as painful symptoms and the patient remains conscious throughout.

Symptoms of a heart attack vary slightly between men and women (although in some cases, patients may experience no symptoms); women are more likely to experience atypical symptoms such as abdominal pain, back pain, and other non–chest-oriented symptoms. Men are more likely to have heart attacks when they are younger, but among older adults, heart attacks are more common among women.

Signs and symptoms of a heart attack may include:

- Crushing or shooting chest pain or pressure
- Numbness in the left arm
- Dizziness
- Nausea
- Dyspnea (shortness of breath)
- Fainting (syncope)
- Heavy sweating

During a heart attack, the priority is to restore a normal heart rhythm as quickly as possible and get emergency help. EMS should be called immediately. If the patient is alert and awake, oxygen should be administered along with nitroglycerin pills. Nitroglycerin pills cause the arteries to relax and expand, thus allowing more blood to flow to the heart. (Always wear gloves when handling nitroglycerin pills as this medication can be absorbed through the skin.) Baby aspirin, which increases blood flow, can also be given to a conscious patient to be chewed.

An unconscious patient may have gone into **ventricular fibrillation** and cardiac arrest, a very dangerous condition in which the heart quivers rapidly instead of beating normally. This can rapidly result in death. These patients require defibrillation with an AED as soon as possible.

Angina Pectoris

Angina is a form of chest pain usually caused by coronary artery disease. During a bout of angina, patients experience chest pains and may become dizzy or have trouble breathing. They may become pale and fearful.

There are two kinds of angina: stable and unstable angina. *Stable angina* occurs at predictable times, such as during exercise or stressful events (like dental visits). *Unstable angina* occurs without warning and is considered much more dangerous. Both types of angina are warning signs of underlying heart disease, but angina is not the same as a heart attack. Angina is a limited event (or *transient*) that does not cause permanent damage to the heart muscle, whereas a heart attack may result in permanent damage to heart tissue.

If a dental patient experiences a bout of angina, all dental work should stop, and the patient should be soothed and made comfortable. The standard treatment for angina is nitroglycerin, which will cause the arteries to relax and expand and hasten the end of the episode. Many patients with stable angina are under the care of a physician and have their own nitroglycerin tablets or spray. If they do not, the emergency kit should be equipped with the drug. The symptoms of angina are similar to those of a heart attack. If the patient is suffering from angina, nitroglycerin will relieve the symptoms. If nitroglycerin does not relieve the pain within a few minutes, the patient may be having a heart attack and emergency services should be called.

Stroke

A **stroke** (also called a *cerebrovascular accident*, or *CVA*) occurs when the supply of oxygenated blood to the brain is disrupted. The brain is extremely sensitive to a lack of oxygen, and even a short period without adequate blood flow can result in brain damage or death. As a result, stroke is one of the leading causes of death and disability among Americans. Strokes are much more likely to affect older Americans. Risk factors for stroke include high blood pressure, blood vessel diseases such as arteriosclerosis (the same underlying process as heart disease), smoking, and a family history of strokes.

There are two types of strokes:

- *Ischemic strokes.* These occur when a blood clot lodges in an artery in the brain, preventing the flow of blood to the tissue beyond. Blood clots can either form in the vessel (thrombus) or travel from another part of the body into the brain (embolism). Ischemic strokes are by far the most common type of stroke, accounting for about 85% of strokes.

- *Hemorrhagic strokes.* These occur when an artery in the brain ruptures, usually due to an aneurysm. Hemorrhagic strokes are less common but more dangerous than ischemic strokes.

Symptoms of both types of stroke are similar and depend on the severity of the event. Patients might walk with an unsteady gait or appear confused. They may experience a sudden and intense headache, along with vomiting, fainting, and nausea. Other symptoms include partial paralysis, vision disturbances, and a sudden loss of the ability to speak clearly. To rapidly assess the possibility of stroke, use the acronym STR: Smile (ask the patient to smile); Talk (ask the patient to repeat a simple sentence); Raise (ask the patient to raise his or her arms above the head).

Speed is essential for stroke patients. The degree of long-term damage caused by the stroke is often directly related to the length of time between the onset of symptoms and the delivery of medical care. Certain drugs are available (called *thrombolytics*) that can help rapidly dissolve blood clots and restore normal blood flow. However, these drugs are not available in dental offices and can be administered only by qualified medical professionals because they can make bleeding strokes worse.

If a patient exhibits symptoms of a stroke in a dental office, all dental work should immediately stop, and the patient should be reclined. Emergency services should be contacted immediately, and oxygen administered until help arrives. Stroke patients should not be given aspirin because it can make bleeding strokes worse.

A lesser form of cerebrovascular disease is known as a **transient ischemic attack**, or *TIA*. A TIA occurs when the patient experiences mild stroke-like symptoms that pass within 24 hours, although the majority pass within 60 minutes. TIAs should be taken very seriously—a significant number of patients who experience TIAs will go on to have a stroke in the near future. If a patient experiences a TIA in the dental office, all work should stop, and emergency medical help should be summoned. Make the patient comfortable while waiting for help to arrive.

Asthma Attack

Asthma is an increasingly common respiratory condition in which affected patients wheeze and sometimes gasp for air. Mucus might also be present, which further constricts breathing. Asthma attacks can be triggered by a variety of factors, including allergens, respiratory infections, and stress.

Experts estimate that about 22 million people in the United States suffer from asthma, and it is the most common cause of childhood hospitalization. Asthma is most common among boys and children; it typically resolves by adulthood.

A DA witnessing an asthma attack needs to be aware of the signs of a developing respiratory emergency. These include a bluish tint to the lips and face; extreme difficulty breathing; pronounced anxiety due to insufficient breath; and rapid pulse, followed by a decreased level of alertness.

If a patient experiences an asthma attack in the dental office, the most common treatment is an inhalation bronchodilator, usually albuterol. If the patient has asthma and is already in the care of a doctor, he or she likely has an inhaler and should be given the opportunity to use it and relieve the symptoms. If not, albuterol from the emergency kit can be used. Patients should be given albuterol in two doses, and symptoms should gradually improve within 10 to 15 minutes. If they do not, or if symptoms worsen, emergency services should be contacted.

Allergic Reactions (Anaphylaxis)

Allergic reactions range in severity from mild, localized reactions to life-threatening systemic reactions called *anaphylaxis*. Allergies are caused when the immune system mistakenly identifies a relatively harmless substance as a threat and mounts an exaggerated immune response against it. These substances, which can include pollens, latex, certain foods, chemicals, and drugs, are known as *allergens*. The severity of the allergy depends on the strength of the immune system reaction—in anaphylaxis, the reaction can be strong enough to cause death.

During an allergic reaction, the symptoms are caused by the immune system as it attacks the body itself. Symptoms of allergic reactions may include inflammation, swelling, hives, sneezing, running eyes, and running nose. In some instances the airway rapidly swells, making it hard for the patient to breathe. Blood pressure can also fall rapidly, leading to fainting.

Treatment for allergy attacks depends on the severity of the episode. The most common treatment for mild allergies is adminstering antihistamines. These drugs block the action of histamines, a component of the immune system that causes swelling. Antihistamines are available over the counter and are usually fairly slow acting.

Severe anaphylaxis, however, is a medical emergency that demands immediate medical attention. The treatment for anaphylaxis is epinephrine, which is typically administered in a self-injecting EpiPen. Many patients who have severe allergies carry EpiPens in case of an emergency. Epinephrine should also be available in the dental office emergency kit. If a patient suddenly exhibits signs of anaphylaxis, epinephrine should be administered as soon as possible. Emergency services should be called and the patient sent to the hospital for monitoring.

Seizure

Seizures occur when the normal electrical brain activity is disrupted. In the past, seizure disorders were referred to as **epilepsy**, but today, the preferred term is **seizure disorder**. A number of conditions can cause seizure disorders, such as head trauma and high fever, but in most people, the cause of the disorder is never diagnosed. A seizure disorder will be diagnosed in persons who have two or more seizures in their lifetime.

About 20% of people who suffer from seizure disorders experience sensations before the seizure, warning them that a seizure is about to occur. The sensations vary, but can include unusual tastes or smells. This is called an *aura*. Seizures typically last between 2 and 5 minutes. After the seizure, the person experiences post-seizure symptoms including headache, sore muscles, exhaustion, memory loss, and confusion.

There are several types of seizures, depending on where the electrical activity is affected in the brain and how strong it is. Most people with seizure disorders experience only one type of seizure, whereas about 30% will experience multiple types.

■ *Simple partial seizures*. Electrical discharges remain confined to a small area of the brain, so symptoms are likewise limited to the functions controlled by that area of the brain. Simple seizures that progress from one part of the body to another are known as *Jacksonian seizures*. During a Jacksonian seizure, for example, shaking or twitching might begin in the forearm and gradually move up to the arm. If the seizure is preceded by an aura and the person begins to lose touch with the surroundings and even passes out, it may be classified as a *complex partial seizure*. Before losing consciousness, the person may stare ahead, utter meaningless sounds, and lose comprehension.

■ *Grand mal seizures*. Grand mal seizures typically start as complex partial seizures, but the abnormal electrical impulses rapidly spread throughout the affected brain region. These seizures rapidly progress into loss of consciousness and convulsions. The patient may experience severe muscle spasms and jerking, along with clenched teeth and tongue. Bladder control may be lost, and the tongue may be bitten. These seizures typically last less than 2 minutes.

■ *Petit mal seizures*. A petit mal seizure is a lesser form of a grand mal seizure. Patients do not lose consciousness, but they may have fluttering eyelids or twitching facial muscles. They are usually unaware of their surroundings. Petit mal seizures are brief, lasting only 2 to 3 seconds and rarely beyond 30 seconds. In many cases, after the seizure is over, the person will resume normal activities with no memory that a seizure just happened.

Long-term treatment for seizure disorders typically involves a class of drugs called *anticonvulsants*. These are effective for the majority of patients. In the dental office, if a patient goes into a seizure, the dental team should remove everything from the mouth, including all tools and devices. The person should not be restrained but allowed to pass through the seizure episode. Do not try to put anything between the patient's teeth. Move any item away from the patient that could cause injury during the convulsions. If the seizure does not resolve in a few minutes, emergency services should be called.

After emerging from the episode, patients may or may not have a memory of what just happened. No matter what the case, patients should be alerted to their seizure, but in a way that does not belittle them or cause embarrassment. Seizure disorders have been stigmatized in the past, and many patients are embarrassed by the disorder. If the patient has a diagnosed seizure disorder, dental work can begin again when the patient has fully recovered. If this was a first-time episode, the patient should be seen by a medical professional.

Diabetic Emergencies

Diabetes is a chronic disorder characterized by abnormally high levels of glucose in the blood. Two forms of diabetes are common: type 1 and type 2. Pregnant women may experience gestational diabetes, a temporary condition. Depending on its severity, diabetes is managed with drugs that sensitize the body to insulin or with insulin injections. Type 2 diabetic patients can also manage their condition through diet, exercise, and weight loss, which lower blood glucose levels. In most cases, the diabetic patient is treated in the dental office the same as a healthy patient—diabetes does not affect routine dental care. Most of the danger posed by diabetes is due to the long-term effect of elevated glucose levels.

However, if the diabetes is poorly controlled or has not been diagnosed, it is possible that glucose levels will rise to potentially dangerous levels during treatment (**hyperglycemia**). If this happens, the patient may need to urinate excessively, may become groggy and confused, and may experience nausea. Because cells need glucose to function but no glucose is being delivered from the blood to the cells, the body will go into panic mode and begin breaking down fat cells and producing ketones. This provides energy, but it also makes the blood too acidic, altering the body's finely controlled pH level. This condition is called *ketoacidosis* and is a very dangerous condition that can rapidly progress into a diabetic coma and death.

Ketoacidosis is very rare among type 2 diabetics, because they usually have some working insulin. It occurs almost exclusively among type 1 diabetics. The standard treatment for ketoacidosis is an insulin shot to help clear glucose from the blood and supply it to the cells. Hospitalization is required, so EMS should be called immediately. Once in the hospital, the patient will be given fluids, electrolytes, and insulin to restore normal levels.

On the other hand, if glucose levels fall too low (**hypoglycemia**), a patient may complain of symptoms that include dizziness, pain, pounding heartbeat, double vision, and fatigue, or may even be rendered unconscious. To treat a hypoglycemic attack, give the patient a food or drink containing sugar; the symptoms should dissipate.

Fainting (Syncope)

Fainting, the most common medical emergency encountered in the dental office, is not a medical condition but a symptom of another problem. In the dental office, it is usually a reaction to the dental treatment itself. Although fainting can be a symptom of a serious underlying medical problem, it is usually caused by stress when it comes to dental treatment. During periods of stress, the body tends to go into "fight-or-flight" mode. Blood moves out of the extremities and the head into the chest cavity, and blood pressure falls. If the blood pressure falls too far, or if patients suddenly change position, they may become faint, dizzy, or weak and then faint.

If a patient faints, all dental treatment should stop, and, if possible, the patient should be laid flat with the feet slightly elevated above chest level. This is called the *Trendelenburg position* and it forces blood to flow back into the head. Administer emergency oxygen and use an ammonia capsule from the dental emergency kit to revive the patient. To use the ammonia capsule, simply break it open and pass it beneath the nostrils once or twice. The strong ammonia fumes will cause the patient to inhale involuntarily, supplying more oxygen to the brain. Do not leave an ammonia capsule under the nose for more than a few seconds—ammonia can be an irritant.

Most patients who faint will revive within a few minutes. If a patient does not revive in a few minutes, or fails to respond to oxygen or ammonia, call emergency services and check for C-A-Bs (see The C-A-Bs of Life Support section earlier in the chapter). Even if the patient revives moments later, unusual or unexplained fainting should receive medical attention.

Fainting itself is usually harmless, but there is a danger that a patient could be injured by falling. If a patient seems unsteady, or breathing is shallow and rapid (**hyperventilating**), ask if he or she is okay and have him or her sit with the head between the knees. Hyperventilation is also caused by anxiety. When people hyperventilate, the carbon dioxide levels in the blood are lowered and they may feel faint, numb, or groggy. If a patient begins to hyperventilate, he or she can slow breathing by timing it against the second hand of a watch, slowing inhalation to last 7 seconds and exhalation to last 11 seconds. Do not begin any treatment until the patient is calm again.

Remember at all times that the dentist's office is a place of extreme stress for many patients. Always treat patient concerns with calm dignity—alarmed or anxious patients will only become more upset if they are belittled or ignored. Speak in soothing tones, explain procedures thoroughly, and, if necessary, reschedule appointments or bring in the dentist to help allay their concerns.

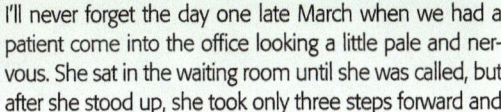

Voice of Experience

I'll never forget the day one late March when we had a patient come into the office looking a little pale and nervous. She sat in the waiting room until she was called, but after she stood up, she took only three steps forward and then collapsed onto the floor. Fortunately, we had thoroughly rehearsed our action plan, so there was only a brief second before everybody fell into their roles. While I checked for a pulse and breathing (fortunately, she was breathing and had a pulse), my colleagues called for help, retrieved the oxygen, and dealt with the other patients. It turned out she was very nervous, but after she revived and had oxygen, she was calm enough to go ahead with her regularly scheduled cleaning!

Dizziness (Orthostatic Hypotension)

Like fainting, dizziness is not a medical condition, but a symptom of an underlying condition. Although many conditions can cause dizziness, including ear conditions and even serious neurological problems, it is often caused by orthostatic hypotension.

Orthostatic hypotension is a rapid shift in blood pressure caused by standing up or changing positions suddenly. This causes a lack of blood flow to the brain, which results in dizziness and possibly even a loss of consciousness (fainting). Although some diseases cause orthostatic hypotension, the most common cause in the dental office is the forced period of lying down. After lengthy procedures, patients might try to sit up suddenly and complain that their head is swimming and they are dizzy, or they may faint back into the treatment chair. This is more likely among patients with circulation problems, including older patients and pregnant women. Additionally, patients who receive nitrous oxide and oxygen are more likely to experience orthostatic hypotension.

To prevent orthostatic hypotension, raise patients in the dental chair slowly and encourage them to remain reclined against the chair for a few minutes. Perhaps engage them in conversation while the blood flow normalizes and until they are able to rise without a loss of blood pressure.

If a patient faints due to orthostatic hypotension, recline the patient if possible. Oxygen can be administered until the patient naturally revives. The loss of consciousness in these circumstances is usually very brief. If it lasts for longer than a minute or two, institute the C-A-Bs of emergency medicine and call for emergency services. In this case, the episode may have been caused by an underlying condition.

Pregnancy Emergencies

Pregnant women are vulnerable to a number of medical problems unique to pregnancy. During pregnancy, the heart is working harder, and, because of concern for the fetus, many drugs should not be used.

Despite these concerns, there is no reason a pregnant woman should avoid the dentist's office. The most common problem with pregnant patients is orthostatic hypotension caused by sudden shifts in position. The woman may become dizzy or even briefly lose consciousness. If this happens, move the patient so she is lying on her left side or sitting upright. This will shift the weight of the uterus from her blood vessels and encourage better circulation.

For any other sudden medical condition, such as vaginal bleeding, call immediately for medical emergency services.

Hemorrhage

A **hemorrhage** occurs when a patient begins to bleed suddenly. A hemorrhage is not a medical condition itself, but a symptom of an underlying problem. Hemorrhages can occur anywhere in the body where there are blood vessels: in the eye, the brain (a stroke), in major organs, and in the major vessels. Symptoms and signs can include pain, light-headedness, decreased blood pressure, vomiting, abnormal urine or stool, and the appearance of bruising. The danger posed by a hemorrhage depends on where it is located. Internal hemorrhages caused by burst aneurysms, such as an abdominal aortic aneurysm, can be life-threatening situations that require immediate emergency medical intervention to prevent collapse and death.

Realistically, there is little the dental team will be able to do in a serious bleeding event, whether internal or external, except for trying to diminish the bleeding, helping the patient relax physically and mentally, providing any emergency lifesaving support necessary, and contacting EMS. It is essential that a thorough medical history has been provided—some drugs, such as anticoagulants, can raise the risk of hemorrhage during medical procedures such as dental operations. This information should be provided to emergency medical personnel as rapidly as possible.

Dental Emergencies

Dental emergencies such as an avulsed or broken tooth are frequently called into the office before the patient arrives in person, so the DA might be expected to handle a phone call with a distressed patient. Although the dentist will perform the treatment—DAs cannot give dental advice on their own or treat any emergencies—it is still helpful to know what types of emergencies might occur. In some less urgent cases, patients may have to schedule an appointment to handle the problem. In others, it is more appropriate for the patient to come in as soon as possible or even be referred to an oral surgeon.

During a phone call, DAs should only give advice under the direction of the dentist, or get the dentist on the phone. In an in-office emergency, the dentist should give all the treatment needed.

Avulsed Tooth

An **avulsed tooth** is one that has been knocked out. Patients often call the dentist's office highly upset and trying to control bleeding. The first step is to calm the patient and assure him or her that, if the tooth can be found and brought quickly to the dentist, it is probable the tooth can be replaced into the empty socket.

Speed is essential when dealing with avulsed teeth. The patient should recover the tooth as quickly as possible and either place it between the teeth and lip (if an adult) or in a glass of milk (if a child, who might swallow or choke on a tooth placed in the mouth). Gauze or cotton can be packed into the empty socket to control bleeding. Pressure may help slow the bleeding; there might seem like a lot of blood because the gingival tissue bleeds readily.

Once the tooth is safely packed, the patient should be advised to come into the office as quickly as possible.

The dentist will reset the tooth into the socket and secure it against the adjoining teeth. Follow-up care is required to perform necessary endodontic treatment, usually after about 8 weeks.

Broken Tooth

Broken teeth are not uncommon, especially anterior teeth. Sharp blows against a steering wheel, hard surface, and even other people can cause portions of the tooth to break off. The treatment depends on the extent of the break, the level of discomfort, the patient's preferences, and whether the broken tooth poses a further risk of injury because of sharp edges. It is not unusual to schedule a patient with a broken tooth for an immediate emergency appointment and provide appropriate follow-up treatment once the dentist has assessed the extent of the injury.

Abscessed Tooth

An abscess occurs when a tooth becomes infected under the gingiva (Figure 18-5). The pocket of infection grows, putting pressure on the tooth's nerve and causing symptoms including pain, swelling, and discomfort when eating. If the abscess is not treated, a fistula may form. A *fistula* is a connection between the infection and the surface of the skin inside the oral cavity. This allows some of the excess fluid to drain away and may somewhat relieve symptoms. Abscessed teeth are treated by cleaning out the infection at the root of the tooth. Fistulas normally close after the infection is gone.

Mouth Injury and Oral Punctures

Mouth injuries occur when patients injure the soft tissues in their oral cavities. There are any number of ways patients can hurt their soft tissues, including teeth puncturing the lips or tongue, falling down, sports injuries, pens or other objects puncturing tissue, or even biting into an electrical cord and causing a burn. Children can suffer from an injury known as a **traumatic intrusion**, which occurs when a young child falls and the blow pushes newly erupted teeth back into their sockets. Soft tissue injuries can also occur in the dental office itself. For example, a patient might twitch unexpectedly and cause an instrument injury.

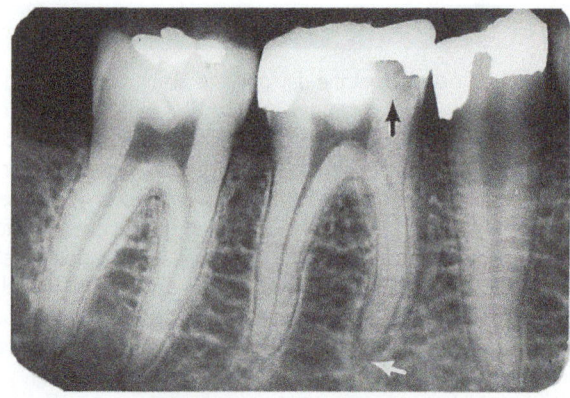

Figure 18–5 Radiograph of acute apical abscess (white arrow).

Treatment for a soft tissue injury depends on the extent of the injury. The best course is for the DA to gather as much information as possible and share it with the dentist, making sure to keep the patient informed. As always, DAs should seek to calm distressed patients. Patients might be called in on an emergency basis, sent to an oral surgeon, or, if the injury is superficial, advised to control the bleeding and set an appointment for a later date.

Broken Prosthesis

Broken prostheses are rarely medical emergencies, but they can be unsightly and reduce the patient's ability to chew food. A patient who calls with a broken dental prosthesis is normally scheduled for a visit at the nearest convenient time so the dentist can assess the prosthesis and, if necessary, send it out for repair. Times for repair vary.

Loose Crown

Crowns sometimes come loose, causing patients to call in for repair. Repair usually consists of recementing the crown in place. The urgency of the situation depends on whether the patient is in pain because the tender pulp is exposed and whether the tooth has sharp edges. In some cases, a loose crown can be held in place with dental wax until the patient can get into the office.

Torn Frenum

There are two frena in the oral cavity: the maxillary frenum and the mandibular frenum. Either can tear due to oral injury. In some cases, if the frenum is constricting, a dentist might choose to resect (snip) it. When a patient calls with a torn frenum, an appointment can be scheduled, although most of these injuries heal on their own without any damage or effects.

The American Dental Association has found an association between a torn frenum in children and child abuse. If a dentist's office suspects child abuse, they should work with local authorities to report the possible situation. See Chapter 4, Ethics and Law, for more information about reporting suspected abuse.

CHECKPOINT

18-5 What is the dental assistant's appropriate role during a phone call with a patient experiencing a dental emergency?

After the Emergency

After the emergency has passed, full documentation of the event is essential. The patient's record should be updated with details of the event, including exactly what happened, the steps taken, and the result. In some states and cities, details of the event might have to also be reported to the controlling body for dentists, such as a state board of dentistry.

Although it might not be the dentist's responsibility, the dentist might choose to follow up after an emergency with the patient, the patient's family, or the patient's personal physician.

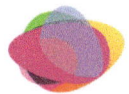

Chapter Highlights

+ Dental assistants need to be prepared for nondental and dental medical emergencies by knowing the symptoms of the most common emergencies and the appropriate responses.
+ All dental office workers should be trained in current cardiopulmonary resuscitation techniques and how to use the automatic external defibrillator.
+ Every office should have an emergency preparedness plan that clearly describes who does what in the case of an emergency. Emergency phone numbers should be posted by every phone.
+ Every dental office should have emergency oxygen available.
+ Every dental office should have an emergency kit stocked with basic medical supplies as well as drugs that might be necessary in a medical emergency. The kit should be checked weekly to make sure everything is current and not expired.
+ All dental assistants should know how to use the contents of the emergency medical kit.

+ Dental offices should stage routine training drills to sharpen the emergency responses of the dental team.
+ Dental assistants cannot offer treatment themselves or advise patients on medical treatment. Only the dentist can fulfill these functions.
+ The current ratio of chest compressions to rescue breaths for cardiopulmonary resuscitation is 30:2 for adults, infants, and children.
+ The *universal distress signal* means a patient is choking. If patients are choking, it is appropriate to use the *Heimlich maneuver*.
+ Be prepared for a variety of medical emergencies that may present themselves in the dental clinic, including dizziness, asthma attack, diabetic emergency, allergic reaction, seizure, stroke, and heart attack. In particular, learn to identify and assist during dental emergencies, including avulsions, abscesses, oral punctures, and loosened crowns.

 **Review Questions**

1. If a patient is acting unusual or seems unsteady or visibly nervous when being led back to the treatment area, the dental assistant should
   a. Cancel the appointment.
   b. Alert the dentist before treatment begins.
   c. Alert the dentist after treatment begins.
   d. None of the above.

2. Which is appropriate for a dental assistant?
   a. Perform cardiopulmonary resuscitation when appropriate in a medical emergency
   b. Tell a worried patient over the phone what's wrong and how to fix it
   c. Replace a broken crown
   d. None of the above

3. What is nitroglycerin used for?
   a. Reviving patients who have passed out
   b. Stopping asthma attacks
   c. Treating allergy attacks
   d. Treating angina

4. What is the current ratio of chest compressions to breaths for adult cardiopulmonary resuscitation (CPR)?
   a. 30:1
   b. 15:1
   c. 15:2
   d. 30:2

5. When is an automatic external defibrillator used?
   a. When a patient is choking
   b. Whenever a patient has fainted
   c. When a patient is unconsciousness and has no pulse
   d. During cardiopulmonary resuscitation

6. What does the acronym C-A-B stand for?
   a. Circulation, Airway, Breathing
   b. Consciousness, Air supply, Breathing
   c. Circulation, Aortic pulse, Breathing
   d. None of the above

7. What is the difference between signs and symptoms?
   a. They are the same.
   b. Signs can be objectively measured, and symptoms cannot.

   c. Symptoms are objective (outwardly evident), and signs are evident only to the patient.
   d. Signs are limited to the skin and major organs.

8. If a patient exhibits the universal distress signal, he or she is most likely
   a. Choking.
   b. Having a stroke.
   c. Having a heart attack.
   d. Having a seizure.

9. The Heimlich maneuver can be used on
   a. Any patient who appears to have something lodged in his or her throat.
   b. Only a conscious patient who can stand under his or her own power.
   c. Any patient who is not pregnant.
   d. Patients only if no emergency services are available.

10. A green cylinder contains
    a. Nitrous oxide.
    b. Carbon dioxide.
    c. Oxygen.
    d. Bronchodilators.

11. A myocardial infarction is also called a
    a. Stroke.
    b. Diabetic coma.
    c. Convulsion.
    d. Heart attack.

12. A transient ischemic attack is different from a stroke because
    a. It does not involve blood flow to the brain.
    b. Symptoms are temporary and resolve without lasting damage.
    c. It is limited to ischemic events.
    d. It is limited to hemorrhagic events.

13. During anaphylaxis
    a. The patient has difficulty breathing due to an allergic reaction.
    b. Patients often pass out and have seizures.
    c. Hallucinations are common.
    d. Patients become lethargic and confused.

14. What is the correct response to a hyperventilating patient?

    a. Bronchodilators

    b. Corticosteroids

    c. Timing slow breaths against a watch's second hand

    d. Repositioning with the knees above the waist

15. Orthostatic hypertension occurs

    a. When patients see a needle or drill.

    b. During anesthesia.

    c. When patients shift position suddenly.

    d. When patients are very stressed out.

16. A dental assistant's role during a dental emergency may include

    a. Observing the patient's condition and taking necessary emergency measures.

    b. Administering cardiopulmonary resuscitation to the patient, if necessary.

    c. Obtaining accurate information from the patient over the telephone and transmitting it to the dentist.

    d. All of the above.

Active Learning Exercises

1. What is the most common medical emergency encountered in the dental office? How is this situation handled? Should a patient receive dental care after such an emergency? Defend your answer.

2. A patient presents for treatment but becomes apprehensive, shaky, and weak; she indicates that she feels dizzy, that her heart is pounding, and that she is experiencing double vision. What condition could this be? What is the treatment for this emergency?

Application Activities

1. Draw up an imaginary emergency preparedness plan, including roles for everybody in the office. Remember to include all the components of the response, such as calling for help and providing lifesaving support.

2. Compile a table listing symptoms and signs of the most common medical disorders that may present in the dental office, along with the appropriate medical response.

3. Use the Internet or the library to locate places in your area that offer cardiopulmonary resuscitation training courses.

> ## PREPARING FOR CERTIFICATION EXAMS
>
> Review the following topics in this chapter to prepare for the Dental Assisting National Board (DANB) exam:
>
> - **Preventing Emergencies**
> - **Emergency Preparedness**
> - **Emergency Equipment and Supplies**
> - **Immediate Life Support**
> - **Responding to Common Medical Emergencies**

Ergonomics

CHAPTER CHECKLIST

On completion of this chapter, students will be able to:

- ☑ Describe the importance of ergonomics for dental assistants.
- ☑ Discuss how to maintain the neutral position.
- ☑ Explain correct and incorrect body mechanics for lifting and reaching.
- ☑ Identity commons types of repetitive stress disorders.
- ☑ Describe strategies for preventing repetitive stress disorders.

KEY TERMS

body mechanics – the study and use of proper muscle movement in daily activities

carpal tunnel syndrome – a condition in which a nerve in the carpal tunnel area of the wrist is compressed and becomes painful; caused by repeatedly extending and holding the wrist in the same position over long periods of time

ergonomics (er-goh-NOM-iks) – the study of how work environments and work tasks can be made safe and comfortable for people on the job

fulcrum (FUL-krum) – a finger rest that allows the muscles of the hand to relax and remain steady

neutral position – best position to maintaining good posture while sitting, standing, or reaching; includes keeping the back straight, legs slightly apart, feet flat on the floor or footrest, lower back pressed against the chair, and ears, shoulder, and hips in a straight line

musculoskeletal (mus-kyuh-loh-SKEL-ih-tul) injuries – injuries to the skeleton and muscles of the body

repetitive stress injuries – injuries that result from performing the same motion repeatedly, especially motions that are awkward for the body

Introduction

Applying the principles of ergonomics has benefits for both dental assistants and patients. Improving both working conditions and methods for performing work makes patient visits shorter and dental practice safer and less strenuous on the dental assistant (DA), in large part by focusing on putting the patient and the DA in positions that offer easy and uninhibited access to working areas. This reduces strain on the muscles, helps prevent injuries, and ensures a safer and more effective process for each patient.

Potential for Injury

It might not seem obvious, but the practice of dental assisting carries some important health risks for DAs. **Musculoskeletal injuries** are those that involve the skeleton and muscles of the body, such as the head, neck, hands (including wrists and fingers), and back. Preventing musculoskeletal injury can help DAs have longer and healthier lives as well as longer and healthier careers.

One of the main reasons why DAs are at risk for musculoskeletal injuries is that they often spend long periods of time sitting or holding their bodies in unusual positions such as when gripping instruments. Performing the same motion repeatedly—especially motions that are awkward for the body—can lead to **repetitive stress injuries**.

In addition to repetitive stress, the physical environment can play a role in causing injuries. The instruments used in dental assisting may require the fingers, wrist, and arm to remain in uncomfortable positions. The vibration of instruments or even the DA's or patient's chairs themselves can place strain on the body. Cold office temperatures also make it difficult for muscles to function easily.

These factors show why working in an ergonomic environment is so important. **Ergonomics** is the study of how work environments and tasks can be made more comfortable for people on the job. For DAs, ergonomics are important when working with patients as well as when performing nonpatient tasks such as sitting at the front desk or at a computer.

Finally, it is important to note personal factors that make injuries more likely. Sitting incorrectly or grasping instruments improperly places extra strain on the muscles and skeleton. Poor physical fitness, lack of rest, and too much stress are other personal factors that can increase or decrease the body's ability to function well.

CHECKPOINT

19-1 What factors put dental assistants at risk for musculoskeletal injuries on the job?

Principles of Body Mechanics

The study of proper muscle movement in daily activities is known as **body mechanics.** This includes the position of muscles while at rest, such as while sitting or standing, as well as while in motion, such as lifting and reaching.

Posture

Keeping good posture is the most powerful tool for preventing injury in the short term and in the future. Good posture must be practiced daily so that it becomes habit. Posture is not just about sitting properly but also includes proper standing and reaching. The best way to keep good posture through the day is to use the **neutral position** (Figure 19-1). This position includes:

- Straight back
- Legs apart slightly
- Feet flat on the floor or on the footrest
- Lower back pressed against the back of the chair
- Ears, shoulders, and hips in a straight line
- Eyes tilted downward at the patient rather than looking directly while bending the neck uncomfortably

The neutral position should also be used when standing, which includes keeping the back straight and feet slightly apart (Figure 19-2). Failure to use the neutral position can cause different types of injuries to the body, including aches, twists, tearing, or overstretching of the muscles (Figure 19-3). In practicing the neutral position, do not:

- Sit on the edge of the chair
- Lean forward excessively

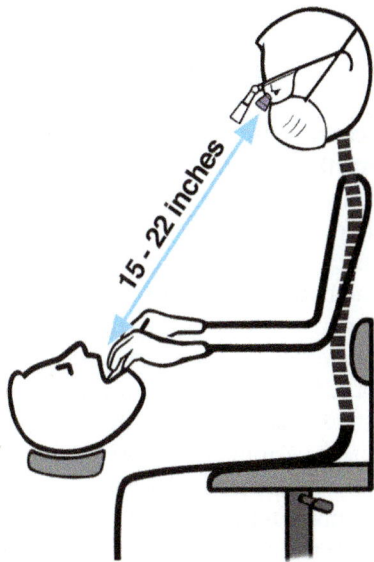

Figure 19-1 Proper working posture and distance. Acceptable positioning shows the patient at the clinician's elbow level and the oral cavity of the patient between 15 and 22 inches from the clinician's eyes.

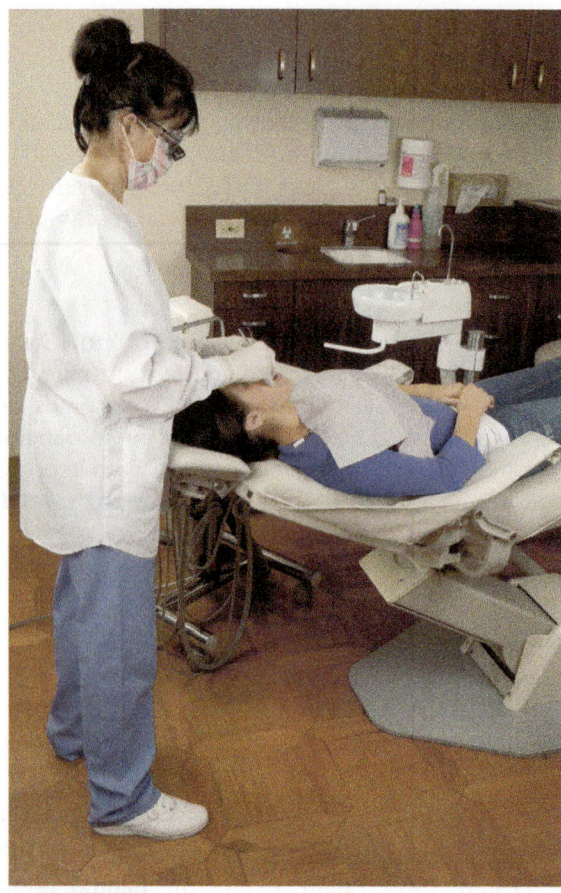

Figure 19–2 **Proper standing posture.** Keep the back straight and feet slightly apart.

■ Hunch the back or shoulders
■ Make quick, jerking movements when reaching or twisting

Body Mechanics for Lifting and Reaching

Lifting and reaching are common movements in the dental office. Sometimes lifting heavy objects or reaching for objects in unusual positions is necessary. Using proper body mechanics while performing these movements can prevent injuries and make the work environment less stressful to the body (Figure 19-4 and Table 19-1).

When using instruments, a fulcrum can be very helpful in maintaining proper body mechanics of the hand, fingers, and arm. A **fulcrum** is a simply a type of finger rest. Some instruments have fulcrums that are detachable. For other instruments, gripping in a specific way can allow the fingers themselves to act as a fulcrum (Figure 19-5). Using a fulcrum is important because it allows the muscles of your hands to remain steady and relaxed while using the instrument. Not only do fulcrums help prevent the hand from becoming overworked or strained, but keeping the instrument steady also prevents the patient from being injured.

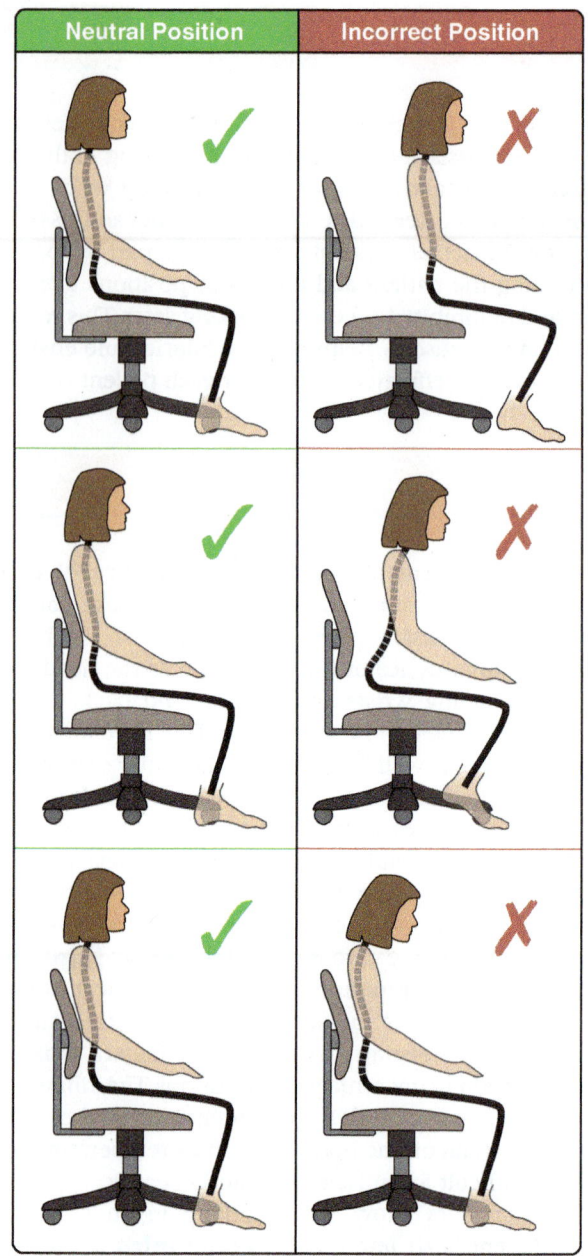

Figure 19–3 **Neutral position vs. incorrect position.** Failure to use the neutral position can be a costly mistake. To keep the skeleton and muscles free from injury, avoid these common mistakes.

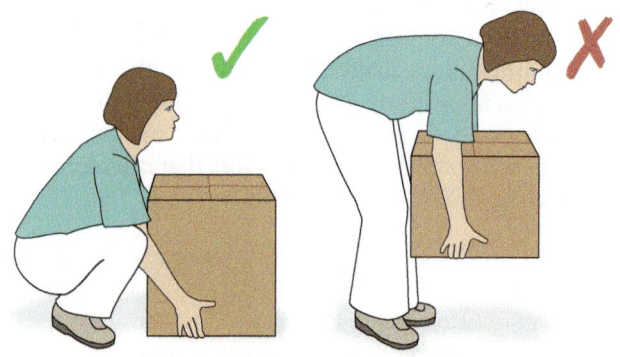

Figure 19–4 Proper vs. poor lifting technique.

TABLE 19-1 How to Lift and Reach without Injuring Yourself

DO...	DON'T...
Keep your back relaxed so the lower back is slightly curved	Keep the back stiff and in a straight line
Hold the object close to your body	Keep the object at arm's length
Squat or kneel on one knee	Bend over at the back from a standing position
Keep feet shoulder-width apart	Place feet close together or too far apart
Use the leg muscles to push yourself up to a standing position	Use the back to pull yourself up
Use a ladder if an object is higher than shoulder level	Try to reach objects higher than the shoulder by yourself
Seek assistance if an object is not easily within reach	Twist your body in awkward positions or rely on shelves or other objects for support while reaching

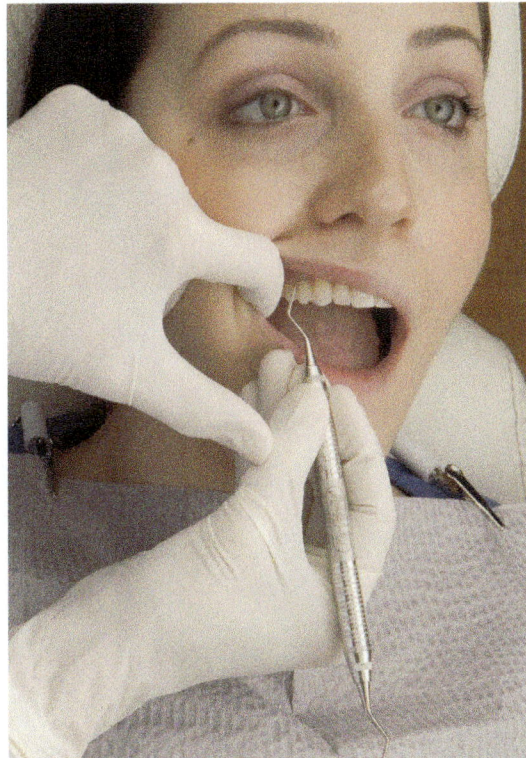

Figure 19–5 Using fingers as fulcrum. Note how the fingers on the working hand are resting against the patient's cheek and jaw, acting as a fulcrum.

CHECKPOINT

19-2 What is the best posture for sitting, standing, and reaching that can help prevent injuries?

Preventing Repetitive Stress Disorders

One of the best ways to prevent repetitive stress injuries is to keep your muscles in good shape. This requires a three-part approach:

- Maintaining proper posture, such as the neutral position, at all times
- Keeping physically fit through a nonsedentary lifestyle outside work, whether through swimming, cycling, hiking, jogging, or other sports and physical activities
- Reducing emotional and physical stress as much as possible

Injury prevention is important no matter what activity is being performed. When working with patients, be sure that both your stool and the patient's chair are at the proper height. Sitting too high above the patient can place strain on the neck, shoulders, and back. Sitting too low can also cause discomfort. When not working with patients, such as sitting at the front desk, be sure your stool is at a height to keep your thighs parallel with the floor. See Chapter 24, The Dental Office, for more details about what to look for in a properly designed stool. If you work at a computer, be sure the top of the computer monitor is at your eye level. Sit approximately 20 to 24 inches from the computer screen, and keep the keyboard below your elbows. Use the armrest so that your wrists can stay relaxed.

Dental Facts

In the past, dentists did not have operator stools and had to work on patients while standing. This is one of the reasons why so many dentists developed back problems.

Make sure to allow for occasional breaks throughout the day so that your muscles have time to relax. In order to maintain good muscle health, simple exercises can be performed both at work and away from the office. These flexing and stretching exercises are designed to work many different muscle groups in the body and should be performed daily. Below are some common types of repetitive stress injuries, followed by suggested exercises in Table 19-2.

TABLE 19-2 Exercises to Prevent Repetitive Stress Injuries

DOING THIS...	HELPS RELAX THESE...	DEPICTION OF EXERCISE
▪ While standing or sitting in the neutral position, interlace your fingers so that your palms face out. ▪ Stretch both arms over your head. ▪ Follow your fingers with your eyes as your hands are raised.	Fingers Hands Arms Neck Back	
▪ While standing in the neutral position, slowly bend forward, rounding your back and bringing your chin toward your chest. ▪ Allow your arms and hands to hang loosely.	Neck Back	
▪ While sitting in the neutral position, tilt your head backward and push your chest forward. ▪ Inhale slowly to the count of 5. ▪ While exhaling to the count of 5, slowly lower your head.	Neck Chest	
▪ While sitting or standing in the neutral position, roll your right shoulder back toward your right ear and down. ▪ Slowly roll your left shoulder back toward your left ear and down. ▪ Do the exercise with each shoulder 10 times, and then reverse the direction to roll each shoulder forward.	Neck Shoulders	
▪ While standing, roll onto the balls of your feet. ▪ Then slowly roll back onto your heels. ▪ Place your hands on a wall for support if needed.	Calves Feet	

Carpal Tunnel Syndrome

Carpal tunnel syndrome occurs when a specific nerve in the wrist, located in an area called the *carpal tunnel*, becomes compressed and damaged from reduced circulation. Repeatedly extending and holding the wrist in position over long periods of time places pressure on the nerve and can cause blood to stop flowing. As a result, numbness and tingling in the thumb, first finger, and middle finger can occur. To reduce the chances of developing carpal tunnel syndrome, allow the hands to rest as much as possible. Use daily exercises to flex the muscles of the hand and wrist, and also be sure to wear properly fitting gloves. Gloves that are too tight can cause swelling, which places added pressure on the muscles of the hand and wrist.

Hand and Finger Stresses

Like carpal tunnel syndrome, hand and finger stress can happen from holding instruments in position for extended amounts of time. Injuries can also come from constantly extending and flexing the fingers. To prevent hand and finger injuries, keep the hand, wrist, and arm in the neutral position while working and resting. Stretch the hands and fingers throughout the day, and use a fulcrum to keep the hand relaxed as much as possible while working.

Back Strain

Back strain is very common in dental settings because DAs spend so much time sitting in the same position. Keeping the back hunched or twisted is a sure way to cause pain and stiffness. To prevent injuries, use proper seating techniques when working with the patient. This includes the following:

- When in the neutral position, there should be about 15 to 22 inches between your eyes and the patient's oral cavity.
- Lower your eyes to view into the patient's oral cavity; do not hunch or roll the back to lean in for a closer view.

- Use the light to see into the patient's cavity.
- When sitting chairside assisting the dentist, sit approximately 4 to 6 inches higher than the dentist.

Remember to take breaks throughout the day to stand up, walk around, and stretch your back as needed. Building up your abdominal muscles through regular exercise will help strengthen the back.

Neck and Shoulder Injuries

Neck and shoulder injuries can come from lowering your head excessively or keeping your shoulders tightened. Again, adjusting both the light and the patient's chair help prevent having to bend your neck too much. A magnifying lens also helps you view inside the patient's oral cavity without having to twist, lean over, or hunch your body uncomfortably. Just as with other injuries, daily stretching and flexing your muscles can help prevent your neck and shoulders from becoming stiff and overworked.

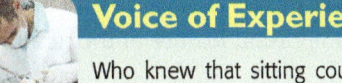
Voice of Experience

Who knew that sitting could be hazardous to your health? I did not realize how much I was slouching and sitting improperly at work until my back and neck began to hurt. At one point, I was taking aspirin regularly and was thinking of visiting a doctor for my pain. It was becoming more difficult to care for my patients because all I could think about was the discomfort I was in. Even desk work became painful! Then a coworker pointed out some easy ways to correct my posture while working. She also showed me some simple stretching techniques. At first, I was unsure whether they would work, but now I take a 10-minute break every afternoon to stretch and relax my body. I may have learned the hard way, but now I know: If you take care of your body, your body will take care of you.

CHECKPOINT
19-3 What are two important ways to prevent repetitive stress injuries?

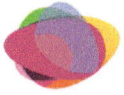
Chapter Highlights

- Dental assistants often sit or are in unusual positions throughout the day, placing them at risk for musculoskeletal injuries.
- Frequently performing the same muscle motions can lead to repetitive stress injuries.
- *Ergonomics* is the study of how work environments and work tasks can be made more comfortable and safer for people on the job.
- The proper movement of muscles in daily activities is known as *body mechanics*.

- Good body mechanics when sitting, standing, reaching, and lifting can help prevent injury and help dental assistants have longer, healthier careers.
- The neutral position is the best posture for sitting, standing, and reaching.
- Poor posture and improper body mechanics can lead to repetitive stress disorders, such as carpal tunnel syndrome, hand and finger stress, back strain, and neck and shoulder injuries.
- Simple exercises can help relieve stress to the muscles and prevent future injuries.

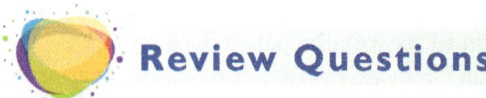

Review Questions

1. Ergonomics
   a. Only matters when working with patients.
   b. Is not an important part of working as a dental assistant.
   c. Is the study of how to make work environments more safe and comfortable.
   d. Is the study of proper muscle movements in daily activities.

2. Which factor increases the risk of musculoskeletal injury to dental assistants?
   a. Hot office temperatures
   b. Exercising daily
   c. Taking breaks throughout the day
   d. Sitting for long periods of time

3. Which of these is an important feature of the neutral position?
   a. Sitting on the edge of the chair
   b. Crossing the legs
   c. Keeping the back against the chair
   d. Propping the elbows on the armrest

4. When lifting an object
   a. Lift with the leg muscles.
   b. Lift by straightening the back.
   c. Keep the object an arm's length away from the body.
   d. Place the feet close together.

5. When reaching for an object
   a. Do not bother coworkers by asking for assistance.
   b. Brace yourself on a shelf, if needed.
   c. Get into whatever position necessary to reach the object.
   d. Use a ladder to reach anything higher than your shoulders.

6. Exercises for repetitive stress disorders
   a. Should never be practiced at work.
   b. Include stretching and flexing different muscle groups.
   c. Are only needed if you become injured.
   d. Have little impact on preventing future injuries.

Active Learning Exercise

1. What repetitive motions are made in dentistry? What modifications can be made to avoid these motions and prevent injury?

Application Activities

1. Make a list of ways you can practice good body mechanics throughout the day. For example, you might practice sitting in the neutral position while in class or proper lifting and reaching while cleaning at home.

2. With other students, form four groups. Each group takes a type of repetitive injury (carpal tunnel, back injuries, hand and finger injuries, and neck and shoulder injuries). Develop three simple exercises that can be performed to prevent that injury, and be prepared to demonstrate the exercises to the entire class.

3. What things do you think might make it hard for a dental assistant to perform injury prevention exercises while at work? How might a dental assistant deal with problems such as feeling too busy, forgetting to perform such exercises, or not knowing how to perform the exercises correctly?

4. Why do you think exercise, stress, and rest are important for musculoskeletal health? How would you go about explaining to another dental assistant the importance of personal factors, such as sleep and relaxation, for maintaining good musculoskeletal health?

Working with Patients

chapter 20

Oral Diagnosis and Treatment Planning

CHAPTER OUTLINE

CHAPTER CHECKLIST

Upon completion of this chapter, students will be able to:

☑ Identify and explain the significance of each part of the clinical examination.

☑ Explain Black's Classification of Cavities.

☑ Identify the four classes of teeth.

☑ Identify the five surfaces of the tooth.

☑ Describe the three main tooth numbering systems.

☑ Identify and use common abbreviations for simple, complex, and compound caries.

☑ Identify and use basic charting terminology.

☑ Identify and use common charting symbols.

☑ Describe the different treatment plan options.

KEY TERMS

anterior teeth – teeth at the front of the mouth: canine to canine

explorer – a slender instrument, sharply pointed at one or both ends, used to detect imperfections in the enamel and to determine the condition of restorations

extraoral – outside the oral cavity

intraoral – inside the oral cavity

mouth mirror – instrument used to see areas within the intraoral cavity that cannot be seen by direct vision

periodontal probe – instrument used to measure the depth of the sulcus

posterior teeth – teeth at the back of the mouth: premolars and molars

Introduction

A thorough understanding of the process of oral diagnosis and treatment planning is necessary for your work as a professional dental assistant (DA). A clinical examination consists of both an **extraoral** examination of the head and neck outside the oral cavity and an **intraoral** examination of the interior of the mouth. During the course of these examinations, the dentist uses a variety of diagnostic techniques and equipment. This chapter explains how to identify each tooth according to its type and numbered location within the mouth, which is important for marking the patient's dental chart accurately and clearly. Classifications of dental caries and variations in treatment plans are also described.

Clinical Examination

As a professional DA, you will see a wide variety of patients in your practice. The process of providing patients with the best possible dental care begins as you escort each patient to the clinical examination area. While doing so, observe the patient's overall appearance, gait, speech, and general behavior. Take note of anything unusual and call anything of concern to the dentist's attention. Once you have seated the patient in the dental chair, secure a paper bib or napkin around his or her neck. As you establish a rapport with the patient and begin to compile or update the patient's medical and dental history, you will learn the reason for the patient's visit.

Whereas some patients are seeking routine assessment and care, others are seeking relief for a sudden painful emergency, returning for a checkup on work done previously, or visiting the practice for the first time. Regardless of the reason for the visit, dental care begins with a thorough examination of the patient's head, neck, and oral cavity.

From the Dentist's Perspective

Dental assistants have to learn a great deal about the whole process of dentistry—the exams, the instruments, and charting. They have to follow along and understand the significance of what we are observing during an exam or doing during a treatment. It is so important, though, never to lose sight of the people connection. I honestly think that might be just as important in some ways. Our dental assistant is great with people from the moment they walk in the door. Our patients know what to expect when they come here. Our dental assistant remembers things about them, their lives, families, work, and more. It makes such a difference to how comfortable patients feel. I really think our patients are more relaxed here than at other practices. Our dental assistant takes the time to know them and stay positive and friendly from the moment she goes to the waiting room to meet them.

Most of this examination is conducted by the dentist and carefully observed by you. As the dentist comments on the patient's dental conditions and health, you will note or chart the findings on specially designed forms for the patient's record. The dentist may later suggest plans for treatment and follow-up care, which you will also note on the patient's chart.

Visual Examination

After a careful review of the medical history, the dental examination begins with an extraoral visual examination of the patient's head and neck and an intraoral examination of conditions within the patient's oral cavity, using magnification as appropriate to better see abnormalities in the tooth. This exam helps determine what type of care the patient previously received, including any problems that have been overlooked or neglected. The dentist will be especially alert for any abnormalities or previous dental restorations.

Cultural Diversity

During dental treatment, it is common for the doctor or the assistant to look into patients' eyes to monitor their comfort status. However, people of some Native American cultures believe that their souls can be stolen by making eye contact with others. They view eyes as the key to the soul. Other cultures do not make eye contact as a sign of respect. In many parts of Asia, for example, it is considered aggressive and rude. Still other cultures, such as Muslim, prohibit male doctors from making eye contact with female patients because it is regarded as a sexual impropriety. Americans, by contrast, view a lack of eye contact as rude or a sign of disinterest or distrust. Being respectful of your patients' practices and beliefs can help you build strong relationships with them.

Soft Tissue Abnormalities

Healthy soft tissue appears light pink throughout without spots of redness, paleness, or swelling. Individuals who have darker pigmentation often have gingival tissue that is darker in appearance, but this is a normal physiological variation. Note on the patient's chart any abnormalities observed by the dentist.

Tooth Structure

The dentist uses a **mouth mirror** to examine areas within the mouth that lie out of sight (Figure 20-1). Examination should reveal teeth that are intact, in sound condition, and of the expected size and shape. Tooth enamel also should be free of chips and discoloration. Note any abnormalities, including missing teeth, on the patient's chart.

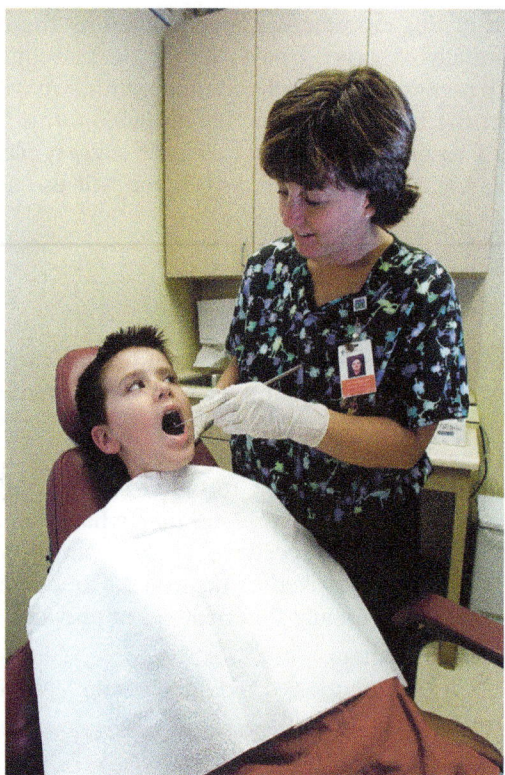

Figure 20–1 Dentist using a mouth mirror.

Restorations

The dentist examines restorations, such as amalgams, composites, crowns, bridges, inlays, or onlays, to ensure that they remain functional and intact. The DA notes restoration type and location, along with any developing problems in the patient's chart.

Examination with Instruments

The use of dental instruments helps the dentist further evaluate areas of the intraoral cavity. Besides the mouth mirror, the dentist typically uses two other instruments during clinical examination.

Explorer

The **explorer**, a slender instrument sharply pointed at one or both ends (Figure 20-2), is used to detect imperfections in the enamel, such as pits or fissures, that may signal the start of caries. A dentist also uses the explorer to check the condition of restorations, such as crowns and amalgam and composite restorations, to make sure they are not loose or otherwise unstable.

Periodontal Probe

The **periodontal probe** is specially marked by millimeters to measure the depth of the sulcus (Figure 20-3), the narrow furrow between the gingiva and the teeth. Regular probing can detect receding gingiva and warn of developing disease.

Examination by Palpation

Palpation, or examination by touch and pressure, is one of the oldest examination techniques in medicine. In dentistry, palpation is used in extraoral examination to determine the size, texture, and consistency of soft tissue by gently squeezing it between the fingers. In many states, DAs examine extraoral soft tissue by palpation. Extraoral swelling, especially of the lymph nodes, most often is detected by palpation. Intraoral tissue is also palpated, including of the floor of the mouth, the vestibules, the edentulous ridges palpated for bony spurs, and so on. A full head and neck examination is recommended when searching for oral cancer in all patients and should include inspection and palpation of extraoral tissues, the temporomandibular joint, the tongue, the floor of the mouth, the palate, the uvula, and the lymph nodes.

Radiographic Examination

In a radiographic examination, radiographs (also known as *x-rays*) are used to assess intraoral development and detect abnormalities such as dental caries, loose or defective restorations, and periodontal disease (Figure 20-4). Radiography may also be used to further investigate extraoral

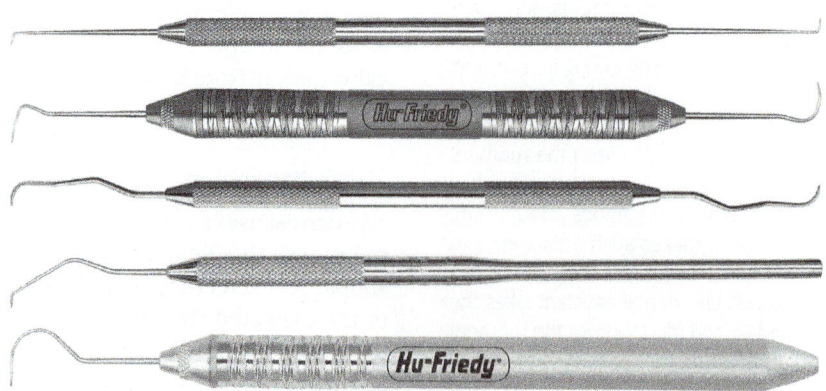

Figure 20–2 Explorers.

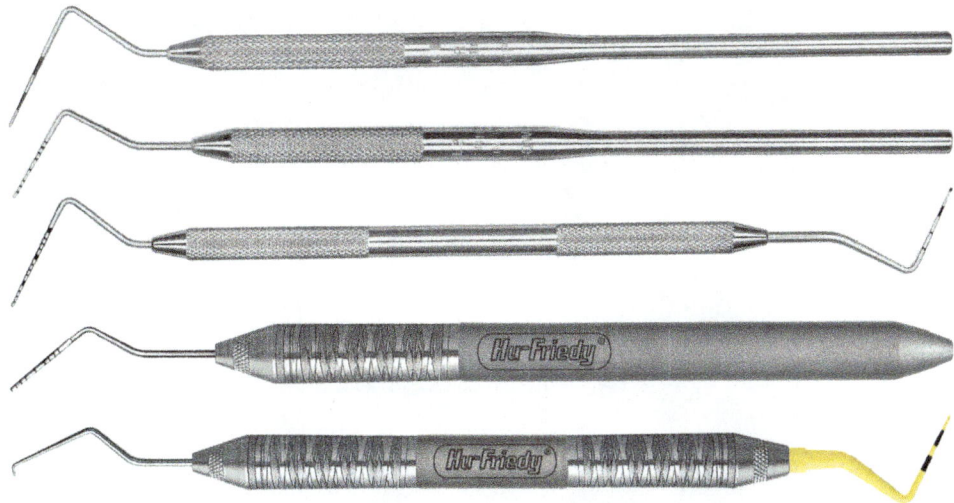

Figure 20–3 Periodontal probes.

abnormalities detected by the dentist or DA. See Part VII, Dental Radiography, for more information about the important role radiography plays in dentistry.

Intraoral Video and Photography

Intraoral video examination uses a very small camera to view the patient's intraoral cavity and displays live video of the examination on a monitor in the same room. Intraoral video has several advantages. It provides access to areas of the mouth that are difficult to view otherwise, offers magnification that allows the dentist to see conditions and abnormalities in greater detail, allows for photographs for patient education and insurance purposes, and provides documentation for the patient's medical history. Small cameras may also be used to photograph and record intraoral conditions with still photographs rather than video (Figure 20-5). Such photography is especially useful in reconstructive or orthodontic dentistry. It provides a before-and-after record of original conditions and the subsequent effects of any procedures, and it helps patients accept treatment by showing them conditions a dentist can otherwise only describe.

Locating Teeth within the Mouth

As described in Chapter 8, Dentition and Tooth Morphology, teeth are described according to their location within the mouth. At their most basic, these distinctions begin with whether teeth are front or back teeth, and whether they are upper or lower.

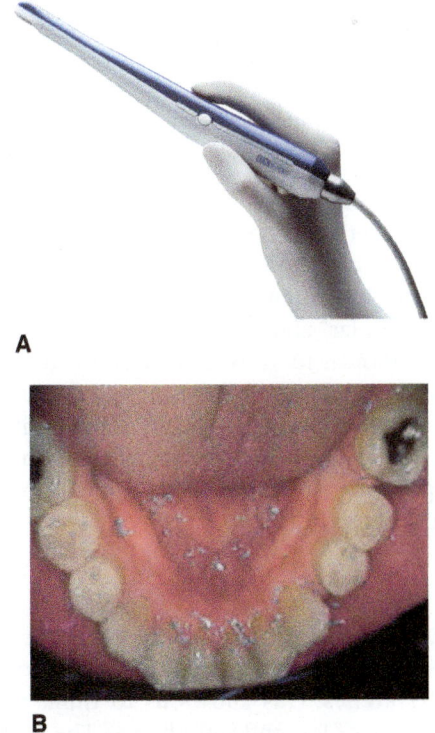

A

B

Figure 20–5 Intraoral photographs. A. An intraoral camera. B. Image from an intraoral camera as viewed on a computer monitor.

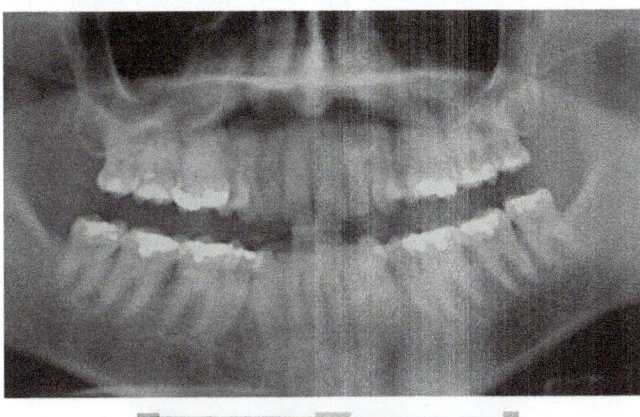

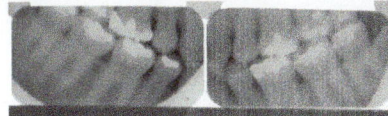

Figure 20–4 Extraoral panoramic radiographic images. Top: of the whole mouth. Bottom: left and right quadrants.

Figure 20–6 Quadrants of the oral cavity.

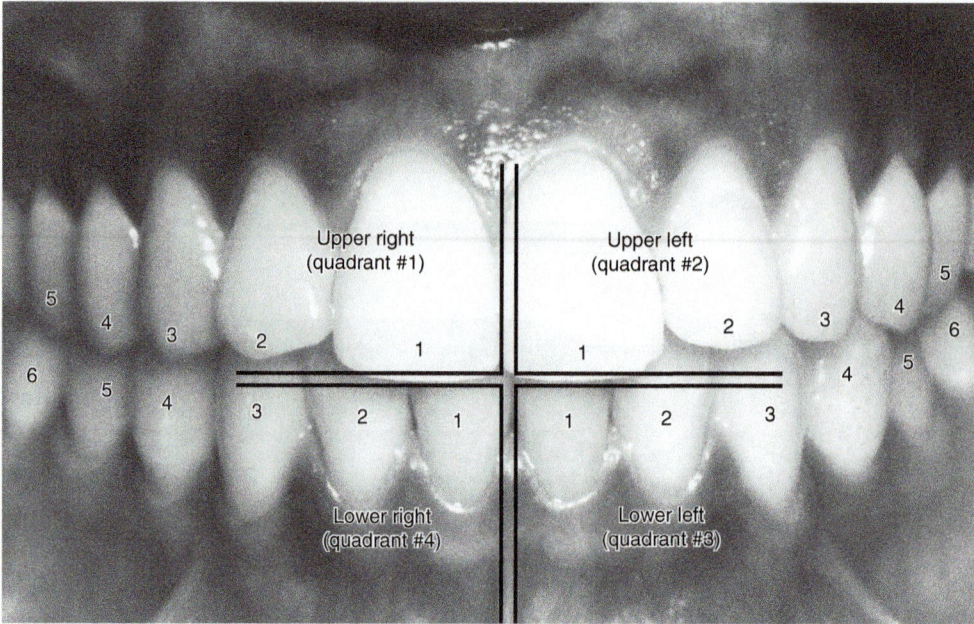

Anterior

Anterior teeth are found at the front of the mouth along both the maxillary and mandibular arches. They include the central incisors, which are found at the midline, followed by the lateral incisors and the canine/cuspid teeth.

Posterior

Posterior teeth are found at the back of the mouth along both the maxillary and mandibular arches. They include the bicuspids/premolars and molars.

Arches

The oral cavity contains two dental arches. The teeth and bone of the mandible, or lower jaw, make up the mandibular arch. The teeth and bone of the maxilla, or upper jaw, make up the maxillary arch. Teeth are identified as being on either the lower jaw or the upper jaw by using the terms "mandibular" and "maxillary" when describing the teeth. A mandibular tooth is located in the lower sections of the mouth; a maxillary tooth is located in the upper section. The maxillary and mandibular arches contain a total of 32 possible permanent teeth, or 16 teeth on each arch. Younger patients may not have developed some or all of their third molars (called "wisdom teeth").

Midline

The midline is an imaginary midsagittal line that runs between the central incisors on both the maxillary and mandibular arches. This allows us to think of the oral cavity in terms of left and right halves. The midline continues on to divide the rest of the body into two equal halves.

Quadrants

Each of the four classes of teeth described under Names of Teeth on the next page is found in each of the four quadrants of the oral cavity: upper right, upper left, lower left, and lower right (Figure 20-6).

Dentition

The word "dentition" refers to the naturally occurring teeth found in the mandibular and maxillary arches. *Primary dentition* (or deciduous dentition) describes the 20 teeth that emerge in early childhood. *Adult dentition* refers to the 32 teeth that emerge later in childhood to replace and supplement the primary dentition. (See Chapter 8, Dentition and Tooth Morphology, for a detailed description of the teeth of primary and adult dentition.)

Sextants

Another way to identify teeth is by dividing the oral cavity into sextants (Figure 20-7). A sextant refers to one-sixth of the dentition; therefore, there are six sextants in the oral cavity, three on each arch organized in the following manner:

- Premolars and molars on the right
- Canine teeth, lateral incisors, and central incisors on the right across to central incisors, lateral incisors, and canine teeth on the left
- Premolars and molars on the left

CHECKPOINTS

20-1 Which of the common dental instruments is used to detect caries?

20-2 Which arch contains the lower teeth?

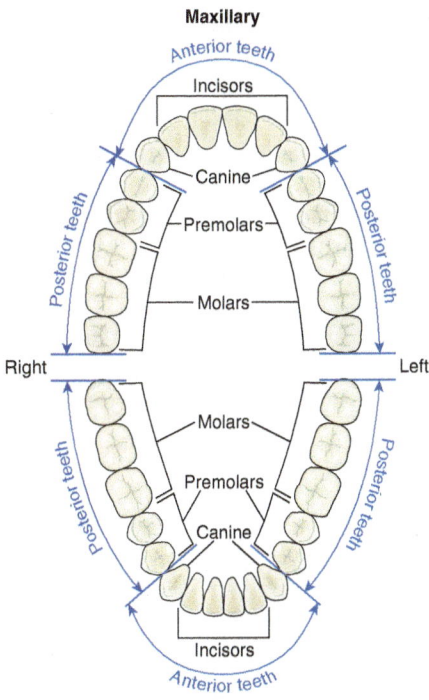

Figure 20–7 Sextants of the oral cavity.

Classification of Cavities

The treatment of caries generally uses a system first developed by 19th-century dental educator and reformer G. V. Black. Known as *Black's Classification of Cavities*, the system takes into consideration the location and pattern of decay, along with the extent of the decay, to decide on the best treatment plan. Table 20-1 describes the five classifications developed by Dr. Black as well as the sixth classification added later.

Dental Facts

Treatments change over time. Today, two cavities on the occlusal surface of a tooth would be filled with one large restoration rather than two smaller ones. Thirty years ago, however, it was not uncommon to see two occlusal pits of decay filled separately on a bicuspid. This type of amalgam restoration was known as "snake eyes" for the way it appeared on a tooth and on a patient's chart!

CHECKPOINT

20-3 Black's Classification of Cavities classifies caries according to what?

Further Classification of Caries

Tooth caries is also classified as simple, compound, or complex. *Simple caries* involves only one tooth surface. *Compound caries* involves two tooth surfaces. *Complex caries* involves more than two tooth surfaces.

Dental Terminology

A thorough knowledge of dental terminology is essential for accurate charting. Defects and treatment plans are described in a patient's chart according to their location and the teeth affected.

Names of Teeth

The names of teeth are determined by tooth morphology as well as the tooth's function (see Chapter 8, Dentition and Tooth Morphology). Recalling the four classes of teeth, we distinguish among them during examination by charting teeth per quadrant. Each type of tooth described below is normally found on both the maxillary and mandibular arches and in all four quadrants of the mouth.

- *Incisors.* The incisors are located at the very front of the oral cavity; central incisors are located on either side of the midline and lateral incisors are located on either side of the central incisors. There are eight incisors: four on each arch, two in each quadrant.
- *Canines.* The canines (or cuspids) are located immediately distal to the lateral incisors. There are four canines: two on each arch, one in each quadrant.
- *Premolars.* The premolars (or bicuspids) are located immediately distal to the canines; first premolars are closest to the midline and second premolars are immediately distal. There are eight premolars: four on each arch, two in each quadrant.
- *Molars.* The molars are located immediately distal to the premolars; first molars are closest to the midline and second molars are immediately distal. Third molars (also known as "wisdom teeth") are immediately distal to the second premolars, if they are present. There are twelve molars (including third molars): six on each arch, three in each quadrant.

The Five Surfaces of the Tooth

Any defects or caries noted during the clinical examination is described according to where it occurs on the surfaces of the tooth. Dental professionals agree on five distinct tooth surfaces: facial, lingual, incisal/occlusal, mesial, and distal (Figure 20-8). These surfaces are named for their relationship or closeness to other intraoral structures, such as the lips and tongue, or according to which direction they face within the intraoral cavity. You must be able to distinguish these five surfaces in order to chart a patient's examination and treatment clearly and accurately.

- *Facial*—the surfaces of the teeth on the outer side of the dental arches that touch the face; *labial* refers to the surface of the anterior teeth that touch the lips, and *buccal* refers to the surface of the posterior teeth that touch the cheek
- *Lingual*—the surfaces of the teeth that face the tongue; also referred to as the *palatal surface* in the maxillary dentition
- *Incisal/occlusal*—the chewing and cutting surfaces of the teeth; the top surface of molars and premolars is described as "occlusal" and the cutting surface of canines and incisors is described as "incisal"
- *Mesial*—the surfaces of the teeth that face the midline of the body
- *Distal*—the surfaces of the teeth that face away from the midline of the body

TABLE 20-1 Black's Classification of Cavities		
CLASS	**DESCRIPTION**	**VISUALIZATION**
I	<ul><li>The pits and fissures of the occlusal surfaces of molars and premolars</li><li>Buccal or lingual pits of molars</li><li>Lingual pits of maxillary incisors</li><li>Restorative treatment is amalgam or composite resins depending on the location of decay and restorative strength needed</li></ul>	
II	<ul><li>Decay is located between teeth, on the mesial or distal surfaces of premolars and molars</li><li>Restorative treatment is silver amalgam or a naturally colored composite resin of adequate strength</li><li>Teeth with extensive decay may be restored with a gold or porcelain crown, inlay, or onlay</li></ul>	
III	<ul><li>Decay is located between teeth, on the mesial or distal surfaces of incisors and canines</li><li>Restorative treatment uses naturally colored composite resins</li></ul>	
IV	<ul><li>Decay is located in the mesial or distal surfaces of the incisal edges of incisors and canine teeth</li><li>Treatment is restoration with a naturally colored composite resin</li><li>Teeth with extensive decay may be restored with a porcelain crown</li></ul>	
V	<ul><li>Decay occurs on the facial or lingual surface of any tooth in the oral cavity</li><li>On the third of the tooth closest to the gingiva (gingival third)</li><li>Decay of this type may result from improper tooth brushing</li><li>Restoration materials used depend on the site of decay</li><li>Posterior teeth may be restored with silver amalgam</li><li>Anterior teeth usually are restored with naturally colored composite resins</li></ul>	
VI	<ul><li>Later added to G.V. Black's Classification of Cavities to account for caries that develop on occlusal cusps or incisal surfaces that have been worn away by abrasion</li><li>Restoration materials and methods depend on the site of caries</li></ul>	

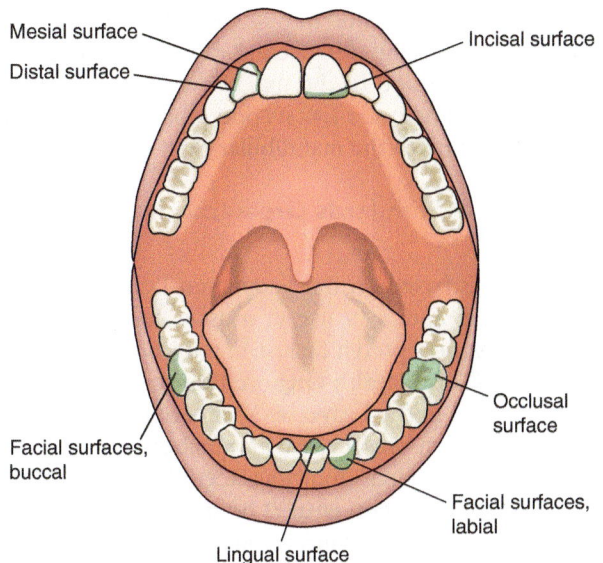

Figure 20–8 Five surfaces of the teeth.

Charting the Examination

Charting the clinical examination provides written documentation of the patient's oral and dental health in much the same way that intraoral photography and video provide a visual record. A variety of different charts are available, but each type will include an area for recording treatment and another area that includes a diagram of the teeth (Figure 20-9). The tooth diagram may show an anatomic depiction of the teeth, or it may use circles to represent the teeth (geometric chart). During the examination, existing conditions and recommended treatments are recorded in the chart. The use of numbering systems, key terms, designated color coding, and charting symbols standardizes charting across the dental profession. Dentists, specialists, DAs, and hygienists can all provide better continuity of care when each visit is recorded thoroughly and accurately.

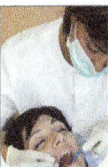

Voice of Experience

When I first started working as a dental assistant, I had a hard time listening to the dentist's comments and charting at the same time. I fell behind a few times and felt embarrassed and frustrated enough to want to do something about it. I decided to practice every chance I got, even as I relaxed after lunch and at home. I invented patients with all sorts of dental problems and restoration work and made up charts for each of them. A friend of mine from my dental assisting training program was feeling frustrated about her charting, too. We decided to practice together, and it really helped us both speed up and keep up with the dentist's comments and chart accurately and clearly.

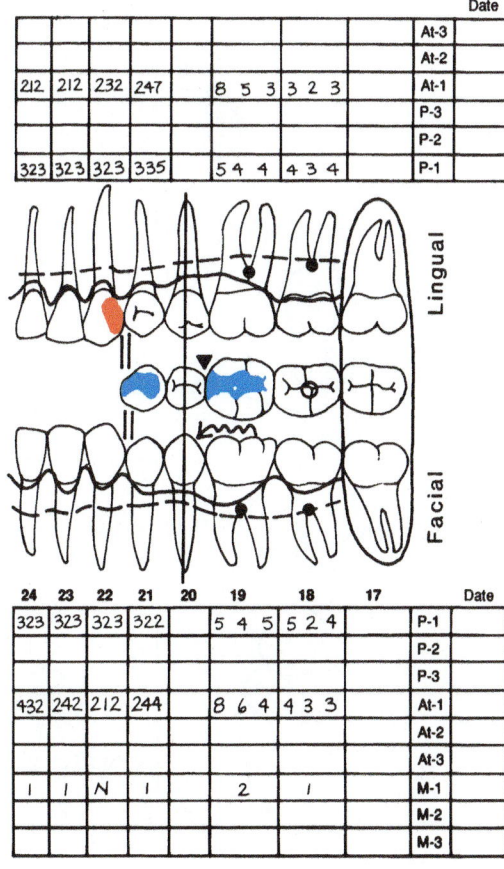

Key

Missing Tooth: | or X
Unerupted or impacted: Encircle tooth
Drift and Migration: 〰
Open Contact: ‖
Food Impaction: ↓ (at occlusal)

Periodental Chart
Gingival Margin: Black line
Mucogingival Junction: Dashed line
Furca involved: ● (in furcation)
Probing depths: (mm) P-1, P-2, P-3
Clinical attachment level: (mm) At-1, At-2, At-3

Dental Chart
Dental Caries: red
Restorations: blue
Defective Restoration: circle with red
Overhang: ▼ (at occlusal)
Mobility: (+, N, 1, 2, 3) M-1, M-2, M-3
Fremitus: F-1 (recorded on maxillary only)

Figure 20–9 Sample of an anatomic chart.

Tooth Numbering Systems

Tooth numbering systems identify individual teeth for charting and descriptive purposes. The main numbering system used on dental charts in the United States is the Universal Numbering System, which was approved by the American Dental Association (ADA) in 1968 and is still accepted by all U.S. insurance companies. Two other numbering systems are also in use: the International Standards Organization (ISO) System and the Palmer Notation System. As a professional DA, you need to be familiar with and capable of using all three systems.

Universal Numbering System

The Universal Numbering System of tooth notation was developed in 1882 by Julius Parreidt, a German dental surgeon. The ADA adopted the Universal system in 1968, and today it is used most commonly by dentists in the United States as well as the American Society of Forensic Odontology.

The Universal system numbers the permanent dentition 1 through 32 (Figure 20-10 and Table 20-2), starting with the right third molar (the patient's right) on the maxillary arch, continuing around to the maxillary left third molar (16), moving down to the left third molar of the mandibular arch, and finishing with the right mandibular third molar as 32. The notation for the primary dentition uses the first 20 letters of the alphabet, A through T. Like the

permanent dentition, numbering begins at the posterior of the maxillary right (the second molar in primary dentition), moves around to the maxillary left second molar, drops to the mandibular left second molar, and continues clockwise around to the mandibular right second molar.

International Standards Organization (ISO) System

This system is based on the Fédération Dentaire Internationale System and is in use in most other countries. In 1996, the ADA accepted it for use in the United States. Also in 1996, the World Health Organization accepted this system in addition to the Universal Numbering System.

The ISO System uses a two-digit number, each digit ranging from 1 to 8, to identify individual teeth (Figure 20-11). This system of tooth notation is used by dentists in most other countries. It is preferred in many countries because it is easily adapted in computerized systems. The first digit represents the dentition, arch, and quadrant on which a tooth is located:

1 = permanent dentition, maxillary right quadrant
2 = permanent dentition, maxillary left quadrant
3 = permanent dentition, mandibular left quadrant
4 = permanent dentition, mandibular right quadrant
5 = primary dentition, maxillary right quadrant
6 = primary dentition, maxillary left quadrant
7 = primary dentition, mandibular left quadrant
8 = primary dentition, mandibular right quadrant

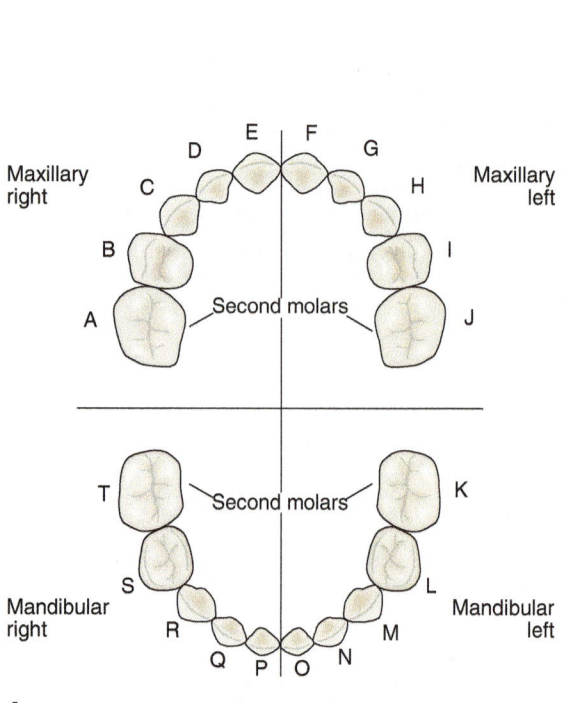

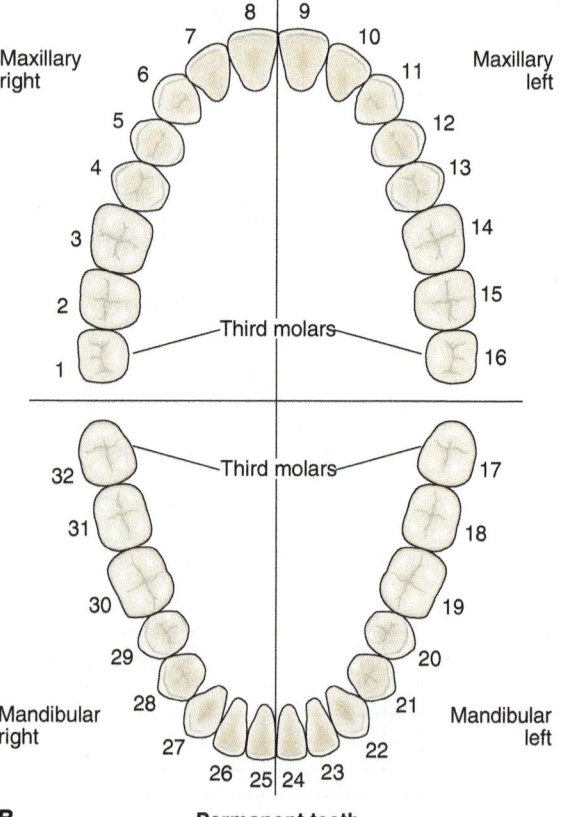

Figure 20–10 **The Universal Numbering System.** (**A**) Primary teeth. (**B**) Permanent teeth.

TABLE 20-2 Universal Notation for the Primary and Permanent Dentitions

	TOOTH	MAXILLARY ARCH		MANDIBULAR ARCH	
Right	Third molar	1	—	32	—
	Second molar	2	A	31	T
	First molar	3	B	30	S
	Second premolar	4	—	29	—
	First premolar	5	—	28	—
	Canine	6	C	27	R
	Lateral incisor	7	D	26	Q
	Central incisor	8	E	25	P
Left	Central incisor	9	F	24	O
	Lateral incisor	10	G	23	N
	Canine	11	H	22	M
	First premolar	12	—	21	—
	Second premolar	13	—	20	—
	First molar	14	I	19	L
	Second molar	15	J	18	K
	Third molar	16	—	17	—

The second digit indicates the tooth's distance from the midline, with 1 being closest (incisor) and 8 farthest (molar).

Numbering moves from the midline to the posterior teeth and, in the adult dentition, begins in the maxillary right quadrant, with the central incisor, tooth 11, and continues to the third molar, tooth 18. Numbering then moves to the maxillary left quadrant, with tooth 21; down to the mandibular left quadrant, beginning with tooth 31; finally ending with the mandibular right quadrant, and its third molar, tooth 48.

Numbering of the primary dentition is done in the same two-digit manner, moving from the midline to the posterior teeth. Numbering of the maxillary right quadrant begins with the central incisor, tooth 51 and continues to tooth 55. Numbering then moves to the maxillary left quadrant, then the mandibular left, ending in the mandibular right with tooth 85.

When ISO numbering is discussed aloud, the dentist and DA should pronounce the digits of the number separately, for example, tooth "five-three," not tooth "fifty-three."

Palmer Notation System

The Palmer Notation System is used in some dental offices in the United States, frequently in orthodontic offices, but its use has diminished significantly with the advent of personal computers, because the notation cannot be typed (for example, on insurance forms), making mistakes common during the recording process (Figure 20-12). Quadrants are represented by brackets, based on your perspective as you face the patient:

⌐ = upper right
L = upper left
⌐ = lower left
⌐ = lower right

Central incisors through third molars are numbered 1 through 8 in each quadrant. The Palmer system charts primary teeth in a similar manner, using letters A through E rather than numbers.

Tooth Surface Abbreviations

When caries or a restoration is noted on a patient's chart, abbreviations are used to indicate the affected surface of the tooth. Each surface—incisal, mesial, distal, buccal, lingual, occlusal, and facial—is abbreviated with a capital letter I, M, D, B, L, O, or F, respectively. For simple caries involving only one surface, a single capital letter is used.

If caries is compound or complex, however, letters are combined to indicate all the surfaces involved. If a mesial surface is involved, the letter M appears first in the abbreviation, followed by letters indicating the other involved surfaces. For example, a mesio-occluso-distal restoration or caries is abbreviated "MOD." This example also illustrates how

PERMANENT TEETH

Q-1
Maxillary right

Q-2
Maxillary left

18	17	16	15	14	13	12	11	21	22	23	24	25	26	27	28
48	47	46	45	44	43	42	41	31	32	33	34	35	36	37	38

Mandibular right
Q-4

Mandibular left
Q-3

PRIMARY TEETH

Q-5
Maxillary right

Q-6
Maxillary left

55	54	53	52	51	61	62	63	64	65
85	84	83	82	81	71	72	73	74	75

Mandibular right
Q-8

Mandibular left
Q-7

Figure 20–11 International Standards Organization (ISO) System.

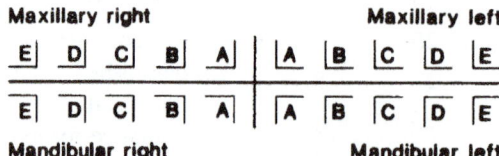

Figure 20–12 Palmer Notation System.

the letters "al" at the end of surface names are changed to the letter "o" when complex or compound caries or restoration is described. Table 20-3 matches surface names with abbreviations for simple, complex, and compound caries and restoration.

Key Charting Terms

Your ability to chart accurately and fully requires a thorough familiarity with the most common characteristics that patients exhibit upon examination. Table 20-4 lists some common charting terms.

TABLE 20-3 Surface Abbreviations

SIMPLE CARIES AND RESTORATIONS	
Incisal	I
Mesial	M
Distal	D
Buccal	B
Occlusal	O
Facial	F
Lingual	L
COMPOUND CARIES AND RESTORATIONS	
Occluso-buccal	OB
Mesio-occlusal	MO
Disto-occlusal	DO
Disto-incisal	DI
Disto-lingual	DL
Mesio-incisal	MI
Linguo-incisal	LI
COMPLEX RESTORATIONS	
Mesio-occluso-distal	MOD
Mesio-occluso-disto-bucco-lingual	MODBL

Symbols and Color Coding

Symbols and colors are marked on the tooth diagrams of the patient chart to indicate dental conditions at the time of examination as well as any recommended or already completed treatments. Symbols used include lines, crossed lines, wavy lines, circles, dots, and letters. Among the most commonly used symbols and abbreviations are those indicating restorations (see Figure 20-9).

Restoration Colors

- The color red indicates conditions that need to be corrected or restoration that is yet to be done.
- The color blue or black indicates work that has been completed.
- The color green may also be used to indicate decay found on a radiograph.

Restoration Symbols

Restorations needed or completed are charted as follows. Treatments needed are indicated in red, whereas treatments completed are indicated in blue.

- Amalgam restorations are represented by solid colors.
- Composite restorations are represented by an outline around the tooth.
- Gold restorations are represented by an outline and diagonal lines across the tooth.
- Porcelain restorations are represented by an outline around the tooth and a capital letter P.
- Stainless steel restorations are represented by wavy lines or by two capital letters S.
- Use of a sealant is represented by a capital letter S on the surface of the tooth where the sealant is placed.
- Implants are indicated by a written comment under the teeth involved.
- Root canals are charted in blue ink, represented by a vertical line through the pulpal area of the root and labeled "RC."
- Veneers are charted in blue ink, with the veneered surface of the tooth outlined and shaded in.

TABLE 20-4 Key Charting Terms

Abscess	An acute, localized infection
Abscess, periapical	An acute infection located at the tip of the root of a tooth
Abscess, periodontal	An acute infection located at the base of a periodontal pocket
Abutment	Existing teeth or implants used to support a partial denture or fixed bridge
Bridge	A permanently cemented dental prosthesis that replaces one or more natural teeth
Bridge, cantilever	A fixed bridge attached to only one abutment
Bridge, Maryland	A fixed bridge that replaces one tooth and is secured to the adjacent teeth with resin or metal-like wings that are cemented on the lingual surfaces of the adjacent teeth
Caries	Tooth decay
Caries, incipient	Beginning caries that has not broken through the enamel; appears as a chalky white area on the tooth indicating that the surface has begun to decalcify or lose calcium (You may be asked to note the word "watch" on such an area of a patient's chart, or use a series of red dots to indicate an area of incipient caries)
Caries, rampant	Widespread or spreading caries
Caries, recurrent	Caries under or near the margins of existing restorations
Crown	Restoration replacing a missing or damaged crown of a tooth; made of gold alloys, porcelain, stainless steel, or other materials
Denture	Removable dental prosthesis that replaces natural teeth in an arch
Denture, partial	Artificial teeth mounted on a removable metal framework; used when a patient's arch still contains natural teeth
Diastema	Space between two teeth in the same intraoral arch
Drifting	Movement of a tooth or teeth into a space created by the loss of an adjacent tooth
Furcation	The point where the roots of a multi-rooted tooth separate
Gold foil	A rarely used restoration that includes several layers of pure gold in the preparation
Impacted	Tooth that is wedged in place within the bone and/or gingiva and unable to erupt
Mobility	Tooth movement and instability caused by trauma or periodontal disease
Overhanging margin	Excess restorative material, such as amalgam or composite, found outside the margins of the restoration
Periodontal pocket	Sulcus depth greater than 3 mm
Pontic	Artificial tooth that replaces a missing natural tooth in a fixed bridge or removable denture
Recession	Reduction or decline in the height of the gingival tissue surrounding a tooth
Restoration	The use of dental materials, such as metal or porcelain, to restore teeth to full function
Root canal	A canal that runs through the roots of teeth and contains a living pulp made of blood vessels, lymph tissue, and nerves that provide the tooth with a sense of touch; also refers to a dental procedure that removes and replaces this pulp when it becomes diseased
Sealant	A resin made of enamel that seals pits and fissures to prevent caries
Supernumerary tooth	Extra tooth that erupts or becomes impacted in the bone
Supragingival	Describes something occurring above the gingival margin
Subgingival	Describes something occurring below the gingival margin
Sulcus	The space between the tooth and the gingiva where the two attach
Unerupted	Teeth still within the gingival tissues, not having erupted into the oral cavity
Veneer	Restorative or cosmetic covering for the facial surface of teeth; made from gold, porcelain, acrylic, or composite resin

- Missing teeth are represented by vertical lines or X's through all tooth surfaces.
- Impacted teeth are charted in red ink, with the facial, occlusal, and lingual surfaces of the tooth circled.
- Drifting or tilting teeth are indicated with blue arrows pointing in the direction of the drift or tilt.

Computerized or Automated Charting

Increasing numbers of dental practices are starting to use computerized or automated dental charting. Some use automated charting in addition to manual written charting, whereas others use computerized charting only. Computerized charting is easy to learn and use, increases efficiency, and helps standardize charting practices.

Some dental practices use voice-activated software capable of recognizing the dentist's voice and recording spoken information onto the computerized chart. Other systems enable the DA to use a keyboard or light pen to record information. Precautions are taken in the clinical area to prevent contamination of keyboards and light pens. Both are covered with special barriers when in use to avoid cross-contamination. Keyboards and light pens allow you to highlight and select symbols and color coding for use in the chart.

Procedure 20–1 **Charting of Teeth**

Materials needed (Figure P20-1-1):

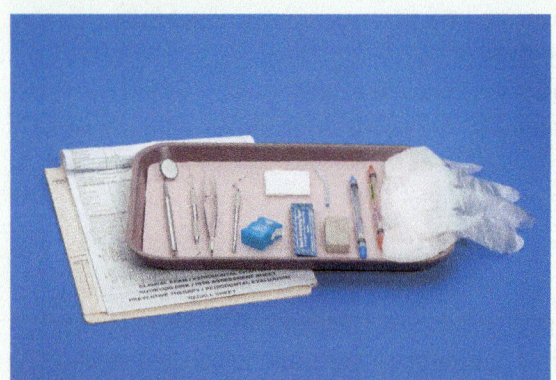

Figure P20-1-1

- Mouth mirror
- Explorer
- Cotton pliers
- Periodontal probe
- Gauze sponges/squares
- Dental floss
- Articulating paper and paper holder
- Air-water syringe and/or HVE
- Red and blue colored pencils
- Eraser
- Clean, unmarked clinical examination form clipped onto the patient chart
- Cover gloves
- Tongue depressor
- Pen

1. Put on appropriate personal protective equipment (PPE).
2. After the patient has been seated and draped with a napkin, position the patient in a supine position in the dental chair. This offers the dentist a better view of and easier access to the patient's entire intraoral cavity.

3. Upon request, transfer the explorer and mouth mirror to the dentist. The dentist uses these instruments to examine each surface of every tooth in the patient's oral cavity.
4. Record on the patient's chart the observations made as the dentist moves through the examination (Figure P20-1-2).

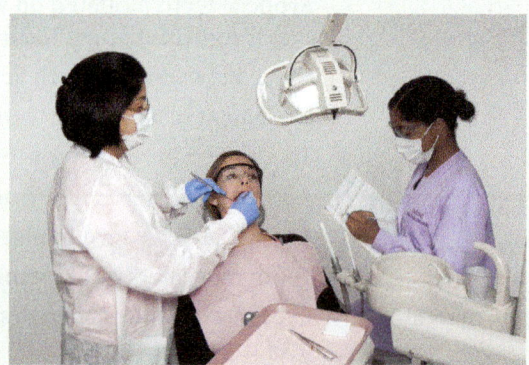

Figure P20-1-2

5. As the procedure progresses, ensure that the mouth mirror is clear, using the air syringe to clear it when necessary.
6. Adjust the operating light above the patient as necessary.
7. When the dentist is ready to examine the patient's occlusion or bite, prepare the articulating paper and holder. Ensure that the paper is positioned correctly in the holder for whichever quadrant of the patient's mouth will be examined first. The holder will be positioned against the cheek with the paper between the teeth.
8. Transfer the paper and holder to the dentist upon request. Any marks made by the paper will remain on the patient's occlusal and incisal surfaces, allowing the dentist to evaluate the patient's bite.
9. At the close of the charting procedure, rinse the patient's mouth with the air-water syringe and suction excess water with either the HVE or the saliva ejector.
10. Make sure all observations made during the examination are charted. Sign the chart.

Procedure 20–2 **Soft Tissue Examination**

Some states allow qualified DAs to complete the soft tissue examination. Otherwise, the examination may be performed by the hygienist or the dentist.

Materials needed (Figure P20-2-1):

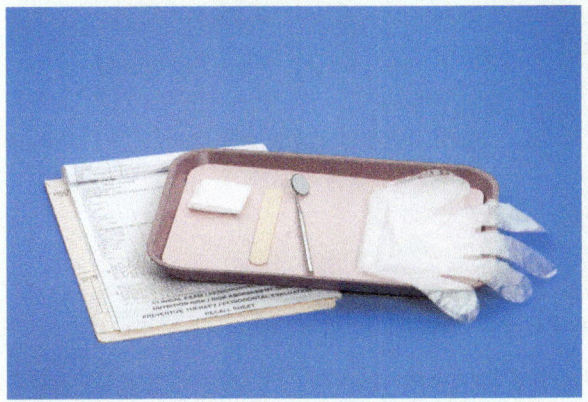

Figure P20-2-1

- Gauze sponges/squares, 2 × 2 and 4 × 4
- Tongue depressor
- Mouth mirror
- Clean, unmarked clinical examination form clipped onto the patient chart
- Cover gloves

Patient Preparation

1. Put on appropriate PPE.
2. Seat the patient comfortably in an upright position in the dental chair.
3. Drape a napkin around the patient's neck.
4. Explain the soft tissue examination to the patient confidently and clearly. A patient who is familiar with the procedure and knows what to expect is more likely to be cooperative and helpful during the examination.

Examination Process

1. Examine the face, neck, and ears for uneven features (asymmetry) or unusual swelling. Be especially alert for signs of scarring, skin discoloration or abrasion that may warrant further evaluation.
2. Examine the lips. Check for any signs of dryness or cracking. Observe the smile line, the contour of the lips when the patient smiles. Evaluate the color, continuity, and texture of the vermillion border. Examine the corners of the mouth for signs of dryness, lumps, or cracking. Do the same for the philtrum.
3. Finish by gently palpating the soft tissues of the face above and below the mandible. Below the mandible, note any abnormality in the submandibular or submental lymph nodes (Figure P20-2-2).
4. Document any findings in the patient's chart.

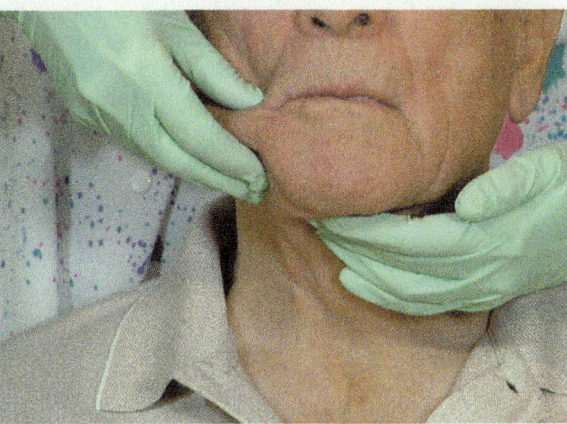

Figure P20-2-2

Examination of Cervical Lymph Nodes

1. Position yourself behind the seated patient. Make sure that you can easily reach the patient's ears.
2. Ask the patient to turn his or her head to the side.
3. To examine cervical lymph nodes on the right side of the neck, position your left hand on the patient's head to steady it. Use the thumb and fingers of your right hand to follow the chain of lymph nodes down the patient's neck from just below the ears to just above the clavicle (collarbone) (Figure P20-2-3). The purpose of your examination is to detect any tenderness, swelling, or abnormality in the nodes.

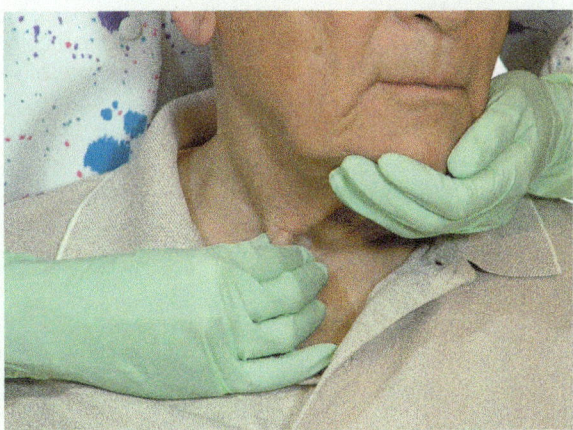

Figure P20-2-3

4. Steady the patient's head with your right hand and perform an identical examination of the lymph nodes on the left side of the neck.
5. Chart any abnormal findings and alert the dentist to them for possible referral.

Examination of the Temporomandibular Joint

1. Begin by asking the patient to open and close his or her mouth normally. Listen carefully for any accompanying noise, such as clicking, as the patient opens and closes the mouth.
2. Then ask the patient to move the lower jaw from side to side.

Procedure 20-2 Soft Tissue Examination (Continued)

3. Next, place your fingers just in front of the tragus of each ear and again ask the patient to open and close his or her mouth normally (Figure P20-2-4). Listen carefully for any accompanying noise, such as clicking, as the patient opens and closes the mouth. Feel for any "catching" as the patient opens the mouth.

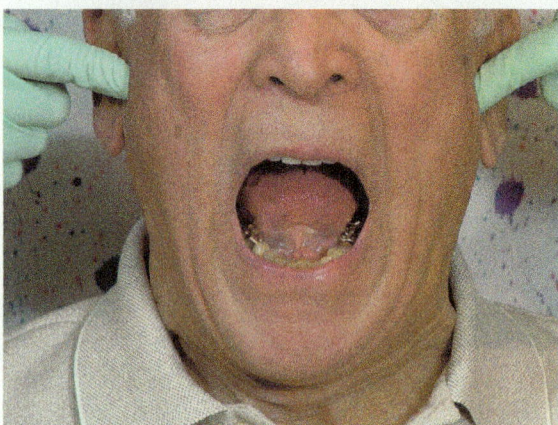

Figure P20-2-4

4. Ask the patient to describe any pain or tenderness.

5. At the end of the examination, examine the patient's teeth for signs of bruxism, such as unusual wear on the teeth.

6. Document your observations or any comments by the patient.

Soft Tissues of the Intraoral Cavity

1. Ask the patient to open his or her mouth completely. Look for any obvious signs of problems, such as lesions in the mouth, abscesses, or dramatic color changes in the oral mucosa.

2. Ask the patient to open the mouth slightly. Examine the interior of the lips by taking the upper lip between your fingers and thumb and gently turning it upward and outward to face you (Figure P20-2-5). Visually examine and gently palpate the mucosa to detect sores, lumps, abrasions, or other abnormalities. Examine the interior of the lower lip by turning it downward in the same manner.

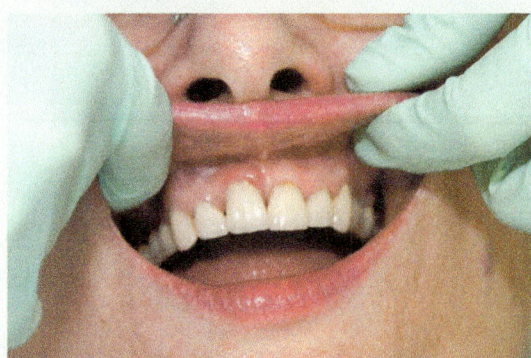

Figure P20-2-5

3. Examine the interior of each cheek by placing the thumb of one hand inside the mouth and the index and middle finger of the other hand on the outside of the cheek. Locate the opening of the Stensen salivary duct and observe the flow

of saliva from it (Figure P20-2-6). Examine the soft tissue covering the hard palate.

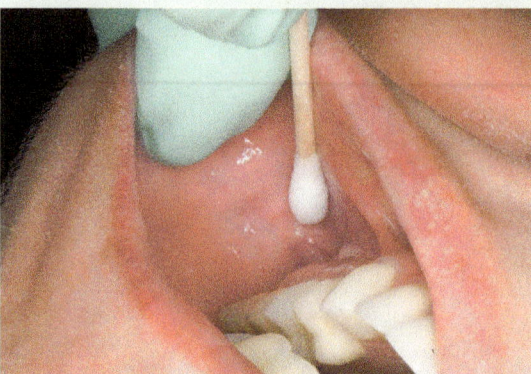

Figure P20-2-6

4. Request that the patient extend his or her tongue and relax it. Using a piece of sterile gauze, gently pull the tongue forward and visually examine all its surfaces (dorsal, lateral, and ventral) (Figure P20-2-7). Observe the tongue's color and note any unusual coatings or other abnormalities. Use a tongue depressor and mouth mirror to view the uvula, the back of the tongue, and the posterior area of the mouth (Figure P20-2-8). Request that the patient say "Ahh" during this portion of the examination to allow you to view the tissues of the oropharynx and ensure that there is no uvula deviation.

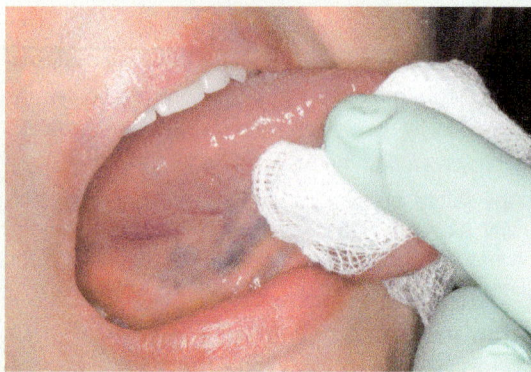

Figure P20-2-7

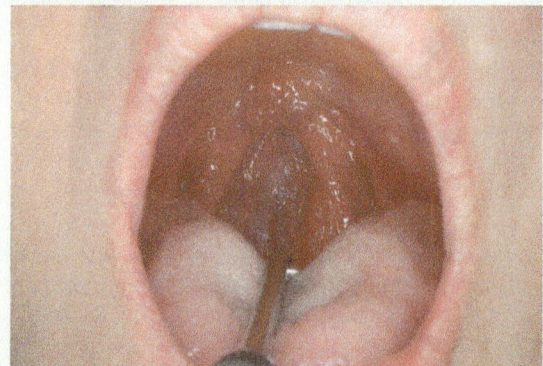

Figure P20-2-8

Procedure 20–2 Soft Tissue Examination (Continued)

5. Remove the tongue depressor and mirror and ask the patient to touch his or her tongue to the hard palate (Figure P20-2-9A). Visually examine the floor of the mouth and salivary ducts.

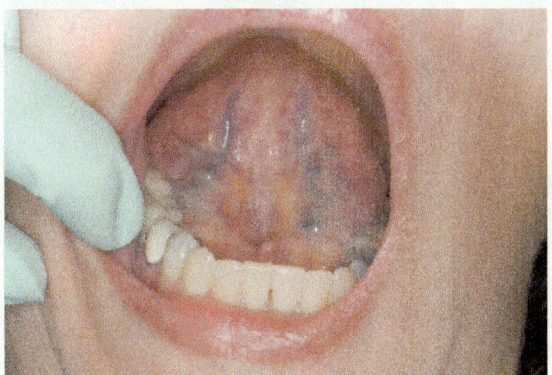

Figure P20-2-9A

Place the index finger of one hand on the floor of the mouth and the fingers of the other hand on the underside of the chin. Proceed to palpate gently (Figure P20-2-9B).

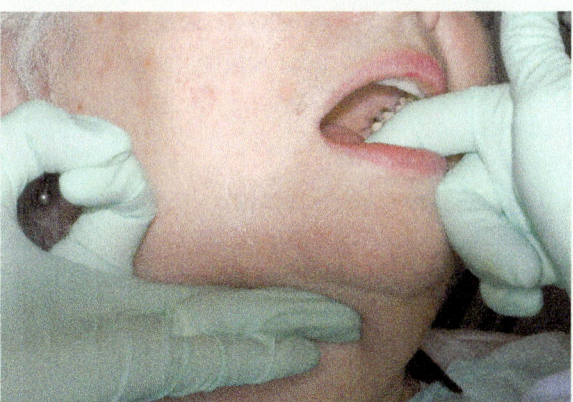

Figure P20-2-9B

Procedure 20–3 Examination and Charting of the Periodontium

Materials needed (Figure P20-3-1):

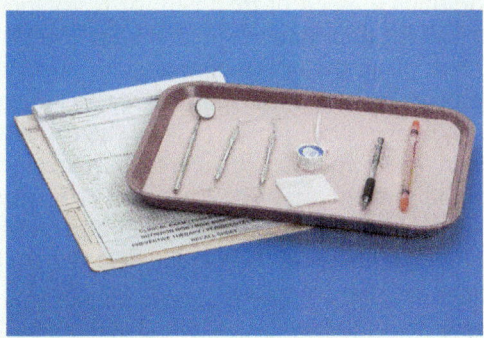

Figure P20-3-I

- Mouth mirror
- Periodontal probe
- Explorer
- Air-water syringe
- Dental floss
- Gauze sponges/squares (2 × 2)
- Black ink pen
- Red pencil
- Clean, unmarked clinical examination form clipped onto the patient's chart

1. Put on appropriate PPE.
2. The dentist or dental hygienist slides the periodontal probe between the tooth and gingiva and "walks" the

probe around the entire tooth in 1-mm steps, noting the deepest measurement for six areas around the tooth (Figure P20-3-2). Transfer instruments as needed and record in the patient's chart the comments and observations dictated by the dentist or dental hygienist.

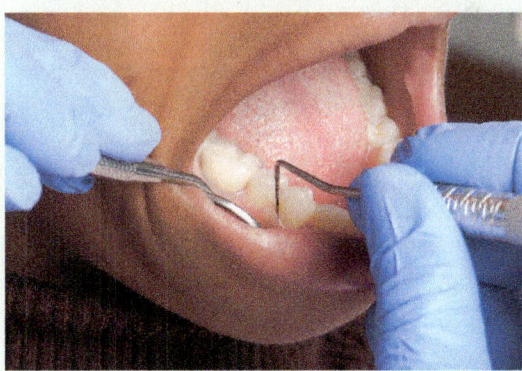

Figure P20-3-2

3. During examination of the periodontium the dentist will check for the following:
   - Overall health of the gingiva
   - Wear on the teeth including evidence of bruxism, or tooth grinding
   - Amount of accumulated plaque or calculus
   - Signs of tissue inflammation
   - Evidence of bleeding
   - Receding gingiva

Procedure 20-3 Examination and Charting of the Periodontium (Continued)

- Unattached gingiva
- Any periodontal pockets measuring more than 3 mm in depth
- Involvement of furcation in disease process
- The presence of exudate, or purulent material, indicating inflammation or infection
- Exposed roots
- Tooth stability
- The progress of any prior treatments for gingival disease

Transfer instruments as needed and record in the patient's chart the comments and observations dictated by the dentist (Figure P20-3-3).

4. In some cases, radiographs may be taken of the alveolar and supporting bone following the initial clinical examination. A patient whose periodontal health raises concerns may be referred to a periodontist, a dentist specializing in treatment of gingival diseases.

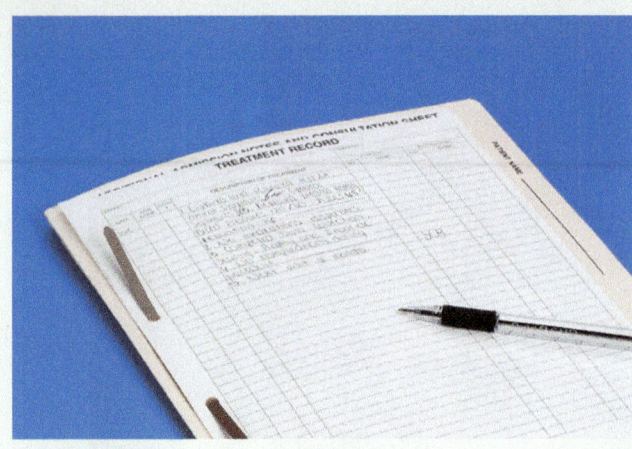

Figure P20-3-3

5. Make a note of the procedure in the patient's record and provide the patient with self-care instructions.

Extra Patient Care

The state where you practice may allow you to complete the soft tissue examination. The information this exam provides is very important to the patient's health and the early detection of any serious developing problems. Much of the exam is conducted using palpation or working with instruments deep within the intraoral cavity. Explain to the patient what you will be doing before you do it. This lets the patient know what to expect and help ease both of you through the exam. Don't rush through or handle the patient in a rushed manner. Not only may you miss something important, but the patient may be startled and move suddenly, upsetting both of you and interrupting the smooth flow of the exam.

CHECKPOINTS

20-4 Using the Universal Numbering System, which tooth is represented by the number 26? Which tooth is represented by the letter H?

20-5 The abbreviation "DO" indicates caries or restoration where?

20-6 The point where the roots of a multi-rooted tooth separate is called what?

20-7 What color in a dental chart indicates caries or other conditions needing treatment?

20-8 What do diagonal lines across a tooth represent in dental charting?

20-9 Marks from articulating paper remain where on the patient's teeth?

The Treatment Plan

A thorough clinical examination may reveal new or neglected conditions in need of treatment or restoration. Many dentists present their patients with a choice of one to three treatment plans: the optimum treatment plan, the standard treatment plan, and the emergency treatment plan. The most desirable plan may be beyond the patient's means. A second, less expensive, plan may be extensive but not as elaborate as the first. The least expensive plan is usually presented last. It normally consists of emergency treatment only. The dentist will thoroughly describe each plan's advantages and disadvantages.

Dentists many times present treatment plans in a private office or other comfortable room away from the clinical treatment area. Enough time is scheduled so that plans can be presented in their entirety and the patient does not feel rushed. You may be asked to prepare the diagnostic materials the dentist needs to have on hand for the discussion. In addition to the patient's chart, these may include

- Radiographs taken
- Casts of teeth needing restoration
- Before-and-after photographs of similar cases
- Models of proposed protheses, such as dentures, bridges, or implants
- Anatomic models of adult or primary dentition that can illustrate the conditions being discussed

After the treatment plan presentation is finished, the dentist or another member of the dental care team will discuss estimated fees and any available payment arrangements with the patient. Further discussion between the patient and the dental care team is encouraged in order to address any questions and concerns the patient may have. When a suitable plan has been selected and financial arrangements made, the patient is scheduled for treatment.

Extra Patient Care

Many treatment plans are complicated and involve a long series of treatments. Patients may need time to decide on a suitable plan for themselves. If you have patient education materials available, such as fact sheets, videos, booklets, or other items, share these with patients as soon as you realize they have questions or concerns. Some patients may have an easier time asking you questions about prospective procedures or treatments. Whenever possible, pass these questions or concerns along to the dentist. The more informed a patient is about upcoming procedures, the easier they will be to treat successfully.

Optimum Plan

An optimum plan restores as much function as possible and results in an appearance that is attractive and pleasing to the patient. Optimum treatment plans commonly include:

- Restorations, such as crowns, inlays, and onlays
- Aggressive treatment of periodontic conditions, such as periodontitis and gingivitis

- Straightening teeth with orthodontic treatments
- Treating diseased roots
- Replacing missing teeth with implants, dentures, or bridges

Standard Care

A standard treatment plan restores as much normal function as possible but is less elaborate than an optimum treatment plan. Standard care commonly includes:

- Restorations, such as amalgams and composites
- Treating diseased roots
- Conservative treatment of periodontic conditions
- Replacing missing teeth with removable protheses

Emergency Care

An emergency care plan relieves immediate discomfort and provides relief to the patient. When possible, emergency care will be followed with either standard or optimum care when the patient's means permit.

CHECKPOINT

20-10 What are the three different treatment plans many dentists present?

Chapter Highlights

- An important role of dental assistants is documenting the dentist's findings during clinical examinations. The findings in addition to plans for treatment and follow-up care are recorded on specially designed forms that go in the patient's record.
- A clinical examination consists of a visual examination of the head and neck area as well as an intraoral examination of the interior of the oral cavity. Typical instruments used during an intraoral examination include the mouth mirror, the explorer, and the periodontal probe.
- A radiographic examination involves the use of radiographs to assess intraoral development and detect abnormalities.
- An intraoral video examination uses a small camera to provide access to areas of the oral cavity that are otherwise difficult to view.
- Black's Classification of Cavities describes six different classes of caries and outlines restorative treatments for each type.
- Specific dental terminology is used to describe teeth according to their position in the oral cavity. Teeth can also be located according to quadrants or sextants in the oral cavity.

- The five distinct tooth surfaces are the facial, lingual, incisal/occlusal, mesial, and distal.
- Charting the clinical examination provides written documentation of the patient's oral and dental health. Existing conditions and recommended treatments are noted in the patient's chart using a standardized numbering system, key terms, designated color coding, and charting symbols.
- Standardized numbering systems are used to identify individual teeth for charting and descriptive purposes. The main numbering system used in the United States is the Universal Numbering System. Two other numbering systems are also in use: the International Standards Organization System and the Palmer Notation System.
- To document dental caries or restoration in a patient chart, abbreviations are used to indicate the affected surface of the tooth.
- Symbols and colors are marked on the tooth diagrams of the patient chart to indicate dental conditions at the time of examination as well as any recommended or already completed treatments.
- Computerized or automated dental charting is becoming increasingly popular.

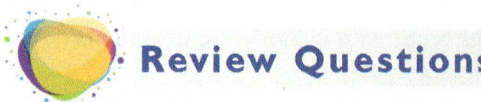

Review Questions

1. A periodontal probe is used to measure
   a. Enamel depth.
   b. Sulcus depth.
   c. Tooth height.
   d. Fluoride level.

2. The explorer detects abnormalities in the
   a. Gingiva.
   b. Sulcus.
   c. Enamel.
   d. Temporomandibular joint.

3. Which tooth surface faces the midline of the body?
   a. Mesial
   b. Distal
   c. Buccal
   d. Occlusal

4. Which class of Black's Classification of Cavities describes dental caries that develops on occlusal cusps or incisal surfaces that have been worn away by abrasion?
   a. Class I
   b. Class III
   c. Class IV
   d. Class VI

5. Caries occurring on two surfaces of a tooth is classified as
   a. Simple.
   b. Complex.
   c. Compound.
   d. Incipient.

6. Using the Universal Numbering System, the maxillary right canine would be numbered as tooth
   a. 3.
   b. 6.
   c. 9.
   d. 13.

7. Using the International Standards Organization System, the maxillary right canine would be numbered as tooth
   a. 3.
   b. 6.
   c. 9.
   d. 13.

8. Which type of caries might require a dental assistant to write the word "watch" across a tooth in a patient's chart?
   a. Rampant caries
   b. Recurrent caries
   c. Incipient caries
   d. Arrested caries

9. An artificial tooth that replaces a missing natural tooth in a fixed bridge or removable denture is
   a. A cantilever.
   b. An abutment.
   c. An implant.
   d. A pontic.

10. Abnormal swelling or tenderness of a patient's cervical lymph nodes could indicate
    a. Inflammation of the temporomandibular joint.
    b. Developing malignancy.
    c. Decreased calcium in the teeth.
    d. Chronic problems with the patient's occlusion or bite.

11. The dentist or dental hygienist slides the periodontal probe between the tooth and gingiva at
    a. Three points on the buccal surface and three points on the lingual surface.
    b. Three points on the distal surface and three points on the mesial surface.
    c. Three points on the facial surface only.
    d. Below each cusp of the molars.

Active Learning Exercises

1. Think of three clinical findings that may be recognized during a clinical examination with the use of digital palpation. How could these findings effect dental treatment or the patient's overall dental health?

2. G. V. Black identified five cavity classifications, with a sixth classification added years later. Draw a diagram of all six classifications and their locations on a tooth surface.

3. What are the three types of tooth numbering systems? Which is most popular in the United States? Which is most predominately used in other countries?

Application Activities

1. Create a set of flash cards to help you study the tooth surface abbreviations. Each card should have an abbreviation on one side and the name of the surface on the other. Use the cards to quiz yourself until you have all the surfaces memorized.

2. Create another set of flash cards to help you memorize the three tooth numbering systems. Each card should have the name of the tooth on one side and the three corresponding numbers used on the other side.

PREPARING FOR CERTIFICATION EXAMS

Review the following topics in this chapter to prepare for the Dental Assisting National Board (DANB) exam:

- **Clinical Examination**
- **Visual Examination**
- **Examination by Palpation**
- **Radiographic Examination**
- **Intraoral Video and Photography**
- **Classification of Cavities**
- **Further Classification of Cavities**
- **Names of Teeth**
- **The Five Surfaces of the Tooth**
- **Charting the Examination**
- **Tooth Numbering Systems**
- **Key Charting Terms**
- **Symbols & Color Coding**
- **Computerized or Automated Charting**
- **The Treatment Plan**

The Patient Record

CHAPTER OUTLINE

CHAPTER CHECKLIST

On completion of this chapter, students will be able to:

- ☑ Identify and describe the elements of a complete patient record.
- ☑ Explain the process of gathering patient information.
- ☑ Understand how to take a dental history.
- ☑ Understand how to take a medical history.

KEY TERMS

clinical examination form – generated during clinical examinations, this form records examination results, diagnoses, and treatments

dental chart – a graphical representation of the teeth that is included in the dental record; it includes areas for notations regarding exam results and lesions; alternatively, the term "dental chart" is sometimes used to refer to the entire dental record

dental history – a patient history of dental care and habits, medications, and lifestyle factors that might affect oral health

medical history – a patient history of medical care, including past conditions, diagnoses, and treatments; medications and substances; family history; and lifestyle factors that may affect health

Introduction

The patient record is the most important patient information maintained at the dental office. This collection of documents includes every piece of information necessary to track and treat a patient.

Because of the complexity of these documents—and legal and privacy issues—the patient record follows a standard format in terms of what information is collected and the way it is organized. A well-maintained patient record records all of the patient's interactions with the dental office, from visits to diagnosis to treatment and follow-up.

From Classroom to Clinic

The dentist relies on a competent dental assistant to help chart a patient's dental treatment plan as well as keep patient records. The skills and techniques you learned in the classroom will help you effectively and accurately perform these daily documentation tasks.

This chapter will discuss the patient record—what it includes, how it is maintained, and the laws that govern its use—as well as how to gather a patient history.

Elements of the Patient Record

A patient record is both a medical and a legal collection of documents and treatment tools. It is maintained by the dental office to keep track of the patient's oral health, including examination progress, test results, diagnosis, and treatments. It also contains legal forms, such as privacy and consent documents and registration forms. In the event that a patient's record is subpoenaed for a court case, any or all of these documents might be required.

The patient record has many uses:

- Records the patient's progress in treatment
- May be used in a lawsuit or settlement case involving the dental office
- May be used to identify an individual in a forensic case
- Used for information purposes by third parties, such as insurance companies or government agencies

The patient record includes any or all of the elements outlined in the following sections. Such elements are increasingly retained not only as hard (paper) copies, but also as digital files accessible via computer.

Patient Registration Form

The patient registration form is a basic information form that is usually kept near the beginning of the record. It includes personal information about the patient, such as demographic information, address, phone number, employer address and phone, date of birth, spousal information, and emergency contact information. The registration form also includes the patient's insurance information, including the name of the insurer and payment information. Many practices require that a copy of the insurance card be attached to the registration form or included in the record for verification. Finally, the patient's signature is required.

Dental History Form

The **dental history** is obtained from the patient at the beginning of their treatment (Figure 21-1). If the dental office already has a completed dental history form, the patient should be given the opportunity to update the form with new information. This should happen with *every new visit*, no matter how closely visits occur. Patients might not be aware of the ramifications of changes in their medications and diet and may not bring them up unless directly asked, "Has anything changed medically since your last visit? Please update your history."

For a more detailed discussion of the dental history, please see the Patient History section later in this chapter.

Medical History Form

The **medical history** contains a record of the patient's past and present medical conditions, including any chronic diseases as well as treatments and medications the patient may be taking (Figure 21-2). It also includes a family medical history. It is essential to have an updated medical history for the following reasons:

- Many chronic diseases, such as diabetes and allergies, can potentially complicate or alter the treatment plan because they affect oral health.
- Medications can affect oral health and may pose the risk of drug interactions with medications used in the dental office.
- In the event of an emergency, the dentist might need to refer to the medical history for information and guidance.

Like a dental history, the medical history should be updated every time the patient visits the office, no matter how recently the previous visit was. Any change in health status can affect oral health and/or a potential treatment plan, even if the patient is not aware of it.

For a more detailed discussion of the medical history, see the Medical History section later in the chapter.

Clinical Examination Form

The **clinical examination form** is the most complicated portion of the patient record. This form includes detailed information from the clinical examination, including

Dental Health Questionnaire

Patient _DONNA D. DOI_ Date _1/30/XX_

Clinician _THALIA JONES_

REASON FOR TODAY'S VISIT - CHIEF COMPLAINT

What is the main reason for your visit today?

CHECK UP

BLEEDING GUMS

How did you hear about our practice? _YELLOW PAGES_

Referred by: _RECENTLY MOVED TO TOWN_

PREVIOUS DENTAL TREATMENT

Have you seen another dentist within the last year? _YES_

When was your last dental visit? _6 MONTHS AGO_

Reason for the above visit? _CHECK UP_

Name of previous dentist? _DR. GLASSCOE ALPINE, COLORADO_

Have you had x-rays of your teeth taken recently? ☒Yes ☐No

TELL US ABOUT YOUR PREVIOUS DENTAL EXPERIENCES

Have your previous dental visits been favorable/comfortable emotionally? ☒Yes ☐No

If no, please explain: _____

In general, do you feel positive about your previous dental treatment? ☒Yes ☐No

If no, please explain: _____

Have you ever had an adverse reaction to dental treatment? ☐Yes ☒No

If yes, please explain: _____

Have you ever had any allergic reactions associated with dental treatment? ☐Yes ☒No

If yes, please explain: _____

Have you ever had difficulty with local anesthetic injections? ☐Yes ☒No

If yes, please explain: _____

Other dental experiences we should know about? _____

TELL US ABOUT ANY DENTAL CONCERNS YOU MAY HAVE

Are you satisfied with your teeth and their appearance? ☐Yes ☒No

If no, please explain: _____

Are you interested in having your teeth a lighter color? ☐Yes ☒No

If yes, please explain: _____

Are you interested in any specific type of dental treatment at this time?
☐ Implants
☐ Cosmetic dentistry
☐ Replacing missing teeth
☐ Dentures
☐ Replacing old fillings
☐ Other _____

A lot can be done to prevent dental diseases (teeth and gum disease). Would you like to know more about preventing dental disease for yourself or your family? ☒Yes ☐No

If yes, please explain: _GUMS BLEED_

Figure 21–1 Sample dental health form.

Dental Health Questionnaire (cont)

EXISTING DENTAL NEEDS/CONDITIONS

Please indicate with a check if you have had or have any of the following:

☐ Sensitive teeth
    ☐ Hot
    ☐ Cold
    ☐ Sweet
    ☐ Pressure
☐ Broken teeth or fillings
☐ Joint pain or popping or clicking of jaw
☐ Gum boils or other infections
☒ Swollen/painful or bleeding gums
☐ Gum recession
☐ Periodontal treatments (gum)
☐ Frequent filling replacement
☐ Discolored teeth
☐ Crooked teeth
☐ Orthodontic treatment (braces)
☐ Injury to the face, jaws, teeth
☐ Root canal therapy

☐ Removal of teeth
☐ Sores or growths
☐ Dry mouth
☐ Pain upon swallowing
☐ Grinding or clenching teeth
☐ Persistent headaches, ear aches, or muscle pain
☐ Bad breath, or bad taste in mouth
☐ Food catches between teeth when you eat
☐ Loose teeth
☐ Denture or partial denture
☐ Your bite is changing
☐ Problems chewing
☐ Sore jaws upon awakening. How frequently:_____
    Do you prefer to breathe through your
        ☐ nose or ☐ mouth?
☐ Abnormal swallowing habit - tongue thrusting
☐ Biting your lip or cheek frequently

DAILY SELF-CARE ACTIVITIES

Do you feel your present daily self-care ☐ Yes ☒ No
is effective in cleaning your mouth?

If no, please explain *MUST NOT BE,*
GUMS BLEED

On a daily basis, how many times do you brush your
teeth? (please circle)

Brush only   0   1   ②   3   4+
Floss only   0   ①   2+
Brush and floss   0   1   2   3+

☐ Do not routinely brush or floss on a daily basis

What type of toothbrush do you use?
☐ Hard
☐ Medium
☒ Soft
☐ Don't know

Do you use any other dental aids on a regular basis?
☐ Bridge cleaners
☒ Stimudents
☐ Rubber tip
☐ Proxabrush
☐ Other_____

DIETARY ACTIVITIES

Please circle:

How many caffeinated beverages do you drink daily?
   0   1   ②   3   4+   less than 2-3/week
How many alcoholic beverages do you drink daily?
   ⓪   1   2   3   4+   less than 2-3/week
How many sugar-containing sodas do you drink daily?
   ⓪   1   2   3   4+   less than 2-3/week
How many "diet" sodas do you drink daily?
   0   ①   2   3   4+   less than 2-3/week
How many "sport/energy" beverages do you drink daily?
   ⓪   1   2   3   4+   less than 2-3/week

How many candy bars or energy/power bars do you
eat daily?
   0   1   2   3   4+   (less than 2-3/week)

Do you regularly eat hard candies or breath mints?
☐ Yes   ☒ No   ☐ Occasionally
Do you regularly use tobacco products?
☐ Yes   ☒ No   ☐ Occasionally
Do you use recreational/street drugs?
☐ Yes   ☒ No   ☐ Occasionally

Signature of Patient ___*Donna Doi*___   Date ___*1/30/XX*___

Reviewed by ___*Thalia Jones*___   Date ___*1/30/XX*___

Figure 21–1 *(Continued).*

ADA. American Dental Association
www.ada.org

Medical Alert:	Condition:	Premedication:	Allergies:	Anesthesia:	Date:

HEALTH HISTORY FORM

Name: DOI   DONNA   D.   Home Phone: (828) SSS-4211   Business Phone: (828) SSS-8716
       LAST   FIRST   MIDDLE

Address: 1401 SPRINGFIELD ST.   City: ARDEN   State: NC   Zip Code: 28711
     P.O. BOX or Mailing Address

Occupation: HIGH SCHOOL TEACHER   Height: 5'5"   Weight: 127   Date of Birth: 27 YRS   Sex: M   F **X**

SS#: 111-11-1111   Emergency Contact: DENNIS DORI   Relationship: HUSBAND   Phone: (828) SSS-2627

If you are completing this form for another person, what is your relationship to that person? _____
                                                    NAME   RELATIONSHIP

For the following questions, please (X) whichever applies, your answers are for our records only and will be kept confidential in accordance with applicable laws. Please note that during your initial visit you will be asked some questions about your responses to this questionnaire and there may be additional questions concerning your health. This information is vital to allow us to provide appropriate care for you. This office does not use this information to discriminate.

DENTAL INFORMATION

	Yes	No	Don't Know
Do your gums bleed when you brush?	X		
Have you ever had orthodontic (braces) treatment?	X		
Are your teeth sensitive to cold, hot, sweets or pressure?		X	
Do you have earaches or neck pains?		X	
Have you had any periodontal (gum) treatments?		X	
Do you wear removable dental appliances?		X	
Have you had a serious/difficult problem associated with any previous dental treatment?		X	

If yes, explain:

How would you describe your current dental problem? CHECK-UP

Date of your last dental exam: 6 MONTHS

Date of last dental x-rays: 1 YEAR

What was done at that time? CHECK-UP

How do you feel about the appearance of your teeth? OK

MEDICAL INFORMATION

If you answer yes to any of the 3 items below, please stop and return this form to the receptionist.

Have you had any of the following diseases or problems?

	Yes	No	Don't Know
Active Tuberculosis		X	
Persistent cough greater than a 3 week duration		X	
Cough that produces blood		X	
Are you in good health?	X		
Has there been any change in your general health within the past year?		X	
Are you now under the care of a physician?	X		

If yes, what is/are the condition(s) being treated?
PREGNANT

Date of last physical examination: LAST WEEK

Physician: DR. M.C. NEWCOMB (828) SSS-2147
NAME   PHONE
540 MARKET ST.   ASHVILLE 28801
ADDRESS   CITY/STATE   ZIP

NAME   PHONE

ADDRESS   CITY/STATE   ZIP

| Have you had any serious illness, operation, or been hospitalized in the past 5 years? | X | | |

If yes, what was the illness or problem?
BROKEN LEG - KNEE REPLACEMENT

	Yes	No	Don't Know
Are you taking or have you recently taken any medicine(s) including non-prescription medicine?	X		

If yes, what medicine(s) are you taking?

Prescribed: SEE LIST

Over the counter:

Vitamins, natural or herbal preparations and/or diet supplements:

	Yes	No	Don't Know
Are you taking, or have you taken, any diet drugs such Pondimin (fenfluramine), Redux (dexphenfluramine) or phen-fen (fenfluramine-phentermine combination)?		X	
Do you drink alcoholic beverages?		X	

If yes, how much alcohol did you drink in the last 24 hours?
In the past week?

	Yes	No	Don't Know
Are you alcohol and/or drug dependent?		X	

If yes, have you received treatment? (circle one) Yes / No

	Yes	No	Don't Know
Do you use drugs or other substances for recreational purposes?		X	

If yes, please list:
Frequency of use (daily, weekly, etc.):
Number of years of recreational drug use:

	Yes	No	Don't Know
Do you use tobacco (smoking, snuff, chew)?		X	

If yes, how interested are you in stopping?
(circle one) Very / Somewhat / Not interested

	Yes	No	Don't Know
Do you wear contact lenses?	X		

PLEASE COMPLETE BOTH SIDES

Figure 21-2 Sample medical health form.

Are you allergic to or have you had a reaction to?

	Yes	No	Don't Know
Local anesthetics	☐	☒	☐
Aspirin	☒	☐	☐
Penicillin or other antibiotics	☐	☒	☐
Barbiturates, sedatives, or sleeping pills	☐	☒	☐
Sulfa drugs	☐	☒	☐
Codeine or other narcotics	☐	☒	☐
Latex	☐	☒	☐
Iodine	☐	☒	☐
Hay fever/seasonal	☒	☐	☐
Animals	☐	☒	☐
Food (specify)	☐	☒	☐
Other (specify) _CATS_	☒	☐	☐
Metals (specify)	☐	☒	☐

To yes responses, specify type of reaction.
SNEEZING, WATERY EYES

Have you had an orthopedic total joint (hip, knee, elbow, finger) replacement? ☒ Yes ☐ No ☐ Don't Know
If yes, when was this operation done? _3 YEARS AGO_

If you answered yes to the above question, have you had any complications or difficulties with your prosthetic joint? _NO_

Has a physician or previous dentist recommended that you take antibiotics prior to your dental treatment? ☐ Yes ☒ No ☐ Don't Know
If yes, what antibiotic and dose?
Name of physician or dentist*:
Phone:

WOMEN ONLY

Are you or could you be pregnant? _5 MONTHS_ ☒ ☐ ☐
Nursing? ☐ ☒ ☐
Taking birth control pills or hormonal replacement? ☐ ☒ ☐

Please (X) a response to indicate if you have or have not had any of the following diseases or problems.

	Yes	No	Don't Know
Abnormal bleeding	☐	☒	☐
AIDS or HIV infection	☐	☒	☐
Anemia	☐	☒	☐
Arthritis	☐	☒	☐
Rheumatoid arthritis	☐	☒	☐
Asthma	☐	☒	☐
Blood transfusion. If yes, date:	☐	☒	☐
Cancer/Chemotherapy/Radiation Treatment	☐	☒	☐
Cardiovascular disease. If yes, specify below:	☐	☒	☐

____ Angina ____ Heart murmur
____ Arteriosclerosis ____ High blood pressure
____ Artificial heart valves ____ Low blood pressure
____ Congenital heart defects ____ Mitral valve prolapse
____ Congestive heart failure ____ Pacemaker
____ Coronary artery disease ____ Rheumatic heart
____ Damaged heart valves disease/Rheumatic fever
____ Heart attack

	Yes	No	Don't Know
Chest pain upon exertion	☐	☒	☐
Chronic pain	☐	☒	☐
Disease, drug, or radiation-induced immunosurpression	☐	☒	☐
Diabetes. If yes, specify below:	☐	☒	☐

____ Type I (Insulin dependent) ____ Type II

	Yes	No	Don't Know
Dry Mouth	☐	☒	☐
Eating disorder. If yes, specify:	☐	☒	☐
Epilepsy	☐	☒	☐
Fainting spells or seizures	☐	☒	☐
Gastrointestinal disease	☐	☒	☐
G.E. Reflux/persistent heartburn _DURING PREGNANCY_	☒	☐	☐
Glaucoma	☐	☒	☐

	Yes	No	Don't Know
Hemophilia	☐	☒	☐
Hepatitis, jaundice or liver disease	☐	☒	☐
Recurrent Infections	☐	☒	☐
If yes, indicate type of infection:			
Kidney problems	☐	☒	☐
Mental health disorders. If yes, specify:	☐	☒	☐
Malnutrition	☐	☒	☐
Night sweats	☐	☒	☐
Neurological disorders. If yes, specify:	☐	☒	☐
Osteoporosis	☐	☒	☐
Persistent swollen glands in neck			
Respiratory problems. If yes, specify below:	☐	☒	☐

____ Emphysema ____ Bronchitis, etc.

	Yes	No	Don't Know
Severe headaches/migraines	☒	☐	☐
Severe or rapid weight loss	☐	☒	☐
Sexually transmitted disease	☐	☒	☐
Sinus trouble	☒	☐	☐
Sleep disorder	☐	☒	☐
Sores or ulcers in the mouth	☐	☒	☐
Stroke	☐	☒	☐
Systemic lupus erythematosus	☐	☒	☐
Tuberculosis	☐	☒	☐
Thyroid problems	☐	☒	☐
Ulcers	☐	☒	☐
Excessive urination	☐	☒	☐

Do you have any disease, condition, or problem not listed above that you think I should know about? ☐ ☒ ☐
Please explain:

NOTE: Both Doctor and patient are encouraged to discuss any and all relevant patient health issues prior to treatment.

I certify that I have read and understand the above. I acknowledge that my questions, if any, about inquiries set forth above have been answered to my satisfaction. I will not hold my dentist, or any other member of his/her staff, responsible for any action they take or do not take because of errors or omissions that I may have made in the completion of this form.

Donna Doe   _1/30/XX_
SIGNATURE OF PATIENT/LEGAL GUARDIAN   DATE

FOR COMPLETION BY DENTIST

Comments on patient interview concerning health history:

Significant findings from questionnaire or oral interview:

Dental management considerations:

Health History Update: On a regular basis the patient should be questioned about any medical history changes, date and comments notated, along with signature.

Date	Comments	Signature of patient and dentist

Figure 21–2 (*Continued*)

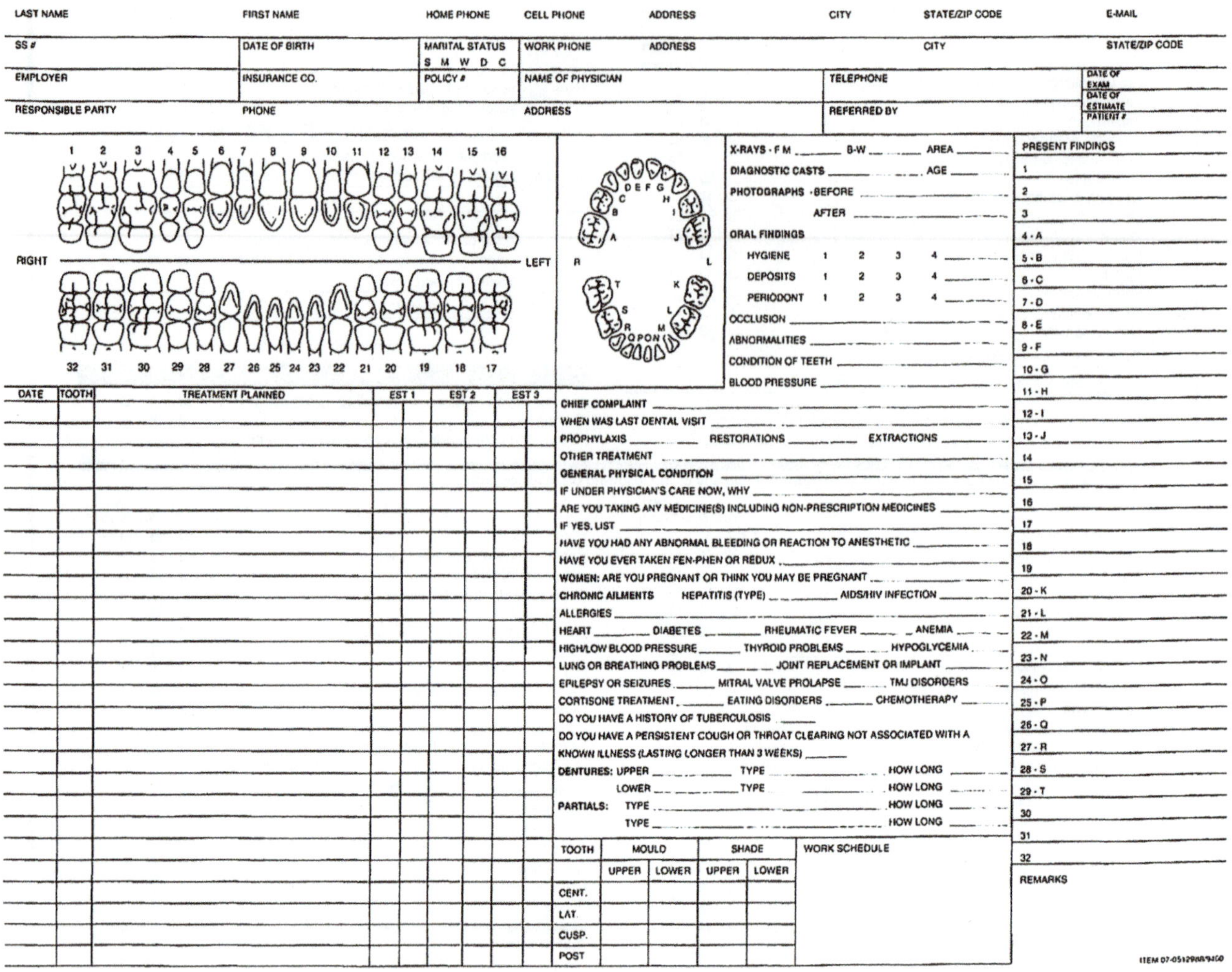

LAST NAME | FIRST NAME | HOME PHONE | CELL PHONE | ADDRESS | CITY | STATE/ZIP CODE | E-MAIL

SS # | DATE OF BIRTH | MARITAL STATUS S M W D C | WORK PHONE | ADDRESS | CITY | STATE/ZIP CODE

EMPLOYER | INSURANCE CO. | POLICY # | NAME OF PHYSICIAN | TELEPHONE | DATE OF EXAM | DATE OF ESTIMATE

RESPONSIBLE PARTY | PHONE | ADDRESS | REFERRED BY | PATIENT #

1 2 3 4 5 6 7 8 9 10 11 12 13 14 15 16

RIGHT LEFT

32 31 30 29 28 27 26 25 24 23 22 21 20 19 18 17

R L

A B C D E F G H I J

T S R Q P O N M L K

X-RAYS - F M ____ B-W ____ AREA ____

DIAGNOSTIC CASTS ____ AGE ____

PHOTOGRAPHS - BEFORE ____

AFTER ____

ORAL FINDINGS

HYGIENE 1 2 3 4

DEPOSITS 1 2 3 4

PERIODONT 1 2 3 4

OCCLUSION ____

ABNORMALITIES ____

CONDITION OF TEETH ____

BLOOD PRESSURE ____

PRESENT FINDINGS

1, 2, 3, 4 - A, 5 - B, 6 - C, 7 - D, 8 - E, 9 - F, 10 - G, 11 - H, 12 - I, 13 - J, 14, 15, 16, 17, 18, 19, 20 - K, 21 - L, 22 - M, 23 - N, 24 - O, 25 - P, 26 - Q, 27 - R, 28 - S, 29 - T, 30, 31, 32

REMARKS

DATE	TOOTH	TREATMENT PLANNED	EST 1	EST 2	EST 3

CHIEF COMPLAINT ____

WHEN WAS LAST DENTAL VISIT ____

PROPHYLAXIS ____ RESTORATIONS ____ EXTRACTIONS ____

OTHER TREATMENT ____

GENERAL PHYSICAL CONDITION ____

IF UNDER PHYSICIAN'S CARE NOW, WHY ____

ARE YOU TAKING ANY MEDICINE(S) INCLUDING NON-PRESCRIPTION MEDICINES ____

IF YES, LIST ____

HAVE YOU HAD ANY ABNORMAL BLEEDING OR REACTION TO ANESTHETIC ____

HAVE YOU EVER TAKEN FEN-PHEN OR REDUX ____

WOMEN: ARE YOU PREGNANT OR THINK YOU MAY BE PREGNANT ____

CHRONIC AILMENTS HEPATITIS (TYPE) ____ AIDS/HIV INFECTION ____

ALLERGIES ____

HEART ____ DIABETES ____ RHEUMATIC FEVER ____ ANEMIA ____

HIGH/LOW BLOOD PRESSURE ____ THYROID PROBLEMS ____ HYPOGLYCEMIA ____

LUNG OR BREATHING PROBLEMS ____ JOINT REPLACEMENT OR IMPLANT ____

EPILEPSY OR SEIZURES ____ MITRAL VALVE PROLAPSE ____ TMJ DISORDERS ____

CORTISONE TREATMENT ____ EATING DISORDERS ____ CHEMOTHERAPY ____

DO YOU HAVE A HISTORY OF TUBERCULOSIS ____

DO YOU HAVE A PERSISTENT COUGH OR THROAT CLEARING NOT ASSOCIATED WITH A KNOWN ILLNESS (LASTING LONGER THAN 3 WEEKS) ____

DENTURES: UPPER ____ TYPE ____ HOW LONG ____

LOWER ____ TYPE ____ HOW LONG ____

PARTIALS: TYPE ____ HOW LONG ____

TYPE ____ HOW LONG ____

TOOTH	MOULD		SHADE		WORK SCHEDULE
	UPPER	LOWER	UPPER	LOWER	
CENT.					
LAT.					
CUSP.					
POST					

ITEM 07-0512988/9460

Figure 21–3 Sample dental chart.

charting (see below), the patient's chief complaint, the results of evaluations, and comments from the dentist. Data for this form is typically dictated by the dentist during the clinical examination, and the dental assistant (DA) makes the proper notations on the form.

A **dental chart** is typically part of the clinical examination form (Figure 21-3). It is a numbered diagram that depicts the teeth and includes notations about oral conditions and the proposed treatments. Standardized symbols and abbreviations are used to represent various conditions and treatments on the chart. Dental charting is covered in greater depth in Chapter 20, Oral Diagnosis and Treatment Planning.

Consent Forms

Most dental offices have new patients sign blanket consent forms to give their consent for dental exams and treatment (Figure 21-4). These forms often also include consent for radiography. For a more extensive treatment, a separate consent form may be required. In this case, the dentist might sit with the patient and explain the proposed treatment, including its risk and benefits. All consent forms require the patient's signature to be valid; they are also often witnessed by the DA and signed by the dentist as well.

Privacy Form

Dental practices are required to have a written privacy policy that is in compliance with the Health Insurance Portability and Accountability Act, or HIPAA. The patient record must include a signed form of acknowledgment that the patient received and understands the privacy policy (Figure 21-5). HIPAA was created in 1996 to protect sensitive medical information and guarantee that patients have access to their own medical records. The law stipulates which types of information are considered privileged medical information and the conditions under which sharing this information is allowed. For example, it is acceptable to share patient treatment information to an insurance company for payment without obtaining prior patient consent. For a closer look at HIPAA, see Chapter 4, Ethics and Law.

NORTH SHORE DENTAL ASSOCIATES

DENTAL TREATMENT CONSENT FORM

Patient Name_____

Please read and initial the items checked below
and read and sign the section at the bottom of form.

☐_____**1. WORK TO BE DONE**
I understand that I am having the following work done: Fillings_____ Bridges_____ Crowns_____
Extractions_____ Impacted teeth removed_____ General Anesthesia_____ Root Canals_____
Other_____

☐_____**2. DRUGS AND MEDICATIONS**
I understand that antibiotics and analgesics and other medications can cause allergic reactions causing redness and
swelling of tissues, pain, itching, vomiting, and/or anaphylactic shock (severe allergic reaction.)

☐_____**3. CHANGES IN TREATMENT PLAN**
I understand that during treatment it may be necessary to change or add procedures because of conditions found while
working on the teeth that were not discovered during examination, the most common being root canal therapy following
routine restorative procedures. I give my permission to the dentist to make any/all changes and additions as necessary.

☐_____**4. REMOVAL OF TEETH**
Alternatives to removal have been explained to me (root canal therapy, crowns, and periodontal surgery, etc.) and I
authorize the Dentist to remove the following teeth_____ and any others necessary for reasons in
paragraph #3. I understand removing teeth does not always remove all the infection, if present, and it may be
necessary to have further treatment. I understand the risks involved in having teeth removed, some of which are pain,
swelling, spread of infection, dry socket, loss of feeling in my teeth, lips, tongue and surrounding tissue (paresthesia)

Figure 21–4 Sample consent form.

NORTH SHORE DENTAL ASSOCIATES

NOTICE OF PRIVACY PRACTICES

THIS NOTICE DESCRIBES HOW HEALTH INFORMATION ABOUT YOU MAY BE USED AND DISCLOSED AND HOW
YOU CAN GET ACCESS TO THIS INFORMATION. PLEASE REVIEW IT CAREFULLY. THE PRIVACY OF YOUR
HEALTH INFORMATION IS IMPORTANT TO US.

OUR LEGAL DUTY
We are required by applicable federal and state law to maintain the privacy of your health information. We are also
required to give you this Notice about our privacy practices, our legal duties, and your rights concerning your health
information. We must follow the privacy practices that are described in this Notice while it is in effect. This Notice takes
effect (09/30/10), and will remain in effect until we replace it.
We reserve the right to change our privacy practices and the terms of this Notice at any time, provided such changes are
permitted by applicable law. We reserve the right to make the changes in our privacy practices and the new terms of our
Notice effective for all health information that we maintain, including health information we created or received before we
made the changes. Before we make a significant change in our privacy practices, we will change this Notice and make
the new Notice available upon request.
You may request a copy of our Notice at any time. For more information about our privacy practices, or for additional
copies of this Notice, please contact us using the information listed at the end of this Notice.

USES AND DISCLOSURES OF HEALTH INFORMATION
We use and disclose health information about you for treatment, payment, and healthcare operations. For example:

Treatment: We may use or disclose your health information to a physician or other healthcare provider providing
treatment to you.

Figure 21–5 Sample privacy form.

Patient Correspondence

Any letters between the patient and the dental office should be included in the patient record. This includes emails, photos, and any other communication that might be pertinent to a patient's dental treatment. Phone calls should also be entered in the chart along with a brief description of what was discussed.

Radiographs

Radiographs are an important part of the dental record. All patient radiographs should be safely stored, including exposed films stored in envelopes and digital radiographs on a hard drive. Dental radiographs are the property of the dentist, and even after a patient leaves a dental office, any radiographs that were taken by that dental office should remain with that office. Patients do have the right to request copies of their films at any time, but the original films should never leave the dental office.

Photographs

Like radiographs, photographs should be stored in the patient's record indefinitely. Photos should be stored in separate sleeves to protect them from light and damage.

Models

Models include diagnostic models or laboratory models. These are often used in orthodontics and other situations that call for a three-dimensional representation of a person's dentition. Models can also be subpoenaed, like other elements of the dental record, and should be stored indefinitely.

CHECKPOINTS

21-1 On which form are details of a patient's examination recorded?

21-2 Where should correspondence between a patient and the dental office be filed?

Gathering Patient Information

Gathering patient information can be a sensitive issue for several reasons. First, legally, patient privacy must be protected, so information must be collected in such a way that it cannot be overheard, read accidentally, or otherwise shared with people who are not privileged to see it.

Second, the patient record is compiled at different stages. The patient provides much of the personal information, usually when enrolling in a new practice. At this point, patients can fill out their registration and dental history forms as well as sign the privacy and consent forms. Information about the responsible party for payment is also provided by the patient at this time.

These forms can be filled out at the patient's home, and some dental practices mail new patients a packet of forms before their initial visit in the interest of saving time. Alternatively, many dental offices ask that patients complete these forms in the reception area, usually using a supplied clipboard.

A patient who cannot fill out the forms should be escorted to a private area in the office. The DA can help by asking pertinent questions and completing the forms and then obtaining the patient's signature. This should never be done in a reception area because of privacy concerns.

During examinations, these forms should be available to the dentist because they supply important clinical information, such as smoking status, that might help guide the dentist during the clinical examination and discussions with the patient.

The clinical examination record is generated during the actual exams. As treatment progresses, the patient's record is continuously updated.

The Initial Visit

Much of the information in a patient record is compiled before or during the initial visit. During the initial visit, it is important to take some time to ask the patient about the following areas:

- Attitude toward dental health and dental treatment
- Use of medications, both prescription and over the counter
- Use of alternative or complementary medicines
- Use of illicit substances
- Any concerns or preferences when dealing with dental care

It is also a good idea to review the medical and dental history forms, which cover a lot of this same information. Sometimes a simple question can prompt important information.

Also during the initial visit, it is common to obtain a full set of current dental radiographs, in addition to examination results and a current dental chart.

Subsequent Visits

On every subsequent visit, patients should be asked to update their medical and dental history. If there is no change to their status—no new medications, complaints, or lifestyle changes—patients should be asked to update their history with a simple "no change" notation, which is signed and dated.

CHECKPOINT

21-3 How often is a patient's medical and dental history updated?

Patient Histories

Dental History

The dental history is valuable because it gives patients the opportunity to communicate their feelings about oral health and their level of concern with their teeth and gingival tissue. If a more complete dental record is not available from another dentist's office, the dental history will provide information about previous dental work and oral problems.

The dental history is a crucial part of the patient record. It should include detailed information about the patient's oral health, with questions such as:

- When was the last time you had your teeth cleaned?
- How often do you typically visit the dentist?
- How often do you brush? Floss?
- Does your gingival tissue bleed? If yes, how much?
- Are you having a specific problem?
- When was the last time you had dental x-rays taken?
- Who was your previous dentist? Do you have his or her address and phone number?
- Have you lost any teeth?
- Do you have any oral appliances?
- Are you happy with the condition of your teeth?
- Are you happy with the appearance of your teeth?
- Have you had orthodontic work?
- Have your teeth been sealed?
- Do you smoke?
- Do you bite your nails or regularly chew on objects such as pen caps or ice cubes?
- Have you ever had a bad experience at a dental office? If so, briefly explain what happened.

Once completed, the dental history form should be signed and dated by the patient.

Medical History

A complete medical history is essential for every patient. It should be available for the dental staff to review before examination or treatment begins. This allows the dental staff to ask questions and adjust the plans based on any medical conditions that might be present.

Legally, patients' medical histories are protected information. When taking a medical history or using one in the office, the information should always remain confidential and hidden. Notations of conditions should never be made on the outside of the folder, and members of the dental team should never discuss patients' medical conditions in public areas.

A thorough medical history, including a family history, serves several purposes by alerting dentists to conditions that might affect treatment, enabling staff to anticipate and better manage medical emergencies, and helping to identify where special treatment may be necessary.

A few of the questions typically asked during a medical history include:

- Who is your primary care physician?
- When was the last time you visited your physician?
- Are you taking any medications or substances?
- Do you regularly take any vitamins, supplements, herbs, or other health-related substances?
- Do you have any allergies, including latex allergies?
- Do you have problems with penicillin, antibiotics, or other medications?
- Have you ever been treated for or diagnosed with heart disease?
- Do you have an artificial heart valve?
- Do you have high blood pressure?
- Do you have human immunodeficiency virus/acquired immune deficiency syndrome?
- Have you ever been diagnosed with or treated for cancer?
- Have you ever been diagnosed with or treated for a sexually transmitted disease?
- Have you ever been diagnosed with an antibiotic-resistant staph infection?
- Have you ever had a total joint replacement?
- Do you use illicit drugs? If yes, which ones and how often?
- Do you drink alcohol? If yes, how many alcoholic beverages do you consume in a week?

If the patient answers yes to any question, the issue should be thoroughly followed up. You should know, for example, not only what medication the patient is taking but *why* he or she is taking it, because some medications have multiple reasons for use.

From the Dentist's Perspective

My practice is successful because we pay careful attention to details. I cannot tell you how valuable it is to have experienced dental assistants do a thorough check of medical records before we start procedures. Some patients forget to mention allergies to medications and anesthetics, so it is invaluable to have a dental assistant catch these critical details before we begin treatment!

Procedure 21-1 Obtaining a Patient History

Standard forms are typically used for both medical and dental histories. These forms become part of the patient's record and should be updated every time the patient returns to the office.
Materials needed (Figure P21-1-1):

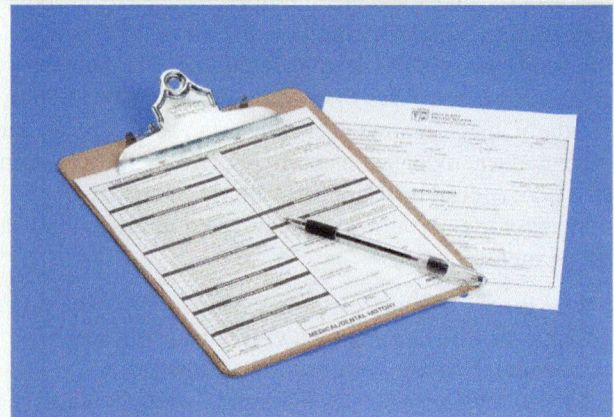

Figure P21-1-1

- Appropriate forms for medical and dental history
- Pen
- Clipboard

1. Supply the patient with the appropriate forms, a pen, and a clipboard. Alternatively, you can mail the forms to the patient so they can be completed before the initial visit.
2. Provide the patient with a private place to complete the forms.
3. Offer to help complete the forms or explain anything that is not clear.
4. Collect the finished forms and review them to make sure they are complete, signed, and dated.
5. Review the forms with the patient briefly, asking pertinent questions. Remember that this is confidential information, so this must be done with an eye toward protecting the patient's privacy.
6. Maintain and update these forms at every new visit.

In some cases, a medical consult may be requested to further clarify the patient's medical history or to verify that the patient is stable for treatment, requires premedication, or for another reason.

Once completed, the medical history should be signed and dated by the patient.

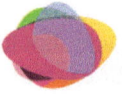

CHECKPOINT

21-4 Which patients are asked to provide a medical history?

Extra Patient Care

Sometimes older patients forget to list every medication they are currently taking, especially if they also take many vitamins and other supplements. If you suspect that a patient might have forgotten to list some, ask him or her to bring in all medication bottles. You can make a list for the patient record—and you can do him or her a favor by providing a copy of the list for other doctors' offices.

Chapter Highlights

- ✦ The patient record contains all relevant information related to the patient's past and current dental care.
- ✦ Elements of the patient record include legal forms, dental and medical history, treatment forms, radiographs, photographs, and correspondence.
- ✦ Portions of the patient record can be subpoenaed in court cases and thus must be current and complete.

- ✦ Patient privacy is protected by the Health Information Portability and Accountability Act of 1996 (HIPAA); dental assistants should be aware of HIPAA regulations and always make sure to protect privacy.
- ✦ Dental and medical histories should be updated with every office visit.

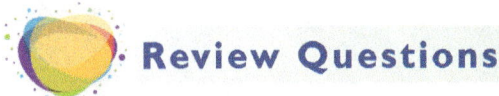

Review Questions

1. The patient record is
   a. A privileged document that may only be viewed by the dentist.
   b. Open to subpoena.
   c. Closed to the patient.
   d. None of the above.

2. Dental histories
   a. Should be updated annually.
   b. Should be updated with new patients.
   c. Should be updated with every office visit.
   d. Should be updated as circumstances change.

3. Dental radiographs should be kept with the patient's record at the dental practice
   a. Indefinitely.
   b. Only until the next set is taken.
   c. For 5 years.
   d. Until the patient changes dentists.

4. Medical histories are important because
   a. Any change in health status can affect oral health.
   b. Patients might not be aware of possible interactions with new medications.

   c. Dentists rely on this information to help diagnose oral conditions.
   d. All of the above.

5. Written correspondence between the patient and the dental office should be
   a. Kept for 60 days and then discarded.
   b. Included in the patient record.
   c. Discarded immediately to save storage space.
   d. Stored separately from the patient's medical forms.

6. In a medical history
   a. Questions regarding private matters such as human immunodeficiency virus status should be avoided.
   b. It is not important to include alternative and complementary medicines.
   c. All substances and diseases should be included.
   d. Potentially incriminating topics, such as illicit drug use, should be avoided.

Active Learning Exercises

1. Discuss the differences between the privacy and consent forms. Why are these forms necessary for every dental office? Who is responsible for ensuring that they are completed?

2. Create a medical history with six "Yes" answers. Using open-ended questions, create a professional dialogue that you could use to ask your patient to elaborate on these answers. Keep in mind that many questions are very personal. You should reassure the patient by explaining the office's policy regarding confidentiality.

3. A treatment plan acts as a guide or a roadmap of when and how each procedure will proceed. Why is a treatment plan necessary for all patients? Can a treatment plan be altered without the patient's consent? Explain your answer.

Application Activities

1. Assemble the needed forms to enroll a new patient.

2. Using a friend or family member as the patient, practice taking a dental history.

PREPARING FOR CERTIFICATION EXAMS

Review the following topics in this chapter to prepare for the Dental Assisting National Board (DANB) exam:

- **Elements of the Patient Record**
- **Patient Registration Form**
- **Dental History Form**
- **Clinical Examination Form**
- **Medical History Form**
- **Consent Forms**
- **Privacy Form**
- **Patient Correspondence**
- **Radiographs**
- **Photographs**
- **Patient Histories**
- **Dental History**
- **Medical History**

Patients with Special Needs

CHAPTER OUTLINE

CHAPTER CHECKLIST

On completion of this chapter, students will be able to:

☑ Describe the purpose of the Americans with Disabilities Act and how it applies to a dental practice.

☑ Describe advance preparations that can be taken to better serve special needs patients.

☑ Explain the importance of having an accurate, current medical and dental history for patients who have special needs.

☑ Describe ways to communicate with various types of special needs patients.

☑ Describe the special tools and education special needs patients may need.

☑ Identify various types of special needs patients and describe specific strategies for providing appropriate patient care.

KEY TERMS

Alzheimer disease – a progressive disease that develops slowly and causes a decline in cognitive functioning; affects memory, movement, language, behavior, judgment, and reasoning

angina (an-JIE-nuh) – recurrent short episodes of chest pain due to restricted blood flow to the heart caused by arteries narrowed from buildup of plaques containing cholesterol and other substances

arthritis – a condition characterized by pain and stiffness caused by inflammation in joints including the knees, wrists, or spinal column; although there are some 22 different types of arthritis, the two main types are osteoarthritis and rheumatoid arthritis

assistive device – a device or modification that helps a person overcome or remove a disability

asthma – a condition that occurs when airways in the lungs become inflamed and constricted and produce extra mucus; symptoms range from mild wheezing to severe attacks

autism spectrum disorders – disorders including autistic disorder, pervasive developmental disorder, and Asperger syndrome that cause significant impairment in communication and social interaction and unusual interests and behaviors; often begins in early childhood and lasts throughout a person's life

cerebral palsy – a group of disorders that affect a person's ability to move and to maintain balance; caused by an abnormality in the part of the brain that controls muscle tone; characterized by spasticity, which involves stiff muscles and awkward movement

chronic obstructive pulmonary disease (COPD) – a group of lung diseases, including emphysema and chronic bronchitis, that restricts airflow and makes breathing difficult; can cause shortness of breath, wheezing, fatigue, chronic cough, and headaches

congestive heart failure – a condition characterized by the heart not being able to pump as much blood as the body needs; can be caused by conditions that weaken the heart, including long-term high blood pressure, coronary artery disease, and diabetes

Down syndrome – a type of mental retardation caused by a chromosomal defect; often accompanied by identifiable physical characteristics, including a flattened back of the head, slanted eyes, and depressed bridge of the nose

emotional disability – a condition not explicable by intellectual, sensory, or health factors and that is characterized by an inability to maintain satisfactory interpersonal relationships, inappropriate behavior or feelings under normal circumstances, and a persistent feeling of unhappiness or depression

hemophilia – a genetic disease in which the body's blood-clotting ability is compromised

hypertension – high blood pressure; a very common condition that is often undiagnosed or improperly managed

hyperthyroidism (hi-per-THIE-roy-dih-zum) – an overactive thyroid that produces too much of the hormone thyroxine, with accompanying symptoms that may include increased appetite, heat intolerance and sweating, anxiety, fatigue, and depression

hypothyroidism – an underactive thyroid that does not produce enough hormones, with accompanying symptoms that may include fatigue, depression, cold intolerance, cramps, weight gain, and constipation

intellectual disability – cognitive disability or mental retardation; may be characterized by a significantly below-average score on a test of intelligence and by limitations in functioning in areas such as communication, self-care, and socialization

mental retardation – a disability characterized by significant limitations both in intellectual functioning and in adaptive behavior, as expressed in conceptual, social, and practical skills

multiple sclerosis (skluh-ROH-sis) – an autoimmune disease in which the body's immune system destroys the protective sheath covering the nerves; can be debilitating and can cause numbness or weakness in the limbs, full or partial vision loss, pain or tingling, unsteady gait, tremors, fatigue, dizziness, and an inability to walk and talk

muscular dystrophy – a group of inherited muscle diseases that causes muscle fibers to be very susceptible to damage; muscles weaken progressively and, late in this disease, are replaced by fat and connective tissue

neurological disorder – any disease or disorder that affects the nervous system, including Alzheimer disease, seizure disorder, Parkinson disease, cerebral palsy, and multiple sclerosis

physical disability – a disability (orthopedic, neuromuscular, cardiovascular, or pulmonary) that may cause a person to depend on a wheelchair, crutches, cane, or another assistive device for mobility; disability may be congenital or the result of an injury, disease or condition, or amputation; some physical disabilities are not apparent to others

psychosocial problem – a problem, including depression, anxiety, bipolar disorder, dementia, addiction, and behavioral problems, that results from background, personality, and social factors and that creates difficulties in a person's external world; some of these conditions are not at first apparent

xerostomia – a condition of dry mouth

Introduction

Dental professionals should strive to maximize the well-being and health of every patient. This goal can involve extra effort when patients have special needs, such as physical or intellectual disabilities. Patients who have special needs may require extra assistance to achieve optimal health, including oral health—an integral part of their overall health and well-being.

"Special needs" refers to mental, emotional, and physical disabilities as well as cultural and language differences. Providing care to these patients may require special attention and awareness to their needs and increased communication with patients and among staff team members.

From Classroom to Clinic

Not everyone is equipped to assist with a patient who has special needs. The dental assistant's specialized education is invaluable in a dental practice. Your extensive training in treating special-needs patients and how to handle them can be essential in your office.

Studies show that people who have intellectual and developmental disabilities generally have higher rates of poor oral hygiene, dental caries, and periodontal treatment needs than the general population. In addition, some disabilities, both mental and physical, are accompanied by health conditions that may complicate dental care. The role of the dental team in treating and educating this patient population in particular cannot be overemphasized. This includes demonstrating techniques of oral hygiene and creative ways to accomplish self-care goals.

Principles of Nondiscrimination

The Americans with Disabilities Act (ADA) of 1990 is a broad civil rights law that prohibits, under certain circumstances, discrimination based on disability—a physical or mental impairment that substantially limits a major life activity. The ADA requires that public buildings be accessible to physically challenged people.

All aspects of patient care must be carried out in a nondiscriminatory way. All members of the staff must be familiar with and comply with the ADA as applicable to dental practices. The ADA prevents discrimination on the basis of a disability. The ADA defines the dental office as a place of public accommodation, which means that dentists—and the whole dental team—need to be familiar and compliant with the regulations. All employers with 15 employees or more must comply with the ADA. The ADA requires that access to medical facilities be manageable by everyone. In addition to the building accommodating patients, the office itself should be free of barriers that would prevent patients who have disabilities from moving about safely. For example, keep passageways and countertops free of obstacles, such as deliveries and packages, chairs, toys, equipment, and stacks of paper. Table 22-1 provides an overview of the ADA requirements for public buildings.

TABLE 22-1 Summary of ADA Requirements for Public Buildings

AREA	REQUIREMENT
Access	Route must be stable, firm, and slip resistant.
	Route must be 36 inches wide.
Ramps	Ramps longer than 6 feet must have two railings.
	Railings must be 34–38 inches high.
	Ramp must be 36 inches wide.
	Ramps and elevators must be available to all public levels.
Entrance and door	Door must be 32 inches wide.
	Door handle must be no higher than 48 inches and must be operable with a closed fist.
	Interior doors must open without excessive force.
Miscellaneous	Carpeting must be no more than 0.5 inch high.
	Emergency egress (exit) system must have flashing lights and audible signals.
	Space for wheelchair seating must be available.
	Tables or counters must be 28–34 inches high.
Restrooms	Tactile signs must identify restrooms.
	Doorway must be at least 32 inches wide.
	All doors (including stall doors), soap dispensers, hand dryers, and faucets must be operable with a closed fist.
	Wheelchair stall is required and must be at least 5 feet by 5 feet.

CHECKPOINT
22-1 What is the name of the civil rights law that prohibits discrimination based on disability?

Preparation

Office visits for patients who have special needs can be made more successful with advance preparation. This includes gathering information before the appointment.

Whenever possible, paperwork should be sent to patients in advance. Completing paperwork, including a medical and medication history, can be time consuming, especially for patients who have more complicated conditions. The dental team must have a thorough and up-to-date medical and dental history for each patient to provide the best possible care. Some information for special needs patient visits can be gathered by phone, including determining if extra time, special equipment, or additional staffing is required for the appointment. Often, extra time is required to provide routine care to patients who have special needs. Sometimes this type of information can be gathered from patients. In other cases, it will come from parents or caregivers. Typically, patients who have special needs and their caregivers are accustomed to sharing this information with appropriate health care providers to accommodate their needs. For example, some patients do better at certain times of the day and should be given appointments accordingly.

When the dentist determines it is necessary, an appropriate staff member may ask the patient or caregiver for the name of the patient's medical provider to gather additional information. Some patients have needs that require checking with a physician before performing certain procedures, such as before having anesthesia. Being familiar with the patient's medical history decreases the chance that a medical condition could be aggravated during dental care.

When a person who has special needs is an existing patient, members of the dental team who have experience with the individual can share with other team members what they have learned about how best to serve and meet the patient's needs. More experienced team members also can share their general experience customizing care to patients who have special needs. A dental practice is enhanced when its team members are familiar with the oral health problems of people who have disabilities. And patients are best served—and, ultimately, their overall health needs are best met—when their individual needs are met through the staff's compassion, patience, awareness, and respect.

Some special needs patients require general anesthesia and an operating room setting for treatment because of their severe limitations. If you have such a patient, the office should refer the patient to a practice or clinic that can provide this service if the dentist does not have a hospital affiliation and privileges. There is nothing out of the ordinary about such a referral, and they are common in severe cases. The patient and caretaker should be advised about the reasons for the referral and given a contact number for the appropriate practice or clinic. This information should also be clearly documented in the patient's record.

✓ **CHECKPOINT**
22-2 What type of important information should be determined in advance for a patient who has special needs?

Communication

According to the ADA, the dental provider must work with a caregiver, guardian, parent, or family member of the patient if communication with the patient is unsuccessful because of a disability. Make every effort to communicate directly with the patient during the dental appointment. When the patient's level of functioning is such that communication is unsuccessful, you can communicate with caregivers or parents and ask for their assistance. Patients must feel they are part of the process, even if their condition requires involvement by family members or other caregivers.

When you have patients whose intellectual functioning is impaired, you may find the training you learned for working with pediatric patients to be helpful. (Pediatric care is covered in detail in Chapter 43, Pediatric Dentistry.) A similar approach includes carefully explaining what will happen during the appointment, showing the instruments that will be used and explaining and demonstrating their roles, using terminology appropriate for the patient's age and intellectual and emotional functioning, encouraging the patient to ask questions, explaining the procedure as it progresses, and breaking up the steps during care into smaller segments to give the patient small breaks. And, of course, do not forget to tell patients when they are doing a good job. Everyone appreciates having their efforts to cooperate noticed. Positive feedback is a behavior modification technique you may want to use during treatment to help ensure success.

Your goal should be to increase the patient's comfort level and decrease fear and apprehension. It is always a good idea to try to look at things from the patient's point of view. For example, how might you feel if you had hearing impairment? How would you want the dental team to accommodate you? How might you feel if you used a wheelchair? How could the dental team make your visits easier? What if you did not speak English? How could the dental team communicate with you?

You are in an important position to make patients' visits easier—more relaxing, more comfortable, and more informative. Patients who feel accommodated and appreciated may be more likely to comply with recommendations to maximize their oral health.

An important point to keep in mind in communicating with or about patients who have special needs or disabilities is to put the person first, and the disability second. That means saying "a person who uses a wheelchair," not "a wheelchair-bound person." Or "a person who has mental retardation," not "a retarded person." Or "a person with a physical disability," not "a disabled person." Thinking "person first, disability second"—and seeing patients in that light—will serve you and your patients well.

As a health care professional, you are expected to treat all patients impartially, guard against discriminatory practices, remain nonjudgmental, avoid stereotypes, and maintain a professional demeanor. In this manner, you communicate to patients that you accept human differences and provide quality care to all those who seek it.

✓ **CHECKPOINTS**
22-3 What does the Americans with Disabilities Act require a dental provider to do if communication with the patient is unsuccessful because of a disability?

22-4 How can the dental assistant make special needs patients' visits easier?

Tools and Education

Patients who have disabilities may need special assistive devices during office visits as well as for their self-care. In-office tools you should be familiar with include transfer boards, backrests, and mouth props. There are many devices that dental practices can use to help accommodate patients' special needs; these are available from vendors and easily viewable in catalogs and on the Internet.

You also can find many products for patients to use in their self-care. Your office may want to keep resources—catalogs, videos, lists of websites, and samples of modified tools—on hand to share with patients and their caregivers.

Dental assistants (DAs) should be familiar with assistive devices, such as grip aids, that help patients manage their oral hygiene (Figure 22-1). In addition to commercially available products, you should be able to explain homemade ways to modify toothbrushes to aid in their use by patients who have disabilities. For example, a toothbrush inserted into a tennis ball and secured with strong tape can provide an easier gripping mechanism for patients who do not have fine motor skills (Figure 22-2).

Use your observation skills and knowledge about physical and intellectual disabilities to recommend the tools necessary to make self-care realistic and achievable. Some patients will find electric toothbrushes and floss holders easier to use. People who have significant physical or intellectual disabilities may need a caregiver to brush and floss

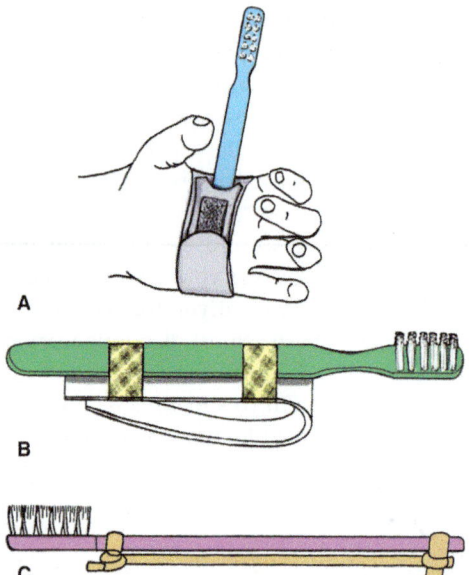

Figure 22–1 Aids for patients who cannot grasp and hold. (**A**) Adjustable Velcro strap around the hand has a pocket designed to hold the toothbrush handle. (**B**) Handle of a fingernail brush is attached to a toothbrush with adhesive tape. (**C**) Rubber tubing attached firmly to toothbrush handle enables patient to hold the brush across the palm of the hand.

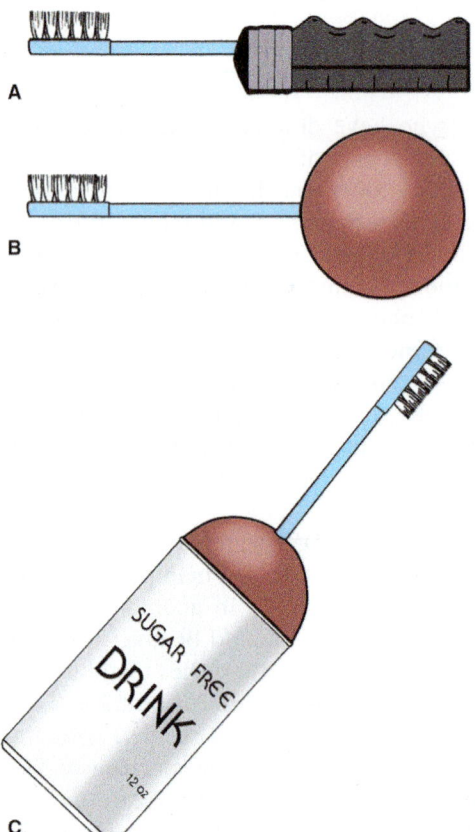

Figure 22–2 Aids for patients with limited grasp. (**A**) Toothbrush inserted into a bicycle handle grip. (**B**) Toothbrush inserted into a soft rubber ball. (**C**) Toothbrush in soft rubber ball inserted into a juice or soda can to provide a handle of appropriate diameter for patients with limited hand closure.

their teeth. In those cases, the caregiver may need you to demonstrate how to perform these tasks on another person. Some organizations have produced videos and brochures demonstrating these tasks. Your office may want to have a lending library to share those materials with patients and caregivers or, at least, refer them to the appropriate resources.

Some patients, including children and those with intellectual or developmental disabilities, may have anxiety about toothbrushing. You play a key role in educating parents and caregivers about ways to help overcome this anxiety. You can recommend they first use a damp washcloth or piece of gauze wrapped around their finger to clean the teeth. When that routine has been accepted, a toothbrush can be introduced, with bristles softened in hot water. When it is age appropriate and safe for the individual, a toothbrush might be suitable for supervised playtime to increase familiarization with it and reduce any negative feelings associated with it. Some patients do not fear toothbrushes but have problems keeping their mouth open long enough for toothbrushing. In these cases a mouth prop may be useful. Regardless, some patients have a serious problem with toothbrushing or being touched around their mouth, despite their best efforts and the caretaker's. Never chastise these patients or humiliate them for their poor oral hygiene. Instead, do your best to reinforce what you can, advise prescription dentifrices or mouthrinses when applicable, and, when appropriate, recommend more frequent cleaning appointments.

Patient education should always include a discussion of diet and how food and beverages affect oral health. Consider being creative when you tell children and patients who have intellectual or developmental disabilities about diet. Your lessons may be more memorable—and fun—if you use visual aids, such as plastic or wooden play food or a doll and a toothbrush.

Patients who have special needs are more likely than others to take multiple prescription medications. Some medications have a negative effect on oral health. Some children's medications contain sweeteners, and medications that older patients take can impair saliva flow. Most dental offices have a *Physicians' Desk Reference* in addition to dental drug reference books that contain information about drug interactions and side effects. Use these resources to determine how your patient's medication may impact dental care and overall oral health. Work with your dentist to inform patients about the effects of the medications they take and ways to combat these effects, including extra brushing and chewing special gums. Prescription toothpastes, mouthrinses, and the use of topical fluorides may also be a boon for those patients who find extra brushing a challenge.

✓ **CHECKPOINT**

22-5 What are some types of education the dental assistant can provide to special needs patients and their caregivers?

Pediatric Patients

Like all patients, pediatric patients should be treated with respect. You should communicate with them appropriate to their age and intellectual and emotional functioning. Children, especially older ones, do not like being condescended to. How you treat them in the initial visit will affect how they feel about future visits. You do not want pediatric patients to think, "That's the place where they talk to me like I'm a baby."

When you greet a pediatric patient in the reception area, call the child by name. Consider kneeling or squatting down to establish eye contact with younger children, or sit in the chair next to the child and introduce yourself. Then greet the parent or guardian. Consider asking the child a couple of questions to establish rapport—the name of his or her favorite sport or some favorite activities.

Note that studies show that children under 50 months of age are more cooperative with a parent present in the treatment room; after that, many offices have the parent sit in the waiting room during actual treatment. This is because several things can happen psychologically if you keep the parent in the room: the child may think that the procedure is so dangerous and risky that the parent is staying to supervise—which could make the child nervous. Furthermore, when two authorities are present in the room—the parent and the doctor—a child may feel that he or she does not need to listen to the doctor.

Accompany the child (and parent, as appropriate) to the treatment room. Some preschool-age patients may welcome the offer of your hand to hold while walking to the treatment room. Use your judgment and observation skills to determine when this is appropriate. Consider asking younger children if they need to visit the bathroom before the exam begins. Lend the child a hand in getting in the dental chair, if necessary. Sometimes the chair will need a booster chair or cushion to raise the child to an appropriate level. If you ask pediatric patients to sit cross-legged in the chair, they will be less likely to slide down.

Explain to the child what will happen during the appointment, and answer questions honestly. Use the communication suggestions mentioned earlier in this chapter when dealing with pediatric patients. The "tell-show-do" method is often helpful here: first tell the child what you are going to do, then show on a model or puppet or something similar, and finally do it. It is a good idea to let pediatric patients know when you are going to touch them, especially if they seem nervous or scared. Some children are sensitive to touch by an adult who is not their parent. Adolescents also may be jumpy about adult touch. Do not take the child's reaction to your touch personally. You can help prevent nervous reactions to your touch by talking out loud about what you are going to do next during the appointment.

After the treatment, explain any steps the child should take to improve self-care. Demonstrate the techniques on yourself, on the child, or on the parent if it would help to make the activity more real to the patient. Ask the child to imitate the technique. If you model the technique first, the child may be less intimidated to do the same. Depending on the child's age and functioning level, ask the patient to repeat back to you how often to brush and floss. The parent or guardian is the backup keeper of information, but try to have as much direct communication as possible with the child.

Accompany the child back to the reception area after the appointment, and confirm any instructions with the parent.

For a detailed look at pediatric dentistry, including techniques for behavior management, see Chapter 43, Pediatric Dentistry.

CHECKPOINT

22-6 What is a way to prevent pediatric patients from sliding down in the dental chair?

Older Adults

The numbers of older adults continues to grow. Throughout the 20th century, the population of people age 65 and over living in the United States grew from 3 million to 37 million in the 2006 Census. The oldest of the older population (those age 85 and over) grew from just over 100,000 in 1900 to 5.3 million in 2006. People are living longer because medicine has progressed and now helps people live longer through treatments and medical advances.

The dental profession currently faces a challenge in the treatment of older adults. Dental professionals must be aware of the physical, psychological, and financial situation of geriatric patients.

Many older adults lack dental care for several reasons:

- Many are no longer employed and are living on a fixed income. Older adults with limited financial resources often find it difficult to meet the basic needs of food, heat, and health care, and can seldom afford preventive dentistry.
- Most no longer have dental insurance provided through an employer.

Most people who speak another language appreciate others' attempts to communicate with them in that language. Anything you can do to make them feel comfortable, welcome, and informed will be appreciated. Think about what you would like if you were in their position. Gestures and other visual cues can help communicate actions you need the patient to take throughout the visit. Pictures can also help communicate important information. Often, patients who do not speak English will be accompanied by a family member or friend who speaks English and can interpret. In those cases, communicate with the patient, not the interpreter.

Cultural Diversity

Patient education and the creation of health goals for all of our patients is our primary concern as dental health care providers. To be truly prepared to educate our patients, we must always be aware of and respect cultural and background differences. Effective communication can be achieved in a variety of ways. Having interpreters in the office will help patients who speak only little or no English. Knowing how and where to obtain an interpreter is essential for communicating with and educating these patients. Pamphlets and videos are other effective tools for patient education. They can be used to demonstrate both self-care and in-office dental techniques to patients who may not fully understand English or dental terminology. Staff training in cultural sensitivity is another essential element of patient education. Workshops and seminars can educate the staff on cultural differences and are a necessary part of any office training. Effective communication and appreciation of cultural, ethnic, and religious differences is key to patient education.

CHECKPOINT

22-8 When a patient brings along an interpreter or another person to help with communication, to whom should the dental assistant direct communication?

Movement-Impaired Patients

Patients whose movement is impaired and who depend on wheelchairs, walkers, crutches, canes, or other devices may need special accommodation to enable them to move easily in public places. Dental practices should make every effort to ensure these patients' visits are easy and unencumbered.

This begins with having handicapped parking close to the building and entry doors and corridors that accommodate wheelchairs. An elevator for offices not on the main floor is necessary as are bathrooms that accommodate wheelchairs.

The office layout itself also must provide space for patients in wheelchairs to move around. The path from the reception area to the treatment rooms should be wide enough and clear to accommodate wheelchairs and walkers (Figure 22-4). In accompanying these patients to

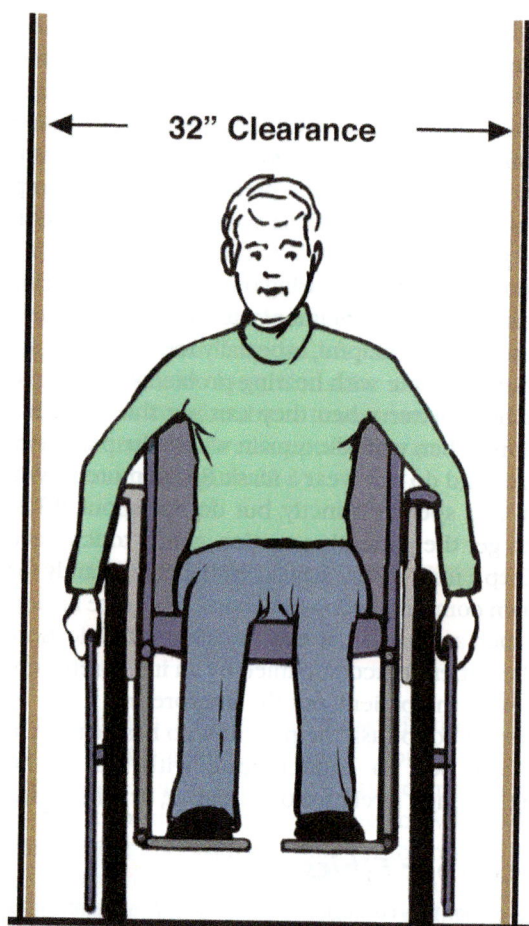

Figure 22–4 Wheelchair accessibility. Wheelchairs designed for adults vary in width from 2 feet 3 inches to 2 feet 8 inches. A clear door width of 32 inches can accommodate these wheelchairs.

treatment rooms, look to them for guidance in signaling if they need assistance.

Make sure the treatment room not only has room for a patient in a wheelchair or walker to enter and be seated but also room for a patient's caregiver to be seated. Some patients who use wheelchairs may need to remain in their special chair during treatment.

Some patients may need help transferring to the dental chair, but they usually are accustomed to speaking up and making their needs known. Talk to these patients just as you do any others to keep open the lines of communication and ensure they are comfortable asking you for help.

Transferring Patients to the Dental Chair

Patients who are in wheelchairs who can temporarily support their weight can be transferred to the dental chair by aligning the two chairs alongside each other and adjusting the dental chair to the same height as the wheelchair, setting the brakes on the wheelchair, and moving the dental chair arm between the two chairs. The patient can move sideways into the dental chair with your help (Figure 22-5).

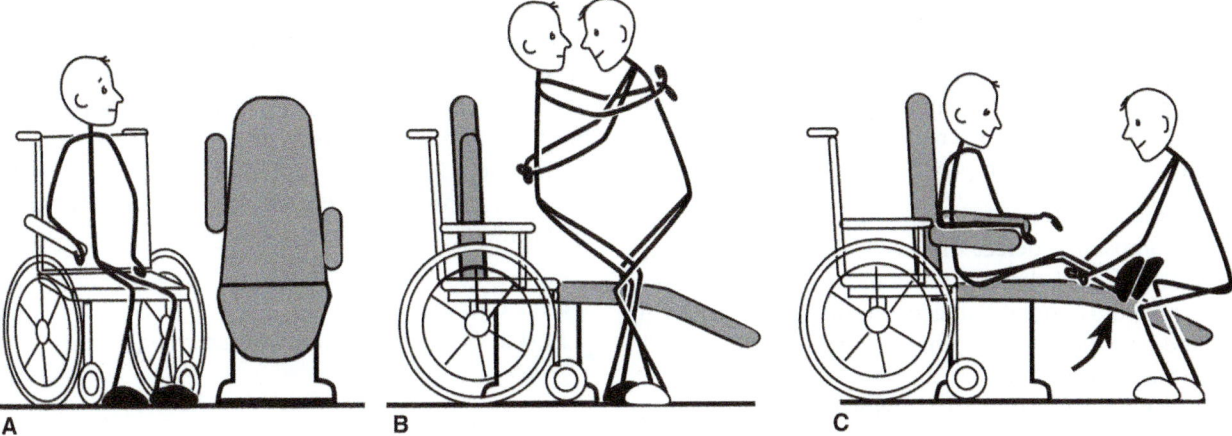

Figure 22–5 Wheelchair transfer for a mobile patient. (A) Position the wheelchair at level of or lower than the dental chair; set wheel locks, remove footrests and armrests, and raise the dental chair arm. **(B)** Clinician places feet outside of the patient's feet, grasps the patient around the waist under the arms, locks hands or grasps belt in back; patient holds clinician around shoulders or neck; patient is lifted up and pivoted to side of dental chair. **(C)** Patient is gently lowered to a sitting position; dental chair arm is lowered; clinician grasps patient's legs together to lift them onto the dental chair.

For patients who are unable to support their weight for this transfer, you and another staff member or a caregiver may be able to make the move. One person should face the patient, with the other behind the patient to make the lift and transfer.

When transferring disabled patients to a dental chair, some dentists use chair boards to slide the patient, or pulley systems to move the patient, from a wheelchair into the dental chair. However, some patients must remain in an upright position to prevent breathing difficulty, so sometimes the dental team will have to perform the move themselves in order to accommodate the patient.

Extra Patient Care

When it is too difficult to transfer a patient from his or her wheelchair, the dental team may need to care for the patient in the wheelchair. When this happens, do not let the patient feel different or as if he or she is inconveniencing the dental team. Putting the patient first and accommodating the patient helps to make the patient feel like every other patient.

Specialty Dental Chairs

One manufacturer, Diaco, makes a dental chair system that allows patients who are in wheelchairs to remain in their chairs yet be moved in the same reclined position as other patients in a traditional dental chair. This system eliminates the need for manual lifting and transfer of patients. The Diaco dental chair is controlled by a joystick and can be moved from room to room. Similarly, some modern dental chairs have reversible headrests that can be positioned as a headrest for a patient who remains in a wheelchair for treatment.

CHECKPOINTS

22-9 What should you make sure there is room for in the dental treatment room, to accommodate caregivers of special needs patients?

22-10 How will you know if a patient needs help transferring into the dental chair?

Patients with Mental Retardation

Intellectual disability is sometimes referred to as a *cognitive disability* or *mental retardation*, and may be characterized by a significantly below-average score on a test of intelligence and by limitations in functioning in areas such as communication, self-care, and socialization.

The American Association on Mental Retardation (AAMR) defines mental retardation as a disability characterized by significant limitations both in intellectual functioning and in adaptive behavior, as expressed in conceptual, social, and practical skills. The AAMR looks at mental retardation as a classification in which individuals have many strengths as well as weaknesses. An individual's level of functioning is based on the amount of support he or she requires to function:

- **Intermittent support**—higher functioning individuals who require little intervention to function; associated with mild retardation.
- **Limited support**—individuals who are trainable but may require additional support to navigate through everyday situations; associated with moderate mental retardation.
- **Extensive support**—individuals who have some communication skills and can complete some self-care

tasks but who rely on daily support to function around the clock; associated with severe mental retardation.

- **Pervasive support** describes daily interventions necessary to help the individual function; this lifelong support applies to almost every aspect of the individual's routine; associated with profound mental retardation.

Down syndrome causes one type of mental retardation. It is a chromosomal defect that often is accompanied by identifiable physical characteristics, including a short nose, slanted eyes, and a round, flat face. People who have Down syndrome may have dental abnormalities such as small, fused, or misaligned teeth.

People with an intellectual disability also may have other disabilities, such as cerebral palsy, seizure disorders, vision or hearing impairment, and attention-deficit/hyperactivity disorder.

Structure your communication with patients who have mental retardation around their level of functioning, not their chronological age. Adults who have mental retardation are not children and should not be treated like children. However, some of the skills you have learned for working with pediatric patients may be helpful, depending on the patient's level of functioning.

✔ **CHECKPOINT**
22-11 What is the type of mental retardation caused by a chromosomal defect and characterized by a flattened back of the head, slanted eyes, and depressed bridge of the nose?

Patients with Developmental Disabilities

Cerebral Palsy

Cerebral palsy is a group of disorders that affect a person's ability to move and to maintain balance. These disorders are caused by an abnormality in the part of the brain that controls muscle tone. The majority of people who have cerebral palsy have spasticity, which involves stiff muscles and awkward movement.

Cerebral palsy does not worsen over time, but an individual's symptoms can change throughout his or her lifetime. Symptoms can range from mild—a person who walks awkwardly but does not need special help—to severe—a person who cannot walk and needs lifelong care. The condition can be accompanied by other disabilities, including seizure disorders, vision impairment, hearing loss, and mental retardation.

Autism

Autism spectrum disorders cause significant impairment in communication and social interaction in addition to unusual interests and behaviors. The abilities of people who have autism spectrum disorders range from gifted to severely challenged. Generally, the condition begins in early childhood, and it lasts throughout a person's life. Boys are more likely to be affected than girls.

Included in autism spectrum disorders are autistic disorder, pervasive developmental disorder, and Asperger syndrome.

✔ **CHECKPOINT**
22-12 Who is more likely to have autism, boys or girls?

Patients with Psychosocial Challenges

Psychosocial problems, including depression, anxiety, bipolar disorder, dementia, addiction, and behavioral problems, can affect a person's ability to communicate. Patients who have a psychosocial problem may be unresponsive to your questions. In those cases, do not force them to communicate. Stay focused on the reason for the visit, and conduct your duties professionally. Tell the patient what to expect, and encourage him or her when appropriate. Never even subtly communicate any judgment about the patient and his or her condition. You do not know how the patient's condition developed or the specifics of his or her lifestyle.

If the patient's behavior is affected by an episode of psychosocial illness at the time, the appointment should be rescheduled. The patient should be stable prior to treatment.

✔ **CHECKPOINT**
22-13 What should you do if a patient who has a psychosocial problem does not respond to your efforts to communicate?

Medically Compromised Patients

Many diseases affect oral health in addition to a particular part of or system in the body. In some cases, it is because the disease compromises the patient's ability to perform self-care.

You should have a general awareness and understanding of major diseases that may affect your patients.

Neurological Disorders

Diseases and disorders in this category affect the nervous system and include Alzheimer disease, seizure disorder, stroke, and multiple sclerosis.

Alzheimer Disease

Alzheimer disease is a degenerative brain disease that develops slowly and grows progressively worse, causing a decline in cognitive functioning. The disease affects behavior, memory, judgment, reasoning, and attention span. The progression from the mild stage to the severe stage varies among individuals. Generally speaking, people who have Alzheimer disease live from 8 to 10 years after diagnosis.

The caregiver of a patient who has Alzheimer disease can advise about the individual's best time of day for a dental visit. Some people who have Alzheimer disease take medications that impair salivation. The dental team should check for this condition and recommend aids to combat this problem.

In the late stage of the disease, a patient with Alzheimer disease who has dentures may not be able to tolerate them. The patient also may not be able to tolerate changes in the mouth such as new crowns or bridges. Treatment must be planned on a case-by-case basis. Patients who wear dentures should have their names inscribed in the dentures (in case they take them out and leave them somewhere), and if financially feasible, a backup pair may be advisable.

Seizure Disorders

Seizure disorders, such as epilepsy, are caused by malfunctioning electrical signals in the brain. Seizures can also be associated with autism and Down syndrome. Seizures can vary from seeming to blank out for a few moments to having convulsions.

At the start of the appointment, before treatment begins on a patient who has a history of seizures, ask if the patient is taking his or her medications, is eating regularly, is well rested, or is under particular stress. These factors can contribute to seizures, and you want to make sure the patient is taking care of himself or herself and does not have a seizure during treatment. You should also ask the patient if he or she has a specific aura that indicates a seizure may be about to occur. This will help the dental team recognize when the patient is about to seize and take appropriate measures.

If a patient does seize in your office, place him or her flat on the floor or chair, remove instruments from the mouth, and move anything potentially dangerous away from the patient. For more information about seizure care, see Chapter 18, Responding to Medical Emergencies.

Stroke

A stroke occurs when the supply of oxygenated blood to a part of the brain is reduced. When the brain tissue is deprived of oxygen, cells begin to die, resulting in brain damage or even death.

A person who has had a stroke may make a full recovery or may have permanent paralysis, loss of muscle movement, difficulty talking or swallowing, memory loss, and trouble understanding.

If the patient's speech is affected and is difficult to understand, be patient. Allow the patient plenty of time to communicate. Consider offering a notepad to help the patient communicate if that seems like an appropriate gesture.

Take special care to make sure patients who have had a stroke are scheduled for the time of day they request, a time when they are most able to tolerate treatment. These patients also may need a slightly longer appointment.

Multiple Sclerosis

Multiple sclerosis (MS) is a progressive autoimmune disease in which the body's immune system destroys the myelin sheath covering the nerve fibers of the brain and spinal cord, causing communication problems between the brain and the rest of the body that can be debilitating. Symptoms, which can appear sporadically, range from mild changes to an inability to walk or talk. Despite the inability to converse, these patients are still aware and should not be spoken to in a demeaning manner. Some people have numbness or weakness in their limbs, full or partial vision loss, pain or tingling, unsteady gait, tremors, fatigue, or dizziness.

MS patients who use wheelchairs may prefer to remain in their chair during dental appointments. Those patients who have muscle tremors that make dental treatment difficult may be able to take medication to make this process easier. Most likely, MS patients will be aware of this but, if they are not, the dentist may want to talk to the patient and his or her medical provider to determine if this is a possibility.

MS patients may benefit from specially tailored oral hygiene implements for their self-care if dexterity issues prohibit them from performing ideal self-care.

> **CHECKPOINTS**
>
> **22-14** For patients who have seizure disorder, what lifestyle factors can affect the likelihood of seizures?
>
> **22-15** If a patient who has had a debilitating stroke has difficulty communicating, what is a way you can help?

Pulmonary Disorders

Allergies

Allergies happen when the immune system encounters foreign substances, such as dust, pet dander, or pollen, and produces proteins to protect the person from the substances. Symptoms of allergies can involve the skin, sinuses, airways, and digestive system. Severity ranges from minor to life-threatening. Many allergy symptoms can be alleviated with over-the-counter or prescription medications.

It is vitally important to ensure that patients do not have a latex allergy, because many of the gloves and barriers used in dentistry contain latex. Non-latex alternatives should then be used. Each patient should be asked about latex sensitivities, and this should be clearly noted in their chart. Chapter 14, Disease and Infection Control, discusses latex allergies in more detail.

Asthma

Asthma occurs when airways in the lungs become inflamed and constricted. Symptoms range from mild wheezing to severe attacks. People who know they have asthma typically take medication to control their symptoms, and carry that medication with them. It is a good idea to have your patients with asthma take their inhaler out of their purse or pocket before beginning the procedure so that it is easily accessible should an attack occur. All offices should nonetheless have a commonly used inhaler such as albuterol accessible in the emergency drug kits, should it be necessary, or should an asthmatic patient forget an inhaler and subsequently need medication. If given a choice, have patients use their own inhaler, for it is prescribed specifically for them and is likely to be newer than the stored inhaler in the kit.

Some patients' asthma symptoms are triggered by stress, so try to keep stress to a minimum. Schedule their appointments earlier in the day or in sessions as short as possible. Be sure to ask the patient who has severe asthma if his or her chair position is comfortable. Also, verify which medications the patient takes and check for any that are contraindicated with those used in the dental office.

Some patients' asthma is triggered by specific allergens. If this is known, note this information in their record and avoid exposing the patient to those allergens if at all possible.

Chronic Obstructive Pulmonary Disease

Chronic obstructive pulmonary disease (COPD) is a group of lung diseases, including emphysema and chronic bronchitis, that restrict airflow and make breathing difficult. Most COPD is caused by smoking and is, thus, preventable.

Symptoms of COPD usually do not appear until significant damage to the lungs has occurred. Symptoms can include shortness of breath, wheezing, fatigue, chronic cough, and headaches.

Mucus may collect in the air passages of patients who have COPD, and this can be difficult to clear. Ask these patients if they need to have the dental chair positioned more upright than reclining. They also may need more frequent drinks of water during treatment. Some COPD patients' breathing may worsen throughout the day, so try to accommodate their possible preference for morning appointments.

The dental team should be aware of medications patients with COPD take and drugs used during dental treatment that may irritate their condition. When a patient has more serious COPD, a member of the dental team may want to communicate with the patient's physician to discuss which medications are advised.

CHECKPOINTS

22-16 What causes most chronic obstructive pulmonary disease?

22-17 Why might patients who have chronic obstructive pulmonary disease need the dental chair to be positioned more upright?

Cardiovascular Disorders

Depending on the severity of their condition, some patients with heart disorders may need special care, including avoiding stress, keeping them in a semi-upright position, monitoring vital signs before and during treatment, and administering supplemental oxygen during treatment. Others may need nitrous oxide or other medication to relieve stress or may take sublingual nitroglycerin immediately prior to treatment. The dentist may want to consult with the patient's physician to determine how best to ensure safety and comfort.

Hypertension

Hypertension, commonly called *high blood pressure*, increases a person's risk of serious health problems, including heart attack and stroke, if it is not controlled with medication or lifestyle changes. A person can have hypertension for years without any noticeable symptoms. Frequently taking your patient's blood pressure provides a valuable service, as it is not unusual for a dental office to be the first to discover that a patient is hypertensive.

Blood pressure is measured by the amount of blood the heart pumps and the resistance to blood flow in the arteries—when the heart has to pump more blood and the arteries narrow, blood pressure increases.

Many offices check each patient's blood pressure at least in the initial visit for a baseline reading and at 6-month recall visits. If your dental office normally checks patients' blood pressure before treatment, be sure to advise patients whose blood pressure is higher than the desired reading (120/80 mm Hg [millimeters of mercury]) to see a health care provider. If the reading is too high, you will have to reschedule the patient—or even have him or her transported immediately to a hospital. In adults who do not have a chronic disease, a reading higher than 120/80 mm Hg is considered prehypertensive. You also may want to tell patients how they can reduce their blood pressure on their own through lifestyle changes, including becoming more physically active, quitting smoking, reducing their weight, reducing their salt and caffeine intake, eating a healthier diet, limiting alcohol, and managing stress. (For more information about blood pressure, see Chapter 17, Vital Signs.)

Angina

Recurrent episodes of chest pain due to restricted blood flow to the heart is called **angina**. Blood flow may become restricted as a result of coronary artery disease, a condition in which arteries that carry blood to the heart are narrowed due to the buildup of plaques containing cholesterol and other substances. An individual who has angina is more likely to experience restricted blood flow and chest pain during exertion.

If a patient does experience chest pain, have the patient lie as still as possible. If the patient is alert and conscious, his or her own nitroglycerin can be administered along with oxygen. If after a few minutes the patient is still symptomatic, the dental team should proceed under the assumption that the patient is suffering a myocardial infarction, or heart attack. Emergency care for heart attack is described in Chapter 18, Responding to Medical Emergencies.

Congestive Heart Failure

When the heart cannot pump as much blood as the body needs, the condition is referred to as **congestive heart failure**. It can be caused by long-term high blood pressure, coronary artery disease, and diabetes—all conditions that weaken the heart. The symptoms of people diagnosed with congestive heart failure can be improved with medication. They also can take steps to improve their quality of life, including exercising, reducing stress, losing weight, and reducing salt use.

People who have severe forms of congestive heart failure are at risk of sudden death. They may need an implantable heart device or a heart transplant.

Many people who have congestive heart failure have difficulty sleeping. When they lie flat in bed, they have trouble breathing. Medication prescribed to prevent their bodies from retaining excess fluid makes them wake up frequently to use the bathroom. This may be important in the dental office, because they may require bathroom breaks during long appointments. Be aware of this, and plan for break times during the procedure during which you can offer the patient the opportunity to use the restroom.

Endocarditis

Endocarditis is an infection of the inner lining or valves of the heart and is caused by bacteria or other germs spreading through the bloodstream into damaged areas in the heart. The condition is most common in people who already have a compromised heart—a damaged heart valve or an artificial valve. Endocarditis can destroy heart valves and cause life-threatening complications. In addition, endocarditis can causes abscesses in the brain, kidneys, liver, and other parts of the body. Treatment for endocarditis includes antibiotics and, sometimes, surgery.

People who have a compromised heart may need to take prophylactic antibiotics prior to dental and medical procedures to prevent bacteria from entering their bloodstream. Be aware of this premedication requirement, and ensure that these patients have taken the right medication in the right dosage at the right time before the appointment.

CHECKPOINTS

22-18 What is congestive heart failure?

22-19 What is it important for patients who have endocarditis to talk to their physicians before dental treatment?

Blood Disorders

Hemophilia

Hemophilia is a disease in which the body's blood-clotting ability is compromised. A person who has hemophilia and gets a cut will bleed for a longer time than would a person whose blood clots normally. The health concerns for people who have hemophilia are deep internal bleeding and bleeding into joints.

It is important for people who have this lifelong disorder to practice good oral hygiene. A tooth extraction, for example, can cause excessive bleeding, which should be avoided. When oral surgery is required, the dentist should consult with the patient's physician to determine necessary steps to protect the patient's health. Always, the patient must be protected from bacterial infection.

Patients who have hemophilia must avoid medications that can aggravate bleeding or thin the blood, including aspirin, nonsteroidal anti-inflammatory drugs, heparin, and warfarin. Acetaminophen is a safer alternative for pain relief.

CHECKPOINT

22-20 What is compromised in a patient who has hemophilia?

Endocrine Disorders

Diabetes

Diabetes mellitus (diabetes) is a group of diseases that affect how the body uses blood glucose (blood sugar, or insulin), the main source of energy for the body's muscle and tissue cells. A person who has diabetes has too much glucose in the blood, which can cause significant health problems.

Patients who have diabetes may have gingival irritation (Figure 22-6), alveolar bone loss, acetone breath, and delayed healing. The dental team should take extra care to

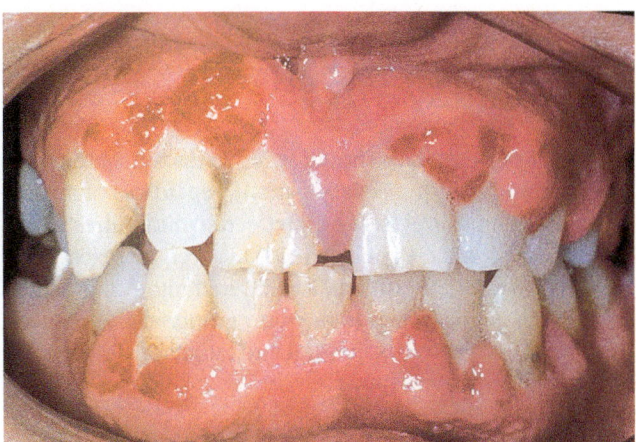

Figure 22–6 Diabetic gingivitis.

minimize risk for infection in patients who have diabetes due to their compromised healing ability. Also, be sure to tell patients who have diabetes to eat normally before a dental appointment to prevent low blood sugar.

Always have a sugar source available should a diabetic go into insulin shock (caused by having insufficient glucose in their system). This can be noted in the patient's behavior as well as appearance. Usually, patients who have diabetes will sense that they are feeling unusual, and you will have time to administer sugar to them. Monitor their vital signs carefully at this point, and determine if further medical intervention is necessary. Chapter 18, Responding to Medical Emergencies, provides more information about care for diabetic emergencies.

Patients with diabetes should also be carefully advised about the importance of oral hygiene, as a link has been increasingly demonstrated between uncontrolled periodontal disease and a worsening diabetic condition.

Thyroid Conditions

Hyperthyroidism, also known as an *overactive thyroid*, is a condition caused when the thyroid produces too much thyroxine. This can cause sweating, weight loss, a fast heartbeat, and nervousness. Hyperthyroidism is usually treated with medications, radiation, or surgery. Patients who have hyperthyroidism may be sensitive to medication, including epinephrine, so it is essential that you have an accurate medical and medication history.

Hypothyroidism, also known as an *underactive thyroid*, results when the thyroid produces insufficient hormones. This can cause weight gain and symptoms such as cold intolerance, depression, and fatigue. Patients suffering from hypothyroidism may be more susceptible to the effects of depressants, narcotic analgesics, or sedatives.

✔ **CHECKPOINT**
22-21 Why is it important to avoid infection in patients who have diabetes?

Other Health Conditions

Arthritis

Although there are 22 different types of arthritis, the two most common are osteoarthritis and rheumatoid arthritis. Both are characterized by pain and stiffness caused by inflammation in joints including the knees, wrists, or spinal column. Other symptoms may include redness, decreased range of motion, swelling, dry eyes and mouth, fatigue, and breathing problems.

Like many chronic diseases, arthritis symptoms may worsen throughout the day. Patients who have arthritis may prefer morning appointments. Be sensitive to the patient's pain, need for assistance getting in and out of the dental chair, comfort level in the chair, and ability to open the mouth and assume other positions as requested. For patients who have severe arthritis, you may want to show them assistive gripping devices to help hold the toothbrush. They may also require bite blocks to help them keep their mouth open during procedures.

Muscular Dystrophy

In **muscular dystrophy**, a group of inherited muscle diseases, muscle fibers are very susceptible to damage. The muscles weaken progressively and, late in this disease, are replaced by fat and connective tissue.

Muscular dystrophy can be slowed with medication and therapy, but the disease is incurable. Symptoms include muscle weakness, lack of coordination, and loss of mobility.

Patients who have muscular dystrophy may lose lung capacity and have a compromised ability to cough or clear their throat. Patients who are affected in this way may not be candidates for sedation or anesthesia. Pay careful attention to the positioning of instruments, because aspiration may be a concern.

✔ **CHECKPOINT**
22-22 Patients with arthritis, like those who have many other chronic conditions, may prefer or do better at appointments at what time of day?

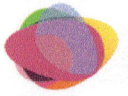

Chapter Highlights

✦ Dental professionals should strive to maximize the well-being and health of every patient, regardless of special needs, such as physical or intellectual disabilities.

✦ Patients who have special needs may require extra assistance to achieve optimal health, including oral health. "Special needs" refers to mental, emotional and physical disabilities as well as cultural and language differences.

✦ Providing care to special needs patients may require extra attention and awareness to their needs and increased communication with patients and among staff team members.

✦ Patient education is often critical for special needs patients, including demonstrating techniques and creative ways to accomplish oral hygiene goals.

◆ The Americans with Disabilities Act (ADA) prevents discrimination based on disability. The ADA requires that access to medical facilities be manageable by everyone.

◆ The dental team should gather as much information in advance to best serve a new patient who has special needs, including mailing medical and medication history forms in advance; determining if extra time or staff or assistive devices are required for the appointment; and talking to the patient's physician if necessary.

◆ The dental provider must work with a caregiver, parent, or family member of the patient if communication with the patient is unsuccessful because of a disability. However, every effort should be made to communicate directly with the patient during the dental appointment.

◆ You play an important role in helping to optimize the patient's visit—making it more relaxing, comfortable, and informative. Patients who feel accommodated and appreciated may be more likely to comply with recommendations to maximize their oral health.

◆ When communicating with or about patients who have special needs or disabilities it is important to put the person first, disability second: "a person with a physical disability," not "a disabled person."

◆ You should be familiar with assistive devices used in the dental office as well as those patients or their caregivers can use for self-care. You should be able to instruct caregivers on how to provide oral hygiene care to another person, and direct patients and their caregivers to where to find these resources and how to modify existing tools for ease of patient use.

◆ Maintain an accurate and current medical and medication status for all patients, especially those who have special needs and may have multiple medical conditions and may take several medications.

◆ Look to patients for guidance about whether they need assistance walking to the exam room or getting in or out of the dental chair.

◆ Make sure the treatment room not only has room for a patient in a wheelchair or walker to enter and be seated but also room for a patient's caregiver to be seated. Some patients who use wheelchairs may need to remain in their special chair during treatment.

◆ Patients who have special needs may have requirements including: appointments at certain times of day when the condition is least aggravating, the dental chair in a more upright position, preventive antibiotics prior to treatment to avoid infection, calming sedation or no sedation at all, and verification that drugs administered are not contraindicated with any prescription medications routinely taken.

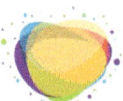 **Review Questions**

1. What is it so important to be attentive to the dental needs of special needs patients?

   a. They may have difficulty with self-care

   b. They may take medications that compromise their oral health

   c. They may have chronic medical conditions that can be worsened by the effects of poor oral health

   d. All of the above

2. Which of these does the Americans with Disabilities Act require of dental practices?

   a. Building entrances accessible by all patients

   b. Special discounts for patients who use wheelchairs

   c. Special lifts that elevate and tilt the patient's wheelchair for ease during treatment

   d. On-site interpreters for patients who speak other languages

3. Why might it be advised for a dental team to contact a special needs patient's physician or medical provider?

   a. To determine if caring for the patient will be a burden

   b. To determine if medications used during dental treatment might be contraindicated with another medication the patient takes or a condition the patient has

   c. To determine if the patient can pay for treatment

   d. To determine how the patient got in his or her current condition

4. What might patients rely on dental assistants for expertise about?

   a. How to adapt existing self-care tools, such as a toothbrush, for patients who are challenged to use them in the traditional way

   b. Where to purchase adaptive products

   c. How to instruct a caregiver in brushing and flossing the patient's teeth

   d. All of the above

5. When you are treating a visually impaired patient, which of these should you not do?

   a. Tell the patient when you enter and exit the room so he or she knows who is present

   b. Tell the patient before you touch him or her during treatment

   c. Whisper or gesture to other staff members in the treatment room

   d. Explain what is happening throughout the procedure so the patient is informed

6. When you are treating a patient who uses a wheelchair, which of these is true?

   a. Assume the patient needs help transferring to the dental chair

   b. Watch for a clue from the patient about whether or not help is needed; when unsure, ask the patient directly if they would like assistance

   c. Ask the accompanying caregiver or family member if the patient needs help transferring to the dental chair

   d. Never help the patient with a transfer to the dental chair, for reasons of liability

7. Which of these statements is true?

   a. People who have mental retardation all have the same level of functioning

   b. You should treat patients who have mental retardation just like children

   c. You are not required to communicate directly with patients who have mental retardation; instead relay information through their caregivers

   d. People who have mental retardation have various levels of functioning, and many of these individuals also have other types of challenges including physical disabilities

8. Patients with which of these condition, in particular, might need the dental chair semi-upright instead of reclining?

   a. Hemophilia

   b. Bulimia

   c. Cardiovascular disease

   d. Alzheimer disease

9. Which of these diseases or conditions causes an inability of blood to clot properly?

   a. Arthritis

   b. Hemophilia

   c. Hypothyroidism

   d. Hyperthyroidism

10. Which of these diseases or conditions is progressive?

   a. Cerebral palsy

   b. Alzheimer disease

   c. Seizure disorder

   d. Hemophilia

11. Which of these is an autoimmune disease in which the body's immune system destroys the protective sheath covering the nerves?

   a. Alzheimer disease

   b. Type 1 diabetes

   c. Down syndrome

   d. Multiple sclerosis

12. Which of these is a group of diseases that affect how the body uses blood glucose?

   a. Down syndrome

   b. Seizure disorder

   c. Autism

   d. Diabetes

Active Learning Exercises

1. What is the significance of the Americans with Disabilities Act? Can you think of three obstacles a patient with a disability might encounter if this act was not recognized or enforced?

2. Patients with mental retardation or other impairment may find it difficult to perform self-care. What are some recommendations you could make to the guardian or caretaker about proper tooth brushing and use of oral aids?

3. When patients who use wheelchairs present to the office, it may be difficult for them to move into the dental chair. Describe the safest way to perform a wheelchair transfer both to and from the dental chair.

CHAPTER 22 PATIENTS WITH SPECIAL NEEDS

Application Activities

1. Make a list of educational resources, including booklets, videos, and online resources, that show patients and caregivers how to do oral self-care. The list should include resources available from advocacy organizations for special needs patients, such as mental retardation and visual and hearing impairment.

2. Make a list of basic sentences you might use to communicate in the dental office with patients who speak the most common non-English language in your geographic area.

3. Think about how you could communicate the basics of oral self-care visually and through play with pediatric patients or those who are developmentally and intellectually at a child's level. Then, assemble a toolkit of materials to use with these patients.

4. Research do-it-yourself ways to modify toothbrushes for patients who have special needs. Prepare some of these ways yourself and try using them so you are familiar with them and can demonstrate them to patients.

PREPARING FOR CERTIFICATION EXAMS

Review the following topics in this chapter to prepare for the Dental Assisting National Board (DANB) exam:

- **Introduction**
- **Communication**
- **Medically Compromised Patients**
- **Neurological Disorders**
- **Pulmonary Disorders**
- **Cardiovascular Disorders**
- **Blood Disorders**
- **Endocrine Disorders**
- **Other Health Conditions**

chapter 23

Communication

CHAPTER CHECKLIST

On completion of this chapter, students will be able to:

- ☑ Describe the elements in the communication process.
- ☑ Describe types of verbal and nonverbal communication.
- ☑ Discuss active listening skills and their importance in the communication process.
- ☑ Discuss strategies for communicating effectively with patients.
- ☑ Discuss how to communicate effectively with other health professionals.
- ☑ Explain how to communicate properly on the telephone, including taking messages.
- ☑ Explain how to communicate properly in writing, including business and electronic communications.
- ☑ Identify ways in which verbal and nonverbal communication is affected by a patient's cultural or ethnic background.

KEY TERMS

active listening – a form of listening that involves giving full attention to the sender and the message communicated

clarification – an understanding of the message communicated

communication – the ways information is sent, received, and responded to

feedback – the receiver's response to a message communicated

kinesics (kih-NEE-siks) – positioning of the body

medium – how communication takes place, such as face-to-face, over the telephone, or in writing

message – the information communicated

nonverbal communication – communication that occurs outside words or language, including body gestures, facial expressions, and eye contact

receiver – the person receiving the message from the sender

sender – the person communicating the message

verbal communication – communication using words or language

Introduction

The dental assistant (DA) is responsible for much of the communication between dental staff and the patient. Effective communication is vital to a successful working relationship both between the dental team and the patient, and within the dental team itself. Learning and using effective verbal and nonverbal communication skills will ensure that you are a valuable and successful part of the dental team. Communication is especially important in our increasingly diverse world. Also important are communications with other health professionals as well as written and telephone communication.

The Communication Process

Communication includes the ways in which we send, receive, and respond to information. In addition to providing information, communication is also important for understanding how others think and feel. For DAs, good communication is necessary for exchanging important information as well as building positive relationships with patients, coworkers, and supervisors.

The communication process includes the following:

- The **message,** or what is being communicated
- The **sender**, or the person communicating the message
- The **medium**, or how communication is made (such as face-to-face, over the telephone, or in writing)
- The **receiver**, or the person receiving the message from the sender
- **Feedback**, or the receiver's response to the message being communicated

During communication, two or more people play different roles as the sender and the receiver. Feedback and **clarification**, or an understanding of the message, are important for both the sender and the receiver. One way to think about communication is to think of a seesaw: both people play different roles (one person providing weight on the ground and one person balancing in the air), but both roles are needed in order to make the seesaw work correctly. The same can be said for communication.

DAs should communicate in a way that conveys professionalism, care, and concern. Conversations will often focus on office procedures, policies, and patient care. Part of good communication includes:

- Clarifying messages to avoid confusion ("Let me explain that again in another way.")
- Confirming the patient's perception ("Yes, we will be sure to call you 24 hours after the procedure to check on you.")
- Adapting messages to the patient's level of understanding (for example, saying *heart attack* instead of *myocardial infarction* when appropriate)

- Asking for feedback to make sure messages are understood by the receiver ("Does what I just explained make sense, or should I go over that again?")

From Classroom to Clinic

Though some students initially consider role-playing or doing skits in school silly, they often find once they reach the clinical setting that such activities have enhanced their ability to communicate. Dental assistants must be able to communicate effectively not only with patients but also with office team members. Classroom training and role-playing can be practice for the "real world."

If your class doesn't include role-playing, you can get together with your peers and run through a variety of scenarios. This preparation will help you navigate potentially difficult situations in the office.

Communication can be both verbal and nonverbal. **Verbal communication** involves exchanging messages using words or language. Strong verbal skills are a necessary part of successfully completing everyday tasks, such as making appointments, educating patients about procedures and policies, making referrals, and sharing information with coworkers and supervisors. Table 23-1 has a list of common issues in verbal communication.

When practicing good communication skills, remember that it is not just what you say but *how you say it* that can make a difference. Along with words and language, verbal communication includes tone of voice, volume, and use of language such as sarcasm. These can send information just as powerfully as the actual words spoken and can make a significant difference in how the receiver hears (or does not hear) the message communicated. For instance, sighing, grunting, and moaning can show boredom, lack of interest, or negative emotions. Smiling and using a happy, upbeat tone can show friendliness and make the receiver feel welcomed. Being mindful of all parts of verbal communication is the only way to make sure communication is successful.

Speaking Skills

Speaking is part of everyday communication and is so common that people are often unaware of just how important it is. The choice of words can make a big difference in whether a message is understood and how it is received. How might someone with little education receive technical, advanced language? How might overly casual language sound in the workplace? Think about how you speak to friends or family compared to how you speak with teachers or supervisors. Speaking skills that are critical to good communication are listed below and in Table 23-2.

- Voice Quality—How does your voice sound? Soothing and quiet? Gruff and short? Make sure the quality of your voice is appropriate for the situation. If you are preparing a patient for a procedure, would you want

TABLE 23-1 Common Dos and Don'ts of Verbal Communication in the Workplace

DO...	DON'T...
Be professional at all times.	Use casual words or phrases inappropriately
Be polite at all times.	Forget to use words like "please" and "thank you"
Say, "Yes, that's correct," and other formal phrases	Say "yup" or "uh-huh"
Say, "No, that's not quite right," and other formal phrases	Say "nope" or "uh-uh"
Say, "Excuse me?"; "Pardon me?"; or, "Could you please repeat that?"	Say "huh?" Or "what?"
Save technical or advanced terms for patients and professionals that have advanced education or knowledge.	Speak down to patients or use words that do not match the patient's level of education or training
Adapt your language to children's needs. For instance, some dental assistants like to use funny names for dental instruments, like calling a polishing brush "Mr. Bumpy." These silly names can help put children at ease, but remember not to use such language with adults.	Expect children to have the same understanding of words and phrases as adults

your voice to be loud and rough or soft and gentle? How might this make a difference to the patient?

- Use of Questions—Asking questions can show interest and warmth. Common questions such as, "How is your day going?" or "Did you have any trouble finding our office?" can put patients at ease. But be careful not to ask inappropriate questions or too many questions. Silence is actually an important part of communicating because it allows the receiver a chance to think about the message and provide feedback. Some people are not comfortable with silence and may feel the need to fill the silence with words. Practice limiting questions and becoming more comfortable with silence.
- Feedback—Giving feedback is critical to good communication because it shows that the receiver is listening and has thought about the message. It also shows basic respect to the message sender.

Listening Skills

Listening is an important part of the communication process. **Active listening** is a form of listening that involves giving full attention to the sender and to the message communicated. This is not always as easy as it seems. In everyday communication, it is not unusual for our minds to wander, or for sounds and objects to distract us from the communication process. However, in order to keep communication strong, it is important to pay attention and focus on the message. In addition to paying attention and ignoring distractions, active listening also involves keeping eye contact with the sender. This can actually help you stay focused and tune out distractions. Good listening means that interruptions are kept to a minimum, and that the receiver actually hears the message being sent rather than being busy thinking of a response.

Nonverbal Communication

Even though it may seem like words are the most important part of communication, what we do not say can be just as important—and powerful. **Nonverbal communication** is communication that occurs without words. It might surprise you to know that nonverbal cues (such as facial

TABLE 23-2 The Five Cs of Effective Verbal Communication

Clear	Make sure the message is easy to understand.
	Speak carefully and clearly.
Concise	Messages should have the necessary information and nothing extra.
	Do not give unneeded or inappropriate information.
Complete	Messages should contain all of the information needed.
	Do not leave out important details.
Courteous	Be polite and deliver messages in a kind manner.
	Be aware of others' feelings and possible reactions to the message.
Consistent	Messages should make sense and be logical.
	Think about what you need to say before you say it.
	Do not drift off topic; stick to the information needed.

TABLE 23-3 Nonverbal Communication

Kinesics, or body movements	■ What is your posture? Are you slouching or sitting upright, at attention? ■ Are the sender and receiver facing one another, or is someone turned away?
Facial expressions	■ Are you smiling? Rolling your eyes? Frowning? ■ Do you have a blank expression on your face?
Hand gestures	■ Do you wave hello when greeting someone? ■ Are your arms crossed across your chest?
Physical distance	■ Are you seated or standing closer than 12 inches to the sender or receiver? ■ Are you backed away at a far distance?

expressions, hand gestures, and posture) make up nearly 70% of your total message! Table 23-3 shows some of the ways you communicate nonverbally.

Nonverbal communication can show thoughts and inner feelings, such as sadness, frustration, anger, nervousness, and lack of interest. For example, making eye contact is one of the most basic forms of nonverbal communication. Looking someone in the eyes can communicate feelings of interest, attention, and respect. However, staring someone in the eyes can also communicate anger or feeling upset. On the other hand, avoiding eye contact can communicate shyness, lack of attention, boredom, or disrespect. It is important to recognize that something as simple as nonverbal communication can actually say quite a lot.

DAs frequently use nonverbal communication because patients are not always able to communicate verbally due to the dental instruments or their dental problems. Also, patients are very aware of the facial expressions and body language of their dental care providers because they spend much of the time facing one another and sitting close to one another. Be sure to pay attention to your own nonverbal communication as well as that of your patient. Table 23-4 shows some of these examples.

Controlling Nonverbal Communication

Just being aware of different types of nonverbal communication is one of the best ways to control nonverbal cues and make sure communication is clear. Practice paying attention to body posture, physical distance, and other nonverbal cues while communicating with friends and family. Notice other people's nonverbal communication and think about the messages they are sending just by how they make eye contact, sit, stand, and gesture. Here are some specific ways to practice being aware of and controlling nonverbal communication skills.

■ Be Attentive—Use body language and gestures to let the person know you are listening. Face the speaker. Use body posture and body language to show that you are paying attention.

■ Make Eye Contact—Make eye contact with the person speaking to you. Do not allow yourself to look away unless you are doing so temporarily such as to take notes. Keeping eye contact while the speaker is talking lets him or her know that you are actively listening.

■ Get Engaged—Engaging with the speaker, such as by smiling or nodding the head, lets the speaker know that you hear and understand the message. Learning how to engage in all conversations helps you listen more actively.

■ Stay Open—Staying open means using body language, eye contact, gestures, and facial expressions that show the speaker that you are interested and engaged. This includes keeping arms at the side or not crossed across the body, making good eye contact, and using friendly and warm facial expressions.

■ Learn Body Language—Body language plays a big role when communicating with others. To let others know you are actively listening, make eye contact, relax the arms and legs, and make sure your facial expression is kind and friendly. Understanding how to "read" other people's body language will help you understand their feelings and state of mind, and make you more aware of your own body language as well.

Cultural Diversity

It is important to remember that the meaning of gestures can differ among cultures. For example, in the United States, the "thumbs up" signal indicates that everything is okay. In some countries, however, such as Thailand, India, and Iran, this sign means the same as what the middle finger means here. In Japan, it indicates a male. Shaking hands, bowing, pointing, and nodding are other gestures that may mean different things to different people. We must not take the meaning of our gestures for granted to avoid offending our patients.

CHECKPOINTS

23-1 What are the five basic parts of the communication process?

23-2 What are some examples of nonverbal communication?

TABLE 23-4 What Your Nonverbal Communication Might Say

IF YOU ARE COMMUNICATING LIKE THIS...	...YOU MIGHT BE SAYING THIS
Arms crossed	■ I am upset with you ■ I am angry ■ I am bored
Slouching or poor posture	■ I do not want to be here ■ Do not take me seriously
Using hands when talking	■ I am excited or happy ■ I am upset ■ Pay attention to what I am telling you
Leaning in close (less than 12 inches) while speaking	■ I want to share something private ■ I feel close to you
Wide open eyes, eyebrows raised	■ I am scared ■ I am surprised

Communicating with Patients

Communicating with patients is among the most important jobs of a DA. Without good patient communication, you cannot perform your job successfully—which means patients cannot receive the oral care they need and deserve. Communication truly is the bridge to good dental health.

However, communication can sometimes be inhibited through no fault of the patient or the DA. Many patients do not speak English as their first language—or may not speak English at all. In such cases, the ideal alternative is translation—enlist the aid of someone, such as a family member, who shares languages with both you and your patient to help you communicate. If you can speak your patient's first language, so much the better. A DA who speaks Spanish, for example, is an invaluable aid in today's dentist office in many areas. See the section on diversity later in the chapter for helpful tips about establishing good lines of communication with non-English-speaking patients.

Not only spoken words are important when communicating with a patient. Although no one is a mind reader, it is important to understand what patients are thinking or

TABLE 23-5 Examples of Effective Patient Communication

Reflecting	■ Repeat what the patient said, but do this only occasionally. Do not be a parrot! ■ Start the sentence, but let the patient finish it; he or she may provide additional information.	"You were saying that it hurts sometimes when …"
Paraphrasing or restating	■ Repeat what the patient said using your own words.	"Let me get this straight: you had two procedures last year, but the most recent one was done in another state?"
Clarifying, or asking for examples	■ When in doubt, ask the patient to give additional information.	"You said that you haven't been feeling well for the past week. What do you mean by that? Can you tell me specifically what's wrong?"
Using open-ended questions	■ Ask questions that allow the patient to answer in greater detail rather than simply saying "yes" or "no." Simple yes-or-no questions may lead the patient to leave out important information.	Rather than asking yes-or-no type questions (such as, "Have you had any teeth removed?"), use an open-ended question, such as, "Tell me about any oral surgeries you have had."
Summarizing	■ Briefly review the information to make sure the message is understood. This gives the patient a chance to give any additional information that might have been forgotten or correct any misunderstandings.	"Overall, you've had one root canal in the past year, but otherwise, you've had no other problems with your teeth."

feeling. Patients may use words to directly tell how they feel or what is on their mind, but often they will not. This is where active listening and "reading" nonverbal cues come in handy. Why is it important to understand patients' thoughts and feelings?

■ *To help patients feel calm and relaxed.* Going to the dentist is not many people's idea of fun. Patients are more likely to keep their appointments and maintain good oral health if they trust and feel respected by their dental care providers.

■ *To help make sure patient education is understood.* If patients are not sure what to do or how to take care of their teeth, their oral health may suffer.

■ *To make DAs aware of patient questions or worries.* Knowing what concerns your patient has will help you know how and when to provide education and reassurance.

Guidelines for Effective Patient Communication

Poor patient communication can lead to confusion and misunderstandings. Be clear and specific when communicating with patients. For instance, giving instructions such as, "Return to the office if you do not feel well" is less clear than saying something as specific as, "Return to

the office if you have any tooth pain, difficulty chewing or swallowing, or notice any bleeding in the next 3 days." See the difference? The clearer the message, the more likely it will be understood. Table 23-5 contains other important tips for successful patient communication.

Good communication starts the moment you say, "hello." Greeting someone properly can set a welcoming and warm tone that makes patients feel at ease. Calling patients by their first names is not appropriate unless they have instructed you to do so. Use proper titles, such as *Mr.*, *Mrs.*, *Ms.* (if you are unsure whether a woman is married or not), or *Doctor.* These show respect and are a courtesy that can go a long way in creating positive relationships with patients. Expressions such as *honey, sweetie,* and *sugar* are not appropriate, no matter how well you know a patient. Also, do not refer to patients by their medical condition. For instance, do not say, "The cracked tooth in Exam 4." Instead, take the time to say, "Mr. Jones, who is here with a cracked tooth, is in Exam 4." Remember: people are people—people are not their medical or dental conditions. Finally, although DAs want be warm and friendly toward patients, it is important to know how to maintain a professional distance and not be overly casual. Always remember to be professional first and friendly second.

And remember that friendliness can take a variety of forms. Before simply taking the lead in conversation, cautiously test the waters to see how your patient responds. Does the patient seem unwilling to engage in conversation? Willing but guarded? Open and talkative? Silent and withdrawn? Instead of forcing the patient to respond to your style of conversation, respond to your patient's. Be a good conversation partner—even if that means staying quiet except for explanations of dental procedures. Do not be afraid of silence if that is what your patient prefers—many DAs try to fill up the silence but doing so may prompt patient complaints. Also note that some offices have particular policies concerning interaction with patients. To help you create the most suitable and helpful environment possible, discuss your office's policy with the dentist to learn his or her preferences.

Is It Possible to be Too Friendly?

Do you:

- Touch your patients inappropriately, such as placing your hand on their back or knee when speaking to them?
- Stand or sit excessively close (less than 12 inches) when not working on patients?
- Ask personal questions about the patient's romantic life, family, or financial situation?
- Speak at length about your own personal life, financial situation, or personal relationships?

Remember: Be friendly, but be professional first!

Communicating with Health Professionals

Health professionals depend on DAs for information to provide quality care to patients. Communication with health professionals should always be proper and never casual. Follow these guidelines when communicating with health professionals:

- Always call a physician or dentist *Doctor* unless he or she tells you otherwise.
- Never call a health professional by his or her first name in front of a patient.
- Use proper medical terms. If you are unsure of the correct term, explain the condition rather than use an inappropriate or casual term.
- Speak confidently to show other health professionals that you are competent and respectful.
- Be honest if you do not know something. It is always better to ask than to make an incorrect assumption.
- When communicating with coworkers, keep the topics professional. Conversations about nonwork subjects should be saved for breaks and should never take place in front of patients. Also, loud talking, joking, and laughing can make the work environment

uncomfortable for patients and other coworkers. When in doubt, be professional!

Extra Patient Care

Communication is key to all relationships but especially those with our dental patients. Recently, a patient who spoke poor English was given a new upper denture. When she complained the next morning that the teeth did not fit, my dental team was confused because we knew it fit perfectly and was measured accurately. When we finally asked what she meant when she said they did not fit, she responded, "They do not fit in my soaking glass!" We were relieved and had quite a laugh, but it just goes to show that you should always ask questions before assuming something is wrong.

CHECKPOINT

23-3 Why is it helpful to use open-ended questions during patient communication?

Telephone Skills

DAs frequently use the telephone as a way of communicating with patients and insurance companies. Telephone skills help create a positive image of the dental office as a professional and friendly environment. However, not being able to communicate face to face can be challenging and requires specific skills. Table 23-6 includes tips on how to handle specific types of calls. Follow these guidelines to practice telephone skills that show respect, professionalism, and care.

- Answer incoming calls quickly—by the second ring, if possible.
- Remember to use a positive and friendly tone.
- Identify the office and yourself by saying, "Dr. Jones' office, this is Mary speaking. How may I help you?"
- Always ask the caller if he or she can be placed on hold; do not immediately place the caller on hold upon answering the phone.
- If a call comes in during the middle of another call, ask the person you are speaking with if you can place him or her on hold. Wait for a reply before placing him or her on hold.
- Explain to the second caller that you are on another line and need to finish that call. Do not take the second call unless:
  - It is an emergency
  - It is a long distance call that cannot be given to another coworker
  - It is a doctor calling to speak with another doctor
- If you cannot take a call off hold after 90 seconds, check back and ask if the caller wants to continue holding.

TABLE 23-6 How to Handle Different Types of Telephone Calls

Billing questions	■ Do not give exact prices; explain that charges depend on the type of procedures and tests performed.
	■ If insurance companies call with questions about billing, make sure to confirm their identity before giving out confidential information about a patient.
Test results	■ If test results are called in by a medical lab, write down the information and place it in the front of the patient's chart.
	■ If the test results are *stat*, this means they are needed immediately. Do not place them in the front of the chart, and instead bring them immediately to the dentist.
	■ Patients may call wanting to know their test results. Some offices give this information over the telephone and some do not. Know your office's policy before giving results over the telephone.
Progress reports	■ Patients may call the office to report how they are feeling. Make a note of these calls and place it in the patient's chart.
	■ The dentist must speak with patients who report that they are not making good progress. Make sure to let the dentist know who the patient is, and if he or she has any new symptoms or worsening conditions.
Prescription refills	■ Dental assistants may handle calls about prescription refills if the patient chart shows that refills are allowed. When in doubt, tell the patient or pharmacist that you will check with the dentist and will call back.
Unidentified callers	■ A caller may not wish to leave his or her name or explain the reason he or she is calling. Politely explain that the dentist is busy, but you will be happy to take a message.
	■ If the caller still does not wish to give you the needed information, ask him or her to call back at a time when the dentist will be available. Then let the dentist know about the call.
Angry callers	■ If a caller is angry, remain calm and do not lose your temper.
	■ Remind the caller that you want to help.
	■ Listen carefully and take notes.
	■ If you cannot take care of the caller's problem, gently explain to him or her that you must speak with your supervisor first and offer to call back as soon as possible.
	■ Always tell the dentist about caller complaints about fees or dental care.

■ If a hold lasts longer than 3 minutes, apologize to the caller and offer to call back as soon as you can.

Taking phone messages is an important part of a DA's daily duties. The office should have notepads specially designed for taking messages (Figure 23-1). At a minimum, the telephone message form should have places to write the following information:

■ The caller's name
■ The date and time of the call
■ The phone number where the caller can be reached
■ A short description of the caller's message
■ The person to whom you are giving the message
■ Your initials, so that the person who receives the call can check with you if he or she has any questions

From the Dentist's Perspective

If I could be in 10 places at once, I would. I sure could get a lot more done! But unfortunately, I cannot, which means I have to rely on my dental assistants to help determine which matters need immediate attention and which can wait. Screening phone calls is an important part of this process because I do not like taking my attention away from the patients in my office unless it is absolutely necessary. When someone calls, I ask my dental assistants to gather some basic information about the call, such as the nature of the problem, whether it is an emergency, and where I can reach the caller. It is also helpful for the dental assistant to let the caller know that, although I am unable to speak with him at that moment, I will return his or her call as soon as possible. No one enjoys waiting, but telephone screening helps me give all patients the attention and care they deserve.

TO Dr. Garcia

DATE 9-28-10   TIME 2:15

MESSAGE

M rs. Horowitz

of

Phone No. (555) 123-4567

TELEPHONED	X	PLEASE CALL	X
WAS IN TO SEE YOU		WILL CALL BACK	
WANTS TO SEE YOU		**URGENT**	
RETURNED YOUR CALL			

Message

Her mouth is swollen and she's in a lot of pain. Please call back.

Operator CM

Figure 23–1 Telephone message.

After taking a message, tell the caller when to expect a return call. Some offices wait until the end of the day to return non-emergency calls and other offices return calls throughout the day. Know your office's policy so you can inform callers.

Make sure you understand the office telephone system. Unlike the telephone you may use at home, office telephones often have features that you might not be used to, including:

- The *hold* feature
- *Call forwarding*, to send a call to another phone in the office
- *Voice messaging* services, including retrieval

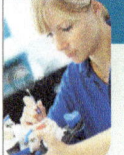

Voice of Experience

No one likes to feel unimportant. That's why when an urgent phone call comes in for the dentist, I use a nifty trick to alert him without making the patient feel as though he or she is less important. Rather than announcing it in front of the patient, I simply write on a piece of paper that there is an urgent phone call and what line the caller is on. I get the dentist's attention by clearing my throat or saying something as simple as, "Excuse me, doctor." After holding up the note, he can excuse himself to take the call without the patient ever knowing. I usually like to reassure the patient that the dentist will be right back and then I stay with the patient until the dentist returns.

- *Three-way calling* to allow a third person to join a phone conversation
- The *intercom* feature, to make an announcement to be heard throughout the office

Most office phones come with user instructions. Be sure to review these before making calls, or practice using some of the features. Accidentally hanging up on a patient or losing a call is learning the hard way. Prepare ahead of time so that you can use the office telephone system confidently.

Writing Skills

The ability to write clearly and accurately is critical to providing patient instructions, recording patient information in medical records, and communicating about appointments, fees, and other office policies. In general, when using written communication, remember that poor writing makes the writer appear unprofessional. No matter what type of written communication is used, it is important to remember three rules of writing—easily remembered as the ABCs of writing:

- A—Always be professional
- B—Be clear in stating the message
- C—Check for errors

Most dental offices have word processing programs for typing letters and office documents. Be sure to review how to use these programs and ask the office manager if you have any questions. Be careful to avoid any spelling or grammatical errors in official written communications, which can make you and the members of the entire dental office appear careless or incompetent, possibly causing the patient to lose confidence in the team. Spreadsheets and office management software are commonly used to organize patient information and appointments. If you are asked to use these programs, sit down with the office manager and make sure you know how to properly open the program, enter information, and save information. If you are using a program and are unsure how to perform an action, such as saving or opening a document, stop and ask someone. Guessing can lead to files being saved incorrectly—or even erased. Many offices now use computers with backup drives; if your office uses a backup system, be sure you are familiar with how to use it appropriately.

Business Letters

Business letters may be sent to patients, insurance companies, drug companies, health care providers, and other businesses. Follow these three steps to make sure business letters are both professional and effective.

1. *Be prepared.* Before you sit down to write the letter, plan out what to say, how to say it, and what you want the reader to do.
2. *Compose your business letter properly by stating your message clearly.* Be short and to the point. Avoid being wordy and using long sentences.
3. *Make sure to edit your letter.* Reviewing the business letter for errors is one of the most important steps. Misspellings and incorrect grammar can appear sloppy and unprofessional. Check your letter for spelling, grammar, punctuation, capitalization, and overall logic and organization of the letter. If possible, have a coworker in the office read it for errors. Also, ask the coworker to make sure the letter makes sense and that the message is clear.

A typical business letter may include the following elements (Figure 23-2):

1. Letterhead—This shows the contact information for the office.
2. Date—Place two to four spaces below the letterhead.
3. Inside address—This is the address of the person to whom the letter will be sent. Place two spaces below the date.

4. Subject line—This shows the reader what the letter is about. This may be optional.
5. Salutation—This is the greeting that starts the letter. It is two lines below the subject line or inside address. Make sure to use the reader's title, such as *Doctor* or *Mrs.*, along with a last name.
6. Body—This is the part of the letter that contains the message.
7. Closing—This ends the letter. Place two lines after the end of the body of the message.
8. Signature and name—Type the name and title of the person signing the letter. Allow four lines after the closing.
9. Identification line—The upper initials tell who composed the letter. The lowercase letters tell who prepared it. This is optional.
10. Enclosure—If something is included with the letter, use the initials *Enc.* to indicate that. If more than one document is enclosed, place the number of enclosures in parentheses.
11. Copy—Use the letters *cc:* to show that a copy of the letter was sent somewhere else.

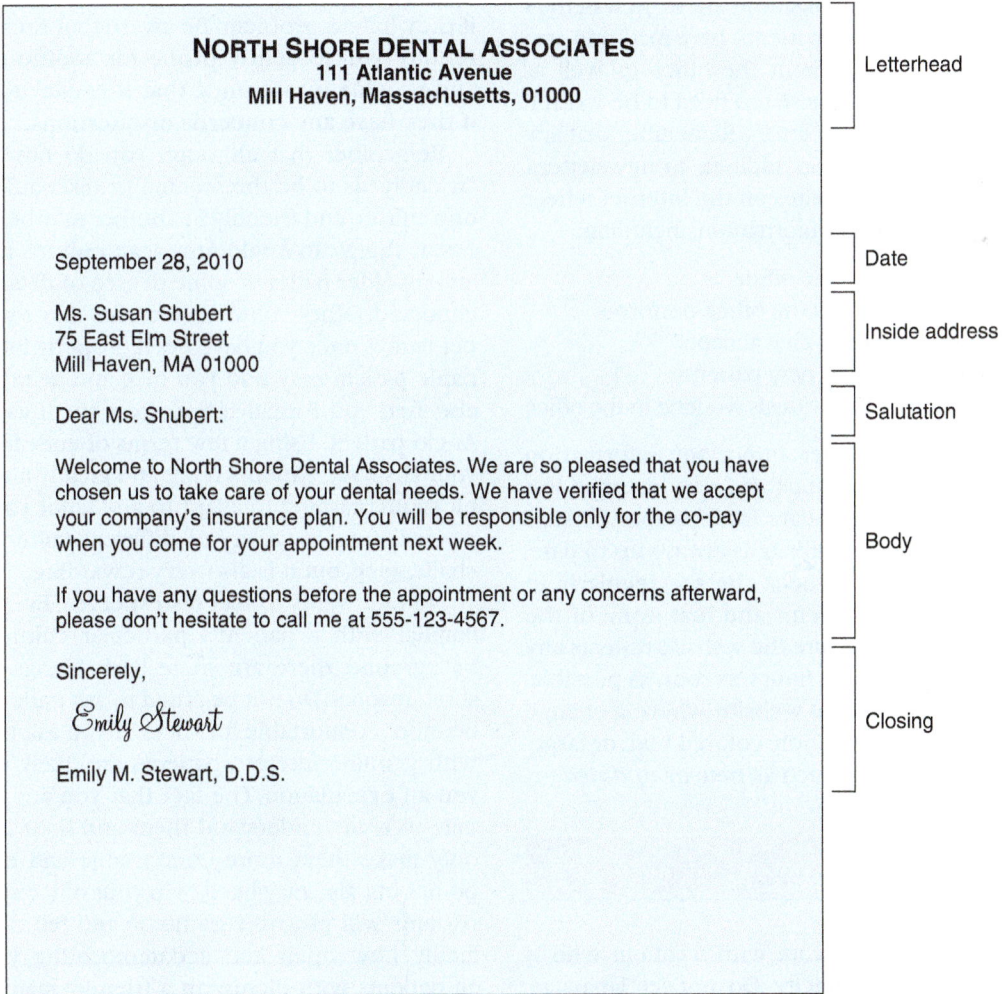

NORTH SHORE DENTAL ASSOCIATES
111 Atlantic Avenue
Mill Haven, Massachusetts, 01000

Letterhead

September 28, 2010

Date

Ms. Susan Shubert
75 East Elm Street
Mill Haven, MA 01000

Inside address

Dear Ms. Shubert:

Salutation

Welcome to North Shore Dental Associates. We are so pleased that you have chosen us to take care of your dental needs. We have verified that we accept your company's insurance plan. You will be responsible only for the co-pay when you come for your appointment next week.

If you have any questions before the appointment or any concerns afterward, please don't hesitate to call me at 555-123-4567.

Body

Sincerely,

Emily Stewart

Emily M. Stewart, D.D.S.

Closing

Figure 23–2 Business letter.

✔ **CHECKPOINTS**

23-4 What important information should be recorded when taking a telephone message?

23-5 What are the ABCs of good written communication?

Electronic Communication

Electronic mail, or e-mail, is one of the most common forms of written communication used today. E-mail is convenient because it allows written communication to be sent and received quickly. However, e-mail is used so frequently in our everyday lives, that it is easy to forget that electronic writing also must be professional and business-like. The same ABCs of written communication also apply to electronic communication. For example, when e-mailing patients, be sure to check for spelling and grammar errors. Most e-mail programs have a spell checker to review misspellings automatically, but many mistakes will not be caught by the spell checker. You still need to review the e-mail yourself and not rely on the computer to catch any mistakes!

More and more offices are using electronic newsletters as a form of patient communication. These newsletters are generally sent directly to patients by e-mail and can provide helpful information about the office as well as general medical information. These too need to be written professionally and reviewed for errors. Remember that any writing reflects on the office. In addition to newsletters, some offices have created websites on the Internet where patients can access important information, including:

- The location and hours of the office
- A description of the services the office performs
- The types of insurance the office accepts
- Whether the office is taking new patients
- Pictures and/or names of individuals working in the office

Websites help patients gather important information about the dental office in a quick and easy manner. But no one likes to receive out-of-date information! Be sure that the information on the website is always up to date. Have someone in the office check the site regularly to make sure there are no problems and that none of the information has changed. Be sure the website reflects any changes, such as new business hours, as soon as possible. It is helpful to indicate on the website where a change has been made by using animation, colored text, or large-sized text, along with words such as *new* or *updated*.

Diversity

Every DA will at some point work with a patient who is from another culture or ethnicity. Do not let language, culture, or ethnicity be a barrier to providing good care. A person's cultural and ethnic background often affects his or her beliefs and values. Understanding differences in cultures and ethnicities can help you give each patient the best care while being sensitive to differences.

Culture and ethnicity affect communication in many ways. For instance, in some cultures, personal questions asked during a medical exam may be seen as offensive and an invasion of privacy. In such cases, the dentist may need to be involved in explaining why the questions are being asked. Some cultures place high importance on making eye contact, whereas others view eye contact as threatening and disrespectful. Also, some backgrounds value having lots of personal space. For these patients, touching, shaking hands, standing closely, or sitting closely may make them extremely uncomfortable. People from many other cultures feel comfortable with less personal space, and may take you as standoffish if you do not greet them warmly. Watch for nonverbal cues to see if patients appear uncomfortable. Finally, realize that culture and ethnicity can also impact how the individual behaves as a patient. In some cultures, it is important not to argue with or question people of authority such as health care providers. These patients may feel shy about asking questions or letting you know if they have a problem. Be aware that these patients may require you to gently probe for additional information and provide reassurance that it is okay to let you know if they have any concerns or questions.

Remember that although you do not want to be so "friendly" as to be threatening or discomfiting, friendly in one culture and friendly in another may be completely different things. In Anglo American culture, and particularly among older patients, some degree of detachment may be expected. Other cultures, however, may expect the use of pet names once you have been properly introduced. A Hispanic patient may find you nice and gentle, but they may also find you formal if you treat them as you would an Anglo patient. Using a few terms of endearment may help your Hispanic patients relax and greatly aid good communication. Learning to adapt to and tailor your approach to patients from a variety of different cultures can be very challenging, but it is also very rewarding.

No one wants to feel disrespected. Even if you are not familiar with a patient's particular culture, ethnicity, or background, there are some basic things you can do to show respect. Do not be afraid to ask patients what would be more comfortable for them. If you ask this politely and with genuine interest, patients are likely to happily give you an explanation. The fact that you are going the extra mile to really understand them and their culture will not only make them more comfortable and earn you bonus points, but also may likely win your office some referrals—patients will probably go home and tell their friends and family how open and accommodating you were. Treat all patients with dignity, in a friendly manner. If a patient appears uncomfortable, do not take offense. Adapt to your patient's comfort level, rather than expect your patient to adapt to you.

Finally, if a patient does not speak English, use gestures and speak slowly. It helps if your office has a foreign language dictionary or if there is someone in the office who speaks multiple languages and can interpret. If your practice happens to be in a city or region where there is a high prevalence of a certain non–English-speaking ethnicity, it is a good idea to have brochures, consent forms, and so forth in that language.

For Spanish in particular, various references are available to help you communicate with your patients and understand them when they communicate with you. Hispanics are one of the largest and most quickly growing demographics in the United States, and many regions have more Spanish speakers than English speakers. Knowledge of Spanish, or at least an ability to convey and understand information in Spanish, is quickly becoming essential in today's workplace.

The United States is more diverse today than ever before, and as our population demographics change, this increasingly prominent diversity will become more prevalent. In the near future, minority populations, in aggregate, are expected to outnumber the Caucasian population, which currently forms the majority. If you are not working with patients from cultures other than your own right now, you soon will be!

Extra Patient Care

When working with patients who speak little or no English, take the time to look up some basic words in their native language, such as *hello, goodbye, open please,* and *close please.* Record these in the patient's record so anyone in the office can use them when the patient comes in. There are also several websites that can translate words and phrases, such as www.freetranslation.com. Bookmark these web pages on your office's Internet browser so they can be reached easily and quickly.

CHECKPOINT

23-6 What are some specific examples of how communication can be impacted by a patient's culture or background?

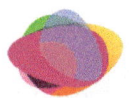

Chapter Highlights

✦ Communication is important for sending, receiving, and responding to information, and is critical for providing good patient care.

✦ Communication can be both verbal—which includes words and language—and nonverbal—which includes body positioning, gestures, facial expressions, and eye contact. Tone, voice quality, and use of language, such as sarcasm, also send important messages.

✦ Effective verbal communication should be clear, concise, complete, courteous, and consistent.

✦ Active listening is a part of communication that involves giving full attention to the speaker and the message communicated and keeping interruptions to a minimum.

✦ Nonverbal communication is especially important for dental assistants because patients are often not able to speak during dental procedures. Be aware of your nonverbal cues, such as body language and eye contact, and the messages they may be sending to patients.

✦ When communicating with patients, always be professional and respectful. Skills such as reflecting, paraphrasing, clarifying, summarizing, and asking open-ended questions can help make communication with patients successful.

✦ Telephone communication should be polite, friendly, and respectful. When placing callers on hold, be sure to use the proper procedure, such as finding out whether the caller has an emergency. Follow proper steps for taking telephone messages.

✦ When communicating in writing, always be professional, be clear in stating the message, and check your writing for spelling, grammar, and other possible errors.

✦ Electronic communications, such as e-mail or websites, are convenient and help reach patients quickly, but should be treated as seriously and professionally as all other types of writing. Remember that written communication from the office that is sloppy and casual make the office appear unprofessional and careless.

✦ Patients have different cultural and ethnic backgrounds, and this can impact their communication style. Pay attention to the patient's nonverbal cues, such as body language, to determine whether he or she is uncomfortable with how you are communicating.

✦ Ways to stay sensitive and respectful of cultural differences include learning about how other cultures and ethnicities communicate, keeping a list of common dental and medical phrases in other languages, and having a foreign language dictionary or office interpreter on hand.

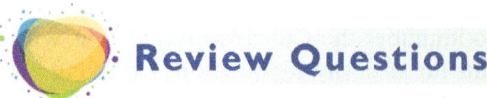

Review Questions

1. In the communication process, the medium is
   a. The person sending the message.
   b. The person receiving the message.
   c. The content of the message.
   d. The way in which the communication is taking place.

2. Verbal communication
   a. Includes words only, but not tone, voice quality, or use of language.
   b. Is more common than nonverbal communication.
   c. Should be lengthy so as to fully explain the message to the receiver.
   d. Should be clear and to the point.

3. Giving full attention to the speaker to show that the message is heard and understood is known as what?
   a. Nonverbal communication
   b. Active listening
   c. Active communication
   d. Attentive communication

4. Looking someone directly in the eyes is communicating what message?
   a. That you are paying attention
   b. That you are shy
   c. That you are bored
   d. Either A or B

5. When communicating with a patient
   a. It is okay to automatically use his first name if he has been a patient for several years.
   b. Open-ended questions may get more information than yes-or-no questions.
   c. Repeat everything he says so you can make sure you understand his message.
   d. It is okay to chat about personal topics, such as relationships or money.

6. When placing a patient on hold
   a. You do not need to ask permission if you truly cannot take the call.
   b. Always first find out if there is an emergency.
   c. Wait 10 minutes before taking a phone number and offering to have someone call back.
   d. Go get the dentist immediately so he or she can speak with the caller.

7. Electronic communication
   a. Is unofficial and does not need to be as serious and professional as a business letter.
   b. Does not need to be reviewed for errors as long as a spell checker is used.
   c. Should always be professional and held to the same standards as other written communication from the office.
   d. Should not be used as a form of patient communication.

8. If a non–English-speaking patient comes into the office
   a. Reschedule the appointment for a time when you can have an interpreter on hand.
   b. Do not attempt to speak in the patient's language unless you already have knowledge of the language.
   c. Use a foreign language dictionary or translation website to help with basic communication.
   d. Speak loudly so that the patient can understand you better.

9. Patients from other cultures or ethnic backgrounds
   a. May use communication skills, such as eye contact or physical distance, differently from those born in the United States.
   b. Will likely use communication skills common to those born in the United States.
   c. Should be instructed on how those born in the United States communicate.
   d. Will often explain to you how they are comfortable communicating.

Active Learning Exercises

1. Manners and professionalism on the telephone are very important. Can you recall a time when you were mistreated on the phone? Describe how you would handle a patient who calls the office while very upset. What could you say to diffuse the situation and help the patient?

2. Although verbal and nonverbal skills are essential, writing skills are equally important. Create a one- or two-paragraph letter welcoming a new patient to your office and highlighting features of the practice. Evaluate your letter for spelling, punctuation, and grammar.

3. Many cultures have different beliefs regarding dental care. Can you think of three cultures that may have differing beliefs regarding dental care? What are they and how could they affect patients' overall health?

Application Activities

1. Go online and search for images of facial expressions. For example, do a Google search using the "images" tab, searching for *faces* or *facial expressions*. Bring some printouts to class and discuss what message each face is "sending" based on its expression. How important are nonverbal cues in the dental office? If this "face" was a patient in your office, how might you communicate based on the message the patient is sending?

2. Do some research on how to greet patients from different countries. Using a map of the world, choose four or five countries. Write down on a small piece of paper greetings from each country, as well as any important nonverbal greetings, such as whether or not cultures from that country shake hands, bow, or make eye contact. Using a stickpin, tack your greeting "cheat sheet" to the country on a classroom map.

PREPARING FOR CERTIFICATION EXAMS

Review the following topics in this chapter to prepare for the Dental Assisting National Board (DANB) exam:

- **The Communication Process**

- **Speaking Skills**

- **Listening Skills**

- **Nonverbal Communication**

- **Communicating with Patients**

Assisting in Basic Procedures

chapter 24

The Dental Office

CHAPTER CHECKLIST

On completion of this chapter, students will be able to:

☑ Identify five factors that affect the environment in a dental office.

☑ Identify three factors that should be considered when designing the layout of a dental office.

☑ Identify the major areas of a dental office, including the purpose of each area and the items that may be found in each area.

☑ Identify and discuss the equipment found in a dental treatment room.

☑ Describe the correct procedures for opening and closing a dental office.

KEY TERMS

amalgamator (uh-MAL-guh-may-tur) – a small, electrical machine that mixes dental materials (amalgams and some cements) by vigorously shaking the ingredients inside of a capsule by a timer device

central air compressor – provides the compressed air needed to operate air-driven handpieces and the air-water syringe

curing light – used to cure (set or harden) light-cured dental materials

dental chair – the chair in which the patient sits during treatment

dental laboratory – a well-ventilated area where various dental devices are trimmed, adjusted, or fabricated outside of the patient's mouth

dental unit – provides the electrical and air-operated components needed to utilize the air-water syringe, dental handpieces, saliva ejector, high-volume evacuator, and ultrasonic scaler

diagnostic cast or study model – positive replica of the form of the teeth and tissues made from an impression; used to study the size and position of the oral tissues

operating light – a bright, moveable, overhead light used to light up the patient's oral cavity during a dental procedure

operatory (OP-er-uh-tor-ee) – a treatment room in which dental work is performed on the patient

photoinitiator – a substance that, when exposed to light, acts as a catalyst to begin the hardening process of dental materials

radiometer – a hand-held device that measures the intensity of a curing light

rheostat (REE-oh-stat) – a round, disk-shaped, foot-operated power control that controls the speed of handpieces attached to the dental unit

sonic scaler – an electronically powered instrument attached to the dental unit that uses rapid energy vibrations of a powered instrument tip (3,000–8,000 cycles per second) to remove calculus (tartar) and other hard deposits from the surface of the teeth

ultrasonic scaler – an electronic instrument attached to a portable unit with an electric generator that uses rapid energy vibrations of a powered instrument tip (18,000–42,000 cycles per second) to remove calculus (tartar) and other hard deposits from the surface of the teeth and to cleanse the environment of a periodontal pocket; some models use water (lavage) to cool the instrument while in use

Introduction

First impressions are everything. The patient's perception of the quality of care that he or she is likely to receive is greatly influenced by the environment established in the dental office. The design and the environment of the dental office should provide a positive experience for the patient from the moment the patient walks in the door until he or she leaves.

The design and environment of the office also needs to be conducive to the work of the dental team. The design needs to be practical, allowing for the most effective and efficient treatment possible by all members of the team. Dental team members spend many hours throughout the day chairside in the treatment rooms. Dental assistants (DAs) need to understand the functions of a wide range of dental equipment.

Office Design and Environment

Decor, lighting, temperature, sound, and smell all affect the environment in an office. They create that critical first impression. The office environment may put patients at ease or may unnerve patients before they even see the dentist.

- The decor of a dental office should calm and relax a patient. It should portray a warm, soothing environment. The colors of the walls, floors, furnishings, or decorations should not be "too loud" or "busy." The decor should reflect the average clientele seen by that office. The entire dental office should be kept clean, neat, and professional looking because the majority of patients equate the cleanliness and neatness of an office with the quality of care that they will receive.
- The lighting in the reception area should be adequate for reading, but not as bright as that used in the business or clinical areas of the office. For example, table or floor lamps work well in the waiting area, whereas fluorescent lighting and dental unit lights are better used in other areas of the dental office.
- A comfortable temperature in the reception area is 72°F; however, a cooler temperature of approximately 68°F to 70°F should be used in the clinical areas of the office because of the smaller size of the rooms and the heat emitted by the dental unit lights.
- The sounds created by dental equipment can be unnerving for those patients waiting to be seen. The layout of the dental office should be such that it minimizes the sound that travels throughout the office. Soft music playing in the background can help to provide a diversion from those sounds and also provide a calming environment.
- Certain smells are produced in dental offices that can result in medicinal odors pervading the office. Fragrance diffusers or candles can be used to help change the aroma in the office.

Areas of the Office

The major areas of a dental office include a reception area, a business area, and treatment and clinical areas. The layout of a dental office should provide for the following:

- Patient privacy, especially when discussing financial matters in the business area or for any discussions between members of the dental team and the patient in the clinical areas
- Open traffic flow, not only allowing easy access to check-in and check-out for patients, but also easy flow of movement for dental team members entering and exiting the different clinical and laboratory areas (Figure 24-1)
- Sound control, minimizing the sounds and conversations from being heard throughout the office

Reception Area

The reception area is the first room that the patient walks into when entering a dental office and where he or she meets the first person in the dental team—usually a receptionist (or administrative assistant). The receptionist answers the phone and enters patient appointments into a computer. The receptionist also greets the patient and lets the operator know that the patient has arrived for his or her appointment.

The receptionist is most often seated at a reception desk with a counter separating the business section of

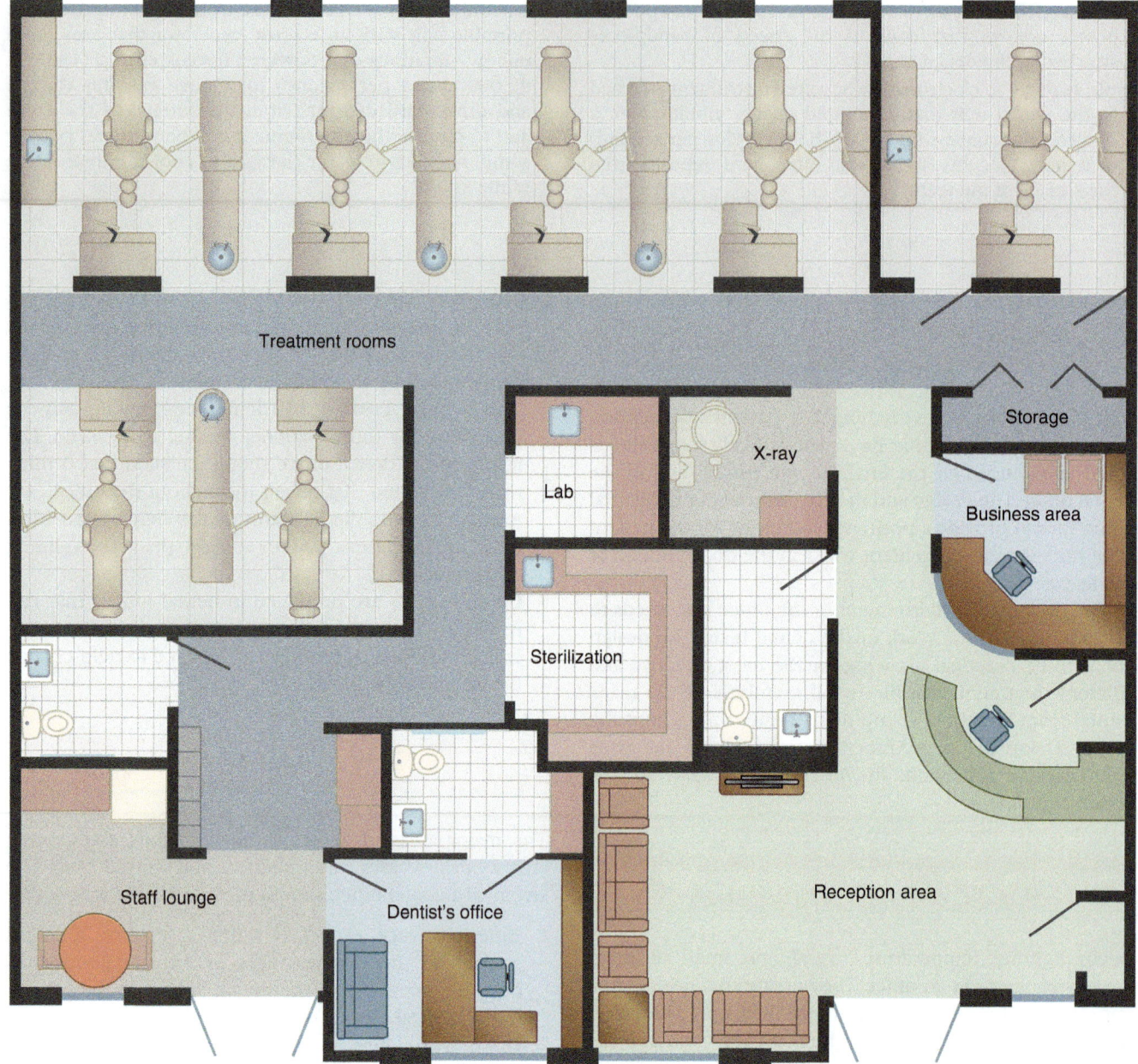

Figure 24–1 Layout of a typical dental office.

the reception area from the patient area. Health Insurance Portability and Accountability Act (HIPAA) privacy regulations require that the design of this separation allows for private interactions between patients and the dental staff, including phone conversations. Sometimes this separation is accomplished by the use of a glass wall or other design element that prevents patients in the patient lounge from overhearing these interactions. The counter incorporated into this separation should be at a level that is comfortable for the average person to be able to stand at the counter to fill out forms, sign papers, or write checks.

Usually included in the reception room is a patient lounge. This area should include:

- Comfortable seating
- Side tables/coffee tables
- Adequate reading light
- Comfortable temperature
- Up-to-date reading material, such as current magazines relevant to the clientele and patient education materials

It may also include:

- Accommodations for hanging coats and umbrellas
- A child-sized table and chairs as well as children's books and a few toys

The waiting area should be checked regularly throughout the day to ensure that it is kept neat and clean.

Business Area

The business area of a dental office may be merged with the reception desk area or it may be in a separate area or room. The business or administrative aspect of the office, including all financial matters, is conducted here. This area will most likely include:

- Patient records
- Business forms and materials
- Storage cupboards containing business supplies
- A desk
- A computer
- A printer/scanner
- A fax machine
- A phone/telecommunications system
- A photocopier
- A filing system

This area should be set up in such a way as to allow for some privacy for the patient while discussing financial matters with the administrative personnel. HIPAA privacy issues need to be considered here.

Treatment and Clinical Areas

The treatment and clinical areas include treatment rooms, a dental laboratory, a sterilizing area, and a radiograph processing room. Some practices also have a separate radiograph room. Each of these areas needs to be kept as neat and clean as possible, not only to maintain an aesthetic appeal, but also to ensure aseptic conditions.

Treatment Room

The treatment room is also known as an **operatory**. A general rule of thumb is that for every dentist in a dental office, at least two of these rooms are used by the dentist for operative dentistry and a third is used by a hygienist. There may be more depending on the size of the practice. Each of these rooms should be similarly designed and arranged, allowing for the most efficient use of the space and equipment. (For a description of the equipment found in a treatment room, see the section titled, "Equipment in the Treatment Room.") Patient privacy should also be considered here. Placing the dental chair so that the foot of the chair is away from the door opening allows privacy for the patient from people walking by the door. Patient comfort, as well as the comfort and ease of movement for members of the dental team, must be considered when designing and arranging these rooms.

Dental Laboratory

The **dental laboratory** is a well-ventilated area in which dental work not performed directly on the patient takes place. Procedures performed in a laboratory can include:

- Creating custom trays
- Pouring impressions
- Creating, finishing, or adjusting prosthodontics, such as crowns, bridges, partials, or dentures
- Polishing removable prosthodontics
- Preparing diagnostic casts

Great care must be taken in a laboratory to ensure aseptic conditions because items prepared here go in and out of patients' mouths. Infection control practices should be strictly followed. Personal protective equipment (PPE), such as protective eyewear, masks, and protective gowns or barrier lab jackets, should also be worn by the staff in this area to ensure their safety. See Chapter 14, Disease and Infection Control, for more information about aseptic conditions and personal protection equipment. The following can be found in a dental laboratory:

- Workbenches or counters
- Storage cabinets, usually mounted on the walls
- A sink
- A heat source, such as a propane or butane torch
- A model trimmer
- A vacuum former
- A laboratory handpiece
- A vibrator
- A dental lathe
- An articulator
- A sandblaster
- Rubber bowls
- Lab knives and spatulas

For a more detailed description of laboratory equipment, see Chapter 35, Laboratory Materials and Techniques.

Sterilization Area

The sterilization area is a well-ventilated area in which patient care items and instruments are cleaned, sterilized, and then stored. There are various types of sterilization equipment resulting in many different methods of sterilization. (For a more detailed description of the various types of sterilization equipment and methods of sterilization, see Chapter 14, Disease and Infection Control.) In addition to the sterilization equipment, this area also usually contains:

- A sink
- A water distiller
- An ultrasonic cleaning machine
- A sharps container

As a DA, you will most likely be the member of the dental team responsible for sterilizing all patient care items and instruments. This area must always be kept neat and clean as well, and infection control practices should be strictly followed here.

Darkroom

The darkroom is a small, well-ventilated room in which radiographs are processed. This room usually contains:

- A counter
- A sink
- An automatic processor/manual processing tank
- Drying racks
- Safelights
- Separation containers for lead liners
- Storage cupboards
- Adequate ventilation

Automatic processors with daylight loaders are being used in more dental offices now. These processors do not require a darkroom. The automatic processor with a daylight loader may be used in treatment rooms or the sterilization area, or even in an open area in a hallway. (For a more detailed description of radiograph processing equipment, see Chapter 32, Film Processing, Mounting, and Evaluation.)

Radiograph Room

A separate x-ray (radiograph) room is used in some offices for taking radiographs. The radiograph machine is found in this room, along with a lead apron and a hanger on which to hang the apron when not in use. Some states require that the walls of this room be lined with lead. The operator always needs to be at least 6 feet away from the primary beam when operating a radiograph machine. The room should be designed in such a way that a 6-foot retractable exposure cord attached to the machine can be used; otherwise, a remote switch, preferrably behind a suitable barrier such as a wall, should be used. State health department safety guidelines protecting both the patient and the operator from secondary and scattered radiation must be followed in this room. (For a more detailed description of dental radiography, see Part VII, Dental Radiography.)

Other Areas

Some dental offices are large enough to include a private office for the dentist, a staff lounge, and a patient education room. These other areas depend on available space, budget, and preferences of the dentist.

Dentist's Office

The dentist may have a room for his or her own private office. The dentist may use this office for:

- Personal business
- Professional business
- Private patient consultations
- Staff meetings

Staff Lounge

A staff lounge is used by members of the staff for breaks and for storing personal items while working. The lounge may include:

- Staff lockers and/or lockable storage cupboards
- A table and chairs
- A coffee maker
- A refrigerator
- A microwave
- A sink/counter
- Dishes
- A washer/dryer

The refrigerator in the lounge, meant for staff food only, should never be used to store refrigerated dental supplies; these must be stored separately in their own refrigerated unit.

Patient Education Area

A patient education area may be part of the reception or treatment areas or it may be in its own room. It may include:

- Dental information pamphlets relevant to the services offered by that office
- A television set with a digital video disc (DVD) player (including educational dental DVDs)
- A table and chairs
- A sink or many sinks
- A counter
- A mirror
- A large mouth model with large toothbrush for brushing demonstrations
- A radiograph view box and/or a computer to display digital images of the tooth/teeth that require work

In addition to being used as a patient education area, this area may also be used as a patient waiting area, consultation area, or an area where a patient can practice home care techniques.

✔ **CHECKPOINTS**

24-1 What is the most important factor to consider when designing the layout of the business area of the dental office?

24-2 What type of radiograph processor does not need a darkroom?

Equipment in the Treatment Room

Whether the treatment areas are in individual rooms or are in a larger open space divided by partial walls, everything in each treatment area is centered around a dental chair in which the patient will sit during treatment. Each treatment area will also include a dental unit, an operating light, an operator's stool, an assistant's stool, storage cabinets, and a counter and sink. (A central air compressor and a central vacuum compressor are two vital pieces of equipment needed for the dental units; however, they are housed in a separate room elsewhere.) Other equipment that may also be found in the treatment area are a curing light, amalgamator, radiograph unit, radiograph view box, office communication system, and a computer. All equipment in each treatment area should be placed in a similar layout allowing for maximum efficiency as the dentist moves from operatory to operatory to see each patient.

Dentists may choose from a variety of styles and designs when selecting the equipment for the office, ranging from economical to very expensive. All equipment, no matter what the cost, can last for many years when it is properly maintained and cared for. Routine cleaning and maintenance of the equipment is usually the responsibility of a specific person in the office, mainly the DA.

The Dental Chair

The patient **dental chair** is designed to provide maximum comfort for the patient and efficiency for the operator and the assistant (Figure 24-2). Many features of the chair are completely adjustable providing ergonomic support of all areas of the patient's body while allowing close proximity for the operator and the assistant to the patient's oral cavity.

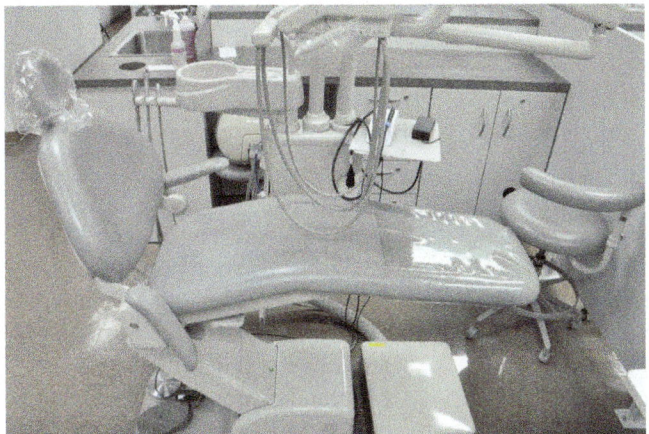

Figure 24–2 **Dental chair**. Note the adjustable head rest and armrests, and the foot control for the operator.

The headrest is adjustable to allow for a patient's height and is formed in such a way as to allow the head to be held comfortably and securely in the correct position for treatment, while at the same time giving support to the neck. Also, the headrest is narrow enough and the upper portion of the chairback thin enough to allow the operator and assistant to get as close as possible to the patient's oral cavity in order to provide treatment. The headrest is covered with an infection control barrier to prevent cross-contamination.

Either finger-operated power controls on the sides of the chair back or foot-operated power controls on the floor are used to adjust the patient's position to the most efficient for the treatment being performed (see Figure 24-2). The following are the ways in which a dental chair can move:

- The headrest and back move as a unit.
- The seat and leg support moves as a unit.
- The chair base permits the chair to be lowered and raised.
- A floor control also allows the chair to rotate left or right.

Foot controls reduce the risk of cross-contamination and get rid of the need for the infection control barriers required on finger-operated controls.

The armrests of the chair are also adjustable, allowing them to be raised or moved to the side to make it more convenient for the patient to be seated and to exit the chair.

The padding being used in many new dental chairs now is "memory foam." This is another design element that adds to the patient's comfort.

The material used to cover the dental chairs must be given consideration because certain disinfectants may discolor or even stain some chair materials. Most dental chairs are covered in vinyl so that they can be cleaned and disinfected properly. Commonly, a color can be chosen that matches the color scheme of the office, adding to the overall aesthetics of the office.

Dental chairs that are specially designed to treat physically challenged patients and that allow easy access for wheelchair patients are also available. (For a more detailed description of these dental chairs, see Chapter 22, Patients with Special Needs.)

The Dental Unit

The **dental unit** provides the electrical and air-operated components needed for use of:

- The air-water syringe
- The dental handpieces
- The saliva ejector
- The high-volume evacuator
- The ultrasonic scaler

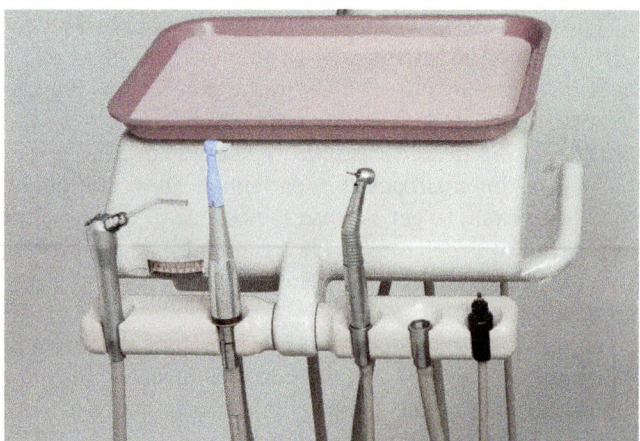

Figure 24–3 Dental unit with handpieces attached.

Dental units are available in a variety of styles and designs (Figure 24-3). The answers to the following questions should be considered when choosing a dental unit:

- What method of delivery does the operator prefer? (See the Types of Dental Units section below.)
- Is the operator right-handed or left-handed?
- Does the operator work with an assistant?
- How much space is available within the treatment areas?
- Is the unit to be attached to a wall, the floor, a cabinet, the side of the dental chair, or a mobile cart?

Types of Dental Units

The types of dental units are:

- Chair-mounted (on the side of the dental chair)
- Mobile cart or cabinet
- Mounted on part of the building structure or a permanent fixture, such as a wall, floor, or built-in cabinet

The type of dental unit chosen may depend on the delivery system preferred by the operator. Table 24-1 details the three types of delivery systems.

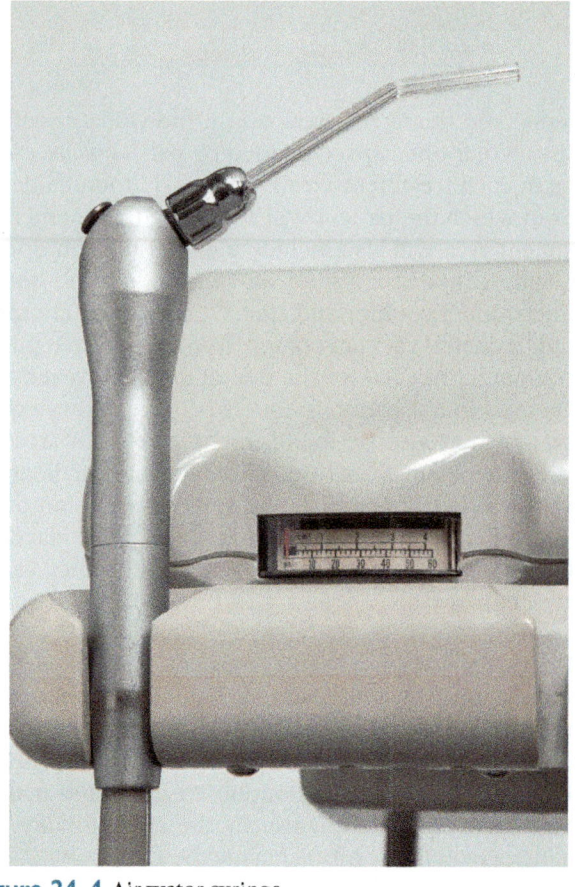

Figure 24–4 Air-water syringe.

Air-Water Syringe

The **air-water syringe** (Figure 24-4) is an essential part of the dental unit that is used for every procedure to keep the oral cavity clean, dry, and protected from the heat produced by the RPMs (revolutions per minute) of the dental handpieces. The air-water syringe can provide:

- A focused stream of air
- A focused stream of water
- A combination spray of air and water

TABLE 24-1 Dental Unit Delivery Systems		
SIDE DELIVERY SYSTEM	**REAR DELIVERY SYSTEM**	**FRONT DELIVERY SYSTEM**
- Positions the unit at either side of the dental chair - Offers separate instrument sections for the operator and the assistant; however, this option may require more floor space - Reduces assistant's access to operative instruments - Keeps instruments out of center view of the patient, allowing only a peripheral view of the instruments	- Positions the unit behind the patient's head - Allows the assistant access to operative instruments - Keeps instruments completely out of the patient's view - Improves infection control because everything is behind the patient and not over his or her body	- Uses a moveable arm to position the unit over the patient's chest - Allows the assistant access to operative instruments - Requires less twisting and movement by operator and assistant - Reduces eye fatigue of operator by not requiring constant adjustment of eyes to oral-cavity distance - Places the instruments in full view of the patient

For infection control, the air-water syringe comes with a removable tip that is made of either disposable plastic or sterilizable metal. It must be replaced after every patient. These tips are angled and come in different lengths to make it easier to use.

The controls of the syringe are found on the shank. The thumb of one hand can be used to operate it. The shank and tubing of the syringe must be covered with new infection control barriers and the syringe flushed with water after every patient.

Waterlines carry water to the syringe and some high-speed handpieces. Many dental units now use self-contained water bottles that are filled with distilled water and that attach to the unit. The water and the air that drives the water in the waterlines are not sterile; therefore, infection control procedures need to be followed with regard to these waterlines. (For a more detailed description of infection control procedures, see Chapter 14, Disease and Infection Control.)

Dental Handpieces

Low-speed and high-speed dental handpieces are attached to hoses on the dental unit (see Figure 24-3), which provides the power to rotate the bur in order to cut or polish tooth structures and castings. (For a more detailed description of dental handpieces, see Chapter 26, Dental Instruments and Equipment.) There are two ways to control the handpieces:

- An on/off switch on the hose attachment; this allows only one handpiece to be turned on at a time
- A **rheostat**; a round, disk-shaped, foot-operated power control on the floor used by the operator to control the speed of the handpiece (Figure 24-5)

As with the air-water syringe, infection control procedures need to be followed after every patient.

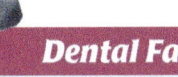

Dental Facts

The first *foot-treadle dental engine* was patented by James B. Morrison in 1871. This machine was able to supply enough power and speed to the dental bur to smoothly cut enamel and dentin, fundamentally and radically changing the practice of dentistry. The first *electric dental engine* was then patented by George F. Green that same year.

Saliva Ejector

The **saliva ejector** is a hollow, perforated suction tube used in the evacuation of saliva or liquid debris from the oral cavity (Figure 24-6). It is also known as a *dental pump*. It uses low-volume suction to comfortably remove excess fluids from the patient's mouth. It is used during less-invasive procedures, such as:

- Routine cleanings
- Fluoride treatments
- Application of sealants

The saliva ejector will only function if it is in fluid, and it can only draw out fluid (unlike the high-volume evacuator, described below, that can also remove solid debris or particles).

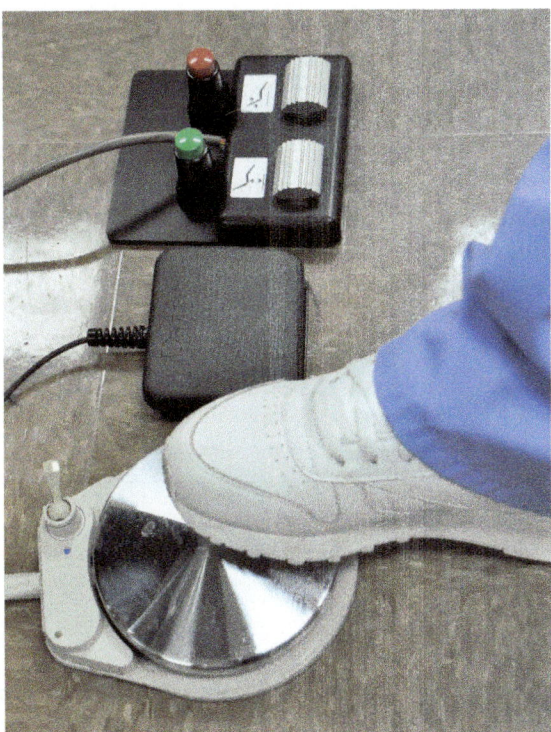

Figure 24–5 Foot-operated rheostat.

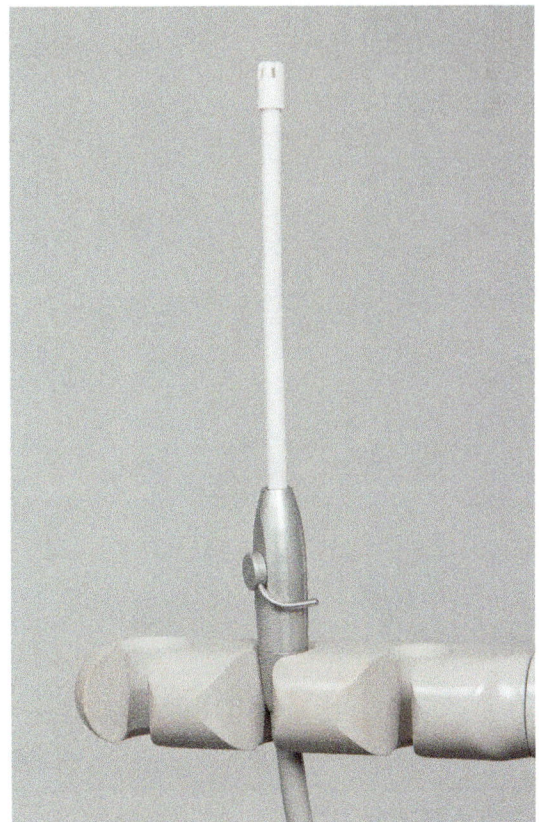

Figure 24–6 Saliva ejector.

The tip of the saliva ejector is a thin, flexible, disposable plastic tube that fits into the opening of the saliva ejector hose attached to the dental unit. This tip must be replaced after every patient and infection control procedures followed.

The saliva ejector contains a filter trap that collects the waste debris created during some dental work procedures. If the trap is disposable, then it must be replaced routinely. If it is metal, it must be removed and cleaned regularly using proper infection control procedures.

High-Volume Evacuator

The high-volume evacuator (HVE) (Figure 24-7) is similar to the saliva ejector; however, it uses high-volume suction to clear the oral cavity of saliva, blood, fluids, and debris in order to maintain a clear field during more invasive dental procedures. It is also known as an *oral evacuator*. As a DA, you will most likely be the one to use the HVE during procedures.

The tip of the HVE is a wider tube than the saliva ejector and is beveled at each end. It fits into the opening of the HVE hose attached to the dental unit. These tips come in a variety of shapes and sizes. Unlike saliva ejector tips, oral evacuation tips can remove fluid and debris even if they are only near fluid and debris; they do not need to be in the fluid

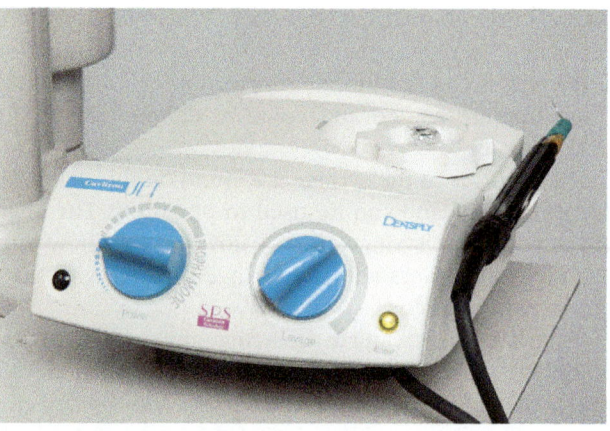

Figure 24–8 Ultrasonic scaler.

to remove it. This tip must be replaced after every patient and infection control procedures must be followed.

The HVE can be vented and also contains a filter trap that collects the solid waste debris created during dental work procedures. If the trap is disposable, then it must be replaced routinely. If it is metal, it must be removed and cleaned regularly using proper infection control procedures. A thorough cleaning of the HVE should be done daily.

Sonic Scaler

The **sonic scaler** is an electronically powered instrument attached to the dental unit that uses rapid energy vibrations (3,000–8,000 cycles per second) of a powered instrument tip to remove calculus (tartar) and other hard deposits from the surface of the teeth.

Ultrasonic Scaler

The **ultrasonic scaler** (Figure 24-8) is an electronically powered instrument attached to a portable unit with an electric generator that uses rapid energy vibrations (18,000–42,000 cycles per second) of a powered instrument tip to remove calculus (tartar) and other hard deposits from the surface of the teeth and to cleanse the environment of a periodontal pocket; some models plug into the water supply on the dental unit in order to use the water to cool the instrument while in use. Antibiotics can be applied using the ultrasonic scaler for patients that have gingivitis or advanced periodontal disease.

CHECKPOINTS

24-3 Name an advantage of the rear delivery system.

24-4 What is the difference between a sonic scaler and an ultrasonic scaler?

Operating Light

The **operating light** is a bright, moveable, overhead light used to light up the patient's oral cavity during a

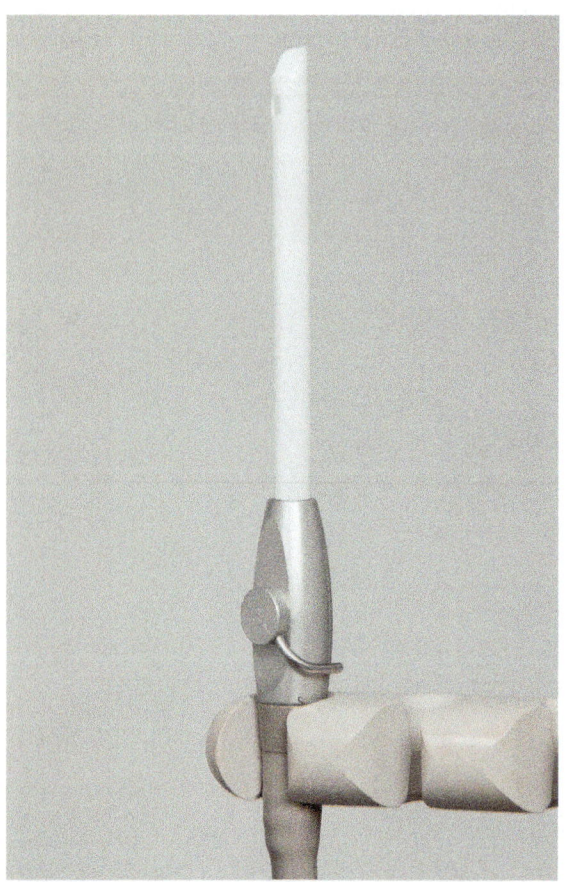

Figure 24–7 High-volume evacuator.

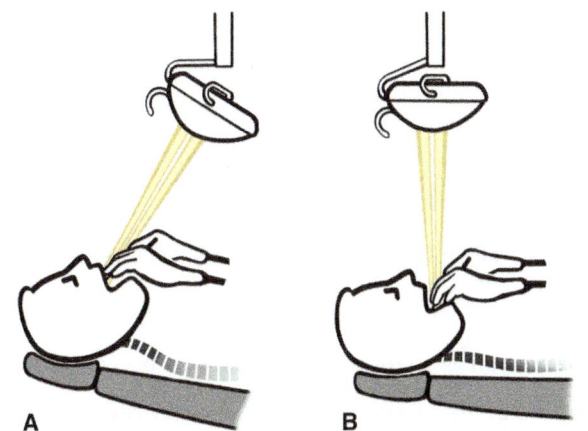

Figure 24–9 **Operating lights.** (**A**) Position for working on the maxillary arch with chin in the up position. (**B**) Position for working on the mandibular arch with chin in the down position.

dental procedure (Figure 24-9). The light is attached to a flexible arm that is mounted on the dental chair, wall, cabinet, track, or ceiling. It has handles on both sides of the light. This allows the operator and the DA to adjust the position of the light regardless of which side of the chair they are on. There is an on/off switch and a control switch to adjust the intensity of the light. The handles and the switches are covered with infection control barriers that must be changed after each patient. The lens should also be wiped between patients, using a soft cloth so as not to scratch the lens.

Additional features that are available on dental operating lights are:

- Color correcting light
- Incandescent or light-emitting diode (LED) bulb (instead of the usual halogen)
- Adjustable focal lengths
- Illumination of various shapes (e.g., horizontal, oval, etc.) and sizes; some with feathered edges
- Various shaped reflectors; shadow-free reflectors
- Adjustable shield
- Third axis of rotation
- Integrated cooling fan; reduced radiant heat emissions
- Removable autoclavable handles
- Touchless activation/deactivation sensor

As the DA, you may be required to position the light over the patient's oral cavity. After the patient is seated, there are several steps that should be taken to do this:

1. Use a gloved hand and a handle on the side of the light to position the light over the patient's chest. The light should be positioned 20 to 30 inches below the patient's chin, depending upon the operator and the light's intensity. Be sure the light is angled down onto the chest.
2. Turn the light on.
3. The light may be adjusted now according to which arch is being worked on—maxillary or mandibular. If working on the maxillary arch with the chin in an up

position, use a handle on the side of the light to slowly tilt the light up toward the oral cavity. The beam of light should be at a 45°–60° angle to the floor (see Figure 24-9A). Be sure not to tilt it up so far as to get it in the patient's eyes. If working on the mandibular arch with the chin in a down position, use a handle on the side of the light to slowly move the light so that the top edge of the light is at the ala of the nose and the light beam almost perpendicular to the floor (see Figure 24-9B).

Following these steps prevents you from accidently turning the light on in the patient's eyes and correctly positions the light so that shadows from the operator's hands or yours are not projected onto the oral cavity.

Most operating lights use halogen bulbs. These bulbs get very hot during use. As a result, the lens of the lamp also gets hot. In order to clean smudges and debris from the lens, you must turn off the light and be sure that it is cool before cleaning it with a soft cloth and a mild disinfectant. If you touch a warm lens with a damp cloth, the lens could crack.

If the bulb needs to be replaced, again you must switch off the light and allow it to cool before replacing it. Extra bulbs should always be kept in stock. You should never touch a quartz halogen bulb with your bare fingers. The oils from your skin dramatically reduce the life of the bulb and could cause it to break. You should use gloves or a lint free cloth to remove and install these bulbs. Be sure to follow the manufacturer's instructions stated on the packaging.

For a more focused lighting, dental spot examination lights are also available as a headband, a portable light on a moveable stand, or can be wall mounted.

The Operator's Stool

Most dental procedures require that the operator be seated in close proximity to the patient for prolonged periods of time; therefore, it is very important that the operator's stool:

- Provides ergonomic support, especially to the lumbar region of the back
- Allows the operator's feet to be flat on the floor in order to maintain proper circulation in the feet and legs
- Provides comfort and prevents fatique
- Does not tip, especially when moving
- Rolls easily, even on carpets, to reduce the need for twisting and stretching
- Is easy to clean and disinfect

As result of these requirements, the operator's stool needs to have:

- A broad, comfortably padded and upholstered seat with no seams

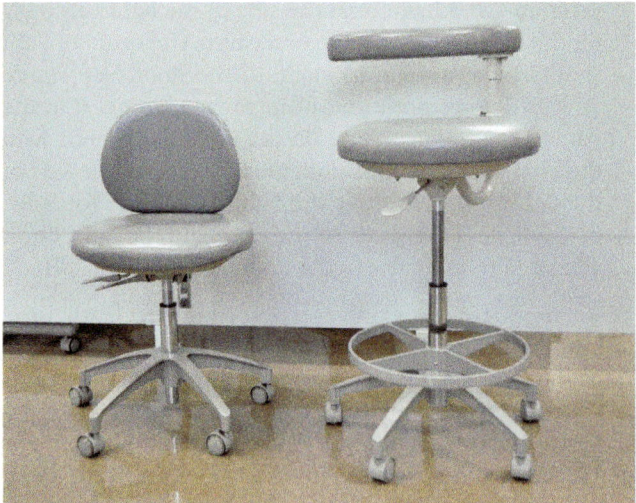

Figure 24–10 Operator's stool (left) and dental assistant's stool (right).

- An adjustment lever for height
- An adjustable backrest
- A broad, heavy base with at least five casters to prevent tipping

The seat should be deep enough to support most of the operator's thighs and have a front edge that curves slightly downward. A seat that tilts slightly downward (5°–15°) has been shown to provide musculoskeletal benefits, especially for the lower lumbar region. Some stools come with one or both arm rests, which can help to reduce strain on the neck, lower back, and arms.

Stool designs range from saddle stools with no back or arm rests to traditional stools with a back and both arm rests (Figure 24-10). Whichever style is chosen, it is very important that the stool be properly adjusted for that operator's body stature in order to maintain good musculoskeletal health.

The Dental Assistant's Stool

Although there are many features of an operator's stool that should also be incorporated into the DA's stool, there are also some differences that need to be noted as well. Similarities with an operator's stool are that it:

- Provides ergonomic support, including the lumbar region of the back
- Provides comfort and prevents fatique
- Does not tip, especially when moving
- Rolls easily, even on carpets, to reduce the need for twisting and stretching
- Is easy to clean and disinfect

Therefore, a DA's stool should also have:

- A broad, comfortably padded and upholstered seat with no seams

- An adjustment lever for height that is easy to operate (a DA may need to raise and lower his or her stool more often than an operator would)
- An adjustable backrest (optional)
- A broad, heavy base with at least five casters

The differences for a DA are that the DA:

- Usually sits 4 to 6 inches higher than the operator during procedures
- May lean or reach more than the operator

Therefore, an assistant's stool should also have:

- An adjustable footrest, usually a metal ring above the casters, to allow the same proper circulation in the feet and legs and ergonomic support of the lumbar region of the back as when the feet are placed flat on the floor
- An extended arm on the side of the chair to provide stability when leaning or reaching (improper leaning on stomach supports have been found to cause abdominal problems and more musculoskeletal problems than benefits and are no longer recommended). The arm extension should be placed at the level of the rib cage and never at the stomach.

As with operator's stools, there are a variety of designs and styles from which to choose (see Figure 24-10), but whichever style is chosen, it is very important that the stool be properly adjusted for the assistant's body stature in order to maintain good musculoskeletal health.

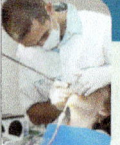

Voice of Experience

One important thing that I've learned working as a dental assistant is to make sure that I have a proper dental assistant's stool that has been correctly adjusted for *me*. Years ago when I first became a dental assistant, I didn't give much thought about the stool I sat on. That was until I started having a lot of pain in my lower back. Then, one day, while assisting the dentist with a procedure, I reached for an instrument and the stool tipped, making me fall onto the patient's lap. It was a simple round stool on four casters that was not very stable. That was it. I did my research and found an ergonomic stool made specifically for a dental assistant, with five casters and a footrest ring. It has an adjustable backrest, an arm rest, and an adjustment lever that easily allows me to adjust the height of the stool so that I can sit a little higher than the dentist while assisting with a procedure. And, I no longer have any lower back pain.

Storage Cabinets, Counters, and Sinks

Storage cabinets, counters, and sinks are just as important as other equipment in the treatment areas. These items also come in a variety of designs, styles, and colors. It will be your responsibility, as the DA, to be sure that the cabinets are well stocked with the appropriate supplies needed in each treatment area.

The size of the treatment areas and the preferences of the dentist will determine the number of storage cabinets, as well as the design and style. Storage cabinets may be:

- Built in
- Freestanding, usually against a wall
- Divider cabinets that divide a larger room into smaller treatment areas; these cabinets allow access to the storage areas from either side of the cabinet

Some cabinets are base units that stand on the floor. This type of cabinetry often comes with a counter top for workspace and many times includes a sink. More storage cabinets may then be mounted on the wall above the counter and sink.

Some cabinets come with hutch-style cabinetry above the base unit. Open adjustable shelving allows for more modern technology needs such as a computer, keyboard and mouse, printer, television with DVD player, videotape recorder, compact disc player and audio speakers, intraoral video camera, video source selector, and communication system.

Some cabinets have dental units mounted on them. These cabinets are often placed against the wall behind the patient's head for dentists who prefer the rear delivery system.

Mobile cabinets come with workspace on top and storage space underneath. Casters on these cabinets allow them to be moved where needed after the patient is seated and then pushed back against the wall when no longer required.

Sinks need to be conveniently located for both the operator and assistant to use. Water controls should be able to be operated using the wrists, knees, or feet, or should contain a motion sensor device that automatically turns the water on and off. This prevents the cross contamination that can occur when using hand controls. Sinks should be easy to clean and disinfect. Soap and towel dispensers should be placed closeby.

Dental Radiograph Unit

A dental radiograph unit is used to take intraoral radiographs. A dental radiograph unit is typically available in each treatment room, along with a lead apron that usually hangs on a hook on the wall. Some practices may have a separate room to house the radiograph unit. The radiograph unit consists of a tubehead with a position indicator device that is attached to a flexible extension arm that is mounted to the wall (Figure 24-11). This allows the tubehead to be extended and positioned where needed. Sometimes the extension arm is mounted inside a cubbyhole of a common wall between two treatment rooms and the tubehead is housed here until needed in one of the rooms. Doors on either side of the cubbyhole can then be opened and the tubehead extended into that room. The control panel is mounted

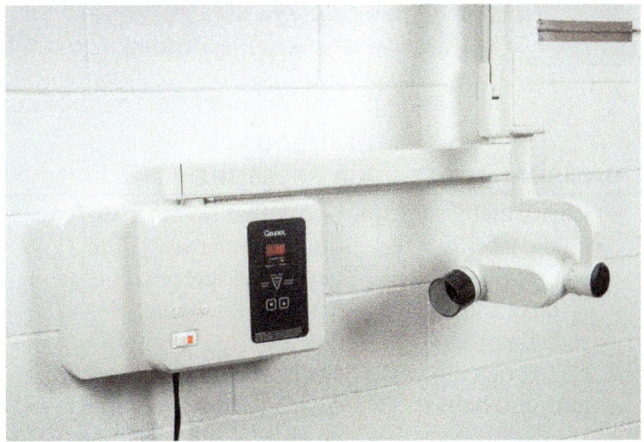

Figure 24–11 Dental radiograph unit.

outside of the treatment room to reduce the radiation exposure to the person operating the unit. Radiation emission occurs only when the exposure timer switch is pushed. (For a more detailed description of dental radiograph units and how they work, see Chapter 29, Basics of Dental Radiography.)

Central Air Compressor

A **central air compressor** provides the compressed air needed to operate:

- Air-driven handpieces
- Air-water syringe

These compressors come in various sizes and horsepower. The size and power chosen to be used is determined by the number of dental units used in the dental office. Air compressors also come with oil-lubricated systems or oil-less systems.

Oil-lubricated air compressors:

- Can cause wear and tear on dental instruments and handpieces due to build-up of oil residue
- Can alter compressive and tensile strength of dental materials, resulting in failure of restorations
- May require more maintenance than oil-less systems
- Force air through the dental tubing, creating oil in the aerosol which is being used in the patient's mouth
- Can inhibit bonding and adhesion if oil has contaminated the tooth surface

Oil-less air compressors:

- Provide dry, oil-free air
- Cause less wear and tear on dental instruments
- Do not need to have oil levels monitored or oil changes performed

The compressor system is usually housed in an area away from the main office due to the noise level and its size.

TABLE 24-2 Air Compressor Troubleshooting

UNUSUAL NOISE	INADEQUATE AIR PRESSURE	COMPLETELY STOPS	COMPRESSOR CYCLES WHEN AIR IS NOT BEING DEMANDED FROM ANY OPERATORY
■ Check that intake filter is not clogged or dirty and is seated correctly. ■ Check that all nuts and bolts are tight. ■ Check that no valves, cooling fans, or other parts are broken. ■ Check for worn parts (e.g., rod or crank shaft bearing).	■ Check that no more than the recommended number of handpieces for that machine are being used at one time. ■ Check that the pressure switch is at the required pressure. ■ Check that no pipes or hoses are leaking or bent. ■ Check that no valves are broken or leaking. ■ Check for loose fittings. ■ Check that the intake filter is not clogged or dirty and is seated correctly. ■ Check that no dust is in the cylinder.	■ Check electrical connections and breakers. ■ Check tank pressure. ■ Check oil level and for oil leaks if compressor uses oil (if oil level is nonexistent, trained office staff or trained maintenance personnel must be called; just adding more oil and trying to restart the compressor could cause more damage). ■ Check for worn or broken parts.	■ Check for leaks. ■ Check moisture monitor or open moisture drain to eliminate any condensation inside.

There are now low noise models, but for safety reasons, these should still be in an area away from the clinical setting.

Although air compressors require routine maintenance services performed by trained maintenance personnel, there are general maintenance procedures that you should do frequently:

■ Check for any unusual noises
■ Check that air pressure meets requirements
■ Check that the pressure switch and safety valve are at the required pressure
■ Check the moisture monitor or open moisture drain to eliminate any condensation inside
■ Check airlines regularly for condensation (condensation in the airlines could potentially produce contaminants, such as algae and sediments, that can destroy handpieces and be blown into a patient's mouth)
■ Check that oil is up to the required level if compressor uses oil
■ Change filters regularly according to the manufacturer's instructions
■ Check that all nuts and bolts are tight
■ Check the tension of any belts

It is very important that the points listed above be followed, because without a properly functioning air compressor, the most basic dental procedures cannot be performed. Most of the maintenance procedures for this equipment are observational in nature. Any major problems or concerns should be handled by an equipment repair technician.

Table 24-2 contains troubleshooting suggestions. If none of these suggestions resolves the problem, you must then call trained maintenance personnel.

Central Vacuum Compressor

A central vacuum compressor is used to provide the suction needed for:

■ The saliva ejector
■ The HVE

As with the air compressor, this compressor is also housed in an area away from the clinical setting. It also must receive routine maintenance services as specified in the manufacturer's instructions. These services keep these two vital pieces of treatment room equipment performing at peak efficiency.

As previously mentioned in this chapter, the saliva ejector and the HVE each contain a chairside filter trap that collects the solid waste debris created during some dental work procedures. There is also a trap in the central vacuum that collects any debris not picked up by the chairside traps, which also must be cleaned frequently. If the trap is disposable, then it must be replaced routinely. If it is metal, it must be removed and cleaned regularly using proper infection control procedures.

Other Treatment Room Equipment

Curing Light

The dental **curing light** is used to cure (set or harden) light-cured dental materials (Figure 24-12). Dental materials used today have some type of photoinitiator in them. A **photoinitiator** is a substance that, when exposed to light, acts as a catalyst to begin the hardening process.

There are many different types of curing lights. The type of dental material being cured determines which features are required in the curing light:

- The light intensity and spectrum
- The heat generation
- The curing speed

Features the dentist considers when choosing a curing light are:

- Ergonomic design
- Portability
- Weight
- Noise level
- Durability
- Reliability

Other features a dentist may prefer are the presence of:

- A wand or tip
- A fan

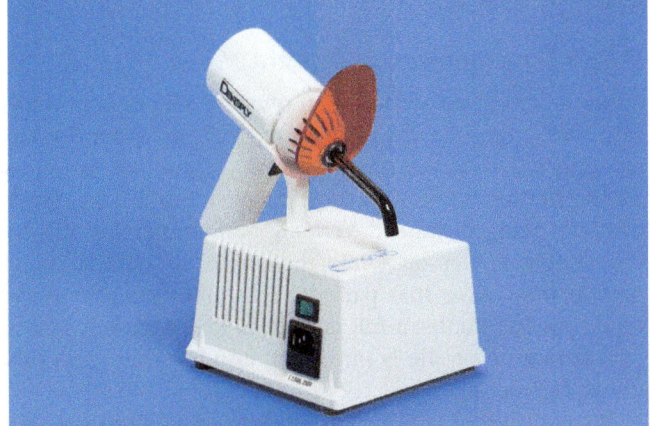

Figure 24–12 Curing light.

- A protective shield
- A filter
- A handle
- An activation trigger
- Cordless
- A digital display countdown timer
- Preset curing times

There are four types of curing light technologies. They are:

- Tungsten halogen
- Argon laser
- Plasma arc (PAC)
- LED

Table 24-3 lists the pros and cons of each type of curing light.

The curing of dental materials can be adversely affected by:

- A dirty or scratched light tip
- Improper positioning of the light tip with regard to the material to be cured
- Ineffective filter
- Incorrect curing time for that particular material

Curing lights, especially those with halogen bulbs, can deteriorate. This can cause the material not to cure properly. A radiometer should be used regularly to test the light. A **radiometer** is a hand-held device that measures the intensity of a curing light. Built-in light meters are a feature in some curing lights. An LED radiometer should be used when testing an LED curing light.

A plastic barrier cover should be used over the light guide to protect it from any material that it may come in contact with during a curing procedure. Follow the manufacturer's instructions when cleaning or disinfecting the light.

It is very important that you never stare directly into a curing light. Eye damage could occur. Eye protectors that filter wavelengths below 500 nm should be worn when using a curing light.

Amalgamator

The **amalgamator** is a small, electrical machine that mixes dental materials (amalgams and some cements) by vigorously shaking the ingredients inside of a capsule (Figure 24-13). Specific speeds and times are required depending on the type of dental material being mixed. There are two main types of amalgamators: manual and computerized. Table 24-4 describes the attributes of each type of amalgamator.

As the DA, you will be responsible for mixing the dental materials before the procedure begins. (For a more detailed description of dental materials, see Chapter 33, Dental Cements, Liners, Bases, and Bonding Agents, and Chapter 35, Restorative Materials.)

TABLE 24-3 Curing Light Technologies

	TUNGSTEN HALOGEN	ARGON LASER	PLASMA ARC (PAC)	LIGHT-EMITTING DIODE (LED)
Pros	■ Durable ■ Cures fairly quickly ■ Broad-spectrum light compatible with all photoinitiators ■ Relatively inexpensive ■ Effective ■ Has a fan to cool unit	■ High intensity light ■ Moderate to fast curing ranges ■ No noticeable heat emissions	■ Powerful ■ Extremely fast ■ Uses multiple setting tips that filter light to be effective with different types of photoinitiators	■ Durable ■ Minimal heat emissions ■ No fan, filter, or bulb ■ Quiet ■ Lightweight ■ Portable ■ Some are cordless ■ Ergonomic designs available ■ Can conserve counter space by mounting on side of counter or integrating into dental unit ■ Newer models are effective with different types of photoinitiators ■ Relatively inexpensive
Cons	■ Emits some heat ■ Have to wait for fan to stop before turning unit off ■ Not portable ■ Filters needed for useless energy emissions ■ Should be tested regularly using a radiometer	■ Not effective with some photoinitiators so will not cure some types of materials ■ Relatively very expensive	■ Emits extremely high levels of heat ■ Some are relatively large and not portable ■ Filters needed for large amounts of useless energy emissions ■ Relatively expensive	■ Batteries need to be checked regularly in cordless units ■ Older models are only effective with the photoinitiator camphorquinone

Radiograph View Box

The radiograph view box has a bright light source inside the box and a frosted glass on the front. Radiographs are mounted and placed on the glass (Figure 24-14). The light shining through them makes the radiographs easy to view so that a diagnosis can be made. A radiograph view box may be mounted to the wall or a cabinet, or it may just be placed on a counter.

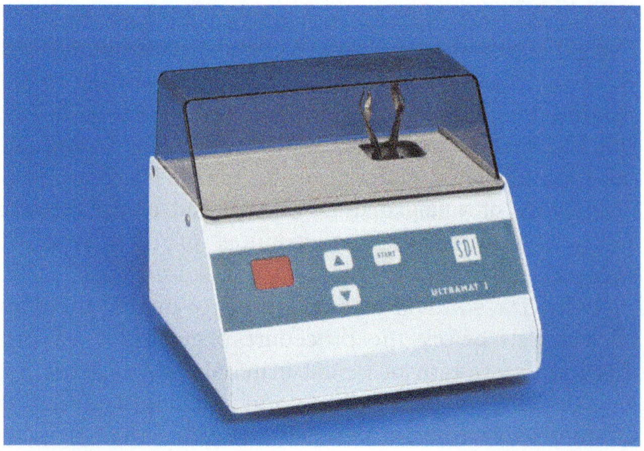

Figure 24–13 Amalgamator.

Office Communication System

All members of the dental team must be able to communicate with each other. A primary example is when the DA has finished an expanded duties procedure and needs to let the dentist know that the patient needs a final check prior to being dismissed. Verbally communicating this to the dentist in person while the dentist is with another patient may make that patient feel unimportant and not receiving the dentist's full attention. Every patient wants to feel that he or she is important and has the operator's full attention.

Many different types of office communication systems are available today and they can be customized to meet the needs and preferences of each dental office. Some systems

TABLE 24-4 Amalgamator

MANUAL	COMPUTERIZED
■ Manual timer; hand dial or digital	■ Fully programmable with preset memories; or programmed control cards for the different types of dental materials being mixed
■ Variable speed control; hand dial or digital	
■ Requires the operator to refer to manufacturer's directions to determine the specific settings required for the different types of dental materials being mixed	■ Touch pad controls
	■ Light-emitting diode display
■ Hand dials make machine harder to clean and disinfect	■ Smooth surface for easy disinfection

come with labelled, light-up buttons that let the operator know where he or she is needed, while others chime softly when a button lights up. Other systems come with a text screen, so that written messages can be sent. Some come with a verbal communication system so that dental team members can speak to each other.

Usually, wall-mounted units are placed in each treatment room, and one is placed on the reception desk. This allows the receptionist to let the operator know when the next patient has arrived. The units in the treatment rooms should be placed in view of the operator while working on a patient. Other units may be placed in the laboratory, the sterilization area, the staff lounge, and the dentist's personal office.

The best units have sealed touchpads that can be cleaned and disinfected easily. If not, they should have protective cover barriers that are replaced regularly.

Computer

Computers are used extensively in dental offices. All staff members should be trained to efficiently and effectively use the computers in the dental office. The receptionist can use the computer to:

■ Book appointments
■ Update patients' personal information
■ Keep track of production
■ Manage the employee time clock

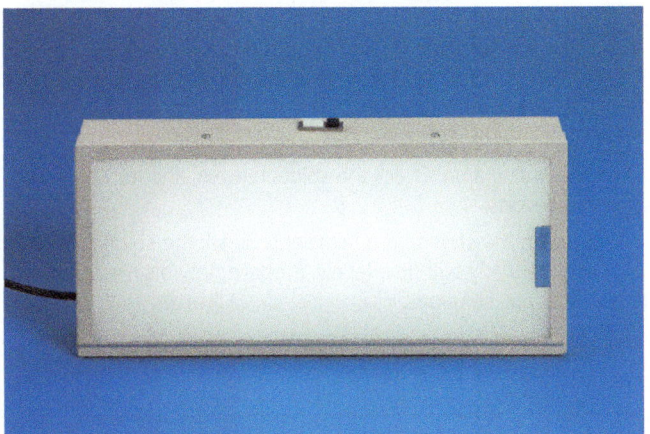

Figure 24–14 Radiograph view box.

The business office can use the computer to:

■ Bill the insurance companies or the patients
■ Maintain financial records
■ Do payroll
■ Keep track of and order supplies

For a more detailed description of using the computer in these areas, see Chapter 47, Office Management.

Computer workstations in the treatment rooms allow the dental team members to:

■ Efficiently update patients' records
■ Print out treatment plans and instructions for the patient
■ Send information to the receptionist regarding patient needs for any further appointments and the charge or bill for that day's services; this negates the need for paper to be taken from the treatment room to the front desk

Television, Video, Video Source Selector

Some dental offices have televisions in their treatment rooms. Usually, they are mounted on the wall at a place where the patient can see the screen while seated and while the operator is performing a procedure. A video source selector can be used to select what should be sent to the television. Many types of electronic equipment can be attached to the selector. They include:

■ A DVD player/video tape recorder; a patient dental education program could be used before a treatment to explain a procedure or afterwards for homecare instructions, or a relaxing nature video or a Disney movie for kids could play in order to distract the patient during treatment; wireless headphones could also be used to provide the sound, not only allowing a quiet work atmosphere for the operator, but also muffling the sound of the dental equipment for a nervous patient
■ Cable or satellite TV/radio (allowing the patient to choose what they want to watch or listen to); again wireless headphones could be used
■ An intraoral video camera; digital images of the patient's mouth can be displayed on the large television screen

to enhance any statements or instructions the operator is making to the patient

■ The treatment room computer; this allows the digital radiographs to be viewed on the large television screen

Office Care and Routines

Routine office care and the opening and closing of the office is often the responsibility of the DA. Although a professional cleaning company is usually hired to maintain the general cleanliness of the office, there are routine maintenance tasks that you will be expected to perform. Some will need to be done daily and some once a week or once a month. These tasks could include:

■ Keeping the dental office tidy in appearance, especially the reception area
■ Ensuring supplies and routine replacement parts are well stocked in treatment areas
■ Regularly changing radiograph processing and ultrasonic solutions
■ Cleaning and testing the sterilizers to ensure that they are in top working order
■ Making small, miscellaneous repairs as needed
■ Opening and closing the office

Consistently and carefully fulfilling these tasks helps ensure that:

■ The office will run smoothly
■ Unnecessary stress for the entire dental team will be avoided
■ The dentist will be able to work efficiently and effectively
■ The patient will not be inconvenienced or made to feel uncomfortable

Procedure 24-1 Opening the Office

1. Turn on all the lights.
2. Turn on the master switches for the central air compressor, central vacuum compressor, dental units, and radiographic equipment.
3. Turn on the computers and the communication system, unlock files, and ensure that the business side of the reception area is organized.
4. Check the answering machine or answering system for messages from patients.
5. Review the appointment schedule of patients to be seen that day. Check that the patient records and radiographs, laboratory cases, and instruments needed for that day's planned procedures are available. Post copies of the appointment schedule where needed.
6. If not already wearing the appropriate clinical clothing, change into the appropriate clothing.
7. Prepare all dental treatment rooms for patients by placing infection control barriers where needed (Figure P24-1-1), filling water reservoirs, flushing handpieces and air-water syringes, and checking that all supplies needed for the day are well stocked. Then, prepare the trays and lab work needed for the first patients of the day.

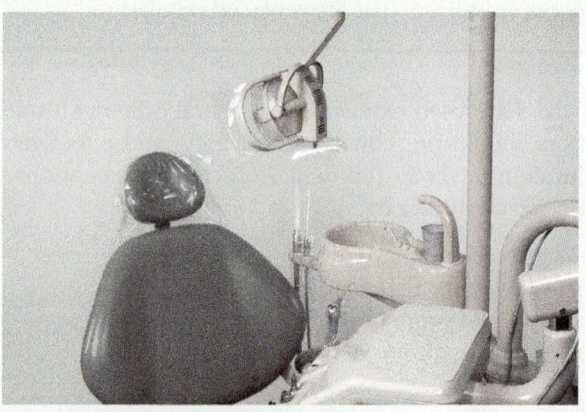

Figure P24-1-1

8. Ensure that the reception area is neat and tidy, and unlock the reception room entry door.
9. Change the water in the processing tanks in the radiograph processing area. Check the solution levels and refill any with low levels.
10. Turn on the sterilizing equipment. Check the solution levels and refill any with low levels. Prepare new disinfection and ultrasonic solutions.

Procedure 24–2 **Closing the Office**

1. Clean all the treatment rooms, following cleanup protocols while wearing the appropriate PPE. Clean all traps and filters (Figure P24-2-1). Flush handpieces and air-water syringes. Run the appropriate solutions through the evacuation hoses (Figure P24-2-2). Clean the dental chair and dental unit. Empty waste receptacles and insert new plastic liners. Clean counters. Restock supplies. Ensure that dental chairs are in the proper position for evening housekeeping. Ensure that all equipment and lights are turned off in all treatment rooms.

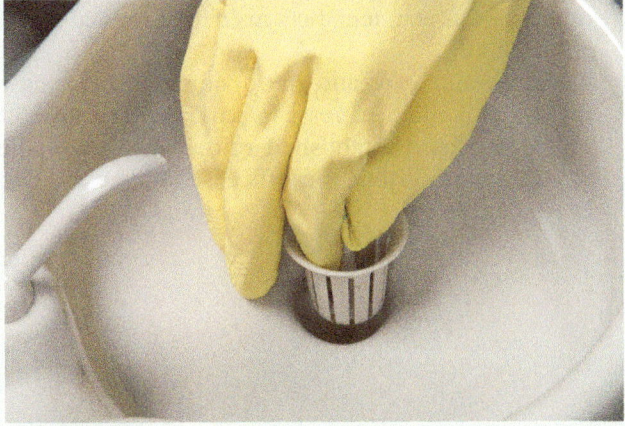

Figure P24-2-1

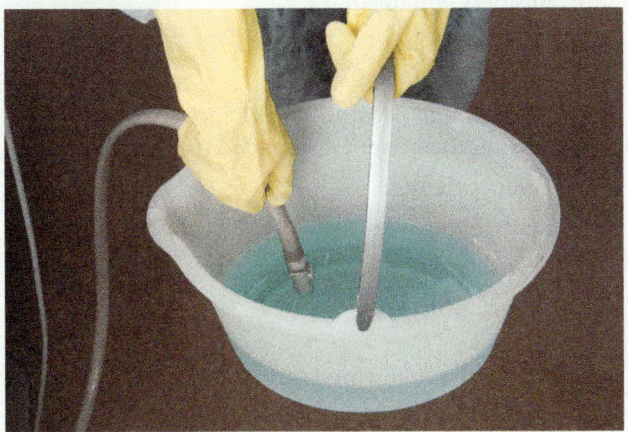

Figure P24-2-2

2. Process, mount, or file any radiographs not yet done. Turn off the water supply to the manual processing tanks and/or shut down the automatic processors. Clean counters and turn off all lights in the radiograph processing room.

3. Sterilize all patient care items and instruments. Turn off all equipment in the sterilization area. Empty the ultrasonic solutions. Rinse out the ultrasonic cleaner with water. Clean counters. Restock supplies. Turn off the lights in the sterilization area.

4. Turn off all master switches (i.e., for the central air compressor, central vacuum compressor, dental units, and radiographic equipment).

5. Ensure that all laboratory cases from that day have been sent to the lab and that any needed early the next day have been received.

6. Be sure that any soiled PPE has been placed into the appropriate containers.

7. If not already completed by the receptionist or business administrative staff, assist in confirming and completing the next day's appointment schedule. Pull any charts needed for the next day. Assist in completing any insurance forms or bookkeeping tasks.

8. Turn off all business area equipment. Lock all business area files. Turn on the answering machine or the answering service. Turn off all lights in the business area.

9. Tidy the reception area. Turn of all lights in the reception area. Lock all doors and windows.

10. Change out of your clinical clothing into street clothes.

 ## Chapter Highlights

◆ The patient's perception of the quality of care that he or she is likely to receive is greatly influenced by the environment established in the dental office. All areas of a dental office must be kept neat and clean.

◆ Decor, lighting, temperature, and sound all affect the environment of an office. Patient privacy, open traffic flow, and sound control should be considered when designing the layout of a dental office.

◆ The reception area is in the first room that the patient walks into when entering a dental office and where he or she meets the first person in the dental team.

◆ The business area should be set up in such a way as to allow for some privacy for the patient while discussing financial matters with the administrative personnel. Health Insurance Portability and Accountability Act privacy issues should be considered here.

◆ Treatment rooms should be designed and arranged for the most efficient use of the space and equipment. Treatment rooms should also be designed for patient comfort and privacy, as well as the comfort and ease of movement for members of the dental team.

◆ Dental work not performed directly on the patient takes place in the dental laboratory where infection control practices should be strictly followed and personal protective equipment worn.

◆ The assistant routinely cleans and maintains the equipment in the treatment and clinical areas.

◆ Everything in a treatment area is centered around a patient dental chair.

◆ The dental unit provides the electrical and air-operated components needed to utilize the air-water syringe, dental handpieces, saliva ejector, high-volume evacuator, and sonic and ultrasonic scaler.

◆ Infection control procedures must be strictly followed regarding all components of the dental unit.

◆ Delivery systems include side, rear, and front designs. The operating light must be correctly positioned.

◆ The ergonomic design and features of the operator's stool and the dental assistant's stool are very important for maintaining good musculoskeletal health. It is critical that each person's stool be properly adjusted for his or her body stature.

◆ The central air compressor and the central vacuum compressor require routine maintenance services as specified in the manufacturer's instructions.

◆ The four types of curing light technologies are tungsten halogen, argon laser, plasma arc (PAC), and light-emitting diode (LED).

◆ Computers are now being used extensively in dental offices, and all staff members need to be trained in their efficient use.

◆ Routine office care and the opening and closing of the office is often, at least in part, the responsibility of the assistant. Established routine procedures for opening and closing the office should be followed every day.

Review Questions

1. How much a patient owes the dentist should only be discussed in the
   a. Reception area.
   b. Business area.
   c. Treatment area.
   d. Patient education area.

2. Where are you most likely to prepare a diagnostic cast?
   a. Treatment room
   b. Business area
   c. Dental laboratory
   d. Sterilizing area

3. What kind of radiographic unit is typically found in a treatment room?
   a. Intraoral
   b. Extraoral
   c. Panoramic
   d. Cephalometric

4. Routine cleaning and maintenance of the treatment room equipment is usually the responsibility of the
   a. Receptionist.
   b. Dentist.
   c. Business administrator.
   d. Dental assistant.

5. The dental unit provides the electrical and air-operated components needed to use the
   a. Model trimmer.
   b. Air-water syringe.
   c. Dental lathe.
   d. Manual processor.

6. Which of the following is an advantage of the front delivery system?
   a. It places the instruments completely out of the patient's view.
   b. It offers a separate instrument section for the operator and the dental assistant.
   c. It allows the assistant access to the operator's instruments.
   d. It's stationary, which reduces the risk of cross-contamination.

7. An air-water syringe provides
   a. A focused stream of air.
   b. A focused stream of water.
   c. A combined air and water spray.
   d. All of the above.

8. Self-contained water bottles can now be found on many
   a. Dental units.
   b. Dental chairs.
   c. Divider cabinets.
   d. Amalgamators.

9. A rheostat is used to control
   a. The flow of water of the air-water syringe.
   b. The amount of suction of the saliva ejector.
   c. The speed of the handpiece.
   d. The amount of power to the ultrasonic scaler.

10. An electronic scaler is used
    a. While creating custom trays.
    b. To trim diagnostic casts.
    c. While manually processing radiographs.
    d. To remove calculus from the surface of the teeth.

11. Which of the following is the correct procedure for positioning the operating light over the patient's oral cavity?
    a. Using a handle on the side of the light, pull the light until it is directly over the patient's mouth and then turn it on.
    b. Position the light over the patient's chest, turn it on, and then using a handle on the side of the light, tilt the light up toward the oral cavity.
    c. Turn the light on above the patient's head, and then move it down towards the patient's mouth.
    d. Position the light to the side of the patient's head, turn it on, and then tilt the light toward the oral cavity.

12. The central vacuum compressor is used
    a. To provide the power for the handpieces.
    b. To provide the suction needed for the saliva ejector.
    c. To provide the suction needed for the air-water syringe.
    d. To harden dental materials.

13. "A lightweight, portable unit with no fan, filter, or bulb" best describes which of the following types of curing lights?
    a. Tungsten halogen
    b. Argon laser
    c. Plasma arc (PAC)
    d. Light-emitting diode (LED)

14. Curing lights should be tested regularly using a
    a. Radiometer.
    b. Rheostat.
    c. Amalgamator.
    d. Photoinitiator.

Active Learning Exercises

1. What is the importance of having a separate business area in the office? Why should the business and reception areas be separated?

2. Create a list of essential tasks that must be followed to open and close the office properly. Who is responsible for performing these daily office routines?

3. Name some distinct differences between the operator's stool and the dental assistant's stool. Is it necessary to have different types of stools? Explain your answer.

Application Activities

1. Recall a recent visit to a dental office, or visit a local dental office. Write each of the four factors that affect the environment in an office as headings across the top of a page. Now identify things that are contributing to the environment in that office and place each thing under the appropriate heading. State whether each thing has a positive or negative effect on the environment of the office. If it is negative, how would you change it?

2. Imagine that a friend has decided to build his own small dental office. Right now, the building space is basically one large square. He asks you how you would design the layout for a dental office that includes a reception area, a business area, three treatment rooms, a dental laboratory, a sterilization area, a radiograph room with a panoramic radiograph machine, a small utility room to house the compressors, a restroom, a small staff lounge, and a personal office. (He will be using automatic processors with daylight loading, so he will not need a radiograph processing room.) Roughly draw the layout of the office, keeping in mind the three factors that should be considered when designing the layout. Describe how these factors affected the layout that you designed.

3. The same friend mentioned in Activity 2 above also asks you to design his treatment rooms. He likes your tastes and style. Each treatment room is to have the same equipment, decor, and layout. The only thing he asks is that you keep in mind that he prefers the rear delivery system. Use the Internet or print resources to research dental products on the market today. Design the layout of the treatment room and choose all the equipment that your friend will need. (Detailed descriptions and/or pictures will help when presenting your ideas to your friend.) You will need to decide on colors and style. Keep in mind that your friend, at the very least, will need cabinets, a counter and sink, a dental chair, a dental unit, an operating light, an operator's stool, a dental assistant's stool, and an intraoral radiograph machine.

PREPARING FOR CERTIFICATION EXAMS

Review the following topics in this chapter to prepare for the Dental Assisting National Board (DANB) exam:

- **Storage Cabinets, Counters, Sinks**

- **Other Treatment Room Equipment**

Preparing for Dental Care

CHAPTER OUTLINE

CHAPTER CHECKLIST

On completion of this chapter, students will be able to:

- ☑ Describe how to prepare for a patient.
- ☑ Describe how to greet and seat a patient.
- ☑ Describe seven things that should be done to prepare the treatment area for the next patient.
- ☑ Identify types of patients that may have special needs and identify strategies for accommodating their needs during a dental visit.
- ☑ Explain the concept of *team dentistry*, identifying the roles played by the entire dental team and outlining the advantages of this method of providing dental treatment.
- ☑ Describe the four positions used for placing a patient in the dental chair and the situations in which each is used.
- ☑ Describe the correct positioning of the operator and of the assistant while performing procedures.
- ☑ Explain the principle of the *efficiency of motion*.
- ☑ Describe the five classes of motion and give an example of each.
- ☑ Describe the four zones of activity as positions on a clock, and explain the benefits of adhering to these zones.
- ☑ Describe the steps that should be followed for dismissing a patient.

KEY TERMS

efficiency of motion – minimizing the size and the number of motions made in order to optimize benefits to the body

four-handed dentistry – the method of providing dental treatment in which the operator and the assistant work together as a team while both are seated in specific positions near the patient; by working as a team, four hands are available to perform one procedure. This method increases the efficiency and productivity of the dental team, while reducing the stress, strain, and fatigue on the members of that team; also known as team dentistry

semisupine position – the position of the dental chair in which the back of the patient's chair is about 45 degrees from the floor; typically used when the operator working on the mandibular arch, or when the operator cannot put the patient back due to medical conditions

six-handed dentistry – a variation of four-handed dentistry that includes the dentist and two chairside assistants, one on the dentist's right and one on the left

Trendelenburg position – the position of the dental chair in which the head is placed lower than the legs and feet; this position is mostly used in emergency situations such as syncope

supine (su-PINE) position – the position of the dental chair in which the patient's body is horizontal with the chest at the same level as the knees, toes, and the top of the patient's head at the top edge of the headrest; the most common position used during dental treatment

upright position – the vertical, seated position of the dental chair in which the back of the chair is tilted back slightly from a 90-degree angle; this position allows the patient easy entrance and exit of the dental chair

zones of activity – specific areas around the patient designated for the different dental team members and equipment; also called operating zones

Introduction

Preparation for patient care is an ongoing responsibility that must be fulfilled not only at the beginning of the day before patients begin to arrive, but also throughout the day in order to ensure the most efficient and effective treatment for each patient. This advanced preparation helps minimize patient discomfort and unnecessary stress for the dental team, while enhancing the flow of patient care.

Preparing for dental care includes preparing for each patient by reviewing the patient record and preparing the treatment area according to individual patient needs and required treatments, as well as greeting and seating the patient, properly positioning each member of the dental team, and dismissing the patient. Preparation may also include calling patients the day before a scheduled appointment to remind them to take their premedications or to check insurance. This will reduce the chance that an appointment will need to be rescheduled.

Preparing for the Patient

It is very important to prepare for the patients that will be seen during the upcoming day. Knowing in advance the schedule for the day and the procedures that will be performed throughout the day allows you to obtain any supplies and prepare equipment that will be needed before the patients begin to arrive. For example, if a patient is scheduled to have a full crown cemented, the day before the appointment you need to be sure that the crown has arrived from the dental laboratory. Always show lab work to the dentist immediately when it arrives; do not wait until the patient's appointment. If the lab work has not arrived or if there is a problem, the patient's appointment can then be rescheduled.

Also, being aware of any patients coming in that day who have special needs allows you to be prepared ahead of time, resulting in the best possible care for each patient.

Reviewing the Patient Record

Before seeing each patient, you should familiarize yourself with the patient's record (Figure 25-1). This will alert you to the patient's premedications. While looking at the patient's record, note

- Any medical concerns that you and the dental team should be aware of
- Any change in dental treatment that should be provided
- Any change in the way in which dental treatments should be performed

Reviewing the patient's record also allows you to prepare any additional equipment or supplies that may be needed (such as nitrous oxide for an extremely nervous patient), or to alert the operator to any symptoms or warning signs that may occur during treatment due to a change in the patient's health. (For a more detailed description of the patient record, see Chapter 21, The Patient Record.) Note any premeds that need to be administered before treatment. Anything that could be harmful to the patient needs to be discussed.

From the Dentist's Perspective

Having a dental assistant who is well-organized and well-prepared is extremely important for the smooth flow of patient care throughout the day. An assistant that knows a patient's history and knows and prepares in advance for any special needs that the patient may have not only makes my job easier, but also provides a much more positive experience for the patient. This results in the office having a satisfied clientele that are more likely to recommend our office to other prospective patients.

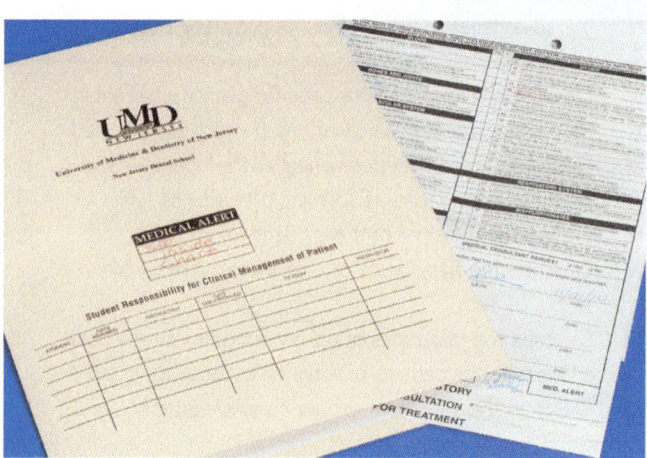

Figure 25–1 Review the patient's record.

Preparing the Treatment Area

There are a number of things that should be done in the treatment area before each patient is invited to that area. They include:

- Cleaning and disinfecting all necessary surfaces, equipment, and instruments, as well as flushing handpieces and air-water syringes for at least 1 minute (see Chapter 14, Disease and Infection Control)
- Placing infection control barriers on items that may become contaminated, such as the dental chair headrest, the arms of the dental chair, the finger-operated controls and tubing of the dental unit, handpieces, air-water syringes, the suction unit, the handles and switches of the operating light, and room light switches (see Chapter 24, The Dental Office, and Chapter 14, Disease and Infection Control)
- Bringing the patient's record, including any radiographs, to the area and reviewing what procedures or treatments are scheduled for that patient's appointment; the patient's record is placed in an area away from the immediate treatment area or covered with an infection control barrier and the radiographs are placed on a view box or the computer screen (if digital)
- Bringing in any lab work or models for that patient
- Bringing in a sterile preset tray and other supplies required for that patient's appointment. (These should be kept covered or out of the patient's view when entering the treatment area. This also allows the patient to feel at ease. Many of the dental instruments can be intimidating.)
- Moving items such as mobile carts, stools, dental light, dental chair arm, and rheostat out of the patient's pathway to the chair
- Positioning and locking the dental chair into the upright position with the chair tilted back slightly and the seat at a good height from the floor (approximately 15 in.); if the dental chair arm can be raised, this should be done before seating the patient to allow the patient to get onto the chair more easily

CHECKPOINT

25-1 What should you look for when reviewing a patient's record?

Greeting and Seating the Patient

As a dental assistant, it is often your responsibility to greet the patient in the reception area and to invite him or her to the treatment area. This is a great opportunity to begin easing any anxiety the patient may be feeling and to develop a long-lasting, comfortable rapport with him or her. Be sure to smile and project a positive attitude, helping the patient to feel at ease.

Cultural Diversity

Patients from some cultures will remove their shoes upon entering the office as a sign of respect and good manners. They also may not wear shoes in their own homes, substituting slippers instead. Typically, indoor footwear is not worn outside the home. Some people of Japan, China, Nepal, and India have adopted these traditions. It is important to respect a patient's right to practice shoe removal in the office.

Escorting the Patient to the Treatment Area

Remember, first impressions are everything. So after entering the reception area and identifying the patient by name, smile, greet the patient courteously while making eye contact, introduce yourself, and politely ask him or her to follow you back to the treatment area. By greeting a patient by name, you will confirm the patient's name and you will also make him or her feel like the staff know who they are. If the patient appears to need assistance, ask if you can assist in any way. Make sure that special needs patients are treated properly; many do not want special treatment. Try to assess this and treat them accordingly.

On the way to the treatment area, walk at the same speed as the patient. Ask how the patient is doing today. This is not only a polite thing to do, but it also may give you an idea if the patient is feeling overly anxious about the appointment.

If your office is large and has many hallways and rooms, tell the patient which room he or she will be in. This will help give the patient a sense of his or her location within the office. You might say, "Come this way, please," and let the patient follow you, or you could say, "The doctor is ready to see you now; please follow me."

Finally, once in the treatment area, point out to the patient where personal items, such as a purse or a jacket, may be placed. Normally a chair that is out of the way but still in full view of the patient while receiving treatment serves this function but an unused shelf or counter, a coat rack, or a hook on the wall may also be used.

Preparing the Patient for Treatment

After the patient has placed his or her personal items out of the way, politely ask the patient to sit down in the dental chair. Follow the steps listed in Procedure 25-1: Seating and Preparing the Patient for Treatment.

It is very important to note that you need to review the patient's medical history at the beginning of every visit, specifically asking the patient if anything has changed medically, as well as dentally, since the last visit. Certain medical conditions may require that the method in which treatment is given be changed from the norm. For example, certain bacterial infections, such as endocarditis (inflammation of the lining of the heart), require that the patient be placed on an antibiotic regimen *before* dental treatment is performed. You should also ask if any of the patient's prescriptions have changed or if new ones have been added since the last medical history update, including any over-the-counter supplements. (For more information regarding medically compromised patients, see Chapter 22, Patients With Special Needs.)

You must be aware, though, that some patients, for one reason or another, may not be as forthcoming as they should when disclosing any medical conditions that have developed recently. They may be:

- Unable to see the relevance to dental care
- Embarrassed
- Concerned with confidentiality
- Fearful of dental treatment being refused
- Limited by comprehension or a language barrier

You should emphasize to patients that there is a direct relationship between their general health and their oral health, and it is very important that your office be kept aware of their current medical condition so that you can maintain an up-to-date medical history in the patient records.

During this time, the patient may ask you questions about specific dental concerns, and while you may provide general information to the patient, specific concerns should be directed to the dentist when he or she comes in to see the patient. The dentist should also handle making modifications to address any uncertain medical conditions. Consider yourself the patient's advocate to the dentist and respond as such.

In the meantime, while preparing the patient for treatment, maintaining a conversation may help keep the patient relaxed. Take your cues from the patient and discuss topics that he or she is comfortable talking to you about. Such topics could include:

- Family
- Work
- Hobbies or sports
- Any trip the patient has taken or is about to take

It is not appropriate to speak with patients about religion or politics. Once you have discovered a topic that the patient seems to enjoy discussing, you could make a personal note in his or her record for the next visit. Knowing topics of interest to bring up at future appointments helps to build a rapport with that patient and helps to put him or her at ease that much sooner after arriving for the appointment. This also lets patients know you have an interest in them and that what they say is important to you.

Procedure 25-1 Seating and Preparing the Patient for Treatment

Materials Needed (Figure P25-1-1):

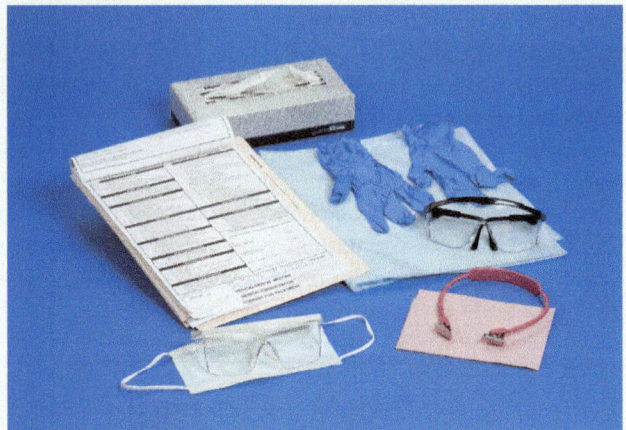

Figure P25-1-1

- Disposable patient napkin with napkin clip
- Tissue
- Patient record
- Patient safety glasses
- Personal protective equipment (mask, protective eyewear, gloves)

1. After ensuring that the dental chair is locked into position with the chair tilted back slightly and the seat at a good height from the floor, politely ask the patient to sit in the chair with his or her back flush against the back of the chair.

2. If the chair has an arm that has been moved out of the way to allow the patient to be seated, position the arm back into its proper place. (Make sure it is secure and locked into place.)

3. Adjust the headrest so that it is properly positioned, allowing for comfortable support for the patient's head and neck. The top of the patient's head should be at the top edge of the headrest.

4. Drape a disposable patient napkin (or bib) over the patient's chest (plastic side down, paper side up, and with the top double-folded so the clips won't slide off), and fasten napkin clips to each outside fold of the napkin in order to hold the napkin in place.

5. If the patient is wearing lipstick or colored lip balm, offer a tissue and ask the patient to remove it.

6. If your office offers patients a lip lubricant to apply, do so now. (If the office doesn't offer this and you notice the patient has dry or cracking lips, you can offer some Vaseline to prevent further damage to the lip area.)

7. Referring to the patient's record, review the patient's medical history, specifically asking if anything has changed since the last time he or she was there, including medications.

Procedure 25-1 Seating and Preparing the Patient for Treatment (Continued)

8. Explain briefly what is scheduled for the appointment today and answer any general questions that the patient may have about the scheduled procedure (Figure P25-1-2). Make sure you understand the patient's questions and the correct answers. If you are unsure, then you should find out the correct information. Take care not to give out misleading or incorrect information.

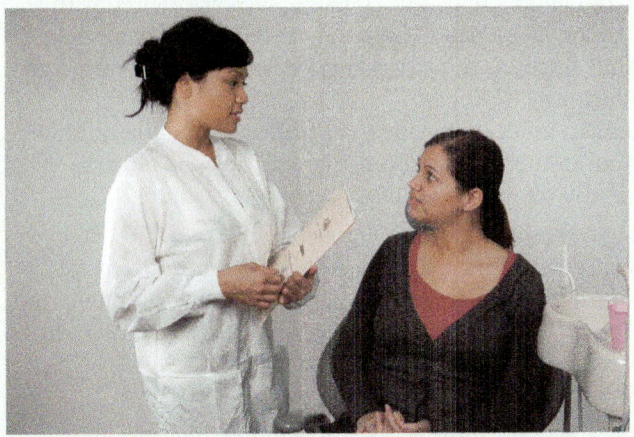

Figure P25-1-2

9. If your office offers patients safety glasses to wear during procedures, do so now. Some offices now offer patients headphones as well.

10. Tell the patient that you are ready to adjust the dental chair in order to position it properly for that appointment's planned procedure or treatment. Inform the patient that you will now lower the back of the chair, and slowly lower the back to the required position. Also, be sure to inform the patient when you are about to raise or lower the height of the entire chair or move any part of it, to avoid startling him or her. The chair must be raised to a proper height that allows the operator to sit comfortably near the patient with the patient's head above the operator's lap. Once the chair is positioned correctly, ask the patient if he or she is comfortable. If not, make any adjustments necessary.

11. Position the operating light correctly. Turn it on to be sure that the field of operation will be well illuminated. Then you may turn it off until the operator is seated and ready to begin. Make sure that if the patient needs to go to the restroom, the light is moved away from the patient's head to prevent injury.

12. Position the rheostat, operator's stool, and assistant's stool in the correct positions.

13. Put on your mask and protective eyewear, and then wash your hands and put on gloves

14. Position tray setup and dental unit equipment. Make sure you have the anesthetic ready and that the topical has been placed if it is needed.

15. Position yourself in an ergonomically correct position. You are now ready to begin the procedure or treatment.

Patients with Special Needs

Some patients have special needs that must be considered when greeting, seating, and treating them. For a detailed description of how to prepare for patients with particular special needs, see Chapter 22, Patients With Special Needs.

Patients who may require adjustments in how they are greeted and seated or positioned include children, pregnant patients, some older patients, mobility-impaired patients who require wheelchairs or walkers, vision- or hearing-impaired patients, patients with a language barrier, and medically compromised patients. Table 25-1 lists the special needs that should be considered with each of these types of patients.

CHECKPOINTS

25-2 Name some topics that are considered inappropriate for conversation with a patient.

25-3 What is the most important thing that should be reviewed with the patient at the beginning of every visit?

25-4 How should the dental chair be positioned in preparation for the patient to arrive?

Positioning

Four-handed dentistry, or team dentistry, is the method of providing dental treatment in which the operator and the assistant work together as a team while both are seated in specific positions near the patient (see Zones of Activity section later in this chapter); this method increases the efficiency and productivity of the dental team, while reducing the stress, strain, and fatigue on the members of that team. This method of providing dental treatment is the most common method used today. A variation of this method, known as **six-handed dentistry**, involves using a second chairside assistant, thus adding another pair of hands.

It is very important that you know the correct positioning of the patient, the operator, and the assistant. Correct ergonomic positioning enhances the comfort and safety of all involved, while allowing efficient access to the patient's oral cavity and the required dental equipment and instruments.

TABLE 25-1 Modifications for Patients with Special Needs

PATIENT	SPECIAL CONSIDERATIONS THAT MAY BE REQUIRED
Children	■ Greet and communicate with children on their level—physically, by kneeling and being eye-to-eye with them; and verbally, by using age-appropriate vocabulary ■ Set the original chair position lower than normal to allow the child to easily be seated ■ Use a cushion or booster chair to elevate the child in the dental chair ■ Reposition the headrest to enhance patient comfort and access to patient for treatment ■ Ask the child to sit with legs crossed to help prevent fidgeting and sliding around on the seat ■ Allow more time for the appointment for children with special issues, such as children with a high gag reflex (schedule in the morning or after a nap to help the procedure run smoothly) ■ Be patient with children who constantly fidget or need reassurance from a parent or guardian, stopping often during the procedure ■ Communicate with the parent or guardian while centering your primary attention on the child (many offices have the parent wait in the waiting room; the child may be more likely to behave better without the parent in the treatment room)
Pregnant	■ Encourage a dental visit to occur during the second trimester, if possible; this is the most comfortable and safe time for a pregnant woman—the first trimester is often accompanied by frequent nausea, and the third trimester can be physically uncomfortable for the woman, requiring frequent restroom breaks and making it difficult for her to breathe when in a reclined position ■ Allow a pregnant patient to remain sitting upright whenever possible ■ Allow frequent restroom breaks for the patient, if needed
Older adult	■ Provide assistance with getting up or sitting down if the patient asks for the help, or politely ask if assistance is needed in any way if the patient seems to be struggling; however, take care not to offend those patients who want to and are capable of doing these things independently ■ Ensure that any changes in the patient's medical condition or medications have been recorded in the patient record (make a copy of a medications list if the patient brings one in so you can put it in the chart and return the original) ■ Allow frequent restroom breaks for the patient, if needed ■ Allow the patient to sit upright whenever possible, if needed
Mobility-impaired	■ Talk openly with the patient to determine what assistance is required and when—some patients using a walker may need assistance getting to and from the treatment area, and being seated and getting up; some patients using a wheelchair may need assistance moving from the wheelchair to the dental chair and back again—these patients know the ways in which you can best assist them; listen to what they ask you to do ■ Make a note in the patient's record about how you were able to assist him or her to provide a reminder for the next appointment
Vision-impaired	■ Talk openly to determine what assistance they require and when; most will be very independent and just need you to explain throughout the procedure what you are doing and what you need them to do
Hearing-impaired	■ Stay in the patient's field of vision as much as possible so that patients can see you ■ Remove your face mask, making eye contact, and speaking slightly slower than normal, so that patients can see your lip movements and facial expressions ■ Ask questions to ensure they understand ■ Learn some relevant words or phrases in sign language for those patients who can sign
With a language barrier	■ Ask if someone that the patient knows or a member of your office staff would be able to act as interpreter for you ■ Learn a few relevant words or phrases in their native language to assist in communicating with them ■ Use pictures and diagrams to help communicate ■ Have available and use translation dictionaries, or translation programs on the computer, when an interpreter is unavailable
Medically compromised	■ Educate yourself and inform the operator about any special conditions that may be required due to the patient's medical condition

Positioning the Patient

Once seated in the dental chair, there are four positions in which the patient may be placed:

- Upright
- Supine
- Semisupine
- Trendelenburg

The **upright position** is the vertical, seated position in which the back of the chair is tilted back slightly from a 90-degree angle (i.e., the original locked position awaiting the patient to be seated). This position allows easy entry and exit from the chair, and is used in the following situations:

- While just talking to the patient
- When taking radiographs
- When a right-handed operator is providing treatment to the patient's lower right side
- When taking impressions

The **supine position** is the position most commonly used during treatment (Figure 25-2). In this position, the top of the patient's head should be at the top edge of the headrest, while the body is in a horizontal position, with the tip of the nose at the same level as the knees. Due to the ergonomics of the chair, the patient's body will not appear to lay completely flat.

The **semisupine position** is typically used when the operator is working on the mandibular arch or when the operator cannot lean the patient all the way back due to a medical condition. The back of the patient's chair is about 45 degrees from the floor, midway between the upright and supine positions.

The **Trendelenburg position** is the position in which the head is placed lower than the legs and feet (Figure 25-3). Although this allows the patient's head to be tilted back further and slightly upwards, making it easier for the operator to see into the oral cavity, this

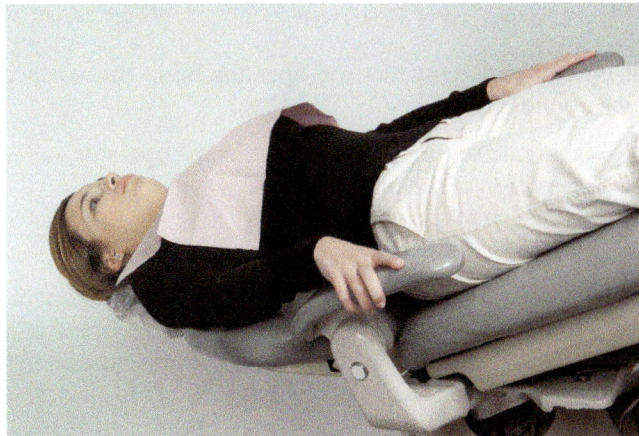

Figure 25–3 Patient in Trendelenburg position.

position is not very comfortable for the patient, and therefore is not used very often during regular treatment. It can be used:

- If the patient is unconscious
- To help treat shock in dental emergencies
- If the patient is hypotensive (experiencing very low blood pressure) or light-headed

After the patient has been properly positioned, the chair may need to be raised or lowered by the operator to get a clear vision of the operating field and to allow ergonomic access to the oral cavity. When placed in the supine position in preparation for treatment, the chair back should be about even with the operator's elbows when close to the operator's body and the operator's face should be approximately 14 inches from the patient's oral cavity (Figure 25-4). The operator may then need to ask the patient to turn his or her head to the left or right, or when working in the mandibular area may need to raise the back of the patient's chair slightly, in order to have better visualization of the operating field.

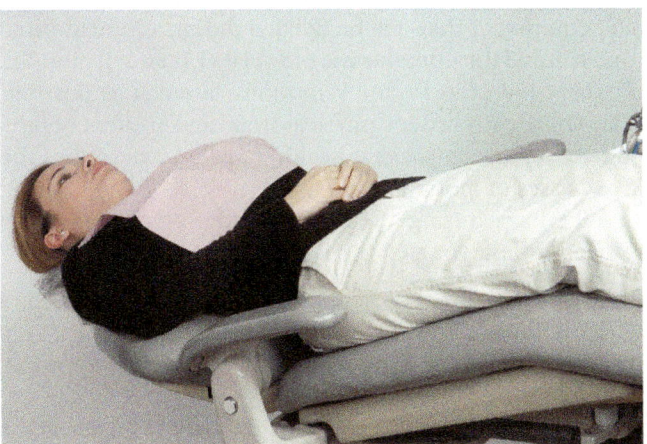

Figure 25–2 Patient in supine position.

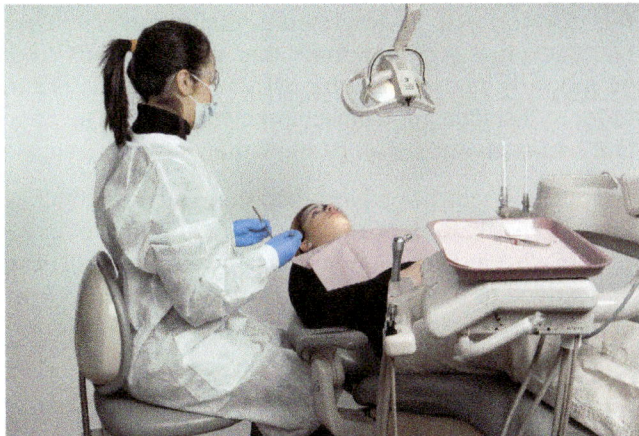

Figure 25–4 Operator correctly positioned to work.

The Operator's Position

It is very important that the operator be in the correct position to ensure:

- Ergonomic support and comfort for the operator
- Clear vision of the operating field
- Easy access to the operating field
- Efficient performance of the procedure

As described in Chapter 24, The Dental Office, the operator's stool should be properly adjusted for that operator's body stature in order to maintain good musculoskeletal health. First, the operator's stool should be set to allow the operator to sit with:

- The feet flat on the floor
- The thighs parallel to the floor
- The back of the knees close to the front edge of the seat
- The back straight and against the back of the chair
- The forearms parallel to the floor
- The elbows close to the operator's sides

Then, the patient's dental chair should be set at a height that allows the operator to sit with:

- Arms bent at the elbow at a 90-degree angle, keeping the forearms parallel to the ground
- A hip angle of 90 degrees

The operator's legs should straddle the dental chair or be placed underneath the headrest (not the back) of the dental chair. The tip of the patient's nose should be below the operator's waist (see Figure 25-4).

The Assistant's Position

The assistant sits on an assistant's stool with knees toward the patient's head. The assistant's position in relation to the operator depends on whether the operator and the assistant are right-handed or left-handed. (For a detailed description of the various positions the operator and the assistant may take in relation to each other and to the patient, see the section titled Zones of Activity in this chapter). Also as described in Chapter 24, The Dental Office, it is very important that the assistant's stool be properly adjusted for that assistant's body stature in order to maintain good musculoskeletal health. The assistant's stool should be set to allow the assistant to sit:

- Four to six inches higher than the operator (to allow clear visualization of the procedure in order to anticipate what instrument or material the operator will need next and to have clear access to the operating field to better assist with the procedure)
- With the thighs parallel to the floor
- With the feet on the footrest
- With the back of the knees close to the front edge of the seat
- With the back straight

- With the left thigh near but not touching the patient's left shoulder (for a right-handed operator)

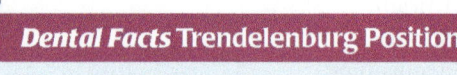

Dental Facts Trendelenburg Position

The Trendelenburg position was first used by a German surgeon named Friedrich Trendelenburg while performing abdominal surgery. It is often used by surgeons while performing operations on organs in the pelvic area, and to help reduce shock. Dentists use this position to reduce shock in dental emergencies.

CHECKPOINT

25-5 What is team dentistry?

Principles of Movement

As the dental assistant, you may do more twisting, turning, and reaching while seated than anyone else in the office. This can lead to fatigue and strain, especially of the lower lumbar region. It cannot be stressed enough that you should do all you can to reduce this fatigue in order to maintain good musculoskeletal health. To do this, you must use ergonomically correct equipment and positioning (see the Zones of Activity section in this chapter), as well as efficiency of motion. Applying the principles of ergonomics in the dental office is discussed at length in Chapter 19, Ergonomics.

Efficiency of Motion

Maximizing **efficiency of motion** by minimizing the magnitude and the number of motions made during every procedure will optimize the ergonomic benefits. Motions have been classified into five classes. You should position yourself, the operator, the dental unit, and all instruments and equipment that will be needed during a procedure so that you and the operator use only class I, II, and III motions. Try to avoid class IV and V motions as much as possible. This will greatly reduce physical strain and ensure continuing good musculoskeletal health. Table 25-2 describes the five classes of motion.

When organizing equipment and instruments for a procedure, ask yourself the following questions:

- Are all instruments, handpieces, and materials needed within reach without having to stretch for them?
- Will I have to turn or twist my body to reach for a specific instrument?
- Does the preset tray contain only those instruments needed for that procedure, and are they in the order that they will be used?

TABLE 25-2 Classes of Motion

CLASS	RANGE OF MOTION	EXAMPLE
I	■ Movement involving only the fingers	■ Moving an instrument on a tooth
II	■ Movement involving the fingers and the wrist	■ Retrieving and transferring the instrument to the operator
III	■ Movement involving the fingers, wrist, and elbow	■ Reaching for and pulling a dental handpiece from the dental unit
IV	■ Movement involving the entire arm and shoulder	■ Adjusting the operating light, or reaching for material on a counter adjacent to the immediate work area
V	■ Movement involving the entire arm and upper torso	■ Twisting or turning in your seat to reach for material on a counter behind you

Even if you can omit class IV and V motions during procedures throughout the day, you could still find your muscles fatigued by the end of the workday. To reduce fatigue and strain during procedures, try to minimize:

- The number and magnitude of motions made during repetitive and routine tasks for both you and the operator
- Jerky movements, by using continuously smooth motions
- Your number of eye movements, especially from objects near and then far away and from brightly lit areas to those areas that are less illuminated; eye strain needs to be avoided just as much as strain on the lower back

It is a good idea to perform regular abdominal exercises, which will help strengthen the back. Well-conditioned muscles have improved control and endurance and reduce the likelihood of strain or injury.

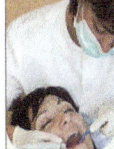

Voice of Experience

Some days can seem very long. There are days when it seems as if we just do the same procedure over and over again, except on different patients. I've learned that if I don't pay attention to the principles of movement and ergonomics, by the end of those days, my entire body will be pretty fatigued, which can lead to an aching lower back, sore neck and shoulders, and eye strain. I've learned, though, that by being organized and arranging everything that is going to be needed during an upcoming procedure in such a way that it reduces the number of motions I need to make during the procedure, I no longer have any of those aches and pains. Suddenly, the days no longer seem so long, and I'm able to enjoy my work again.

Zones of Activity

Zones of activity, also called *operating zones*, are specific areas around the patient designated for the different dental team members and equipment (see Table 25-3). In four-handed, or team, dentistry there are four zones of activity centered around the patient:

- Operator's zone
- Assistant's zone

- Transfer zone
- Static zone

The efficiency of motion is dependent on the operator and the assistant respecting and using these four zones of activity. When positioned correctly, both the operator and the assistant:

- Have good visualization of the operating field
- Have easy access to the patient's oral cavity
- Have ergonomic access to all instruments, equipment, and materials needed for the procedure
- Have efficient transfer of instruments
- Have a reduction in the amount of physical fatigue and strain
- Avoid each other's legs
- Have increased productivity

The zones of activity are described as positions on a clock. When the patient is lying in the supine position, picture the patient's oral cavity as the center of the clock and the area above the top of the patient's head as 12 o'clock. The different zones are defined differently depending on whether the operator is right-handed or left-handed. Basically, the zones are reversed or the "clock" presents as a mirror image for the left-handed operator compared to the right-handed operator (Figure 25-5A,B).

Essentially, the left-handed operator works from the upper left side of the patient, and the right-handed operator works from the upper right side of the patient. Then, the assistant normally works across from the operator on the opposite side of the patient.

Some versatile chairs can be rotated to accommodate a left-handed operator and dental assistant. Left-handed operators who work in a right-handed chair may find that the cuspidor and suction equipment will be in the way of their work flow. A left-handed assistant must learn to adapt; the working conditions depend on the operator's or the dentist's hand preference. Some dental chairs are not adaptable for left-handed operators; others are. Newer dental units (particularly rear-delivery units) have a handpiece station that can be positioned either right or left so

TABLE 25-3 Zones of Activity

ZONE OF ACTIVITY	PURPOSE	CLOCK POSITION	
		RIGHT-HANDED OPERATOR	LEFT-HANDED OPERATOR
Operator's Zone	■ Best area for the operator to visualize and access the oral cavity ■ Allows some flexibility in positioning of the operator depending on which area of the oral cavity the operator is working	7 o'clock to 12 o'clock	12 o'clock to 5 o'clock
Assistant's Zone	■ Best area for assistant to assist operator with tasks such as suctioning and passing instruments ■ Minimal area in which to be positioned in order to minimize motion ■ Dental unit and mobile cart with instrument tray and dental materials may be positioned within this zone for easy access by the assistant	2 o'clock to 4 o'clock (ideally 3 o'clock)	8 o'clock to 10 o'clock
Transfer Zone	■ Best area for transferring instruments between assistant and operator ■ Areas under patient's chin and above the patient's chest (never rest instruments or handpieces on the patient's chest) ■ Front delivery systems are positioned within this zone	4 o'clock to 7 o'clock	5 o'clock to 8 o'clock
Static Zone	■ Rear delivery systems are positioned here for easy access by the assistant (and operator, if needed) ■ Other portable equipment, such as nitrous oxide, portable curing light, or blood pressure equipment, may be positioned here ■ Also may use this area to pass a local anesthetic syringe to the dentist if working with a squirming child	12 o'clock to 2 o'clock	10 o'clock to 12 o'clock

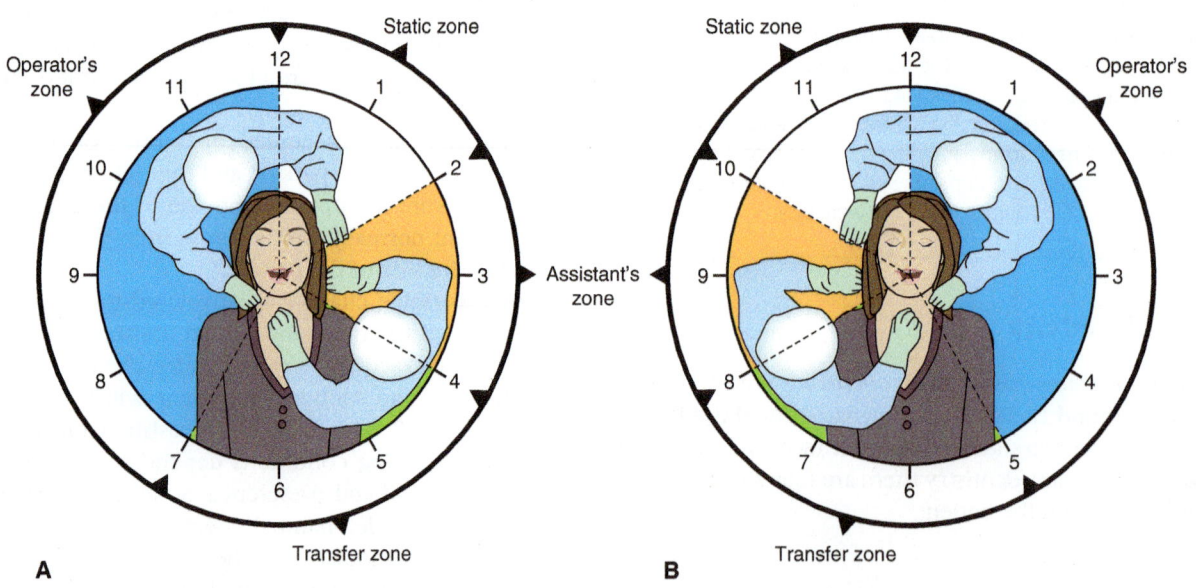

Figure 25–5 **Zones of activity.** (**A**) For right-handed operator. (**B**) For left-handed operator.

the unit can be adjusted for the operator. A dental assistant assists a right-handed dentist by always passing instruments with the left hand and suctioning with the right hand. A dental assistant assists a left-handed dentist by passing instruments with the right hand and suctioning with the left.

A left-handed chair design has everything the operator needs on the opposite side of the chair. The assistant needs to learn to work on the opposite side to work with a left-handed operator.

Ergonomics

It is very important that all aspects of the working environment be as ergonomically sound as possible in order to reduce fatigue and maintain good musculoskeletal health, as well as improve efficiency and productivity.

Principles for the Operator

In order to maintain good musculoskeletal health, the ergonomic principles the operators should follow include:

- Positioning themselves in the operator's zone close to the patient with the back/headrest of the patient dental chair lowered over the operator's knees and at a level even with the operator's elbows
- Distributing weight evenly on the seat of the operator's stool with the feet flat on the ground, the back of the knees close to the front edge of the seat, the back straight and all the way back in the chair, and the arms bent at the elbow at a 90-degree angle, keeping the forearms parallel to the floor and close to the side of the body

- Following the principles of efficient instrument transfer as outlined in Chapter 26, Dental Instruments and Equipment
- Following the principles of efficiency of motion by restricting hand and arm movement to the transfer zone and eye focus to the operating field

Figure 25-6 demonstrates incorrect and correct operator positioning.

Principles for the Assistant

In order to maintain good musculoskeletal health, the ergonomic principles the assistant should follow include:

- Positioning yourself in the assistant's zone close to the patient with knees facing toward the wall behind the patient or toward the rear-delivery dental unit
- Positioning yourself four to six inches higher than the operator
- Positioning your left thigh near the patient's left shoulder (for a right-handed operator)
- Distributing your weight evenly on the seat of the assistant's stool with your feet on the footrest, the back of your knees close to the front edge of the seat, and your back straight against the back of the chair, *not* using a stomach rest, and leaning forward from your hips rather than bending your neck
- Following the principles of efficient instrument transfer as outlined in Chapter 26, Dental Instruments and Equipment
- Following the principles of efficiency of motion by having dental equipment, instruments, and materials as close as possible in order to avoid twisting, turning, and overextending your arms

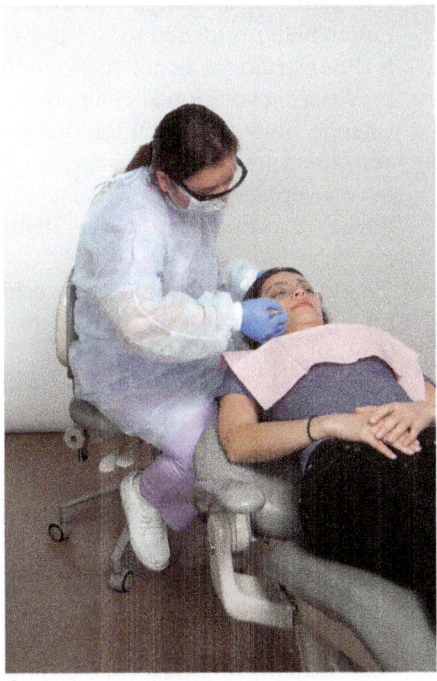 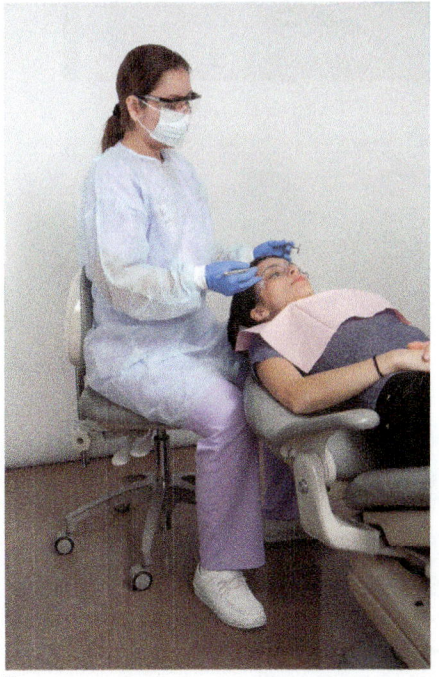

A **B**

Figure 25–6 **Operator positioning.** (**A**) Operator seated incorrectly. (**B**) Operator seated correctly.

Figure 25-7 demonstrates incorrect and correct assistant positioning.

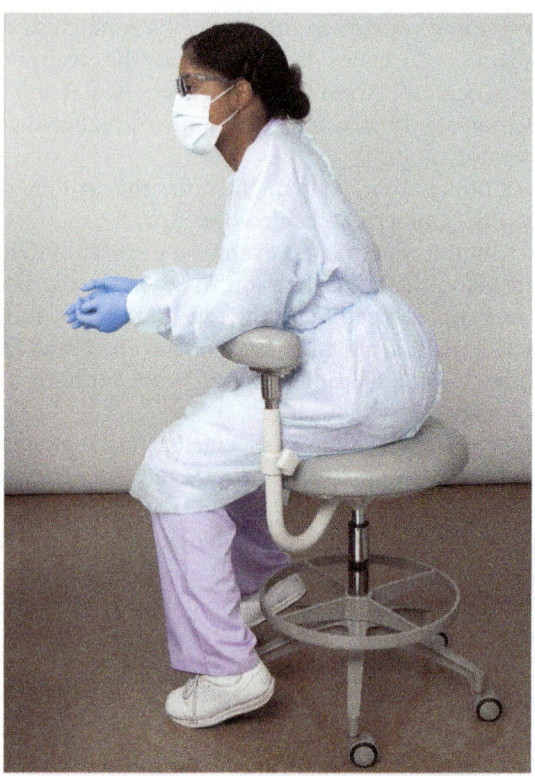

A

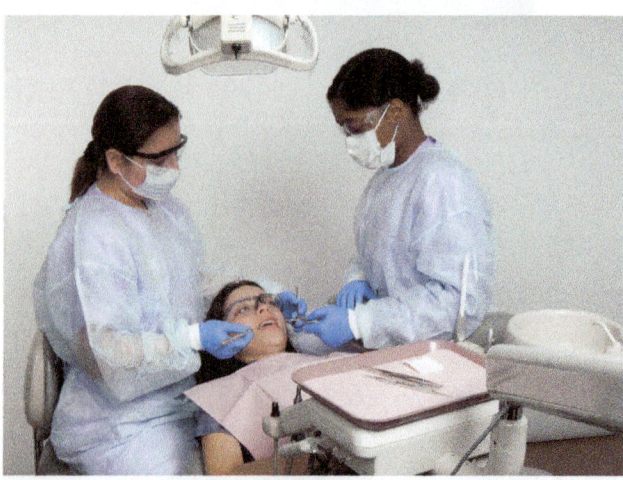

B

Figure 25-7 Assistant positioning. (**A**) Assistant seated incorrectly. (**B**) Assistant seated correctly.

The Dental Assistant's Chairside Role

The dental assistant's main responsibility is to efficiently and effectively assist the operator during dental procedures. In order to accomplish this, you need to be able to perform the following functions:

- Thoroughly understand any procedure in which you will be assisting. (If you are unsure of the proper way to perform a procedure, ask for assistance until you feel comfortable.)
- Cooperate with the operator in developing a standardized routine for basic dental procedures, as well as a predictable instrument transfer protocol. (For a more detailed description of instrument transfer protocol, see Chapter 26, Dental Instruments and Equipment.)
- Recognize when a change is needed in a procedure.
- Recognize when a patient or a member of the dental team needs to be repositioned in order to improve visibility, access, ergonomics, or efficiency of motion.
- Anticipate the operator's needs during a procedure and be ready at all times to transfer any instruments, materials, or equipment needed.
- Learn to recognize nonverbal signals given by the operator indicating a need to exchange an instrument.
- Transfer instruments to the operator only in the transfer zone.
- Maintain the order of the instruments in the preset trays according to the order in which they will be used, as well as the dental materials that will be used. Be sure to return them to that position after use so that if they are needed again, they can be easily located.
- Use gauze or a sponge to remove debris from instruments being returned to the preset tray, if time allows; if the instrument is not to be used again, place it in a precleaning solution at chairside.
- Change burs on dental handpieces as needed. (Make sure the burs that are on the bur block are not dull—have a replacement sterile backup in case one breaks during a procedure or the dentist requests a new one.)
- Maintain the operating field by using appropriate moisture control practices (see Chapter 27, Moisture Control and Isolation).
- Follow any verbal directions given by the operator without delay.
- Keep the immediate work area clean and orderly.
- Recognize a patient's needs by noting nonverbal communication such as body language in order to ensure the patient's comfort and safety.

Dismissing the Patient

When the procedure is complete, do a final rinse and evacuation of the patient's oral cavity and, if the operator has not done so already, turn off the dental light and position it out of the patient's way. Then follow the steps listed in Procedure 25-2: Dismissing the Patient.

Procedure 25-2 Dismissing the Patient

Materials Needed:

- Tissue
- Hand mirror
- Patient record

1. Inform the patient that you will now raise the back of the chair, and slowly raise the back to the upright position. If the patient has been lying back for an extended period of time, raise the chair in two stages to avoid any dizziness caused by postural hypotension (Figure P25-2-1). Also, be sure to inform the patient if you need to raise or lower the height of the entire chair.

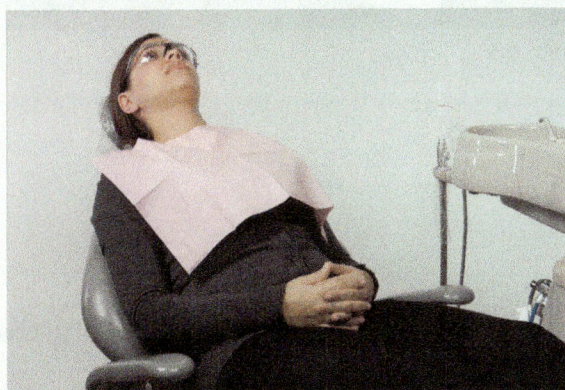

Figure P25-2-1

2. Wipe any debris from the patient's face, or offer a tissue and a mirror if the patient would prefer to do it (Figure P25-2-2).

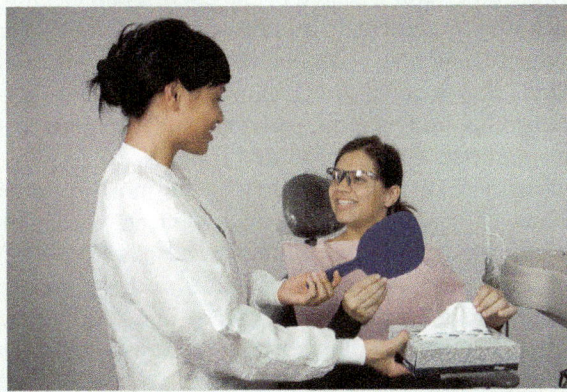

Figure P25-2-2

3. Ask the patient to remain seated for a moment while you update his or her record. This gives the patient the opportunity to adjust to being raised to an upright position, allowing any light-headedness that he or she may be experiencing to subside.

4. Remove the air-water syringe, saliva ejector, and oral evacuator tips and place them on the tray.

5. If safety goggles were used by the patient, ask for those back and place them on the tray.

6. Remove the patient napkin and place it over the tray, covering everything on the tray.

7. Remove and dispose of your gloves. Then wash your hands and remove goggles.

8. Update the patient's record by documenting the procedure either in the patient's chart or using the computer workstation in the treatment area. If x-rays are on an x-ray view box, gather those and place them with the patient's chart.

9. Provide any postoperative instructions that the patient may need.

10. Ask the patient if he or she has any questions.

11. Move items such as the mobile cart, stools, and rheostat out of the patient's exit path from the dental chair.

12. Move the arm of the chair out of the patient's way and assist the patient, if needed, in getting out of the chair (Figure P25-2-3).

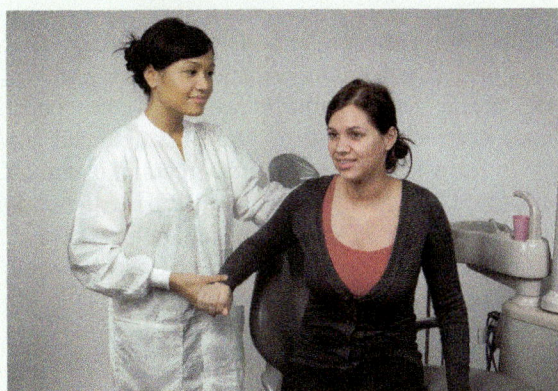

Figure P25-2-3

13. Remind the patient to retrieve all personal items.

Procedure 25-2 Dismissing the Patient (Continued)

14. Escort the patient to the reception area, taking the patient's chart (with the x-rays) with you. If the patient had nitrous oxide, make sure he or she sits for a minimum of 5–15 minutes. Administer plain oxygen for 5 of those minutes. (Nitrous oxide should be off.) If the patient had sedation, make sure you never leave his or her side until you get to the waiting area, where a responsible adult should be waiting to drive the patient home safely. (This should never be a cab or a shuttle.)

15. Give the patient's chart to the receptionist and explain when patient's next appointment should be and what treatment will need to be provided (Figure P25-2-4). Then inform the patient that the receptionist can help schedule the next appointment and complete the financial aspect of the visit. Ask the patient to contact the office with any questions or concerns and say that someone will respond as soon as possible.

16. Politely wish the patient a good day and good-bye (Figure P25-2-5).

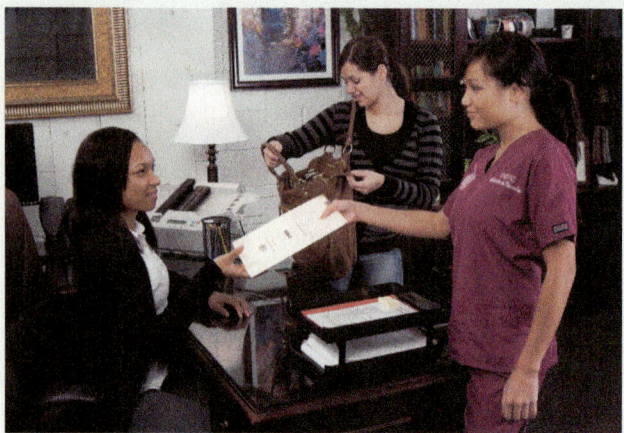

Figure P25-2-4

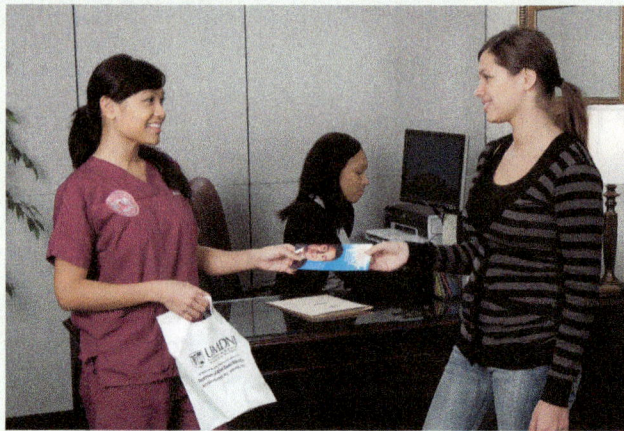

Figure P25-2-5

Chapter Highlights

✦ Preparation for patient dental care is an ongoing responsibility from the beginning of the day, before patients begin to arrive, throughout the day to ensure the most efficient and effective treatment for each individual patient.

✦ Reviewing the patient's record before seeing that patient will alert you to any medical concerns that you and the dental team should be aware of, any change in dental treatment that should be provided, and any change in the way in which dental treatments should be performed. It also allows you to prepare any additional equipment or supplies that may be needed and to alert the operator to any symptoms or warning signs that may occur during treatment due to a change in the patient's health.

✦ Greeting the patient in the reception area and escorting the patient to the treatment area offers a great opportunity to begin easing any anxiety the patient may be feeling and to develop a long-lasting, comfortable rapport.

✦ The most important thing that should be reviewed with a patient at the beginning of every visit is the patient's medical history, specifically asking if anything has changed *medically* as well as dentally since the last visit.

✦ A dental assistant may provide general information in response to a patient's questions, but specific concerns should be directed to the dentist.

✦ Patients that may require adjustments in the way that they are greeted and seated or the circumstances under which the treatment is performed include children, pregnant patients, older patients, mobility-impaired patients that require wheelchairs or walkers, vision- or hearing-impaired patients, patients with a language barrier, and medically compromised patients.

✦ Four-handed, or team, dentistry is the most common method of providing dental treatment, in which the operator and the assistant work together as a team while both are seated in specific positions near the patient; this method increases the efficiency and productivity of the dental team, while reducing the stress, strain, and fatigue on the members of that team.

✦ The four positions for the patient in the dental chair are the upright position, supine position, semisupine position, and Trendelenburg position.

◆ The most common position for the patient during procedures is the supine position.

◆ The principle of efficiency of motion is minimizing the magnitude and the number of motions made during every procedure in order to optimize the ergonomic benefits.

◆ There are five classes of motion; avoiding class IV (movement involving the entire arm and shoulder) and class V (movement involving the entire arm and upper torso) as much as possible will greatly reduce physical strain and ensure continuing good musculoskeletal health.

◆ To reduce fatigue and strain during procedures, try to minimize the number and magnitude of motions made, jerky movements, and the number of eye movements.

◆ The four zones of activity centered around the patient in team or four-handed dentistry are the operator's zone, the assistant's zone, the transfer zone, and the static zone, and are described as positions on a clock.

◆ The operator and the assistant should follow specific ergonomic principles to maintain good musculoskeletal health.

◆ The dental assistant's main responsibility is to efficiently and effectively assist the operator during dental procedures in a chairside role.

 **Review Questions**

1. How should the dental chair be positioned in preparation for the next patient?

   a. The supine position

   b. The semisupine position

   c. The Trendelenburg position

   d. The upright position

2. Which of the following positions is most commonly used for dental procedures?

   a. The upright position

   b. The supine position

   c. The semisupine position

   d. The Trendelenburg position

3. Medically compromised patients that are predisposed to bacterial infections, such as endocarditis, should

   a. Never undergo any dental procedures.

   b. Be placed on an antibiotic regimen *before* dental treatment is performed.

   c. Be placed on an antibiotic regimen immediately *after* dental treatment is performed.

   d. Be placed on an antibiotic regimen only if an infection develops after the dental treatment is performed.

4. Which of the following statements is true?

   a. There is a direct relationship between a patient's general health and his or her oral health.

   b. A patient's general health does not affect his or her oral health.

   c. A patient's general health is none of the dental office's concern, only his or her oral health.

   d. The dental assistant should ask a patient about his or her medical history only if there are obvious signs that the patient is medically compromised.

5. The best time for women who are pregnant to undergo dental treatment is

   a. Never.

   b. The first trimester.

   c. The second trimester.

   d. The third trimester.

6. In which position is the patient placed when taking radiographs?

   a. The upright position

   b. The supine position

   c. The semisupine position

   d. The Trendelenburg position

7. In which position is the patient placed to help treat shock in dental emergencies?

   a. The upright position

   b. The supine position

   c. The Trendelenburg position

   d. The lotus position

8. The dental assistant should sit with his or her knees toward the

   a. Operator's knees.

   b. Patient's side.

   c. Patient's feet.

   d. Wall behind the patient's head.

9. Which of the following motions should the dental assistant avoid while assisting in procedures?

   a. Movement involving only the fingers

   b. Movement involving the fingers and the wrist

   c. Movement involving the fingers, wrist, and elbow

   d. Movement involving the entire arm and upper torso

10. Which of the following is an example of a class V motion?

    a. Picking an instrument off the tray

    b. Reaching for and pulling a dental handpiece from the dental unit

    c. Twisting or turning in the seat to reach for material on a counter behind the seat

    d. Reaching for material on a counter adjacent to the immediate work area

11. In which clock position should the assistant be positioned when working with a right-handed operator?

    a. 12 o'clock to 2 o'clock

    b. 2 o'clock to 4 o'clock

    c. 4 o'clock to 7 o'clock

    d. 7 o'clock to 12 o'clock

12. In which zone of activity would a front delivery system be positioned?

    a. Operator's zone

    b. Assistant's zone

    c. Transfer zone

    d. Static zone

Active Learning Exercises

1. Describe the Trendelenburg position. When would it be necessary to place a patient in this position?

2. Create a diagram of the zones of activity for both a right- and left-handed operator and dental assistant. Why are these zones important?

3. Imagine that a patient is having an amalgam filling placed. How does the dental assistant prepare for this treatment? How is the patient prepared for the treatment? What are some things the patient should know?

Application Activities

1. Partner with another student to role-play a situation in which one of you is the dental assistant and one of you is a new patient with special needs, such as a hearing-impaired patient. Remember, the patient cannot hear anything the assistant is saying, but may be able to read lips. Go through the process of greeting, seating, and preparing the patient for treatment. When finished, write a short report describing the experience, specifically noting any difficulties or discomforts either of you experienced. Explain how these situations could have been handled differently. Now, each of you reverse roles implementing the solutions you devised and write how this experience was different from the first. This activity may be repeated role-playing a patient with a different special need.

2. In groups of four students, choose one student to be the operator and one student to be the assistant. First, presume the operator is right-handed. Have the operator and the assistant sit on their respective stools in preparation of beginning a procedure on an imaginary patient in the supine position. The remaining two students should scrutinize both the operator's and the assistant's positioning and identify where changes should be made. Pay attention to all details of their ergonomic positioning, as well as their positions within the zones of activity. Then have the "operator" and the "assistant" reverse roles and position themselves presuming that the operator is now left-handed. Again, the remaining two students should scrutinize their positioning and identify where changes should be made. Now, the two students who originally assumed the roles of the operator and the assistant should observe as the other two students repeat the entire activity.

PREPARING FOR CERTIFICATION EXAMS

Review the following topics in this chapter to prepare for the Dental Assisting National Board (DANB) exam:

- **Preparing for the Patient**
- **Greeting and Seating the Patient**
- **Positioning**
- **Zones of Activity**
- **The Dental Assistant's Chairside Role**
- **Dismissing the Patient**

chapter 26

Dental Instruments and Equipment

CHAPTER OUTLINE

CHAPTER CHECKLIST

On completion of this chapter, students will be able to:

- ☑ Identify the three parts of a dental instrument.
- ☑ Describe the various instrument classification systems.
- ☑ Identify dental hand instruments and describe their functions.
- ☑ Describe how trays are assembled, including systems for organizing and positioning instruments.
- ☑ Identify rotary dental instruments by number and function.
- ☑ Describe the proper way to grasp dental instruments.
- ☑ Describe how to correctly transfer dental instruments to an operator.

KEY TERMS

amalgam carrier – an instrument used to transfer mixed amalgam into a cavity preparation until the restoration is completely filled

angle former – a hand instrument with angled and beveled blades used to create line angles inside the cavity preparation

articulating forceps – a device used to hold articulating paper for the patient to bite down on

articulating paper – used to determine tooth contacts when the patient bites on it; synonymous with occluding paper or carbon paper

blade – the working end of an instrument with special shapes or designs used to create and cut lines or grooves on or in a tooth surface

burnisher – an instrument for smoothing and polishing surfaces or margins of a dental restoration

carver – a dental hand instrument, available in a wide variety of end shapes, used to form and contour wax as well as temporary and permanent restoration materials

chisel – a single beveled end-cutting blade instrument with a straight or angled shank used for cutting or splitting dentin and enamel

dappen dish – a heavy, double-ended glass dish or plastic disposable cup device with a variety of uses in dentistry

excavator – a dental hand instrument, generally a small, spoon-shaped instrument used for cleaning out and shaping a carious cavity preparatory or other materials from a tooth or restoration

fulcrum – the point of stabilization for holding dental instruments or handpieces with the ring finger

gingival margin trimmer – an angulated, chisel-like curved-blade instrument used to bevel the gingival margin of a tooth in cavity preparation

handpiece – a hand-held powered dental instrument, used to hold rotary cutting, grinding, or polishing tips; can be low-speed or high-speed

hatchet – a dental instrument with a curved shank and a flat, single-beveled blade, used to smooth cavity walls in preparation for a restoration

hoe – a single-beveled dental excavator, with a blade at an angle to the axis of the handle and a cutting edge perpendicular to the plane of the angle

nib – the portion of a condensing instrument that comes into contact with the restorative material being condensed into the tooth; usually blunt and not bladed

shaft – the handle of an instrument

shank – the portion of the instrument that connects the cutting or functional portion to a handle; with rotary instruments, it connects burs and drills into the chuck of the handpiece

spatula – a flat blade, like a knife blade without the sharp edge, used for mixing impression materials, cements, and plaster, as well as some ointments

tactile sensation – using the sensation of touch to gain information when performing a dental stroke or procedure; "reading" the information gained by the touch

transfer zone – the space where instrument transfer occurs during four-handed dentistry, usually below the patient's chin and directly over the throat and upper chest

tray – a flat receptacle with a lipped edge and compartments; in the preset tray system, trays are organized with all the dental instruments and armamentarium needed for a particular procedure before the procedure begins

working end – the part of an instrument used to perform a task or procedure

Introduction

Dental instruments come in a wide variety of shapes, sizes, and purposes. Typically made of stainless steel, rubber, plastic, or anodized aluminum, dental instruments are designed for specific jobs. New dental instruments are continually introduced as material technologies and procedures create demand for new instrumentation.

Dentists typically choose the instruments they are most comfortable with, or they rely on instruments that are specifically designed for the procedure they are performing. Dental assistants are responsible for setting up instrument trays, often according to the dentist's preference or sequence of the procedure, and providing chairside assistance, including instrument transfer.

Understanding Instruments

It is essential that dental assistants understand how dental instruments operate and how they are classified. Although there are variations in instrument ergonomics to suit personal preferences, dental instruments are generally standardized and follow the same design from one manufacturer to the next.

Instrument Parts

Dental instruments are generally about six inches long and designed to fit easily within a working hand. They are either single- or double-ended, and generally have the following parts (Figure 26-1).

The Working End

As the name implies, the **working end** of the instrument is the specially designed portion that is used to accomplish the instrument's unique function. Single-ended instruments have one working end, while double-ended instruments have two working ends.

The nature of the working end varies, depending on the nature of the instrument. Working ends can be blades, points, or nibs. Each of these is used for a different purpose:

- **Blades** are used for cutting. Blades can be single-ended or double-ended, curved or straight.
- Points are used for prodding and exploring.
- **Nibs** are blunt surfaces that can be serrated or smooth and may be made from rubber or another material more forgiving than metal, such as plastic or Teflon.

The working end of a dental instrument may also be a mirror.

The Shank

The **shank** is the portion of the instrument that connects the working end to the handle. It is like the narrow part of a piece of silverware that connects the spoon, fork, or knife to the handle. Shanks are shaped to make it easier to access certain portions of the oral anatomy. They can be straight, for work on anterior areas, or have a single-, double- or triple-angle design to reach anterior regions.

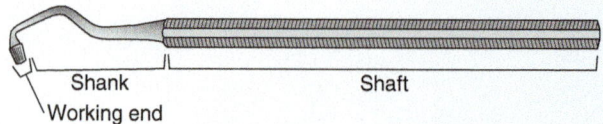

Shank   Shaft
Working end

Figure 26–1 Instrument parts.

The shank is usually tapered, made from metal, and sometimes flexible. Its flexibility determines how much pressure can be put on it.

The Shaft

The **shaft** (or handle) is the longest and thickest portion of the dental instrument. This is where the operator holds the instrument during use. Handle design varies between different manufacturers and lines of instruments. Handles may be smooth or textured to improve grip. They can be round or hexagonal. Some handles are larger in diameter, while others are fitted with rubber or plastic grips to make gripping easier and less stressful on the fingers and hands. A few handles are equipped with a cone socket that allows for replacement of the shank and working end.

Dental Facts

Early dental instruments were barbaric compared to the elegant devices we use today. Between the 14th and 18th centuries, a popular extraction device was known as the pelican, because it resembled a pelican's beak. A later generation of extraction instruments were inspired by and shaped vaguely like door keys. It wasn't until the 19th and 20th centuries that dental instruments began to resemble today's hand instruments.

Instrument Classification and Identification

Because there are so many different types of dental instruments, and smooth communication is essential during dental procedures, it is important that everyone involved in the process is able to quickly identify which instruments are needed. Thus, a number of classification systems have been developed to help dental professionals identify and describe dental instruments.

In general, dental instruments are classified by:

- *Working ends.* They may be referred to as single- or double-ended instruments.
- *Purpose.* Instruments may be referred to as basic examination instruments, hand cutting instruments, restorative instruments, or accessory hand instruments.
- *Number.* Dental instruments typically include a manufacturer's number on the handle, which is sometimes used to identify the instrument during a procedure.
- *The Black formula.* Invented by Dr. G. V. Black, this system is used to describe dental instruments based on the number of angulations and size of various instruments. It is covered in greater depth below.

The Black Formula for Dental Instruments

Black's formula is used to describe many types of dental instruments, including cutting instruments, chisels, and others. The system is based on a series of numbers, each with a special meaning (Figure 26-2). For cutting instruments, the system is as follows:

- First number. This describes the width of a cutting blade in tenths of a millimeter. For example, if the number is 10, the blade is 1 mm wide; the number 20 indicates a blade that is 2 mm wide.
- Second number. The length of the blade in millimeters. For example, a number 10 would indicate a blade that is 10 mm long.
- Third number. This describes the angle of the blade in relation to the long axis of the handle. Thus, if the number is 90, the blade is positioned at a 90-degree angle to the long axis of the handle, while a number of 14 would indicate a 14-degree angle from the long axis of the handle. The number 0 indicates that the blade is in line with the long axis of the handle.

An alternative to the three-number Black system uses four numbers. In this case, the system is modified as follows:

- First number. The same as the three-number system, with the first number indicating the width of the blade in tenths of a millimeter.
- Second number. This number represents the degree of the *cutting edge* of the blade in relation to the handle, so a number 85 would indicate that an 85-degree angle is formed between the cutting edge of the blade and the handle. This is useful if the cutting edge is not aligned with the axis of the blade itself.
- Third number. The same as the second number in the three-number system, meaning that it indicates how long the blade is in millimeters.
- Fourth number. The same as the third number in the three-number system, meaning that it indicates the angle of the blade in relation to the long axis of the handle.

CHECKPOINTS

26-1 What are the three parts of dental hand instruments?

26-2 What do the three numbers in the Black formula stand for?

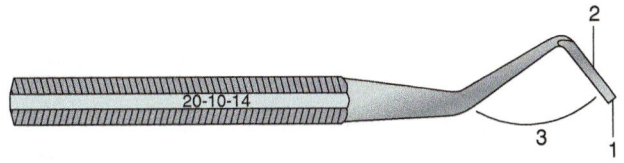

Figure 26–2 Black's formula. This instrument has a Black formula of 20-10-14.

Dental Hand Instruments

There are many variations among dental instruments, and new instruments are constantly being introduced to meet the needs of new procedures. The following sections describe the most common hand instruments found in the dental office.

In a typical examination, dental hand instruments are organized on a tray, which is used during the procedure itself. Trays are covered in greater depth later in this chapter, but in general, trays contain instruments specific to the procedure being performed, in the sequence and order they will be used. Any of the following instruments might be included on a tray, depending on the procedure to be performed and the operator's preference.

Basic Examination Instruments

Basic examination instruments are the most fundamental, and most common, hand instruments used during dental procedures. These instruments are not specialized for particular procedures, as some other instruments are, but are useful in a variety of situations, including oral examinations and evaluations. Basic instruments are typically included in every tray set-up.

Mirrors

Mirrors are available as single-ended instruments (Figure 26-3). Mouth mirrors are used throughout dentistry and are considered a staple instrument in any instrument tray.

Mirrors include a shaft and a slightly angled shank that allows the operator to see obscure angles in the oral cavity. There are a variety of sizes available, although most dental offices rely on the no. 4 or no. 5 size mirror. Mirrors may be disposable instruments or reusable instruments that are sterilized in the autoclave.

Mirrors are available as flat plane mirrors or with concave surfaces, which provide slight magnification to the image. Regular mirrors feature reflective coating on the back of a glass, which yields a ghost image as the light is reflected off both the glass surface and the reflective coating. Front surface mirrors have a layer of reflective coating on top of the glass to eliminate the ghost image so the operator experiences less distortion.

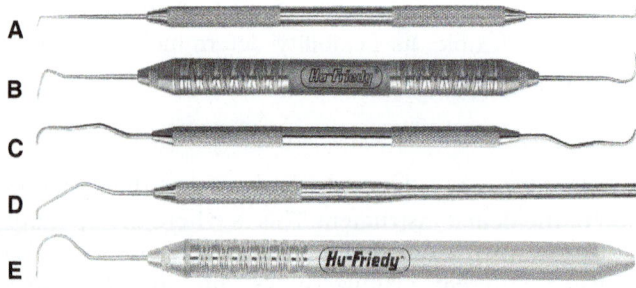

Figure 26-4 Explorers. (**A**) Pigtail. (**B**) Cowhorn. (**C**) ODU 11/12. (**D**) TU 17. (**E**) Shepherd's hook/no. 23.

Explorer

Explorers are available in a few configurations, but their basic design is the same (Figure 26-4). The working end of the explorer is a thin, flexible, and pointed section of steel that allows the operator to probe and test the teeth. They can be single-ended or double-ended.

Explorers are used for a variety of purposes, including identifying calculus deposits and decay on the tooth surface, scraping away excess material during dental procedures, and checking restorations for structural problems.

The most common shapes for explorers include the right angle (no. 17), the pig tail, and the shepherd's hook (no. 23). The combination of a shepherd's hook and no. 17 (Tufts-Wilkins) is referred to as a no. 5 explorer. Other explorer shapes include the cowhorn and no. 11-12 ODU (Old Dominion University).

Cotton Pliers

As the name implies, cotton pliers are used to manipulate cotton rolls, swabs, or other materials in the oral cavity. These instruments look like large tweezers, often with a slightly angled end to make it easier to grab and hold cotton rolls (Figure 26-5). Aside from cotton, these instruments are often used to manipulate any small objects in the oral cavity.

Cotton pliers are available as locking or nonlocking models. Locking models can be locked into position and will not release until the operator unlocks them. They are also available with plain tips or serrated tips. Sometimes these instruments are referred to as "college pliers."

Periodontal Probes

Periodontal probes are available as single- or double-ended instruments that are used to measure the depth of periodontal pockets (Figure 26-6). This depth is used as an indicator of gingival health, with deeper pockets indicating less healthy gingival tissue. Because periodontal pockets are

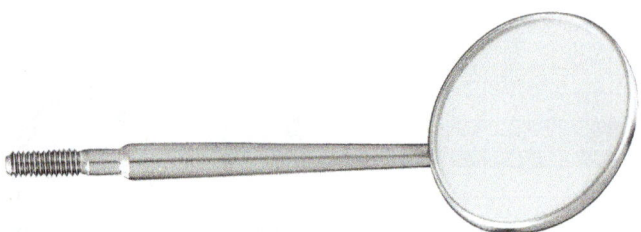

Figure 26-3 Mouth mirror.

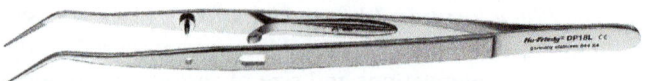

Figure 26-5 Cotton pliers.

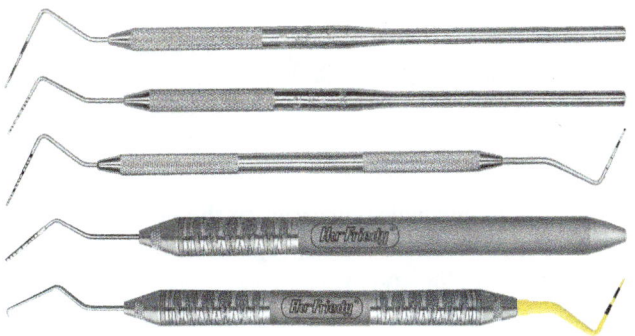

Figure 26–6 Periodontal probes.

measured in millimeters, periodontal probes are marked with millimeters on the working end. Some probes are color-coded to enhance reading them. Some probes are round or cone-shaped, and others are flat sided.

Combination explorers/periodontal probes are available. These instruments are known as *expros*.

Hand Cutting Instruments

Hand cutting instruments are sharp or pointed instruments that are used during cavity treatment to remove decayed tooth material, smooth and prepare the cavity walls, and place retention grooves or bevels to make the restorative material more stable within the tooth. Hand cutting instruments are typically used in conjunction with rotary instruments.

There are six basic hand cutting instruments, any of which may be included in a dental tray.

Chisels

Chisels feature a straight cutting blade with a single bevel. They are used to prepare the cavity before the procedure. Chisels are available as single- and double-ended instruments. Double-ended chisels typically feature the same working head with reversed bevels to make it easier for the operator to switch back and forth between cutting edges.

Chisels typically have either a straight or an angled shank. The angle of the shank determines the type of chisel and its use:

- *Straight chisel.* No angle in the shank; used on mandibular and maxillary teeth for class III or class IV caries (Figure 26-7A).

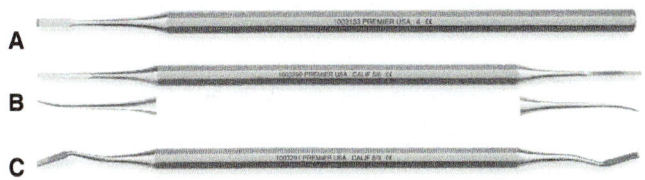

Figure 26–7 Chisels. (**A**) Straight chisel. (**B**) Wedelstaedt chisels. (**C**) Binangle chisel.

- *Wedelstaedt chisel.* A slightly angled or curved shank, used for class III and class IV caries (Figure 26-7B).
- *Binangle chisels.* A double-angled shank, used in class II caries (Figure 26-7C).

Hatchets

Hatchets are typically double-ended instruments with a curved shank and a flat, single-beveled blade (Figure 26-8). They are used to smooth cavity walls in preparation for a restoration. Some hatchets are marked with "left" and "right" indicators to let the operator know which side the blade is on.

Hoes

Hoes are shaped like garden hoes (Figure 26-9). They have either straight or angled shanks and a straight blade. They are used to prepare the cavity floor in preparation for a restoration, just as one would till the soil with a garden hoe.

Angle Formers

Angle formers are used to create angles and points within the cavity. Angle formers are double-ended instruments that are shaped like hoes, except they have angled and beveled blades (Figure 26-10). The opposite working ends of angle formers are complementary, with each side facing a different direction so they can be used on the right and left side of the cavity.

Excavator

Excavators are used to remove material from caries, including both debris and carious material (Figure 26-11). There are two basic types of excavators: straight-blade, or smooth, excavators and spoon-billed excavators. Although these instruments have blades, they are not sharp. The edges are usually rounded to make scooping and scraping motions easier.

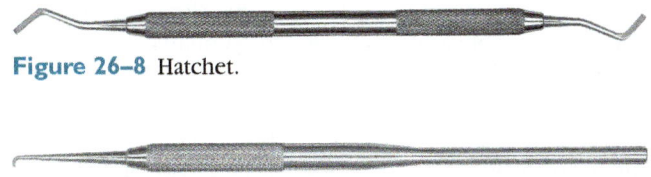

Figure 26–8 Hatchet.

Figure 26–9 Hoe.

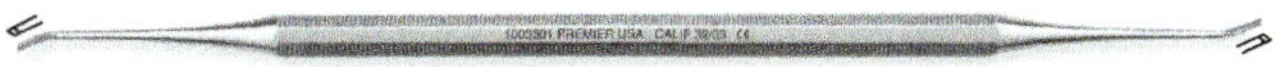

Figure 26–10 Angle former.

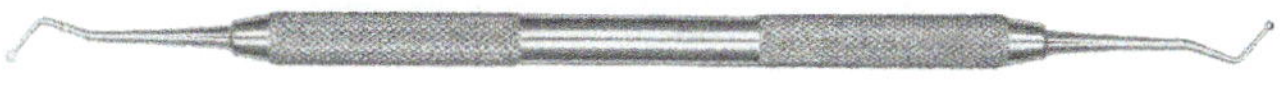

Figure 26–11 Excavator.

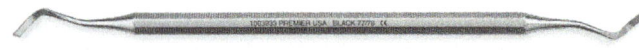

Figure 26–12 Gingival margin trimmer.

Gingival Margin Trimmers

Gingival margin trimmers feature an angled shank with a curved blade that has an angled cutting edge (Figure 26-12). These are double-ended instruments, with opposing curves on each end. One blade curves to the right, while the other blade curves to the left. Thus, gingival margin trimmers are designed for ease of use in the left and right side of the oral cavity; trimming both the mesial and distal margins. These instruments are used to prepare the gingival margin of a cavity.

CHECKPOINTS

26-3 What are the four basic examination instruments?

26-4 Name the six basic hand cutting instruments.

Restorative Instruments

Restorative instruments are used during restoration procedures to shape, mold, and carve the dental material to follow the natural contour of the tooth. The exact order of these instruments on a prepared tray depends on the sequence of the dental procedure and the dentist's preference.

Composite Placement Instruments

Composite placement instruments are used to place composite material. These instruments are typically double-ended and made from either anodized aluminum or Teflon plastic to prevent discoloration of the composite material, which can happen when using steel instruments. A typical composite placement instrument might have a paddle at one working end and a condenser shape at the other end (Figure 26-13A). These are known as "plastic" instruments. In addition to the regular plastic instrument, there is also a Woodson plastic instrument with a bulkier, boxier condensing end and a flat paddle end (Figure 26-13B). It can be made from plastic or stainless steel. These instruments are also available as single-ended instruments.

Amalgam Carriers

Amalgam carriers are used to transport amalgam in an amalgam well to the tooth for placement (Figure 26-14). These double-ended instruments feature wells on both ends—usually one larger and one smaller well. To transport the amalgam, the dental assistant fills the well and

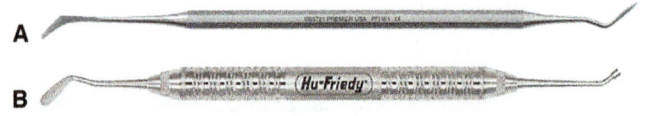

A

B

Figure 26–13 **Composite placement instruments.** (**A**) Plastic instrument. (**B**) Woodson instrument.

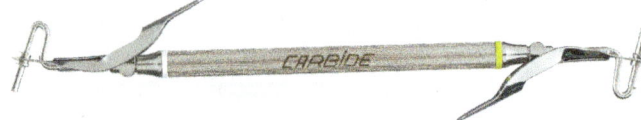

Figure 26–14 Amalgam carrier.

either hands the amalgam carrier to the dentist or places the amalgam directly into the prepared tooth. Carriers can be single or double ended.

Carvers

Carvers are used to contour and remove excess restorative material and carve tooth anatomy into the amalgam before the material hardens. Depending on the type of carver, they can also be used in crown procedures, or to carve wax inlays and onlays.

There are a number of carver shapes available—the type required often depends on the operator's preferences. Carver shapes include:

- *Cleoid-discoid.* The working ends resemble a tiny arrow or spade on one side (cleoid) and a rounded circle or disc on the other (discoid). These are used to carve occlusal surfaces (Figure 26-15A).
- *Hollenback.* This carver features sharp, oblong, oval-shaped working ends that are often used to remove excess restorative material (Figure 26-15B).
- *Ward.* The working ends on a Ward carver are long, flat blades. One side features a more sharply angled shank, while the other is gently angled.
- *Interproximal (globin).* This sharp, double-ended bladed instrument is used to carve the mesial and distal surfaces of a restoration (Figure 26-15C).
- *Tanner.* A double-ended instrument that is used to carve occlusal anatomy.
- *Frahm.* The working ends are square-bladed on one side and diamond-shaped on the other side.

Burnishers

Burnishers are smooth instruments used to smooth and shape the margins of restorative material and to manipulate metal matrix bands (Figure 26-16). They are single- or double-ended instruments, available in a variety of shapes, including the ball, the football, the T-ball, the beavertail, and the acorn/anatomical burnisher.

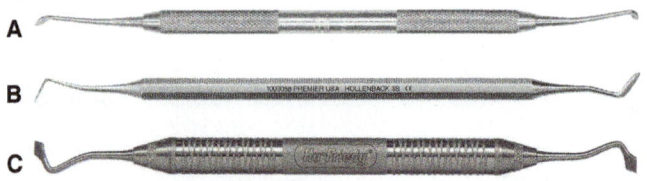

A

B

C

Figure 26–15 **Amalgam carvers.** (**A**) Cleoid-discoid carver. (**B**) Hollenback carver. (**C**) Frahm carver.

Figure 26–16 Burnisher.

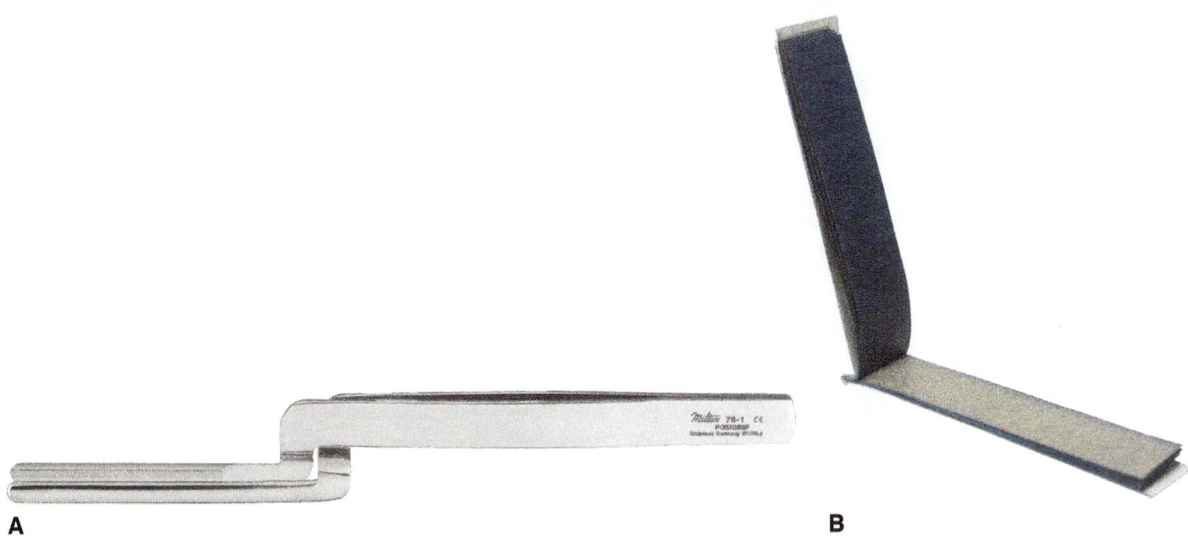

Figure 26–17 Articulating forceps (**A**) and paper (**B**).

Articulating Paper and Articulating Forceps

Articulating forceps and **articulating paper** are used together to check the patient's occlusion after the restoration is in place (Figure 26-17). To use them, the operator grips the ends of the stainless steel forceps around the blue paper and asks the patient to gently bite down on the articulating paper. Articulating paper is made from carbon paper that marks the patient's bite. Articulating forceps are often used in other procedures also, so they might be included on various trays.

Accessory Hand Instruments

Accessory hand instruments are sometimes used on restorative trays, as well as a variety of additional dental procedures. Their inclusion depends on the dentist's preference.

Spatulas

Spatulas are commonly used in procedures that require restorative material (Figure 26-18). *Cement spatulas* are single-ended instruments that are used to mix cements, bases, and liners. They are available in a variety of shapes and sizes. *Plastic spatulas* are used with plastic and resinous materials; they are typically double-ended and often disposable because of the challenge involved with cleaning plastic. Finally, *laboratory spatulas* are used to mix plaster and impression materials. They are frequently made from rigid or flexible metal, but may also be made from plastic.

Scissors

Dental scissors used during restorative procedures are crown and bridge scissors (Figure 26-19). Their short, sharp blades may be straight or curved and come in various sizes. They are used to cut many materials, including retraction cord, stainless steel crowns, dental dam material, and for a variety of other purposes.

Dappen Dish

The **dappen dish** is a heavy, double-ended glass dish that features a cup on either end. Dappen dishes are used to mix materials for restorations. Today, many disposable dappen dishes are made from plastic and have different size wells (Figure 26-20).

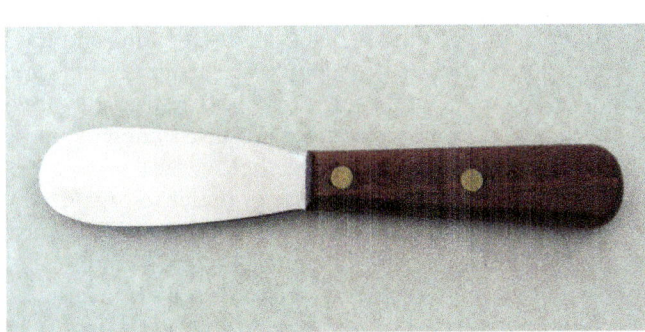

Figure 26–18 Plaster spatula.

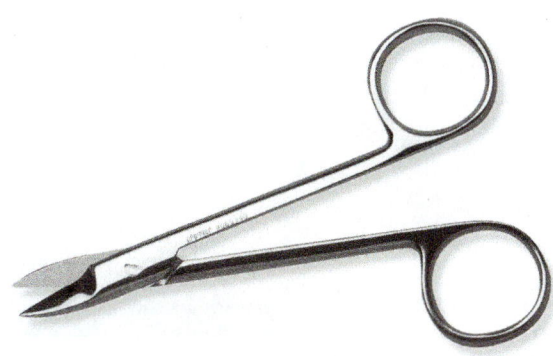

Figure 26–19 Dental scissors.

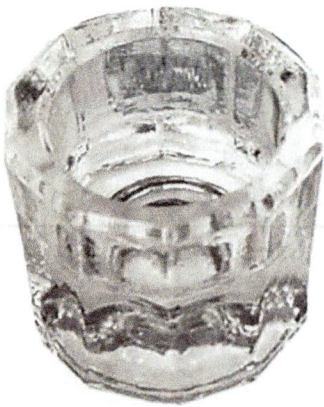

Figure 26–20 Dappen dish.

Liner Applicators

Liner applicators are used to apply cavity preparation liner-materials to restorations as a protective liner before the cement base or the restorative material is placed. These are supplied by the manufacturer and should be used according to the manufacturer's instructions. Dycal is a popular brand, and you may hear liner applicators from this manufacturer referred to simply as "Dycal applicators" (Figure 26-21).

Applicators and Brushes

Plastic disposable brushes and applicators are commonly used in a variety of dental procedures. One popular brand, the Benda brush, features stiff, chemical resistant bristles that are designed to carry and apply restorative material (Figure 26-22). They are available in single- or double-ended styles, with straight or curved shanks. Other types of applicators and brushes feature spongy ends and soft bristles.

✓ CHECKPOINTS

26-5 What are the six basic carver shapes?

26-6 What is articulating paper used for?

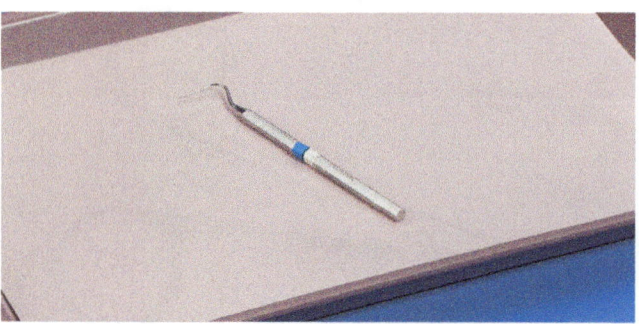

Figure 26–21 Liner (Dycal) applicator.

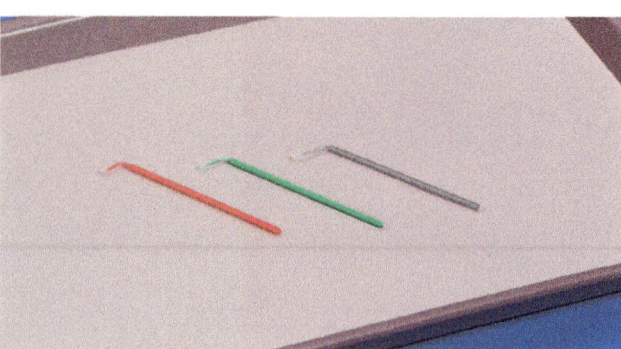

Figure 26–22 Benda brushes.

Tray and Tub Systems

Trays are assembled before a procedure and carried into the treatment room ready to use. This system, known as the preset tray or tub system, makes it easier to correctly assemble instruments and armamentarium needed for the procedure and helps the office run more efficiently.

Dental trays are assembled based on the procedure being performed and the operator's instrument preference. Some instruments—such as mouth mirrors—will be included in virtually every tray assembled in the office, while others—such as specialized cutting instruments—might only be included if they are needed.

The trays themselves are made from either plastic or metal, and they have a variety of configurations. The most common types of trays are plastic tubs with dividers. Additionally, trays are usually color-coded to help in identification and organization. Most practices color code the trays and tubs according to procedures.

Before placing instruments on a tray, the trays are often covered with tray paper or plastic barriers to make disinfection easier.

Color Coding Trays and Instruments

Color coding is used to help the dental office stay organized and allow employees to rapidly identify instruments. There is no standard color-coding scheme, so it will differ from office to office, depending on how that office operates and its unique needs and layout.

Color coding schemes include:

- *By procedure.* In this scheme, all instruments and trays used for particular procedures are assigned the same color. So, for example, trays, tubs, and instruments used during composite restorations are all assigned the same color and are always kept together.
- *By treatment room.* Some offices prefer to organize by treatment room, so all the instruments, tubs, and trays used in one treatment room are assigned a color.
- *By operator.* Instruments sets and trays can also be color-coded based on the operator, so each dentist or

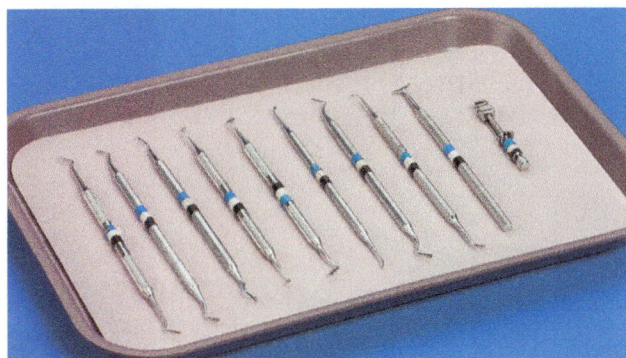

Figure 26–23 Color-coded tray with color-coded instruments.

hygienist might maintain his or her own color-coded instrumentation. This is especially helpful to keep the dentist's and hygienist's trays separate.

- *By sequence.* Instruments are sometimes color-coded based on their sequence of use during a procedure.

Dental instruments, trays, and tubs are not sold with color-coding. This is done in the office with the use of bands or tape (Figure 26-23).

Positioning Instruments on Trays

Instruments are generally lined up on a tray in the order in which they will be used, however, each operator may have a different preference (Figure 26-24). There are some general guidelines when it comes to assembling trays:

- Use tray barriers to separate instruments if they are not already included in the tray design.
- Position the instruments to be used first on the left side of the tray. This includes the basic examination instruments (e.g., mouth mirror, explorer, cotton pliers, and periodontal probe).
- Keep instruments together based on their function. In other words, if multiple hatchets are required, keep all the hatchets together.
- Cotton products are kept together, along the top of the tray.
- Hinged instruments, such as scissors, are often positioned to the far right for easier access.

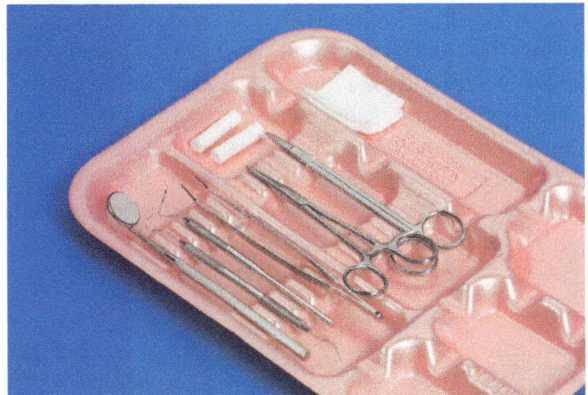

Figure 26–24 Completed tray.

- After an operator is done with an instrument, replace it in the same place it was originally located. This helps minimize instrument confusion during hand-offs.
- If possible, wipe instruments clean with a gauze sponge before returning them to the tray, removing any debris, restorative material, and/or blood. This will help make sterilization easier.

The Cassette System

Cassettes have a number of positive attributes. They allow for the easy organization of preset trays; they reduce the likelihood of puncture wounds during instrument transport; and they make it possible to transport sterilized equipment through the office without fear of contamination.

Cassettes include the assembled trays, which are then wrapped in paper and color-coded. Before a procedure, the cassette is carried into the treatment room and opened when it is needed. After the procedure is over, the cassette is carried back to the sterilization area, where it is prepared for sterilization. Instruments are placed back into the cassette in order, and the entire unit can be placed in the ultrasonic unit. After it is washed, the sealed cassette is rinsed, wrapped in a new covering and labeled, and sterilized. Once sterilization is complete, the unit can be safely stored until it is needed again.

✓ CHECKPOINTS

26-7 Which order should instruments be positioned in trays?

26-8 Can cassettes be sterilized as a unit?

Dental Rotary Instruments

Dental rotary instruments were introduced in the 1940s and continue to be refined. The predecessor to the modern air-powered rotary instrument was introduced in the 1950s.

These rotary instruments operate on the same principle as power instruments like drills: a rotary device is used with a combination of tips to accomplish work needing more pressure than hand instruments. They can include tips for cutting, grinding, polishing, and abrading dental surfaces. Dental rotary instruments operate at much higher speeds, and with greater precision and power, than is possible with hand instruments. Thus, they have enabled dentists to perform procedures of greater complexity on harder tooth material.

Dental Handpieces

The dental **handpiece** is ubiquitous. Dental handpieces are similar to the body of a power drill. They are used throughout restorative dentistry to prepare teeth for filling; to polish teeth; to finish and polish restorations; and to cut, finish, and polish dental appliances. During the same

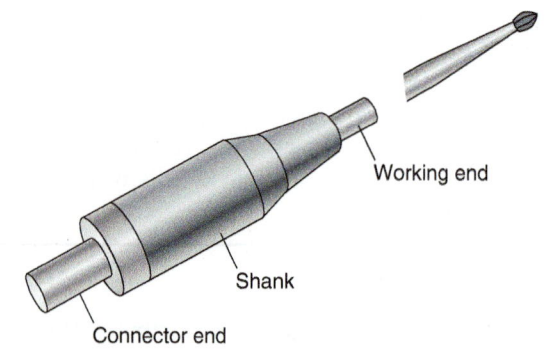

Figure 26–25 Handpiece.

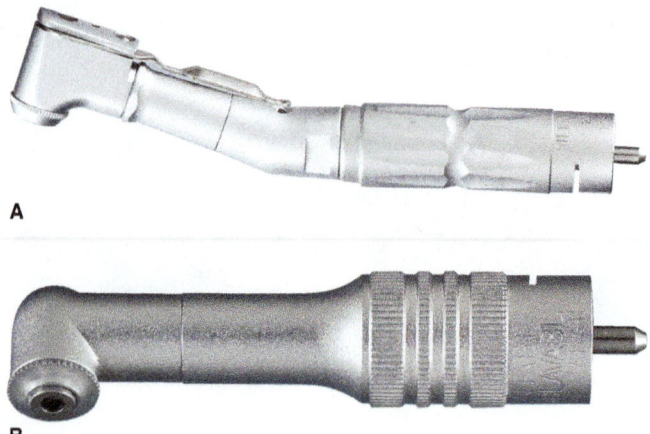

Figure 26–26 Low-speed handpiece attachments. (**A**) Contra-angle attachment. (**B**) Right-angle attachment.

procedure, the dentist might switch between hand instruments and the dental handpiece.

The two most common types of handpieces are low-speed handpieces and high-speed handpieces—both types have the same basic design.

Handpiece Design

Handpieces all have the following parts (Figure 26-25):

- *Working end.* This is the working end of the handpiece that rotates around an axis and contains a connector where different rotary instrument attachments can be inserted. Rotary instruments include burs, cutting discs, stones, and polishing instruments.
- *Shank.* This is the handle portion of the handpiece. Shanks can be straight or bent at the end, depending on their purpose.
- *Connector end.* This is where the handpiece attaches to the power source. The controls are typically located here (e.g., forward and reverse controls).

Low-Speed Handpieces

Sometimes called straight handpieces, low-speed handpieces are extremely versatile instruments. They are used both in the treatment room and dental laboratory. Uses for the low-speed handpiece in the treatment room include polishing teeth and dental restorations, defining cavity margins and walls, treating root canals, and removing softer carious material in preparation for restorations. In the laboratory, the low-speed handpiece is used to finish restorations, trim and contour crowns, and trim and reline removable partials and dentures.

There are two sizes of low-speed handpieces: standard length and the "shorty" handpiece. They generally operate at 10,000 to 30,000 rotations per minute (rpm), in either direction (e.g., forward or backward).

To increase the low-speed handpiece's versatility, a number of attachments are available (Figure 26-26):

- *Straight Attachment.* This standard attachment locks into place over the motor. It is used with long-shank rotary instruments such as burs, discs, and stones.
- *Contra-Angle Attachment.* This attachment fits to the end of the motor and is slightly angled near the working

end. This allows the operator better access to the posterior oral cavity and makes it easier to work on occlusal surfaces. Contra-angle attachments usually work with latch-type burs, although they are also available with friction grip burs. Instruments used with the contra-angle attachment include rubber cups, burs, stones, brushes, discs, and mandrels.

- *Right-Angle, or Prophy-Angle, Attachment.* These attachments are used during polishing procedures with rubber cups or brushes.

High-Speed Handpieces

High-speed handpieces are air-driven power instruments that operate at speeds of up to 450,000 rpm (Figure 26-27). These devices are a single unit and do not have attachments. The shank of the high-speed handpiece is slightly angled, similar to the contra-angle attachment of the low-speed handpiece.

High-speed handpieces are designed to accommodate a variety of rotary instruments, including burs. These instruments fit into the end of the handpiece by means of a shank that fits into the chuck, or end, of the handpiece, which grips them tightly as they rotate. This is called a *friction-grip design.* The principle is very similar to the way power drills operate. Instruments are removed and installed in the chuck using either a chuck key or, in more modern units, a button that releases tension on the instrument's shank. Burs are covered in greater depth later in this chapter.

High-speed handpieces are used to cut away hard material during restorations, including tooth material and defective or faulty restorations. They are also used to prepare the cavity for a new restoration, as well as polishing and finishing restorations and during dental surgeries.

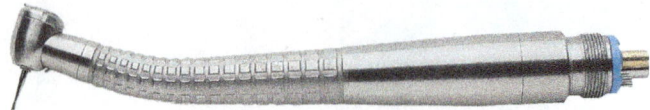

Figure 26–27 High-speed handpiece.

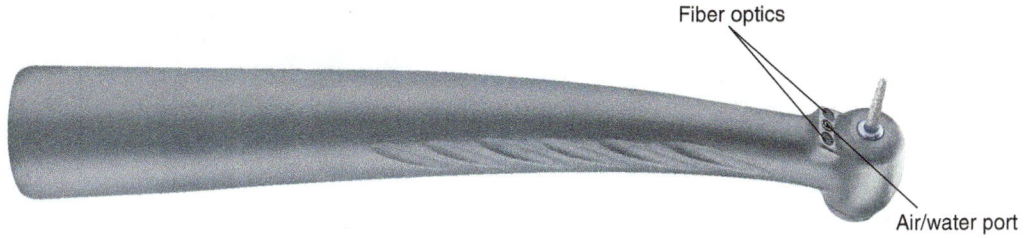

Fiber optics

Air/water port

Figure 26–28 Fiber optic lighting and water coolant system.

High-speed handpieces are typically equipped with the following features:

- *Water Coolant System*. Because high-speed handpieces operate at such high speeds, they generate a considerable degree of heat friction. This heat can cause damage to tooth pulp. To prevent heat damage, high-speed handpieces are equipped with water coolant systems, which bath the bur and the target tooth in a spray of cool water to reduce temperatures (Figure 26-28).
- *Fiber Optic Lighting*. High-speed handpieces are equipped with fiber optic lighting to help illuminate the working field. The light emanates from the head of the handpiece, directly behind the bur. The light is carried along fiber optic bundles in the device itself, from a light source in an external unit (see Figure 26-28).

Electric Handpiece

Electric handpieces are an increasingly popular alternative to the air-powered handpieces commonly used today (Figure 26-29). Electric handpieces are quiet, vibration-free, sterilizable, and efficient. They are available in both low-speed and high-speed models, although the top speed of the electric high-speed handpiece does not yet equal the air-powered version.

Like their air-powered counterparts, electric handpieces can be used with a variety of attachments and rotary instruments. Low-speed electric handpieces are available as both straight-line and contra-angle instruments. High-speed electric handpieces operate much like their air-powered versions, with friction-grip design and fiber optic

lighting. The advantage of an electric handpiece is that it does not need to be connected to an air compressor and dental unit and is therefore much more portable.

Ultrasonic Handpiece

Ultrasonic handpieces (Figure 26-30) are used during the prophylaxis procedure to remove calculus and stain or to remove bonding materials after orthodontic appliances are removed. Although powered by electricity, ultrasonic handpieces generate pulsating waves of water and sound to perform their function. They are frequently outfitted with instruments similar to scaling instruments.

Laser Handpiece

Laser handpieces (Figure 26-31) operate by means of a tightly focused laser that is used to vaporize decayed tooth structure or cauterize soft tissue. The device itself resembles a standard handpiece, including the use of water and air to cool the target tooth. However, the laser handpiece is connected by a fiber optic cable to a console that generates and controls the laser.

Laser handpieces offer one major benefit over other treatments: no anesthesia is necessary with the laser handpieces. This is faster and more comfortable for patients and dentists alike. However, laser treatments cannot be performed on teeth with existing restorations, they take longer than traditional procedures, and the technology is still limited in its availability.

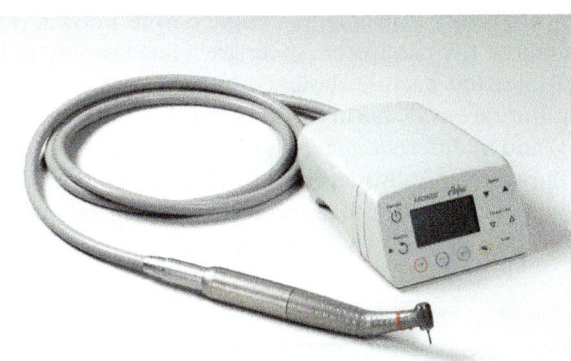

Figure 26–29 Electric handpiece.

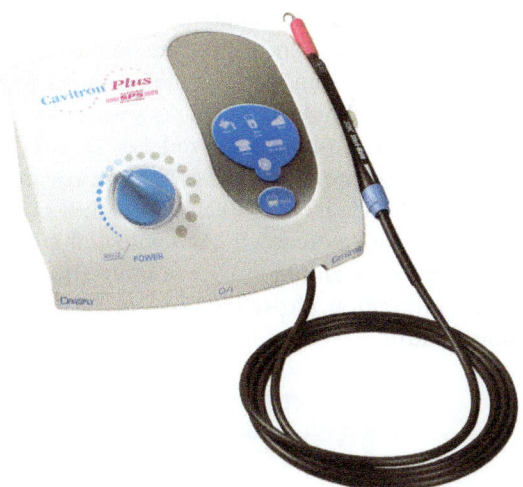

Figure 26–30 Ultrasonic handpiece.

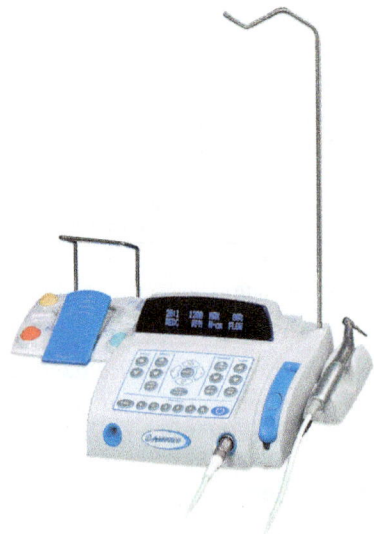

Figure 26–31 Laser handpiece.

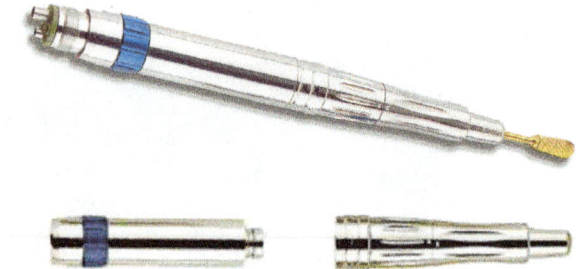

Figure 26–32 Laboratory handpiece.

Laser handpieces also require special care when dealing with the fiber optic cable. The cable should not be bent or twisted because it might cause the unit to burn or function improperly. Similarly, operators should not touch exposed fiber optic cable or the fiber optic cable connector.

Laboratory Handpiece

A laboratory handpiece is a specialized type of low-speed handpiece that is designed for use in the laboratory (Figure 26-32). These devices operate much like standard low-speed handpieces, with a range of attachments and instruments available. However, they are built with greater torque, which is necessary during construction of appliances, when operators are grinding and manipulating hard dental materials.

Care of Handpieces

Because of the variety of handpieces available, it is important to acquaint yourself with the manufacturer's instructions for cleaning and maintaining any particular handpieces. Improper maintenance, lubrication, and sterilization can result in debris accumulating in the working parts of the handpiece, which reduces its working life and may void the manufacturer's warranty.

All handpieces must be sterilized before being used. Disinfection is not enough, because handpieces are designated as critical instruments, which means they come into direct contact with potentially contaminated substances such as bone, saliva, and blood. For a more thorough discussion of sterilization, please see Chapter 14, Disease and Infection Control.

Proper lubrication is also essential to maintain a good, working handpiece. Both under- and over-lubrication are potentially harmful, and it is important to lubricate the handpiece at the proper time (e.g., before, after, or before and after sterilization). Specific guidelines should be available from the manufacturer.

In general, principles of proper handpiece maintenance include:

- Flush the handpiece for 20 to 30 seconds while the bur is still in place and the tubing is still attached. If the manufacturer has specific instructions for flushing, follow those.
- The handpiece should be wiped free of visible debris after flushing.
- Do not use disinfectants on handpieces prior to sterilization. Mild soap and water should be sufficient. Disinfectants might damage the handpiece, and it is unnecessary because the device will be sterilized. Never submerse the handpiece in water.
- Only use the ultrasonic cleaner if the manufacturer suggests it. Never submerse the handpiece in the ultrasonic cleaner bath.
- Follow the manufacturer's instruction for sterilization, including wrapping and sterilization technique. The most common forms of sterilization for handpieces include the use of an autoclave or chemical vapor sterilizer.
- Lubricate the handpiece according to the manufacturer's instructions, making sure not to obscure the fiber optic port with lubricant.

Dental Burs

Burs are rotary instruments designed to fit into the working end of the handpiece. There are a huge variety of burs available, and each is designed to accomplish a specific task. Burs are available in different shapes (e.g., round, cone, etc.) and in different materials (e.g., diamond, steel, etc.).

Burs are typically identified by their structure and form, as well as their length. Specific numbering schemes are covered in the following sections.

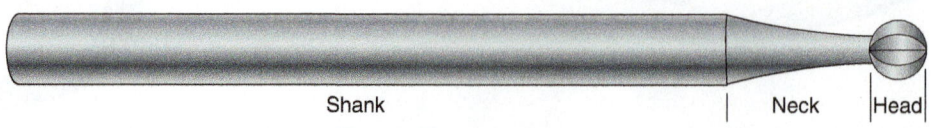

Shank | Neck | Head

Figure 26–33 Dental bur.

Bur Structure

Generally speaking, all burs have the same basic parts: shank, neck, and head (Figure 26-33).

The bur *shank* is the portion that is inserted into the handpiece. There are three general styles of shank:

- *Straight.* This is most often used with low-speed hand-pieces fitted with a straight-line attachment.
- *Latch type.* This type of shank has a grooved end that locks into the contra-angle end on the low-speed handpiece.
- *Friction grip.* The friction-grip shank is smooth, without any grooves to hold it in place. This shank is slid into the chuck of a high-piece handpiece and held in place by the friction generated through rapid rotation. Friction grip instruments are also sometimes used in contra-angle attachments on low-speed handpieces.

The *neck* of the bur is the short section that connects the head to the shank.

The bur *head* is the portion that performs the work. Bur heads are designed to finish, polish, or cut material. Burs are typically classified by their head size and shape.

Cutting Burs

Cutting burs are used to excavate caries in preparation for restoration. These burs are typically made from tungsten-carbide, with cutting blades on the surface of the bur.

Cutting burs are identified in three ways: by head shape, size, and length of shank.

There are nine basic head shapes in cutting burs, and each is offered in a variety of sizes (Figure 26-34). When requesting a particular bur, the dentist will often ask for it by head shape, followed by number to designate size, and possibly by the length of shank. Table 26-1 lists the basic cutting burs and their sizes, along with the typical use for each bur. Shank length is typically identified by one of the following letters: *L* for long; *S* for short; and *P* for pedodontic.

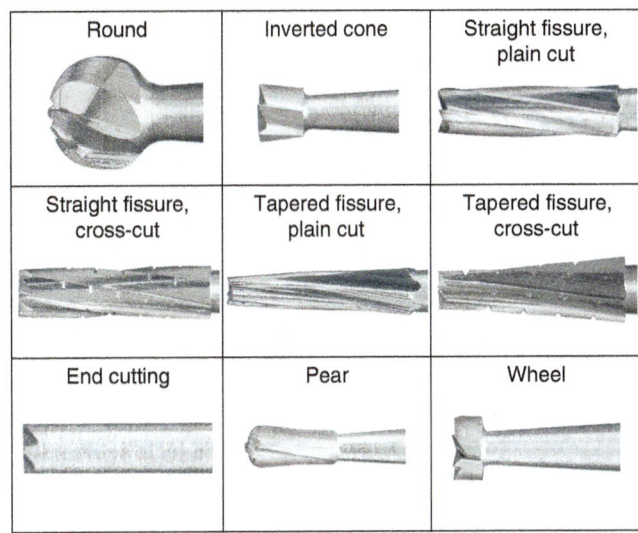

Figure 26-34 Cutting burs.

Finishing Burs

Finishing burs resemble cutting burs, but they have more blades on their surfaces, which enables them to better polish surfaces (Figure 26-35). Finishing burs are used to smooth and polish restorations, both metal and natural tooth-colored. The range of finishing burs is similar to cutting burs in shape and size—the most commonly used finishing burs include round, tapered, and flame-shaped. They are identified by manufacturer's number. Additionally, some finishing burs are color-coded to indicate how many blades are on the bur's surface:

- Red band = 8 and 12 blades
- Yellow band = 16 and 20 blades
- White band = More than 30 blades

Diamond Burs

Diamond burs are used for many of the same purposes as tungsten-carbide burs. These rotary instruments feature a metal base that has been coated with a fine grit of industrial

TABLE 26-1 Cutting Burs		
BUR SHAPE	**SIZE RANGE**	**USES**
Round	1/4, 1/2, 1–8, 10	Open cavities initially and remove caries
Inverted cone	33-1/2, 34–39, 36L, 37L	Remove caries and cut retention grooves
Straight fissure, plain cut	55–60, 57L, 58L	Open cavities initially and form cavity walls in preparation
Straight fissure, cross-cut	556–560, 567L, 568L	Prepare cavity walls
Tapered fissure, plain cut	169–172, 169L, 170L, 171L	Form angled cavity walls
Tapered fissure, cross-cut	699–703, 699L, 700L, 701L	Form angled cavity walls
End cutting	957, 958	Open cavities initially and provide the shoulder for crown preparations
Pear	330–333, 331L	Open cavities initially and extend preparation
Wheel	14	Form retention

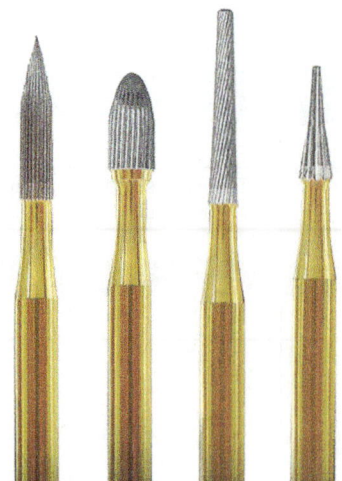

Figure 26–35 Finishing burs.

diamonds. The result is a very hard cutting edge that can be used to cut carious material, tooth material and bone, restorations, and appliances.

Diamond burs are available in a variety of shapes (Figure 26-36). They are classified by their grit: extra fine, fine, and coarse. They are frequently color-coded to help quickly distinguish between the different grits. Alternatively, the coarseness might be indicated by a letter at the end of the bur's designation number. This varies from manufacturer to manufacturer.

Diamond burs are important instruments, but they do lose some of their effectiveness over time. After repeated use and sterilization, the diamond flecks embedded in the bur's head begin to dislodge, causing the bur to lose some of its grit. Older diamond burs need to be replaced.

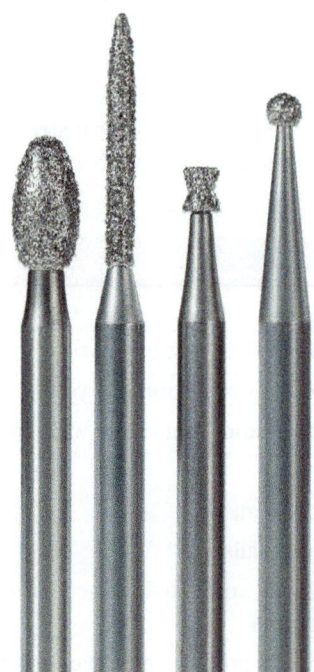

Figure 26–36 Diamond burs.

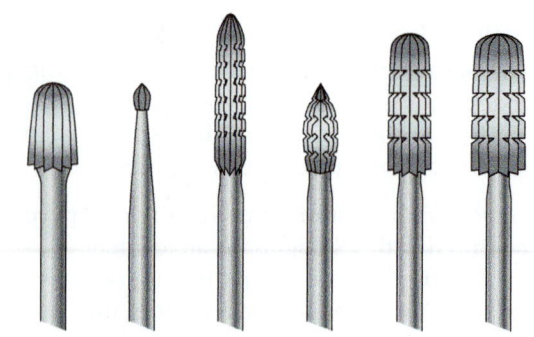

Figure 26–37 Surgical burs.

Surgical Burs

Surgical burs have long shanks and are designed to shape and contour alveolar bone and tooth structure. They are designed for use with the low-speed handpiece. Surgical burs are available in a variety of shapes and sizes that can be used only in a surgical handpiece (Figure 26-37).

Laboratory Burs

Laboratory burs are larger and longer than burs designed for use in the oral cavity. These burs are designed for use with the low-speed handpiece or the laboratory handpiece. They are used for forming and polishing dental appliances. A specialized acrylic bur is designed to cut and shape acrylic. Laboratory burs are available in various shapes and sizes (Figure 26-38).

Fissurotomy Burs

Fissurotomy burs are very small devices (0.33 mm) that are used to explore the occlusal surface of healthy teeth. They do not cut into the tooth structure, but leave behind a smooth groove. Fissurotomy burs are used to help diagnose caries in suspicious fissures and grooves on the tooth surface. By leaving the tooth intact, but providing access to fissures, these specialized burs allow the dentist to visualize hard-to-see areas without causing lasting damage.

Abrasive Instruments

Abrasive instruments are most often used to finish restorations, although some can be used for cutting. They lack cutting blades, but instead feature a variety of abrasive materials on a variety of bases and shapes. Abrasive instruments are classified by their shape (e.g., wheel, disc, etc.) and their material (e.g., rubber, stone, etc.). A variety of types are outlined below.

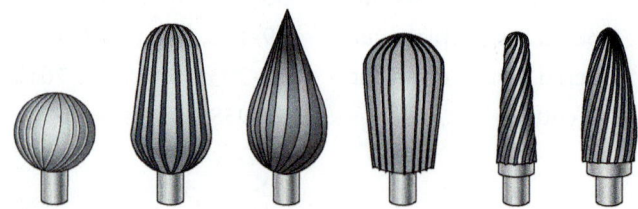

Figure 26–38 Laboratory burs.

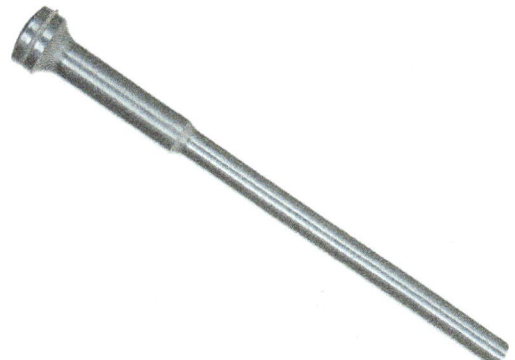

Figure 26–39 Mandrel.

Mandrels

Mandrels feature a shank and head that is attached to an abrasive substance (Figure 26-39). Some mandrels come with the abrasive material permanently placed (mounted), while others allow operators to attach the abrasive material (unmounted). Mandrels are used in low-speed handpieces; they are available with straight, friction grip, screw-on, or latch shanks.

Discs

Discs are typically attached to the end of mandrels, either by a snap-on or a screw-type device. Their function depends on their design: discs are available as sandpaper, diamond, or carborundum. They are rigid or flexible, available in various sizes, and come with different grits. It is important when ordering discs to make sure the discs you are ordering will work with the mandrels available in your dental office.

The following types of discs are available (Figure 26-40):

- Sandpaper discs feature an abrasive material bonded to one side of the disc. They are used to finish and polish restorations, and they are available with a wide range of abrasives, including sand, emery, and cuttlefish.
- Diamond discs feature industrial diamond chips coating both sides of a steel disc. They are used for rapid cutting, much like diamond burs.

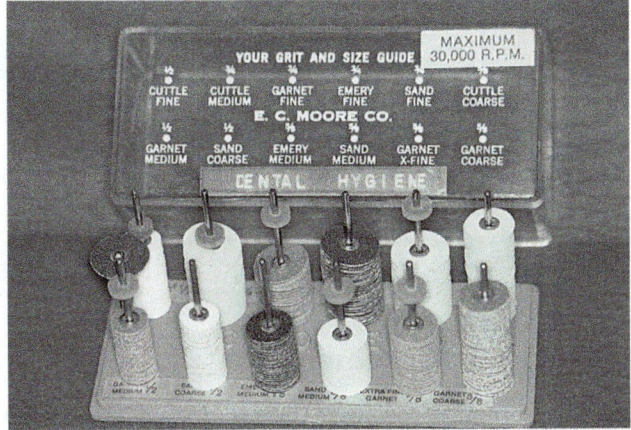

Figure 26–40 **Discs**. Assorted discs coated with sand, cuttle, garnet, and emery.

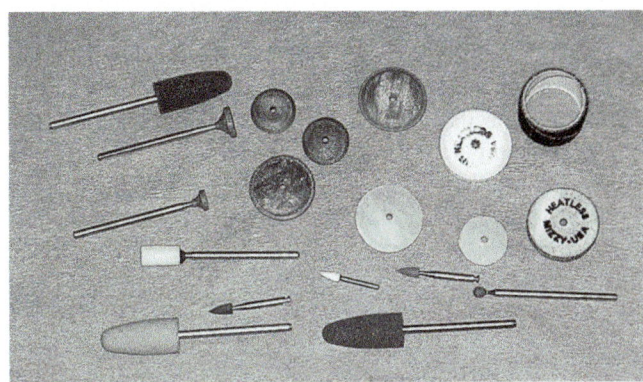

Figure 26–41 **Stones and rubber instruments**. Assorted stones, rubber wheels, and rubber points.

- Carborundum discs are primarily used in the laboratory. Sometimes called Jo-dandy discs, they are thin and brittle and break easily; they are used to cut and finish fold restorations.

Stones

Stones are used in both the treatment room and the laboratory to cut, polish, and finish dental materials. Many sizes, grits, and shapes of dental stones are available (Figure 26-41). They are available as both mounted and unmounted instruments, and some stones are heatless, which reduces the amount of friction heat generated during use. The stone's function depends on its shape and grit.

Rubber Instruments

Rubber instruments are available as both wheels and points (see Figure 26-41). Rubber instruments are used for polishing and finishing. They have material embedded in their surface to yield different grits.

Air Abrasion

Air abrasion is a specialized technique that uses the air abrasion handpiece (Figure 26-42). The principle of air abrasion is similar to sand-blasting paint from houses: the unit shoots a high-pressure stream of aluminum oxide particles at the tooth surface to gently remove stains and other materials without damaging the underlying tooth surface.

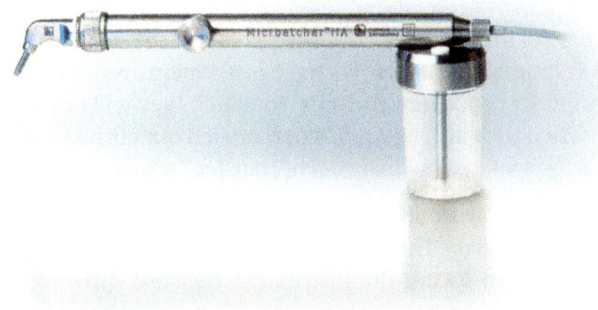

Figure 26–42 Air abrasion handpiece.

Air abrasion is most effective when used to remove sealants, stains on tooth enamel, class I through class IV preparations, endodontic access, and crown margins. It is also effective in preparing the tooth surface for cementation.

Air abrasion is not a replacement for conventional abrasion instruments—it is used mainly in support of other restorative procedures. Its main advantage lies in the fact that dentists can remove material on the tooth surface without the use of anesthetics.

CHECKPOINTS

26-9 Name the three attachments for low-speed handpieces.

26-10 Some high-speed handpieces can operate at how many rpms?

26-11 What are the advantages of electric handpieces?

26-12 What is the major advantage to a laser handpiece?

26-13 What is the proper method to clean handpieces between patients?

Instrument Transfer

Four-handed dentistry relies on the smooth transfer of instruments between the dentist and the dental assistant. In this approach to dentistry, the dental assistant sits across from the dentist and hands instruments across the transfer zone to the dentist as they are needed. The **transfer zone** is the invisible area where the actual exchange of instruments takes place—it is typically below the patient's chin, over the chest.

Smooth instrument transfer is more than simply handing off instruments as they are needed. A well-trained assistant/dentist team will function as one unit, wordlessly and efficiently passing instruments as they are needed. The dental assistant will anticipate which instruments are needed and make them available to the dentist at the exact moment they are needed.

Goals for Successful Instrument Transfer

Successful instrument transfer requires that the dental assistant is intimately familiar with the instruments required for a particular procedure, the order in which they will be used, and when they are required. When carried out correctly, the goals for a successful instrument transfer include:

- Allowing the dentist to keep his or her eyes focused on the oral cavity. The dentist should not have to look up or away to locate the instrument because this breaks concentration.
- Making the right instruments available at precisely the right time.

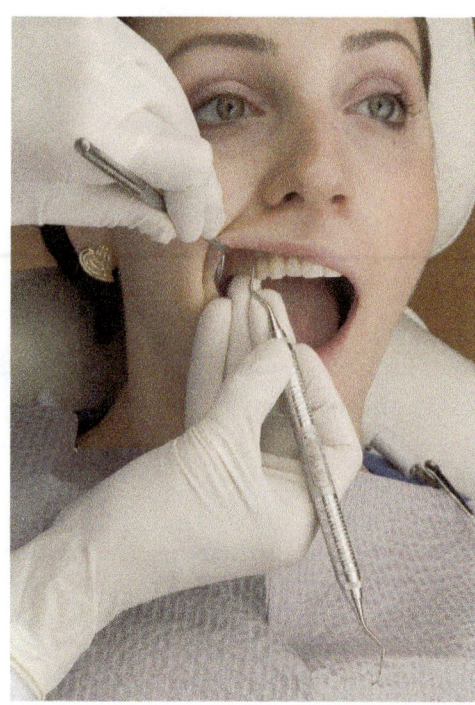

Figure 26–43 **Fulcrum.** Upper hand is using the patient's cheek as a fulcrum. Lower hand is using the patient's teeth as a fulcrum.

- Maintaining the dentist's fulcrum. A **fulcrum** describes a hand position in which the fingers are stabilized so the hand can easily pivot and perform work within the oral cavity (Figure 26-43). This might mean the fingers are resting on the patient's teeth, providing a strong support for the rest of the hand. A solid fulcrum is important, so successful instrument transfer should not interfere with the fulcrum.
- Transferring instruments with the proper hand, while still performing tasks such as suctioning.
- Making the instruments easily available for the dentist to grasp and begin using immediately without repositioning.

All of this should be accomplished within a few seconds. The remainder of this chapter is devoted to the methods used to accomplish these goals.

From the Dentist's Perspective

When my assistants and I are working well together, it's almost like magic: the instruments simply appear when I need them to, and I can provide faster and more efficient treatment for our patient. I call this "anticipation," and it means the assistants' ability to predict which instrument I'll need and wordlessly provide it. It's an invaluable skill.

Grasping an Instrument

Instruments are grasped with the appropriate hand as they are passed and used. The dental assistant should know when the dentist has a firm grip on the instrument by feel, or **tactile sensation**. A number of grasps are used

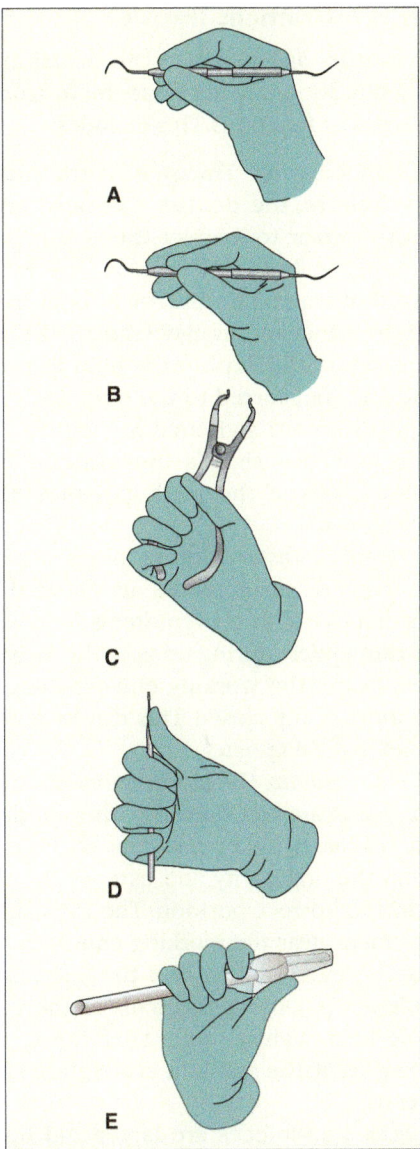

Figure 26–44 **Grasping.** (**A**) Pen grasp. (**B**) Modified pen grasp. (**C**) Palm grasp. (**D**) Palm-thumb grasp. (**E**) Modified palm grasp.

throughout dentistry to ensure smooth instrument transfers and more efficient use (Figure 26-44).

Pen Grasp

When using the pen grasp, the instrument is held in the same way a pen is held, between the thumb and the fleshy part of the index finger and stabilized by the side of the middle finger (Figure 26-44A). This grasp is used to hold instruments with angled shanks. It is also know as the "wand grasp."

Modified Pen Grasp

The modified pen grasp is similar to the pen grasp with one important difference: instead of being placed opposite the thumb, the pad of the middle finger is placed atop the instrument, along with the index finger (Figure 26-44B). The use of either the pen grip or the modified pen grip is a matter of personal preference. Some operators prefer the

modified pen grip because it enables them better control of the instrument. This grip is used with bent-shank instruments, the same as the pen grasp is.

Palm Grasp

The palm grasp is when the instrument is held firmly in the palm, with the fingers wrapped around the instrument shank (Figure 26-44C). This grasp is commonly used with forceps and pliers, which require greater hand strength to use effectively. Depending on how the instrument is used, the palm can be either facing up or facing down. When working on maxillary teeth, the palm is facing up; when working on mandibular teeth, the palm is facing down.

Palm-Thumb Grasp

The palm-thumb grasp is a modification of the palm grasp. The instrument is held in the palm in the same manner, with the fingers wrapped around the instrument handle, except that instead of being lined up with the fingers, the thumb extends upward along the instrument shank (Figure 26-44D). This grasp is used with straight-line instruments where both precision and strength are necessary, such as chisels and hoes. This grasp can also be used to hold a suction tip.

Modified Palm Grasp

The modified palm grasp is often used with the evacuator. This grip is the mirror image of the palm-thumb grasp. The hand is held in the same position, with the thumb along the straight axis of the instrument, but instead of facing the patient, the operator's thumb faces backward, toward the dental assistant (Figure 26-44E). This allows the operator to manipulate the evacuator without the obstruction of a thumb. This grasp is sometimes called the thumb-to-nose grasp.

Evacuator Versus Instrument Grasps

In four-handed dentistry, one of the assistant's hands is frequently occupied with holding the high-volume evacuator (HVE) while the other is passing instruments. The HVE can be held with the pen grasp, but is usually manipulated with one of the palm grasps. Which one is used depends on where the HVE tip is placed:

- The pen or modified pen grasp is used most often for anterior teeth.
- The modified palm, or thumb-to-nose, grasp is used more often for posterior teeth.

Transfer Techniques

Transferring instruments should be a smooth act that happens almost as second nature. Of course, this will take some experience, as every dentist and every assistant is different, but there are broad guidelines you can use to make it as easy as possible.

One-Handed Transfer Versus Two-Handed Transfer

The one-handed instrument transfer is the standard instrument transfer. It allows for the dental assistant to pass necessary instruments to the dentist while also performing tasks such as holding the HVE or using the air-water syringe. For example, when working with a right-handed operator, the assistant will pass instruments with the left hand and hold the suction tip with the right hand.

During a one-handed instrument transfer, the assistant picks up the next instrument from the tray to pass to the operator, and with the same hand, prepares to receive the instrument the operator just finished using. This process is covered and illustrated in Procedure 26-1.

The one-handed transfer is also used to rotate a double-ended instrument so the operator can switch sides without a break in his or her concentration.

The two-handed transfer requires both of the assistant's hands. It is usually used to transfer forceps or scissors. In this method, the assistant picks up the next instrument with one hand and receives the instrument the operator just finished using with the other hand. For example, when working with a right-handed operator, the assistant will retrieve an existing instrument from the operator with his or her left hand and pass the new instrument, such as a forceps or scissor, with the right hand.

Basic Principles of Instrument Transfer

Although these principles may be modified from office to office, you should be aware of the following rules for a basic instrument transfer:

- During a transfer the assistant grasps the instrument from the opposite end the operator will use. In single-ended instruments, this will be the end of the handle opposite the shank. In double-ended instruments, this will be the end nearer the working head that is *not* needed.
- The working end of the instrument should be presented in the same orientation as it will be used. For maxillary work, the working end should be positioned facing upward. For mandibular work, the working end should be positioned facing down.
- The instrument should be held in the transfer space, parallel to the instrument currently being held by the operator. The instruments should be as close as possible without causing conflict.

Voice of Experience

Many dental instruments have sharp points or cutting blades, which can easily pierce examination gloves and result in possible contamination. So you should always keep your eyes on the operator during instrument transfer—if they are not looking while they are transferring the instrument, it is easy to end up with a puncture wound! And remember: it is your job to stay alert!

Variations in Instrument Transfer

The previous rules apply to standard dental instruments, but a few modifications are necessary for instruments with different shapes or functions. This includes:

- *Mirror and Explorer Transfer.* At the beginning of every procedure, the dentist will need an explorer and mouth mirror to inspect the area being treated. In this transfer, both the mirror and explorer are transferred at once. The mirror is held in the assistant's right hand and transferred to the operator's left hand, while the explorer is held in the assistant left hand and transferred to the operator's right hand (these positions are switched for left-handed operators). The operator signals the assistant by placing his or her hands at the ready position next to the patient's mouth.
- *Cotton Pliers Transfer.* Cotton pliers are frequently used to remove small pieces of material from the patient's oral cavity. To prevent items from slipping out of nonlocking pliers during transfer, the assistant grasps the pliers nearer the working end, pinching the pliers to keep them firmly closed. This can be accomplished with a one-handed transfer.
- *Hinged Instruments.* Hinged instruments such as scissors and pliers are transferred with a modified grasp. To signal readiness, the operator moves his or her hand away from the oral cavity and extends the thumb and fingers in the correct position. The assistant picks up the instrument near the working end, with the fingers grabbing the hinge, and places the instrument in the operator's grasp. During the transfer, the instruments should be held slightly open. After the instrument is done being used, the assistant again grasps it from the hinged end.
- *Handpieces.* Handpieces are larger and bulkier than hand instruments, and they are attached by a hose. However, a one-handed instrument transfer can still be accomplished, with a little experience and practice. Make sure not to tangle the hose during the transfer.
- *Air-Water Syringe Transfer.* To transfer the air-water syringe, the assistant holds it from the nozzle end, with the working top of the syringe in the palm. The handle is presented to the operator.

CHECKPOINTS

26-14 Which grasp is commonly used with forceps and pliers?

26-15 Which grasp is commonly used with the evacuator?

26-16 When transferring an instrument, which end of the instrument should you grasp?

Procedure 26–1 **Instrument Transfer**

The following steps are used in the one-handed instrument transfer.

1. Put on appropriate PPE.
2. Pick up the instrument from the tray. Typically, a pen grasp is used to pick up the instrument to be transferred (Figure P26-1-1).

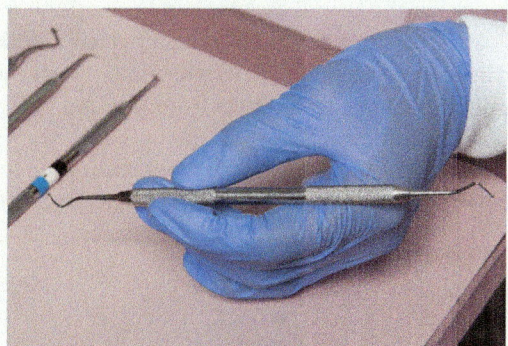

Figure P26-1-1

3. Grasp the instrument with the end to be used positioned away from you, so your hand is at the far end of the instrument from the working end the operator will be using.
4. Hold the instrument in the transfer zone, making sure it is positioned parallel to the instrument the operator is currently using (Figure P26-1-2).

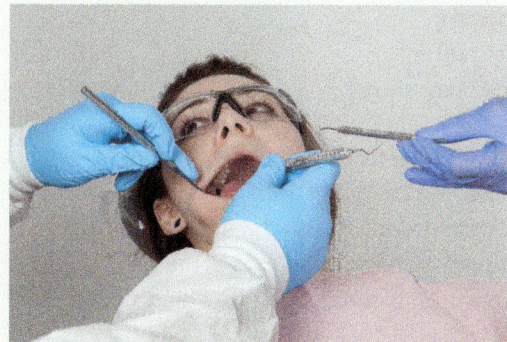

Figure P26-1-2

5. When the operator signals it is time to transfer, first retrieve the instrument the operator just finished using. To do this, extend the last two fingers of your hand and grab the used instrument with these fingers. In the meantime, continue to grip the next instrument in your thumb, index, and middle finger (Figure P26-1-3A).

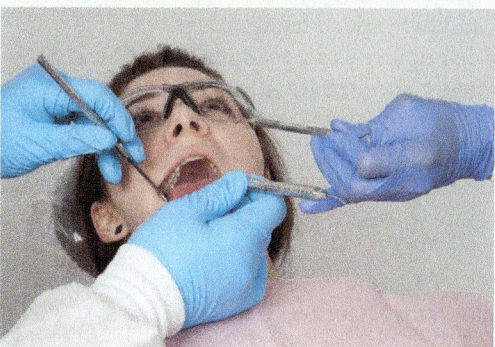

Figure P26-1-3A

6. Roll the used instrument toward your palm while firmly pressing the new instrument into the operator's fingers, using your sense of touch and signals from the operator to know when the instrument has been successfully grabbed (Figure P26-1-3B). Most operators will slightly withdraw their hand after transfer.

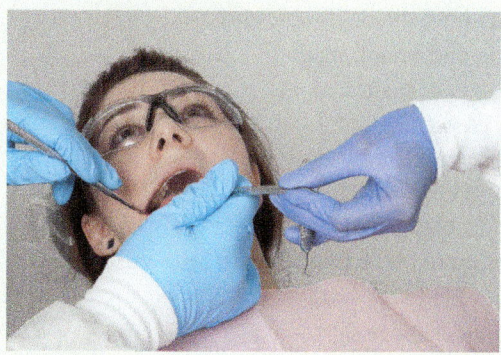

Figure P26-1-3B

7. Place the used instrument back in the tray in its original position.

 ## Chapter Highlights

- ✦ Hand dental instruments include a shaft, shank, and working end. The working ends and shank styles vary, depending on the instrument's function.
- ✦ The Black formula for dental instruments is used to quickly identify needed instruments. It comprises three numbers that describe the width of the blade, the length of the blade, and the angulation of the blade.

- ✦ Basic examination instruments include the mouth mirror, explorer, cotton pliers, and periodontal probe.
- ✦ Hand cutting instruments include chisels, hatchets, hoes, angle formers, excavators, and gingival margin trimmers.
- ✦ Restorative instruments include composite placement instruments, amalgam carriers, carvers, burnishers, articulating paper and articulating forceps, and plastic instruments.

- Accessory hand instruments include spatulas, scissors, dappen dishes, applicators, and brushes.
- Hand instruments are often organized on trays before procedures, and the sterile tray is carried into the examination room and opened just before the procedure.
- Trays should be assembled with the instruments to be used first on the left; there are also compartments for cotton and other materials used during a procedure.
- The most common handpieces in the dental office are low-speed and high-speed handpieces.
- Low-speed handpieces can accommodate three different attachments: the straight, the contra-angle, and the right-angle, or prophy-angle, attachment. Each has a different purpose.
- High-speed handpieces are used with burs and other grinding, cutting, and polishing instruments during restorations.
- Other types of handpieces include electric, abrasion, laser, and laboratory handpieces.
- Handpieces must be sterilized and lubricated between patients.
- Dental burs are classified by their shape, size, and function. Cutting burs, the most common variety, are assigned numbers.
- A wide variety of abrasive instruments are used to cut, finish, and polish, including discs, stones, wheels, and rubber instruments.
- Four-handed dentistry relies on smooth instrument transfer between the dental assistant and the operator.
- The goal of successful instrument transfer is to provide the right instrument at the exact right moment, so the operator does not have to look up from the oral cavity or break concentration.
- Dental assistants should know the proper technique for both one-handed and two-handed instrument transfers.

Review Questions

1. What are the three parts of dental instruments?
   a. Working end, rotary cuff, shank
   b. Working end, shank, double end
   c. Working end, shank, shaft
   d. Working end, shaft, scalpel

2. In the three-number Black formula, what does the third number stand for?
   a. Length of blade
   b. Angulation of blade in relation to long axis of handle
   c. Width of blade
   d. None of the above

3. Which of the following is not a basic examination instrument?
   a. Hoe
   b. Explorer
   c. Periodontal probe
   d. Cotton pliers

4. Which of the following is not a type of carver?
   a. Hollenback
   b. Ward
   c. Tanner
   d. Wedelstaedt

5. Which of the following is not a typical color-coding system?
   a. By procedure
   b. By operator
   c. By assistant
   d. By treatment room

6. When positioning instruments on a tray
   a. Place them from right to left, in order of use.
   b. Place them from left to right, in order of use.
   c. Line up all working ends.
   d. Rotate working ends, depending on order of use.

7. Which of the following is NOT a use for low-speed handpieces?
   a. Polishing restorations
   b. Preparing cavity margins
   c. In the laboratory
   d. Cutting with diamond burs

8. Between patients, high-speed handpieces
   a. Must be disinfected.
   b. Must have all disposable parts replaced.
   c. Must be sterilized.
   d. Must be covered with protective material.

9. What is the major disadvantage to electric high-speed handpieces?
   a. They are costly
   b. They are painful for patients
   c. They are not as fast as conventional high-speed handpieces
   d. They require extra training for use

10. Handpieces should always be lubricated
    a. According to manufacturer instructions.
    b. Before sterilization.
    c. After sterilization.
    d. Monthly.

11. What are the three styles of shanks for dental burs?
    a. Straight, latch, friction grip
    b. Straight, angled, friction grip
    c. Angled, crooked, latch
    d. Friction grip, latch, dappen

12. What are fissurotomy burs used for?
    a. Cutting dentin
    b. Trimming gingival margins
    c. Exploring the tooth surface
    d. Preparing cavities

13. What is the fulcrum?
    a. A stabilization point based on finger placement for better instrumentation
    b. The space where successful instrument transfer takes place
    c. The point where an instrument is gripped and balanced during transfer
    d. None of the above

14. What is the most common grasp used with the high-volume evacuator when working on posterior teeth?
    a. Pen grasp
    b. Thumb-to-nose grasp
    c. Two-handed grasp
    d. Modified pen grasp

Active Learning Exercise

1. Explain the differences between an explorer and a probe. What is the function of each? When would each be utilized and for what particular procedures?

Application Activities

1. Develop a color coding scheme for organizing a standard instrument tray. First make a list of all the instruments that are used in a basic tray. Then review the organizational methods that are described in the text. Choose one of the methods and organize your tray by assigning a color to each of the instruments on your list.

2. Using a pen, a toothbrush, or a similar item, practice the pen grasp and the modified pen grasp described. Write a paragraph or two describing how each grasp feels. Does the grasp feel like it will make movements accurate or awkward? Which grasp do you prefer using?

PREPARING FOR CERTIFICATION EXAMS

Review the following topics in this chapter to prepare for the Dental Assisting National Board (DANB) exam:

- Introduction
- Tray and Tub Systems
- Positioning Instruments on Trays
- Dental Rotary Instruments
- Dental Handpieces
- Dental Burs
- Abrasive Instruments
- Instrument Transfer
- Transfer Techniques

chapter 27

Moisture Control and Isolation

CHAPTER OUTLINE

CHAPTER CHECKLIST

On completion of this chapter, students will be able to:

☑ Identify the methods for maintaining the operating field.

☑ Describe the two main rinsing techniques.

☑ Identify the two main instruments available for oral evacuation, and describe their use.

☑ Identify equipment maintenance steps that can reduce the risk of contamination.

☑ Describe the devices available for tooth isolation.

☑ Explain the purpose of a dental dam, including appropriate circumstances for use.

☑ Describe the basic components of a dental dam.

☑ Describe the procedure for placing and removing a dental dam.

☑ Describe adjustments that can be made to the dental dam to accommodate special circumstances.

KEY TERMS

air-water syringe – a dental device that provides focused streams of air and water, or a combination of both, to produce water spray

anchor tooth – during placement of a dental dam, the tooth the clamp is fastened to (as well as another tooth); used to keep the dam material in place

dental dam – a device consisting of a frame and sheet of thin, pliable material that is used to isolate teeth during dental procedures

high-volume evacuator (HVE) – a dental device that provides a strong suction, used to remove large amounts of fluid and debris from the oral cavity during dental procedures; also called an oral evacuator

interseptal dam – in a dental dam, the part that is placed between the teeth (the area of the dam between the punched holes)

key punch hole – in a dental dam, the largest hole in the dental dam, meant to be used with the bow on a dental clamp to securely hold the dental dam material in place

operating field – during a dental procedure, the area where the work will be performed, including the oral cavity and the transfer space where instruments are transferred between the operator and the dental assistant

saliva ejector – a dental device that provides low-strength suction and is meant to remove excess saliva during a procedure; it does not remove debris

template – a dental device that contains the imprint of the dental arch used for marking hole positions on the dental dam

Introduction

Moisture control and tooth isolation are important elements of modern dentistry. A well-prepared operating field, with effective moisture control, allows the procedure to be done more quickly and efficiently, and provides superior infection control for the dental team.

A dental assistant is an important part of the moisture control and tooth isolation team. In some states, tooth isolation techniques with dental dams are considered expanded functions, but all dental assistants should be familiar with tooth isolation. Moisture control is a universal task for dental assistants. This chapter is devoted to the devices and techniques available for both moisture control and tooth isolation.

Maintaining the Operating Field

The **operating field** is the area where the procedure is actually being performed. During the procedure, it has to be well lit, free from debris and moisture, and easily accessible to the instruments needed to perform the procedure. This is not just for aesthetics: a crowded or poorly defined operating field represents a danger to the patient and can result in harm.

The operating field differs from procedure to procedure. The requirements for a root canal, for instance, differ from those of a dental restoration. The dental assistant should know beforehand where his or her help is needed and be prepared to assist in any way. During the procedure, dental assistants are called on to:

- Transfer instruments and devices to the operator's hands so the operator does not have to break concentration
- Keep the operating field free of fluid and debris that might disrupt the operator or be aspirated or swallowed by the patient
- Keep the working lines clear, so the operator's hands, arms, and legs do not become entangled in tubes, wires, or cables attached to dental instruments

There are a number of methods used to accomplish these tasks.

From the Dentist's Perspective

It's hard to overestimate the importance of a clean operating field during a tricky procedure. Proper use of the air-water syringe to rinse and dry the field, coupled with the evacuator to keep it clean, means that I can do my job faster and more efficiently, with better results for the patient. So when it comes to moisture control and isolation, I really count on my assistants to help me deliver superior patient care.

Lighting

Lighting is essential for a safe, clear operating field. Once the procedure has begun, it falls to the dental assistant to make sure the dental light is positioned at all times to ensure that maximum light falls on the operating field. Light may also be provided by the handpiece LED, an illuminated mouth mirror, or even lights on the operator's eye gear. Ideally, the top glow of light should rest at the ala of the patient's nose. Dental lights are extremely intense (the equivalent of 1200 candles), so adjust the light upward starting at the patient's chest, not on the face moving downward. This prevents blinding the patient and making him or her uncomfortable. Chapter 24, The Dental Office, details how to correctly position the operating light.

Retraction

During a dental procedure, it is often necessary to move obstructing tissues, including the tongue, lips, cheeks, and any other tissue. This can be accomplished with a number of instruments, which are used to gently push or pull and hold the tissue out of the line of vision, including mouth mirrors (Figure 27-1), evacuators, the rubber dam, tissue retractors, cotton products (e.g., rolls and swabs), and tongue depressors.

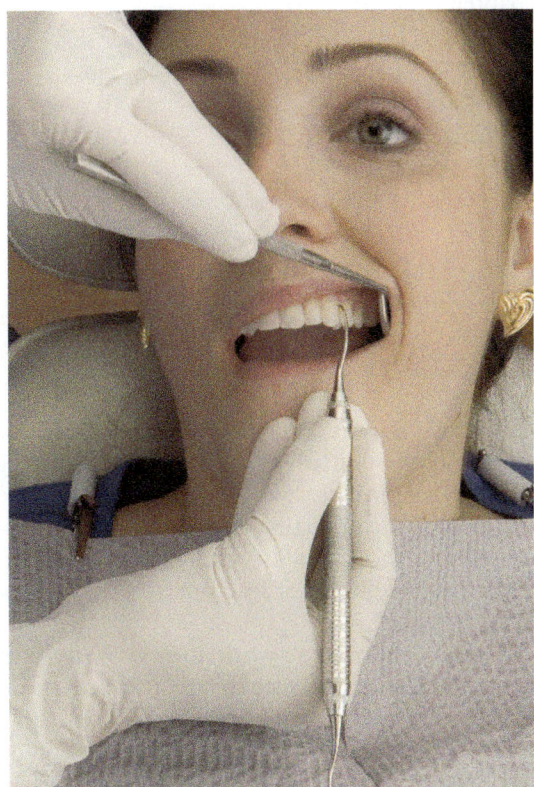

Figure 27–1 Retraction. Operator using a mirror to retract the lip and cheek.

Use of Mouth Props

In addition to tissue retraction, some patients might require the use of mouth props during longer procedures. These devices are designed to help patients keep their mouths open by giving them something to hold between their teeth.

Mouth props can be rubber or plastic devices that are held between the maxillary and mandibular arches, or they can take the form of forceps-like metal ratchet devices with rubber-coated ends that are held between the jaws. During placement, care should be taken that the patient is comfortable and relaxed—mouth props should not be uncomfortable for the patient. Rather, they should make it easier for the patient to keep his or her mouth open without strain.

Evacuation

Evacuation is typically accomplished through use of the **air-water syringe** in conjunction with the high-volume evacuator or the smaller saliva ejector.

The **high-volume evacuator** is a powerful suction instrument that is used to remove saliva, blood, and debris from the oral cavity. In contrast, the saliva ejector is used during less-intensive procedures to remove saliva and water; it does not have the suction strength to remove debris.

Use of these devices is covered in greater depth later in this chapter.

✓ **CHECKPOINTS**

27-1 What is the operating field?

27-2 What is a mouth prop used for?

Rinsing

The air-water syringe is used simultaneously with an evacuator to clear the oral cavity of unwanted saliva, blood, and debris. Oral rinsing should be performed frequently in order to keep the operating field clear. Because this procedure requires the dental assistant to be working in the same space as the dentist or lead operator, careful coordination is necessary.

Rinsing is performed with the air-water syringe (Figure 27-2). This device is actually a three-way device that sprays air, water, or a combination of both to flush the operating field and dry it. Some equipment companies call three-way syringes *triplex syringes*. Air-water syringes are equipped with disposable aseptic tips that must be discarded between patients. Alternatively, they may be

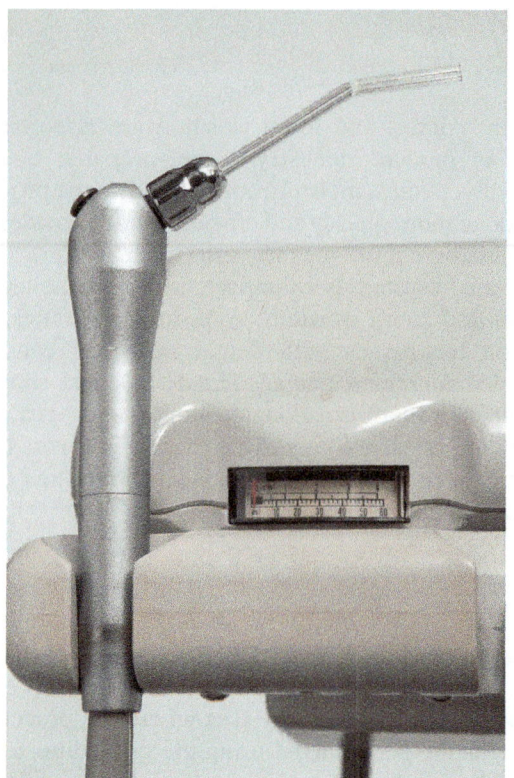

Figure 27–2 Air-water syringe.

equipped with metal tips that can be sterilized between patients. Air-water syringes are connected to the dental unit by tubing or a hose. The handle contains buttons to control the air and water.

Rinsing Techniques

There are two rinsing techniques used with the air-water syringe:

- *Limited Rinse.* Limited rinsing is designed to clean only the area around the immediate operating field. It is frequently performed during short breaks in the procedure, such as when the dentist inspects the field. During a limited rinse, a relatively small amount of water or combined water and air is sprayed quickly on the area and the result is immediately evacuated.
- *Complete Oral Irrigation.* During this procedure, the full oral cavity is refreshed and rinsed with the air-water syringe. This may be done after a long procedure, after dental prophylaxis, or whenever the dentist feels it is necessary. Complete oral irrigation is covered in Procedure 27-1.

✓ **CHECKPOINT**

27-3 Which instrument is used for rinsing?

Procedure 27-1 Complete Oral Irrigation

Complete oral irrigation requires the air-water syringe and evacuator to be used in tandem. A saliva ejector may also be used in tandem with this procedure. It is placed at the lowest point in the oral cavity, where moisture will pool. For example, if the patient's head is turned to the left, place the saliva ejector in the lower left section of the oral cavity.

Materials needed (Figure P27-1-1):

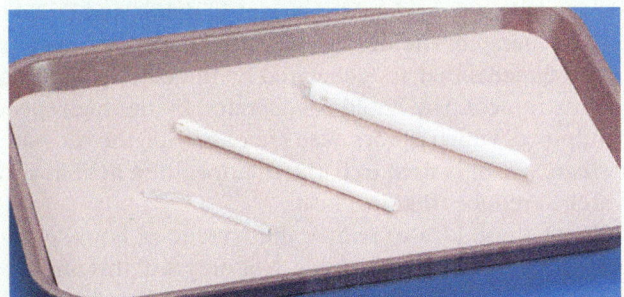

Figure P27-1-1

- Air-water syringe
- Evacuator
- Saliva ejector

1. Put on appropriate PPE.
2. Ask the patient to turn his or her head toward you. This encourages water to pool in one area of the mouth, where it can be more easily evacuated.
3. Turn on the high-volume evacuator or saliva evacuator and position it. The air-water syringe should be held in the dominant hand during this procedure, so right-handed assistants will hold it in their right hands (Figure P27-1-2).

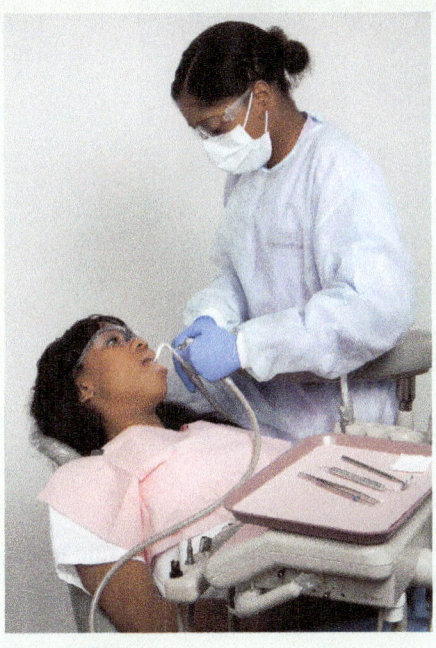

Figure P27-1-2

4. Spray the patient's oral cavity with water in quadrants, beginning with the maxillary arch and progressing to the mandibular arch. Depending on the patient position and the procedure, you can progress from the left to the right or the right to the left, making sure the evacuator is correctly positioned to remove all liquid.
5. After the rinsing is done, use the high-volume evacuator to remove all liquid from the patient's oral cavity so they do not accidentally swallow or aspirate fluid.

Oral Evacuation

Evacuation refers to the practice of removing saliva, blood, water, and debris from the patient's oral cavity during dental procedures. Effective evacuation serves two major purposes: (1) it keeps the operating field clear so the dentist can perform the procedure, and (2) it helps prevent the patient from swallowing or aspirating any byproducts of the procedure.

There are two main devices used during evacuation: the saliva ejector and the high-volume evacuator.

Cultural Diversity

Among some cultures and faiths, such as Judaism, it is forbidden to swallow blood. The dental assistant must make every effort to ensure that the saliva ejector and high-volume evacuation are used accordingly to suction blood for these patients. Knowledge of these kinds of cultural and ethnic beliefs can help to avoid misunderstandings in treatment and better meet your patients' needs.

Saliva Ejector

The **saliva ejector** is a low-volume evacuator used to remove fluids from the patient's oral cavity. This device is usually made from a flexible, narrow-gauge plastic tube with a plastic tip (Figure 27-3). It is connected to the dental unit by a hose and features an enlarged handle so the operator can manipulate it if necessary.

The working end of the saliva ejector is made from thin, pliable plastic that can be easily bent into the appropriate position and positioned within the patient's oral cavity to remove pooled saliva. Saliva ejectors are frequently bent into candy cane shapes and "hung" from the patient's mandibular arch during a procedure.

Saliva ejectors are not strong enough to remove debris and should not be used for this purpose. Likewise, they should not be used during procedures that generate copious amounts of fluids, such as oral fluoride treatments. Saliva ejectors work only when the tip is immersed in water or saliva. Patients should never close their mouth around the saliva ejector, as studies have shown that a

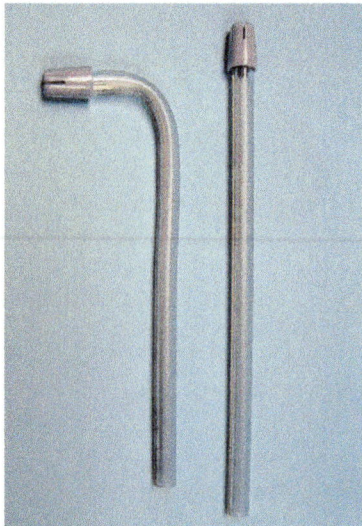

Figure 27–3 Saliva ejector.

backflow can be created, thus allowing some liquid in the hose to be forced back into the patient's mouth.

High-Volume Evacuator

The high-volume evacuator, or HVE, is a larger, more powerful suction device (Figure 27-4). It is used to remove large amounts of liquid and debris from the oral cavity during dental procedures. It will vacuum out water and debris

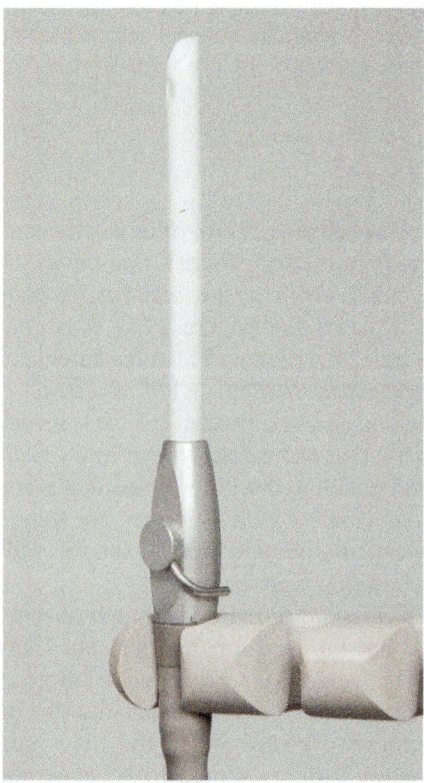

Figure 27–4 High-volume evacuator (HVE) with disposable plastic tip.

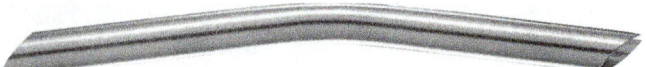

Figure 27–5 Steel HVE tip.

when placed near water; the tip does not need to be in the water or saliva to remove the water and debris. It can also be used to retract tissues during procedures.

During high-speed cutting with the dental handpiece, for example, a considerable amount of debris and liquid is often generated. The debris consists of tooth and restoration fragments that are generated by the cutting action of the instrument. The liquid is generated by the high-speed handpiece, which sprays water, along with the air-water syringe, which is used to bathe the operating field in cool water to reduce frictional heat.

It is a good idea to reduce the volume of liquid in the oral cavity as much as possible. Not only will this improve the operator's ability to perform the procedure, but when water comes into contact with the high-speed handpiece, it may be vaporized into a potentially contaminated mist.

Properly used, the HVE dramatically reduces the amount of liquid, vapor, and debris generated during use of the dental handpiece.

The HVE unit consists of several parts:

- *The hose.* The hose or tubing connects the HVE to the dental unit. Hoses must be long enough to reach from the dental unit to the treatment chair, allowing the dental assistant to easily work with the HVE. During procedures, it is up to the dental assistant to make sure the dentist or instrument operator does not become entangled in the HVE hose.
- *The tip.* The tip is the portion of the HVE that is actually inserted into the oral cavity. Unlike the saliva ejector tips, HVE tips are not flexible. They come in a variety of lengths, and some are straight while others have a slight bend (Figure 27-5). HVE tips commonly have beveled, or angled, ends so the operator can more easily reach into corners during evacuation. Tips are made from plastic or steel, and they may be disposable or reusable. Reusable tips must be sterilized between patients.
- *The handle.* The handle is where the operator holds the HVE and where the controls are located. Depending on the manufacturer, controls may be included in a switch, dial, or push button. Controls are operated with one hand. The hose connects to the base of the handle. The lower portion of the HVE handle also contains a small wire trap. This v-shaped wire will prevent accidental suction of a dropped crown or larger object, which could clog or obstruct the hose or unit.

Grasping the HVE

In four-handed dentistry, the HVE is held in one hand while the other hand is occupied passing instruments

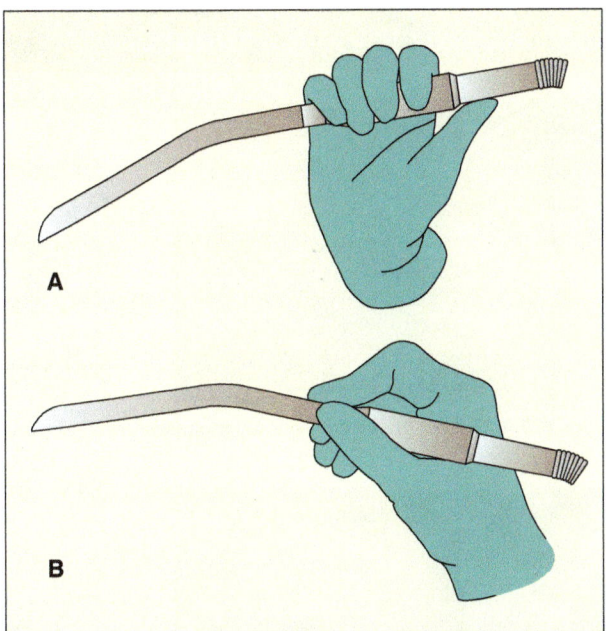

Figure 27–6 Grasping the HVE. (A) Thumb-to-nose grasp. (B) Pen grasp.

or performing some other task. The exact grasp used to manipulate the HVE depends on where the tip needs to be positioned in the patient's oral cavity and the angle the assistant is working from. Typically, the HVE is grasped with a thumb-to-nose grasp or a pen grasp (Figure 27-6), which allows for precise manipulation of the tip, but other grasps may be appropriate. Instruments grasps are covered in greater depth in Chapter 26, Dental Instruments and Equipment.

Principles for HVE Use

HVE placement and use falls to the dental assistant. These general principles guide HVE use:

- The HVE should be placed in the patient's oral cavity *before* the operator positions the high-speed handpiece or hand instruments, including the mouth mirror. The HVE is then repositioned as needed depending on where the operator has the handpiece.
- The HVE tip should be placed on the surface of the target tooth closest to the dental assistant, with the beveled edge parallel to the occlusal plane of the tooth surface and slightly distal.
- The suction tip edge should be slightly elevated from the occlusal plane of the tooth being worked on, thus exposing the target tooth to the maximum suction power.
- The HVE should be stabilized by hand during operation of the high-speed handpiece or hand instruments.
- If the HVE is to be in place for a long time, the tip can be positioned against cotton rolls. It should not be rested directly on gingival tissue.

CHECKPOINTS
27-4 What is the saliva ejector used for?

27-5 What is the HVE used for?

27-6 What are the most common grasps for holding the HVE?

27-7 When should the HVE be placed in the patient's oral cavity?

Procedure 27–2 Positioning the High-Volume Evacuator (HVE)

Materials needed (Figure P27-2-1):

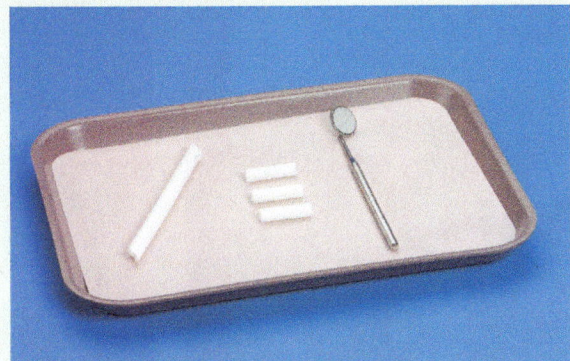

Figure P27-2-1

- High-volume evacuator (HVE)
- New tip
- Mouth mirror
- Cotton rolls, if needed

1. Put on appropriate PPE.
2. Prepare the HVE by pushing a new tip onto the handle.
3. Depending on the angle, use the mouth mirror or HVE to retract mucosal tissue or the tongue. Position the HVE before the operator places the handpiece or hand instruments.
4. Position the HVE tip as close as possible to the target tooth. One good rule of thumb is to position the HVE tip within one tooth's length of the target tooth.
5. Position the beveled end of the HVE parallel to the buccal or lingual surface of the tooth.
6. Position the HVE so the edge of the tip extends just beyond the occlusal plane of the target tooth. Correct positioning for suctioning of various surfaces is shown in Figures P27-2-2A through P27-2-2H.
7. Rest the HVE tip on cotton rolls for a fulcrum, not the gingival surface.

Procedure 27–2 Positioning the High-Volume Evacuator (HVE) (Continued)

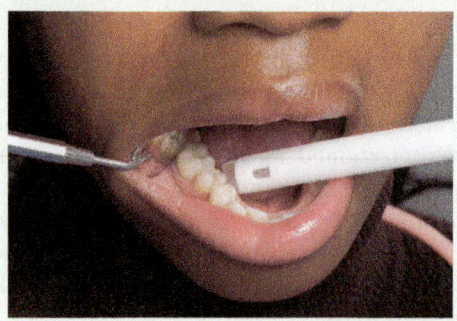

Figure P27-2-2A HVE placement for a posterior mandibular tooth, lingual surface.

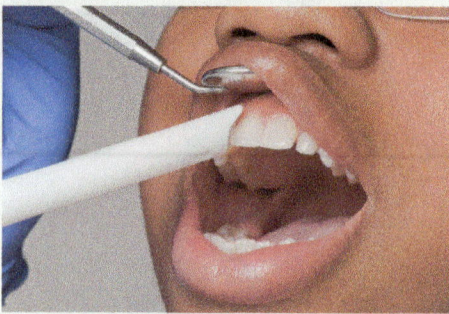

Figure P27-2-2E HVE placement for an anterior maxillary tooth, labial surface.

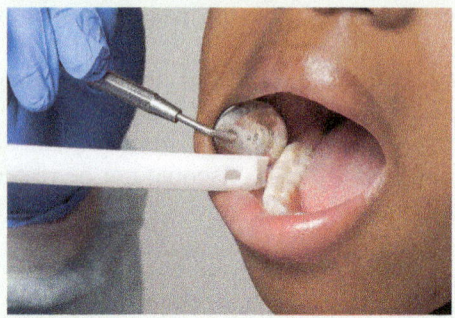

Figure P27-2-2B HVE placement for a posterior mandibular tooth, buccal surface.

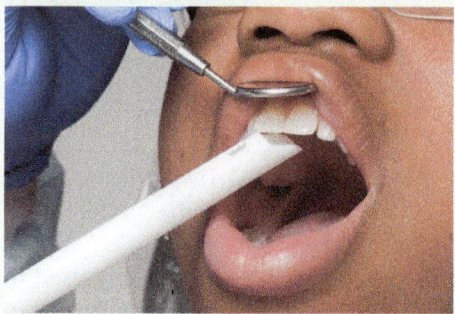

Figure P27-2-2F HVE placement for an anterior maxillary tooth, lingual surface.

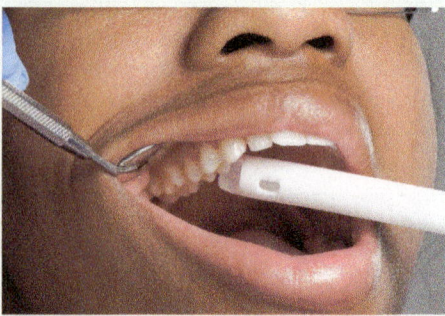

Figure P27-2-2C HVE placement for a posterior maxillary tooth, lingual surface.

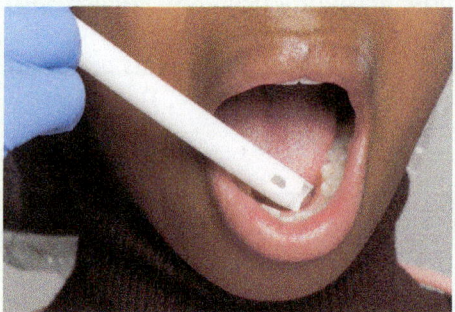

Figure P27-2-2G HVE placement for an anterior mandibular tooth, lingual surface.

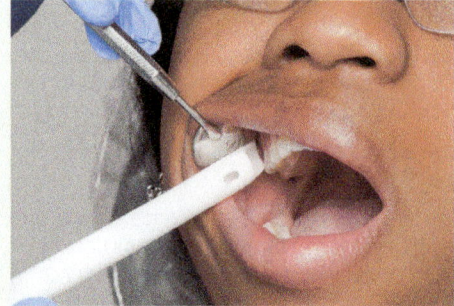

Figure P27-2-2D HVE placement for a posterior maxillary tooth, buccal surface.

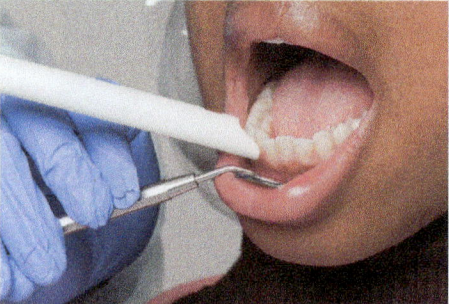

Figure P27-2-2H HVE placement for an anterior mandibular tooth, labial surface.

Care of Equipment

Like all dental equipment, the air-water syringe, saliva ejector, and HVE require regular care and maintenance to function at peak levels and reduce the risk of contamination. For a detailed discussion on infection control, please see Chapter 14, Disease and Infection Control.

In general, the following factors should be kept in mind:

- In years past, dental workers routinely told patients to close their mouths around the saliva ejector to clear the oral cavity. *However, this is no longer standard operating procedure. When patients close their mouth around the saliva ejector, this potentially causes a vacuum that allows possibly contaminated liquid from the saliva ejector to backflow into the mouth.*
- The water lines from the dental unit should be flushed at the end of every day with a disinfectant.
- The disposable traps in the dental unit should be cleaned and checked daily for any residual debris.
- The saliva ejector tubing should be cleaned daily and the screens should be checked and replaced as needed.

CHECKPOINT

27-8 Should patients close their mouths around the saliva ejector during use? Why or why not?

Tooth Isolation

Tooth isolation is the practice of isolating a single tooth, a specific area, or even an entire quadrant, during a dental procedure. The isolated area should be kept clean and dry and well lit, allowing the dentist or equipment operator to deliver the highest quality patient care possible.

A number of instruments and devices are used in tooth isolation. They are usually positioned before the procedure begins, although sometimes tissue retraction is an ongoing process throughout the procedure. Effective tooth isolation should be:

- Easy to implement and not too time-consuming
- Comfortable for the patient
- Not obstructing for the dentist
- Able to provide full tissue retraction without placing undue strain on the patient or the dental assistant

The dental assistant is largely responsible for tooth isolation. The next sections will deal with the techniques and instruments used to accomplish effective tooth isolation.

Cotton Rolls

Cotton rolls are an essential part of tooth isolation. Cotton rolls are small, tightly bound cotton products that are used to isolate teeth, hold tissues away from teeth, balance the

HVE tip, place materials, and provide something for the patient to bite during procedures. Cotton rolls are available in a variety of sizes. A properly prepared tray should contain all the appropriate cotton rolls for a specific procedure. Cotton rolls are used during restorations, examinations, application of sealants, and cementation of castings.

Although cotton rolls are easy to place, adaptable, and widely useful, they do have certain drawbacks. They are not typically used as the only isolation device during more complicated or longer procedures because they do not provide complete isolation, nor do they protect the patient from accidentally aspirating or swallowing liquids or materials. Additionally, cotton rolls must be replaced frequently because of saturation.

Cotton rolls are placed and removed with either gloved fingers or with cotton pliers. If multiple cotton rolls are required, and there are not enough hands available to place and maintain them, a device called a *cotton roll holder* can be used. This metal or plastic device holds multiple cotton rolls and is used to place cotton rolls on either side of the mandibular arch (Figure 27-7). To use it, the cotton rolls are slid onto the device's rods or points and then placed in the patient's oral cavity. The metal device features a clamp that extends down the chin and under the jaw. After the rolls are comfortably in place, the operator slides the clamp until it is firmly held in place. There are also plastic cotton roll holders that simply fit over the arch without the chin strap.

During removal, dry cotton rolls will sometimes adhere to mucosal surfaces. To prevent these, dry rolls should be slightly moistened before they are removed. It can be uncomfortable and even painful for patients to have dry cotton rolls forcibly peeled from tender tissue after a dental procedure. Direct a stream of water under the cotton roll, against the gingival tissue and the cotton roll, to moisten it before removal.

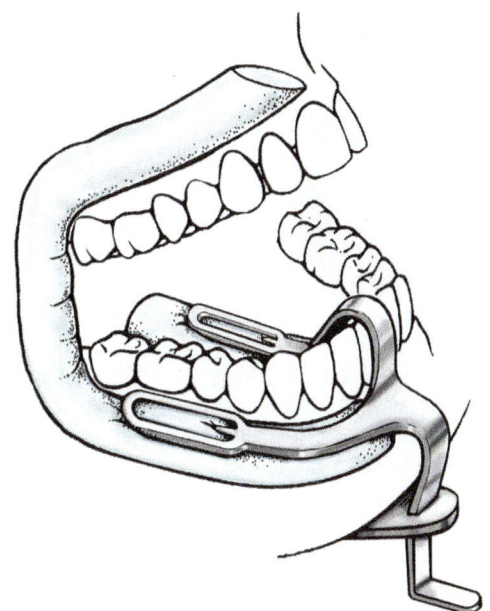

Figure 27–7 Cotton roll holder. Cotton roll holder used to treat two quadrants simultaneously.

Procedure 27–3 **Using Cotton Rolls**

Materials needed (Figure P27-3-1):

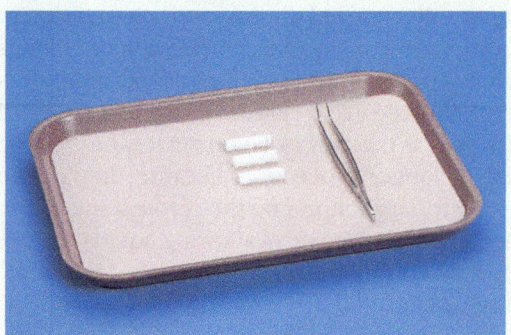

Figure P27-3-1

- Cotton roll(s)
- Cotton pliers
- Air-water-syringe and tip
1. Put on appropriate PPE.
2. Ask the patient to face you with his or chin raised for maxillary placement or lowered for mandibular placement.
3. Pick up the cotton roll with the cotton pliers, with the beaks of the cotton pliers placed in the direction of the arch on which you are working, but not extending beyond the cotton roll, which might pinch gingival tissue.
4. If necessary, retract the tissue (e.g., tongue or buccal tissue) and place the cotton roll in the correct alignment (Figure P27-3-2). In anterior placements, it may be necessary to bend the cotton roll before placement so it fits comfortably around the arch of the mouth. The long access of the cotton roll should be parallel to the long axis of the arch being worked on.

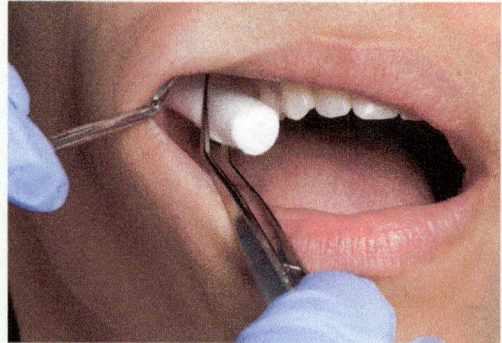

Figure P27-3-2

5. Make sure the cotton roll is securely in place with a gloved finger and tucked into the vestibule of the tissue. Correct placement for various positions is shown in Figures P27-3-3A through D.
6. Prior to removal, wet the cotton roll.

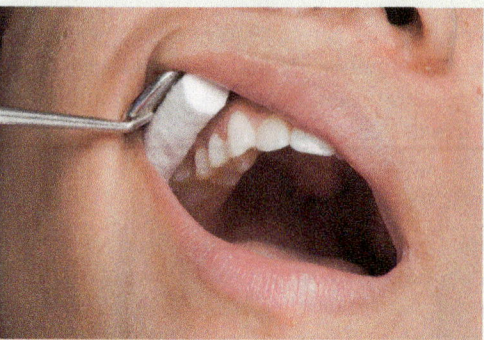

Figure P27-3-3A Cotton roll in position in the maxillary posterior buccal region.

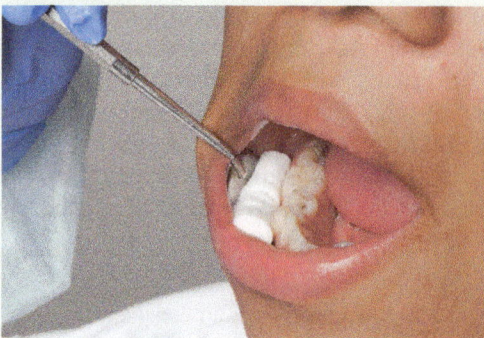

Figure P27-3-3B Cotton roll in position in the mandibular posterior buccal and lingual region.

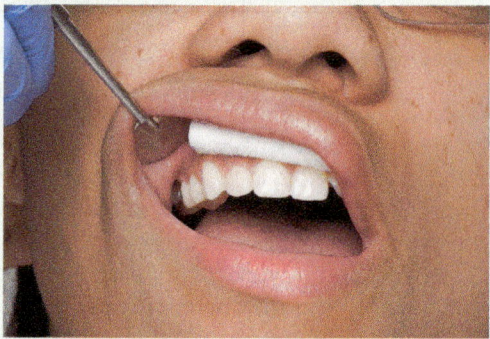

Figure P27-3-3C Cotton roll in position in the maxillary anterior labial region.

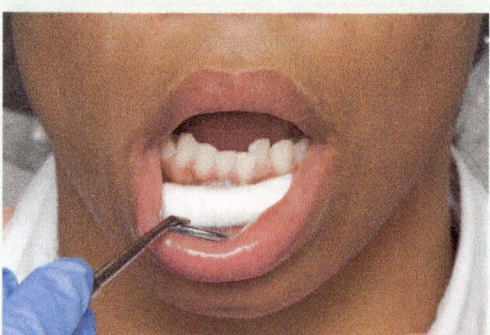

Figure P27-3-3D. Cotton roll in position in the mandibular anterior labial region.

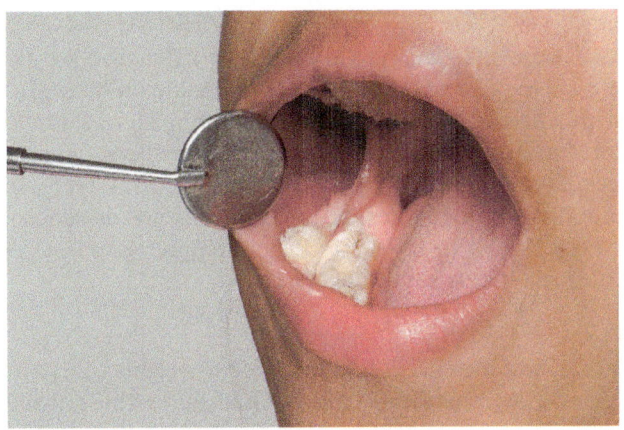

Figure 27–8 Dry angle placed in oral cavity.

Dry Angles

A dry angle is another aid used to prevent excess saliva in the oral cavity and aid in tissue retraction. These triangular, absorbent pads are designed to be placed directly against the buccal tissue in the posterior area of the maxillary and mandibular arches. This is where Stensen duct empties saliva from the parotid gland into the oral cavity. The duct opening is located approximately at the maxillary second bicuspid area. Dry angles are placed with cotton pliers with the narrow end of the triangle placed toward the back of the mouth and the wider end toward the lips (Figure 27-8). Dry angles may become saturated during the procedure and need to be replaced. To remove a dry angle, moisten it with water from the air-water syringe and use cotton pliers to gently remove it from the oral cavity, then place a new angle if needed.

✓ CHECKPOINTS

27-9 What is the appropriate procedure for removing a dry cotton roll?

27-10 What are dry angles used for?

Dental Dams

Dental dams are thin, pliable sheets of latex or latex-free material that are used in conjunction with specially designed frames to completely isolate teeth during procedures. Once properly placed, only the target tooth or target teeth will be visible, and the dental dam will prevent liquid and debris from falling into the patient's oral cavity to be swallowed or aspirated. Other advantages of the dental dam include:

- Excellent moisture control as the dental dam prevents saliva from reaching the target area. This is especially important during use of materials such as bonding agents, etchants, and other restorative materials that cannot be exposed to moisture during placement.

- Better visibility and accessibility by aiding in tissue retraction.
- Protection of sensitive mucosal tissue during procedures such as acid-etching.
- Decrease in the amount of potentially contaminated aerosol spray generated during the procedure, thereby protecting the patient from inhaling or ingesting harmful bacteria or contaminated materials.
- Decrease in the risk of contaminants traveling from infected teeth into the oral cavity during endodontic procedures.
- Deterrent for conversation by the patient, which can increase operator efficiency and allow procedures to be performed much faster.
- Prevention of aspiration of materials or small instruments.

Dental dams are placed after the local anesthetic is administered. Typically, it should take less than 5 minutes to prepare and place a dental dam.

Responsibility for creating and placing dental dams varies from state to state. In some states, the dental assistant with expanded functions training can place the dental dam alone. In other states, dental assistants should assist the dentist or hygienist in placement of the dental dam. No matter what your state allows, it is important to know how dental dams function and how they are placed.

Dental Facts

Dental dams are not new, but they certainly have changed since their early days. One early dental clamp, known as a Woodbury-True clamp, features large clips on the frame and straps that stretched behind the patient's head. It looked barbaric!

Indications and Contraindications

Dental dams can be used on almost any appropriate patient, including pediatric patients, during any appropriate procedure. To some degree, use of the dental dam depends on the dentist's preference—some dentists use them frequently, while others reserve their use for specific procedures.

Some patients, however, are not good candidates for dental dam use. Dental dams should not be used if:

- The patient has physical conditions that would make it uncomfortable or induce anxiety. Such conditions include asthma, respiratory illnesses such as COPD, herpetic lesions around the mouth or painful canker sores, and conditions affecting the corners of the mouth
- The patient is severely claustrophobic or truly phobic about dental devices or procedures.

Materials and Equipment

With experience, preparing and placing dental dams should take only a few minutes. Although they are extremely versatile, all dental dams are made from the same basic components: the dam material and the dental dam frame. Other armamentarium are used to help prepare the dental dam and increase patient comfort. All components are chosen specifically for the tooth or area being isolated. Knowledge of the types of materials and equipment used is crucial for successfully placing a dam for isolation.

Dental Dam Materials

Dental dams are typically made from sheets of pliable, thin latex or latex-free material. Latex allergies can result in a medical emergency, so it is important to review the patient's medical history before installing a latex dental dam. If there is any question of an allergy to natural rubber latex, it is recommended that latex-free dental dam material and gloves be used during treatment. Make sure not to cross-contaminate latex-free products with products containing latex or items that have come into contact with latex (i.e., the dental dam template or stamp). Always store latex-free materials separately from latex products. For more information on latex allergies, see Chapter 14, Disease and Infection Control. Dental dams are available in various sizes, thicknesses, and colors (Figure 27-9).

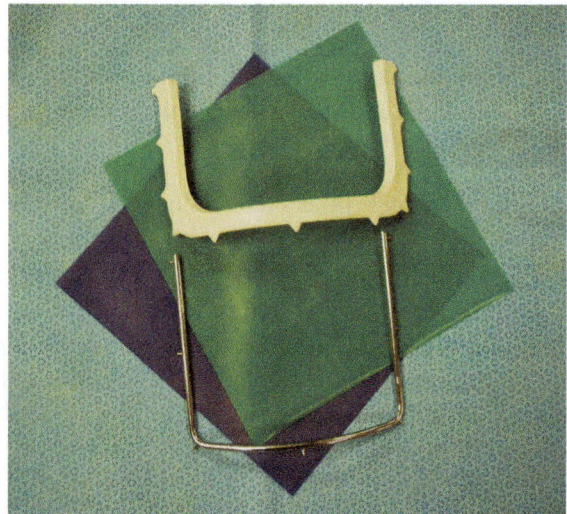

Figure 27-9 Dental dams and dental frames.

Size

Standard dental dams are made from 5 × 5-inch, 6 × 6-inch, or 8 × 8-inch squares of material, depending on their placement. The 6 × 6-inch sheets are used in posterior applications and on adult teeth. The 5 × 5-inch sheets are used for primary teeth, anterior applications on adult teeth, and endodontic procedures. Material squares are usually sold in boxes of 50, or the material can be purchased in a continual roll that is cut to fit.

Thickness

Dental dam material is sold in different weights (e.g., thicknesses) to accommodate different procedures. These include:

- *Thin.* Thin material is used most often for endodontic procedures and in situations where only one tooth needs to be exposed. This material stretches readily and tears easily and does not effectively retract tissues.
- *Medium.* Medium material does not tear as easily and is often used during procedures in which more than one tooth is isolated.
- *Heavy.* Heavy material is used when tissue retraction is important and a more tear-resistant material is required. Procedures that might call for a heavy dental dam material include crowns, fixed bridges, or restorations on areas with tight contacts.

Color

Dental dam materials are available in a variety of colors, from grey to green and dark blue to ivory, including pastels in pink, purple, and pale blue along with bright colors. Experience has shown that patients are more accepting of brightly colored dental dams, although some operators prefer dark grey because it enhances contrast, making it easier to see the teeth. The darker the dam material, the better the visibility for the operator.

Besides pleasing colors, scented and flavored dental dams are also available to make the patient's experience more comfortable.

Dental Dam Frames

Dental dam frames are used to stretch and tightly hold the dental dam in place, thus isolating the operating area and ensuring that the dental dam will not interfere with the procedure.

Frames are typically made from plastic or metal and are sterilizable (see Figure 27-9). Plastic frames are radiolucent, so they do not need to be removed during dental radiographs.

There are several styles of frame available, depending on the procedure. They include:

- *Ostby frame.* Ostby frames are circular or oval plastic frames that fit on the contours of the lower face. The frame is equipped with sharp projections along the outer edge to hold the dental dam in place. Ostby frames are radiolucent.

- *Young frame*. The Young frame is a U-shaped metal frame with sharp projections along its outer edge to hold the dental dam in place.
- *U-frame*. The U-frame is similar to the Young frame, except it is made from radiolucent plastic. One benefit of using a plastic frame is that is does not have to be removed for radiographic exposure; all metal frames must be removed if a radiograph is to be taken.

Dental Dam Napkins

Dental dam napkins are disposable, absorbent, fabric-like napkins that fit between the frame and the patient's face, thus preventing direct contact between the patient's face and the dental dam material. Napkins are designed for the patient's comfort and to absorb liquids and moisture. Dental dam napkins are precut by the manufacturer.

Lubricants

Three types of lubricant are often used with dental dams: shaving cream, cocoa butter, and K-Y Jelly. A small amount of lubricant may be applied to the patient's lips for his or her comfort. Next, a water-based lubricant is applied to the underside of the dental dam. This makes it easier to slide the dental dam over the teeth. A petroleum-based lubricant should not be used for this because it may leave a film on the teeth, interfering with some materials used during restorations. Also, petroleum-based lubricants can degrade the dental dam material.

Dental Dam Templates and Stamps

Templates and stamps are used to help the operator punch holes in the correct place on the dental dam material (Figure 27-10).

Dental stamps are rubber stamp pads used with ink pads to mark the dental arches on the dental dam material. Once the arches are marked, the operator can line up the punch and perforate the dam material.

Templates operate on a similar principle. A template is a printed card that is laid under the dental dam material, which is then marked with a pen to show the correct location for punching holes.

Both stamps and templates are general guides. They show ideal pediatric and adult dental arches, but they are not custom-designed for individual patients. Thus, variations might have to be made to accommodate each patient's unique dentition. Over time, as they become more comfortable using dental dams, many assistants cease using templates and stamps.

Dental Dam Punch

A dental dam punch is an instrument used to punch holes in the dental dam material. The instrument resembles a standard paper punch, but it is much more specialized. The working end of the dental dam punch includes a sharp *stylus* that works in conjunction with the *punch table* or *punch plate* to produce the right size hole (Figure 27-11). The punch plate is a rotating wheel with holes of various sizes to accommodate different teeth. Punch plates have five holes, numbered from 1 to 5, with 5 as the largest and 1 as the smallest. The two styles of dental dam punches are the Ainsworth and the traditional style.

To correctly operate the dental dam punch, the punch plate is rotated into position and then the operator gently squeezes the handles to make sure the stylus and the punch plate line up. If the punch plate has not firmly clicked into position, it can result in damage to either the punch plate or the stylus, or it can result in ragged margins on the holes of the dental dam. Uneven holes in the dental dam allow moisture to escape beyond the dam. These are called "tags."

Dental Dam Clamps

Dental dam clamps are used to securely fasten the dental dam in place, allowing for the procedure to take place. They are not placed on the target teeth, but one or two teeth distal to the target tooth. The tooth used for the dental clamp is called the **anchor tooth**.

Dental clamps are made from stainless steel or chrome. They come in various shapes and sizes to accommodate different teeth and different procedures. Parts of the dental clamp include:

- *Bow*. The bow is the arched metal portion of the clamp that provides tension and holds the dental dam material

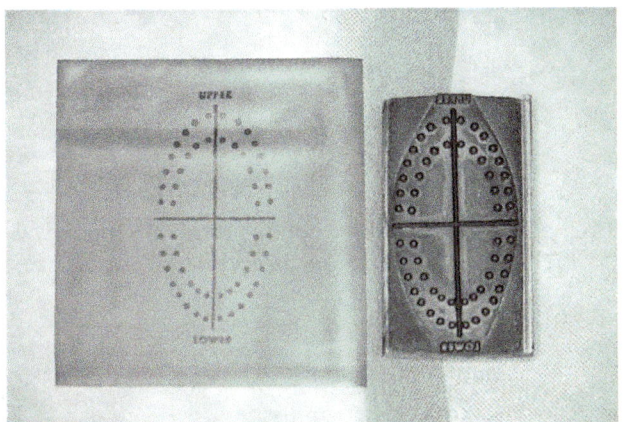

Figure 27-10 Dental dam template and rubber stamp.

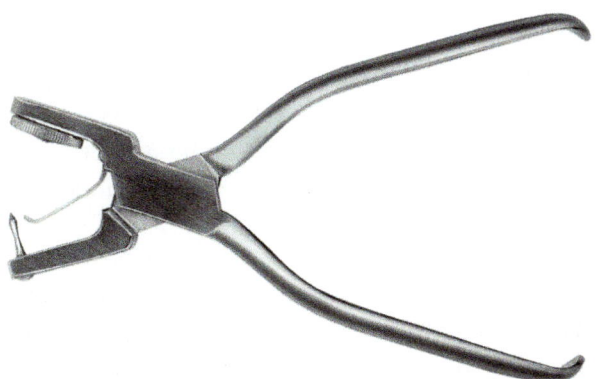

Figure 27-11 Dental dam punch.

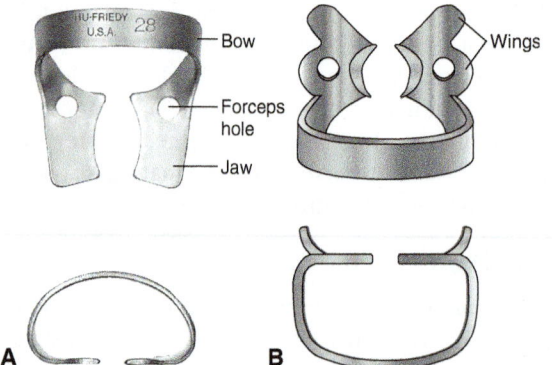

Figure 27–12 **Dental clamps**. **(A)** Wingless clamp. **(B)** Winged clamp.

in place during the procedure. The bow should always be placed so the arch is distal to the target tooth.

■ *Jaws*. The jaws are the portion of the clamp that actually encircle and grip the anchor tooth. Jaws should be matched to tooth size. To obtain a solid fit, all four points of the jaws should be firmly positioned against the anchor tooth, at the level of the cementoenamel junction (CEJ).

■ *Anchor* or *forceps holes*. Located on the jaws of the clamp—or in the case of a winged clamp, on the wings—the anchor holes are where the dental dam forceps grip the clamp, allowing the operator to position, open, and close the clamp; ligature floss is also placed here.

Common types of dental clamps include (Figure 27-12):

■ *Winged clamps*. These clamps feature small metal extensions from the jaws, near the anchor holes. They are used for increased stability.

■ *Wingless clamps*: These clamps have the letter W before the clamp number on the clamp and also have no winged projections on the clamp.

■ *Cervical clamps*. These clamps are double-bowed clamps and are used for anterior teeth. Besides holding the dental

dam in place, they also help retract gingival tissue. These clamps are often referred to as "butterfly" clamps.

■ *Pediatric clamps*. These are designed for smaller, pediatric teeth.

Table 27-1 describes the types of clamps and their particular uses.

Ligating the Dental Clamp

Before placing a dental clamp, it is essential to first attach an arm's length of dental floss to the clamp. This is a safety device that allows for rapid recovery of the dental clamp if it should break in the patient's mouth or snap off and go down the throat.

To correctly ligate a dental clamp, the dental floss should be doubled and passed through one anchor hole, looped across the bow several times, and then passed through the next anchor hole on the buccal surface of the tooth (Figure 27-13). Once the dental dam is in place, these cords should be pulled through the dental dam so they are attached to the outside of the dam frame and remain easily accessible to the dental assistant. It is important to ligate dental clamps through both anchor holes in case the dental clamp breaks in half and either or both halves must be retrieved separately.

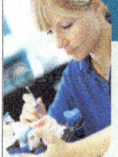

Voice of Experience

Although it is a small job, learning how to tie floss to a dental clamp is a critical responsibility. Clamps are under pressure, and they do sometimes spring loose and come off in the patient's mouth. Only quick thinking and a correctly tied floss string can help prevent a major problem!

Dental Dam Forceps

Dental dam forceps are instruments used to place and remove dental clamps (Figure 27-14). The working end of dental dam forceps is equipped with beaks that fit into the anchor holes on the dental clamps.

TABLE 27-1	Selecting the Appropriate Clamp	
TOOTH	**CLAMP NO.**	**CLAMP CHARACTERISTICS**
Anterior tooth	No. 9	Double bowed
Premolar	No. 2; no. 00	Small, flat jaws
Maxillary premolar	No. 1	Curved jaws
Mandibular molar	No. 3; no. 7	Flat jaws
Maxillary molar	No. 8; no. 4; no. 56	Curved jaws
Partially erupted tooth	No. 2A; no. 8A; no. 14; no. 14A	Curved jaws with points placed in subgingival direction; choose clamp suitable to the size of the anchor tooth
Structurally compromised tooth	No. 12A; no. 13A	Serrated jaws
Class V restoration	No. 212; no. B5; no. B6	Gingival retractor
Placement of sealant	No. B2; no. B3	Will not impinge on tissue

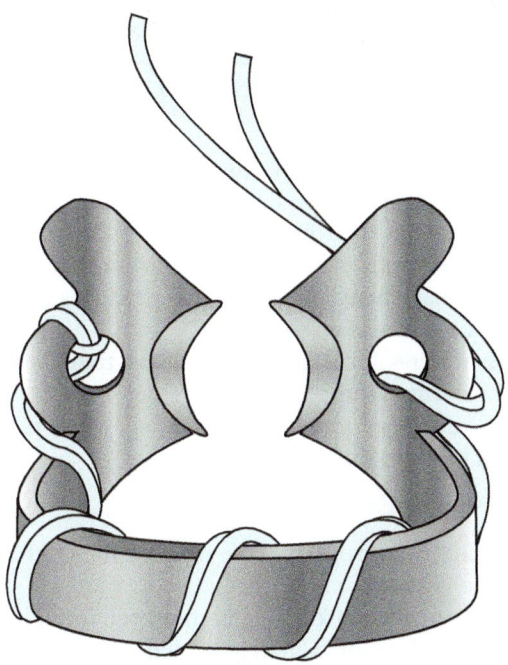

Figure 27–13 Ligated dental clamp.

To use forceps, the beaks are inserted into the anchor holes and gentle pressure is used to pry open the clamp's jaws. Once the jaws are opened, a sliding bar is used to lock the forceps in position during placement on the anchor tooth. To release the forceps, they are squeezed gently again and the sliding lock is released. Once the clamp is placed, the forceps's beaks can be removed from the anchor holes and the forceps removed from the oral cavity.

Forceps should always be inserted into the oral cavity with the curve of the beaks facing toward the target arch and the bow toward the distal surface of the anchor tooth. This prevents them from having to be rotated in the oral cavity.

Dental Floss

Dental floss serves a number of purposes during placement of dental dams.

1. It is used as a safety measure to ligate dental clamps. Make sure the length of floss is long enough to span the clamp from hole to hole and then come through the dental dam and rest on the patient's chin or cheeks.
2. It is used to work the dental dam material into place through close contacts.
3. It is sometimes used to stabilize dental dam material on the opposite tooth from the anchor tooth. To perform this procedure, the clamp should be placed first, then the dental dam, then floss is looped through the interproximal space to secure the dental dam in place; dental stabilization material may also be used for this purpose.
4. It is used to help invert the dental dam material around teeth to add an additional layer of protection against leakage. A stream of air from the air syringe helps accomplish this.

Dental Dam Stabilization Cord

Dental dam stabilization cord is another way to secure dental dam material into place. The cord is a thick, disposable, stretchable cord that is positioned in the interproximal space to help hold dental dam material in place. Stabilization cord is available in various sizes (e.g., small, medium, large) to accommodate different-sized interproximal spaces.

To place stabilization cord, stretch the cord until it thins and slide it into the interproximal space, making sure it is deep enough to firmly secure the dental dam material. Then release the cord so it springs back to its original diameter.

Preparation

Although dental dams are very useful armamentarium, many patients find the experience to be intimidating. As with all dental procedures, it is important to gain the patient's trust by fully explaining the reasons for using a dental dam and demonstrating how it will work.

Patient Preparation

Before placing dental dams, introduce patients to the concept of a dental dam and ask if they have any questions. Some patients might be worried they will not be able to breathe while it is in place, and others might be concerned that it will hurt during placement or removal although most patients should have a local anesthesia for this procedure. Patients are typically told they will feel some pressure.

It is worth it to take the extra minute or so to put the patient at ease. You can instruct the patient to breathe through his or her nose while the dental dam is in place. Additionally, prepare them for the sensation of pressure on the anchor tooth, but assure the patient that the utmost care will be taken with placement and removal of the dental dam. Remind the patient that the dental dam is a safety precaution that makes it less likely that unwanted liquid and debris will fall into the oral cavity. Patients may be concerned that they will not be able to communicate with the dentist during the procedure, should the need arise. You can propose a simple communication strategy, such as a raised finger, in the event that the patient wants to communicate during the procedure.

Ultimately, the point of patient preparation is to gain acceptance and increase trust. It often helps to point out that dental dams generally make dental work go more quickly and efficiently.

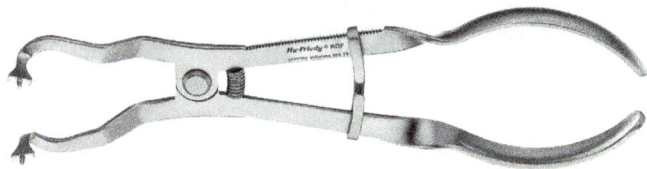

Figure 27–14 Dental dam forceps.

Dental Dam Preparation

Before the dam is placed, it must be prepared. This involves dividing the dam and marking it for punching, then punching it.

The first step is to identify the area that needs to be isolated, whether it is on the maxillary or mandibular arch, and locate the anchor tooth. The anchor tooth is typically distal to the target tooth. The area of isolation depends on the procedure and operator's preference. Some dentists prefer just one or two teeth to be isolated, while others prefer for several teeth to be isolated. Additionally, the procedure might call for specific teeth to be isolated. When exposing multiple teeth, it is best to expose between six and eight teeth so the dental dam is not warped by the curvature of the arch.

It is also important at this time to note individual factors such as wide or narrow arches and misaligned teeth. Dental dam templates do not account for misaligned teeth, missing teeth, or different arch structures, so this is left to the person who is preparing the dental dam.

Problems can arise when working with dental dams. Following these tips will help prevent some of the more common errors, such as tearing and leakage. To avoid tearing the dental dam:

- Make sure the dental dam product has not expired. Check the expiration date on the box.
- Store dental dam material below 80°F (avoid storing above a sterilizer or near a sunny window).
- Use a sharp punch. A dull punch produces tags or nicks that cause the dam to tear.
- Use water-soluble lubricant on the tissue side of the dam during its application.
- Use knife-edge and loop techniques when placing the dam interproximally.

To prevent dental dam leakage:

- Punch the appropriate hole sizes for the teeth included in the isolation.
- Maintain adequate spacing between punched holes (3.5 mm, or approximately ¼ inch).
- Make adjustments for malposed or missing teeth.
- Make sure the dam doesn't snag on the wings of the clamp.
- Seal small leaks with OraSeal® dental dam caulking.

Finally, before placing the dam, floss the patient's teeth to identify any possible tight contacts.

Once these steps have been taken, the dental dam is selected and divided, then punched. This is covered in greater depth in Procedure 27-4.

Procedure 27-4 Preparing a Dental Dam

Materials needed (Figure P27-4-1):

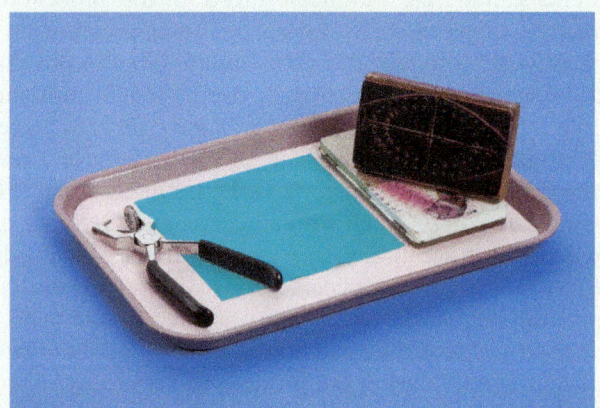

Figure P27-4-1

- Dental dam material
- Template or rubber stamp (if needed)
- Dental dam punch

1. Put on appropriate PPE.
2. Identify the tooth or teeth that need to be isolated.
3. Select the appropriate dental dam, in terms of thickness, size, and color.
4. Divide the dental dam into quadrants. To do this, fold the dental dam in half and crease it to mark the mandibular and maxillary arches. Next, fold the dam from the long ends, further dividing it into thirds or quarters. The creases will provide guidance while actually punching the holes.
5. Unfold the dental dam and mark it using the template or rubber stamp, if you're using it. This will show a typical mandibular and maxillary arch (Figure P27-4-2).

Procedure 27-4 **Preparing a Dental Dam** (Continued)

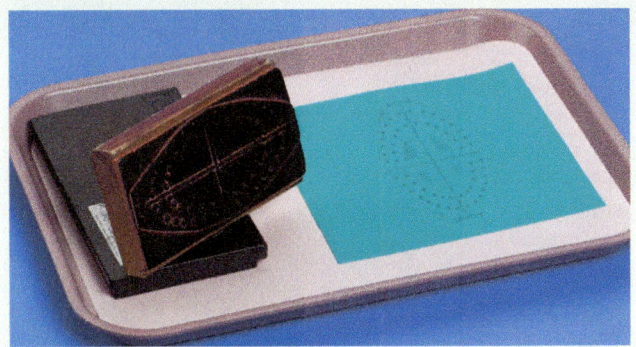

Figure P27-4-2

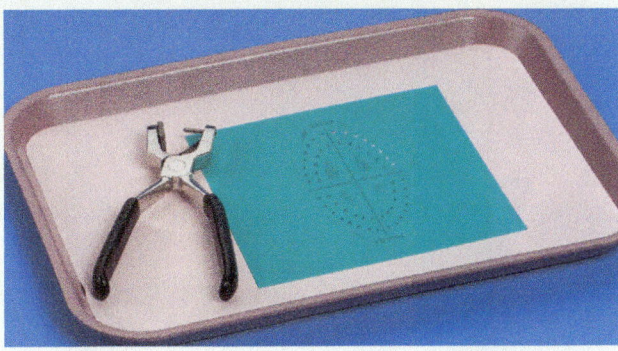

Figure P27-4-3

6. Punch the **key punch hole** first. Use the no. 5 setting on the dental dam punch.

7. Punch the holes for individual teeth, moving forward from the key punch hole. Make sure to use the appropriate sized hole for each tooth, which will prevent moisture leakage around the dam. Leave about 3.0 to 3.5 mm of space between the edges of the holes (Figure P27-4-3).

8. During punching, follow the patient's teeth, including misaligned teeth. Remember, if a tooth is either lingually or facially malpositioned, the hole should be punched 1 to 3 mm in either direction to avoid bunching of the material. Skip over missing teeth and bridges. Missing teeth do not require holes to be punched.

9. Punch a hole in the upper right-hand corner of the dam last, so that you will always keep your perspective of the dam.

Dental Dam Placement

After the dental dam material is prepared, there are several options for placement:

- Placement of the clamp first, followed by the dental dam and then the frame
- Placement of the clamp and dental dam simultaneously, followed by the frame
- Placement of the clamp, dental dam, and frame simultaneously

Some types of dental clamps (e.g., cervical clamps) might need to be held in place with adhesive stick compound. This compound must be heated before application, usually with a butane torch or Bunsen burner. To use the compound, soften the stick gently over the flame until the tip bends, then place it in hot water for 5 seconds. Dental compound resembles a hot glue stick. Twist off the soft portion of the stick compound and shape it into a cone, then reheat the cone. Work the softened cone around the bow of the clamp on the occlusal surface. Repeat the procedure with the second bow for cervical clamps. After the procedure is done, remove the compound before removing the dental dam and the clamp.

Dental dam placement is covered in Procedure 27-5.

Procedure 27-5 **Assisting with Dental Dam Placement**

In some states, dental assistants are allowed to place a dental dam as an expanded function after meeting additional training and licensing requirements.

There are several variations in dental dam placement, and placing pediatric dental dams is also slightly different. This general procedure is meant to cover the basics, but details might vary among different offices.

Materials needed (Figure P27-5-1):

- Prepared dental dam
- Lip lubricant
- Mouth mirror
- Dental floss
- Dental dam lubricant

Procedure 27–5 Assisting with Dental Dam Placement (Continued)

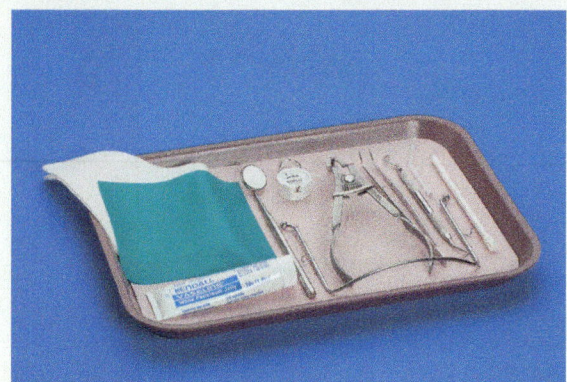

Figure P27-5-1

- Dental dam clamp (winged or wingless)
- Dental dam frame (Young frame)
- Dental dam forceps
- Cotton pliers
- Dental dam stabilization cord (if needed)
- Dental napkin
- Spoon excavator (if needed)
- Air-water syringe
- Saliva ejector

1. Put on appropriate PPE.

2. Prepare the patient by asking about any questions or concerns. Take this time to explain the benefits of a dental dam and prep the patient on what to expect. You can say, "You may feel some pressure on your tooth as we attach the dental dam. The dam will help prevent liquid and debris from entering your mouth, and it will make the whole procedure go faster."

3. Assist the dentist with administration of anesthetic or any other pre-procedure steps necessary.

4. After the anesthetic has taken effect, apply lubricant to the patient's lips using a cotton swab.

5. The dentist uses the mouth mirror to examine the site where the dental dam will be placed, making sure it is free from plaque and debris. The dentist flosses all contacts and makes note of tight contacts for later.

6. Transfer the prepared dental dam to the dentist. If using latex dam material, the powdered side of the dam goes toward the patient's face. There is no powder on latex-free dam material.

7. The dentist lubricates the back side of the dam material to ease the dam in between the interproximals.

8. Select an appropriate clamp. The clamp should be the right size to fit securely at the CEJ of the anchor tooth.

9. Tie a safety line of dental floss to the clamp by doubling it and running it through one anchor hole, across the bow, and through the next anchor hole. Use a long enough piece of floss that it can be strung through the dental dam and left to be attached to the dam frame (Figure P27-5-2).

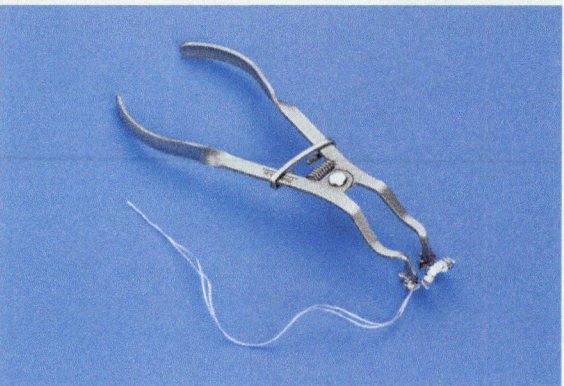

Figure P27-5-2

10. Transfer the clamp to the dentist.

11. The dentist grips the clamp with the forceps by inserting the forceps beaks into the clamp and uses gentle pressure to spread the beaks of the forceps. If the dental dam is already in place, the dentist inserts the forceps through the dental dam material. If the clamp and dental dam are being placed simultaneously, the dentist slides the key hole over the bow at this time. The dentist places the clamp by sliding it over the anchor tooth. The lingual side of the clamp is placed first, which allows for better visibility, followed by the buccal side. The clamp should not be pinching gingival tissue but should be firmly placed at the CEJ (Figure P27-5-3).

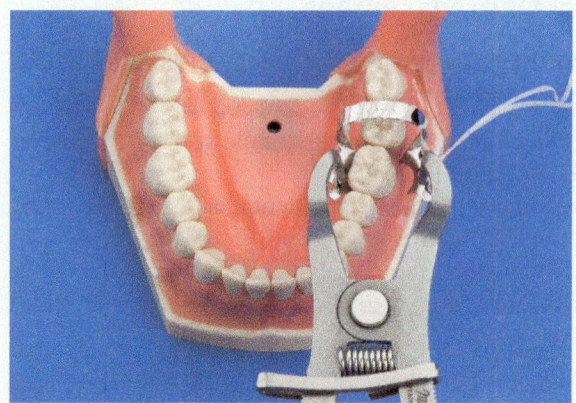

Figure P27-5-3

12. Confirm with the patient frequently that there is no discomfort. The patient should only experience pressure.

13. The dentist gently releases the forceps and removes the beaks from the anchor holes.

14. If the dentist has not already placed the dental dam, the dentist slides the key hole over the bow of the placed clamp.

15. The dentist retrieves the dental floss ligature with cotton pliers and slides it through the dental dam.

16. The dentist secures the dental dam to the opposite tooth (typically the opposite canine), using either a double loop of dental floss, a small slit of dental dam material, or dental dam stabilization cord (Figure P27-5-4).

Procedure 27-5 Assisting with Dental Dam Placement (Continued)

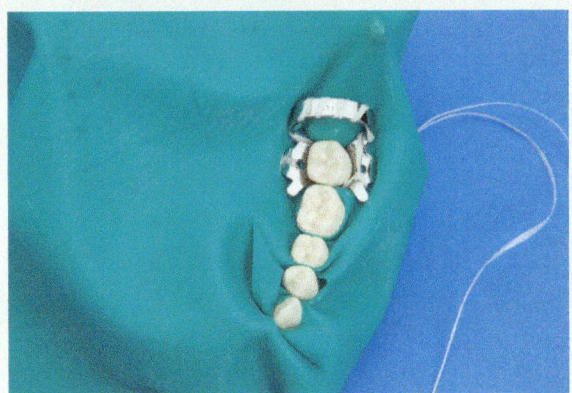

Figure P27-5-4

17. The dentist places the dental napkin around the patient's oral cavity and slides the frame into position, hooking the dental dam material on the frame to hold it steady. Frames can be placed over or under the dental dam material (Figure P27-5-5).

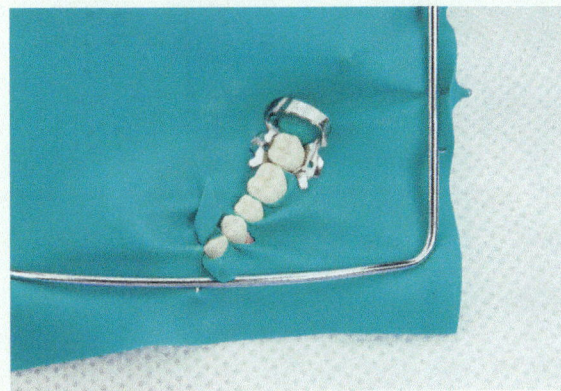

Figure P27-5-5

18. Using fingers and dental floss, the dentist works the remaining teeth to be isolated through the punched holes in the dental dam material. The dentist works the dental dam ligature in between the tooth contacts, using floss if necessary to ensure that the dental dam is located below the contacts (Figure P27-5-6).

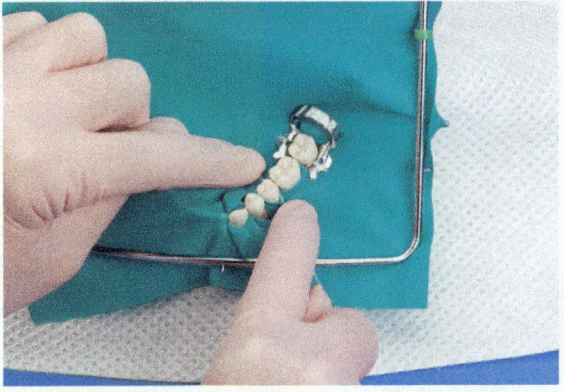

Figure P27-5-6

19. When the dental dam is placed, the dentist inverts (or tucks) the material.

20. Use the air-water syringe to dry the isolated teeth (Figure P27-5-7).

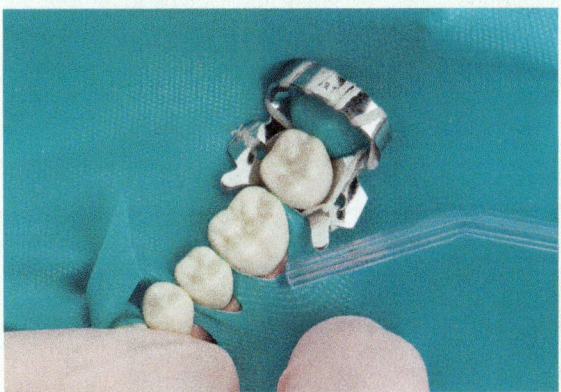

Figure P27-5-7

21. Place a saliva ejector and/or bite block for patient comfort. If the patient is having trouble breathing through the nose, a small hole is cut in the dental dam to facilitate breathing.

22. The dentist confirms that the dental dam is well placed, with all the edges inverted, and secure.

Dental Dam Removal

After the procedure is over, the area should be rinsed and cleared of debris, using the air-water syringe and evacuator. At this time, remove the saliva ejector from the patient's oral cavity and prepare to remove the dental dam itself. This is covered in Procedure 27-6.

Quickdam

A quickdam is an alternative to a full dental dam. Used either by itself or with a clamp, the quickdam provides a faster way to isolate teeth.

The quickdam is an oval dental dam that comes with its own frame and punching guides. To prepare the dental

Procedure 27–6 Dental Dam Removal

Materials needed (Figure P27-6-1):

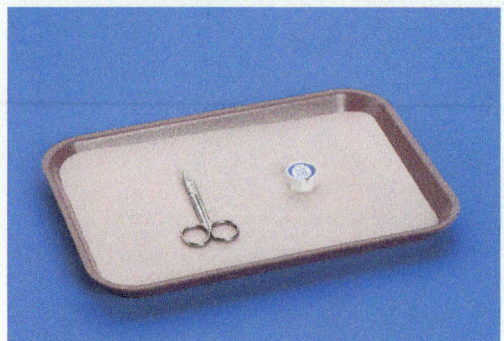

Figure P27-6-1

- Crown and bridge scissors
- Dental floss

1. Put on appropriate PPE.
2. Prepare the patient by saying that it's time to remove the dental dam and cautioning him or her not to bite down on the dental dam during removal.
3. Remove the clamp and any ligature or stabilization cord that was used to secure the dental dam (Figure P27-6-2).

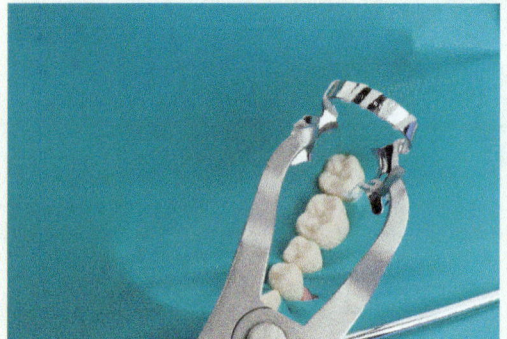

Figure P27-6-2

4. Pull the dental dam material away from the teeth. This stretches the material so the septa can be seen and accessed.
5. Clip the **interseptal dam** material with scissors, moving from anterior to posterior and holding the scissors away from the gingiva. Keep one finger behind the dam while cutting (Figure P27-6-3).

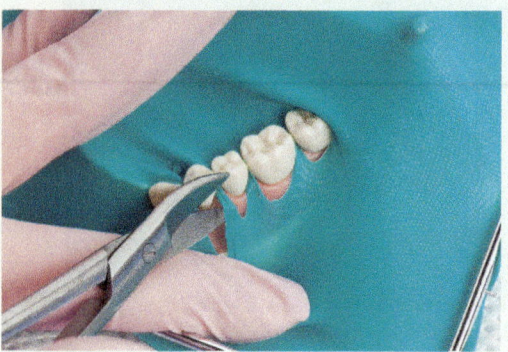

Figure P27-6-3

6. Pull slightly on the dam lingually to ensure it's free from the interproximal space.
7. Remove the dam and frame in one motion (Figure P27-6-4).

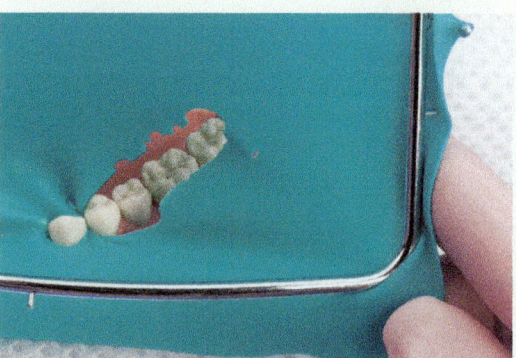

Figure P27-6-4

8. Remove the napkin, if used, and wipe the patient's mouth and face clean.
9. Inspect the dental dam by placing it flat on a counter to ensure that no part of it has been left inside the patient's oral cavity. If any of the septa are still in between the patient's teeth, remove them with floss.
10. Floss teeth after removal to ensure that no piece of the dam has been left behind, which would cause a gingival problem for the patient.

dam, the holes are punched using the same equipment as with a conventional dental dam. To place the quickdam, the plastic frame is folded in half and the dam is inserted into the patient's oral cavity. The dam material is positioned around the teeth in the same manner, and the plastic frame is released to provide tension and hold the quickdam in place. Quickdams can also be used with dental clamps or stabilizing cord for anchoring.

Special Considerations for Dental Dams

Pediatric Patients

Dental dams are frequently used with pediatric patients. In fact, some of the advantages inherent in dental dams are even more pronounced among pediatric patients, especially when it comes to isolating the teeth and protecting the lips and tongue, which children sometimes have a harder time keeping still than adults.

One of the main considerations with a pediatric dental dam is patient preparation. Children often respond very well to the dental dam, provided they understand beforehand what to expect and what it looks like. Try to explain the dental dam's purpose in simple, child-friendly language. You can even demonstrate how the device protects them from water and other fluids.

When it comes time to prepare the dental dam, use a 5 × 5 dental dam and pediatric arches for marking. Examine the child's teeth beforehand and make note of any missing or partially erupted teeth, as well as mixed dentition. Generally, no holes are punched for partially erupted teeth, and missing teeth are treated the same as with adult missing teeth. Holes should be punched slightly closer together for pediatric teeth to allow for smaller contacts.

When placing the dental dam, use bicuspid clamps on partially erupted teeth and a floss ligature to hold the dental dam in place. Wooden wedges can be used to move the gingiva and tuck the dental dam down into position.

Fixed Bridges

Fixed bridges are permanent dental prosthetics used to replace missing teeth. Because they lack interproximal spaces, a conventionally punched dental dam cannot be used—there is no room for the septum to slide between the teeth.

However, dental dams can still be used with fixed bridges. During the hole punching, simply skip the fixed bridge. Then, when placing clamps, place a clamp on the distal portion of the bridge. It might also be necessary to place a clamp on the mesial portion of the bridge. These clamps will hold the dental dam in place during the procedure. Otherwise, the preparation and placement of a dental dam follows the normal procedure.

CHECKPOINTS

27-11 At what point in the sequence of performing a restoration should a dental dam be placed?

27-12 Can dental dams be used during radiography?

27-13 What is the tooth (or teeth) called to which the dental clamp(s) is attached?

27-14 Name two uses of dental floss during a dental dam procedure.

Chapter Highlights

+ Moisture control is an essential part of dentistry because it improves the operator's ability to perform the procedure. Moisture control is critical for success when using some types of dental materials.
+ Tooth isolation is widely used during dental procedures to make the procedure easier, more efficient, and safer for the patient.
+ Tissue retraction can be accomplished with hand instruments such as a mouth mirror, the HVE, or cotton rolls.
+ Saliva ejectors are low-suction instruments used to remove saliva during procedures; they are often left in place during the procedure.
+ HVE, or high-volume evacuators, are high-powered suction devices used to remove debris or copious amounts of fluids.
+ The HVE should be held using a fulcrum at all times; it should never be rested against the patient's tissues. It can be placed on a cotton roll. The HVE should be positioned in the patient's mouth before the high speed handpiece or hand instruments are placed.

+ The air-water syringe is used to rinse the oral cavity during dental procedures. Its use is accompanied by an evacuator.
+ Instruments used in tooth isolation include cotton rolls, dry angles, and dental dams.
+ Dental dams can be used for almost any procedure on a wide range of patients; these devices consist of a thin sheet of material that fits snugly around the tooth or teeth being worked on.
+ Equipment used to place and hold a dental dam in place includes templates, stamps, punches, frames, clamps, forceps, stabilization cord, and floss.
+ Many patients are unnerved by the rubber dental dam, so it is essential to work with patients before the procedure to gain their trust and acceptance.
+ Dental dams are placed just after the local anesthetic is administered.
+ Dental dams can be effectively used on pediatric patients as well as adults.
+ A quickdam is a simple dental dam that takes less time to install than the traditional variety.

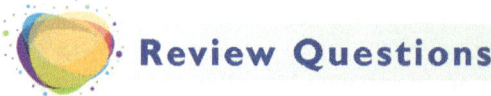 **Review Questions**

1. Evacuation devices include
   a. HVE and air-water syringe.
   b. HVE and dental dam.
   c. Saliva ejector and air-water syringe.
   d. Saliva ejector and high-volume evacuator.

2. The saliva ejector
   a. Should never touch mucosal tissue.
   b. Can be left in the patient's oral cavity during a procedure.
   c. Is used to remove debris.
   d. Must be used with the HVE.

3. The HVE tip
   a. Is curved for better retraction.
   b. Is non-replaceable.
   c. Can be angled for better evacuation.
   d. Is sharp.

4. The HVE should be in place
   a. After the procedure starts.
   b. Before the high speed handpiece and instruments are placed.
   c. Throughout the procedure, resting in the patient's oral cavity.
   d. After the procedure finishes.

5. What is NOT an advantage of dental dams?
   a. Reducing potential contaminated spray
   b. Making dental procedures easier for the operator
   c. Making it easier for patients to breathe during procedures
   d. Aiding in tissue retraction

6. Who is not eligible for a dental dam?
   a. Pediatric patients
   b. Patients with fixed bridges
   c. Patients with missing teeth
   d. None of the above

7. Which type of dental dam frame is incompatible with radiography?
   a. Ostby
   b. Young
   c. U-frame
   d. Plastic

8. Which is the largest hole size on a dental dam punch?
   a. 2
   b. 3
   c. 4
   d. 5

9. Dental dam templates
   a. Are drawn for each patient.
   b. Are not for use with pediatric patients.
   c. Are standard sizes.
   d. Do not depict both arches.

10. Where or what is the anchor tooth?
   a. Isolated by the dental dam
   b. Opposite the clamp
   c. Used to hold the clamp
   d. None of the above

11. Which type of dental clamp often requires the use of sticking compound?
   a. Winged
   b. Standard
   c. Pediatric
   d. Cervical

12. Which is NOT a use for dental floss during dental dam procedures?
   a. Perforating the dental dam
   b. Ligating the dental dam
   c. As a safety cord for clamps
   d. Checking for tight contacts

Active Learning Exercises

1. What is the purpose of using high-volume evacuation?
2. Other than for isolation purposes, name four other reasons why a dental dam may be needed.

Application Activities

1. Write a paragraph or two comparing and contrasting the use of cotton rolls and dry angles, noting the strengths and drawbacks of each.
2. Practice handling the HVE using the thumb-to-nose grasp and the pen grasp.
3. Using the method outlined in the text, practice tying safety floss ligature to a dental clamp. Be sure the floss is tied through both anchor holes.

PREPARING FOR CERTIFICATION EXAMS

Review the following topics in this chapter to prepare for the Dental Assisting National Board (DANB) exam:

- **Maintaining the Operating Field**
- **Cotton Rolls**
- **Dental Dams**
- **Materials and Equipment**
- **Preparation**
- **Dental Dam Placement**
- **Dental Dam Removal**

Anesthesia and Pain Control

CHAPTER OUTLINE

CHAPTER CHECKLIST

On completion of this chapter, students will be able to:

- ☑ Describe the various types of local anesthesia, including their composition and use.
- ☑ Identify and describe the equipment used to administer local anesthesia.
- ☑ Identify and describe the methods for injecting local anesthesia.
- ☑ Describe the use of nitrous oxide in sedation, including indications and contraindications, equipment needed, methods for administration, necessary safety measures, and patient monitoring.
- ☑ Describe the use of oral sedatives, intravenous sedation, and intramuscular sedation.
- ☑ Describe the use of general anesthesia, including the four stages of consciousness.
- ☑ Describe how to document anesthetic administration.

KEY TERMS

anesthesia – a temporary loss of feeling induced by medication

anesthetic – a medication that produces a temporary loss of feeling

anxiolytic (ang-zee-oh-LIT-ik) – a medication to relieve anxiety

aspirating syringe – the most commonly used type of syringe in a dental practice, it allows the dental professional to ensure the needle has not been placed in a blood vessel

conscious sedation – a state of sedation in which patients remain awake, relaxed, responsive, reflexive, and able to cooperate

field block anesthesia – one of the three most common dental injections, this type of local infiltration anesthesia is injected near the apex of the tooth, near larger terminal nerve branches, to prevent impulses from passing from the tooth to the central nervous system

gauge – thickness of a needle

general anesthesia – a medication-induced state in which the patient loses feeling and enters an unconscious state

infiltration anesthesia – one of the three most common dental injections, this method puts the anesthetic solution into tissues near the small terminal nerve branches

local anesthetic – a liquid medication injected into the soft tissues that comes into contact with sensory nerve fibers and blocks sensations from registering a feeling of pain in the brain

nerve block anesthesia – one of the three most common dental injections, this is given near a main nerve trunk to prevent pain sensation from passing to the brain; eliminates sensation over a large area; also known as mandibular block injection

paresthesia (par-us-THEE-zha) – a condition that occurs when numbness induced by local anesthesia does not wear off as it should; numbness may last for days, weeks, years, or permanently

tidal volume – the amount of air inhaled and exhaled with each breath

topical anesthetic – a solution that is applied to oral mucosa to numb the mucosa and nerve endings to prevent pain during injection

vasoconstrictor (vay-zoh-kun-STRIK-ter) – a medication that narrows blood vessels in the area where the drug is administered; prolongs the effects of an anesthetic and slows down the flow of blood in that area

Introduction

For thousands of years, various substances have been used to ease pain during medical procedures. Early treatments for pain relief involved opium. Later, cannabis, alcohol, coca leaves, and morphine were used. Nitrous oxide was discovered in 1769 and its anesthetic qualities were revealed in 1799. In the 1840s, American dentist Horace Wells first used nitrous oxide as an inhaled anesthetic in a dental procedure.

Many modern dental procedures are possible, in large part, due to the availability of pain-control and anxiety-reducing methods. Recognizing and managing a patient's pain and anxiety is an important part of dental care. Use of a medication to manage pain and anxiety depends upon the treatment being given and the patient's overall health.

Cultural Diversity

Pain is perceived and handled differently among those of different cultures and backgrounds. Some Japanese and Chinese patients, for example, may internalize pain because they believe that showing pain indicates weakness and is frowned upon in their culture. Patients from other countries, such as the Philippines, believe the complete opposite and feel free to yell out or scream when pain presents. As health care providers, we must proceed carefully during potentially painful procedures because not all patients will alert us that they are in pain, whereas others may seem to exaggerate the pain. In both situations, it can be difficult to provide adequate pain management. Knowledge of a patient's culture may help you better understand his or her pain behavior.

Medications that produce the temporary loss of feeling—**anesthesia**—are called **anesthetics**. Dentists use various ways to control pain and reduce anxiety. A dentist must be trained, following American Dental Association guidelines, in the types of anesthesia and sedation he or she can administer. A dentist may employ a nurse anesthetist or anesthesiologist to provide general anesthetic to patients in lieu of having this training. Dental assistants may assist with the equipment used for anesthesia and should understand the processes and procedures involved.

Local Anesthesia

With a local anesthetic, the medication blocks the nerve action, which causes a loss of feeling in the area of the application. The patient remains conscious and only the area being treated is affected. Local anesthesia is appropriate for many dental procedures because it is safe, fast-acting, and effective at eliminating pain for the duration of a treatment. These qualities make local anesthesia the most commonly used type of dental pain control.

Indications and Contraindications

Local anesthesia is indicated for treatments that may cause pain or discomfort. Anesthesia also helps to ward off the patient's anticipation of pain, which can help with relaxation and overall comfort during treatment.

In addition to providing pain control in restorative dentistry, local anesthesia is also used with dental hygiene procedures, including:

- Scaling and root planning in areas with probing depths of 4 mm or greater
- Extensive instrumentation with manual or externally powered instruments
- Areas of challenging pocket topography, furcations, or other difficult root anatomy
- Instrumentation of sensitive root surfaces
- Instrumentation in areas of painful, inflamed soft tissue
- Treatments that involve soft tissue manipulation, such as gingival curettage, suture removal, and removal of subgingival overhanging margins of restorations
- Areas of excessive hemorrhage

Local anesthesia is safe for almost all patients, although fear of needles may prevent some patients from receiving local anesthetic injections. Others may have medical conditions that prevent the use of local anesthesia. Medical contraindications include allergy to amide anesthetics—a rarity—or to ester anesthetics, which is more common. Patients who are allergic to ester anesthetics also cannot have topical anesthetics. Patients who are allergic to sodium metabisulfite, acetone sodium bisulfite, and sodium or potassium bisulfite—the preservatives in vaso-constrictors—should not be given anesthetics that contain vasoconstrictors.

Additional medical contraindications exist for patients with:

■ The potential for heart failure during treatment
■ Coronary disease, heart attack, recent heart surgery, angina pectoris, hypertension, and stroke; avoid or limit use of vasoconstrictors, depending on the individual patient's condition
■ Uncontrolled hyperthyroidism; avoid solutions containing vasoconstrictors
■ Severe liver or kidney function impairment; avoid local anesthetics
■ Pregnancy; avoid elective drug administration, especially during the first trimester
■ Methemoglobinemia, a congenital or acquired condition
■ Malignant hyperthermia
■ Hemophilia

In addition, some medications are contraindicated with local anesthetics and vasoconstrictors. For that reason, check all drugs that patients list in the medical history to ensure their safety for interaction with local anesthetics. A comprehensive, accurate medical history for every patient, updated for every procedure, is an essential part of a safe dental practice.

Topical Anesthetics

Topical anesthetics are typically used to block pain in areas being prepared for an injection. Available as liquids, sprays, ointments or gels, and patches, topical agents numb nerve endings in the skin and oral mucosa so the patient does not feel the needle stick. Each of these forms is applied differently and takes a prescribed amount of time to effectively numb the treatment area.

Some states allow dental assistants to apply topical anesthetics. To apply a topical ointment:

■ Dry the site with a gauze pad. This will help the anesthetic penetrate better, without being diluted by saliva.
■ Place a small amount of the anesthetic on a cotton-tipped applicator and place it on the injection site, holding it in place for several minutes before the injection is administered. Remove the applicator immediately before the dentist gives the injection.

If the patient needs more than one injection, repeat this process at each site. Never dip a used applicator back into the ointment container. Doing so could lead to contamination of the anesthetic medication. Some forms of topical anesthesia are available in single-dose packaging.

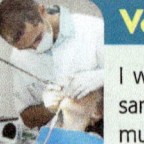

Voice of Experience

I worked with a very busy dentist who dipped the same cotton-tipped applicator in the topical anesthetic multiple times. I threw the jar of ointment in the trash when I realized what he'd done. Later, I saw that same jar on the counter. I approached the dentist and expressed my concerns. Busy and distracted, he told me that supplies were expensive and that it wasn't a big deal. When I told him I had concerns about infection control issues, he stopped what he was doing and listened to what I had to say. He ended up thanking me for my commitment to patient safely and agreed to dispense the topical differently.

A newer topical agent is a patch, which acts within 10 seconds. It is generally used to alleviate pain from injections or discomfort from existing sores. Topical ointments are slower acting and take several minutes for maximum numbing effect. Spray agents require greater attention. Generally applied to the throats of patients who have a strong gag reflex, sprays are highly concentrated and can cause an overdose reaction if used in excess. For that reason, the spray form is metered to ensure an appropriate amount is used.

Popular topical anesthetics include benzocaine, tetracaine, dyclonine hydrochloride, and lidocaine. Numbing usually takes effect within a few minutes after application and lasts for up to 30 minutes.

Regardless of the topical anesthetic used, it is important to be aware of possible allergic and toxic reactions. The dentist should decide the type, concentration, and administration of a topical anesthetic, and the dental assistant and entire dental team should review the patient's medical and allergy history at every appointment.

Local Anesthetics

Local anesthetics are commonly used to control pain for dental procedures. These liquid medications are injected into the soft tissues, coming into contact with the sensory nerve fibers and blocking sensations from registering a feeling of pain in the brain.

Local anesthetics come in premeasured cartridges or carpules available in blister packs or tins.

Anesthetic Agents

Local anesthetics can be divided into two main groups, esters and amides (Table 28-1). Esters are widely used in topical anesthetic agents. Common esters include propoxycaine HCl and procaine HCl. Except for topicals, all currently used local anesthetic agents are amides. Common amides include lidocaine HCl, mepivacaine HCl, prilocaine HCl, articaine HCl, etidocaine HCl, and bupivacaine HCl (Table 28-2).

For some patients, a certain anesthetic may be more effective than another. If a patient has had either a positive

TABLE 28-1 Major Groups of Anesthetic Drugs

GROUP	GENERAL CHARACTERISTICS
Esters	■ Widely used in topical anesthetic agents ■ Have a higher incidence of allergic reactions; are less effective and are shorter acting compared with amides ■ Metabolized in the blood plasma by the enzyme cholinesterase. The medical condition atypical plasma cholinesterase may result in the slow removal of the drug from the body
Amides	■ Extremely low incidence of allergic reactions ■ Potential for toxicity or drug overdose makes attention to detail in technique of administration and total drug dose critical ■ Metabolized by the liver ■ Causes vasodilation of local blood vessels

process—or the patient's return to a normal state—is referred to as *duration*.

How long a local anesthetic lasts depends on whether it includes a vasoconstrictor. A **vasoconstrictor** is a medication that can be added to an anesthetic to prolong its effects. Vasoconstrictors work by narrowing blood vessels in the area where the drug is administered, which slows the rate at which the medication is absorbed into the bloodstream. With less blood flowing in the area, bleeding during a surgical procedure is minimized. Another positive effect of less blood flow in the area is less local anesthetic in the bloodstream and a lower risk of a toxic reaction. Clinically, there is also a reduced blood flow in the area where the dentist is working, making visibility better.

The most common vasoconstrictor used with local anesthetics, in very small amounts, is epinephrine. Vasoconstrictors usually are not warranted for patients who have a history of a heart condition, including high blood pressure (hypertension), because they can strain the heart. These patients should only have anesthetics that do not contain a vasoconstrictor. This contraindication between heart problems and vasoconstrictors emphasizes the importance of having an up-to-date, accurate medical and medication history for each patient.

Some medications that patients take can interfere with vasoconstrictors so it is important to ensure patients' medical and medication histories are up to date.

or negative reaction to a medication, note it in the chart for future reference.

The time period between injection and the area being effectively numbed is referred to as *induction*. The time period from induction to completion of the reversal

TABLE 28-2 Characteristics of Specific Amide Drugs

DRUG	BRAND NAME	GENERAL CHARACTERISTICS
Lidocaine	Xylocaine, Octocaine, Lignospan	■ First amide and still most widely used dental anesthetic; also available as a topical ■ Used with vasoconstrictor to give adequate working time
Mepivacaine	Carbocaine, Polocaine, Isocaine	■ Causes less vasodilation than lidocaine; therefore, can be used for short procedures without vasoconstrictor ■ Mepivacaine 3%, also called Mepivacaine Plain, is often the drug of choice when vasoconstrictors or their sulfite antioxidants are contraindicated
Prilocaine	Citanest Plain, Citanest Forte	■ Metabolic by-products can cause transient methemoglobinemia, a condition that reduces the blood's oxygen-carrying capacity ■ Can be used without vasoconstrictor because it causes limited vasodilation ■ When injected into tissues with limited vascularity, the duration of action is similar with and without vasoconstrictor
Articaine	Septocaine, Septanest, Ultracaine	■ Reported to diffuse through soft and hard tissues better than other amides ■ Metabolized primarily in plasma; has shorter half-life so reinjection may occur sooner
Etidocaine HCl	Duranest	■ Long-lasting anesthetic with a duration of action of 5 to 10 hours ■ Used for long procedures or for postcare pain management
Bupivacaine HCl	Marcaine	■ Long-lasting anesthetic with an extended period of analgesia for postcare pain management ■ May have delayed onset of action

28-1 What is the most commonly used type of pain control in a dental practice?

28-2 What effect do local anesthetics have and how is it accomplished?

28-3 What are two common types of conditions for which local anesthetics may be contraindicated?

28-4 What is the function of topical anesthetics?

28-5 What is the name for the time period between injection and the area becoming numb?

28-6 What is the name for the time period from induction to reversal of the numbing process?

28-7 What can be added to a local anesthetic to increase how long it lasts?

28-8 How does a vasoconstrictor work?

Injection Equipment

Local anesthesia is typically administered using a needle, a syringe, and a cartridge or carpule of anesthetic. The tray for local anesthetic administration should include (Figure 28-1):

- Anesthetic syringe
- Two carpules of anesthetic (as determined by the dentist)
- Long and short needles
- Alcohol sponge to wipe anesthetic diaphragm/aluminum cap (especially necessary if carpule is dispensed from a can rather than a blister pack of anesthetic)
- Cotton gauze to wipe injection site
- Tongue depressor (optional: can be used to retract tongue and cheek to avoid injecting them)
- Needle recapping device
- Sharps disposal system
- Topical anesthetic
- Cotton applicator on a clean cotton gauze
- Air-water syringe tip.
- Oral evacuator.

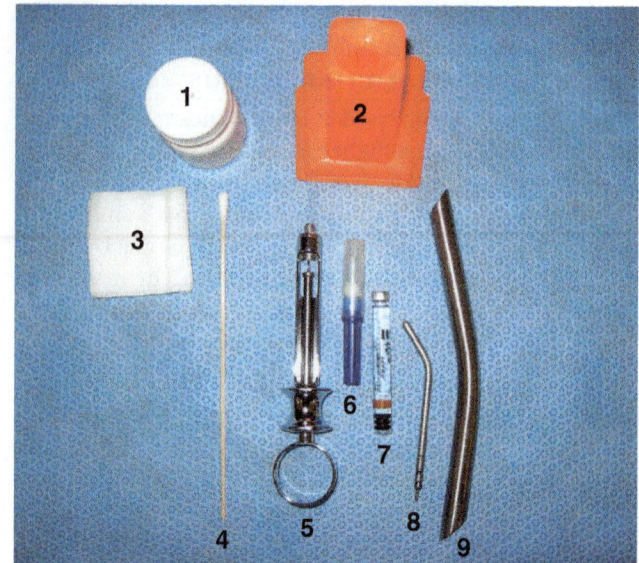

Figure 28–1 Setup for local anesthetic administration. (**1**) Topical anesthetic. (**2**) Needle recapping device. (**3**) 2 × 2 gauze. (**4**) Cotton applicator. (**5**) Aspirating syringe. (**6**) Anesthetic needle. (**7**) Anesthetic cartridge. (**8**) Air-water syringe tip. (**9**) Oral evacuator.

Anesthetic Syringe

The most common type of syringe in dental procedures is the **aspirating syringe**. This syringe features a harpoon on the end of the piston to penetrate the rubber end of the cartridge, and a thumb ring for retracting the anesthetic. The dentist or anesthetist places the needle in the patient's tissues, then retracts the thumb ring. This creates negative pressure. A thin line of blood will be drawn into the cartridge if the needle penetrates a blood vessel. In that case, the professional repositions the needle and repeats the process to make sure the needle is not placed in a blood vessel, which can be potentially harmful to the patient.

A syringe used in local anesthesia typically includes these parts (Figure 28-2):

- *Thumb ring*—a ring located at one end of the syringe designed for placement of the operator's thumb
- *Finger bar*—supports operator's fingers to prevent slippage while in the finger rest
- *Finger rest*—area designed to support the operator's fingers
- *Piston rod*—the rod pushes the rubber stopper of the anesthetic cartridge, forcing the anesthetic through the needle; also known as the plunger

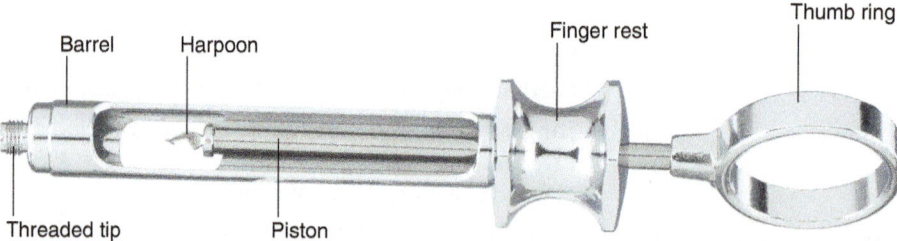

Figure 28–2 Anesthetic syringe.

- *Harpoon*—this hook is at the end of the piston and locks into the rubber stopper of the cartridge, enabling the stopper to be retracted when the dentist pulls back on the thumb ring
- *Barrel*—the anesthetic cartridge is loaded into the syringe mechanism through the open side of the barrel, which then secures the cartridge in place. The operator can check for bleeding during aspiration via a window on the other side of the barrel.
- *Threaded tip*—the cartridge end of the needle goes through the smaller opening in the middle of this tip and punctures the rubber diaphragm of the cartridge; the needle hub attaches to the syringe on the tip. Also known as the needle adaptor, hub of the syringe, or syringe tip.

Anesthetic Cartridges

Local anesthetics are packaged in glass carpules or cartridges (Figure 28-3A). Every cartridge also has a thin, plastic label with identifying information from the manufacturer, including brand name, volume of anesthetic, solution concentration, vasoconstrictor ratio, lot number, and expiration date.

Anesthetic cartridges should be stored away from direct sunlight and at room temperature. Temperature extremes and sunlight can render the solutions ineffective. Before dispensing the anesthetic, always first check that the carpule has not expired; has not been frozen, cracked, chipped, or damaged; is not cloudy or discolored; and that the aluminum cap is not rusted, the stopper is not pushed out, and there are no large air bubbles in the cartridge. Do not load the cartridge into a syringe until you are ready to use it.

The metal from the needle can affect the solution and cause swelling in the area of the injection. After a cartridge has been loaded into a syringe and needle, the solution must be used or thrown away. A cartridge is not reusable later.

The American Dental Association (ADA) Council on Scientific Affairs developed the color-coding system that is standard on injectable anesthesia products (Figure 28-4). This system helps to make an anesthetic solution easily identifiable by its color band, located near the stopper end of the cartridge. Manufacturers that want to display the ADA seal of acceptance must conform to this uniform system.

Disposable Needles

Injections are made with a sterile needle, usually stainless steel and disposable. A two-part plastic covering protects the needle (see Figure 28-3B). If the seal on this outer casing is broken, do not use the needle and dispose of it in a sharps container.

The shorter end of the needle, the cartridge end, fits through the threaded tip of the syringe. This end, protected by a plastic cap, punctures the anesthetic cartridge.

The mechanism to attach the needle to the threaded tip of the syringe is the needle hub, which is made of self-threading plastic or pre-threaded metal.

A needle guard protects the injection end of the needle, which is 1 inch for a short needle, or 1 5/8 inch for a long needle. Generally, a shorter needle is appropriate for infiltration anesthesia and other instances where little penetration of the soft tissues is required. A longer needle is appropriate for nerve block anesthesia and other instances that require penetration of multiple layers of tissue. Needle

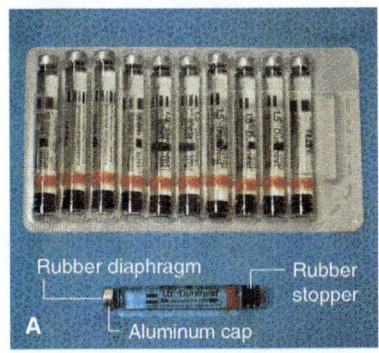

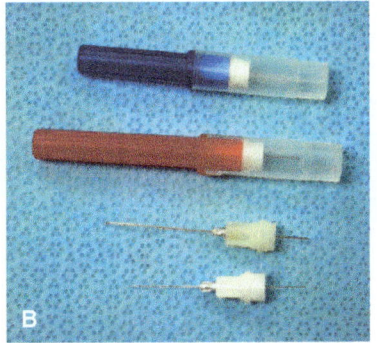

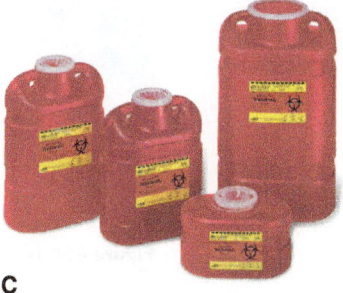

Figure 28–3 Local anesthesia accessories. **(A)** Anesthetic cartridges. **(B)** Anesthetic needles. **(C)** Sharps containers.

Anesthesia color codes

PRODUCT	COLOR
Lidocaine 2% with Epinephrine 1:100,000	▬
Lidocaine 2% with Epinephrine 1:50,000	▬
Lidocaine Plain	▬
Mepivacaine 2% with Levonordefrin 1:20,000	▬
Mepivacaine 3% Plain	▬
Prilocaine 4% with Epinephrine 1:200,000	▬
Prilocaine 4% Plain	▬
Bupivacaine 1.5% with Epinephrine	▬
Articaine 4% with Epinephrine 1:100,000	▬

Figure 28–4 ADA color coding system for anesthetics.

diameter, or thickness, is measured by the needle **gauge**, with the smaller numbers indicating a larger diameter. Commonly used sizes are 25-, 27-, and 30-gauge needles.

After a needle has been used, dispose of it in a sharps container (see Figure 28-3C). Any needle used to penetrate a patient's tissue more than four times during a procedure should be changed due to possible dullness. Everyone involved in dental procedures should be aware

of the location and position of the uncovered needle tip to prevent needlesticks. Needles that are not being used should be protected with covers.

Another safeguard is the needle cap or a stick shield. A plastic or metal cap should be located near the needle operator and assistant for convenient capping. A shield, a rectangular piece of cardboard, fits onto the needle cap to protect the assistant from a needlestick with a used needle.

Voice of Experience

During a procedure, the dentist accidentally placed a needle back on the tray without a cover or shield. I reached for a gauze pad, and the used needle punctured my glove and grazed my skin, drawing blood. I panicked. I froze for a moment. I made eye contact with the dentist. She saw what had happened. My training kicked in. I got up calmly and asked one of my colleagues to assist the dentist with the patient. Then I went to a sink in another room, away from the patient. I removed my gloves and washed my finger with soap and hot water. After the patient left, I met with the dentist, who reviewed the patient's chart to check for any medical conditions that would be a concern. The patient would be contacted and asked to be tested for hepatitis B and HIV. In the meantime, I went to the emergency department of our local hospital to begin preventive treatment. It's important to begin such treatment very soon after exposure.

I was relieved that the patient appeared to be healthy. I learned a lot that day. I became much more careful around needles. Our entire dental team discussed the issue at a meeting the next morning. This incident increased everyone's awareness of the importance of using covers and shields to prevent needlesticks. I felt proud that I didn't gasp out loud or say anything to alarm the patient.

Procedure 28–1 Preparing and Handling a Local Anesthetic Syringe

Materials needed (Figure P28-1-1):

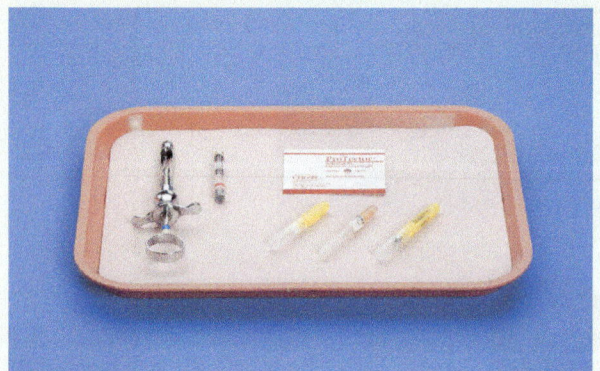

Figure P28-1-1

- Syringe
- Anesthetic cartridge
- Needle (different gauges and lengths)
- Needle recapping device (optional)

1. Put on appropriate PPE.
2. Pull back on the syringe's thumb ring (Figure P28-1-2). Because the thumb ring can loosen, it should be tightened before each use.

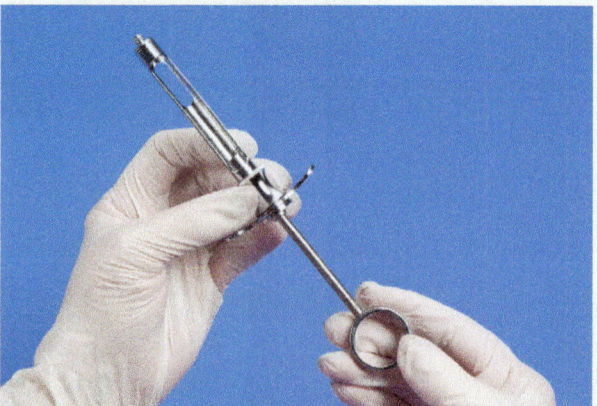

Figure P28-1-2

3. Insert the anesthetic cartridge, rubber stopper end first, toward the end of the thumb ring, then the diaphragm end toward the needle opening (Figure P28-1-3).

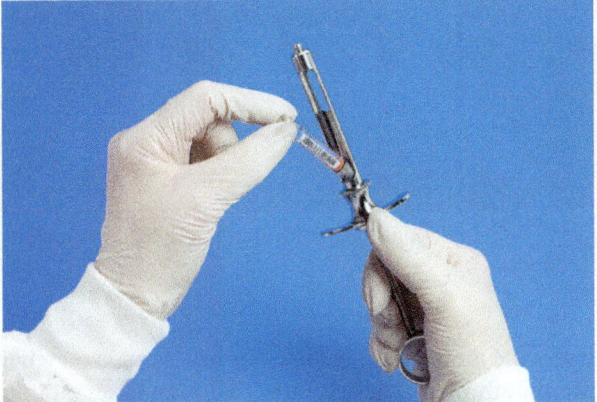

Figure P28-1-3

4. Set the harpoon and test for lock into the rubber stopper. Press or gently tap the harpoon to engage the harpoon into the rubber stopper (Figure P28-1-4).

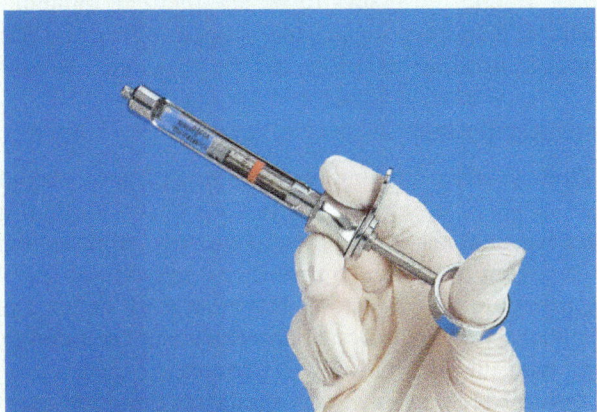

Figure P28-1-4

5. Remove the safety cap from the needle (Figure P28-1-5).

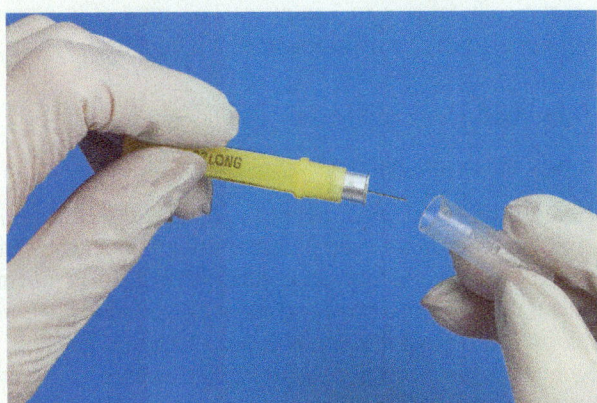

Figure P28-1-5

6. Screw the needle onto the syringe, making sure that it is properly aligned and attached (Figure P28-1-6).

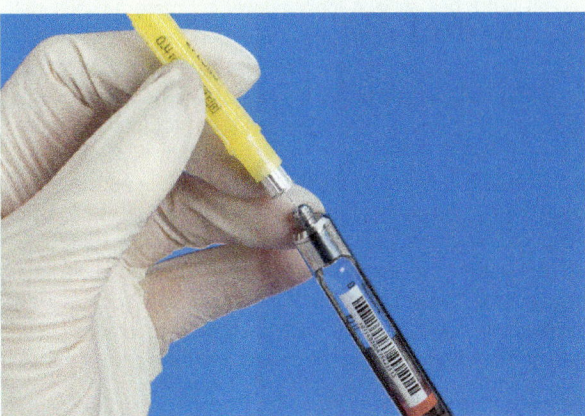

Figure P28-1-6

7. Check the syringe before handing it to the dentist. Remove the needle guard and express two drops of anesthetic onto clean gauze.

8. After use, recap the needle using the one-handed needle recap technique mandated by the Occupational Safety and Health Administration (OSHA) (Figure P28-1-7A) or use a needle recapping device (Figure P28-1-7B).

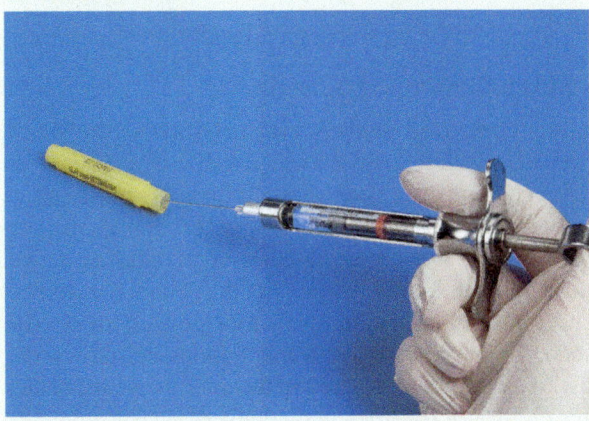

Figure P28-1-7A

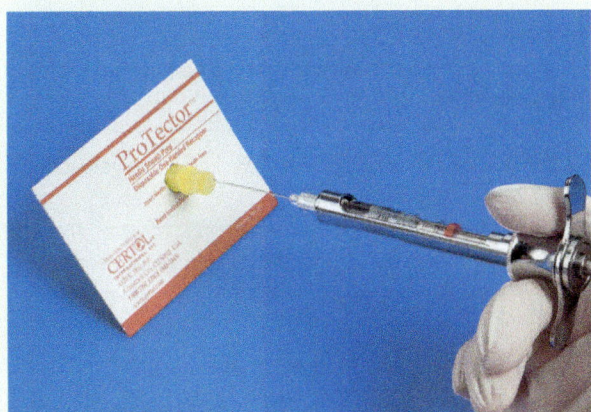

Figure P28-1-7B

Needleless Systems

A needle-free system can help reduce a patient's fear and trauma associated with traditional needles and syringe injections. Needle-free devices include the MadaJet, which uses compression to inject a very fine stream of anesthetic into the tissue. The system, which is appropriate for many procedures, injects the anesthetics into palatal and soft tissues with virtually no pain.

Computer-Controlled Systems

Computer-controlled delivery systems, such as the Wand, can be used to administer local anesthesia. This system provides controlled pressure and delivery of anesthesia at a rate below the pain threshold. Standard anesthesia cartridges fit the system as do needles of any size or gauge. Plastic tubing links the system to the Wand handpiece, which contains the needle, and a foot pedal controls the delivery. The design of the Wand handpiece allows the dentist to grasp closer to the needle and gives him or her greater control of the anesthesia delivery.

CHECKPOINTS

28-9 What determines the length of the needle used in a local anesthetic injection?

28-10 If you load an anesthetic cartridge into a syringe but do not use it, can you use it later?

28-11 Of 25, 27, and 30, which is the thinnest gauge needle?

Injection Sites and Techniques

Injection Sites

Most dental procedures use one of three types of injections—local infiltration, field block, or nerve block.

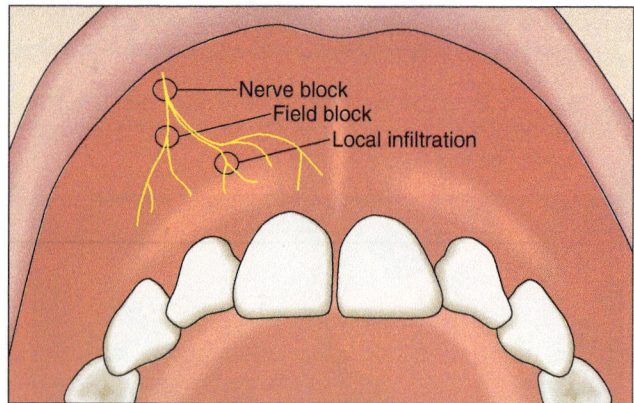

Figure 28–5 Injection sites for local infiltration, field block, and nerve block.

The specific method the dentist chooses is based on where in the mouth he or she will inject and the innervation of that area or tooth (Figure 28-5).

Infiltration Anesthesia

For **infiltration anesthesia**, anesthetic is injected directly into or around the tissues to be anesthetized. Infiltration anesthesia is appropriate for procedures involving maxillary premolars, maxillary anteriors, and the mandibular incisors.

Block Anesthesia

A kind of local infiltration anesthesia, **field block anesthesia** is injected near the apex of the tooth, near larger terminal nerve branches, to prevent impulses from passing from the tooth to the central nervous system. It is appropriate for procedures involving teeth or bone on the maxillary and mandibular anterior areas. The numbing effect typically takes only 2 to 3 minutes.

Nerve block anesthesia eliminates sensation over a larger area than either of the other two types of injections. These injections are given near a main nerve trunk to prevent pain sensation from passing to the brain. The numbing effect typically takes 4 to 5 minutes. This type of injection is also referred to as a mandibular block injection.

Safety and Precautions

Possible Complications

The mouth tissues of most people tolerate the medications used in local anesthesia. Even then, the tissue may show slight changes. Some people may get contact dermatitis, an inflammation of the tissues caused by an allergic reaction, from these solutions. This type of reaction is called a localized reaction.

More widespread reaction to the solution is called a systemic reaction and can depend on the medication administered, the amount given, the rate of administration and rate of absorption, and other medications the patient may have taken.

When numbness induced by local anesthesia does not wear off as it should, the condition is called **paresthesia**, and it may be temporary or permanent. In most cases, the condition clears up within 8 weeks with no treatment. If a nerve has been severed, the condition can be permanent, although this is rare. The nerve can be damaged if the injection or a surgical procedure injures the nerve sheath or causes bleeding into or around the sheath. Another cause of paresthesia can be contamination of the anesthetic solution, usually with alcohol or a sterilizing solution used to disinfect the medication cartridge.

A patient who contacts your dental office complaining of numbness after it should have worn off should talk to the dentist and be seen as soon as possible.

Patient Monitoring and Safety

Always stay in the room with the patient after an injection and observe the patient carefully for signs of an adverse reaction. Adverse reactions are most likely to occur during or shortly after the injection.

Dental Office Personnel Safety

To guard against needlestick injuries, use needles that include safety devices, such as a self-sheathing safety needle (Figure 28-6) or safety syringe. Disposal containers for contaminated sharps should be readily accessible and located as close as possible to the area where they are being used.

If a needlestick injury occurs, wash the injured area with soap and water, and report the injury to the dentist immediately.

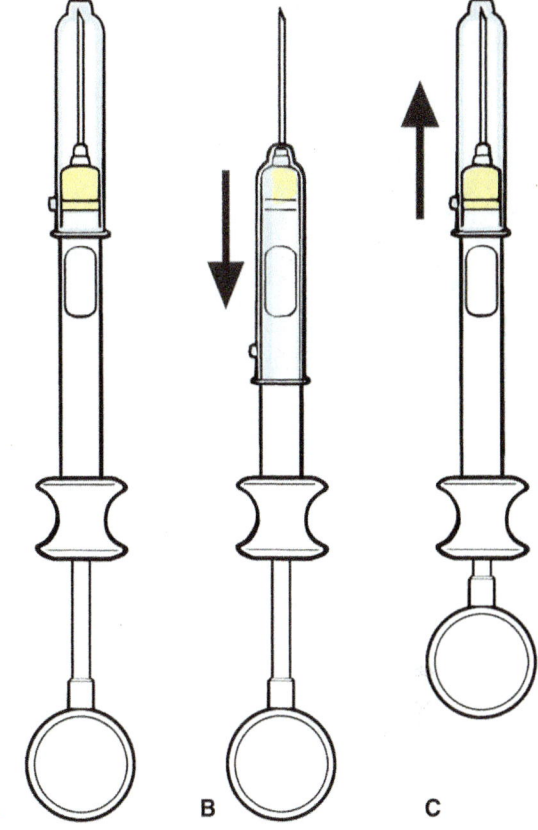

Figure 28–6 Self-sheathing safety needle. (**A**) Syringe with sheath over needle. (**B**) Sheath slides back as injection is made. (**C**) After injection, sheath returns to cover the needle.

Procedure 28–2 Assisting with Administration of Local Anesthetics

Materials needed (Figure P28-2-1):

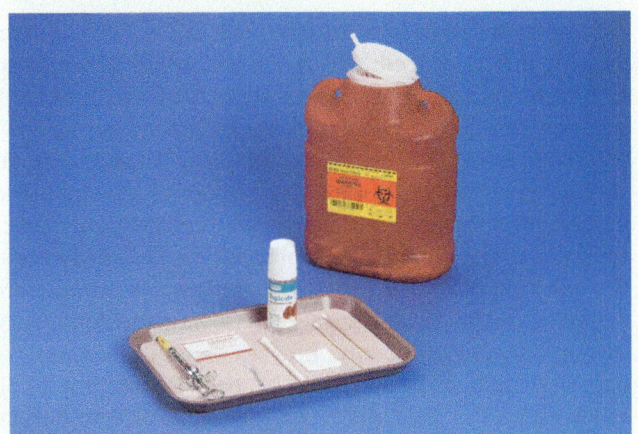

Figure P28-2-1

- Loaded anesthetic syringe
- Needle guard
- Air-water syringe
- Saliva evacuator
- Sharps container
- Medical waste container
- Topical anesthetic
- Cotton applicator
- Gauze

1. Put on appropriate PPE.

2. When the dentist is ready to give the patient an injection of a local anesthetic, the DA or the dentist should apply a topical anesthetic to the injection area. To do this, apply a small amount of topical anesthetic onto the cotton applicator. Dry the injection site with a gauze square, then place the topical anesthetic onto the injection site for 3–5 minutes. Wipe excess topical anesthetic off with a gauze square prior to the dentist administering the local anesthetic

3. Loosen the needle guard and give the syringe to the dentist, placing the thumb ring over his or her thumb and the index and middle finger under the finger bar. Ideally, this exchange will take place high on the patient's chest, in the transfer zone, near the chin and out of the patient's sight line (Figure P28-2-2). Occasionally with pediatric patients, the syringe transfer may take place behind the patient's head, with the dentist bringing the syringe around and under the chin.

Procedure 28-2 **Assisting with Administration of Local Anesthetics (Continued)**

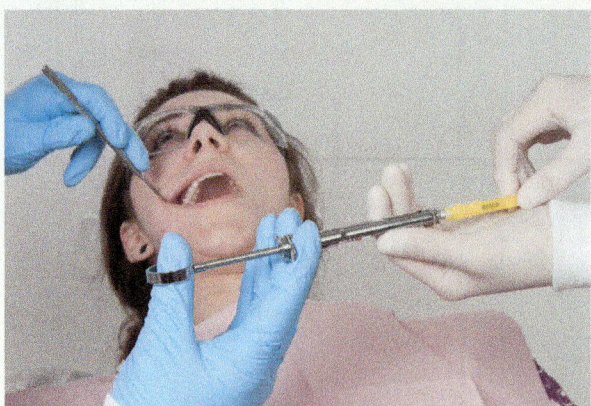

Figure P28-2-2

4. During the injection process, monitor the patient for side effects. You can help keep the patient relaxed by maintaining a calm demeanor.

5. After the injection is given, the dentist will place a needle guard on the syringe to prevent an accidental needlestick injury. This should be done using the one-handed needle scoop technique.

6. Instruct the patient to turn toward you for a mouth rinsing with the air-water syringe and saliva evacuator.

7. Staying chairside, monitor the patient the entire time. At the conclusion of the procedure, remind the patient about the effects of numbness and the need to be aware of not biting his or her lips or cheeks.

8. Be sure to dispose of the used needle in a sharps container (Figure P28-2-3), and dispose of the anesthetic cartridge in a medical waste container. (If the anesthetic cartridge has become contaminated with blood or other bodily fluids, discard in a sharps container.) The syringe should be placed with items that require sterilization.

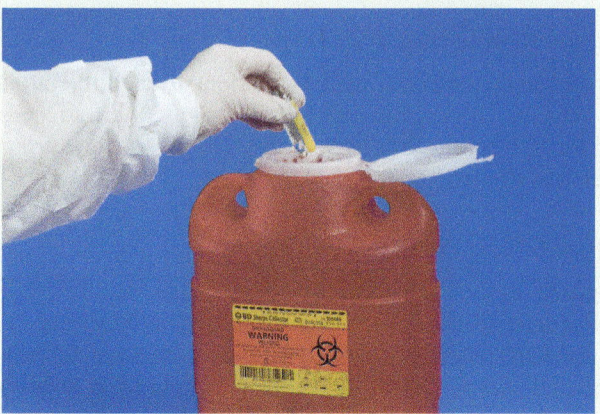

Figure P28-2-3

Electronic Anesthesia

An electronic system can be used to administer anesthesia, although it is more effective when combined with nitrous oxide inhalation sedation. It may be appropriate when local anesthesia is contraindicated due to allergy or extreme fear of injections.

This type of system uses low-current electricity to block pain. Pads are placed on the backs of the patient's hands, and another pad is placed on the area involved in the procedure. This pad, called the intraoral receptor, is placed to the lingual side near the gingival margin. The patient helps to control the system by increasing the level of the signal that blocks pain.

This type of local anesthesia does not involve needles or chemicals, does not cause numbness or swelling after a procedure, and involves the patient in reducing anxiety and controlling pain.

CHECKPOINTS

28-12 Of local infiltration, field block, and nerve block, which provides numbness over the largest area?

28-13 What is the condition called when numbness does not wear off?

General Anesthesia and Sedation

Inhalation Sedation: Nitrous Oxide

Inhalation sedation is considered the safest form of sedation for dental procedures, and it is easy for a dentist to administer to patients of all ages. The patient inhales a combination of nitrous oxide (dinitrogen monoxide or N_2O) and oxygen (O_2) through a face mask, a laryngeal mask airway, or an endotracheal tube. The two gases are combined in a reservoir bag from which a hose extends and carries the gases to the patient's nosepiece. The relaxing effects of the sedation from this tasteless, colorless gas mixture are almost immediate, and the patient is awake and responsive throughout the procedure. Inhalation anesthetics relieve pain and induce drowsiness. The patient may not recall much about the procedure. The patient returns to normal within minutes, usually without adverse side effects.

The gases nitrous oxide and oxygen (N_2O/O_2) (also known as "laughing gas"), in combination, are widely used in dental practices to produce a safe state of **conscious sedation**—especially for patients who are very fearful of dental procedures. Patients remain awake, relaxed, responsive, reflexive and able to cooperate. To a point, patients given nitrous oxide are insensitive to pain. Sometimes nitrous oxide is used in concert with a local anesthetic to further alleviate pain.

Nitrous oxide is considered a safe sedative because it is not metabolized in the body—it enters and exits almost entirely through the lungs. Patients typically recover quickly from its sedative effects. They report having felt tingly or as if they were floating.

Combined with oxygen, nitrous oxide, a stable, non-flammable gas, is one of the safest anesthetic agents. The patient wears a nosepiece to breathe in the anesthesia, which moves from the nasopharynx and oropharynx into the body to the circulatory system. The gas is transported to the brain, where it takes effect on the central nervous system, raising the pain threshold while retaining consciousness.

Indications and Contraindications

Nitrous oxide is appropriate when a patient fears dental treatment, has a long appointment, has an unusually sensitive gag reflex, or has a heart condition that would benefit from the increased oxygen and stress reduction. A patient who receives nitrous oxide must be able to breathe through his or her nose.

There are no clear-cut medical conditions that make N_2O/O_2 an inappropriate choice for sedation. However, you may want to choose an alternative for some patients, including those who have nasal obstruction, those who have breathing difficulties related to emphysema or multiple sclerosis, those who may have a neurological condition, those undergoing in vitro fertilization treatment, and those who may have an adverse reaction due to emotional instability or drug use or a psychiatric condition. Additionally, patients who are pregnant should only have N_2O/O_2 after the first trimester and only with permission from an obstetrician.

As a precaution, always review a patient's medical and medication history before administering N_2O/O_2.

The effects of N_2O/O_2 can inadvertently enhance the effects of other medications.

Equipment

Some dental offices have built-in N_2O/O_2 equipment. Others have portable units. Installation and storage of this equipment is regulated by each state and OSHA. States also control supplies and require a dentist's signature and license number when ordering.

N_2O and O_2 cylinders must be stored upright, held stable in position, and be stored away from heat sources (Figure 28-7). The cylinders used with built-in equipment should be chained to a wall, and those used with portable units should be chained to the unit. These precautions help to ensure that the cylinders cannot fall on their valve stems and explode.

Cylinders are color-coded—blue for N_2O and green for O_2. Every cylinder has a valve to control the release of the gas, and a meter on the equipment shows the rate of flow. Every flow meter has safety features that prevent the flow of N_2O/O_2 if the concentration of O_2 falls below 30% or if the concentration of N_2O/O_2 is greater than 70%. These safety features have been standard since 1976.

Nosepieces or masks through which the patient inhales the gas are available in sizes to fit adults and children and in a single-use disposable style and a multiple-use rubber style that is sterilized after each use. Tubing connects the patient's nosepiece to the gas tanks. The excess gas and that which the patient exhales flow through a secondary mask. This outside mask is connected to a reservoir bag and vacuum system that carry away this excess gas, protecting the patient and dental team.

Administration

Some states permit dental assistants to monitor nitrous oxide under the direct supervision of a dentist.

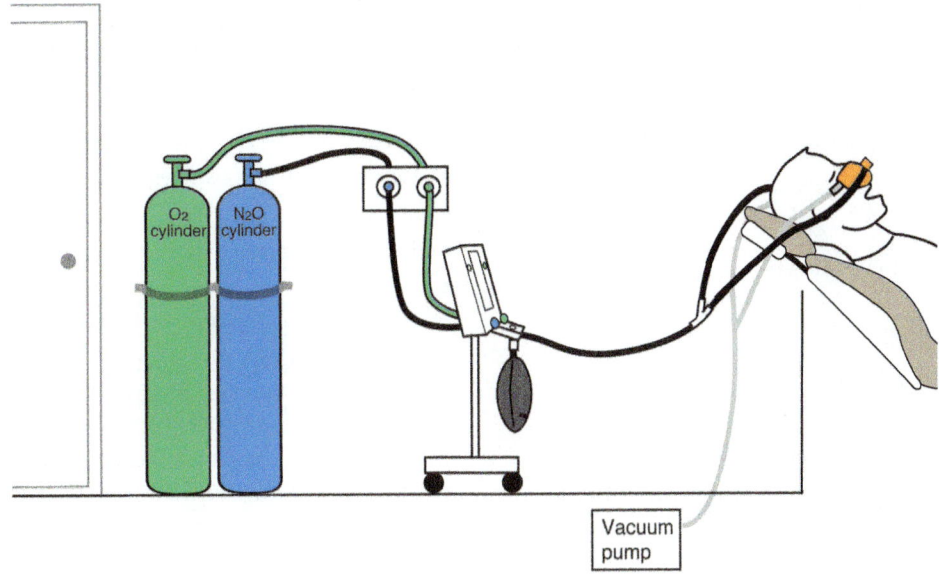

Figure 28–7 Nitrous oxide system.

Sedation with N_2O/O_2 begins and ends with giving the patient pure O_2. At the start of the process, the operator establishes the patient's **tidal volume**, the amount of air inhaled and exhaled with each breath, and then slowly titrates the concentration of N_2O until the appropriate level is achieved for the individual patient at the particular visit. The amount of sedation a patient may require can vary from visit to visit, and the dental team should not rely on a past experience documented in the patient's record as an indication of the amount needed for another visit. At the end of the sedation process, 100% O_2 should be given again, for several minutes. Ask the patient about symptoms such as dizziness, headache, or tiredness. When the patient reports feeling normal, check vital signs again and compare them to those taken before the procedure began. Naturally, advise patients who do not feel well after having inhalation sedation to have a friend or family member drive them home.

Safety and Precautions

Prior to a patient receiving N_2O/O_2, you should explain what to expect from this form of sedation. Of course, tell the patient that he or she will remain awake and responsive at all times. Emphasize the importance of breathing through the nose and keeping the mask snug during treatment. Describe the feeling the patient is likely to experience, often expressed as warm and tingly.

N_2O is toxic when used other than appropriately for patient treatment, and the gas can harm members of the dental team if large amounts of the gas escape into the atmosphere over time. The maximum allowable amount of N_2O released into the treatment area is 50 parts per million. Occupational risk can be avoided by using a scavenger system, which reduces the N_2O that escapes and is inhaled. It is also important to make sure the patient's nosepiece or mask fits firmly to prevent gas leakage, discourage patients from talking during gas administration, inspect equipment and hoses for leaks, and vent gas outside the building.

Monitoring the Patient

The dental team must monitor, assess, and record the vital signs—blood pressure, pulse, and respiration—of patients receiving N_2O/O_2. Postoperative readings are compared to preoperative readings to indicate the patient's recovery from the sedative.

Procedure 28-3 Assisting with Nitrous Oxide Administration and Monitoring

Make sure you're familiar with N_2O/O_2, the equipment involved, and vital sign measurement and assessment. Not all states allow dental assistants to administer nitrous oxide, even under the direct supervision of a DMD. Be aware of the laws regarding nitrous oxide administration and monitoring in your state.

Materials needed (Figure P28-3-1A and B):

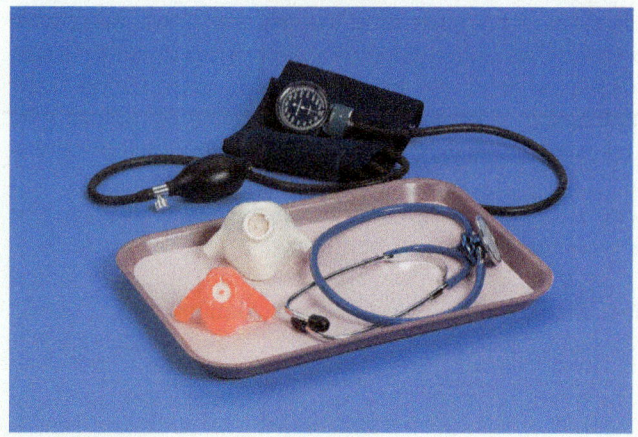

Figure P28-3-1B

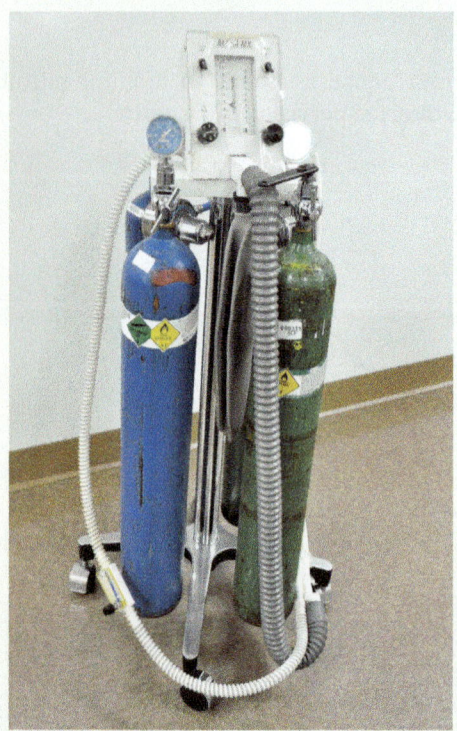

Figure P28-3-1A

- Nitrous oxide/oxygen (N_2O/O_2) equipment
- Nasal hoods of various sizes
- Tubing
- Blood pressure cuff
- Stethoscope
1. Put on appropriate PPE.
2. When preparing for a patient, first check the tanks for appropriate supplies of gases. Prepare the correct nasal hood size for the patient and attach it to the tubing.
3. After you've placed the patient in the chair and reviewed the medical history, record the patient's vital signs.
4. Talk to the patient about the sedation to be provided and its effects, and have the patient provide informed consent.

Procedure 28–3 Assisting with Nitrous Oxide Administration and Monitoring (Continued)

5. Recline the dental chair into the supine position and fit the sterile nasal hood on the patient (Figure P28-3-2). Once the fit is right, tighten the tubing behind the patient to prevent leaking of gases, and drape the tubing on each side. If the nasal hood irritates or pinches the patient's skin, place a piece of gauze next to the skin. Direct the patient to breathe slowly through the nose.

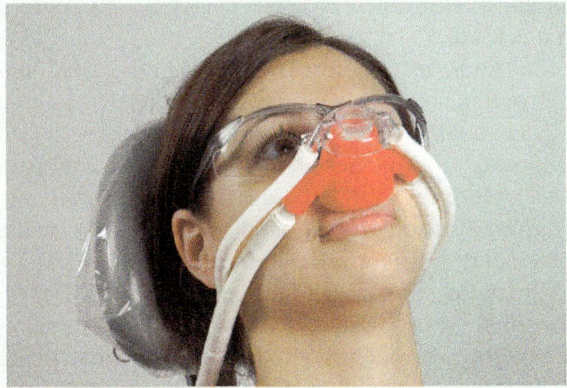

Figure P28-3-2

6. The dentist will adjust the flow meter for O_2 only. The patient should receive pure O_2 for at least 1 minute. The dentist then adjusts the N_2O flow by increments of 0.5 to 1 liter per minute, and reduces O_2 flow by the same amount. (Some current equipment does this automatically.) The dentist continues to adjust the N_2O flow by the increments described here, and reduces O_2 flow in 1-minute intervals until the patient shows signs of sedation. Monitor the patient for 3 minutes and titrate .5 L of N_2O if the patient needs additional sedation.

7. Record the patient's baseline level, remaining close to the patient to allow you to do close monitoring. Periodically, ask the patient how he or she feels, and monitor the rise and fall of the reservoir bag and the patient's chest.

8. As the treatment ends, the dentist will begin oxygenating the patient with O_2 turned on 100% and the N_2O turned off. Doing this for at least 5 minutes helps to prevent diffusion hypoxia, a condition that causes lightheadedness.

9. When the dentist indicates that oxygenation is complete, remove the patient's nasal hood and turn off the O_2. Gently and slowly change the patient to a seated position. Doing this too quickly could cause fainting.

10. Again ask the patient how he or she feels and ask the patient to remain seated for a couple of minutes. When the patient reports feeling normal, you can dismiss him or her.

11. Record the patient's baseline N_2O and O_2 levels and response to the sedation. This documentation is important for reasons including the patient's future care and future sedation, and it serves as a legal record of care should it ever be necessary.

CHECKPOINTS

28-14 Is nitrous oxide metabolized by the body?

28-15 Which of the body's systems does nitrous oxide act on to produce its effects?

28-16 What is administered at the beginning and end of the process to the patient who is receiving nitrous oxide?

28-17 How can you tell when a patient has recovered from nitrous oxide administration?

Dental Facts

Nitrous oxide became popular for use in dental practices because they did not typically have access to anesthesiologists. Nitrous oxide allowed patients to feel no pain but remain responsive to verbal commands.

Oral Sedatives

Sometimes a dentist will prescribe sedating medication in pill form for the patient to take at home 30 to 60 minutes before a procedure. These medications to relieve anxiety are called antianxiety drugs or **anxiolytics**. Taken in large amounts, they can cause sleep, sedation, and anesthesia. Antianxiety medication is most typically used when the patient is extremely anxious about the procedure, or is very young and the treatment is extensive. Antianxiety medication also may be used when the patient has a mental disability, or when a procedure will be difficult or long. Methods of administration include oral, intravenous, and inhalation. Dentists must have specialty training in various classes of medication they wish to administer.

One common medication used in this way is benzodiazepine (diazepam). This dual-function medication can be used for anxiety relief—to calm and relax the patient—or as a sedative hypnotic—to calm the patient and induce drowsiness. Other medications in this category include barbiturates (pentobarbital, secobarbital). All of these medications depress or slow the central nervous system. Another medication, chloral hydrate (Noctec), may be used with pediatric patients.

Because these medications cause drowsiness, patients should be instructed to have someone else drive them to and from the appointment.

Intravenous Sedation

Sedative medication provided directly into the patient's blood system through an intravenous line into a vein is called intravenous (IV) conscious sedation. The IV remains in place throughout the procedure, and the patient's vital signs are monitored.

Some states allow certified dental assistants who have completed a board-approved course to help with IV conscious sedation, specifically monitoring the patient and removing IV lines. Typically, most of the process involved in IV sedation is performed by an oral surgeon or periodontist. These individuals must be trained and certified in intravenous sedation techniques.

Before a patient receives IV sedation, these steps must be completed:

- Physical exam, including weight to determine dosage
- Medical history
- Signed consent (parent's or guardian's written consent for pediatric patients)
- Baseline vital signs, level of consciousness, and motor function
- Oximetry (blood oxygen concentration)
- Electrocardiogram

To create the minimally depressed level of consciousness achieved through IV sedation, the patient is slowly given antianxiety medication through a vein in the hand or forearm. The patient maintains the ability to respond to commands and breathe normally.

The skin is cleaned with an antiseptic and a small needle is inserted into a vein made more prominent by a tourniquet wrapped around the upper arm. The tourniquet, a flexible rubber tube, restricts blood flow in the lower arm and plumps the veins up for easier access by needle.

An IV must be monitored throughout the dental procedure, including the recovery period, to check for inflammation or pain at the site of needle insertion, and to ensure the needle remains in place and functioning appropriately. If you observe a potential problem with an IV, notify the surgeon or another dental professional immediately.

Vital signs, including blood pressure, heart rate, respiration, oximetry, cardiac rhythm, and level of consciousness, should be measured and recorded at least every 15 minutes. The dental practice should have on hand supplemental O_2, suction, and a defibrillator for emergencies.

Intramuscular Sedation

Intramuscular sedation involves an in-office injection of a sedating medication into the muscle of the upper arm or thigh. This form of sedation is sometimes used with pediatric patients. It takes 20 to 30 minutes for the full effect to kick in. The medication produces total relaxation and minimizes fear and anxiety. Often, the patient will remember little of the procedure.

General Anesthesia

Medications used in **general anesthesia** affect the central nervous system, and the patient loses feeling and enters an unconscious state. This form of sedation is appropriate for some patients and some surgeries and treatments. General anesthesia requires close monitoring by a professional trained in anesthesia administration, usually in a hospital setting but sometimes in offices of oral and maxillofacial surgeons.

A dental assistant is not involved with administering general anesthesia but may assist during a procedure in which it is used.

General anesthesia differs from conscious sedation in that the patient is unconscious, not responsive to commands, and unable to keep an open airway for breathing. This state of anesthesia is induced with a mixture of gases, including N_2O/O_2, halothane, or enflurane mixture, and medications introduced intravenously, including thiopental and methohexital. General anesthesia is provided by an anesthesiologist and is typically given at a hospital or a facility that has a higher level of equipment for emergency situations than most dental practices.

Medications used for anesthesia can produce four different stages of consciousness, and the patient can move from one stage to the next:

- Stage 1—In this stage, analgesia, the patient is conscious but relaxed and able to respond to commands. Along with relaxation, the patient feels euphoric and less pain. The patient's vital signs are normal.
- Stage II—In this stage, excitement, the patient may begin to become unconscious and less aware of his or her surroundings. This is not a desirable stage, and nausea and vomiting may occur and the patient may be unmanageable.
- Stage III—When stage II has passed and calm has set in, the patient is in this stage, general anesthesia, and does not feel pain. Because this stage includes unconsciousness, it is achieved only under the control of an anesthesiologist in a setting such as a hospital.
- Stage IV—This stage is definitely undesirable and occurs if the patient's heart and lungs slow down or stop functioning. This leads to cardiac arrest or respiratory failure. If not reversed immediately, the patient could die.

Before having general anesthesia, a patient must have a physical examination and laboratory tests and must sign a consent form.

No food or drink are allowed for 8 to 12 hours before having general anesthesia, and the patient must be driven home by a friend or family member afterward. The dentist and anesthesiologist will explain the risks of anesthesia to the patient before the procedure. The patient is monitored after the procedure until the anesthesia wears off, which is characterized by a return of reflexes, coherent speech, and response to commands.

Documenting Anesthetic Administration

All aspects of the care provided in your dental office should be meticulously recorded including, of course, medications provided to relieve pain or anxiety. Among the details to document include:

- Review of the patient's medical history
- Preoperative and postoperative vital signs
- The patient's tidal volume, if inhalation sedation was provided
- The time anesthesia was commenced, the time when the peak concentration was administered, and the time when administration was ceased
- The time elapsed during patient's recovery after the procedure
- Any patient concerns or adverse events

CHECKPOINT

28-18 During conscious IV sedation, how often should a patient's vital signs be measured and recorded?

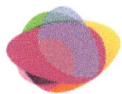

Chapter Highlights

- Awareness of and compassion for patients' anxiety about pain and fears about needles and injections are an important consideration for any dental professional. Work to develop a chairside manner that projects calm and does not unnecessarily provoke nervousness.
- A current, comprehensive medical and medication history for every patient is always important, even more so when considering medications to relieve anxiety and pain.
- Local anesthesia is the most commonly used type of pain control in dental practices.
- Dental assistants play an important role in preparing anesthetics, talking to patients about medications they will receive for pain and anxiety, helping to keep patients calm, and monitoring patients throughout procedures. In some instances, dental assistants may assist in administering anesthetics and sedatives.
- Dental assistants should be very familiar with syringes used in dental injections, including the parts of the syringe; how to assemble the parts; how to add the

anesthetic cartridge and needle to the assembly; and how to sterilize, maintain, and dispose of this equipment.
- Dental assistants play an important role in the safety aspects of anesthesia and sedation administration, including infection control and patient safety and well-being. Documenting any adverse reaction helps ensure the patient has a better experience the next time.
- Dental assistants should check and recheck details related to medications, including asking the dentist the desired ratio of an anesthetic solution and checking for a patient's condition that might contraindicate a chosen drug.
- Patients deserve and need to be informed about medications they will receive and should be told about what to expect, possible side effects, how long the effects will last, warning signs of an adverse reaction, and medical conditions that might contraindicate a particular medication.
- Dental assistants also play an important role in helping to ensure the safety of members of the dental team, including preventing needlestick injuries, exposure to nitrous oxide, and properly storing gas canisters.

Review Questions

1. Which of these anesthetics is not metabolized by the body?
   a. Amides
   b. Esters
   c. Nitrous oxide
   d. None of the above

2. What can be added to local anesthetic solutions to prolong their effects?
   a. Nitrous oxide
   b. Vasoconstrictors
   c. Oral sedatives
   d. Anxiolytics

3. For which of these conditions might local anesthetics be contraindicated?
   a. First trimester of pregnancy
   b. Heart problems, including recent heart surgery
   c. Severe kidney or liver function impairment
   d. All of the above

4. Which of these is not an effect of a vasoconstrictor?

   a. It slows the rate at which the medication is absorbed into the bloodstream.

   b. The patient will be rendered unconscious.

   c. Bleeding during a surgical procedure is minimized.

   d. There is less risk of a toxic reaction.

5. Which of these does not render an anesthetic cartridge useless?

   a. It has been frozen.

   b. It has expired.

   c. It has been shaken.

   d. It is cloudy.

6. What is numbness induced by local anesthesia that does not wear off as it should?

   a. Contact dermatitis

   b. Systemic reaction

   c. Induction

   d. Paresthesia

7. Which of these is not one of the three common types of dental procedure injections?

   a. Innervation

   b. Local infiltration

   c. Field block

   d. Nerve block

8. Which system in the body does nitrous oxide affect?

   a. Central nervous system

   b. Limbic system

   c. Lymphatic system

   d. Musculoskeletal system

9. Which of these conditions is not a contraindication for nitrous oxide administration?

   a. Emphysema

   b. Pediatric patient

   c. First trimester of pregnancy

   d. A sensitive gag reflex

10. Nitrous oxide canisters should be chained to a wall or to a portable unit. Why?

   a. To avoid someone stealing and abusing the gas

   b. To avoid them falling on someone and hurting them

   c. To prevent them from being shaken

   d. To prevent them from falling on their valve stems and exploding

Active Learning Exercises

1. Pain reduction is essential in the dental office. What is the difference between topical and local anesthetics?

2. Prior to placing a topical anesthetic, the tissues should be dried with gauze. What is the purpose of drying the tissue? Why is this technique necessary?

3. Anesthetic can be very dangerous if not administered properly. What type of patient observations should be made for a patient under local anesthetic? Under nitrous oxide sedation? Under IV sedation? Under general anesthesia?

PREPARING FOR CERTIFICATION EXAMS

Review the following topics in this chapter to prepare for the Dental Assisting National Board (DANB) exam:

- **Introduction**

- **Local Anesthesia**

- **Topical Anesthetics**

- **Injection Equipment**

- **Procedure 28-2: Assisting with Administration of Local Anesthetics**

- **Inhalation Sedation: Nitrous Oxide**

- **Intravenous Sedation**

- **Intramuscular Sedation**

- **General Anesthesia**

Dental Radiography

Basics of Dental Radiography

CHAPTER OUTLINE

CHAPTER CHECKLIST

On completion of this chapter, students will be able to:

- ☑ Describe the history of radiation and the development of the dental radiograph.
- ☑ Describe the structure of the atom.
- ☑ Describe the forms and properties of radiation.
- ☑ Describe the effects of radiation on the human body.
- ☑ Identify patient-selection criteria for dental radiography.
- ☑ Explain the safety concepts and equipment used to protect both patients and operators from radiation hazards.
- ☑ Identify and describe all the parts of dental x-ray units, including their function.
- ☑ Describe the composition of dental x-ray film.
- ☑ Explain the steps involved in taking a radiograph.
- ☑ Describe intraoral and extraoral film, including properties, sizes, and types.
- ☑ Describe the different kinds of digital radiography, including the advantages and disadvantages of digital radiography.

KEY TERMS

ALARA – when dealing with radiation, using the lowest amount of radiation possible to achieve the objective; stands for As Low As Reasonably Achievable

analog – in radiography, a non-digital image that is comprised of continuous shades of grey obtained by traditional x-ray film

anode (AN-ode) – the positively charged end of an x-ray tube containing the tungsten focal spot where x-rays are generated after being bombarded with electrons from the cathode end

atoms – basic units of matter, atoms are made of electrons orbiting a nucleus

cathode – the negatively charged end of an x-ray tube where electrons are created by heating a tungsten filament before being shot across the vacuum tube to the anode end

cell senescence (sih-NES-ens) – cell death

cephalometric (sef-uh-loh-MEH-trik) film – a radiograph of the jaws and cranium that allows their measurement and diagnosis of conditions

chromosomes – large strands of DNA within the cell nucleus, susceptible to radiation damage

collimator (KOL-uh-may-ter) – a lead-based safety device in the x-ray tubehead that focuses and targets the x-ray beam as it emerges from the x-ray tube

contrast – describes the quality of a radiograph; contrast is determined by the different densities of the areas radiographed, with denser areas showing up as white or grey and less dense areas as black

control panel – a component on a dental x-ray machine where the operator can control the unit's kilovoltage (kV), milliamperage (mA), and other settings; control panels vary by manufacturer and type of machine

crests – the length between the peaks on a wave; x-rays are short-wavelength waves and thus high-energy, penetrating energy

definition – describes the clarity of a radiograph; determined by the film speed and motion

density – the compactness of a substance; in radiography, it describes the opacity of an object to x-rays, with denser objects appearing more opaque

disclosure – the act of telling a patient the reasons, risks, and benefits of a procedure, including radiography; disclosure is a legal requirement to obtain informed consent

electromagnetic energy spectrum – the array of electromagnetic radiation, organized by wavelength, and including gamma rays, radio waves and visible light, and x-rays

electrons – a negatively charged subatomic particle that orbits a nucleus as part of an atom; flowing electrons constitute electricity and are used to generate the energy that creates x-rays

energy – in physics, defined as the ability to perform work; energy has no mass

film badge – a device worn by employees in dental offices to measure exposure to radiation

film-holding device – special device that is designed to hold film steady in a patient's mouth during radiography; reduces exposure to radiation by preventing the need to manually hold film

focal spot – the spot in the anode where x-rays are generated after being hit with a stream of electrons; the focal spot is made from tungsten and precisely aimed to direct the x-ray beam out of the x-ray tube

focusing cup – a component in an x-ray tube head, made from molybdenum; a heated tungsten filament creates an electron cloud that remains within the focusing cup until the exposure button is pressed, at which time the electron cloud shoots across the vacuum to a tungsten target called a focal spot, thus creating x-rays

genetic cells – reproductive cells, or cells that carry half as many chromosomes as regular cells, and are very sensitive to radiation exposure; examples include sperm and egg cells

grey scale – in digital imaging, the number of shades of grey that an image possesses; most computers recognize about 256 shades of grey, while the human eye recognizes about 32 shades of grey; the greater the number of shades of grey, the more detailed the radiograph

halide (HAL-ide) crystals – used in the manufacture of dental x-ray film; halide crystals are suspended in a gelatin coating on the film surface, they are sensitive to x-rays and form a latent image when struck by x-rays during exposure

Hittorf-Crookes (HIT-orf Kruks) tube – an early x-ray tube based on a cathode/anode design

ion (EYE-on) – an unstable atom in which one electron has been removed or added through exposure to energy, including x-rays; ions are attracted to surrounding atoms and can cause biological damage

ionization (EYE-uh-nih-ZAY-shun) – the process of creating an ion through exposure to energy

kilovolts (KIL-oh-vohlts) (kV) – a unit of electrical potential, equal to 10^3 volts; in dental radiography, a measure of the power of the dental x-ray unit

latent image – a radiographic image stored on dental film after exposure but before processing; the latent image cannot be seen with the naked eye and is only visible after it has been processed

latent period – the period between radiation exposure and its biological effects; the latent period may be years

lead apron – a protective device used in dental offices to shield patients from excess radiation exposure during radiography; lead aprons extend from the neck to below the reproductive organs

leakage radiation – radiation that escapes from an improperly functioning x-ray tubehead; equipment should be regularly tested to guard against leakage radiation

matter – a substance that has form and shape and occupies space

maximum permissible dose (MPD) – according to the National Council on Radiation Protection and Measurements, the maximum permissible dose of radiation a body can receive in a given time frame without causing biological damage

milliamperage (mil-ee-AM-per-ej) (mA) – one thousandth of an amp; in dental radiography, a measure of how many electrons are contained in an x-ray beam

mitochondria (my-toh-KON-dree-uh) – a cell structure where energy is generated for use by the cell

mitosis (my-TOH-sis) – the process of cell division by which one cell is split into two exact copies of itself

molecule – unit of matter comprised of atoms arranged in a predictable pattern; a water molecule, for example, includes two atoms of hydrogen and one atom of oxygen

natural radiation – environmental radiation caused by the sun and emitted from radon within the earth; exposure to natural radiation is unavoidable

nucleus – a cell center; in a biological cell, the nucleus is home to the DNA; in a non-biological cell, the electrons orbit the nucleus in predictable patterns

panoramic radiograph – a radiograph of the complete jaw structure

penumbra (pih-NUM-bruh) – a partial shadow around an object; in dental radiography, penumbra reduces detail in the image and can be reduced by a tight focal spot

position indicator device (PID) – a device on the x-ray tubehead that aims the x-ray beam; PIDs are available in cylindrical and rectangular shapes, with rectangular shapes reducing radiation exposure

primary radiation – direct exposure to x-ray beams from their source

radiation absorbed dose (RAD) – a unit for measuring the dose of absorbed radiation; 100 RAD = 1 Gy

radiolucent (ray-dee-oh-LOO-sunt) – the quality of being penetrable by x-rays; radiolucent objects show up as dark areas on a radiograph

radiopaque (ray-dee-oh-PAKE) – the quality of being impenetrable by x-rays; radiopaque objects absorb x-ray energy and show up as lighter areas on a radiograph

radiosensitive – the quality of being sensitive to radiation; radiosensitivity of different organs varies, with reproductive organs, the thyroid gland, and non-specialized cells being more radiosensitive than other kinds of cells

roentgen (RENT-gen) – a unit of measure for ionizing radiation, named after the discoverer of x-rays, Dr. Wilhelm Roentgen; one roentgen is the amount of radiation needed to ionize one cubic centimeter of dry air

roentgen equivalent man (REM) – a unit for measuring how much radiation was actually absorbed in a human; REM varies based on the kind of radiation and how easily it is absorbed into tissue; 100 REM = 1 Sv

scatter radiation – radiation caused when the primary radiation beam bounces off obstructing objects, such as bones and tissues; scatter radiation is weaker than primary radiation

secondary radiation – radiation that has been deflected or leaked from a source other than the primary source; scatter radiation is a form of secondary radiation

somatic (soh-MAT-ik) cells – nonreproductive cells that contain 46 chromosomes and are present in tissues, organs, and other biological structures

thermoluminescent (thur-moh-loo-muh-NES-unt) device (TLD) – a device worn by employees in dental offices that measures radiation exposure; thermoluminescent devices emit light energy when exposed to radiation and are very accurate measures of exposure

thyroid collar – a protective device worn by patients during radiography to protect the thyroid gland in the neck; thyroid collars are made from lead and can be either separate devices or incorporated into a lead apron

tubehead – the portion of the x-ray unit containing the x-ray tube, collimator, and PID, where x-rays are actually generated

wavelength – in the electromagnetic spectrum, a measure of the length of each wave of energy; the shorter the wavelength, the more penetrating and higher energy the wave; x-rays have a very short wavelength and are very penetrating, high-energy waves

x-ray tube – the portion of the dental x-ray unit where the x-rays are generated; a vacuum tube containing the anode and cathode; x-ray beams are directed from the x-ray tube, through the PID, and toward the patient

Introduction

Understanding dental radiography, including the equipment and films used in the process, is essential for dental assistants. Dental radiographs are indispensable tools used to diagnose a wide variety of conditions that often cannot be seen with the naked eye. Most dental offices recommend that patients receive regular dental radiographs to ensure healthy teeth and gingival tissue. Dental radiographs enable dentists to:

- Locate dental caries
- Evaluate bone formation and growth
- Track a patient's health over time
- Evaluate bone loss
- Aid in forensic identification

However, dental radiographs, like all radiographs, use ionizing radiation to capture images of bones and internal structures. Overexposure to this form of energy may cause long-term detrimental effects. In fact, many of the pioneers of dental radiographs died from radiation exposure. Today, the industry has developed detailed safety protocols to protect those who work in dental offices and their patients.

History of Radiology

The world's first x-ray was captured in 1895 by Wilhelm Conrad Roentgen. Roentgen, a professor of physics at the University of Wurzberg in Germany, had been experimenting with cathode rays. These rays produced streams of electrons. He was using a kind of cathode tube called the **Hittorf-Crookes tube**, which consisted of a glass vacuum chamber with electrodes at either end. When electricity was passed through the tube, a stream of visible light was observed. Roentgen installed special fluorescent screens near the cathode tube to study the properties of this light. These screens glowed when exposed to the cathode tube light.

In late 1895, Roentgen was working in a darkened laboratory when he made a startling observation. Although the visible rays in the cathode tube could not travel far from the device itself, a number of fluorescent screens were glowing even though they were located on a table several feet away. He realized that the cathode tube must be emitting some kind of unknown ray. He called it an x-ray, using the common mathematic variable x for unknown.

Roentgen shifted the focus of his experiments to these unusual rays. He learned they could travel further than cathode tube rays, and he switched from a fluorescent screen to photographic film. He quickly learned that he could capture shadow images of objects by placing objects between the rays and the photographic film. The intensity of these images depended on the density of the object. Wood, for example, caused a darker image than metal because metal blocked the rays.

On November 8, 1895, he placed his wife Berta's hand on the photographic plate and exposed it to 15 minutes of x-ray. The resulting image showed the bones in her hand, which were denser than the surrounding soft tissue. This was the world's first x-ray (Figure 29-1).

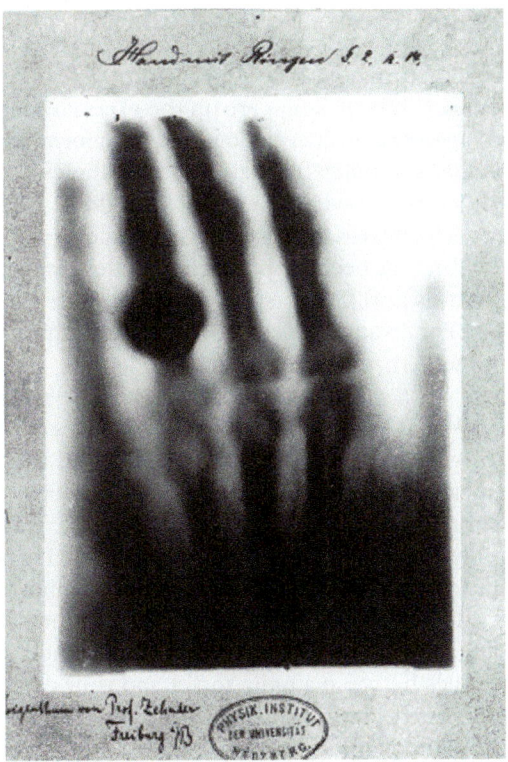

Figure 29–1 **Early x-ray**. Wilhelm Roentgen took an x-ray of his wife's hand in 1895. He presented this print of the x-ray to a colleague in early 1896.

In 1901, Roentgen's discovery would earn him the first Nobel Prize ever awarded in physics and revolutionize the practice of medicine. X-rays were the first noninvasive technology that allowed physicians to glimpse inside the human body. For many years afterward, x-rays were known as "roentgen rays" and radiographs were called "roentgenographs."

Interestingly, however, Roentgen's work was not universally recognized at first. In Victorian England, he was originally vilified for having created a machine that could see through women's dresses.

The Development of Dental Radiographs

Radiography was applied almost immediately to dentistry. In 1895, the same year Roentgen captured the first radiograph image, Dr. Otto Walkoff inserted a small glass plate coated with photographic emulsion and rubber into his own mouth and subjected himself to 25 minutes of x-ray exposure. Again that same year, a physician in New York captured a dental radiograph from a skull.

A year later, in 1896, Dr. C. Edmond Kells incorporated dental radiographs into his practice. He was the first dentist in the United States to take pictures of the oral cavity with an x-ray machine. Dr. Kells used himself to experiment on, holding his hands in front of the x-ray tube until he could see the bones in his own hand. No one at the time was aware of the dangers of prolonged x-ray exposure, and Kells paid a steep price for his experiments. His hands

soon developed cancerous lesions, and he first lost three fingers, then his hand, and finally his arm. In 1928, at the age of 72, Kells committed suicide rather than face an additional surgical amputation scheduled for the next morning.

Highlights in the development of dental radiographs include:

- In 1896, Dr. William Rollins of Boston, Massachusetts, invented an early dental x-ray unit. This unit still relied on a cathode ray tube. Like other early pioneers, Dr. Rollins suffered radiation burns and recommended lead shielding for the cathode tube and the patient.
- In 1913, Dr. Frank Van Woert in New York was among the first to use the new Kodak dental film as opposed to glass plates. That same year, Dr. William D. Coolidge invented a hot cathode x-ray tube that emitted variable x-rays and did not rely on residual gas, instead relying on a filament inside the tube. This general principle is still in use today.
- In 1920, Frank McCormack developed the right-angle technique, which was further developed by Gordon M. Fitzgerald and William J. Updegrave. Together, this group is credited with developing the long cone technique and designing devices that helped dentists place and aim x-rays. The long cone was later replaced by open-ended cylinders and rectangular tubes, which are more accurate yet.
- In 1923, the Victor X-Ray Corporation (later General Electric Corporation) developed an x-ray machine based on the Coolidge cathode ray that was cooled by oil immersion.

Dental Facts

The first dental radiology textbook was introduced in 1925. It was titled *Elementary and Dental Radiology*, by Professor Howard Riley Raper of Indiana Dental College. Professor Raper also introduced the bite-wing radiograph.

Types of Dental Radiographs Used Today

Over the past few decades, dental radiographs have continued to advance in safety and technology. Panoramic radiographs are now achieved using multiple exposures from very specific angles. Modern x-ray film has dramatically reduced the amount of exposure time for patients. And in 1987, digital imaging was introduced. Digital images have a number of advantages. They do not require film processing, and images are obtained instantly and can be easily incorporated into paperless charts or e-mailed to specialists or insurance companies. Finally, they make chairside consultations easier because the dentist is able to quickly and simply show the patient areas of concern.

Radiation Physics

To understand why x-rays work, and why they are dangerous, it is important to understand some basic physics. The universe is broadly made up of **matter** and **energy**. X-rays are a form of energy that interacts with, and alters, matter. Matter is defined as an object that has form and shape and occupies space. Stones, bones, water, metal—these are all examples of matter. Matter can range from the very large, like planets or moons, to the very small subatomic particles that scientists study.

Structure of Atoms

All matter is composed of basic building blocks called **molecules**. Chemically speaking, a molecule is the smallest unit of any matter that still retains the qualities of that substance. The water molecule, for instance, contains hydrogen and oxygen (Figure 29-2). Individually, hydrogen and oxygen do not possess the characteristics of water. Combined, however, they form a water molecule.

Molecules themselves are made up of smaller units called **atoms** (Figure 29-2). In the example above, the water molecule is made up of two atoms of hydrogen (H) and one atom of oxygen (O), all linked together. This is expressed as the familiar H_2O. Chemically speaking, atoms are made up of a central **nucleus** (containing both protons, which have a positive charge, and neutrons, which have no charge) around which **electrons** (which have a negative charge) orbit like planets in a solar system—meaning that they orbit the nucleus in a predictable and stable pattern.

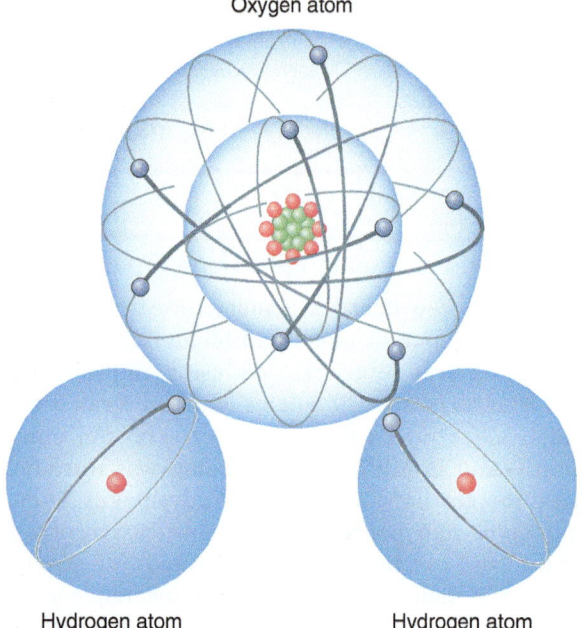

Oxygen atom

Hydrogen atom   Hydrogen atom

Figure 29–2 Molecules and atoms. Water molecules are composed of two atoms of hydrogen and one atom of oxygen.

Forms and Properties of Radiation

As opposed to matter, x-rays are a form of energy. Like light, sound, and heat, x-rays are on the **electromagnetic energy spectrum**. Energy does not have form or shape, but it follows predictable patterns nonetheless. Electromagnetic energy travels in straight lines from its source in waves. The waves themselves are made up of atoms that are vibrating because of the interaction with energy. Energy travels at different speeds through different kinds of atoms. For example, heat energy travels much faster through metal than it does through wood.

Energy waves are measured by their **wavelength** (Figure 29-3). If you picture a wave, with its **crests** and valleys, a wavelength is the distance between the crests. When measuring electromagnetic energy, shorter, faster waves carry more energy. For example, radio waves are low-energy waves with a very long wavelength. This means that radio waves are easily deflected from solid objects. That is why it takes very powerful transmitters to send weak radio waves even a relatively short distance, such as the few miles between a radio tower and your car.

By contrast, x-rays are considered very high-energy waves. Unlike visible light, radio waves, and heat energy, x-rays cannot be seen, heard, or felt. But they are actually much more powerful. Their natural energy enables them to easily penetrate bone and other objects.

Ionization

When an x-ray passes through matter, it carries enough energy to interact with the atoms of the matter itself. Once again, consider the example of an oxygen molecule, with its eight electrons orbiting a nucleus in a predictable and stable pattern. These electrons are held in place by a force similar to gravity known as electron binding energy. However, the power of this force varies from atom to atom. If a sufficiently strong energy force interacts with the molecule, it is possible to knock an electron out of its orbit.

These electrons are then considered free-floating, and they will immediately search for a new atom to bind to. In this way, atoms can gain or lose electrons. This process is

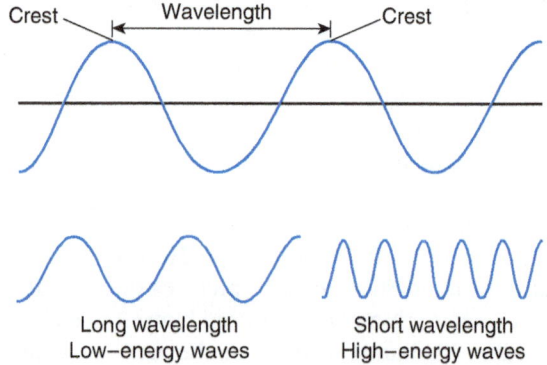

Crest   Wavelength   Crest

Long wavelength   Short wavelength
Low–energy waves   High–energy waves

Figure 29–3 Wavelengths are measured from crest to crest. Low-energy waves, such as radiowaves, have a very long wavelength. High-energy waves, such as x-rays, have short wavelengths.

known as **ionization**. An atom that has gained or lost an electron is known as an **ion**. Ions are often unstable and can interact with other atoms, binding to them and changing the molecule structure.

Radiation Biology

Almost immediately after discovering radiation, scientists began to suspect that it had negative effects on the human body. After the discovery of x-rays, Thomas Edison began experimenting with x-rays in New Jersey. In fact, one of Edison's assistants was the first person to die from radiation exposure, and Edison himself observed redness around his eyes after experiments. Eventually, Edison developed a lifelong fear of radiation.

Direct and indirect effects of radiation can range from headache and lowered immune response to nausea, hair loss, and cancer. Although the radiation produced in the tubehead is chiefly Bremsstrahlung radiation (which is emitted when electrons rapidly change direction, specifically while decelerating), the tubehead also emits minor characteristic radiation, or low-level radiation produced in a unique form by each element.

Radiation Effects on Cells and Tissues

Radiation causes biological damage through ionization. X-rays are frequently called ionizing radiation because of their ability to interact with, and change, atoms. Thus, x-rays are capable of changing the molecular structure of an organ. This can happen in a number of ways, depending on which cell was affected and how much radiation it was exposed to.

Somatic and Genetic Effects

The human body is made up of hundreds of kinds of cells. Cells in the body include blood, muscle, and bone cells, as well as many others. Biological cells are unique and complicated structures (Figure 29-4). They are surrounded by a semipermeable cell wall that allows some substances to pass through, into the cell itself. Within the cell, there are structures that produce energy to keep the cell alive, called **mitochondria**, and a cell nucleus that acts as the cell's control center. At the heart of the nucleus is the DNA. DNA is organized into long chains called **chromosomes**. These chromosomes contain the unique genetic blueprint for every individual.

Normal cells have a limited lifespan. New cells are first formed by division, just like the original fertilized egg, which divides rapidly. These new cells perform their duty, whatever it may be, and then depending on their type, they either die or divide again. Cell death is referred to as **cell senescence**. Cell division is known as **mitosis**.

Cells are divided into two groups:

- **Somatic cells**. These cells make up the organs and tissues of an organism, such as lungs, blood, bone, and skin

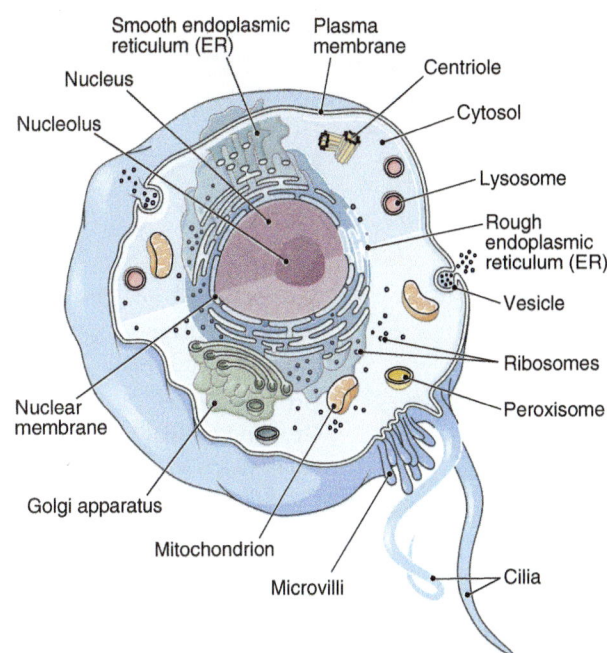

Figure 29–4 Biological cell.

cells—essentially all body cells except for reproductive cells. A normal somatic cell has 46 chromosomes.
- **Genetic cells**. Sometimes called germ cells, these cells are related to reproduction. Egg cells and sperm cells are genetic cells. Genetic cells carry only 23 chromosomes.

At high levels or prolonged exposure, x-rays cause immediate cell death, no matter what kind of cell. At lower levels or reduced exposure, the effect on cells, and therefore health, depends on the cell type. Radiation exposure can cause damage to the DNA located within somatic cells. Cell division may be prevented or compromised, resulting in damage to the organism.

In contrast, genetic cells experience damage to the chromosomes carried within the cells. The exposed individual might suffer somatic effects or might appear to be in perfect health. However, should these damaged germ cells be used to reproduce, the damage will be passed onto the offspring. Genetic mutations can cause potentially serious conditions in children of people exposed to radiation.

Radiosensitive Organs

Just like different cells react differently to radiation exposure, not all organs are affected the same way. Some organs are less susceptible to damage from radiation than others. Scientists say these organs are less **radiosensitive**. Highly radiosensitive organs, on the other hand, are more easily damaged by radiation. A number of factors influence whether an organ is radiosensitive or not, including:

- *Rate of cell division*. Some cells reproduce and replace themselves more quickly than others. Cells that divide more frequently, such as lung cells and the outermost

TABLE 29-1 Radiation Sensitivity of Tissues and Organs

Low	Liver
	Kidney
	Muscle
	Nerve
Moderately low	Salivary gland
	Mature bone
	Mature cartilage
	Thyroid gland tissue
Moderate	Growing bone
	Growing cartilage
	Small vasculature
	Connective tissue
	Optic lens
Moderately high	Oral mucosa
	Skin
High	Bone marrow
	Reproductive cell
	Intestine
	Lymphoid tissue

layer of skin cells, which slough off regularly, are more vulnerable to radiation exposure.

- *Immature cells.* This includes embryonic cells. Special consideration is always given to exposing pregnant women to x-ray radiation because of potential damage to the babies they are carrying. Embryos exposed to radiation may be born with congenital birth defects or malformations or may die. Because of this risk, x-rays are only administered to pregnant women if it is medically necessary.
- *Non-specialized cells.* Cells that are less specialized are more sensitive to radiation.

In dental practice, the most sensitive organ of concern is the thyroid gland. Located in the neck area, this gland has a number of important functions, including regulating metabolism. To protect the thyroid gland, all patients should wear lead thyroid collars during x-rays, as well as the lead body aprons that protect reproductive cells and internal organs. The lens of the eye is also more sensitive to radiation, but today's x-ray devices allow for very precise control of the weakest x-ray beam possible (see Limiting Exposure, below), so the eye should not be exposed.

Table 29-1 summarizes radiosensitivity levels of different organs.

Radiation Exposure

Radiation exposure is measured in units known as **roentgens** (R). This measure was established in 1937 by the International Committee for Radiological Units. A roentgen is the amount of radiation it takes to produce 1 electrostatic unit of electricity in one cubic centimeter of air. In other words, a roentgen measures how much radiation is necessary to alter the air, or ionize it, and produce an electric charge.

Other terms used with measuring radiation include:

- *RAD, or radiation absorbed dose.* Also known as a gray (Gy), this unit is used to measure how much actual radiation was absorbed by an object or substance. It is a measure of dose.
- *REM, or roentgen equivalent man.* This is a measure of how much radiation was actually absorbed in a human, taking into account its biological effects. Different kinds of radiation have different REM numbers, depending on how easily they are absorbed into the human body. This number is known as the quality factor, or QF. To determine risk, scientists multiply the QF by the RAD, so REM = QF × RAD.

Table 29-2 lists the terms used to measure radiation and their metric equivalents. Both RAD and REM generally have been replaced by their metric equivalent.

Radiation exposure is not always damaging. In fact, each of us is exposed to a certain amount of environmental radiation on a daily basis. This kind of radiation is often referred to as **natural radiation.** The sun emits radioactive energy, and radiation is emitted from the earth in the form of radon. In most cases, cells can recover from whatever damage has been caused by mild exposure to natural radiation.

However, damage occurs when individuals are either exposed to high levels of radiation suddenly (e.g., acute exposure) or exposed to low levels of radiation over a very long time (e.g., chronic exposure). Acute exposure can cause immediate cell death. However, dental x-rays do not use high levels of radiation, so acute exposure is less of a concern.

Chronic exposure is a greater concern, for both patients and dental office workers. However, by following proper radiation safety procedures, the risk of harm from chronic exposure can be dramatically reduced. For more information, see Chapter 15, Safety Regulations.

Finally, radiation exposure is cumulative. That is, cell damage slowly builds up before the effects are noticed.

TABLE 29-2 Measuring Radiation

STANDARD	METRIC, OR SYSTEM INTERNATIONALE (SI)
Roentgen (R) (measures exposure)	Coulomb per kilogram (c/kg) (1 c/kg = 3.88 × 10R)
RAD (measures dose)	Gray (Gy) (1 Gy = 100 RADs)
REM (measures dose equivalent in humans)	Sievert (Sv) (1 Sv = 100 REMs)

This is why it frequently takes many years for people who live in very sunny areas to get skin cancer. The damage to their rapidly dividing skin cells builds up over time, and eventually, a cancerous lesion is formed.

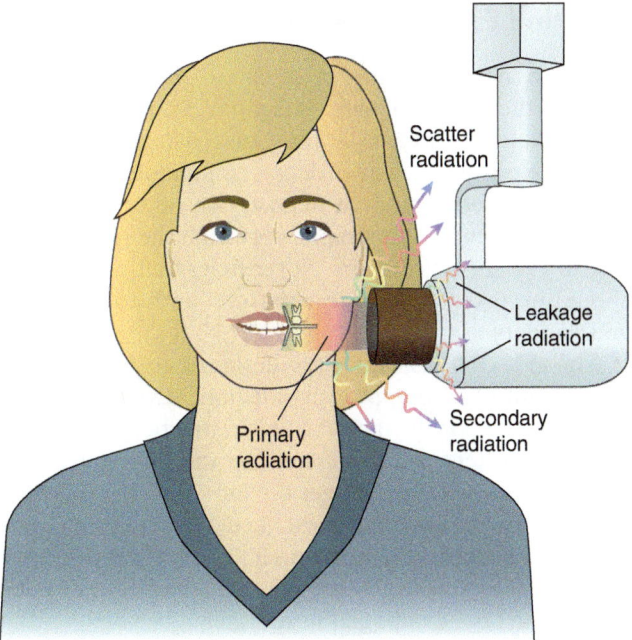

Figure 29–5 Types of radiation.

CHECKPOINTS

29-1 Who took the first radiograph?

29-2 What year was the first dental radiograph taken?

29-3 When was digital imaging introduced?

29-4 Where do x-rays reside on the electromagnetic energy spectrum? What qualities do they possess?

29-5 Through what process does radiation damage biological tissues?

29-6 Name three kinds of cells that are very radiosensitive.

29-7 What does RAD stand for?

Radiation Safety

Dental radiographs are an essential tool in the modern dentist's office, but this kind of energy must be handled carefully to protect both the employees in the office and the patients.

Types of Radiation

X-rays are classified by the way they behave after they have left the x-ray tube. There are several recognized kinds of radiation (Figure 29-5):

- **Primary radiation**: These are x-rays that came directly from the x-ray tube where they are generated. These are high-energy, short-wavelength beams that travel in a straight line from their source. In practice, this is often referred to as the useful beam.
- **Secondary radiation**: This is created when the x-ray beam interacts with another substance, in this case, the patient's tissues. Secondary radiation has less energy and longer wavelengths than primary radiation. It is not considered useful because it creates foggy or cloudy dental radiographs.
- **Scatter radiation**: Scatter radiation is a form of secondary radiation, and the terms are sometimes used interchangeably. This occurs when the radiation beam is deflected by a substance; it scatters in all directions. Scatter radiation has longer wavelengths and less energy than primary radiation, but it is dangerous to operators. To avoid scatter radiation, operators must stand six feet

away from the patient, or remain behind some kind of shielding during exposure.
- **Leakage radiation**: This form of radiation escapes from the x-ray unit itself. It is not useful and potentially harmful. Dental x-ray units should be inspected regularly to make sure the device is not leaking radiation.

Finally, the effects of radiation exposure are cumulative, meaning they add up over time. The higher the dose, the more serious the effect. This is why people who live in very sunny areas and spend a lot of time outdoors eventually develop rough, brown skin. This is the same reason that people who suffer from serious sunburns as teenagers are more likely to develop skin cancer in adulthood. The period between radiation exposure and its biological effect is known as the **latent period**.

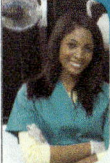

Voice of Experience

Since I've been working in dental offices, I've noticed that many more people show up with concerns about radiation exposure than ever before. I certainly understand their concern, as no one wants more radiation than necessary! So whenever possible, I always take time to explain that dental x-rays are very safe, and that we have many layers of safety devices that reduce exposure significantly, especially compared with other x-ray procedures, like CT scans. I also carefully explain the legal issues surrounding dental x-rays, including all the risks and benefits, and make sure they understand the concept of informed consent. Ultimately, though, dental x-rays are an invaluable tool to help us diagnose many conditions while they're still easily treatable, so I always try to reassure patients that we only take x-rays when it's medically necessary, and we do everything we can to reduce their exposure to the lowest level possible.

Limiting Exposure—The ALARA Concept

Although not all forms of radiation are equally dangerous, there is no safe radiation. Even low-energy, long-wavelength radiation can cause damage with prolonged exposure. However, dental radiographs are also an invaluable tool in modern dentistry. In other words, the benefits of dental radiographs outweigh the risks, so the risk to benefit ratio is low. Nevertheless, all precautions should be taken to reduce exposure, both to operators and patients.

The **ALARA** concept was designed to help people understand how to approach radiation. ALARA stands for "as low as reasonably achievable." In practice, this means exposing patients and operators to the lowest possible dose of radiation that will get the job done. Dental radiographs should never be prescribed on a routine basis. Their use should be based on clinical need. Today, most state regulatory agencies require documentation of need rather than taking radiographs routinely.

Maximum Permissible Dose

In contrast to ALARA, which deals with the smallest exposure to accomplish the task, the **maximum permissible dose** (MPD) is concerned with how much radiation is safe. This concept was developed by the National Council on Radiation Protection and Measurements (NCRP). MPD is defined as the maximum dose equivalent that a body is permitted to receive in a specified period of time without causing any damage. Remember that dose equivalent, or REM, measures the biological effects of a particular dose of radiation.

Protective Equipment for Patients

The dental x-ray unit itself has built-in safety features that make it possible to precisely control and shield the x-ray. See the section Dental X-Ray Units later in this chapter for a complete discussion of these features.

A number of items are used to protect patients from unnecessary radiation exposure. There are also different considerations to keep in mind when dealing with pediatric and pregnant patients. The most important items used to limit exposure include:

- **Lead apron** (Figure 29-6). Radiation cannot penetrate lead, so the lead apron is a standard safety feature when dental radiographs are obtained. Lead aprons are made from 0.25 mm lead or lead-equivalent materials. The lead apron should cover the patient completely from the neck to the upper legs to protect from scatter radiation. It is important that the reproductive area is covered because this region is home to radiosensitive genetic cells. Use of a lead apron may be mandatory, depending on state law.
- **Thyroid collar** (Figure 29-6). The thyroid gland is located in the neck, and it is particularly sensitive to

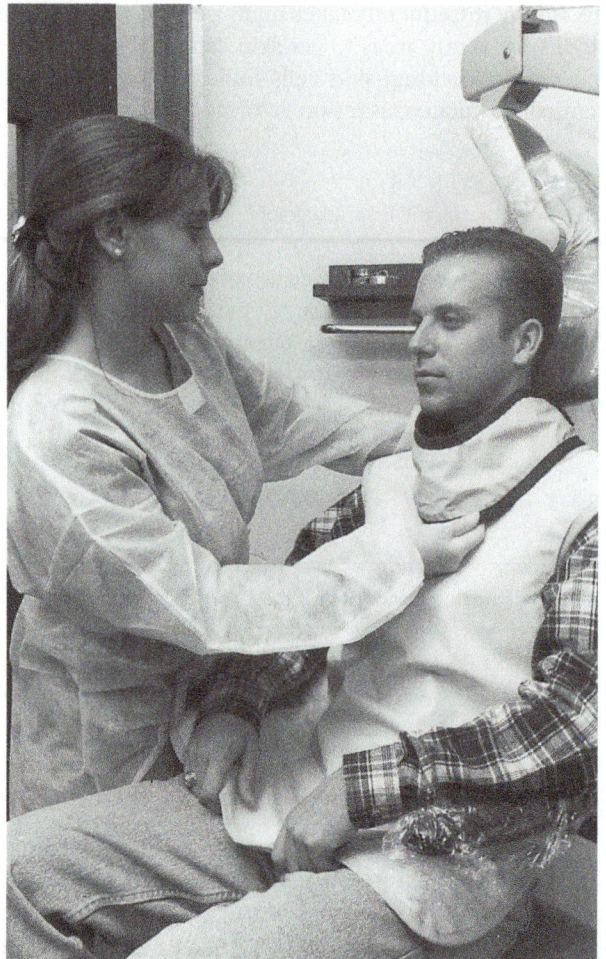

Figure 29–6 Lead apron and thyroid collar.

radiation. Thyroid collars are flexible lead shields that wrap around the patient's neck and protect the thyroid gland from scatter radiation. Thyroid shields may be built into the lead apron, or they may be separate devices. If patients are concerned, it is helpful to mention this is a safety precaution. Radiation exposure has been known to cause thyroid disease, but not at the low levels used in dental radiographs.

- **Film-holding devices** (Figure 29-7). These devices hold the film in place in the patient's mouth. Film holders can be used with external aiming devices that allow the operator to take more precise pictures. This is in keeping with the ALARA concept because patients do not have to hold the film in place with their fingers, which would expose their fingers, and it reduces the number of exposures due to misalignment.

Lead aprons should be worn every time a radiograph is taken. It is important to note that lead aprons should never be folded in storage, creased, or cut. Any break in the lead shielding will allow radiation to break the protective barrier and seep through to the patient below. The apron therefore should be hung on apron hooks designed to keep the apron straight, or hung over a towel bar.

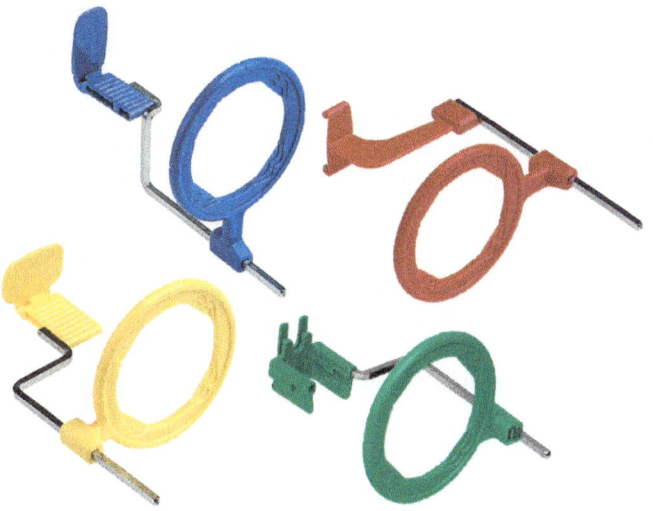

Figure 29–7 Film-holding devices.

Pregnant and Pediatric Patients

Among pregnant women, dental radiographs can be an alarming idea. Many pregnant women have heard that x-rays should be avoided, and popular pregnancy books often counsel pregnant women to avoid x-rays. A patient's concerns over dental radiographs should always be taken seriously, and if it is possible to avoid radiographs on pregnant patients, this may be preferable for many dentists.

However, both the American Dental Association (ADA) and the U.S. Food and Drug Administration (FDA) say that dental radiographs are safe for pregnant women if precautions are taken. During the radiograph procedure, the lead apron should extend below the pelvic region to provide protection to the mother's reproductive organs and the fetus. When the apron is applied correctly, studies have shown that radiation exposure is close to zero.

Children, too, can be safely radiographed as long as the safety measures are followed. If a child is uncooperative and will not stay still or will not hold the film still, the child can be seated on a parent's lap during the radiograph. Both parent and child should be covered with lead aprons, and the parent can manually hold the film in place. The damage to the parent is minimized because it is a single exposure.

Protective Equipment for Operators

The risk for x-ray operators is somewhat different than the risk for patients, as x-ray operators are not exposed to the primary radiation. However, repeated use of x-rays raises the risk of cumulative, long-term exposure to scatter or secondary radiation, and poorly sealed x-ray units can expose assistants to leakage radiation. There are three important factors of operator safety:

- Time. Radiation exposure is cumulative, even at low doses. So it is very important for operators to limit their exposure whenever possible. This means the operator should never try to stabilize patients or the x-ray device manually. If the tubehead is drifting, for example, the

operator should discontinue that series of radiographs and stop using that machine until it can be serviced. An x-ray tube should never be held manually because leaked radiation can dramatically increase exposure. Similarly, if patients are difficult to stabilize, including young children, the operator should not volunteer to hold them in place during the radiograph; a guardian can do so. Finally, if the operator is having trouble with film-holding devices, manually holding the film in place should not be an acceptable option. Instead, the operator should work with different-sized or shaped devices or use a different technique to achieve the same results.

- Shielding. Just as the patient is shielded with a lead apron, the operator should take care to avoid radiation exposure. Most dentist's offices are built with some form of structural shielding where the operator can take refuge during exposure. Structural shielding includes walls made from cinderblock, thick drywall, steel, or even lead. The exposure button is permanently mounted behind this protective barrier.

- Distance. If shielding is not an option—for example, in an older practice with open bays—the operator should remain as far away as possible from the x-ray unit. Ideally, *the operator should stand at least 6 feet away,* behind the bulkiest part of the patient's head, and between 90 degrees and 135 degrees out of the primary beam. This will reduce exposure to scatter radiation from the patient's head. Additionally, x-rays lose strength and energy with distance.

From the Dentist's Perspective

In my office, it's important that every dental assistant is licensed and knowledgeable—and not just because it happens to be state law here. The office functions better, and I have more confidence in my assistants, when I know that they have received specialized training in the use, safety issues, and benefits of dental radiographs. As a dentist, it's my responsibility to make sure everyone is current with training and licensure. And it's up to my assistants to bring that knowledge to the practice every day, to the benefit of our patients and themselves.

Determining Radiographic Exposure

Dental radiographs are an important part of modern dentistry, but they should not be prescribed on a routine basis. The decision to take a set of dental radiographs should be guided by clinical need. This is consistent with the ALARA concept, which states that patients should be exposed to the lowest possible radiation dose.

There will, however, be times when dental radiographs are essential tools. The ADA issued guidelines in 2004 to guide dental offices on patient selection (see Table 29-3). Before any radiographs are ordered, a complete oral examination should be conducted and a patient history should be taken, including any medical conditions as well as previous exposure to x-rays. This information should weigh into the decision to prescribe x-ray imaging.

TABLE 29-3   ADA Indications for Dental Radiographs

Positive Historical Findings	Previous periodontal disease History of pain or trauma Family history of dental anomalies Postoperative evaluation Remineralization monitoring Implants or evaluation for implants
Positive Clinical Signs/Symptoms	Evidence of periodontal disease Large or deep restorations Deep lesions Malposed or clinically impacted teeth Swelling Facial or dental trauma Sinus fistula, or tract Sinus pathology Growth abnormalities Oral involvement in systemic disease Positive neurologic findings in head or neck Evidence of foreign objects Pain in temporomandibular joint Facial asymmetry Abutment teeth for fixed or removable partial prosthesis Bleeding Sensitivity of teeth Unusual eruption, spacing, or migration of teeth Unusual tooth morphology, calcification, or color Unexplained absence of teeth Clinical erosion
Increased Risk of Dental Caries	High level of caries or demineralization History of recurrent caries Higher titers of carcinogenic bacteria Existing restoration of poor quality Poor oral hygiene Inadequate fluoride exposure Prolonged nursing (bottle or breast) High sucrose content in diet Poor family dental health Enamel defects (developmental or acquired) Disability (developmental or acquired) Xerostomia Genetic abnormality of teeth Many multisurface restorations Chemo/radiation therapy Eating disorders Drug/alcohol abuse Irregular dental care

From: American Dental Association, U.S. Food & Drug Administration. The Selection of Patients for Dental Radiograph Examinations. Document created November 2004. Available on www.ada.org.

Once the decision has been made to prescribe radiographs, the following practices should be used to reduce overall exposure:

- The operator should use the fastest film possible
- The operator should use proper film exposure and processing techniques
- The patient should be protected with a lead apron and thyroid collar (see Protective Equipment for Patients above)

Occupational Exposure

Government agencies have set guidelines for occupational radiation exposure. According to the NCRP guidelines, the maximum permissible dose (MPD) for occupational exposure to radiation is 0.05 Sv (50 mSv, or 5.0 REMs) per year. For people who are not exposed to radiation at work, or pregnant women, the MPD is 0.001 Sv (0.1 REM) per year.

Although these guidelines are widely accepted, alternative guidelines have been issued by the International Commission of Radiological Protection. This limit for occupational exposure has been set at 20 mSv (2.0 REMs) per year.

Check Your Ethics

Although there are many indications for dental radiography (see Table 29-3), radiographs should never be prescribed on a routine basis. If a patient asks for radiographs, however, what is the proper course of action?

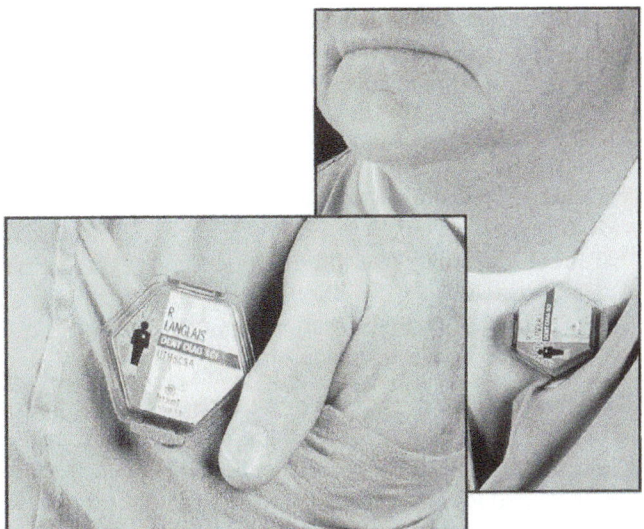

Figure 29–8 **Thermoluminescent device (TLD).** For monitoring radiation exposure.

Radiation Monitoring

Because radiation is invisible and odorless, it is important to use the appropriate monitoring devices to detect unwanted radiation. There are a few approaches to monitoring radiation, including area monitoring, personnel monitoring, and equipment monitoring.

Area monitoring is typically conducted by special companies that are equipped to detect radiation in the dental operatory and to determine if radiation is passing through screening enclosures.

Personnel Monitoring

Only a few states mandate personnel monitoring for radiation exposure, but more and more dentists are voluntarily adopting measures to safeguard their employees. Remember that personnel monitoring devices do not actually protect an operator from radiation exposure. They merely alert the operator that he or she has been exposed to radiation. A number of devices are available, and the various devices measure different factors. Some will only tell if radiation exposure had occurred, some will tell what kind of radiation exposure has occurred, and some will measure both the kind and the dose.

Radiation monitoring for personnel is often contracted out by the dental office. An outside firm provides the devices and analyzes them off-site, then provides a report to the office about the level of radiation exposure in the office.

Personnel monitoring devices include:

■ The **film badge**. This is the most common device in use. This device contains a piece of film similar to a dental radiograph film, along with the employee's name and an ID number. The same technology is also used to make rings and bracelets for employees whose hands might be exposed to radiation. Film badges are typically worn for a month before being returned to the monitoring service. Film badges should not be worn outside the office or into strong sunlight, as this will skew the results of the monitoring. Film badges only record exposure to the part of the region of the body where the badge is located.

■ The **thermoluminescent device** (TLD) (Figure 29-8). Sometimes called a thermoluminescent dosimeter, this device is also worn as a badge. These devices are worn for three months before they are returned to the monitoring company. TLDs are made with special crystals, usually lithium fluoride, that are sensitive to radioactive energy. When exposed to radiation, they heat up and emit visible light. The brighter the light, the greater the exposure.

Equipment Monitoring

Dental x-ray units are machines, and like any other machines, they are subject to breaking down or working improperly. In this case, however, a leakage from the x-ray tube can cause radiation exposure, so it is very important that machines are maintained in top operating shape.

In 1974, the U.S. government established the Federal Performance Standard for Diagnostic X-Ray Equipment. This law required certain safety features on every dental x-ray unit sold in the United States. For more information, see the section on Safety Devices later in this chapter.

Rules for the inspection and monitoring of existing dental x-ray machines is largely left to the states, so different standards exist from state to state. In some cases, dental x-ray registration and inspection is included in the state's licensing procedures. Dental x-ray units should also be calibrated at least annually. This requires the services of a specialized technician, who makes sure the machine is operating correctly and producing high-quality radiographs.

The American Academy of Oral and Maxillofacial Radiology further recommends annual testing of dental x-ray machines. Tests should cover the following eight elements:

- X-ray output
- Focal spot size
- Collimation-beam alignment
- Half-value layer (HVL)
- Tubehead stability test
- Timer test
- Milliamperage test (see section on Control Panel)
- Kilovoltage test (see section on Control Panel)

These tests can be performed by a dentist, a dental hygienist, a dental assistant, or a service representative from the manufacturer. The tests require radiography film, testing materials, and logs to record results. Instructions on how to conduct these tests can be found in a pamphlet called *Quality Control Tests for Dental Radiography,* published by the Eastman Kodak Company, Rochester, New York (Kodak Publication No. ME-504a). This pamphlet can be located online.

Responsibilities for Safety

Responsibility for maintaining dental x-ray safety is spread among equipment manufacturers, dentists, dental assistants, and patients.

Equipment Manufacturer

Since 1974, the federal government has mandated certain safety features on dental x-ray units. These include:

- The unit must have a "dead man" switch. This switch is a separate control that cuts electricity to the machine after a preset time when the switch is released. This prevents the machine from continuing to run if the switch malfunctions.
- The PID must be lead-lined; the x-ray tube must be sealed in an oil-immersion casing.
- The **control panel** must have displays for the **kilovolts** (kV), **milliamperage** (mA), and impulses per exposure time.
- The unit must be outfitted with a collimator that fits over the opening where the x-ray beam emerges from the machine. The collimator must be made from lead, and the opening must not be more than 2.75 inches in diameter.
- Any unit that operates at a higher level than 70 kV must have aluminum filtration of 2.5 mm built into its head. Total filtration of 1.5 mm is required for units that operate at 70 kV or less.

Dentist

The dentist's responsibilities include the following:

- The dentist is responsible for the installation and maintenance of the equipment in the office, including

x-ray units. This includes the design of the operatory and the placement of shielding walls to protect x-ray unit operators. Similarly, the dentist is responsible for making sure the x-ray unit is calibrated, inspected, and tested regularly. In some states, this is mandated by law.
- The dentist is responsible to patients and should only prescribe radiographs when it is clinically necessary. Radiographs should not be part of the routine dental exam; rather, the dentist should follow the guidelines set forth by the ADA.
- The dentist is responsible for having x-ray machines repaired promptly if necessary and discontinuing the use of broken or leaking machines.
- The dentist is responsible for providing the appropriate prescription for patient exposure and evaluating radiographs.

Dental Assistant

The dentist assistant's responsibilities include the following:

- Dental assistants should be trained in radiation safety, aseptic techniques, and quality assurance.
- Dental assistants should understand radiation, understand how the dental x-ray unit works, and thoroughly understand the risks associated with radiation exposure.
- Dental assistants need to be properly educated regarding the ALARA principle and adhere to it whenever they are taking radiographs.
- Dental assistants are responsible for processing, labeling, and storing patient radiographs.

Extra Patient Care

In the early years, dental radiography could be extremely uncomfortable—and even dangerous—for patients. Fortunately, those days are gone. Today, dental radiology is safer and more comfortable for patients than ever before. Digital radiography can reduce the amount of radiation exposure by 50%, while newer film packs and sensors are thinner and more flexible, and the sensor edges are more rounded than ever. Film-holding devices are also being designed to make x-rays more comfortable. And finally, there are steps dental assistants can take to make radiography even easier. Simple breathing techniques can relax patients, and topical anesthetic eliminates even mild discomfort during the radiographs.

Patient

Patients are responsible for communicating their complete medical history and status to the dental office. This includes pregnancies, previous radiographs, systemic diseases that might be affected by exposure to radiation, and any other conditions that might affect the dentist's clinical judgment.

Legal Issues in Dental Radiography

A number of legal issues are involved in dental radiography, ranging from the manufacture of the dental x-ray unit to interactions with patients and privacy laws.

In 1974, the U.S. government established the Federal Performance Standard for Diagnostic X-Ray Equipment. This law required certain safety features on every dental x-ray unit sold in the United States. For more information, see the section on Safety Devices in this chapter.

Many states also mandate the registration and regular inspection of dental x-ray machines. Laws vary, but inspections are often required every 2 to 4 years.

In 1981, the federal government passed the Consumer-Patient Radiation Health and Safety Act, which required that states develop minimum licensing standards for x-ray operators. However, adoption of the law's provisions is voluntary, so not all states have adopted licensure. Among the states that do, people who operate dental x-ray equipment must be certified and obtain either a registered dental hygienist (RDH) or certified dental assistant (CDA) credential. Certifying bodies include the National Board of Dental Hygiene Examiners (NBDHE) and the Dental Assisting National Board (DANB). Additional state rules and examinations may also be required.

In states where licensure and certification is not required, there may be a direct supervision law. This states that an unlicensed operator can take dental radiographs, but only under the direct supervision of the dentist.

Legal Issues Concerning Patients

A dentist cannot compel a patient to undergo dental radiographs. All patients have the right to self-determination (in the case of minors, this right rests with parents or legal guardians). This means that patients have the right to refuse treatment, including radiographs. If a patient refuses radiographs, he or she should be asked to sign a release clearly stating their refusal and their understanding of its possible consequences. They should also be informed that the dentist can refuse to continue seeing them as a patient if they continue to refuse radiographs.

Before radiographs are administered, the operator or dentist should obtain informed consent. Most dental offices include consent for radiography in the general consent form the patient signs upon their initial visit to the office. Informed consent means the patient is aware of the risks of radiographs and also understands why they are being prescribed. This process is called **disclosure**. Elements of informed consent include:

- Why the radiographs are necessary (purpose)
- The benefits of the radiographs
- Possible risks associated with radiation

- Number and type of radiographs that will be taken
- Possible risks of refusing the radiographs
- Who will actually perform the procedure
- Alternative diagnostic procedures that may be applicable

Whoever provides disclosure, the supervising dentist is technically liable for the interaction and outcomes. This means the dentist can be held responsible for the actions of the x-ray operator.

Dental assistants can also be held legally responsible for their own actions. Just like dentists, they can be sued for negligence or malpractice.

After the set of dental radiographs has been obtained, they become part of the patient's dental records. Dental records are maintained by the dentist or under the supervision of the dentist. These records should include:

- A statement of the patient's informed consent
- The number and type of radiographs, including retakes
- The date the radiographs were obtained and the name of the operator
- The reason they were prescribed
- The diagnostic interpretation of the radiographs

Like all medical records, dental records are covered by federal privacy laws to protect the patient's privacy. In 1996, the federal government passed the Health Insurance Portability and Accountability Act (HIPAA). This law gives patients greater control over their own medical records, including the right to reasonable access to their records. In 2003, the federal government strengthened this law, which includes radiographs. Under these laws, radiographs are considered confidential information and should never be shown to anyone outside the dental practice without first obtaining a patient release. Patient release forms spell out clearly how the information will be used and who is allowed to see it.

Ownership of Dental Records

Finally, many patients assume they own their own dental radiographs. This is not true. The courts have decided that dental radiographs are the property of the dentist, even though the patient pays to have them taken and interpreted. These dental records can be used in malpractice and negligence court cases. Under HIPAA, however, patients should have reasonable access to their dental records. If a patient transfers to a new dental office, he or she can request that a copy of his or her radiographs be forwarded to the new office.

Dental records, including radiographs, should be carefully stored and retained indefinitely. Some sources recommend that dental records are stored for seven years after the patient ceases to be a patient of that office. However, the statute of limitations on legal action varies from state to state, and this can be a complicated question. As a result, it is prudent to store dental records forever.

✓ **CHECKPOINTS**

29-8 Which kind of radiation is most useful in dental radiography?

29-9 What does ALARA stand for?

29-10 Can pregnant women be safely radiographed?

29-11 How far should operators stand from an x-ray unit during exposure to minimize radiation exposure?

29-12 What does a thermoluminescent device detect?

29-13 Who owns dental radiographs?

Radiographic Equipment

The manufacture and design of x-ray units is standard throughout the United States. Digital units are equipped with sensors for producing digital images, but the fundamental concept behind both film-based radiography and digital radiography remains the same.

Radiograph Image Production

Radiograph images are produced through the interaction of the x-ray beam and the substance it is passing through. Modern dental x-ray units enable the operator to precisely control the characteristics of the x-ray beam. The image is created when this beam encounters tissues and structures with different densities. Organs and structures in the body are considered radiolucent or radiopaque, depending on how easily x-ray beams pass through them.

Radiolucent structures are low-density objects through which radiation beams can easily pass. These appear dark on the final radiograph as the film is exposed to greater radiation. Radiolucent structures include air, soft tissues, abscesses, decay, and dental pulp.

Radiopaque structures are ones through which radiation does not easily pass through. These images appear light on the final radiograph because the film is exposed to less radiation. Radiopaque objects include metal, tooth enamel, and dense bone.

Radiograph Image Characteristics

X-ray beams are measured in terms of their quality, quantity, and intensity (see Factors Affecting the Image). These characteristics determine the final quality of the radiograph itself. Radiographs are defined by their density, contrast, definition, magnification, and distortion. All these factors determine the quality of the final radiograph and its clinical usefulness.

- **Density**. Density is the most important factor in determining radiograph contrast. Objects that are less dense appear grey or black on the final radiograph. Radiation beams pass easily through these objects and expose the underlying film. Objects that are more dense appear light grey or white on the final radiograph. These objects absorb radiation beams, so the underlying film is not exposed.

- **Contrast**. Contrast is defined as the visible difference between objects on the radiograph. A number of factors affect contrast, including the radiograph subject, the quality of the beam, and the film itself. X-ray beams are deliberately kept as small as possible through the use of devices called collimators to prevent local scatter radiation from the patient's head. Local scatter radiation reduces contrast because it exposes all parts of the film equally. Contrast is also affected by the type of film used, the length of exposure, and the processing technique (this does not apply to digital images, which are computer generated).

- **Definition**. Definition is the degree to which objects on the radiograph are distinguishable from one another. Clear, easy-to-read radiographs have good definition. Definition is determined by geometric factors and, in traditional radiography, the film quality. There are several geometric factors that influence definition, including:

  - Focal spot size. This describes the region on the x-ray machine where electrons are converted into x-ray beams. The tighter, or smaller, the focal spot size, the smaller the **penumbra**, or partial shadow around the object to be pictured. This increases sharpness and reduces unwanted magnification.

  - Movement. Movement of any kind will reduce definition. This includes movement of the x-ray tubehead, the film, or the patient.

  - Film quality. Traditional x-ray film is coated with special crystals that respond to radiation. The larger these crystals are, the faster the film is, thus reducing radiation exposure. However, faster films with larger crystals yield less defined images. This does not apply to digital images (see below).

  - Distortion. Distortion occurs when the angle of the x-ray beam is not exactly perpendicular to the film or electronic sensor, or the object is not parallel to the film. This results in images that are elongated or shortened and not proportional to their true size.

  - Magnification. All dental radiographs are slightly magnified. To reduce magnification and increase sharpness, the distance between the film and the tooth should be as small as possible, whereas the distance between the x-ray beam and the tooth should be as great as possible. (Note that x-rays behave according to the inverse square law, whereby their intensity upon reaching their target changes by a factor that is the square of the change in the distance of their source from the target.) Completed radiographs can be magnified, either in the darkroom or using a computer, for diagnosis.

Dental X-Ray Units

Dental x-ray units still follow the same basic design and principles of the original devices. However, they are much more precise and safer than the first models. Modern x-ray units contain an x-ray tube and tubehead, position indicator device, arm assembly, and control panel (Figure 29-9).

The X-Ray Tube and Tubehead

The x-ray **tubehead** (Figure 29-10) is where the x-rays are generated. It contains several components:

- A metal housing on the outside, which is lined with lead or made from lead to prevent radiation leakage.
- An oil bath inside the metal housing that absorbs heat generated by the x-ray tube.
- Transformers to convert the electrical charge into the form needed to produce usable x-rays. A step-up transformer produces the kilovoltage (kV), which determines the energy and penetrating power of the x-ray beams. A step-down transformer reduces the voltage to produce the milliamperage (mA), which is used to control the numbers of electrons produced. Both kV and mA are discussed in greater detail later in the chapter.
- The **x-ray tube** where the x-ray beam is generated. An x-ray tube is a small glass vacuum tube, usually about 6 inches long. This device includes a **cathode**, or negative electrode, at one end, and an **anode**, or positive electrode, at the opposing end.
- An aluminum filter just outside the x-ray tube that filters out the nonpenetrating, longer wavelength beams.
- A **position indicator device** (PID) at the end of the unit. This device is lined with lead and contains an aperture through which the primary x-ray beam passes as it leaves the device and heads to the patient. The PID can be either cylindrical or rectangular; it limits the size of the x-ray beam by its shape. X-ray beams cannot be larger than 2.75 inches in diameter. Rectangular PIDs reduce the size of the x-ray beam to the size of a piece of dental film, thus reducing radiation exposure to the patient.

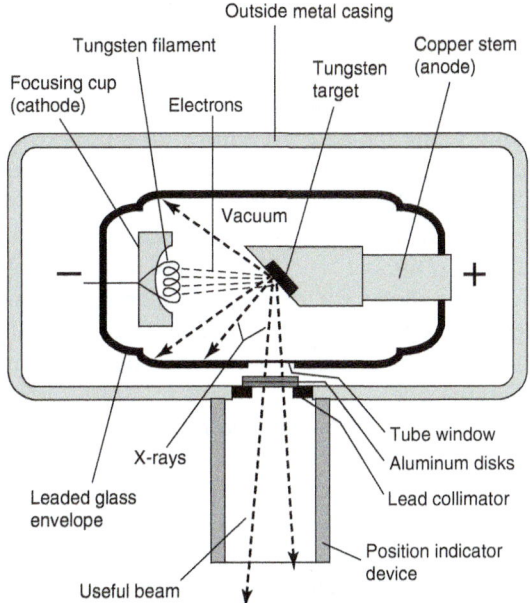

Figure 29–10 **X-ray tubehead.** High-speed electrons flowing from cathode to anode hit the tungsten target and create x-ray photons. The x-rays exit through the tube window and position indicator device.

The Control Panel

Usually located outside the x-ray room, the control panel is where the operator stands while the radiographs are taken (Figure 29-11). The control panel allows the operator to adjust the power of the x-ray beam, as well as turn the dental x-ray unit on and off. Elements of the control panel include:

- A *master switch* to turn the unit on and off. X-ray units can be left on all day without danger because x-rays are only generated when the exposure switch (see next bullet point) is pressed.

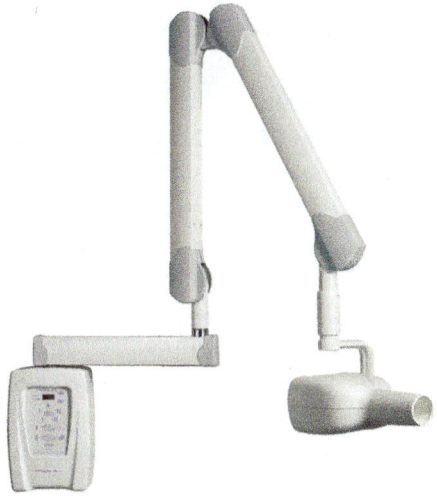

Figure 29–9 Dental x-ray unit.

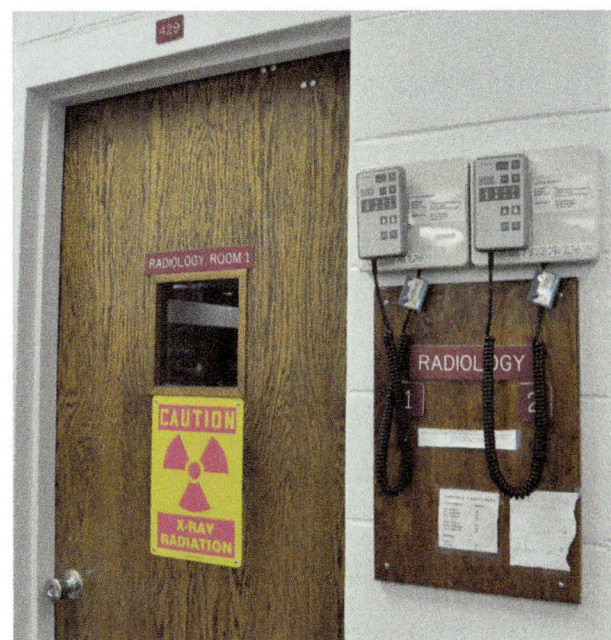

Figure 29–11 X-ray unit control panel.

■ An *exposure switch,* which signals the machine to produce x-rays. Modern digital machines have built-in timers that determine how long the x-rays will be produced, depending on the size of the subject. Simple icons indicate a child or an adult. X-rays are not constant, but produced in impulses. The number of impulses depends on the number of cycles in the electric current. Thus, a 60-cycle alternating current emits 60 pulses of x-ray per second. Older units have a dial that allows the operator to manually adjust the exposure cycles. However, these manual dials are notoriously imprecise and may not be up to current radiation code.

■ A *kilovoltage peak (kVp) selector.* Kilovolts are a measure of the penetrating power of the x-ray beam. The higher the kV, the more powerful and faster the x-rays, resulting in less exposure time needed. Modern x-ray units operate from 70 kV to 90 kV. On modern digital machines, kV is sometimes automatically adjusted based on the area to be x-rayed.

■ A *milliamperage (mA) selector.* Milliamperage is a measure of the quantity of electrons generated inside the x-ray tube. The more electrons, the greater the amount of radiation. Some modern machines are preset for 7 mA for all x-rays. In older machines, it might be set for 10 mA or 15 mA, and the milliamperage switch doubles as the master switch.

The Arm Assembly

The arm assembly is firmly attached to the wall in the room where the patient sits and the radiographs are taken. The tubehead is located at the hanging end, with the PID ready to be precisely positioned to take the radiographs. Arm assemblies allow for the tubehead to be positioned in the optimal position for radiograph exposure.

Generating Radiographs

To take a radiograph, the operator first sets the control panel to the correct kV, mA, and exposure time, if necessary. Newer digital devices are often automated, and the operator need only enter the size of the patient to be x-rayed (e.g., adult or child) and the area to be x-rayed. The machine will handle the rest.

The process of taking a radiograph begins when the unit is first turned on at the master switch. This begins the flow of power from the control panel through electrical wires in the assembly arm and to the tubehead.

Inside the tubehead, the electrical charge goes into the step-down transformer, where the standard 120 volts from the outlet are transformed into 3 or 4 volts. This small charge is used to heat the *tungsten filament* at the cathode end of the x-ray tube. Tungsten is the material of choice for x-ray tube filaments because it has a very high melting point, can be spun into very fine wires, and generates a great number of electrons when heated.

As it is heated, the filament gives off a cloud of electrons that are gathered in a **focusing cup** made of molybdenum. The electron cloud stays in the focusing cup, around the filament, until the exposure button is pressed.

When the exposure button is pressed, a high-voltage circuit is activated that shoots the cloud of electrons across the vacuum tube to a tungsten target on the positive, or anode, side of the x-ray tube. The tungsten target on the anode side of the tube is known as the **focal spot**. The vacuum inside the x-ray tube allows the electrons to travel at the speed of light without encountering oxygen to slow them down.

During this process, an intense amount of heat is generated at the tungsten target. This heat is conducted through a copper stem attached to the tungsten target to a heat radiator that dissipates the heat into the cooling oil bath. About 99% of the energy used to generate x-rays is lost as heat energy; only 1% is converted into usable x-rays.

The tungsten target is precisely angled to deflect the x-rays through a small window in the anode. Immediately after leaving the anode, the x-rays go through a solid metal aluminum filter that filters out all but the short-wavelength, powerful x-rays.

The x-rays next go through a safety device called a **collimator**. The collimator is a piece of lead that reshapes the size of the beam and further filters out low-wavelength beams.

Finally, the beams travel down the PID and toward the patient.

Factors Affecting the Image

Together, the kV, mA, and exposure time dictate the characteristics of the x-ray beam, including its quality, quantity, and intensity (see Table 29-4). These, in turn, affect the quality of the resulting radiographs.

TABLE 29-4 Factors Influencing Radiograph Images

FACTOR	AFFECT ON RADIOGRAPH
Milliamperage (mA)	Higher mA = increased density
	Lower mA = decreased density
Kilovoltage peak (kVp)	Higher kVp = increased density, long-scale contrast, low contrast
	Lower kVp = decreased density, short-scale contrast, high contrast
Time	Longer time = increased density
	Shorter time = decreased density

Safety Devices

Many of the components on dental x-ray units are designed to make the machine safer. When used in conjunction with patient and operator safety devices (e.g., lead aprons and structural blockage), the risk of dangerous radiation exposure is very low.

The aluminum filter in the tubehead is designed to filter out long-wavelength x-rays that are damaging but do not contribute to the radiograph. According to federal law, x-ray machines that operate at 70 kVp or greater require aluminum filtration of at least 2.5 mm.

The collimator is a small device that shapes the x-ray beam. It can be rectangular or cylindrical. Rectangular collimators significantly reduce the amount of radiation the patient is exposed to because they restrict the beam to the size of the film

The position indicator device (PID) is at the end of the tubehead; it is used to help precisely position the beam. PIDs are available in two sizes: 8-inch and 16-inch. The longer the PID, the less radiation exposure because it keeps the beams more tightly focused.

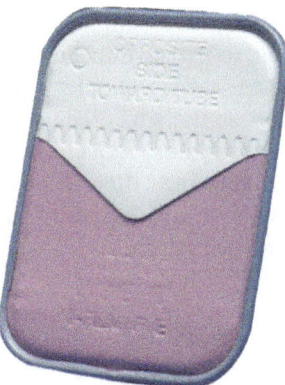

Figure 29–12 Photo dental film.

is taken, the dental film is positioned behind the object to be x-rayed. During exposure, an image is imprinted on the film that is then made visible through processing. Dental x-ray film is similar to photograph film, except that instead of being sensitive to visible light, it is sensitive to x-ray radiation.

CHECKPOINTS

29-14 What color do radiolucent structures appear on a radiograph?

29-15 Do dense objects appear lighter or darker on radiographs?

29-16 Name the components of the x-ray tubehead.

29-17 What does the collimator do?

Dental X-Ray Films

In the early days of dental radiography, dental film consisted of glass plates or film that had been cut into pieces, coated with a radiosensitive material, then hand-wrapped in black paper or rubber by the dentist. The packets were square and hard, and they were relatively large. Dental radiography was uncomfortable.

The first commercial, prepackaged dental x-ray film was introduced in 1913 by the Eastman Kodak Company. Since then, film design has steadily progressed (Figure 29-12). Today's films measure exposure time in fractions of a second as opposed to as many as 8 seconds. This means much less radiation exposure for patients. At the same time, today's films deliver higher quality radiographs with improved contrast and detail.

Although many dental offices are switching to digital imaging, it is still important to have a basic understand of traditional dental film and the way it works. When a radiograph

Composition of Dental Film

Dental film has several layers, including:

- The base. The film base is a 0.2 mm piece of cellulose acetate. It is clear, with a slight bluish tint to enhance the quality of the final radiograph.
- The adhesive layer. Both sides of the film base are covered with a thin layer of adhesive material that attaches the film emulsion (see next bullet point) to the film base.
- The film emulsion. The film emulsion is a fine layer of particles that are sensitive to x-rays. Film emulsion is composed of gelatin and silver **halide crystals**. The gelatin serves two purposes: it evenly spreads the silver halide crystals in a uniform layer, and during processing, it absorbs chemicals and allows them to interact with the silver halide crystals. The silver halide crystals are sensitive to x-rays. There are two kinds of silver halide typically used, either silver bromide (AgBr) or silver iodide (AgI). Most dental films have between 1% and 10% silver halide in the emulsion; the rest is gelatin.
- The protective layer. This thin layer covers the film on both sides. It protects the emulsion from handling and damage.

Formation of Latent Images

During exposure, the film is exposed to radiation, which excites the silver halide crystals. The crystals are excited to differing degrees, depending on how much radiation they are exposed to. Crystals that are exposed to a greater degree of radiation absorb more energy. Crystals that are exposed to less radiation absorb less energy.

The amount of radiation that reaches any part of the film depends on the material between the film and the source of the x-rays (the x-ray unit). Denser materials, like an amalgam filling, for example, will block a significant degree of radiation, so the silver halide crystals on the film behind the amalgam absorb less. By contrast, air absorbs very little radiation, so the silver halide crystals behind an open space will absorb more radiation.

After the exposure is over, the silver halide crystals have been imprinted with various degrees of radiation, forming a pattern on the film. The pattern, however, is not visible to the naked eye. This invisible image is called a **latent image**.

The latent image will not be visible until the film is processed.

Film Speed

Film speed is a measure of the film's sensitivity to radiation. Film speed is determined by the size of the silver halide crystals, the thickness of the emulsion, and radiosensitive dyes in the film. The most important of these factors is the size of the silver halide crystals. Film speed determines how much radiation, or mA, will be needed to adequately expose the image.

Faster films are more sensitive to radiation and thus require less mA for exposure. Slower films are less sensitive to radiation and require more mA for exposure. No slow-speed film is made today, but there are various kinds of fast-speed film on the market. Fast films are sometimes labeled "lightning" or "ultra speed."

Film speed is designated by the American National Standards Institute (ANSI). The ANSI has assigned a letter classification system to the various films, ranging from A through F. A is the slowest film, while F is the fastest film. The ADA and the American Academy of Oral and Maxillofacial Radiology recommend that only the E-speed or F-speed films be used. Currently, no film speed less than D-speed is used. E-speed film is twice as fast as D-speed film, which reduces radiation exposure by 50%. F-speed film is 20% faster, thus requiring 20% less radiation exposure than E-speed film and 70% less radiation exposure than D-speed film.

Intraoral Film Sizes and Packets

Intraoral film is placed inside the mouth during the radiograph (*intra* means inside). Intraoral film is used to take pictures of teeth and other structures inside the mouth. It has emulsion on both sides of the film base to decrease exposure time.

Intraoral film comes in five sizes (Figure 29-13):

- Child size: no. 0, for children younger than 3 years of age
- Narrow anterior: no. 1, for anterior views
- Adult size: no. 2, for use in bilateral bitewing and periapical images
- Large bitewing size: no. 3, for bitewing images
- Occlusal: no. 4, for use with occlusal images

Dental film comes wrapped in packages known as *packets*. In practices, the terms "dental film" and "film packets" are often used interchangeably.

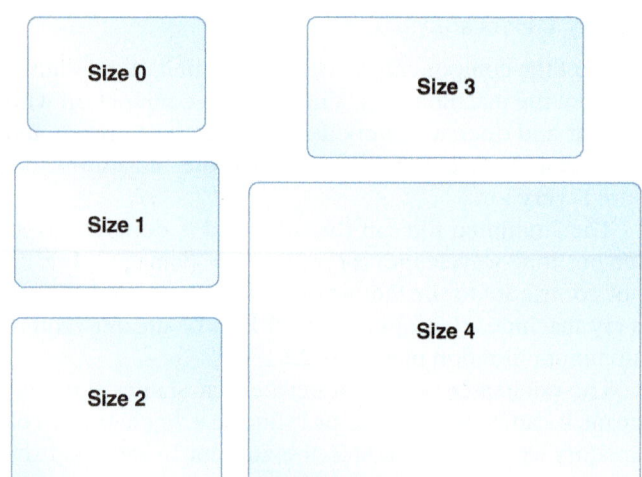

Figure 29–13 Sizes of dental film.

Intraoral film typically comes in boxes that contain either 25, 100, or 150 film packets. Film packets typically contain either single or double film packets in each wrapping. Double film packets are used when duplicates are needed, such as for referral to a specialist. Boxes of intraoral film are labeled with the type of film, film speed, film size, number of films per packet, number of films in the box, and the film's expiration date.

Each film packet has the same basic components: (1) a waterproof outer package to protect the film; (2) black paper on either side of the film itself; (3) the radiograph film; and (4) a lead foil backing. Film packets can also be purchased with a clear plastic outer barrier to protect against contamination.

Intraoral radiograph film is covered in greater depth in Chapter 30, Producing Intraoral Dental Radiographs.

Film Holders

Film holders are special devices used to hold dental film stable in patients' mouths during exposure (see Figure 29-7). Film holders reduce radiation exposure by eliminating the need for patients or operators to manually hold the film in place during exposure. Film holders also help the operator line up the PID correctly.

Basic intraoral film holders are made from plastic or polystyrene and contain a bite block, a slot for holding the film, and a backing plate for the film to rest against. The patient gently bites down on the bite block to hold the film in place. The PID is then positioned, either with or without PID-positioning rings, at the appropriate angle to obtain a diagnostically sound radiograph. There are a variety of basic film holders available.

Rectangular collimators are also available. These devices restrict the size of the primary beam to a rectangle that is only slightly larger than a no. 2 film. This reduces the overall amount of radiation exposure for the patient.

Intraoral film holders and techniques for using them are covered in greater detail in Chapter 30, Producing Intraoral Dental Radiographs.

Extraoral Film

Extraoral film is placed outside the oral cavity during exposure. Extraoral radiography may be necessary in the following situations:

- Patients who cannot or will not open their mouths. This includes patients with illnesses, such as trismus or temporomandibular joint (TMJ) ankylosis, or mental disability.
- When a larger image is needed than can be supplied with intraoral techniques. Sometimes dental images may be needed of large areas of bone and jaw structure. This includes a **panoramic radiograph**, which shows wide-angle exposures of both the upper and lower jaws on a single film, and **cephalometric film**, which shows the bony and soft tissue areas of a facial profile.

Extraoral radiographs and film are covered in greater detail in Chapter 31, Extraoral Radiography and Other Imaging Systems.

Handling Dental Films

Like any kind of film, dental films should be stored carefully to prevent early exposure or film degradation. Dental film should be protected from stray radiation, moisture, temperature extremes, chemicals, and light. Ideal temperatures for dental film storage range between 50°F and 72°F, with a relative humidity from 30% to 50%. Dental film should not be refrigerated, however, because of the risk of condensation and water damage.

When storing dental film, it is best to store newer boxes toward the back, so older boxes with a more recent expiration date are pulled first. Pay careful attention to the expiration dates on the boxes to make sure that all dental film is within its expiration date.

Exposed and processed film should be mounted and stored in a protective envelope. Just as the processed radiographs are part of the patient's dental records, exposed film is considered part of the dental record and can also be used in a legal proceeding.

CHECKPOINTS

29-18 Name the layers that make up traditional x-ray film.

29-19 What does the term *film speed* refer to?

29-20 Which film is faster, E or F?

29-21 How does use of a film holder reduce exposure to radiation?

Digital Radiography

Introduced in 1987, digital radiographs are revolutionizing the way dental practices operate. They allow for instantaneous diagnosis, much easier record-storage, and less exposure to radiation.

Basics of Digital Radiography

Digital radiographs (Figure 29-14) differ from traditional film-based radiography in several key areas:

- There is no film. Instead of dental film, patients hold special sensors in their mouths that detect radiation. Thus, instead of "taking a radiograph," dentists may say they are "acquiring an image" when using digital equipment.
- Digital x-ray units need to be equipped with electronic timers. This only affects older machines that use impulse timers, which are notoriously unreliable and cannot control impulses at the very fast rates used in digital imaging.
- Digital radiographs are displayed on a computer. After the image is acquired, the sensor is fed into a computer that has been equipped with the proper software to read the image. The images are then instantly displayed on the screen; no processing is required.

Although the final product looks similar, digital images are fundamentally different from traditional images. In film-based radiography, images are **analog**. Analog images are created by transitioning smoothly from black to white, with various shades of grey between. The degree of black or white depends on the film's exposure to radiation.

By contrast, digital images are created by arranging tiny pixels into a coherent image. A pixel is a tiny dot of color,

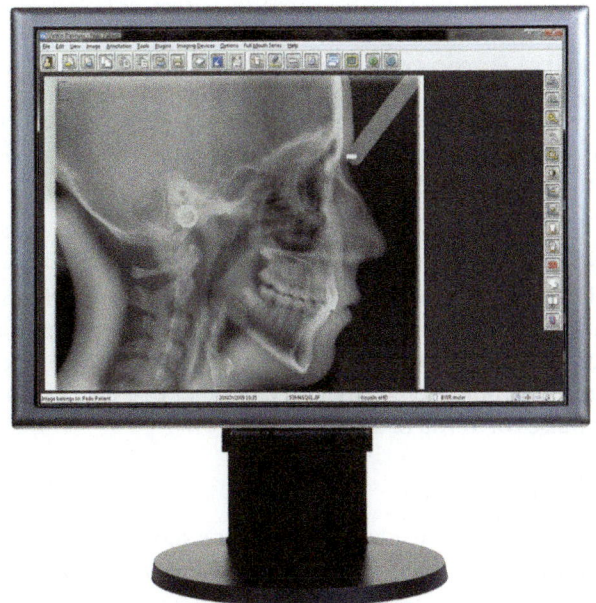

Figure 29-14 **Digital x-ray.**

or in this case, of black, white, or grey. The quality of digital images is determined by how many pixels are used and how many shades of grey are available.

The number of pixels is often referred to as the resolution. The more pixels in an image, the higher the resolution, which translates into greater contrast and clarity.

The number of shades of grey is called the **grey scale**. The more shades of grey, the better the quality of the image. Some high-end digital radiographic systems claim to produce 65,500 shades of grey, but modern computer monitors can only display 256 shades of grey, and the human eye can only discern about 32 shades of grey. However, this does not mean that higher-quality systems are wasted. Imaging software uses this information to produce higher quality images.

Direct Versus Indirect Digital Imaging

There are two methods to obtain a digital image: direct and indirect imaging.

Indirect imaging is the process of converting traditional radiographs to digital images. This is done by using a scanner or camera to take a picture of the image, then uploading it to a computer. A special device called a transparency adapter is used to scan radiographs on traditional scanners. Transparency adapters are sometimes included automatically on flatbed scanners. There is usually some image degradation when a radiograph is scanned, so this method is not used frequently.

Direct digital imaging is the process of obtaining an image directly from a digital sensor placed in the patient's mouth instead of film or a phosphor sensor. When the x-ray beam hits the sensor, it produces a charge of varying intensity, depending on how much radiation is actually reaching the sensor. This charge is converted into digital data, which is transmitted along a wire from the sensor to a computer and instantly displayed on the computer's screen.

Digital Radiograph Equipment

Direct digital images can be acquired with several pieces of equipment, including an x-ray machine, a sensor, and a computer and software to manage the image.

X-Ray Machine

Digital radiographs can be obtained with a standard x-ray machine, provided the machine is capable of operating at very low kilovoltages (70 kV or less) and low milliamperage (5 mA or less) and has a precise timer that can measure impulses of 1/100 of a second.

Sensor

The sensor is placed in the patient's mouth in place of traditional film (Figure 29-15). Digital sensors are specially

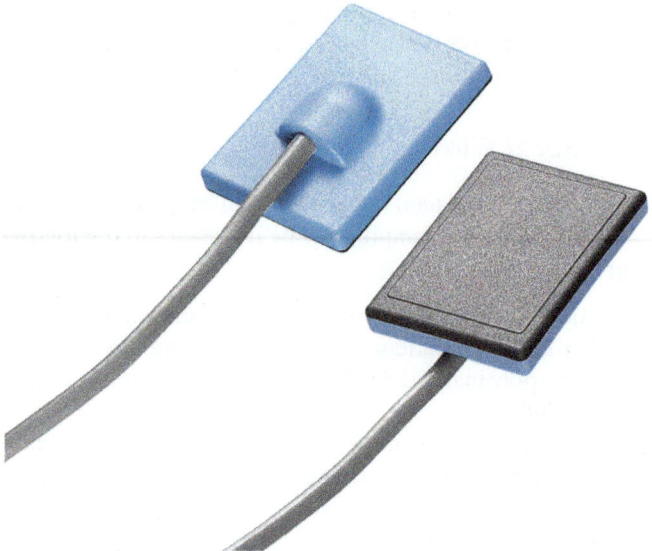

Figure 29–15 Digital x-ray sensor.

coated plates that covert x-rays into electronic patterns. Digital sensors are available as wired devices or wireless. The wires connecting wired sensors to the computer range between 8 feet and 35 feet long. Wireless sensors communicate with the computer using radiofrequency signals.

Digital sensors are sized to approximate film, and improvements are being made all the time to their design and comfort level. Newer sensors are very thin (3 mm) and flexible, with contoured edges, to make them easier for patients to use.

Varieties of sensors include:

- Charge-coupled device (CCD). This is the most common sensor used in digital radiography. These devices were invented in the 1960s and originally used in a wide variety of consumer applications, including video cameras and fax machines. The surface of the CCD is a solid-state detector whose surface is covered with a grid of tiny transistor elements that convert x-rays to electrons. The electrons generated on the grid are then deposited into pixels. Each CCD contains 640 by 480 pixels. After exposure, the pixels are translated into a digital radiograph.
- Complementary metal oxide semiconductor (CMOS). This chip is similar to a CCD, except that it allows for smaller pixels and requires less computer power. CMOS chips are cheaper and can be used on a laptop connected to the chip by a conventional, low-speed Universal Serial Bus (USB) cord. Currently, CMOS chips are available, but not as widely accepted as CCD sensors.
- Photostimulable phosphor (PSP). This relies on a completely different technology than CCD or CMOS

sensors. In this method, a special plate coated with rare earth phosphor (barium europium fluorohalide) in inserted into the patient's mouth. During exposure, the phosphor stores energy from the x-ray beams, much like silver halide crystals on conventional film. After exposure, the image on the plate is converted into a traditional radiograph on a high-speed laser scanner, which transmits the image to a computer. This extra step can take up to several minutes. After exposure, the phosphor plates can be cleared in a light box and reused.

Computer and Software

Many types of computers are capable of working with digital radiographs, as long as they are compatible with the software used to decode and manipulate the images. The main things to consider with a computer that works with large graphics is the amount of memory, which determines its speed, and the amount of storage, which will determine how many radiographs can be stored on the machine. The monitor is also critically important, as a larger monitor will make it easier to display and view radiographs. If the computer has an Internet connection, and the software is compatible, radiographs can be quickly transferred to other offices or specialists.

Digital radiograph software is available from several manufacturers. These software suites typically include some in-office training or some other kind of access to training so staff can learn how to use the program.

Advantages and Disadvantages of Digital Radiography

Like any new technology, digital radiography has a number of advantages and disadvantages compared to the traditional film-based radiography.

Advantages of digital radiography include:

- Much less radiation exposure for the patient and operator, even when compared to F-speed film.
- No harsh chemicals and no need for chemical disposal.
- Images are available instantly.
- Storage is more efficient because the images can be stored electronically.
- Digital images may be e-mailed to specialists, other dentists, and legal professionals, should the need arise.

Disadvantages of digital radiography include:

- Initial cost of equipment, including computers and software, can be prohibitive for smaller practices.
- Training is required to use imaging software.
- Digital sensors may not be as comfortable for patients as traditional film packets.

CHECKPOINTS

29-22 What is used in place of traditional film when taking a digital radiograph?

29-23 Name some of the benefits of digital radiography.

Chapter Highlights

- The world's first radiograph was taken in 1895 by Wilhelm Conrad Roentgen. That same year, radiography was applied to dentistry by Dr. Otto Walkoff.
- In 1913, the hot cathode ray tube was invented. Modern dental x-ray units are still based on this same design.
- Digital imaging was introduced in 1987 and has revolutionized dental radiography. Digital imaging operates at much higher speeds and dramatically reduces radiation exposure.
- X-rays are small wavelength, high-penetrating waves. They are known as ionizing radiation for their ability to ionize molecules, a process that is very damaging to biological tissues.
- Reproductive cells, non-specialized cells, and fast-dividing cells are especially vulnerable to x-ray damage.
- Primary radiation is the form of radiation that comes directly from the x-ray tube. This is the most important form of radiation. Secondary radiation is deflected from another object and contributes to the overall radiation

burden without helping to create better radiographs. Scatter radiation is a form of secondary radiation.
- The ALARA concept stands for As Low As Reasonably Achievable. This means that the patient should be exposed to the absolute least amount of radiation needed to accomplish the desired outcome.
- The use of safety devices such as lead aprons, thyroid collars, and film-holding devices reduces radiation exposure for patients.
- It is safe to administer x-rays to pregnant women and children using appropriate safety devices. However, many pregnant women will opt not to undergo dental x-rays.
- Dental x-ray operators are protected from unnecessary radiation exposure by standing behind structural walls during exposure, limiting their time, and remaining at least 6 feet away from the tubehead during exposure.
- Dental radiographs should never be routine, but only prescribed when medically necessary.

+ Film badges and thermoluminescent devices measure radiation exposure. They are important safety devices that should be worn by all operators.
+ The American Academy of Oral and Maxillofacial Radiology recommends annual testing of dental x-ray machines. Rules for inspection and monitoring of dental x-ray units are left to the individual states.
+ Dental radiographs are legally owned by the dentist.
+ Denser objects appear light on the radiograph as they absorb more x-ray energy. Less dense objects appear darker on the radiograph.
+ Radiographs are measured by their density, contrast, and definition.
+ Dental x-ray units include a tubehead and x-ray tube, control panel, and arm assembly.

+ Kilovoltage (kV) determines the penetrating power of the x-ray beam. The higher the kV, the more power and faster the x-rays.
+ Milliamperage (mA) determines the amount of radiation contained in the x-ray beam.
+ Dental film is coated with a layer of silver halide crystals that store a latent image after exposure. The latent image only becomes visible after processing.
+ Digital radiography uses electronic sensors or phosphor plates to store x-ray energy and convert it to digital images. It requires less radiation and the images are immediately available.

 **Review Questions**

1. What kind of tube is used to produce x-rays?
   a. A photon tube
   b. An anode tube
   c. A cathode tube
   d. A Roentgen tube

2. The first person to use radiography in dentistry was
   a. Dr. William Rollins.
   b. Frank McCormack.
   c. Dr. C. Edmond Kells.
   d. Dr. Otto Walkoff.

3. X-rays are what kind of energy?
   a. Short wavelength, powerful rays
   b. Short wavelength, weak rays
   c. Long wavelength, powerful rays
   d. Long wavelength, weak rays

4. When a molecule is ionized, what has happened?
   a. It has split in half.
   b. It has died.
   c. It has lost or gained an electron.
   d. Its nucleus has been replicated.

5. Which are examples of somatic cells?
   a. Sperm, bone cells, red blood cells
   b. Red blood cells, brain cells, skin cells
   c. Lung cells, egg cells, eye cells
   d. Sperm and egg cells

6. In radiology, what does REM stand for?
   a. Rapid eye movement
   b. Round energy magnetics
   c. Radiation energy mass
   d. Roentgen equivalent man

7. Which kind of radiation is most useful in dental radiology?
   a. Primary radiation
   b. Leakage radiation
   c. Secondary radiation
   d. Scatter radiation

8. Which would violate the ALARA principle?
   a. Taking radiographs annually, whether they are medically necessary or not
   b. Retaking images with small flaws
   c. Asking a patient to hold loose film in place
   d. All of the above

9. Lead aprons should be stored
   a. In the refrigerator.
   b. Carefully folded in a dark place.
   c. Flat or draped.
   d. None of the above.

10. Who legally owns dental records?

    a. The dentist

    b. The court

    c. The patient

    d. They are part of the public record

11. A radiopaque object will appear as what color on the radiograph?

    a. Black

    b. Purple

    c. White

    d. Gold

12. Digital radiographs are preferred over conventional film due to

    a. Reduced radiation exposure.

    b. Absence of chemical developers.

    c. Ease of storage.

    d. All of the above.

13. Which would increase magnification?

    a. Faster film

    b. More powerful x-ray beams

    c. Greater distance between the tooth and the film

    d. Less distance between the tooth and the film

14. The oil bath in the x-ray tubehead is designed to

    a. Lubricate the moving parts.

    b. Balance and level the tubehead.

    c. Absorb excess heat.

    d. Filter out low wavelength x-rays.

15. Milliamperage is a measure of what?

    a. The penetrating power of the x-ray beam

    b. The distance between crests of x-rays

    c. The amount of radiation in the x-ray beam

    d. The amount of electricity needed to generate the beam

16. Which piece of the dental x-ray unit shapes the x-ray beam, reducing the amount of radiation the patient is exposed to?

    a. Collimator

    b. Position indicator device (PID)

    c. Aluminum filter

    d. Focal spot

17. A latent image is

    a. The unseen image stored on silver halide crystals on exposed dental film.

    b. An older image from an exposed radiograph that has faded.

    c. An overlapping image on a radiograph that was taken incorrectly.

    d. The exposed image that appears after a radiograph is processed.

18. The fastest dental film is

    a. B.

    b. C.

    c. D.

    d. F.

19. How many shades of grey can the human eye recognize in a digital image?

    a. 256

    b. 32

    c. 65,000

    d. 5

20. Photostimulable phosphor plates

    a. Are reusable.

    b. Are disposable.

    c. Are uncomfortable.

    d. Taste funny.

Active Learning Exercises

1. Patients often question the use of the lead apron. What is the best explanation you can give to a patient regarding the importance of using the lead apron?

2. Imagine that a radiation, or film, badge has come back positive for the presence of radiation exposure in a particular room. What is your state's protocol for thermoluminescent devices? What government agency will assist in this process?

Application Activities

1. The Consumer-Patient Radiation Health and Safety Act of 1981 requires states to develop minimum licensing standards for x-ray operators, though compliance is voluntary. Using the Internet or your local library, look up what regulations your state has in place for minimum licensing standards for x-ray operators.

2. Develop scenarios that violate the ALARA principal. How can film handling, film placement, and PID placement affect ALARA?

3. Create a timeline of all the milestones in dental radiography, from the invention of the x-ray tube to the introduction of digital radiography.

PREPARING FOR CERTIFICATION EXAMS

Review the following topics in this chapter to prepare for the Dental Assisting National Board (DANB) exam:

- **Introduction**
- **Radiation Physics**
- **Radiation Biology**
- **Radiation Effects on Cells and Tissues**
- **Radiation Safety**
- **Limiting Exposure—The ALARA Concept**
- **Determining Radiographic Exposure**
- **Radiation Monitoring**
- **Radiograph Image Production**
- **Dental X-Ray Units**
- **Dental X-Ray Films**
- **Formation of Latent Images**
- **Film Speed**
- **Intraoral Film Sizes and Packets**
- **Handling Dental Films**
- **Digital Radiography**

chapter 30

Producing Intraoral Dental Radiographs

CHAPTER OUTLINE

CHAPTER CHECKLIST

On completion of this chapter, students will be able to:

☑ Describe the steps involved in setting up and conducting a full mouth series.

☑ Describe techniques for helping patients suppress the gag reflex during radiography.

☑ Describe the steps involved in setting up and conducting the paralleling technique.

☑ Describe the steps involved in setting up and conducting the bisecting techniques.

☑ Describe the steps involved in setting up and conducting a bitewing series.

☑ Describe the steps involved in setting up and conducting the occlusal technique.

☑ Describe the steps involved in setting up and conducting the endodontic technique.

☑ Identify common errors made during radiographic exposures and discuss how to avoid them.

☑ Describe how to obtain diagnostic radiographs among pediatric populations and people with special needs.

☑ Describe correct infection control procedures.

☑ Describe the elements in a quality assurance program.

KEY TERMS

ala (A-luh) – a winglike anatomic structure; used in radiology to describe the nostril when aligning the PID

automatic processing – a technique of exposing radiographs that relies on a machine to automatically produce visible radiograph images from the latent images on exposed x-ray film

bisecting (bi-SEKT-ing) technique – a dental x-ray technique in which the primary x-ray beam is directed at a perpendicular angle to an imaginary plane created by bisecting the plane of the long axis of the teeth and the film

bisector – a line that divides an angle into two even, smaller angles, for example, a 90-degree angle into two 45-degree angles; used in radiography to determine the angulation of the primary x-ray beam in the bisecting technique

bitewing exposure – a radiograph that includes the crowns of teeth on both the mandible and maxillary bone

canthus (KAN-thus) – the angle of the eye

coin test – a test used to measure safelights in radiology darkrooms

cone cut – section of a radiograph that appears clear due to improper alignment between the film and the PID

double image – results from accidentally exposing the same dental x-ray film twice, so it shows one image laid over the top of another

edentulous (ee-DEN-chuh-lus) – without teeth

elongated (ee-LONG-gate-ed) image – an x-ray image in which the teeth appear stretched in relation to their roots; results from insufficient vertical angulation in the bisecting technique

foreshortened image – an x-ray image in which the teeth appear shortened with rounded roots; results from excessive vertical angulation in the bisecting technique

herringbone pattern – an x-ray image with an irregular pattern across the surface of the image, caused by reversing the film in the patient's mouth before exposure so the x-rays must pass through the embossed lead foil; a nondiagnostic image

horizontal angulation – the angle of the PID on a horizontal plane around the patient's head during exposure

interproximal (in-ter-PRAWK-sih-mul) decay – decay that occurs where adjoining teeth touch each other

interproximal radiograph – a radiograph that images the region where teeth come into contact with one another; used to diagnose interproximal decay

long axis of the tooth – an imaginary line drawn from the end of the root to the incisal or occlusal surface of a tooth

midsagittal plane – an imaginary line that divides the body into right and left halves, used in radiology to help determine angulation

occlusal (uh-KLOO-zul) exposure – an x-ray technique used to show large areas of the maxillary and mandibular arches

occlusion (uh-KLOO-zhun) – the act of closing or being closed; any contact between the incising or masticating surfaces of upper and lower teeth; the relationship between the occlusal surfaces of the maxillary and mandibular teeth when in contact

overlapping image – a dental x-ray in which the images of teeth improperly overlap on the final image, obscuring the interproximal area; results from incorrect horizontal angulation

paralleling technique – a dental x-ray technique in which the film is held parallel to the long axis of the tooth and the primary x-ray beam strikes the film at a perpendicular angle

periapical (per-ee-A-pih-kul) exposure – at or around the apex of a tooth; used in radiology to describe radiographs that show the tooth from its apex to its root

sublingual (sub-LING-gwul) – below the tongue

topographic technique – an exposure technique used in occlusal imaging in which the primary x-ray beam is directed at a perpendicular plane created by bisecting the central axis of the teeth and the film

tragus (TRAY-gus) – a tonguelike projection of the cartilage of the auricle in front of the opening of the external acoustic meatus and continuous with the cartilage of this canal

transitional mixed dentition – describing the dentition of a child who has both primary and adult teeth

vertical angulation – the angle of the PID on a vertical plane around the patient's head during exposure

Introduction

Intraoral radiographs are the most common kind of radiograph taken in dental offices. The traditional dental x-ray unit has been improved steadily to allow for greater precision and better radiographs with less radiation exposure. In recent years, digital radiography has transformed the practice by eliminating the need for film and developing chemicals and further reducing radiation exposure.

The ability to take high-quality radiographs is within the reach of any dental assistant who is familiar with the equipment and techniques and can apply them to various settings. The approach to different patients will vary, based on their age and size, their level of comfort and cooperation, and the radiograph prescription ordered by the dentist. In each case, a thorough understanding of the scenario and the best approach will result in clinically valuable, or diagnostic, radiographs.

The Full-Mouth Radiographic Survey

The full-mouth radiographic survey, or FMX, is the standard technique used to obtain a complete set of images from a patient's mouth. It is the cornerstone of a complete radiographic dental record, and all patients should have a current FMX in their record.

An adult FMX (Figure 30-1) typically consists of 18 to 20 films showing the patient's entire dentition. The number and kind of films used in an FMX varies depending on the dentist's preferences and the patient's

Using the Paralleling Technique

The paralleling technique is the standard technique used to obtain periapical and bitewing images. To obtain high-quality images, the following factors must be taken into account:

- Film placement. The film must be placed in a manner that will completely cover the teeth to be imaged.
- Film position. The film must be parallel to the long axis of the tooth.
- **Vertical angulation**. The central beam of the x-ray must strike the film at a perpendicular angle. This is accomplished by swiveling the tubehead up and down so that the PID is raised or lowered until it is brought into line at a perpendicular angle. On most x-ray machines, angles are marked on the yoke where the tubehead is connected. The 0 marking means the PID is parallel to the floor. *Positive angulations* occur when the PID is tilted toward the floor. *Negative angulations* occur when the PID is tilted toward the ceiling. In the paralleling technique, vertical angulation is typically within 10 degrees of zero, as opposed to +40 or +50 degrees in the bisecting technique.
- **Horizontal angulation**. The central beam should pass directly through the interproximal spaces between the teeth, otherwise **overlapping images** of the same tooth structure will appear on the film. This is accomplished by swiveling the tube head from side to side in a horizontal plane.

- Central ray. The x-ray beam must be centered on the film so that all areas of the film are exposed. Partial images are referred to as **cone cuts** (Figure 30-8). A cone cut is the result of the PID not being positioned evenly to the film, resulting in an image that leaves a partial blank space on the exposed film.

Film and Sensor Holders in the Paralleling Technique

Film holders (Figure 30-9) are used during parallel radiography to hold the film still in the patient's mouth and, in some cases, to help the operator obtain the correct angulation. Film holding devices include:

- Hemostat devices with bite blocks
- Bite blocks
- Rinn XCP instruments
- RAPD
- Precision
- Intrax

Film holding devices that include *localizing rings* make vertical and horizontal angulation easier. The PID can be placed in direct contact with the localizing ring. If there are any gaps in the contact, the operator can adjust the angulation until the PID is flush against the ring.

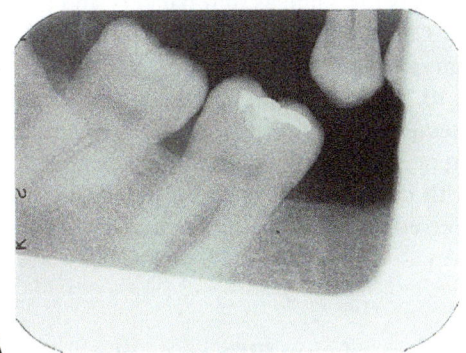

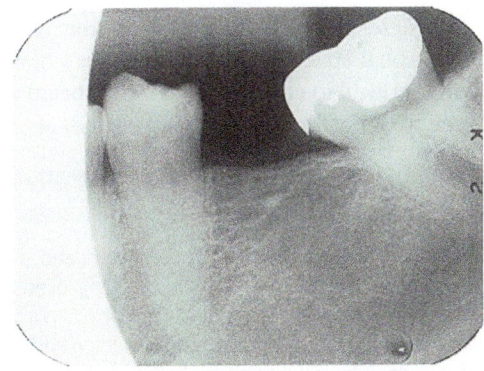

Figure 30–8 Cone cut is the result of the PID not being positioned correctly over the film. (**A**) Cone-cut with rectangular PID. (**B**) Cone-cut with round PID.

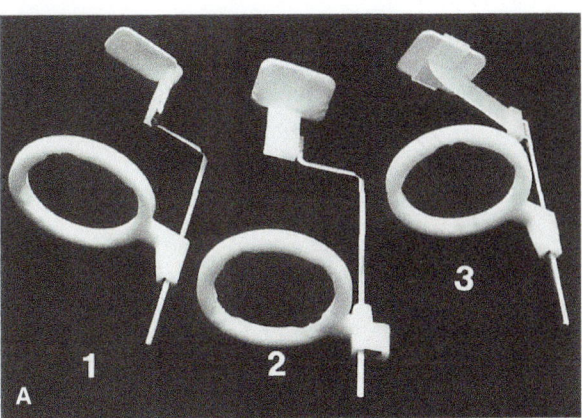

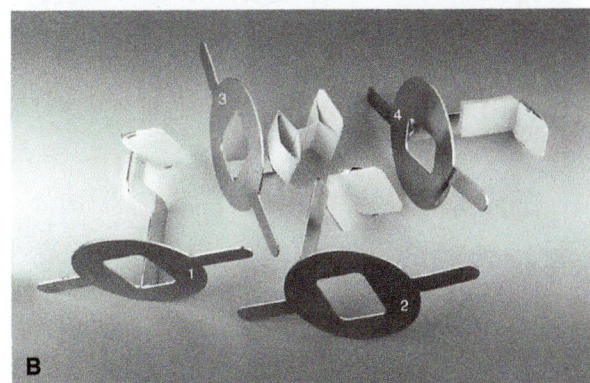

Figure 30–9 Paralleling instruments. (**A**) Rinn XCP instruments used with the paralleling technique. (**B**) Masel Precision rectangular instruments used with the paralleling technique.

Versions of these film-holding devices are available for digital sensors and phosphor plates. Digital sensor holding devices often feature a notch for the cable.

Without Film Holders

Although the use of film holders with external localized rings is strongly recommended, they might not always be available. In these situations, the patient's relative position to the floor and the *points of entry* become crucial tools in helping to achieve the proper angulation. Points of entry are the areas of the face where the x-ray beam will enter the tissue; they are located along the apices of the teeth, or the ends of the roots.

Although this technique is more difficult than using a localizing ring, it is still possible to obtain high-quality radiographs. Points to consider include:

- For maxillary radiography, the horizontal plane is located along an imaginary line extending from the **tragus** of the ear to the **ala** of the nose (Figure 30-10). To obtain the correct angle, the PID of the tubehead is rotated around the patient's head along this horizontal plane, according to the following points of entry:
  - The tip of the nose for incisor radiographs
  - The depression at the ala of the nose for canines
  - Directly below the pupil of the eye for premolars
  - Below the **canthus** of the eye for molars

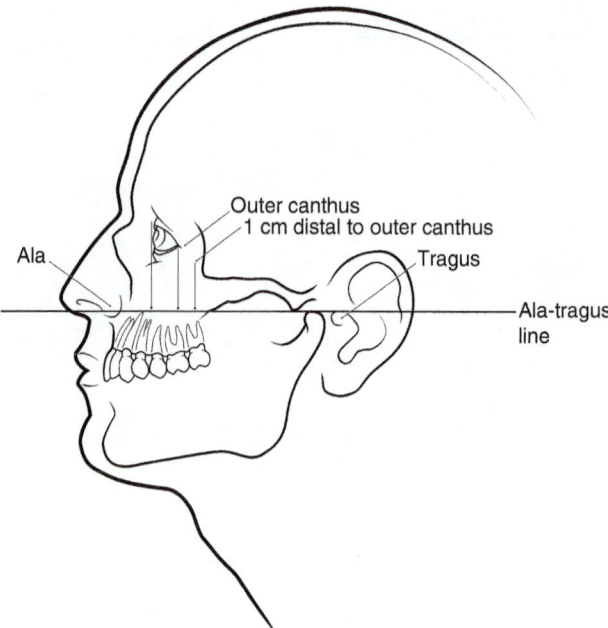

Figure 30–10 **Locating apices of teeth.** To localize each maxillary tooth apical region, use the imaginary line from various landmarks on the face to the ala-tragus line. The landmarks for the maxillary second molar, first molar, second premolar, canine, and incisors are shown on the drawing. In the mandible, the root apices can be established by estimating the points of entry from the lower border of the mandible. This is usually the width of the thumb (0.5 inches).

- During these radiographs, the PID should be almost touching the face and the primary beam should be directed through the middle of the teeth rather than the apices to prevent cone cutting errors.
- For mandibular radiographs, the horizontal plane is located about 1/2 inch above the lower border of the mandible. The same points of entry are used in relation to the different teeth.

Film or Sensor Placement in the Paralleling Technique

Film placement within the patient's mouth is critical for obtaining successful parallel radiographs. The film should be placed away from the teeth, toward the middle of the mouth. For anterior projections, the film should be held with its long side vertical, and for posterior projections, the long side should be horizontal. The edge of the film should extend 1/8 inch beyond the occlusal plane. The dot on the film packet should be facing the occlusal/incisor tooth surface. One helpful hint is to make sure the dot is always placed in the slot of the bite block, or the "dot in the slot." Care should also be taken to guarantee that all the teeth to be exposed are in front of the film. Finally, the white surface of the film packet should be facing the tubehead to prevent distortion from the lead shield in the film packet.

The placement procedure for digital sensors and phosphor plates is the same as film packets, and they are sized the same. Care should be taken to keep the patient relaxed and calm, as some digital sensors are thicker and more difficult to hold in the mouth than film packets. See the earlier section on gagging for advice on handling patients who gag or have trouble with film placement.

As with conventional film, the paralleling technique is the preferred exposure with digital and phosphor sensors and plates.

Angulation of the PID

Angulation describes the position of the PID in the three-dimensional space around the patient's head. Vertical angulation is critical to ensure that the x-ray beam strikes the bisector angle of the film and tooth's long axis at 90 degrees.

> ### *From the Dentist's Perspective*
>
> My practice depends on competent and knowledgeable radiographers. Often, I'll ask a prospective employee to bring in an FMX series so I can see his or her work for myself. I'll be looking for clear useful images that are free from distortion and processing errors. If they don't have existing films to bring in, I might ask them to come in for a working interview, and you can be sure that the working interview will include at least one radiograph series!

Patient Preparation and Exposure Sequence Using the Paralleling Technique

When an FMX has been ordered, the dental assistant must perform a number of tasks quickly and efficiently to deliver safe and clinically useful radiographs. FMX series consist of both periapical and bitewing images. The preferred technique is the paralleling technique whenever possible.

To prepare the room and patient, the following steps should be included:

1. Review the patient's chart and history.
2. Put on appropriate PPE, except for gloves.
3. Wash and dry hands, then pull on appropriate gloves.
4. Prepare the room with the necessary infection control techniques and equipment to be used, including the lead apron, tissues or paper towels, and a cup. Do not store unexposed film in the room with the x-ray unit. Unprotected dental film that is stored in a room in which radiographs are frequently obtained will be subjected to secondary radiation, which may compromise the film. Some dental offices have lead-lined receptacles for unexposed and exposed film. These can be safely used in the same room as the dental x-ray unit.
5. Set the mA, kVp, and exposure time on the x-ray machine. Digital machines often use pictographs to make setting the machine easier.
6. Seat the patient in the chair and position the chair for the initial radiographs. The occlusal line of the jaw being x-rayed should be parallel to the floor and the head should be firmly supported. This may be more difficult in some newer chairs. Remember to ask the patient to remove anything that might interfere with the radiographs, including jewelry, earrings, appliances, nose studs, eyeglasses, and any objects in his or her mouth.
7. Secure the lead apron and thyroid collar in place. Answer any questions the patient may have about the procedure.
8. Discard gloves, wash and dry hands again, and pull on appropriate gloves.
9. Assemble the sterile film-holding devices according to the manufacturer's instructions.
10. Take the radiographs. See below for an example of an effective exposure sequence of periapical films using the paralleling technique. After film is exposed, remove it from the patient's mouth, wipe it clean of saliva, and properly store it. If a plastic film is used, remove the barrier from the film and place the clean film in a cup for processing. Films that cannot be processed immediately should be labeled and set aside in a safe place until they can be developed.

The number and types of exposures will vary, depending on the patient. An adult FMX typically includes 14 periapical radiographs and four to six bitewing radiographs, for a total of 18 to 20 radiographs. However, this may vary if the patient is missing teeth.

Once the patient is prepared and the equipment is assembled, you can begin taking the radiographs. There is no established sequence for obtaining the periapical radiographs, so you can develop whatever protocol makes sense or use one mandated by the dentist. However, it is a good idea to always follow the same radiograph sequence to help minimize mistakes in case you are interrupted during the sequence.

Ideally, the film should remain in the patient's mouth for as little time as possible to obtain a good exposure. This will reduce the tendency to gag. Once a gag reflex begins, it is often hard for the patient to stop, even on exposures that normally would not have stimulated a gag reflex.

A typical sequence follows.

Anterior Exposures

Anterior exposures are often recommended as a beginning point for FMX surveys (Figure 30-11). They use smaller film (no. 1) and patients are less likely to gag. This is a good way to relax the patient into the radiography series. The number of anterior exposures depends on the size of the film used. If no. 1 film is used, seven exposures may be necessary, with four maxillary exposures and three mandibular exposures. If no. 2 film is used, only six exposures may be necessary. Some dental offices, however, use no. 1 film.

The Rinn XCP instrument sequence is:

1. Begin with the maxillary right canine and expose all the maxillary canine teeth from right to left. You will be moving from tooth no. 6 to tooth no. 11.
2. Move the mandibular arch.
3. Begin with the mandibular left canine, this time moving from left to right. You will be moving from tooth no. 22 to tooth no. 27.

This orderly sequence minimizes extra movement of the PID. After each exposure, the film should be removed from the patient's mouth, cleaned of saliva, and either stored in a clearly marked lead container in the x-ray room or, if such a container is not available, away from the dental x-ray unit. Take care to separate exposed and unexposed film.

Posterior Exposures

After the anterior exposures have been obtained, move onto the premolars (Figure 30-12). Once again, this will reduce the patient's likelihood of gagging. A total of eight exposures are typically taken for the posterior regions. The size of the film depends on the patient's mouth and his or her ability to hold it. For very small mouths, or for difficult placements, a size no. 0 or no. 1 film may be desired. The typical film size, however, is no. 2.

(*Text Continued on page 552*)

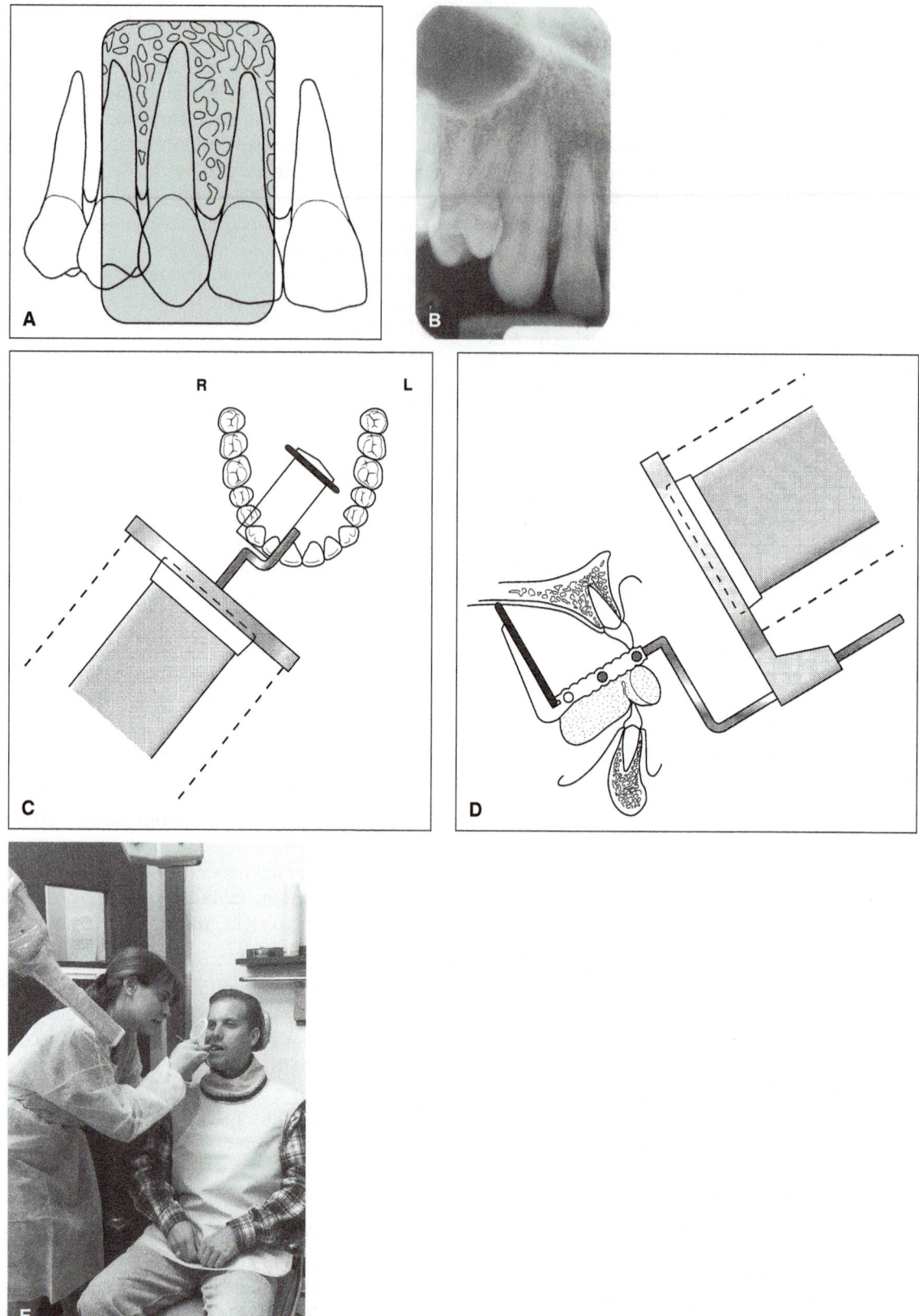

Figure 30–11 **Begin exposures with the maxillary right canine and expose all of the maxillary anterior teeth from right to left.** (**A**) Region coverage for maxillary canine region. (**B**) Resultant radiograph. (**C**) Horizontal film and PID placement. (**D**) Vertical film and PID placement. (**E**) Placement of Dentsply/Rinn XCP instrument.

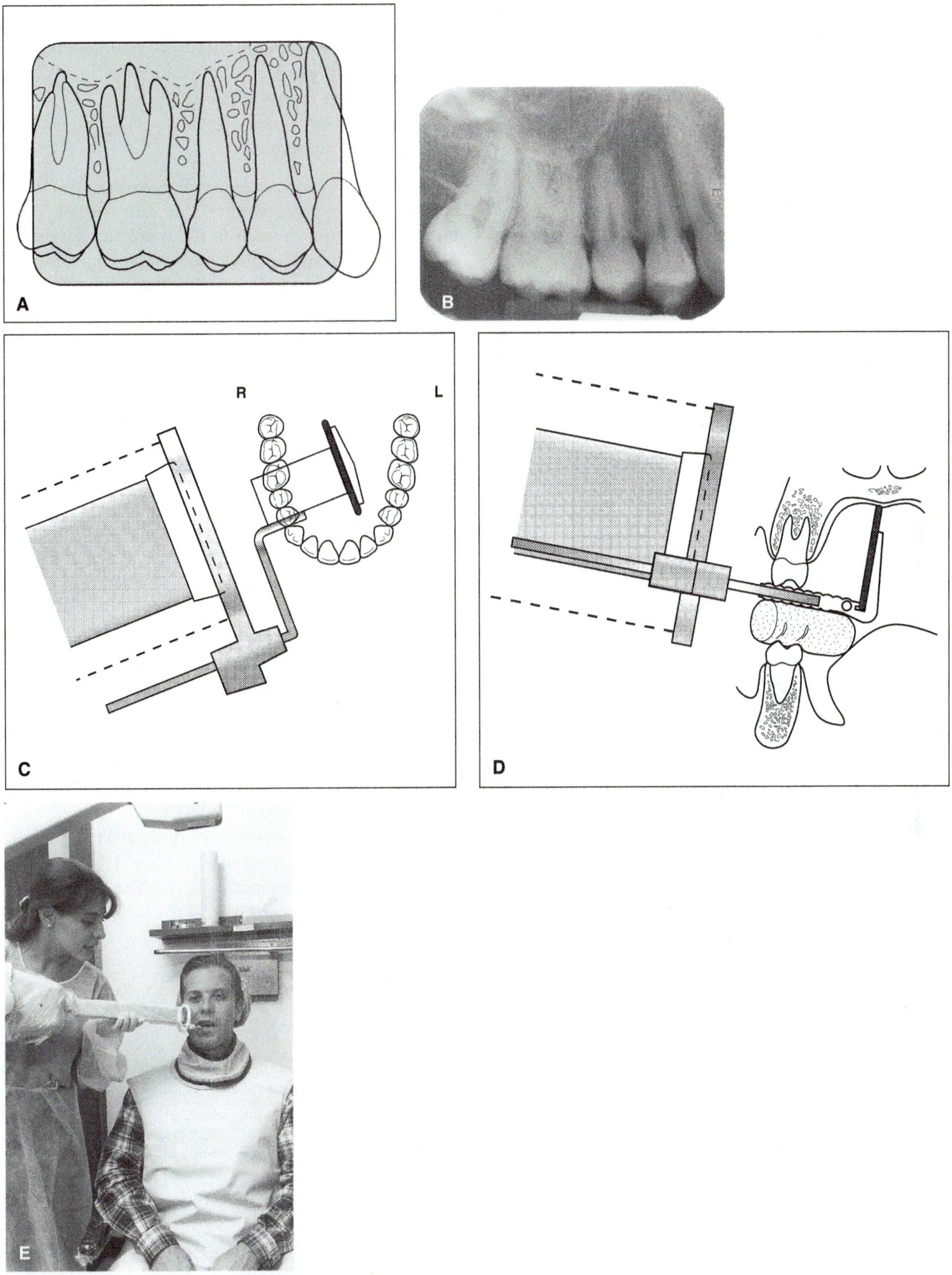

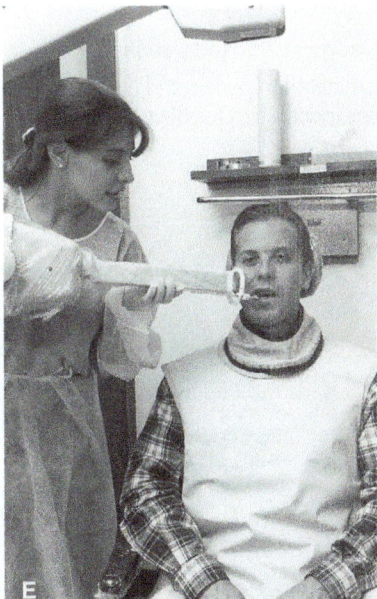

Figure 30–12 After the canines are complete, continue the series with the maxillary right premolars, then molars. (A) Region coverage for maxillary premolar region. (B) Resultant radiograph. (C) Horizontal film and PID placement. (D) Vertical film and PID placement. (E) Alignment of PID with XCP instrument.

Film for posterior exposures is typically placed horizontally in the film holder to maximize its coverage. However, a vertical orientation is sometimes requested for a periodontal exam.

The suggested Rinn XCP sequence for posterior exposures is:

- Maxillary right premolars
- Maxillary right molars
- Mandibular left premolars
- Mandibular left molars

These exposures are obtained without reassembling the XCP instrument, thus reducing the overall time needed to obtain the sequence. After this sequence is completed, the XCP instrument is reassembled, and the following sequence is suggested:

- Maxillary left premolar
- Maxillary left molars
- Mandibular right premolars
- Mandibular right molars

Although this is one suggested sequence, you may find another that is more comfortable and natural. The most important factors to keep in mind are the patient's comfort, obtaining high-quality radiographs, and minimizing the risk of double exposures. Once you have developed a sequence, you should follow it every time.

Procedure 30–2 Using the Paralleling Technique for a Full-Mouth Survey (FMX)

In some states, dental assistants who perform radiological procedures must complete additional training and pass a certification examination. Requirements and expanded functions vary from state to state. Check the regulations governing your state for more information about the specific duties dental assistants are allowed to perform.

Materials needed (Figure P30-2-1):

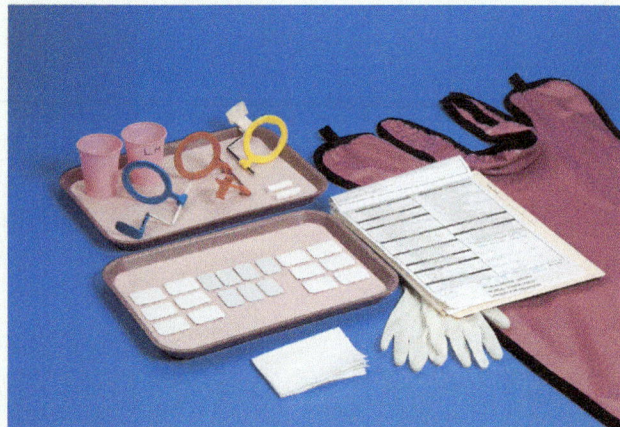

Figure P30-2-1

- Radiographic films
- Film-holding devices (assembled anterior, posterior, and bitewing XCPs)
- Paper cup labeled with patient's name
- Paper cup for trash
- Paper towels
- Lead apron
- Thyroid collar
- Cotton rolls
- Gloves
- Patient chart

General Preparation:

1. Prepare the x-ray room and patient.
2. Put on appropriate PPE.
3. Open and assemble the sterile film-holding devices.
4. Follow the specific instructions for each area of the oral cavity, as described below, to obtain each exposure.
5. After each exposure, remove the film-holding device, remove the film, wipe away any saliva, and place the film in cup to await development. Exposed film should be stored outside of the x-ray room to avoid secondary radiation.
6. When all exposures are complete, remove your gloves, then remove the lead apron and thyroid collar from the patient. Return the lead apron to its hanging position. Escort the patient out of the x-ray room.
7. Return to the x-ray room, wash hands, and reglove.
8. Dispose of all contaminated materials and disinfect the x-ray room. Transport the exposed film for development.

Maxillary Canines

1. Insert a no. 1 film packet vertically into the film-holding device (Figure P30-2-2A and B).

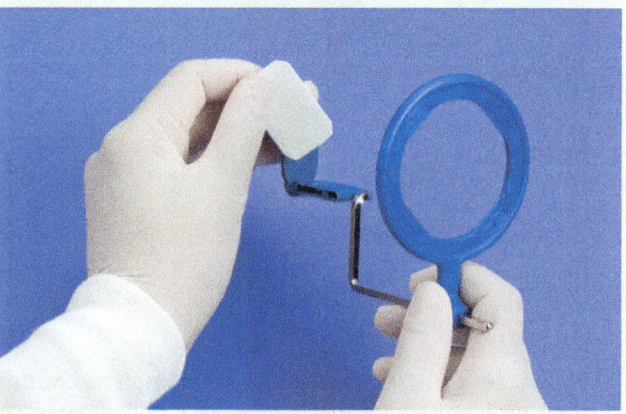

A
Figure P30-2-2A

Procedure 30–2 Using the Paralleling Technique for a Full-Mouth Survey (FMX) (Continued)

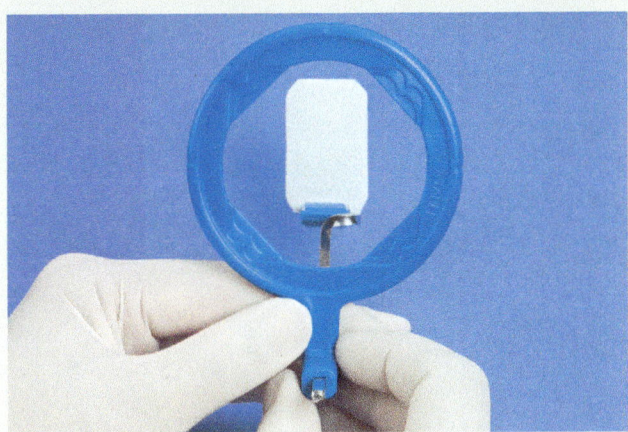

B

Figure P30-2-2B

2. Position the film packet with the canine and first premolar centered and as far posterior as possible. Instruct the patient to close his or her mouth.
3. Align the localizing ring and PID (Figure P30-2-3).

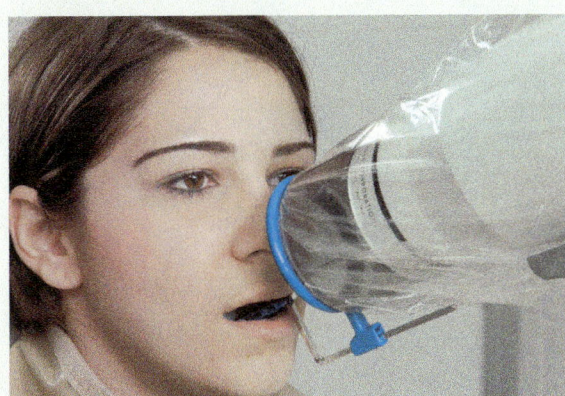

Figure P30-2-3

4. Expose the film.

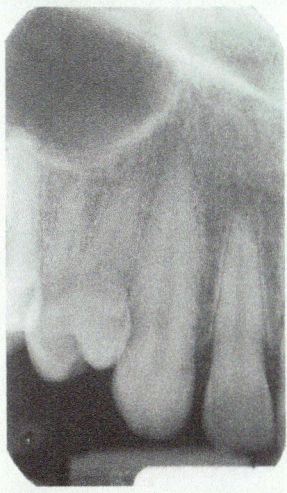

Figure P30-2-4. Resulting radiograph.

Maxillary Central/Lateral Incisors

1. Insert a no. 1 film packet vertically into the film-holding device.
2. Position the film packet centered between the central and lateral incisors, as far posterior as possible. Instruct the patient to close his or her mouth.
3. Align the localizing ring and PID (Figure P30-2-5).

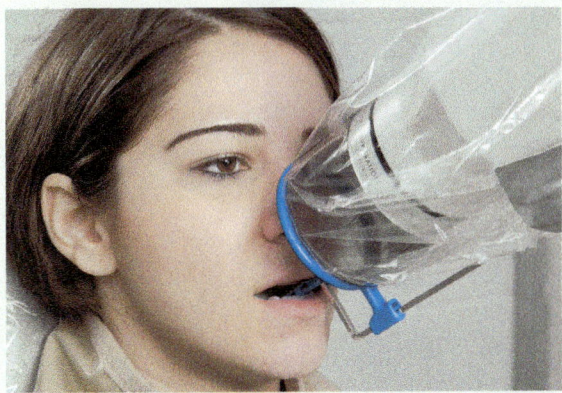

Figure P30-2-5

4. Expose the film.

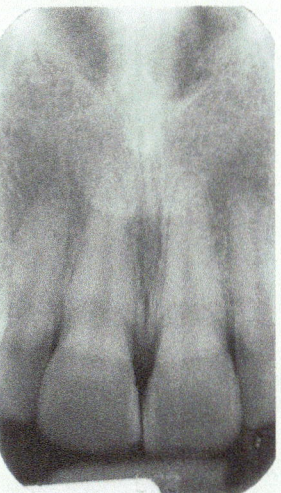

Figure P30-2-6. Resulting radiograph.

Mandibular Canines

1. Insert a no. 1 film packet vertically into the film-holding device.
2. Center the film packet on the canine, as far in the lingual direction as possible. Place a cotton roll between the teeth and film-holding device, if necessary, to prevent movement of the device and for patient comfort. Instruct the patient to close his or her mouth.
3. Align the localizing ring and PID (Figure P30-2-7).

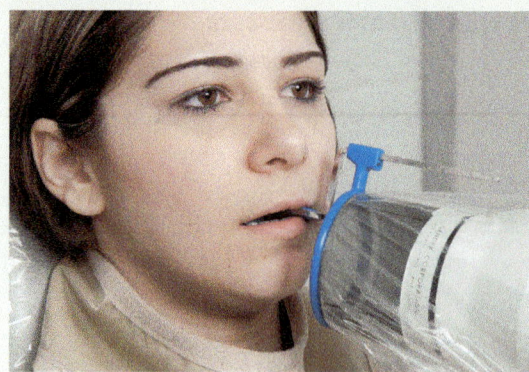

Figure P30-2-7

4. Expose the film.

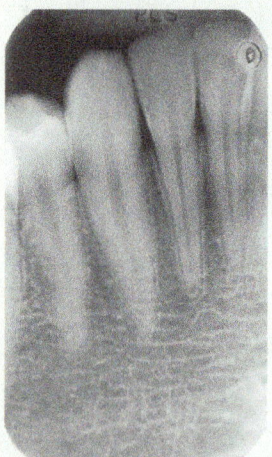

Figure P30-2-8. Resulting radiograph.

Mandibular Incisors

1. Insert a no. 1 film packet vertically into the film-holding device.
2. Center the film packet between the central incisors, as far in the lingual direction as possible. Instruct the patient to close his or her mouth.
3. Align the localizing ring and PID (Figure P30-2-9).

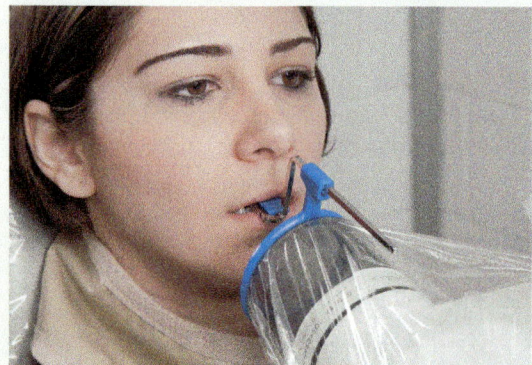

Figure P30-2-9

4. Expose the film.

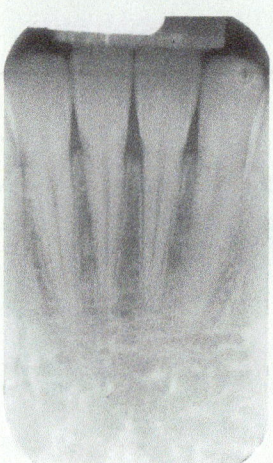

Figure P30-2-10. Resulting radiograph.

Maxillary Premolars

1. Insert a no. 2 film packet horizontally into the film-holding device (Figure P30-2-11).

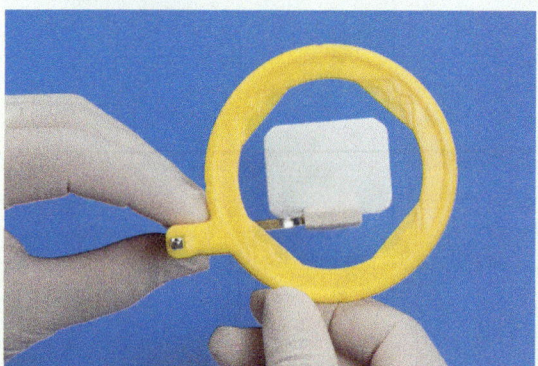

Figure P30-2-11

2. Center the film packet on the second premolar and position the film in the midpalatal area. Instruct patient to close his or her mouth.
3. Align the localizing ring and PID (Figure P30-2-12).

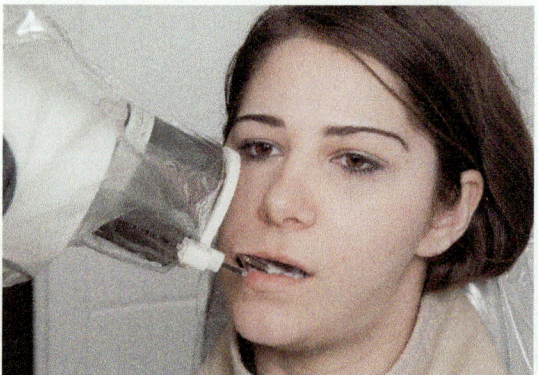

Figure P30-2-12

Procedure 30–2 Using the Paralleling Technique for a Full-Mouth Survey (FMX) (Continued)

4. Expose the film.

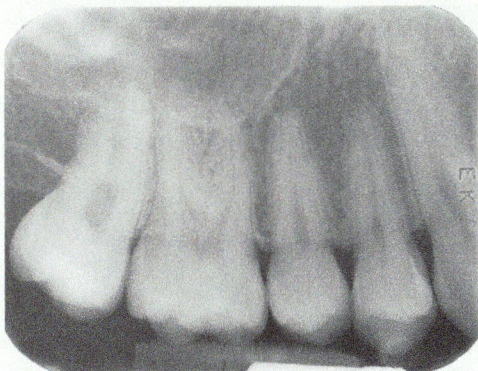

Figure P30-2-13. Resulting radiograph.

Maxillary Molars

1. Insert a no. 2 film packet horizontally into the film-holding device.
2. Center the film packet on the second molar and position the film in the midpalatal area. Instruct patient to close his or her mouth.
3. Align the localizing ring and PID (Figure P30-2-14).

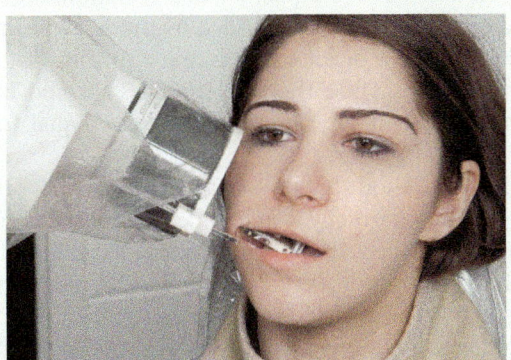

Figure P30-2-14

4. Expose the film.

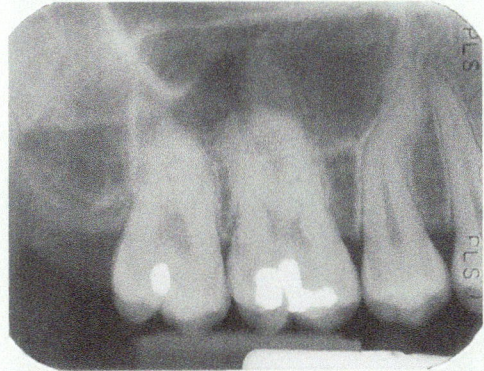

Figure P30-2-15. Resulting radiograph.

Mandibular Premolars

1. Insert a no. 2 film packet horizontally into the film-holding device.
2. Center the film packet on the contact point between the second premolar and the first molar, as far in the lingual direction as possible. Instruct the patient to close his or her mouth.
3. Align the localizing ring and PID (Figure P30-2-16).

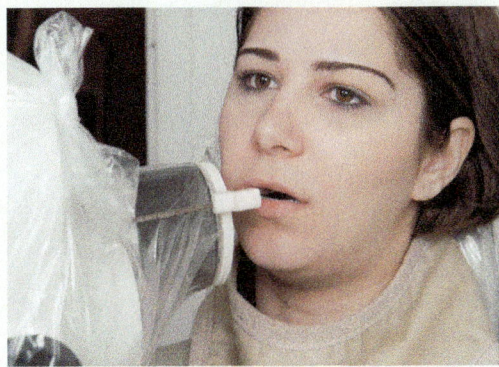

Figure P30-2-16

4. Expose the film.

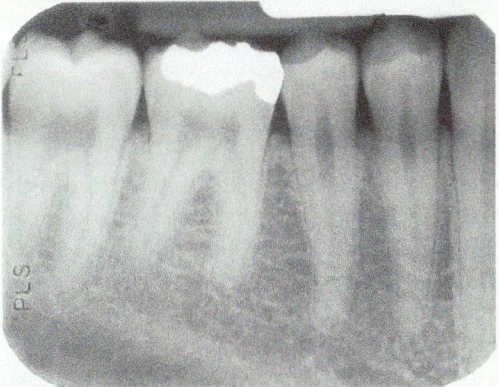

Figure P30-2-17. Resulting radiograph.

Mandibular Molars

1. Insert a no. 2 film packet horizontally into the film-holding device.
2. Center film packet on the second molar, as far in the lingual direction as possible. Instruct the patient to close his or her mouth.

Procedure 30-2 Using the Paralleling Technique for a Full-Mouth Survey (FMX) (Continued)

3. Align the localizing ring and PID (Figure P30-2-18).

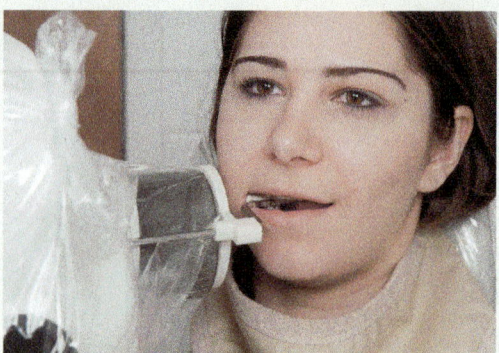

Figure P30-2-18

4. Expose the film.

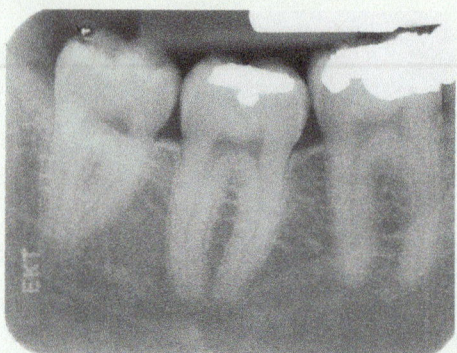

Figure P30-2-19. Resulting radiograph.

✓ **CHECKPOINTS**

30-3 What is seen during a bitewing exposure?

30-4 What is an occlusal exposure?

30-5 What is the paralleling technique?

Using the Bisecting Technique

Although the paralleling technique is the preferred technique for most periapical radiographs, some situations call for the bisecting technique. This technique is based on a geometric principle known as the rule of isometry. The rule of isometry states that two triangles are equal if they share two equal angles and have a common side.

Using this rule, the film is placed against the lingual surface of the tooth so the plane of the film intersects the long axis of the tooth. An imaginary line is drawn midway between these two planes, bisecting the angle of the film and the tooth axis. This imaginary line is sometimes called the **bisector** and represents a common side to the two triangles (Figure 30-13).

The bisected angles are equal, for one common angle. The second common angle is provided by the x-ray beam, which is directed at a perpendicular angle to the imaginary bisecting angle. Thus, the two triangles formed by the film, the tooth and the bisecting angle, are equal triangles.

Although this method sounds complicated, it is easier to visualize. If it is used correctly, it yields accurate radiographs with minimal or no distortion. The bisecting technique is also sometimes called the *short cone technique*, although it can be used with either the long or the short PID.

The bisecting technique is used when the paralleling technique will not work, including with children, adults with small mouths, and patients with shallow palates or high palatal vaults that may not easily accommodate some film packets.

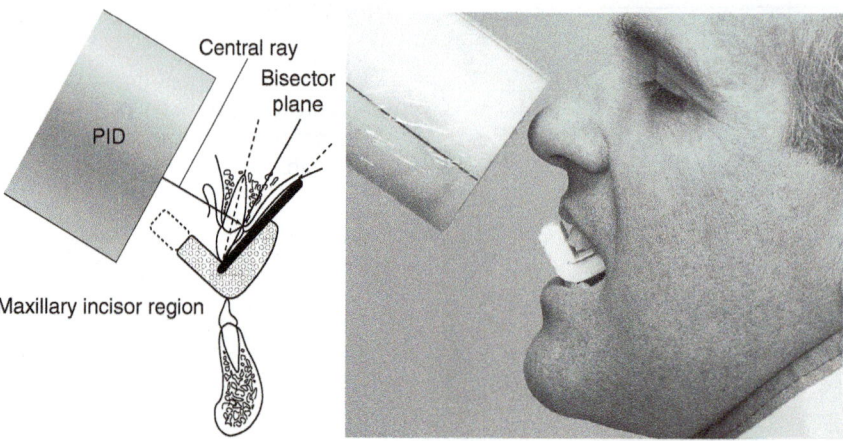

Figure 30-13 Maxillary incisor Stabe bisecting technique.

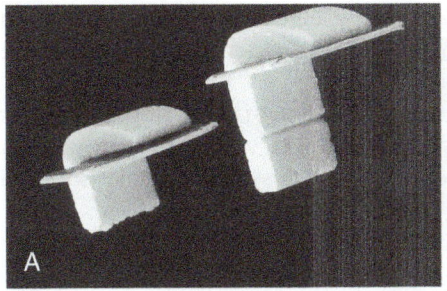
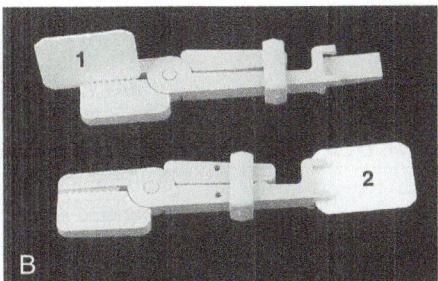
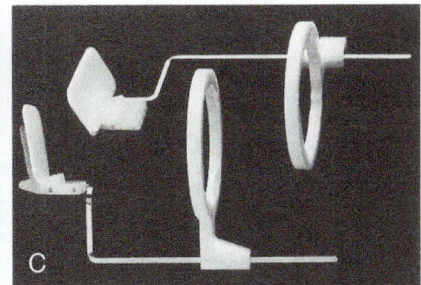

Figure 30–14 **Dentsply/Rinn bisecting angle instruments (BAI)**. (**A**) Stabe disposable bite blocks. (**B**) EEZEE-Grip film holders: posterior projection (1) and anterior projection (2). (**C**) Posterior (*upper*) and anterior (*lower*) Rinn BAI instruments. Note that these instruments are identical to the Rinn XCP instruments except that the bite block is angled.

Film and Sensor Holders in the Bisecting Technique

In the bisecting technique, the film is placed directly against the patient's tooth. Dentists and radiographers sometimes ask the patients to hold the film in place with their fingers during exposure. *This is not recommended* as it is not consistent with ALARA principles.

A variety of film holders are used with the bisecting technique (Figure 30-14), including:

- Rinn BAI. The Rinn BAI (bisecting angle instruments) are designed for bisecting radiographs. This system includes plastic bite blocks, plastic aiming rings, and metal indicator arms. Snap-on collimators are available to attach to the plastic aiming rings to further reduce the radiation burden on the patient.
- Stabe bite block. Bite blocks can be used with either the parallel or the bisecting technique. To use in the bisecting technique, the scored front section is removed to allow film placement as close to the teeth as possible. Stabe bite blocks are made of Styrofoam and are disposable.
- EEZEE-Grip film holders. This piece of equipment was formerly known as the Snap-A-Ray. It can be used in either the bisecting or paralleling technique.

Digital film sensors are treated the same as film in the bisecting technique, although special sensor holders are needed to hold them steady. Digital sensor holders, such as the EEZEE-Grip, have a notch in the bite block to accommodate the wire.

Film or Sensor Placement in the Bisecting Technique

Film placement in the bisecting technique depends on the teeth being radiographed. The film should be in direct contact or close to the crown of the tooth and extending at an angle into the oral cavity. For maxillary radiographs, the film will extend toward the roof of the mouth. For mandibular radiographs, the film will extend toward the floor of the mouth.

As with the paralleling technique, the film should extend beyond the incisal or occlusal surface of the tooth by about 1/8 in.

It is important when using the bisecting technique to make sure the film is carefully lined up with the PID to prevent cone cutting or exposure errors.

Angulation of the PID

Vertical angulation is critical to ensure that the x-ray beam strikes the bisector angle of the film and tooth's long axis at 90 degrees. (The approach used to determine horizontal angulation is the same for both the parallel and bisecting techniques.)

Either an 8-inch or a 16-inch PID can be used with the bisecting technique. The shorter PID is typically preferred because it reduces the degree of distortion in the final radiographs.

Horizontal Angulation

Correct horizontal angulation ensures that the x-ray beam passes through the contact areas of the teeth. If the PID is positioned to either side of horizontal, overlapping shadow images may occur on the final radiograph. These films cannot be used and must be taken again.

Vertical Angulation

Vertical angulation is crucial to taking usable radiographs. To correctly orient the patient, the occlusal line of the jaw being radiographed should be parallel to the floor, or at zero degrees vertical angulation. Unfortunately, this represents a drawback because it is very hard to orient patients in this position in some of the newer dental chairs.

The bisecting technique uses much greater vertical angles (as marked on the tubehead) than the paralleling technique (see Table 30-1). For maxillary radiographs, the PID is aimed at the floor (positive angulation). For mandibular radiographs, the PID is aimed at the ceiling (negative angulation).

Improper vertical angulation will result in either foreshortened or elongated images.

- *Foreshortened images* (Figure 30-15A) are radiographs in which the teeth appear to be shorter in proportion to their true length. This type of image results from excessive vertical angulation, when the PID is aiming too high (maxillary) or too low (mandibular) to the

TABLE 30-1 Vertical Angulation for Bisecting Technique

TOOTH TYPE	MAXILLARY ANGULATION	MANDIBULAR ANGULATION
Canines	+45 to +55	−20 to −30
Incisors	+40 to +50	−15 to −25
Premolars	+30 to +40	−10 to −15
Molars	+20 to +30	−5 to 0

tooth being radiographed. It also occurs if the central x-ray beam strikes the film at a perpendicular angle, rather than the imaginary bisector line.

■ *Elongated images* (Figure 30-15B) are radiographs in which the teeth appear to be stretched in proportion to their true length. This type of image results from insufficient vertical angulation. It also occurs if the central x-ray beam strikes the tooth at a perpendicular angle, rather than the imaginary bisector line.

Patient Preparation and Exposure Sequence Using the Bisecting Technique

Patient preparation for the bisecting technique is the same as preparing a patient for the paralleling technique, as described previously.

When seating patients for bitewing exposures, the **midsagittal plane** should be perpendicular to the floor. For maxillary films, this means the patient's head should be upright. For mandibular films, the patient's head should be tipped back slightly.

A film exposure sequence must be developed before you start taking radiographs. The sequence takes into account the prescription, the patient's needs, and any special requests or circumstances. It provides you with an easy game plan to follow to keep track of the procedure and prevent mistakes.

The FMX typically consists of 14 to 18 periapical films for an adult. This number can vary for different patients. Children and patients who are missing teeth may not need the entire series.

When performing an FMX with the bisecting technique, always start with the anterior teeth (the canines and incisors). Patients are less likely to gag during anterior exposures. Once a patient's gag reflex has been stimulated, he or she may be unable to suppress it, even on radiographs that would not normally cause a problem.

Anterior exposures with the bisecting technique typically use a size no. 2 film, placed vertically in the oral cavity, with three exposures each for the maxillary arch and the mandibular arch. Patients with smaller arches may require no. 1 film, in which case four anterior exposures may be necessary.

The exact sequence of the exposures is up to the operator. However, once you have found a sequence that works, it is a good idea to always use the same sequence. This reduces the likelihood of unnecessary exposures.

One recommended exposure sequence is:

■ Begin on the right maxillary side at tooth no. 6, and move across, from *right to left*, to tooth no. 11.
■ Move to the mandibular arch and start on the left side with tooth no. 22. Shoot from *left to right* and finish with the right mandibular canine, or tooth no. 27.

This sequence reduces movement of the PID, so it can be accomplished more quickly and efficiently. It also exposes the teeth in numerical order, making it easier to read the resulting radiographs. The sequence is the same for the digital sensors and phosphor plates.

After completing the anterior sequence, move to the posterior teeth. Again, a no. 2 film is recommended, but this time the film is horizontally aligned in the oral cavity. Begin with the premolar teeth and move to the molars. This will reduce the gag reflex and make it easier and more comfortable for the patient.

In all, eight posterior exposures are usually recommended: four maxillary exposures and four mandibular exposures. A recommended exposure sequence for anterior exposures is:

■ Right maxillary premolars (teeth no. 4 and no. 5)
■ Right maxillary molars (teeth no. 1, no. 2, and no. 3)
■ Right mandibular premolars (teeth no. 28 and no. 29)
■ Right mandibular molars (teeth no. 30, no. 31, and no. 32)
■ Left maxillary premolars (teeth no. 12 and no. 13)
■ Left maxillary molars (teeth no. 14, no. 15, and no. 16)
■ Left mandibular premolars (teeth no. 20 and no. 21)
■ Left mandibular molars (teeth no. 17, no. 18, and no. 19)

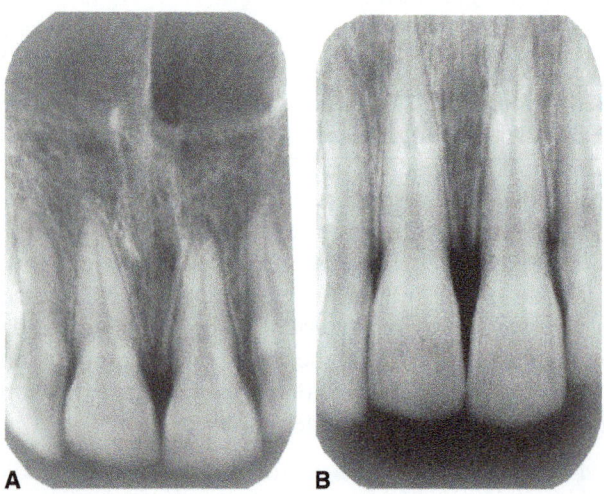

Figure 30–15 Radiographic results of improper vertical angulation. (**A**) Foreshortening occurs when too much vertical angulation is used. (**B**) Elongation occurs when not enough vertical angulation is used.

The most important factors to keep in mind during exposure are the patient's comfort, obtaining high-quality radiographs, and reducing the amount of radiation received by the patient.

Procedure 30–3 Using the Bisecting Technique for a Full-Mouth Survey (FMX)

In some states, dental assistants who perform radiological procedures must complete additional training and pass a certification examination. Requirements and expanded functions vary from state to state. Check the regulations governing your state for more information about the specific duties dental assistants are allowed to perform.

Materials needed (Figure P30-3-1):

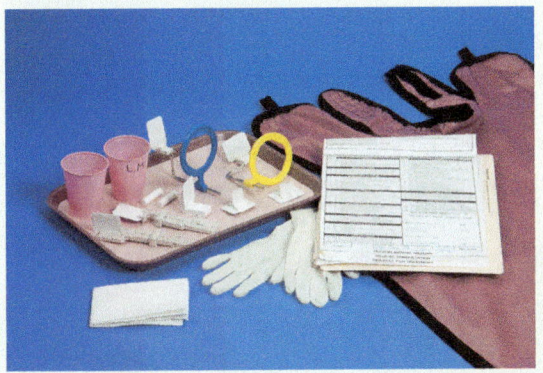

Figure P30-3-1

- Radiographic films
- Film-holding devices with films inserted and labeled anterior and posterior
- Paper cup labeled with patient's name
- Paper cup for trash
- Paper towels
- Lead apron
- Thyroid collar
- Cotton rolls
- Gloves
- Patient chart

General Preparation

1. Prepare the x-ray room and the patient.
2. Put on appropriate PPE.
3. Open and assemble the sterile film-holding devices.
4. Follow the specific instructions for each area of the oral cavity, as described below, to obtain each exposure.
5. After each exposure, remove the film-holding device, remove the film, wipe away any saliva, and place the film in a cup to await development. Exposed film should be stored outside of the x-ray room to avoid secondary radiation.
6. When all exposures are complete, remove your gloves, then remove the lead apron and thyroid collar from patient. Return the lead apron to its hanging position. Escort the patient out of the x-ray room.
7. Return to the x-ray room, wash hands, and reglove.
8. Dispose of all contaminated materials and disinfect the x-ray room. Transport the exposed film for development.

Maxillary Canines

1. Insert a no. 2 film packet vertically into the film-holding device.
2. Position the film packet centered on the canine. Instruct the patient to apply light pressure to the lower edge of the film-holding device.
3. Set vertical angulation between +45 and +55 degrees as appropriate.
4. Set horizontal angulation by aligning the central ray between the contacts of the canine and the first premolar.
5. Center the PID on the film (Figure P30-3-2).

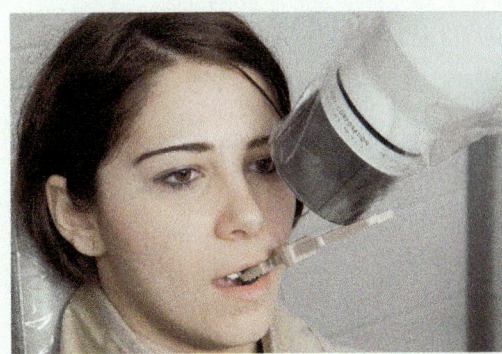

Figure P30-3-2

6. Expose the film.

See Figure P30-3-10 for a typical full radiographic survey taken by bisecting angle technique.

Maxillary Incisors

1. Insert a no. 2 film packet vertically into the film-holding device.
2. Position the film packet on the incisal edge of the incisors, as close as possible to the lingual surface. Instruct the patient to bite lightly on the edge of the film-holding device.
3. Set vertical angulation between +40 and +50 degrees as appropriate.
4. Set horizontal angulation by aligning the central ray between the contacts of the central incisors.
5. Center the PID on the film (Figure P30-3-3).

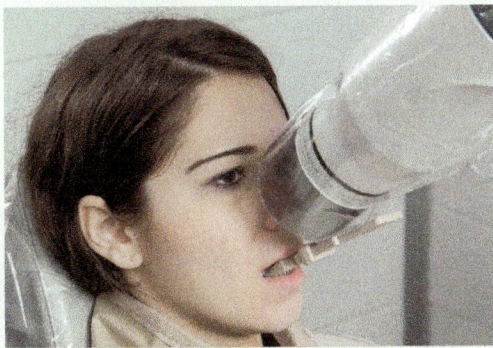

Figure P30-3-3

6. Expose the film.

Mandibular Canines

1. Insert a no. 2 film packet horizontally into the film-holding device.
2. Position the edge of the film packet on the incisal edge of the canine. Instruct the patient to bite lightly on the edge of the film-holding device.
3. Set vertical angulation between –20 and –30 degrees as appropriate.
4. Set horizontal angulation by aligning the central ray between the contacts of the canine and first premolar.
5. Center the PID on the film (Figure P30-3-4).

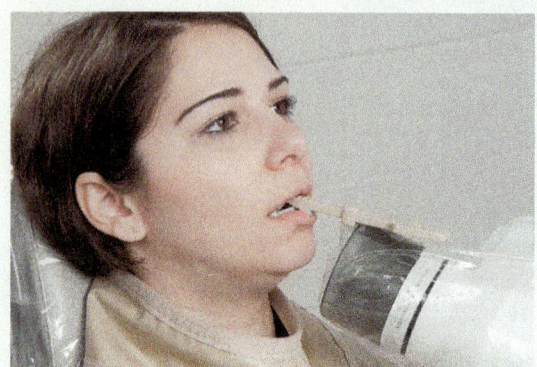

Figure P30-3-4

6. Expose the film.

Mandibular Incisors

1. Insert a no. 2 film packet vertically into the film-holding device.
2. Center the film packet on the contact between the two central incisors and against the lingual surface. Instruct the patient to bite lightly on the edge of the film-holding device.
3. Set vertical angulation between –15 and –25 degrees as appropriate.
4. Set horizontal angulation by aligning the central ray between the contacts of the central incisors.
5. Center the PID on the film (Figure P30-3-5).

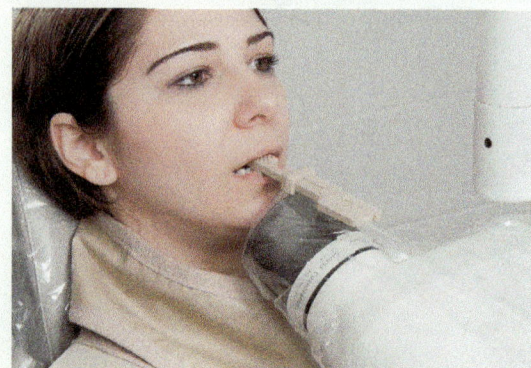

Figure P30-3-5

6. Expose the film.

Maxillary Premolars

1. Insert a no. 2 film packet horizontally into the film-holding device.
2. Center the film packet on the second premolar, against the lingual surfaces of the teeth.
3. Set vertical angulation between +30 and +40 degrees as appropriate, directing the central ray at the most anterior part of the cheekbone.
4. Set horizontal angulation by aligning the central ray between the contacts of the premolars.
5. Center the PID on the film (Figure P30-3-6).

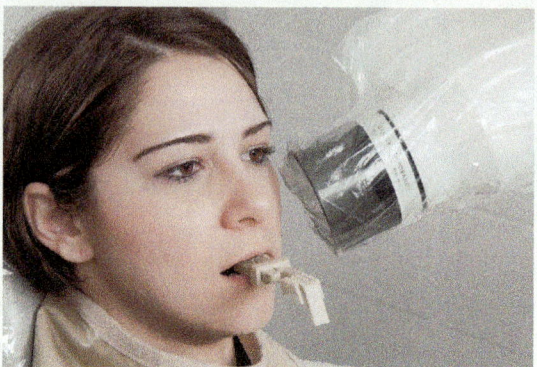

Figure P30-3-6

6. Expose the film.

Maxillary Molars

1. Insert a no. 2 film packet horizontally into the film-holding device.
2. Center the film packet on the second molar, against the lingual surfaces of the teeth.
3. Set vertical angulation between +20 and +30 degrees as appropriate, directing the central ray through the zygomatic arch, toward the center of the film.
4. Set horizontal angulation by aligning the central ray between the contacts of the molars.
5. Center the PID on the film (Figure P30-3-7).

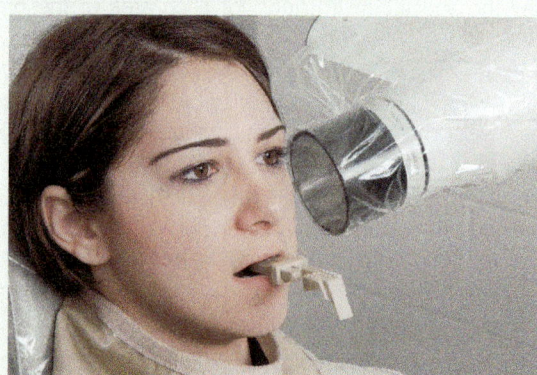

Figure P30-3-7

6. Expose the film.

Procedure 30–3 Using the Bisecting Technique for a Full-Mouth Survey (FMX) (Continued)

Mandibular Premolars

1. Insert a no. 2 film packet horizontally into the film-holding device.

2. Center the film packet on the second premolar, aligning the front edge of the film packet with the mesial aspect of the canine, and positioning the film packet against the lingual surfaces. Instruct the patient to bite gently on the film-holding device.

3. Set vertical angulation between −10 and −15 degrees as appropriate, directing the central ray at the mental foramen, aimed at the center of the film.

4. Set horizontal angulation by aligning the central ray between the contacts of the premolars.

5. Center the PID on the film (Figure P30-3-8).

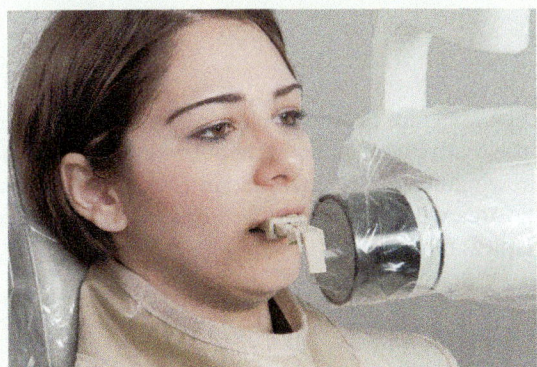

Figure P30-3-8

6. Expose the film.

Mandibular Molars

1. Insert a no. 2 film packet horizontally into the film-holding device.

2. Center the film packet on the second molar, aligning the front edge of the film packet with the midline of the second molar. Instruct the patient to bite gently on the film-holding device.

3. Set vertical angulation between −5 and 0 degrees as appropriate, directing the central ray at the roots of the molars.

4. Set horizontal angulation by aligning the central ray between the contacts of the molars.

5. Center the PID on the film (Figure P30-3-9).

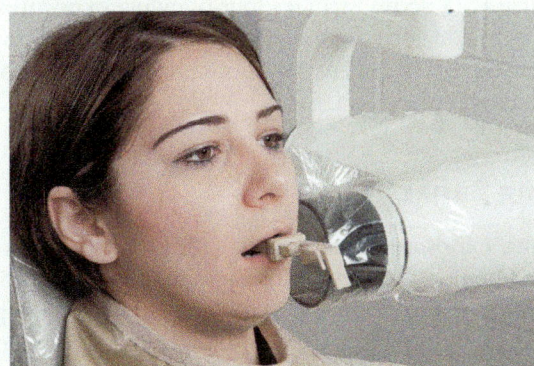

Figure P30-3-9

6. Expose the film.

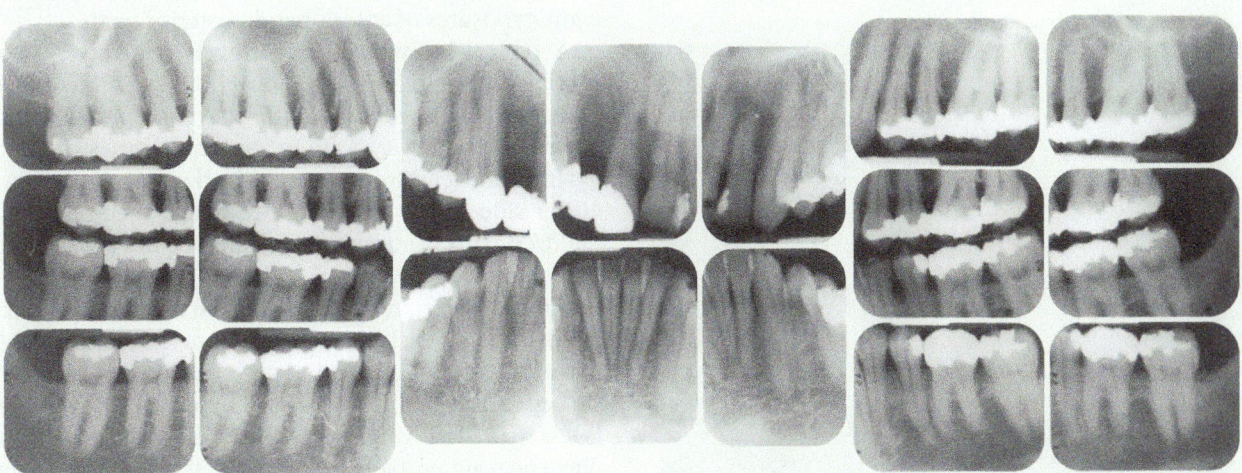

Figure P30-3-10. Full-mouth survey using the bisecting technique.

Using the Bitewing Technique

A bitewing exposure shows the crowns and alveolar bones of the mandibular and maxillary arch on one exposure. Bitewing exposures are probably the most common exposures in dental practice. They are sometimes referred to as **interproximal radiographs** because they are especially effective at showing the area where teeth come into contact with each other.

Bitewing radiographs are most commonly used to detect dental caries in posterior teeth and alveolar bone crests between teeth. They can detect carious lesions that are not yet clinically visible, particularly in premolars and molars, making bitewing radiographs a powerful diagnostic tool (Figure 30-16).

A typical FMX series includes four bitewing exposures, two on each side, for a total of 18 to 22 exposures. However, bitewing exposures are also routinely taken as part of a bitewing series.

Bitewing Basics

A bitewing exposure is taken with a film packet that is positioned behind the teeth to be radiographed. It is positioned close to the teeth, unlike film in the paralleling technique, and covers the crowns and alveolar crests on both the maxillary and mandibular arch. The central x-ray beam is directed through the contact areas where opposing teeth touch (Figure 30-17).

A properly placed bitewing film is nearly parallel to teeth on both the mandibular and maxillary arches. Because of

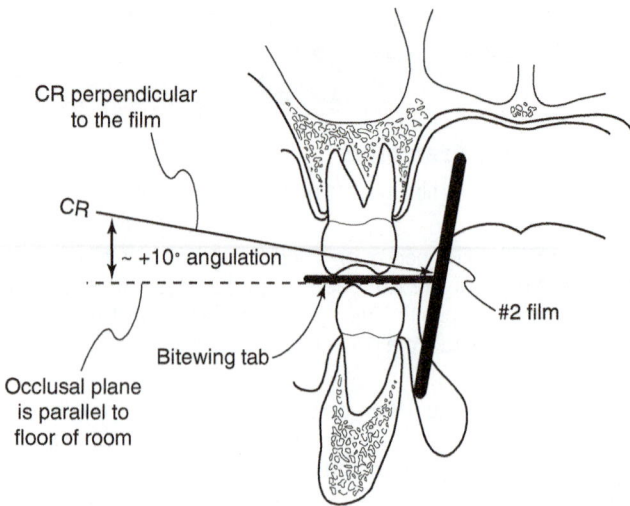

Figure 30–17 Using the bisecting technique for posterior bitewings, the central ray is directed perpendicular to the film positioned behind the teeth to be exposed.

this close, parallel film position, bitewing radiographs tend to image the teeth better, making them more sensitive. This is why bitewing images are included in FMX surveys, even though the area will have already been radiographed once with periapical films.

Bitewing Film Selection

Bitewing radiographs are taken with size no. 0 through size no. 3 film. The films are typically positioned horizontally, but they may be positioned vertically for patients with periodontal issues. These patients may require up to eight exposures of anterior and posterior teeth.

A typical bitewing series, however, involves two to four posterior exposures. The choice of film depends on a few factors, including the size and curvature of the patient's oral cavity. Among patients with smaller oral cavities and children, a single horizontal no. 2 film on either side might be enough to image the area. Smaller children with primary teeth might require a size no. 0 or no. 1 film.

For adults, a standard bitewing survey requires four no. 2 films, two on each side. A no. 3 extra-long horizontal film is available for adult bitewing surveys. This allows the entire survey to be taken with just two exposures. However, this is less than ideal and there are serious disadvantages to this film. The main problem lies with the shape of the posterior arches. Often the premolar and molar arches are slightly different, so imaging them on a single film increases the odds of overlapping images. Also, because the film is narrower than the standard no. 2, it does not show as much of the alveolar crest.

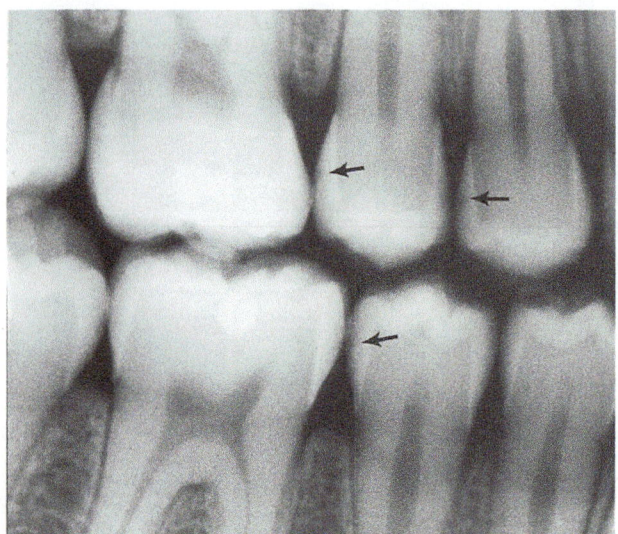

Figure 30–16 Bitewing/interproximal radiograph revealing incipient enamel caries (*arrows*).

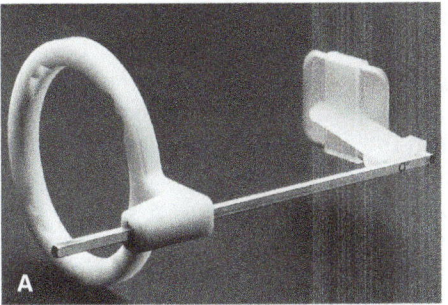 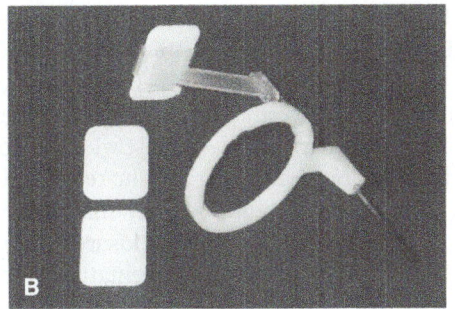 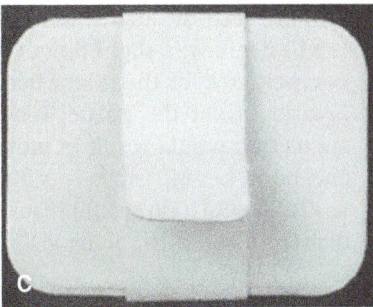

Figure 30–18 **Instruments used for bitewing exposures**. (**A**) Dentsply/Rinn horizontal posterior bitewing instrument. (**B**) Dentsply/Rinn vertical anterior and posterior bitewing instruments. (**C**) Size 2 intraoral film with bitewing tab.

Film and Sensor Holders in the Bitewing Technique

There are two ways to hold film in place for bitewing exposures:

- Bitewing film holders. These systems (usually the Rinn XCP bitewing film holder) include plastic bite blocks, aiming rings, and metal indicator arms (Figure 30-18A and B). A plastic collimator can be snapped onto the aiming ring to help the operator properly angulate the PID and reduce radiation exposure.
- Bitewing tabs. The simplest option, a bitewing tab, is a paper tab that extends from the film, which the patient clamps between his or her teeth. It is attached via a sticky side—like a sticker—on the white portion of the film. Bitewing film packets are offered for sale with the tabs pre-attached. Alternatively, bitewing tabs can be looped around standard periapical films to create bitewing films. Bitewing tabs are also sometimes called bite tabs or bite loops (Figure 30-18C). These loops are available in various sizes to accommodate different-sized films, as well as digital sensors and phosphor plates.

Film or Sensor Placement in the Bitewing Technique

Film placement is standardized in a regular bitewing series. Thus, the films used and their positions are the same from one practice to another for each of the oral regions. Film should be placed so that the teeth being imaged are centered against the film. However, it is important to note that when placing bitewing film, care should be taken to include partial teeth on either side of the target in the image. This will allow for high-quality images of the proximal surfaces of these teeth.

The best way to accomplish this is by visually inspecting the patient's oral anatomy, then lining up the edge of the film with the central line of one of the partial teeth.

If bitewing tabs are used, it often helps to insert the film into the patient's mouth in a flat position. Once the film is in, flip the bite-tab out and rotate the film until it is vertical or horizontal (depending on what is needed). The tab is then pressed against the occlusal surface of the mandibular teeth and the patient is instructed to bite down firmly to hold it in place. Patients should close their jaws normally and maintain light pressure on the bitewing tab until the exposure is completed.

Angulation of the PID

Angulation describes the orientation of the PID along horizontal and vertical planes around the patient's head. Proper angulation with the bitewing technique is essential to prevent overlap or shadow images on the final radiograph. Use of the Rinn XCP bitewing film holder with plastic aiming rings makes angulation considerably easier. The PID should be pressed flat against the plastic aiming ring to achieve the right angulation. If bite-tabs are used, angulation is determined by the position of the patient's head and the film packet.

- *Horizontal angulation.* Horizontal angulation is the position of the PID on a horizontal plane around the patient's head. In correct horizontal angulation, the central x-ray beam is directed through the *contact areas* of the teeth, in an angle that is perpendicular to the curvature of the arch. Incorrect horizontal angulation results in overlapping images from adjacent teeth, obscuring the interproximal contact areas. These radiographs cannot be used, because bitewing radiographs are usually taken to examine potential caries in this area.
- *Vertical angulation.* Vertical angulation is the position of the PID on a vertical plane around the patient's head. Vertical angulation is marked in degrees on the tubehead, with 0 degrees being parallel to the floor. Positive angulation means the PID is aiming at the floor. Negative angulation means the PID is aiming at the ceiling.

Proper vertical angulation for bitewing exposures is +10 degrees (a slight downward tilt of the PID). This compensates for the minor bend of the film caused by pressure from the palate. Too much positive vertical angulation would result in more of the maxillary teeth and bone being visible. Too little positive, or negative, vertical angulation would result in more of the mandibular teeth and bone being visible.

Patient Preparation and Exposure Sequence for a Bitewing Series

Patient preparation for a bitewing series is similar to patient preparation for other series.

As with periapical exams, an exposure sequence should be in place before the patient is seated and exposures begin. A full bitewing series might only involve two exposures, but a periodontal bitewing series might require seven exposures. The number of exposures will depend on the size of the film or sensor being used and the prescription ordered by the dentist.

If bitewing tabs are used, all the film should be prepared before exposure begins, just as film holder instruments would be prepared.

Note that bitewing exposures are part of an FMX series. However, it is not a good idea to interrupt the periapical exposure sequence to take bitewing exposures. Instead, save the bitewing exposures until the periapical exposures are completed. Bitewing exposures are usually better tolerated, so even a patient who has been having trouble

with the periapical exposures will be more tolerant of the bitewing series.

Bitewing radiographs are the most common radiographs in dentistry. They are frequently used to diagnose preclinical carious lesions in the premolars and molars, as well as evaluate the health of the alveolar bone crest.

A full bitewing series typically involves two or four exposures, depending on the size of the film used and its orientation. Vertical bitewing series usually require four to six exposures. As with periapical series, it is best to follow the same exposure sequence every time to prevent reexposures. A typical exposure sequence for an adult bitewing series includes:

- Right premolar exposure
- Right molar exposure
- Left premolar exposure
- Left molar exposure

If the bitewing series calls for seven or eight films, again start with the anterior exposures (premolars) before moving to the posterior exposures. This series is often used with patients who have periodontal issues. The film is always aligned vertically, so it captures more of the alveolar bone. Do all exposures on one side before moving to the other side. This reduces the need to move the PID around, which takes longer.

It should also be noted that most digital programs are set with an automatic advance that dictates the order of exposure. However, this exposure sequence can be modified to fit the needs of any particular operator.

Procedure 30-4 Using the Bitewing Technique

In some states, dental assistants who perform radiological procedures must complete additional training and pass a certification examination. Requirements and expanded functions vary from state to state. Check the regulations governing your state for more information about the specific duties dental assistants are allowed to perform.

Materials needed (Figure P30-4-1):

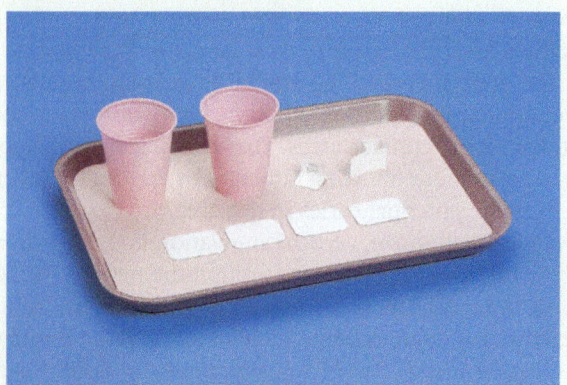

Figure P30-4-I

- Four size no. 2 films
- Paper cup labeled with patient's name
- Paper cup for trash
- Paper towels
- Lead apron
- Thyroid collar
- Bitewing tabs
- Gloves
- Patient chart

General Preparation:

1. Prepare the x-ray room and the patient.
2. Put on appropriate PPE.
3. Follow the specific instructions for each area of the oral cavity, as described below, to obtain each exposure.
4. After each exposure, remove the film, wipe away any saliva, and place the film in a cup to await development. Exposed film should be stored outside of the x-ray room to avoid secondary radiation.

Procedure 30-4 Using the Bitewing Technique (Continued)

5. When all exposures are complete, remove your gloves, then remove the lead apron and thyroid collar from the patient. Return the lead apron to its hanging position. Escort the patient out of the x-ray room.

6. Return to the x-ray room, wash hands, and reglove.

7. Dispose of all contaminated materials and clean the x-ray room. Transport exposed film for development.

Premolars

1. Set vertical angulation at +10 degrees.

2. Place the lower half of the film packet between the tongue and the mandibular teeth, with the anterior border at the middle of the canine. Press the tab over the occlusal aspect of the mandibular teeth to hold the film packet in place.

3. Ask the patient to close the mouth slowly, holding the film in place until the teeth have met the tab and are holding the film packet in place.

4. Set the horizontal angulation by standing in front of the patient and placing your index finger along the premolar area, then aligning the PID parallel with your index finger and the curvature of the arch of the premolar area (Figure P30-4-2).

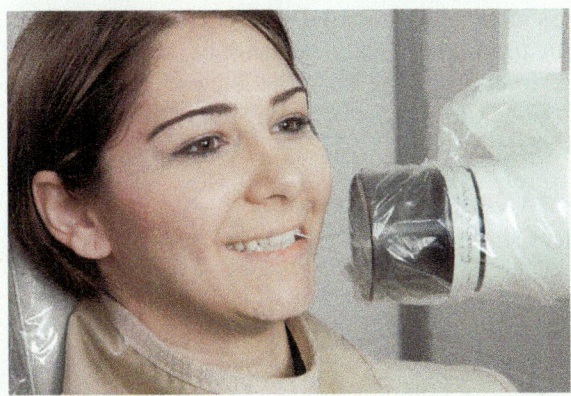

Figure P30-4-2

5. Expose the film.

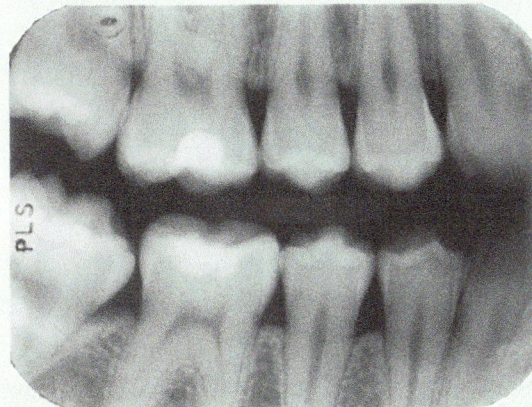

Figure P30-4-3. Resultant radiograph.

Molars

1. Set vertical angulation at +10 degrees.

2. Place the lower half of the film packet between the tongue and the mandibular teeth, centering the film on the second molar and aligning the front edge of the film with the middle of the mandibular second premolar. Press the tab over the occlusal aspect of the mandibular teeth to hold the film packet in place.

3. Ask the patient to close the mouth slowly, holding the film in place until the teeth have met the tab and are holding the film packet in place.

4. Set the horizontal angulation by standing in front of the patient and placing your index finger along the premolar area, then aligning the PID parallel with your index finger and the curvature of the arch of the premolar area.

5. Position the PID far enough forward to cover the maxillary and the mandibular canines to avoid a cone cut, directing the central ray through the contact areas (Figure P30-4-4).

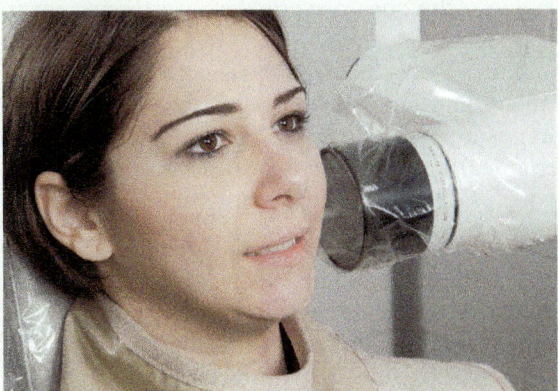

Figure P30-4-4

6. Expose the film.

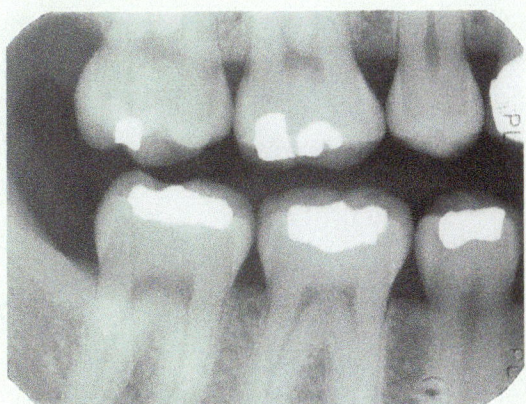

Figure P30-4-5. Resultant radiograph.

30-6 What is the bisecting technique?

30-7 Which is the preferred PID in the bisecting technique?

30-8 If the vertical angulation is excessive in a radiograph, what will happen?

30-9 What does it mean when overlapping images appear in a radiograph?

30-10 How many exposures does a typical adult bitewing series require?

Using the Occlusal Technique

The occlusal technique is used less often than periapical and bitewing techniques. Nevertheless, it is important to master this technique.

Occlusal exposures are used to visualize large areas of the maxillary and mandibular arches (see Figure 30-5). These exposures are sometimes taken in conjunction with periapical and bitewing exposures. A dentist might request occlusal images for the following reasons:

- Locate extra, unerupted, or impacted teeth
- Locate foreign bodies in the maxilla or mandible
- Locate salivary stones in the submandibular gland
- Locate lesions in the maxilla or mandible
- Visualize fractures in either the maxilla or mandible
- Visualize dental structures in patients who cannot open their mouths

- Visualize cleft palates
- Measure changes in the shape or size, or growth patterns, of the maxilla or mandible

During an occlusal exposure, the film is placed against the occlusal surface of the teeth, and the patient gently bites down on it to hold it in position during exposure.

Occlusal Exposure Techniques

Three techniques are used during occlusal exposures:

- **Topographic technique.** The topographic technique yields large images of the maxillary or mandibular arch that somewhat resemble periapical images, but it yields more information about the surrounding areas than periapical exposures. Topographic exposures are also used to examine the palate. This technique can be used with both the mandibular and the maxillary arches (Figure 30-19A).
- Lateral technique. In this technique, the PID is positioned to either side of the patient's head (right and left) to visualize the palatal roots of the molars, or to locate foreign bodies or biological abnormalities of the maxillary. The lateral technique is used only with maxillary radiographs.
- Cross-sectional technique. The cross-sectional technique produces an elliptical image of the mandible. It is used to examine the floor of the mouth, including the area under the tongue (**sublingual**) (Figure 30-19B).

Film or Sensor Placement in the Occlusal Technique

The occlusal technique uses larger film and sensors. In adults, a size no. 4 film is used; in children, a no. 2 film is used.

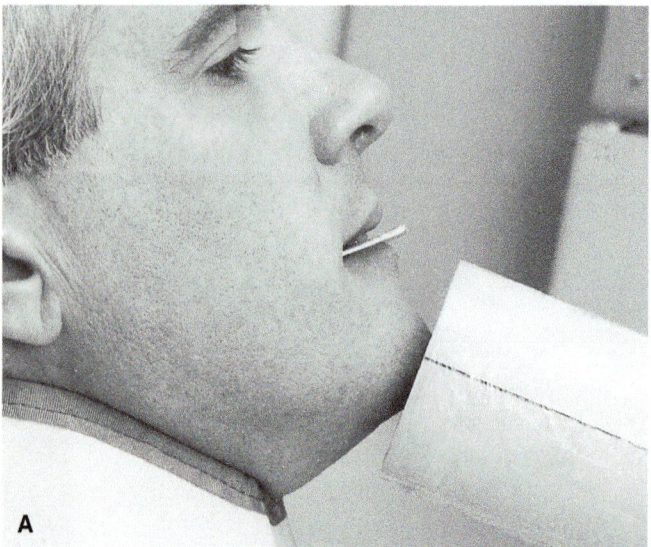
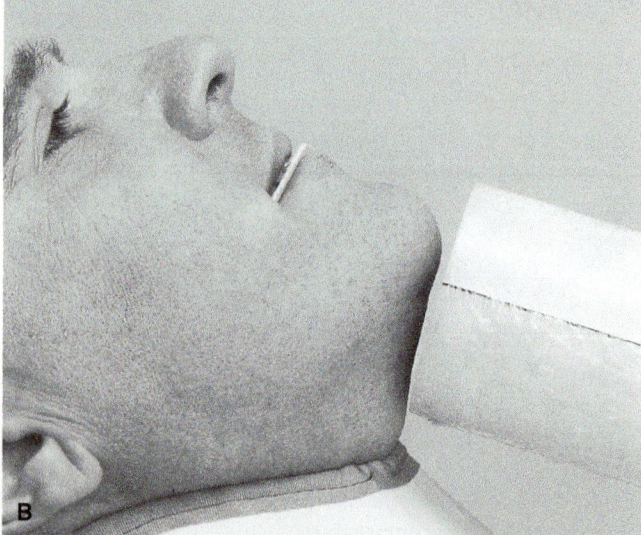

Figure 30–19 PID and film placement for occlusal radiographs. (**A**) Placement of PID and film for maxillary occlusal topographic radiograph. (**B**) Placement of PID and film for mandibular cross-sectional occlusal radiograph.

With the occlusal technique, the film is placed in between the patient's jaws and held in place with light pressure between the jaws. The white surface of the film should be facing the structure that is being visualized. For a mandibular radiograph, for example, the white side should be aimed at the mandible.

Angulation of the PID

Angulation in the occlusal technique depends on the image type.

Topographical images. Because the orientation of the film packet to the x-ray beam is not perpendicular, the theory behind PID placement in topographical images is similar to the bisecting technique in periapical exposures. The central beam of the x-ray is directed at an angle perpendicular to the imaginary bisector between the central axis of the teeth and the plane of the film. The patient should be seated with the occlusal plane (and thus the film) parallel to the floor. The angulation varies slightly for anterior and posterior exposures. See Table 30-2 for typical angulation for topographical films.

Cross-sectional images. During a mandibular cross-sectional exposure, the central beam of the x-ray is directed at a perpendicular angle through the plane of the film. To achieve this, the patient should be reclined. Take care to make sure the occlusal plane of the teeth (where the film is gripped) is at a 90-degree angle (perpendicular) to the floor. The PID is then positioned horizontally level (0 degrees angulation) under the chin for the exposure.

An 8-inch PID is preferred for occlusal radiographs. This length is easier to use and reduces the magnification and distortion associated with the larger 16-inch PID.

Patient Preparation and Exposure Sequence Using the Occlusal Technique

Patient preparation for occlusal radiography is the same as it is for periapical and bitewing images. Once again,

TABLE 30-2 Angulation in the Occlusal Technique	
EXPOSURE	**ANGULATION**
Maxillary topographical, anterior	+65
Maxillary topographical, posterior	+45
Mandibular topographical, anterior	–55
Mandibular topographical, posterior	–45

all the necessary films and equipment should be set out beforehand.

The vertical angulation can be preset for topographical images, since it does not vary among exposures.

Endodontic Technique

Endodontic radiographs are taken during a root canal procedure. They are sometimes required by the dentist to check the progress of the procedure. However, because the patient cannot close his or her mouth during the radiograph, it is essential to work quickly.

The correct procedure for an endodontic radiograph is:

- The paralleling technique should be used, as opposed to the bisecting technique. The idea is to minimize the slight distortion associated with bisecting radiographs.
- The film may be held in place with endodontic film holders or a hemostat (Figure 30-20). Preferably, a specialized endodontic holding device called an EndoRay can hold the film in place and includes a plastic positioning ring to aid in PID placement.
- The tooth should be centered on the film, with at least 5 mm of bone beyond the tooth apex visible on the film.

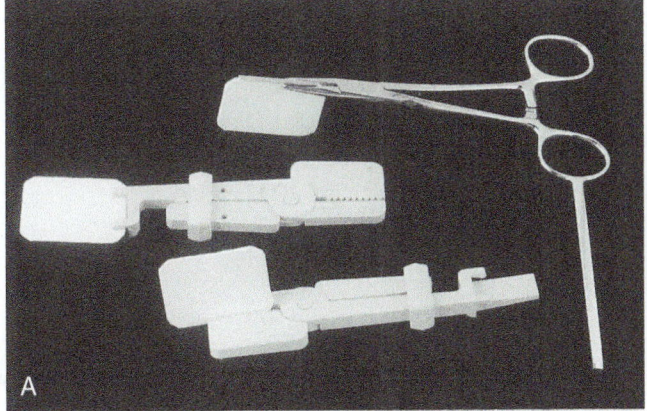
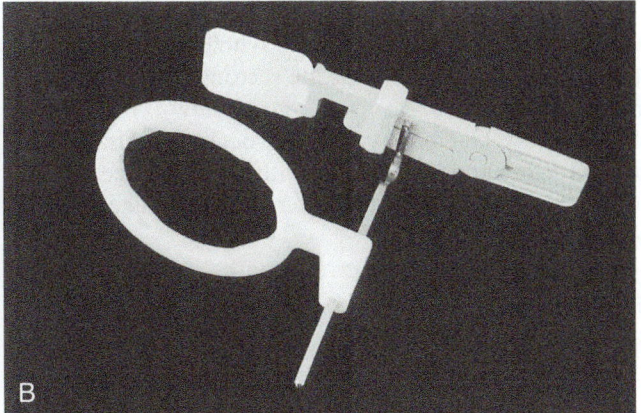

Figure 30–20 Dentsply instruments used for endodontic exposures. (**A**) EEZEE-Grip film holders (lower) and a hemostat (upper). (**B**) Snapex film holder.

Avoiding Common Technique Errors

Radiographs are meant to have *diagnostic value*. To have value, the radiograph must result from a properly placed film or sensor, the right exposure, and correct processing techniques. A diagnostic radiograph is useful to the dentist. It yields information that helps inform the dentist's medical opinion regarding treatment. A nondiagnostic radiograph is one that has errors in the film placement, exposure, or processing. These films cannot be used, and they have to be retaken. Retaking radiographs increases the radiation burden on the patient and is not consistent with the ALARA principle.

Although the dentist reads radiographs, it is essential that the dental assistant knows how to recognize errors and quickly correct them. This means dental assistants need to know what a good radiograph looks like. The image should capture the teeth and bone structures, showing all the relevant areas. It should be a clear image with minimal distortion or none at all. Images should not be elongated, foreshortened, magnified, or distorted in any way. There should be a clear contrast on the film between light and dark areas.

Some errors that look the same can have different causes. For instance, an image that is too light might be caused by underexposure, film handling problems, or underdevelopment. It is important, then, that the operator be able to quickly figure out what is causing the error. Multiple retakes are to be strenuously avoided.

Errors with radiographs generally fall into one of three categories: placement, exposure, and processing.

Placement Errors

No matter what kind of technology is used (film, digital sensor, or phosphor plate), correct placement is essential to obtaining a diagnostic radiograph. Placement errors are the most common problem with radiographs.

Periapical Films

A periapical film should show the whole tooth, including the root and tooth apex, plus the surrounding tissues. The image should extend at least 2 mm below the root and show the alveolar bone crest. The occlusal/incisal plane of the teeth should be parallel with the film edge, with a border of 6 mm (1/4 inch) between the film edge and the occlusal/incisal edge.

Common placement errors with periapical films include:

- *Absence of apical structures* (Figure 30-21). The film packet was not placed either high enough (maxillary) or low enough (mandibular) during exposure. To correct

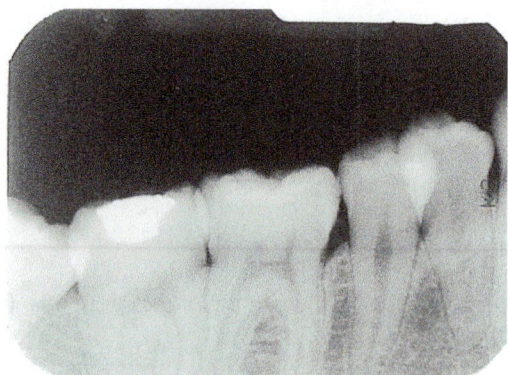

Figure 30–21 Apices are not visible due to poor film placement.

this, make sure that no more than 2 mm of film extends beyond the occlusal/incisal edge of the tooth. However, this can also be caused by insufficient vertical angulation. If film placement errors are not to blame, it is most likely an angulation problem. This kind of problem can occur with both the parallel and bisecting technique.

- *Absence of crown structure* (Figure 30-22). The film was placed either not low enough (maxillary) or high enough (mandibular) during exposure. A lip of film measuring 2 mm should extend beyond the occlusal/incisal edge of the tooth to correctly expose the crown. The use of film holders and the correct size film can prevent this. Once again, this error can also be caused by vertical angulation. In this case, excessive vertical angulation is the culprit. To correct this problem, make sure the film extends 2 mm beyond the occlusal/incisal edge and is firmly held in place during exposure.

- *Tilted image or dropped film corner* (Figure 30-23). This results in a radiograph with a tilted occlusal plane. It is caused when the film edge is not placed parallel to the occlusal/incisal edge of the tooth. This most often occurs when an inferior or broken film holder is used.

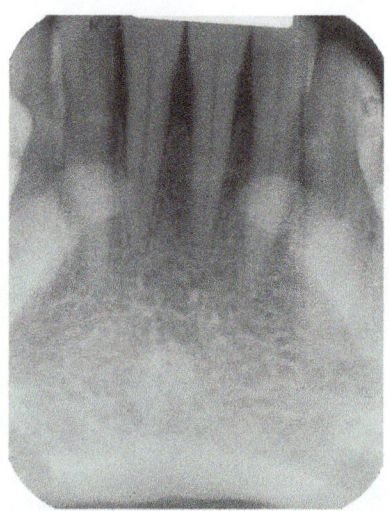

Figure 30–22 Crowns are cut off due to excessive vertical angulation.

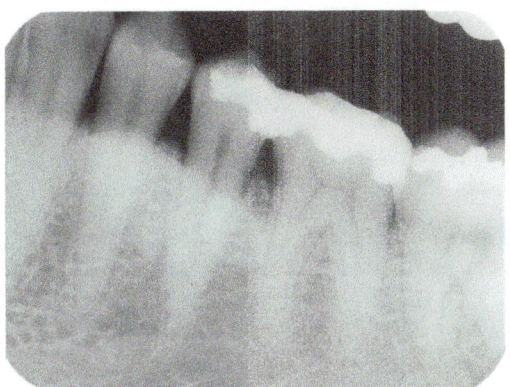

Figure 30–23 Slant is due to film not being placed parallel to the occlusal/incisal edge of the teeth.

Also, the finger-holding technique results in tipped films. To fix, use a proper film holder. The finger-holding technique for film should not be used because it results in increased radiation exposure.

■ *Angulation problems* (Figure 30-24). Angulation describes the position of the PID along the horizontal and vertical planes around the patient's head. Angulation varies between the parallel and bisecting techniques. A detailed explanation of these techniques can be found earlier in this chapter. Some common problems resulting from incorrect angulation include:

  ■ Overlapping contacts (see Figure 30-24A). This occurs when the x-ray beam is not directed straight through the contact areas of the teeth. It is an error in horizontal angulation.

  ■ Foreshortened images (see Figure 30-24B). The teeth appear short, with rounded roots. This is caused by excessive vertical angulation in the bisecting technique.

  ■ Elongated images (see Figure 30-24C). The teeth appear stretched, and the teeth appear longer than their actual roots. This is caused by insufficient vertical angulation in the bisecting technique.

Bitewing Films

A bitewing film should show the crown of both the maxillary and mandibular teeth in the image, and provide a good view of the interproximal contact spaces between the teeth. The image should depict an equal portion of the maxillary and mandibular teeth, with the occlusal/incisal plane of the teeth parallel to the film edge. The radiograph should also show the intended teeth.

Bitewing radiographs can suffer from the same problems as periapical radiographs in terms of a tipped occlusal plane, overlapping interproximal contacts, distortion, and missing regions.

Common placement problems with bitewing films include:

■ *Improper placement.* Bitewing images are designed to show a specific section of the mandibular/maxillary arches. In a premolar bitewing, the film should be placed so the radiograph clearly shows the contact areas between the canines and the premolars. To achieve this, the film should be positioned so its leading edge is parallel with the mandibular canine. Incorrect placement will obscure the distal canine surface. For the molar bitewing, the image is supposed to show the third molars. To achieve this, the film should be placed so its front edge is parallel with the midline of the second premolar. This is the proper position whether or not the third molars are present.

■ *Angulation problems.* The correct horizontal angulation sends the primary x-ray beam *directly through* the contact areas of the teeth. If the x-ray beam is shifted to either side, there will be overlapping contact areas on the radiograph, rendering it useless. A correctly aligned image will show a thin dark line (radiolucent) between the contact areas. The correct vertical angulation for bitewing radiographs is +10 degrees. Excessive vertical angulation will result in foreshortening of the teeth, while insufficient angulation will result in elongation of the teeth.

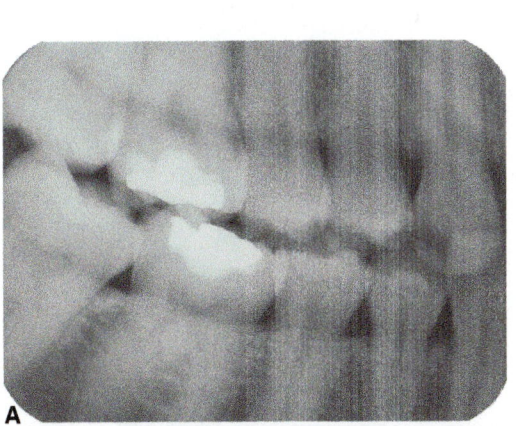 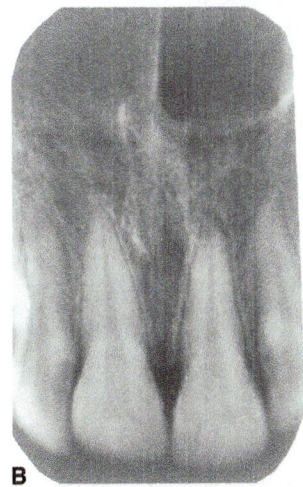 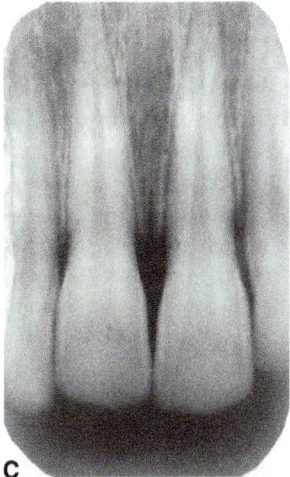

Figure 30–24 (A) Incorrect horizontal angulation will cause the overlapping of teeth. The x-ray beam must be directed between the contact areas. **(B)** Excessive vertical angulation will cause the teeth to appear shortened. **(C)** Insufficient vertical angulation will cause the teeth to appear long.

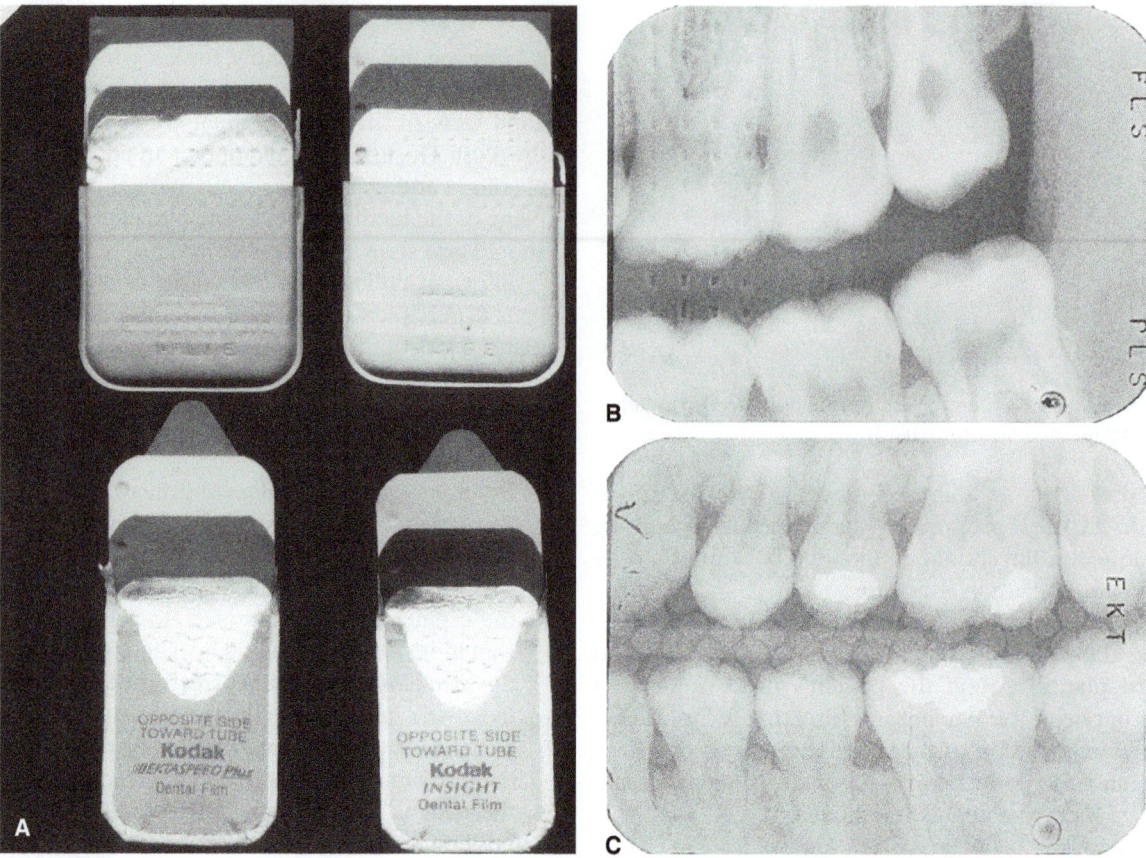

Figure 30–25 Backward film. (**A**) A herringbone pattern (top) or "ping-pong ball" pattern (bottom) is caused by placing the film packet reversed in the patient's mouth during exposure, leading to embossed patterns on the lead foil. (**B**) Radiograph with a herringbone pattern. (**C**) Radiograph with a "ping-pong ball" pattern.

General Placement Problems

Placement problems generally fall into one of the following categories:

- *Cone cuts* (see Figure 30-8). Cone cuts appear as clear areas on the film. This happens when the PID is aligned incorrectly and the central x-ray beam does not expose the entire surface of the film. Cone cuts also occur with the use of rectangular PIDs, which reduce the amount of radiation exposure by more tightly focusing the central x-ray beam, but require additional care in placement. To correct this error, make sure the PID is carefully aligned with the placement ring on the film holder.

- *Herringbone and ping-pong ball patterns* (Figure 30-25). A **herringbone pattern** or "ping-pong ball" pattern across the surface of the radiograph means that the film was reversed in the patient's mouth during exposure. These patterns are created by the embossed lead foil backing on the film. These films are also significantly underexposed. To correct this, make sure that the film is facing the correct way, with the tube side toward the teeth and x-ray beam.

- *Film bending* (Figure 30-26). If the film is bent excessively during exposure, the teeth will appear rounded or stretched. This typically occurs when the curvature of the palate is excessive and pressure from the patient's

mouth is bending the film. To prevent this, cotton rolls can be used with the paralleling technique to release pressure on the film. Film-holding devices are also helpful in preventing this.

- *Film creasing* (Figure 30-27). If the film is creased during or before exposure, a thin, dark (radiolucent) line will appear across the image at the point of the crease.

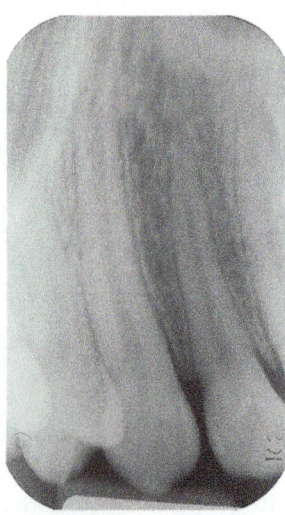

Figure 30–26 Film bending can cause the teeth to appear rounded or stretched.

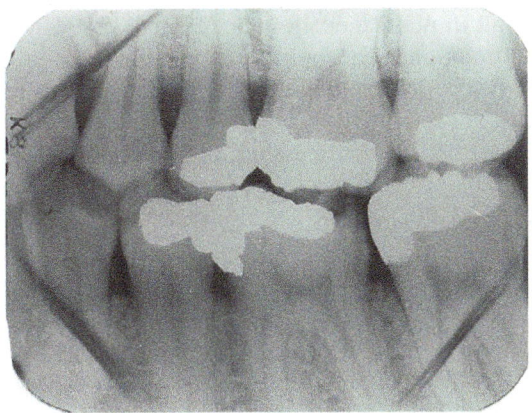

Figure 30–27 Black marks will occur on a film if the edges were creased during exposure.

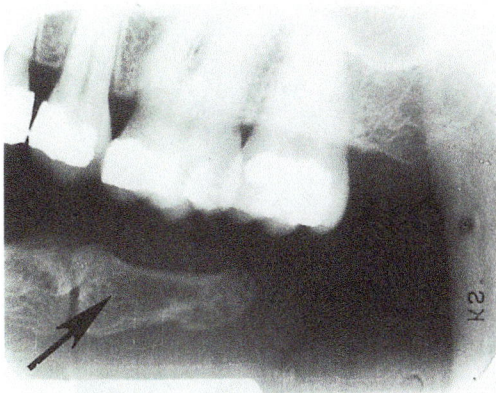

Figure 30–29 The patient's finger(s) (***arrow***) might appear in the radiograph if asked to hold the film during an exposure.

To prevent this, handle film carefully and soften the corners before putting it into the patient's mouth.

- *Movement* (Figure 30-28). Patient movement during exposure will result in blurry radiographs. To prevent this, the patient should be stabilized in a comfortable position, with his or her head firmly supported, before exposure. The operator should also be aware of the patient and refrain from pressing the exposure button if the patient is moving.

- *Phalangioma* (Figure 30-29) (patient's fingers appear in radiograph). This occurs when the patient is asked to hold film and his or her fingers are accidentally exposed. In general, the finger-holding method is discouraged because it exposes the patient to unnecessary radiation. If, however, it is unavoidable, the patient's finger should be placed *behind* the film, not in front of it.

Exposure Errors

Exposure errors commonly occur because of improper settings on the x-ray control panel. Radiographs with exposure errors are nondiagnostic. Exposure errors include:

- *Underexposure* (Figure 30-30). Underexposure results in a light image. Underexposure can be caused by

inadequate exposure time, kilovoltage, or milliamperage, or by too much distance between the film and the PID. This can also be caused by placing the film backward, which is a placement error. To prevent this, make sure the kilovoltage, milliamperage, and exposure time are set correctly, and that the exposure switch is held down for the full cycle.

- *Overexposure* (Figure 30-31). Overexposure results in a dark image. This can be caused by excessive exposure time, kilovoltage, or milliamperage. To prevent this, reduce exposure time, kilovoltage, or milliamperage to their correct levels.

- *No image.* A clear film indicates that the film was never exposed. This can happen because the x-ray machine is still off, there are electrical problems, or the machine itself is malfunctioning. If this happens, check the machine carefully and, if necessary, call for service.

- *Black image.* This happens when x-ray film is exposed to white light. See the section on processing errors for a more complete discussion on how to handle x-ray film.

- *Double image* (Figure 30-32). A **double image** is the result of accidentally exposing the same film twice. To prevent this, make sure exposed film is immediately

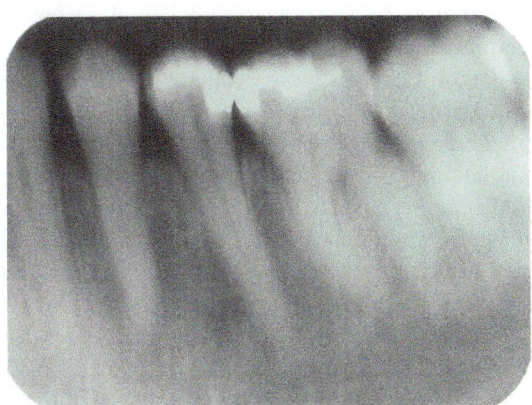

Figure 30–28 A blurry radiograph can occur if the patient moved while the film was exposed.

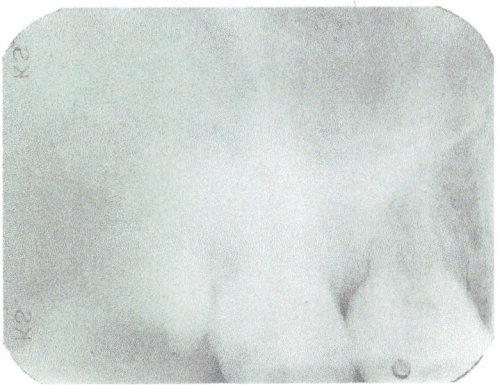

Figure 30–30 Inadequate exposure time, kilovoltage, or milliamperage, or too much distance between the film and the PID, can result in a light image.

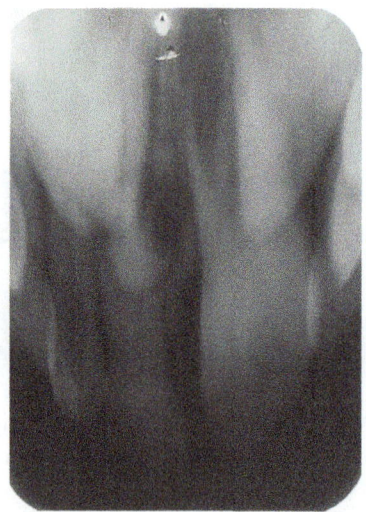

Figure 30–31 Excessive exposure time, kilovoltage, or milliamperage can result in a dark image.

placed in the proper spot, whether it is a film container in the room or outside of the room. Develop a procedure and follow it every time.

Processing Errors

After exposure, the method used to process radiographs depends on whether a traditional film-based or a digital system is used. Digital radiographs do not require processing. These images appear almost instantly on the computer monitor and are immediately available for diagnosis. This is one of the great advantages of digital radiography.

Film, on the other hand, needs to be processed. **Automatic processing** machines for film have made this task much easier, but processing errors are still possible and

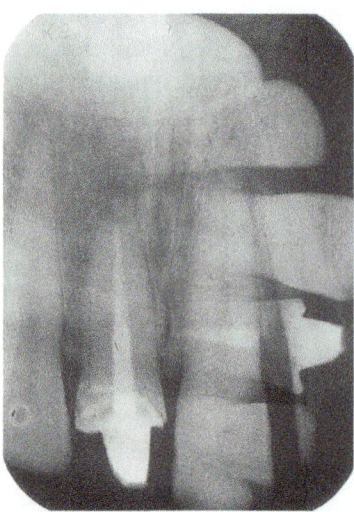

Figure 30–32 A film that has been accidently exposed twice will have a double image.

can result in nondiagnostic film. Many dentist offices still rely on traditional darkroom processing.

For a more complete discussion of film processing techniques and errors, as well as how to handle exposed films, see Chapter 32, Film Processing, Mounting, and Evaluation.

CHECKPOINTS

30-11 What is the cross-sectional technique used for in occlusal exposures?

30-12 When might a dentist require endodontic exposures?

30-13 If no apical structures appear in a periapical film, what most likely went wrong?

30-14 What is a cone cut?

30-15 A herringbone image on a radiograph indicates what?

Patients with Special Needs

Depending on the practice setting, radiograph operators might frequently come into contact with patients who have special needs or require a specialized approach. This can include pediatric patients, patients with no teeth, or those with mental or developmental disabilities. Because radiography is an important tool for these patients as well as healthy adults, operators must learn how to approach these patients. For a detailed discussion of patients with special needs, see Chapter 22, Patients with Special Needs.

Radiography in Pediatric Patients

Dental radiography is an important part of pediatric dentistry. Children have the same basic needs as adults for excellent oral health, and in fact, the best time to establish a life-long awareness of dental health is during childhood. During the first 6 years of a child's life, his or her teeth are developing rapidly. At the same time, however, children are more vulnerable to fast-developing dental caries. Dental radiographs are used to evaluate development and growth issues, diagnose caries, and evaluate the child's overall bone and dental structures.

Dental radiography does not differ significantly between adults and children, but there must be allowances made for the child's smaller oral cavity size. This means using smaller film (usually ranging between no. 0 and no. 2, depending on the patient's size). Typically, the pediatric patient also requires less kilovoltage, milliamperage, and exposure time. Fortunately, many modern machines include easy-to-use icons that automatically set these factors for pediatric patients. On older machines, the manufacturer's instructions should be followed.

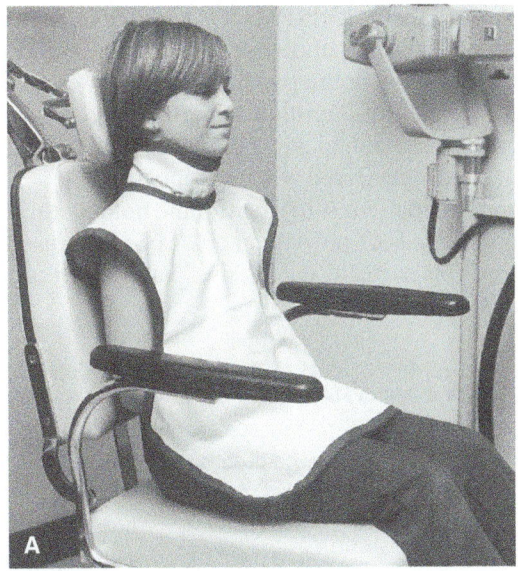
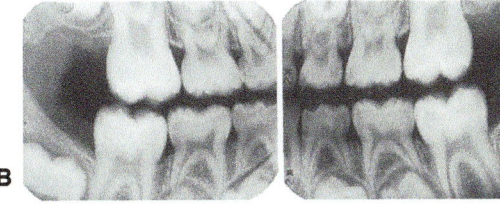

Figure 30–33 (**A**) Child with a lead apron waiting to have x-rays performed. (**B**) Bitewings of a child with mixed dentition.

Among children with **transitional mixed dentition**, or a mixture of adult and primary teeth, the most common film size is no. 2 (Figure 30-33). This allows for a larger area to be imaged. The number of exposures depends on the individual case. During a bitewing series, for example, often only two exposures are needed prior to eruption of the permanent second molar, while four are used after eruption of the permanent second molar.

One of the major concerns with pediatric patients, especially younger ones, is fright, gagging, or other behavioral obstacles. It is essential that a radiographer working with children remain calm, encouraging, and kind during exposure. It is best to escort children back into the operatory without their parents, encouraging them throughout that they will do a great job.

Radiographers can use the "Show-Tell-Do" procedure to help the children better understand the procedure. Children should be allowed to handle a packet of film and film holders so they can see and feel the items themselves. Then the radiographer can explain the technique, answering any questions the child may have, and finally go ahead with the exposure.

For children who are particularly difficult, or whose behavior represents a serious problem, a parent or older sibling should be involved in the process. The technique can be modeled on the older patient, and if necessary, the parent or guardian can hold the child. As always, the parent or guardian should wear an apron and gloves to reduce their radiation exposure.

Patients with Developmental Disabilities

Many different disabilities, both mental and physical, can complicate the process of performing radiography. These include physical disabilities, developmental disabilities, and mental disorders. A developmental disability is defined as a "substantial impairment of mental or physical functioning that occurs before the age of 22 and is of indefinite duration." Developmental disabilities include autism, cerebral palsy, and others.

When dealing with a patient with a development disability, it is essential for the radiographer to understand the disability. The patient's medical records should be carefully reviewed before the exposures begin. It is equally important that operators exercise respect when dealing with developmentally disabled patients. An operator can offer help, for example, with a wheelchair, but should not ask intrusive personal questions about living with the disability.

During the exposure, the operator should work within the patient's limitations. Some patients, for example, may be unable to hold film holders in their mouths, or they may experience involuntary movement that causes errors during exposure. In this situation, exposure time can be reduced and milliamperage increased to reduce the overall exposure time.

If it is impossible to take quality intraoral radiographs, then intraoral radiographs should not be attempted. Instead, the operator should turn to extraoral films.

Patients with Sensory Impairments

Sensory impairments include hearing and visual impairments. In these cases, the patient's oral health needs are exactly the same as someone without the disability, but communication is key. In a patient with visual disabilities, dental assistants should communicate with clear verbal instructions and refrain from gesturing at other people in the room silently. This is considered rude. Remember that eyewear should be removed prior to exposure. During exposure, patients might be allowed to handle film packets so they can better understand the procedure, and clearly communicate each time before film needs to be placed in or removed from the patient's mouth.

With people with hearing impairments, it depends on the patient's preferred form of communication. Some people will prefer to read lips, in which case the assistant should remember to always face the patient while speaking. In other cases, written instructions will work, and in still other cases, an interpreter or caregiver can serve as a go-between, using sign language. Remember that interpreters should never be exposed to additional radiation. During panoramic radiographs, hearing aids may have to be removed.

Patients with Mobility Impairments

Patients with mobility impairments include those who are in wheelchairs; those who may have lost the use of their legs, arms, or both; or those who are unable to raise or lower themselves into the dental chair for whatever reason.

If it is possible to transfer a patient into the dental chair, this is the preferred approach to radiography. It is easier for operators to work with patients in a familiar position. However, this may not always be possible. In this case, radiographs can be taken with a patient still seated in a wheelchair. The challenge here will be getting the patient close enough to the PID to take quality radiographs.

Edentulous Patients

Edentulous patients are those with no teeth. However, the lack of teeth does not mean that radiographs are unnecessary (Figure 30-34). For these patients, radiographs are used to:

- Detect objects embedded in the bone
- Inspect retained root tips, impacted teeth, or lesions below the surface
- Assist in the construction of dentures or preparation for implant surgery
- Inspect the alveolar bone

Despite the lack of teeth, it is possible to perform occlusal, periapical, and panoramic radiographs. Additionally, either the bisecting or the paralleling technique can be used. Due to the lack of dentition, there is more leeway with vertical and horizontal angulation. The paralleling technique is generally preferred whenever possible.

If the patient is having trouble holding the film in place, cotton balls or polystyrene blocks can be used. This is also true for partially edentulous patients, or those who are missing a few teeth.

✓ CHECKPOINTS

30-16 What film size is commonly used for pediatric patients with a transitional mixed dentition?

30-17 If a patient in a wheelchair cannot be transferred to the dental chair, what arrangement should be used for seating the patient to take radiographs?

Infection Control During Radiography

During any kind of dental procedure, there is the risk of transmission of infectious diseases. Diseases can be transmitted from patient to dental personnel, from dental personnel to patient, or even from patient to patient.

Infection control is a very important part of modern dentistry. At every step of the process, every care should be taken to prevent the spread of disease by following established infection control protocols.

Diseases of concern include:

- AIDS, which is caused by HIV
- Viral hepatitis
- Tuberculosis
- Herpes viruses
- Influenza
- Cold viruses

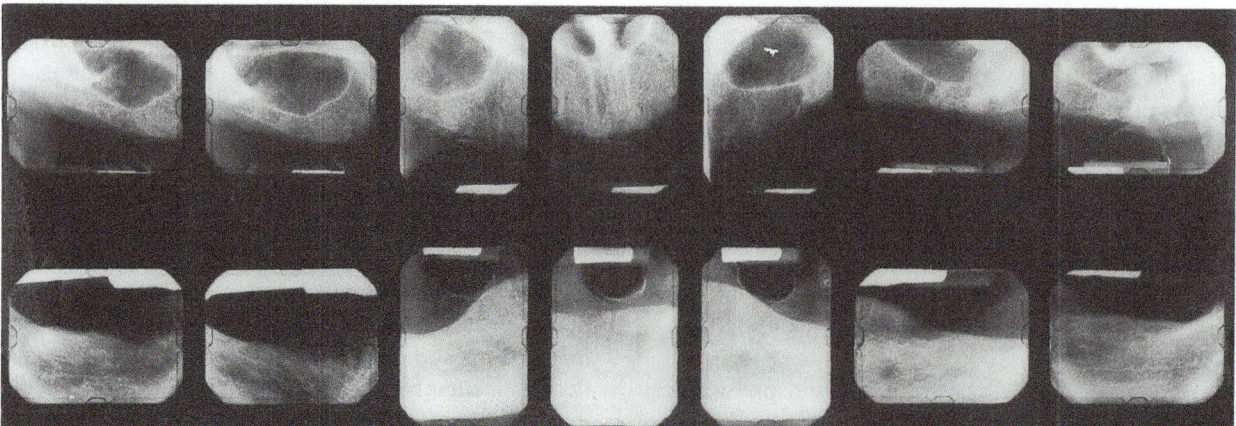

Figure 30–34 An FMX of an edentulous patient. Note that there are no bitewings.

These diseases can be transmitted through a number of routes, including:

- Direct contact with pathogens, usually in saliva or blood, respiratory excretions, or lesions
- Direct contact with airborne pathogens found in aerosol oral or respiratory excretions (e.g., sneezing)
- Indirect contact with contaminated objects, such as instruments that have been improperly cleaned

In order for transmission to be successful, the following three conditions must be present:

1. A susceptible host is available, meaning that the host is not already immune
2. A pathogen is available with adequate infectivity and numbers to cause infection
3. A portal of entry is available through which the pathogen can enter the host

Infection control is aimed at blocking one or all of these conditions to prevent the spread of infectious diseases. For a more complete discussion of infection control in general, refer to Chapter 14, Disease and Infection Control.

Centers for Disease Control and Prevention (CDC) Guidelines

The CDC published practices for infection control in 2003. The publication, *Guidelines for Infection Control in Dental Health Care Settings,* covers every area of dental treatment, including radiology. Because many people are unwilling to admit to infectious diseases, the CDC recommends that *all* patients be treated as if they are potentially infectious. This applies even to patients for whom a thorough medical history has been obtained and there is no indication of an infectious disease. It only takes one break in the protocol to result in a potential disease transmission.

The CDC's guidelines cover:

- Using barrier techniques and protective clothing
- Using heat-tolerant or disposable film-holding devices
- Cleaning and sterilizing film holders between patients
- Transporting and handling exposed film packets in a manner that reduces risk of infection
- Cleaning and sterilizing digital sensors and other equipment

Infection control can be easily broken down into three steps: before, during, and after exposure.

Infection Control Before Exposure

Before the radiographs are taken, the dental assistant should prepare himself or herself, the treatment area and equipment, and the patient using aseptic techniques. The following steps are crucial:

- Preparation of the treatment area. Any surface that is likely to be touched must be covered with impervious, disposable barriers, including plastic wrap, aluminum foil, or plasticized paper. This will eliminate the need for cleaning and disinfecting between patients. If disposable coverings are not used, then all the surfaces must be thoroughly disinfected between patients. Items to be covered include the x-ray unit, the dental chair, the work area, and the lead apron. Preparing the treatment area includes preparing any supplies to be used during the procedure. This includes film holders, film-holding devices, and any other items. Film can be prepared with the use of barrier envelopes. These plastic barriers slide over intraoral film packets and help to minimize contact with potential contaminants after exposure. Film-holding devices should be packaged in sterilized bags. Finally, any other items—cotton rolls, paper towels, and so forth—should be collected beforehand.
- Preparation of the patient. After the treatment area is prepared and all the supplies are gathered, the patient can be seated in the dental chair. The chair should be adjusted for that particular patient and the lead apron placed on the patient. Any obstructing objects, such as eyeglasses, should be removed at this point.
- Preparation of the dental assistant. At this point, the patient is seated in the chair and the treatment area has been prepared. It is now time for the radiographer to prepare himself or herself for exposure. This includes wearing protective attire and barrier clothing, such as gowns, lab coats, gloves, masks, and protective eyewear. The assistant's hands should also be washed before gloving and after removing gloves. Once the radiographer is gloved, it is safe to remove any sterilized objects, such as film holders, from their sterile packaging.

Infection Control During Exposure

By the time of exposure, there should be little risk of infection, based on the preparation. The radiographer should be gloved and gowned, taking care to only touch surfaces that are protected themselves. It is best to touch as few surfaces as possible. If, however, it is impossible to avoid unprotected surfaces—if a drawer needs to be opened, for example—the radiographer should remove his or her gloves, wash his or her hands again, and get new gloves.

After each exposure, the film should be removed carefully from the patient's oral cavity. Any saliva should be removed immediately by gently swiping the film with a disinfectant premoistened paper towel. The film can then be dropped into a paper cup labeled with the patient's name for transport. Do not touch the edges of the cup with either gloved hands or the film to prevent the spread of potentially infectious saliva.

If barrier envelopes are used, they should be wiped off and held over the plastic cup when they are opened so the film can slide directly into the cup. These films can be safely handled with clean, dry hands, or with newly gloved hands. Films should always be held by the edges to prevent fingerprint artifacts on the final image.

Remember that exposed film should never be left in the same room as the dental x-ray unit during exposure. For more information on processing films, see Chapter 32, Film Processing, Mounting, and Evaluation.

Film holding devices should be transferred during exposure from a protected work surface to the patient's mouth. After exposure, they should be moved back to the protected work surface.

Infection Control After Exposure

After exposure, the radiographer's gloves should be removed and the hands washed again. The lead apron is then removed from the patient and the patient is dismissed from the radiology area.

After the patient is gone, the operator returns to the radiology area, dons a new pair of gloves, and disposes of all contaminated objects, such as used barrier film envelopes and disposable film-holding devices. Uncovered surfaces should be decontaminated. Make sure to collect everything that was used during the radiographs, including barrier protections, cotton rolls, bitewing tabs, cups, bags, and paper towels. These items should be discarded following the rules established by the Environmental Protection Agency and local state laws.

Nondisposable objects should be placed in an area for contaminated objects.

Procedure 30–5 Infection Control Steps Before, During, and After Intraoral Radiography

Materials needed:

- Antibacterial soap
- Gloves
- Plastic or foil barriers for x-ray room equipment
- Disinfectant
- Paper towels

1. Wash hands, following hand-washing procedures, and pull on gloves.

2. Disinfect all surfaces in the radiology room that might come into contact with the patient (e.g., PID, x-ray tube head, dental chair, lead apron). *Note:* Do not spray the machine head or the control panel directly, as moisture may damage the wiring inside. Instead, spray the disinfectant on a paper towel and wipe the equipment with the wet paper towel.

3. Discard gloves and wash hands again, then pull on clean gloves.

4. Cover all the exposed surfaces in the room with plastic or foil barriers, including the PID, x-ray tubehead, control panel, light handle, dental chair, and film packets (if using protective barriers) (Figure P30-5-1).

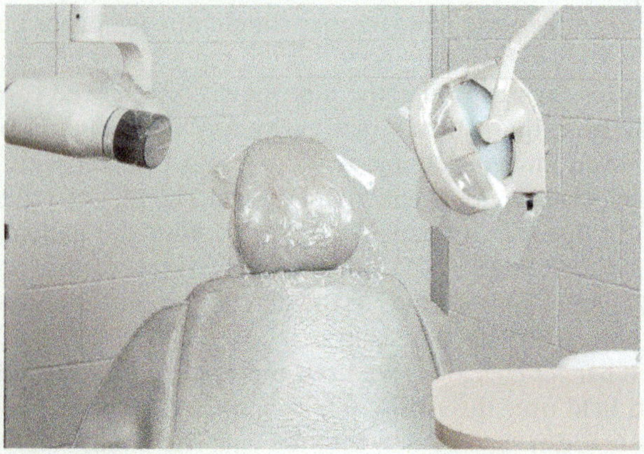

5. Gather all the supplies needed for taking intraoral radiographs.

6. Soak a paper towel with disinfectant for use during film removal.

7. Remove gloves and follow hand-washing procedures. Put on clean gloves.

8. Seat the patient and pull on overgloves. Place lead apron. Remove overgloves and place on the counter for disposal.

9. Begin exposures. *If using films without barriers,* after each exposure, wipe the films or protective envelope with a paper towel or gauze that has been lightly sprayed with disinfectant. Place the film in a paper cup or bag labeled with the patient's name. *If using films with barriers,* wipe the films with a dry paper towel and then open the barrier (Figure P30-5-2A and B). Drop the film packet into a cup with patient's name without touching film packet. After the exposures are complete, escort the patient out of the x-ray room.

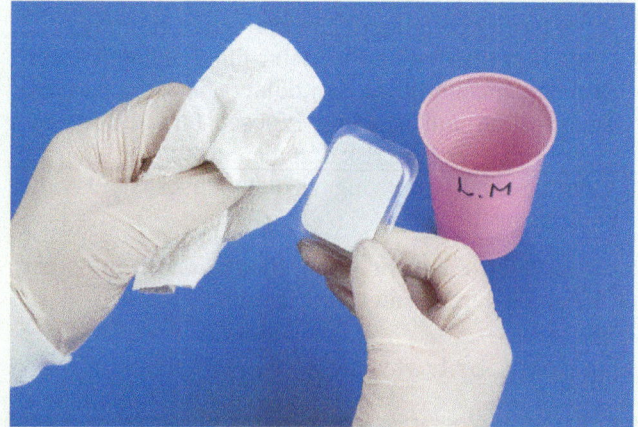

Figure P30-5-2A

Figure P30-5-1

Procedure 30–5 Infection Control Steps Before, During, and After Intraoral Radiography (Continued)

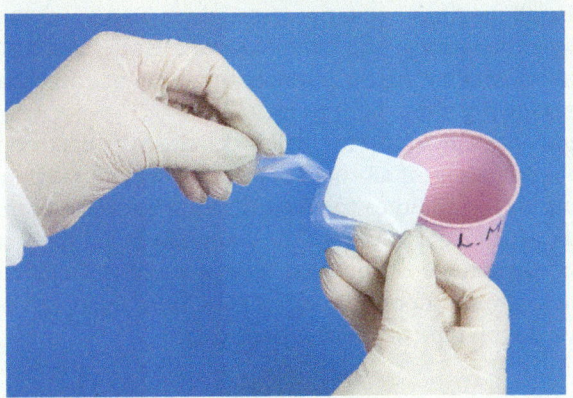

Figure P30-5-2B

10. Return to the treatment area, wash hands, and reglove.
11. Collect all the disposable items for disposal and collect all the contaminated equipment for sterilization. Remove all the barriers for disposal, and disinfect the surfaces underneath.

✔ CHECKPOINT

30-18 What surfaces are covered with infection control barriers during a radiography procedure?

Quality Assurance in Radiography

A quality assurance program is designed to guarantee that the highest-quality radiographs are produced under the best possible conditions, including the lowest possible radiation exposure. Every dental office should have a quality assurance program for its radiology program. This program should cover the tests used to monitor the machines used in the office (e.g., x-ray unit, film processing machines), film storage system, darkroom, documentation and record maintenance, and competency.

Some elements of a quality assurance program may be mandated by local or state laws. For example, maintenance and testing of the x-ray machine is frequently required by local regulatory agencies. There are a number of tests that should be conducted on the x-ray machine annually, including:

- Kilovoltage (kVp) output
- Milliamperage (mA) accuracy
- Exposure timer accuracy
- Radiation output
- Focal spot size
- Beam alignment and beam size
- Tube head stability
- Half-value layer

These tests may be conducted by a qualified health physicist as part of a licensing or registration program. Comprehensive test records should be maintained, and should include the name of the person conducting the test, the date, and the results.

Using the Step Wedge

A step wedge is a device made of layered metal steps of varying thickness. They are available for commercial purchase or can be made by soldering overlapping foil layers from film packets (Figure 30-35). These devices can be used to check both the radiation output and the processing solution.

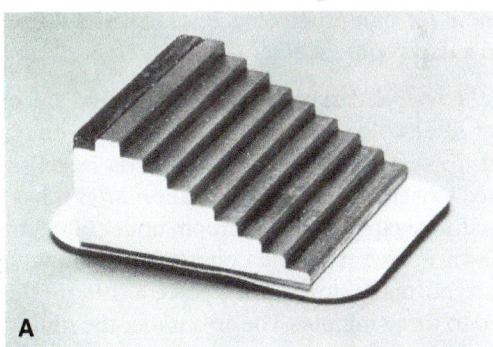

A

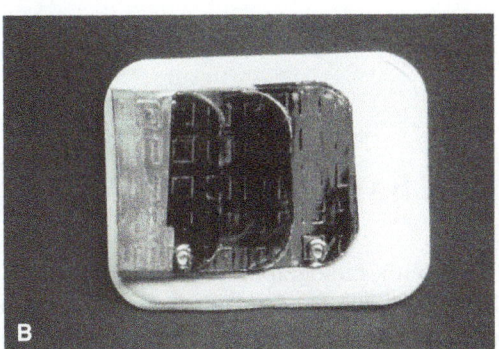

B

Figure 30–35 Step wedges. These may be (**A**) made of layered metal available for commercial purchase or (**B**) made by soldering overlapping foil layers from film packets.

To check the radiation output, set the step wedge on a no. 2 film and expose the film with preset exposure factors. Store this film somewhere safe. Then, at intervals determined by the practice, expose new films in the same way with the same exposure factors. For example, exposures can be made in the morning, in the afternoon, and again just before the practice closes. When all the exposures are made, process all the film at the same time and compare the radiographs. A consistent x-ray tube will produce three identical radiographs. A failed test will yield three different radiographs, meaning that the x-ray output varied over the course of the day. A failed test should trigger a service call.

Step wedges can also be used to test the processing solution in a darkroom or automatic film-processing machine. To conduct this test, place the step wedge on film packets and expose 20 consecutive radiographs. Do this on the day the processing solution is first changed. Process the first film and store it somewhere cool and dry. Then, every day or every other day, process another film packet and compare it to the radiograph processed on the first day. The bands created by the step wedge should be identical in every radiograph. Varying darkness means the processing solution is not working correctly. In this case, check the processing solution, including its temperature, the time of processing, and whether the solution has been contaminated.

Darkroom Testing

Although many dental offices are switching to digital radiography, and thus doing away with darkrooms, it is still important to know how to maintain a proper darkroom environment for film processing. Tests that should be conducted in a darkroom include:

- *Safelight test.* A darkroom safelight should be of the correct filter color and wattage for the film being processed. To test this, use a film that has been slightly exposed to a small amount of radiation. After it has been exposed, unwrap it in the darkroom under safelight conditions and place it on the counter where unwrapped films are normally stored. Then place a coin on the film for two to three minutes. The area under the film will be protected from light exposure, while the rest of the film is vulnerable. This is called a **coin test**. After a few min-

utes have elapsed, process the film as normal. If the coin is visible on the film, the darkroom has failed the test. This means the film is fogging due to less than optimal light conditions in the darkroom, which will compromise all the films being processed there. To correct this, check the wattage and filter color of the safelight. Also, make sure there are no cracks in the safelight cover that are allowing white light to escape.

- *Light leak test.* To test for light leaks, close the darkroom door and turn off all the lights, including the safelight. Wait for five minutes to allow the eyes to adjust to the dark. If any light is visible, the room has failed the test. Find the source of the light leak and seal it, including cracks around doors or ceiling tiles. Light leaks can be sealed with tape or weather stripping.

Elements of a Quality Assurance Program

A good quality assurance program includes a deliberate series of protocols that are carefully followed, including a written plan. This plan will include the purpose of the quality assurance program, assign authority for its implementation, list all the equipment that needs testing, list the tests to be conducted on this equipment, and contain a log of all the previous tests. In addition, periodic evaluations of the program should be included.

Operator competency is an important part of quality assurance and should also be included. A log should be kept of all retakes, including the operator and the reason for the retake. Retakes are highly undesirable because they expose patients to unnecessary radiation. A consistent pattern of retakes or errors should be addressed and corrected.

Additionally, programs and educational opportunities should be offered to help radiographers stay current in their skills. Participation in these programs should be noted in the log as well.

CHECKPOINTS
30-19 What is the purpose of a step wedge?

30-20 Why is it crucial to minimize the number of retakes when performing radiography procedures?

 **Chapter Highlights**

- The full-mouth radiographic survey, or FMX, is the standard technique used to obtain a complete set of images. It contains between 18 and 20 images, including 14 periapical films and four to six bitewing films.
- An FMX series can be obtained in adults, pediatric patients, and patients with special needs or no teeth.

- All exposure sequences begin with anterior teeth to reduce the risk of gagging during exposure. Patients who gag can be soothed and distracted, or in bad cases, given an anesthetic mouth rinse or throat lozenge to reduce the gag reflex.

◆ A periapical exposure pictures teeth from the apex to the occlusal/incisal surface, including the root and surrounding tissues.

◆ A bitewing exposure shows the crowns and occlusal surfaces of both mandibular and maxillary teeth on one film. It is especially useful to diagnose interproximal decay.

◆ An occlusal exposure shows either portions of or the entire maxillary or mandibular arch. It is used to show large areas of the bone structure and teeth.

◆ The paralleling technique, which is preferred by the American Dental Association, aims the central x-ray beam at a perpendicular angle to the long axis of the tooth.

◆ The bisecting technique aims the central x-ray beam at an imaginary bisector of the angle formed by the plane of the film and the long axis of the tooth. Some minimal distortion is inevitable.

◆ Vertical angulation describes the orientation of the PID in a vertical plane around the patient's head. Positive vertical angulation means the PID is pointing toward the floor. Negative vertical angulation means the PID is pointing toward the ceiling.

◆ Horizontal angulation describes the orientation of the PID in a horizontal plane around the patient's head. The central x-ray beam should be aimed *directly through* the spaces between the patient's teeth.

◆ Film holders with specialized localizing rings are used to help determine the correct angulation.

◆ The same sequence exposure should always be followed to minimize mistakes.

◆ The endodontic technique is used during a root canal procedure.

◆ Technique errors during radiography include film placement errors, exposure errors, and processing errors. In some cases, these look the same. Therefore, the radiographer needs to be familiar with every step of the process to prevent errors.

◆ Infection control is a major part of dentistry. According to the CDC, all patients should be treated as infective risks, and infection control protocols should be followed every time.

◆ A quality assurance program helps guarantee the highest quality radiographs and the lowest radiation exposure by establishing a schedule of testing and record-keeping for all office equipment, procedures, and personnel.

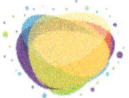 **Review Questions**

1. How many films, of which variety, are in a typical adult FMX?

   a. 18–20 films, including 14 periapical and 4–6 bitewing

   b. 18–20 films, including 12 periapical and 6–8 bitewing

   c. 20–22 films, including 14 periapical and 6–8 bitewing

   d. Depends on the patient

2. A typical apron includes which of the following components?

   a. A 1/2-inch lead barrier

   b. A thyroid collar

   c. A shin guard

   d. Oil to absorb x-ray heat

3. To reduce the risk of gagging, which exposures should be taken first?

   a. Periapical

   b. Posterior

   c. Bitewing

   d. Anterior

4. A periapical exposure shows what?

   a. The crowns of teeth on the mandible and maxillary jaw

   b. The surface of teeth on both the mandible and maxillary jaw

   c. The whole tooth on either the mandible or maxillary jaw from the apex to the occlusal/incisal surface

   d. Roots and surrounding tissues of both mandibular and maxillary teeth

5. A bitewing exposure shows what?

   a. The crowns of teeth on the mandible and maxillary jaw

   b. The surface of teeth on both the mandible and maxillary jaw

   c. The whole tooth on either the mandible or maxillary jaw from the apex to the occlusal/incisal surface

   d. Roots and surrounding tissues of both the mandibular and maxillary teeth

6. An occlusal exposure shows what?

   a. The crowns of teeth on the mandible and maxillary jaw

   b. The surface of teeth on both the mandible and maxillary jaw

   c. The whole tooth on either the mandible or maxillary jaw from the apex to the occlusal/incisal surface

   d. Roots and surrounding tissues of both the mandibular and maxillary teeth

7. At what angle should the central x-ray beam strike the long axis of the tooth in the paralleling technique?

   a. 45 degrees

   b. 90 degrees

   c. Depends on the film angle

   d. A 90-degree angle to the bisector

8. How do you calculate vertical angulation in the bisecting technique?

   a. Divide the parallel angulation by half

   b. It is a right angle to the plane of the film

   c. It is a right angle to the plane of the tooth

   d. It is a right angle to the bisector formed by the tooth and the film

9. Excessive vertical angulation results in what?

   a. Overlapping images

   b. Artifacts

   c. Foreshortened images

   d. Elongated images

10. Which film size is typically used in an adult bitewing series?

    a. no. 4

    b. no. 3

    c. no. 2

    d. no. 1

11. How many millimeters beyond the occlusal or incisal surface should film extend in the periapical exposure to guarantee a good image?

    a. 2 mm

    b. 1 mm

    c. 4 mm

    d. 5 mm

12. The topographic technique in occlusal exposures shows what?

    a. A narrow image of the mandibular arch

    b. A narrow image of the maxillary arch

    c. Large sections of either the mandibular or maxillary arch

    d. Large sections of only the maxillary arch

13. Which film size is typically used for an occlusal exposure on an adult patient?

    a. no. 1

    b. no. 2

    c. no. 3

    d. no. 4

14. A cone cut occurs under what circumstances?

    a. The PID is not aligned with the angulation correctly.

    b. The vertical angulation is too steep.

    c. The PID is too narrow.

    d. The PID is not aligned correctly with the film.

15. According to the CDC's infection control procedures

    a. Patients should be treated as infective risks according to their medical histories.

    b. All patients should be treated as potentially infective.

    c. Antibiotics should be administered to all patients before radiography.

    d. Only patients with blood-borne diseases represent a serious health risk.

16. If the patient moves during exposure, which of the following errors may occur?

    a. A thin dark line appears on the radiograph.

    b. The teeth appear distorted.

    c. A herringbone pattern appears on the radiograph.

    d. The entire image is blurry.

Active Learning Exercises

1. Gagging is a common patient reflex, especially during radiographic exposures. What are some techniques you can use to alleviate the gag response?

2. Radiographic diagnosis is essential for the clinical examination. What are some differences between the horizontal and vertical bitewings? Which dental specialty would use one or the other more often?

3. Proper angulations for the bisecting technique are crucial. What are some common errors made when using this technique and how could they be corrected?

Application Activities

1. Using the Internet or your local library, research any state and local laws that define the required elements of a radiological quality assurance program.

2. Draw a diagram showing the bisecting technique, including the bisector and the central x-ray beam.

PREPARING FOR CERTIFICATION EXAMS

Review the following topics in this chapter to prepare for the Dental Assisting National Board (DANB) exam:

- **The Full-Mouth Radiographic Survey**
- **Preparing the Equipment**
- **Preparing the Patient and During Exposure**
- **The Gag Reflex**
- **Intraoral Exposure Types**
- **Overview of Techniques**
- **Using the Paralleling Technique**
- **Using the Bisecting Technique**
- **Using the Bitewing Technique**
- **Using the Occlusal Technique**
- **Avoiding Common Technique Errors**
- **Placement Errors**
- **Exposure Errors**
- **Patients with Special Needs**
- **Infection Control During Intraoral Radiography**

chapter 31

Extraoral Radiographs and Other Imaging Systems

CHAPTER CHECKLIST

On completion of this chapter, students will be able to:

- ☑ Identify the types of exposures obtained through extraoral radiography.
- ☑ Identify the equipment and materials used in extraoral radiography.
- ☑ Explain the purpose of panoramic radiographs.
- ☑ Describe the process involved in panoramic radiography.
- ☑ Identify the equipment and materials used in panoramic radiography.
- ☑ Describe the steps involved in setting up and conducting a panoramic radiograph.
- ☑ Identify common errors that occur in panoramic radiography.
- ☑ Describe the main advantages and disadvantages of panoramic radiography.
- ☑ Describe additional types of extraoral radiographs and the purpose of each.
- ☑ Explain the process involved in computed tomography (CT) scanning and its use in dentistry.
- ☑ Explain the process involved in magnetic resonance imaging (MRI) and its use in dentistry.

KEY TERMS

cassette – a device used in extraoral radiography that holds the screen film and two intensifying screens in a light-safe environment during exposure

cephalometer – an instrument used to position the head to produce oriented, reproducible lateral and posteroanterior head films; also called a cephalostat

computed tomography – a form of x-ray imaging that uses multiple sensors placed around the patient and a computer program to yield high-quality diagnostic images of thin slices of tissue or organs; this same principle is used in panoramic dental radiography

condylar neck – condyles located in the neck bones

condyle – a rounded articular surface at the extremity of a bone

extraoral radiography – a technique of obtaining dental radiographs in which the film is placed outside the patient's oral cavity during exposure

fluoresce – to glow or emit light, in this case under the influence of radiation

focal trough – in panoramic radiography, the curved, narrow region where the x-ray beam is focused to yield clear images; it is created by the movement of the x-ray tubehead in relation to the film

Frankfort plane – an imaginary plane that extends from the orbital ridge directly under the eye to the top of the ear canal

grid – in extraoral radiography, a device used to reduce the amount of scatter radiation produced during exposure

intensifying screen – device used in extraoral radiography to convert x-ray beams into visible light, which is used to expose the screen film; an intensifying screen reduces the amount of radiation needed to create a diagnostic exposure

magnetic resonance imaging – a technique of medical imaging that uses powerful magnetic waves to create high-quality images of internal structures and organs

occipital protuberance – the raised and tangible lump in the base of the neck caused by the occipital bone, which is located in the back of the head

panoramic radiography – the practice of obtaining extraoral radiographs using a special x-ray unit that rotates around the head and visualizes both the maxilla and mandible in one large film

ramus – a part of an irregularly shaped bone that forms an angle with the main body, e.g., ramus of the mandible

rotational center – in panoramic radiography, the imaginary point around which the tubehead and film cassette rotate

screen film – film used in extraoral radiography; screen film is larger than intraoral films and must be exposed with intensifying screens enclosed in a cassette to yield a diagnostic image

skull radiograph – an x-ray image of a portion of the skull

temporomandibular joint – a synovial articulation between the head of the mandible and mandibular fossa and articular tubercle of temporal bone; a fibrocartilaginous articular disc divides it into two cavities

tomogram – an x-ray projection of the temporomandibular joint

tomography – the practice of obtaining tomograms

zygomatic arch – arch formed by temporal process of zygomatic bone that joins zygomatic process of temporal bone

Introduction

Although intraoral radiographs are the essential core of dental radiography, there are times when it is not possible to take them or when another type of image is more appropriate to the clinical circumstances. In these cases, extraoral radiographs are often necessary.

Extraoral radiographs are obtained by placing the film *outside* the patient's mouth (Figure 31-1). These films are commonly used when an image of a large portions of the patient's jaw or skull is needed, or when a patient cannot tolerate intraoral radiographs. This includes patients who suffer from jaw fractures, impacted teeth, or large oral lesions and patients who cannot or will not open their mouth. Extraoral radiographs are also used in orthodontics.

Extraoral radiographs are sometimes used in conjunction with intraoral radiographs. Pediatric patients may also tolerate extraoral radiographs better than intraoral, as long as they can hold still during the extended exposure time.

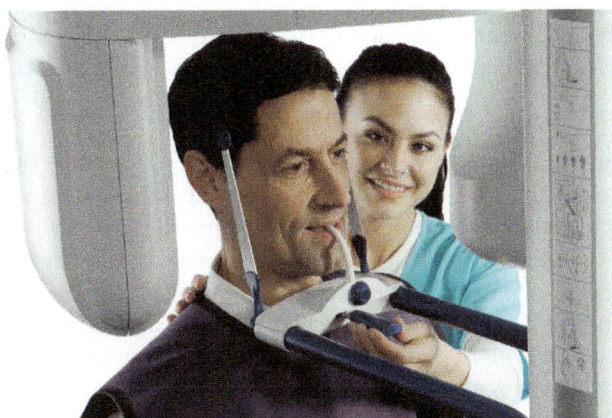

Figure 31–1 Patient having an extraoral radiograph taken.

In general, extraoral radiographs are used to:

- Examine large areas of the skull and jaws
- Evaluate growth and development
- Evaluate impacted teeth
- Evaluate fractures and jaw and skull trauma
- Diagnose diseases and lesions in the jaw and skull
- Evaluate the temporomandibular joint

Because some dental offices are not equipped with the machines needed to make extraoral radiographs, some dental assistants may never use these specialized techniques. However, a basic knowledge in extraoral radiography and other radiographic techniques is still an important part of the dental assistant's complete education.

Basics of Extraoral Radiography

The most common form of **extraoral radiography** is known as **panoramic radiography** (Figure 31-2). This kind of radiograph produces a large image of the maxilla and mandible on a single piece of film. It uses a special type of film and a special x-ray unit that rotates smoothly around the patient's head while the exposure is being taken. Panoramic radiography is also sometimes called *rotational panoramic radiography*.

Extraoral projections can also be obtained with a standard intraoral x-ray unit, in conjunction with special head-positioning devices, beam-alignment devices, and film. These types of nonpanoramic projections, however, have been replaced by panoramic radiography in some cases. Exposures that can be obtained by this method include:

- *Lateral jaw radiographs.* These images expose the posterior section of the mandible. It is especially useful for children or patients who cannot open their jaws.

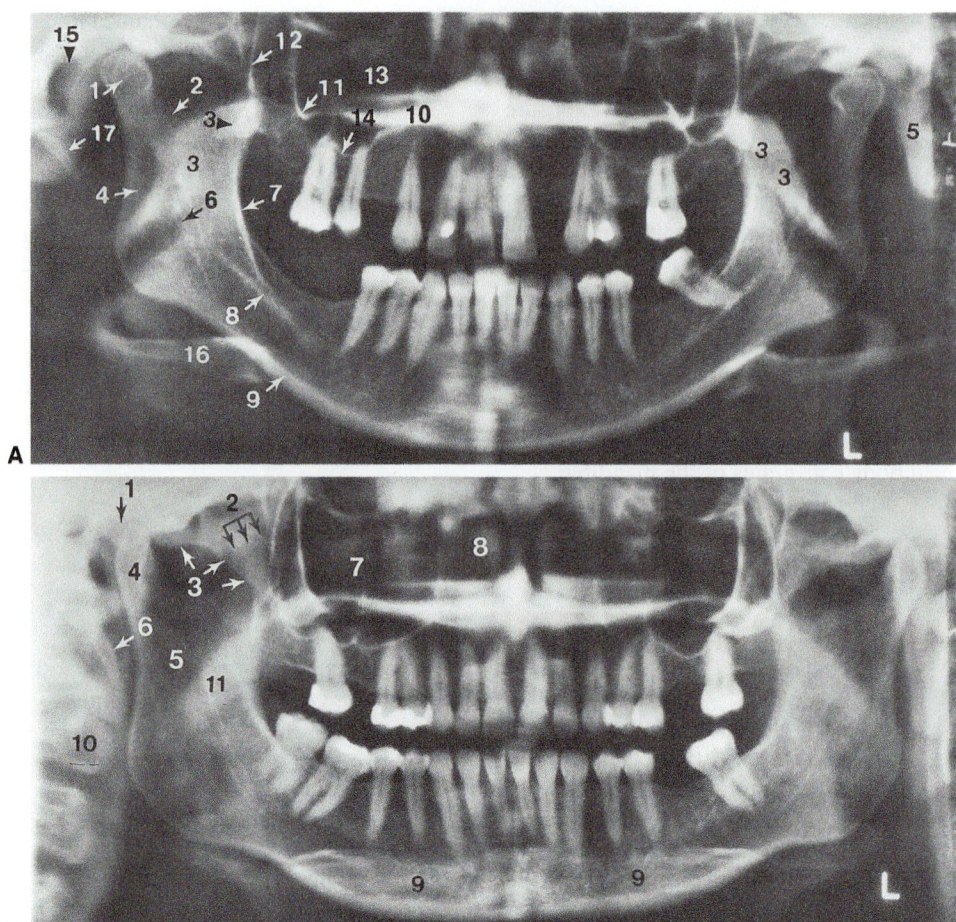

Figure 31–2 Panoramic radiographs with common anatomical structures labeled. **(A)** (1) Condyle. (2) Nasopharyngeal air space. (3) Soft palate. (4) Oropharyngeal air space. (5) Soft tissue of ear. (6) Glossopalatal air space. (7) External oblique ridge. (8) Mylohyoid (internal oblique) ridge. (9) Lower border of mandible. (10) Hard palate. (11) Lower border of zygomatic bone. (12) Posterior wall of maxillary sinus. (13) Maxillary sinus. (14) Lower floor of maxillary sinus. (15) External auditory meatus. (16) Hyoid bone. (17) Stylohyoid process. **(B)** (1) Glenoid fossa. (2) Nasopharyngeal air space. (3) Zygomatic arch. (4) Condyle. (5) Oropharyngeal air space. (6) Stylohyoid process. (7) Maxillary sinus. (8) Inferior turbinate. (9) Ghost of hyoid bone. (10) Spinal column. (11) Soft palate.

■ ***Skull radiographs***. These radiographs expose larger sections of the skull, including the bones of the face. Some exposures require a special device called a **cephalometer**, which stabilizes and positions the head during exposure. Cephalometric radiographs are typically used by orthodontists and oral surgeons.

■ ***Temporomandibular radiographs***. These radiographs are used to examine the temporomandibular joint (TMJ). They are used to diagnose ankylosis (a stiffening of the TMJ), as well as other disorders involving the TMJ.

Each of these techniques, including the various exposures, is discussed in this chapter.

Equipment Used in Extraoral Radiography

With all types of extraoral radiographs, the basic principles are the same. During an extraoral exposure, the primary x-ray beam is directed through the patient's jaw or skull to strike the film or digital sensor behind it. Film and sensors for extraoral radiography are much larger than those used for intraoral radiography, because the areas being visualized are much larger. However, special devices called intensifying screens are used to minimize radiation exposure.

Film Types

Extraoral radiographs use **screen film** to produce diagnostic images. Screen films are paired with intensifying screens that are housed within the film cassette.

Unlike intraoral films, extraoral films are extremely light sensitive and must be packaged into the film cassettes under safelight conditions in a darkroom. Check the manufacturer's instructions to make sure the filter used in the darkroom is appropriate for the specific type of extraoral film being used. The same darkroom filters that are used for intraoral films may not be appropriate for extraoral films.

Extraoral films are either sensitive to green light (Kodak T-Mat G and Ortho G) or blue light (Kodak X-Omat RP and Ektamat G). They must be used with intensifying screens that emit the same color light for a proper exposure. In other words, a blue-sensitive screen film must be paired with blue-emitting intensifying screens, and a green-sensitive film must be paired with green-emitting intensifying screens.

The most common extraoral film sizes are 5 × 7 inch and 8 × 10 inch. Film sizes are slightly different for panoramic cassettes. Extraoral film comes in boxes of 25, 50, or 100 pieces of film. These boxes should be opened only under safelight conditions to avoid ruining the film. Extraoral film should be handled with clean, dry hands and held carefully by the edges. Touching extraoral film with latex or vinyl treatment gloves should be avoided because of the risk of static electricity. A static charge will leave an artifact on the radiograph, possibly rendering it nondiagnostic.

In some cases, traditional no. 4 size intraoral occlusal film can be used to obtain extraoral radiographs. These films are typically used with either lateral jaw or transcranial projections. These films do not require the use of intensifying screens, but they do have several drawbacks. Because of their smaller size, they do not allow for large projections. And, most important, because they are not used with intensifying screens, it takes longer to obtain a good exposure. This increases the radiation burden on the patient.

Film Cassettes

The film **cassette** is designed to hold the screen film and the two intensifying screens in close contact and protect the screen film from white light. Cassettes should always be assembled with film and intensifying screens in a darkroom safelight environment to protect the integrity of the film. Once the cassette is sealed, it is safe to move it into white light.

Cassettes are available in either rigid or flexible shapes, either flat or curved. They come in a number of sizes that fit the various types of films available. Rigid cassettes are typically 5 × 7 inch or 8 × 10 inch. Flexible cassettes, which frequently are used for exposing panoramic films, are typically 5 × 12 or 6 × 12. It is imperative that all cassettes are completely light safe to prevent contamination of the film.

Cassettes have a designated front and back side. The front is made from a plastic covering that allows x-rays to penetrate to the film below. The back is made from metal that absorbs any remnant x-rays.

Once a cassette has been assembled, it can be marked with R or L, indicating the patient's right or left side, and labeled with the patient's name, the dentist's name, and the date. Film should also be clearly marked upon removal to prevent errors.

Like all radiographic equipment, cassettes should be inspected regularly to ensure they are working properly. The Velcro straps or hinges that hold the sides of cassettes together are possible light pollutants that should be monitored regularly. Also, warped cassettes result in improper contact between the film and intensifying screen, which yields blurry images.

Intensifying Screens

Intensifying screens are designed to reduce the amount of radiation a patient is exposed to during the relatively longer exposure times involved with extraoral radiography. These special screens convert x-ray energy into visible light, which then exposes the screen film. Each film cassette contains two intensifying screens, one in front of the film and one behind (Figure 31-3).

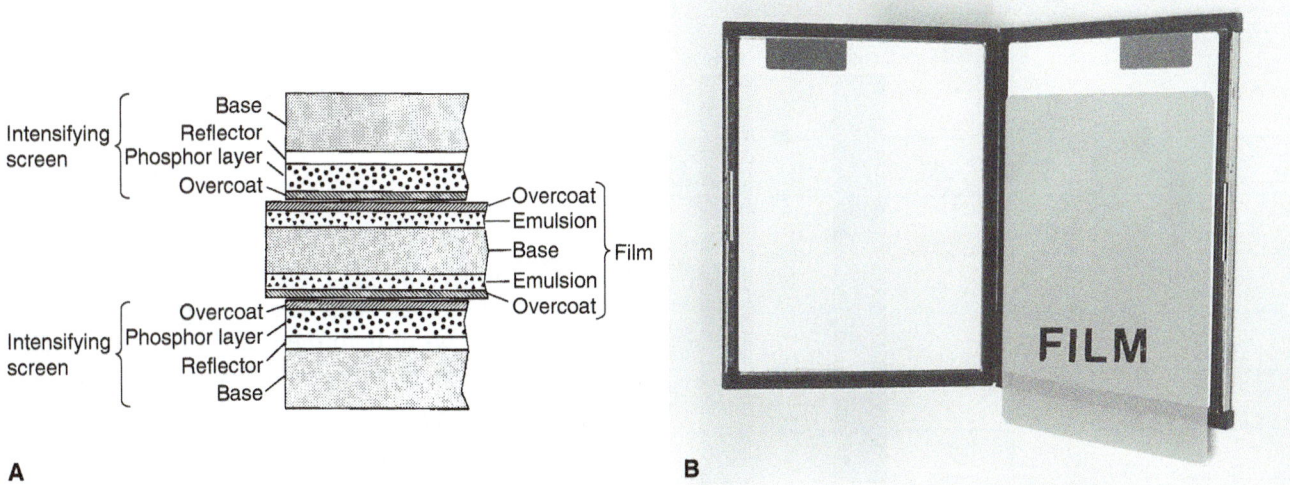

Figure 31–3 Intensifying screens. (**A**) Illustration of double-coated film sandwiched between two intensifying screens. (**B**) Photo of 8 × 10 inch film cassette with two white intensifying screens.

Intensifying screens are covered with phosphors within a binding medium. Phosphors are tiny crystals that **fluoresce**, or absorb x-ray energy and then emit it as fluorescent light. There are two basic types of intensifying screens:

- *Green screens.* These screens are covered with rare earth crystals. They must be paired with green-sensitive film.
- *Blue screens.* These screens are covered with calcium tungsten and must be paired with blue-sensitive film.

The number and pattern of the crystals affect the final quality of the radiograph. Other factors that influence the final image include:

- *Crystal size.* Larger crystals require less radiation to produce an image because they emit more light. However, larger crystals also yield less sharp images.
- *Emulsion thickness.* Thicker emulsion allows for more crystals, which produces more light and requires less radiation to obtain an exposure. Again, however, this results in less sharp images.
- *Crystal type.* The rare earth (green) crystals require less radiation than the calcium tungsten (blue) crystals.

Just as with conventional intraoral films, a number of speeds in both film and intensifying screens are available. Faster films, which use larger crystals and thicker emulsions, are recommended by the American Dental Association. These screens do result in less sharp images, but the trade-off—less clarity in exchange for less radiation exposure—is considered acceptable in most cases.

Grids

Grids are special devices designed to reduce the amount of scatter radiation that reaches the film cassettes. They are placed between the patient's head and the film (Figure 31-4).

Grids are made up of thin lead strips laid out in a grid and encased in plastic. As the central x-ray beam passes through the patient's head, a certain amount of scatter radiation is generated, which could cause film fog on the resulting radiograph by reducing the contrast.

A grid works by intercepting the scatter radiation beams, which are generally traveling at angles and are intercepted by the lead. The primary x-ray beam, however, passes directly through the plastic at a perpendicular angle and strikes the film.

The lead strips in the grid, however, do reduce the amount of radiation that ultimately reaches the film. To compensate for this, a slightly higher exposure time is required.

The use of grids results in higher contrast and better images at the cost of increased radiation exposure. Thus, the decision to use a grid must be weighed carefully. For example, if the idea is simply to measure growth and development, then use of a grid is probably not warranted. If, however, the radiograph is prescribed to diagnose a tumor, then a grid might be warranted.

Extra Patient Care

Patients are sometimes intimidated by the unfamiliar equipment used in extraoral radiography. With panoramic units, it is very important to explain and illustrate how the moving parts work, and with cephalometry, it is very helpful to briefly illustrate why and how the positioning rods work. To put the patient at ease, make sure you explain exactly what is being done throughout.

CHECKPOINTS

31-1 What is the difference between panoramic and nonpanoramic projections?

31-2 What are the two colors used in extraoral radiography? What makes them significant?

31-3 What are the two types of film cassettes?

31-4 What is the purpose of an intensifying screen?

31-5 What is the purpose of a grid?

Panoramic Radiography

Panoramic projections are by far the most common form of extraoral exposures. These large radiographs are used to image broad views of both the maxilla and the mandible. Panoramic radiographs are used to examine:

- Impacted third molars and root tips
- Large areas of the face and jaw
- Large lesions in the posterior mandible
- Growth and development of the bones in the jaw and face
- Trauma

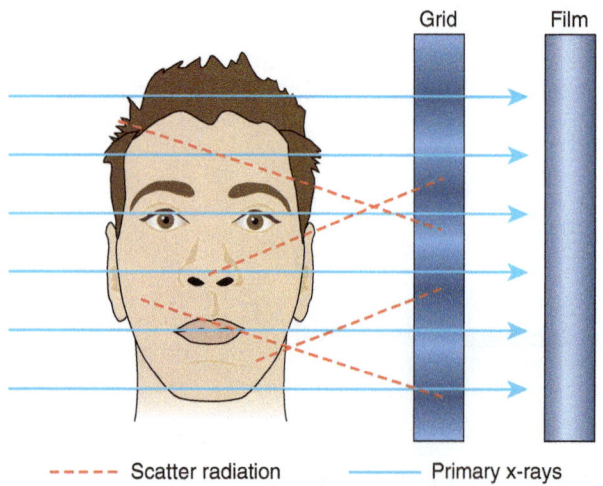

- - - - - Scatter radiation ———— Primary x-rays

Figure 31-4 Use of a grid to reduce radiation scatter.

Although panoramic imaging technology has improved, it is still inferior to intraoral radiography. Thus, it is often used in conjunction with intraoral radiographs.

Basics of Panoramic Radiography

During a panoramic projection, the patient's head remains still while the x-ray tube rotates in one direction and the film rotates in the opposite direction (see Figure 31-1). Patients may be sitting or standing.

Panoramic radiography works on a principle called **tomography**. This principle is used to image selected layers of tissue while deliberately blurring other layers or sections of tissue. The same principle is used in computed tomography scanning, or CT scanning. Radiographs obtained in this way are known as tomographs.

In panoramic radiography, the shape of the tomographs corresponds to the dental arches. This is made possible by the corresponding movement of the film and x-ray tubehead, which result in a constantly rotating x-ray beam around an imaginary axis located between the tubehead and the film. Terms used to describe this movement include rotational center and focal trough.

Rotational Center

The **rotational center** is the axis point around which the film and the x-ray tubehead rotate (Figure 31-5). The rotational center moves as the tubehead and film rotate around the patient's head. Two things are accomplished with the rotational center:

1. The amount of radiation is reduced because the central x-ray beam is reduced to a narrow vertical opening on

the tubehead. This beam passes through the patient and then into a narrow opening on the film cassette before exposing the film.

2. The device can obtain an image of the slice of tissue and bone in the dental arches. The curve made by the beam as it moves around the rotational center is the same shape as the dental arches.

Not all panoramic machines have the same rotational center. Machines are built with one of three rotational centers:

- *Double-center*. Panoramic exposures taken with a double-rotational center appear as split images on the final film. During this kind of exposure, the tubehead begins to rotate around one side of the dental arch. When it reaches the middle of the arch, the radiation is temporarily shut off and it shifts to a new rotational center. Afterward, the radiation begins again to film the second half of the dental arch.

- *Triple-center*. Instead of two rotational centers, the camera uses three rotational centers. These smaller shifts in rotational centers allow for a continuous image on the final film.

- *Moving-center*. This is the most common arrangement. In this exposure, the rotational center shifts in a smooth arch throughout exposure. This allows for a continuous image on the film and constant magnification of the upper and lower dental arches. Additionally, the size of the arch can be adjusted based on the patient's dental arches.

Focal Trough

The **focal trough** is a three-dimensional curved area where the x-ray beam clearly exposes structures and tissues. The size and location of the focal trough vary depending on the machine being used. Most panoramic x-ray units are set for standard dental arches, but can be customized depending on the patient.

The depth of the focal trough is determined by the distance from the rotational center. The further away the rotational center is from the target area, the deeper the focal trough will be. The closer it is, the narrower the focal trough will be. This measure can be controlled by varying the speed of the moving cassette. It is important to position the patient's jaws exactly right to obtain the best image.

- Double rotation systems are wider in both the front and back of the dental arches, but do not image the temporomandibular area as well.

- Triple and continuous moving units have wide troughs in the posterior and anterior regions, with better imaging of the TMJ.

Panoramic Equipment

Various types of panoramic units are available, with double-, triple-, and moving-rotational centers. Accordingly, the different brands have varying focal troughs and use different

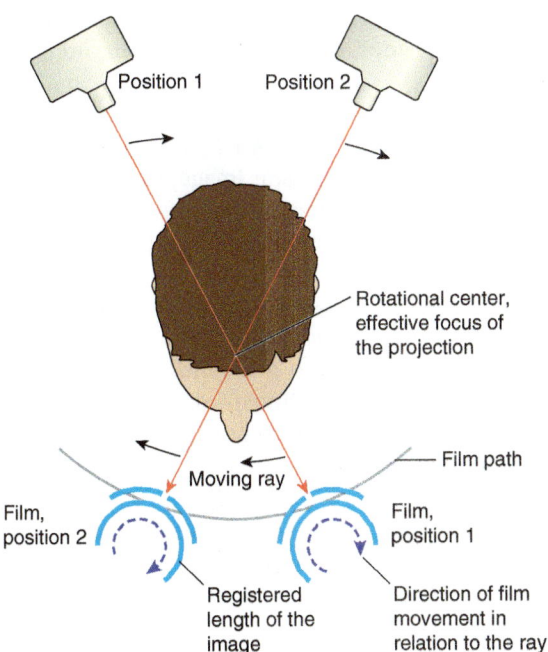

Figure 31–5 **Rotational center.** This is the access point around which the film and x-ray tubehead rotate.

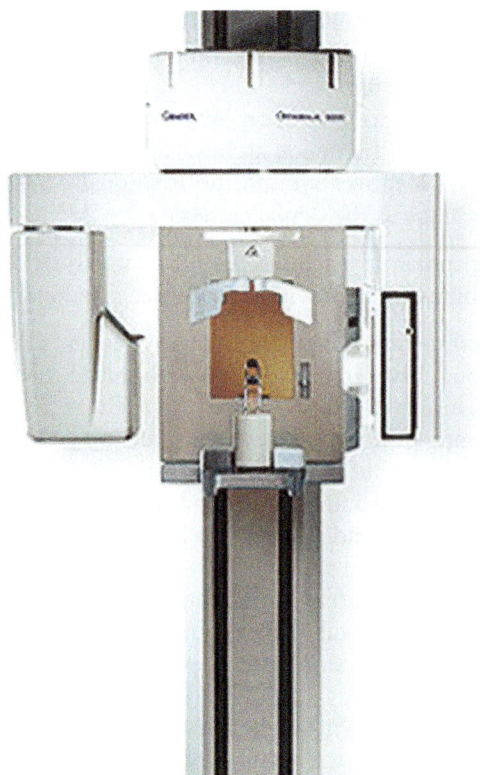

Figure 31–6 Panoramic x-ray unit.

types of film transports. Despite this, panoramic x-ray units all share the same basic components (Figure 31-6):

- X-ray tubehead
- Cassette holder
- Head positioner guide
- Exposure panel

Although some of these are familiar components, there are a number of differences between a panoramic x-ray unit and a traditional x-ray unit.

The collimator on a panoramic x-ray unit (Figure 31-7) is different from the collimator on a traditional x-ray unit.

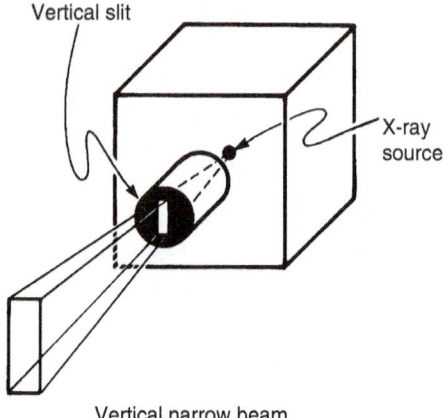

Figure 31–7 Collimator on a panoramic x-ray unit. Note the vertical slit.

In a traditional unit, the collimator is rectangular or cylindrical. This device shapes the beam and directs it as it exits the tubehead. In the panoramic x-ray unit, however, the collimator is a narrow vertical slit. This narrow beam passes through the patient's head and enters a corresponding narrow slit on the film cassette.

Additionally, in a panoramic x-ray unit, the tubehead is positioned behind the patient's head, while the film cassette rotates in front of the patient's head during exposure. Also unlike a traditional x-ray unit, the tubehead in a panoramic unit is in a fixed position, pointing slightly upward. Thus, vertical angulation is not an issue with a panoramic x-ray unit.

Because of the fixed tubehead position, it is essential for the patient's head to be properly positioned during exposure. Panoramic x-ray units are all equipped with head positioners. A head positioner includes a forehead rest, a chin rest, a bite block, and side supports or guides. Using these guides allows the radiographer to correctly position the patient. Some units are equipped with beams of light that are directed onto the patient's face to indicate proper positioning.

Finally, the exposure panel on panoramic units allows the operator to adjust the kilovoltage (kVp) and milliamperage (mA), depending on the size of the patient. Larger patients typically require greater kVp. The exposure time, however, is fixed and cannot be changed. Exposure times in panoramic radiography are much longer than traditional radiography, ranging from 15 to 20 seconds.

Preparing the Patient

Before exposure, the radiographer must prepare the equipment and the patient. See Procedure 31-1, Preparing for a Panoramic Radiograph, for step-by-step instructions.

It is essential during patient preparation to correctly position the patient's head. An incorrect head position will result in a nondiagnostic image. Correct head positioning depends on a number of factors, including the area being imaged and whether it includes the TMJ, the teeth and jaws, or the sinuses.

Each manufacturer issues guidelines with its machine that indicate how to position patients to obtain diagnostic images. Patient position is essential because the focal trough on each machine is fixed—it cannot move. Thus, it is important to situate the patient so the desired structures are within the focal trough.

Patients are positioned according to facial landmarks. Different panoramic machines use different landmarks; the manufacturer's instructions will offer a guide on which ones to use with its particular machine. Common landmarks (Figure 31-8) include:

- *Midsagittal plane.* This imaginary line divides the patient's face into right and left halves on a vertical

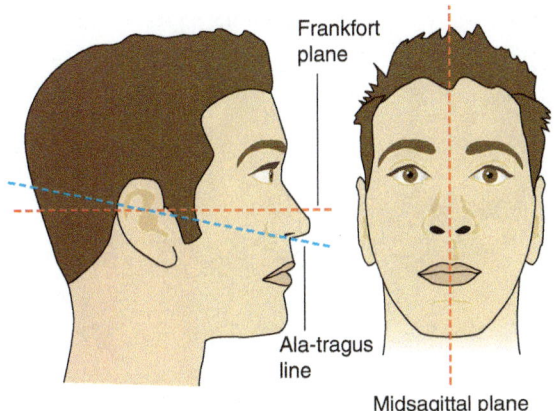

Figure 31–8 Common facial landmarks for positioning patients. Ala-tragus line, Frankfort plane, and midsagittal plane.

axis. The midsagittal plane must be perpendicular to the floor; that is, the patient has to be standing or sitting straight up with the chin resting securely on the chin rest.

- *The ala-tragus line.* This imaginary line extends from the ala (a wing-line projection of the nostril) back along the cheek to the tragus (a projection of cartilage in front of the acoustic meatus of the ear). Correctly positioned, the ala-tragus line should be angled toward the floor about 5 degrees.

- *The Frankfort plane.* This imaginary plane extends from the orbital ridge directly under the eye to the top of the ear canal. Correctly positioned, the **Frankfort plane** will be parallel to the floor.

Procedure 31-1 Preparing for a Panoramic Radiograph

Materials needed:
- Extraoral film
- Cassette
- Infection control barriers
- Double-sided lead apron (without a thyroid collar)

Preparing the Equipment

1. Load the film into the film cassette in a darkroom, making sure that the film is matched to the appropriate intensifying screen. To avoid fingerprints, handle the film by the edges only.

2. Prepare the panoramic x-ray unit by covering or disinfecting all surfaces that will come into direct contact with the patient (e.g., forehead rest, chin rest, lateral head positioner guides, and support handles). Make sure to use a sterile or disposable bite block.

3. Load the film cassette into the cassette holder.

Preparing the Patient

1. Review the patient's medical records and the prescription.

2. Explain the procedure to the patient and answer any questions he or she might have about the procedure or the prescription.

3. Put on appropriate PPE.

4. Ask the patient to remove anything that might obstruct or degrade the image, including eyeglasses, jewelry, implants, hair-holding devices, piercings, and studs.

5. Outfit the patient with a lead apron without a thyroid collar. A double-sided apron is recommended.

Positioning the Patient

1. Guide the patient into the unit. Patients should be instructed to stand or sit straight up.

2. Ask the patient to bite on the bite block and slide the upper and lower teeth into the grooves on the end of the bite block to align the teeth in the focal trough (Figure P31-1-1).

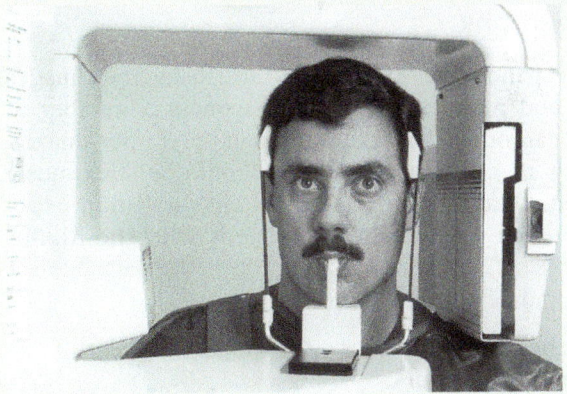

Figure P31-1-1

3. Close the lateral guides and position the patient so the midsagittal plane is perpendicular to the floor and the Frankfort plane is parallel to the floor. Some units have special light beams that help with patient positioning.

4. Tell the patient to position his or her tongue on the roof of the mouth and keep it there during the exposure.

Exposure

1. Set the exposure factors according to the manufacturer's instructions for the size of patient and the exposure.

2. Tell the patient to remain absolutely still during the exposure.

3. Get behind a protective barrier or far enough away from the machine to be safe. Press the exposure button and hold it down for the entire exposure cycle. During exposure, monitor to make sure the patient does not move and the lead apron does not interfere with the machine. If anything happens, release the exposure button and stop the exposure.

4. After exposure, release the patient from the machine, return the machine rests to a normal position, and follow infection control procedures.

5. Document the procedure in the patient's record.

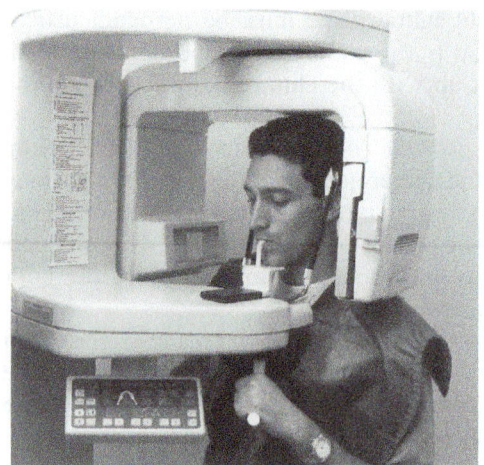 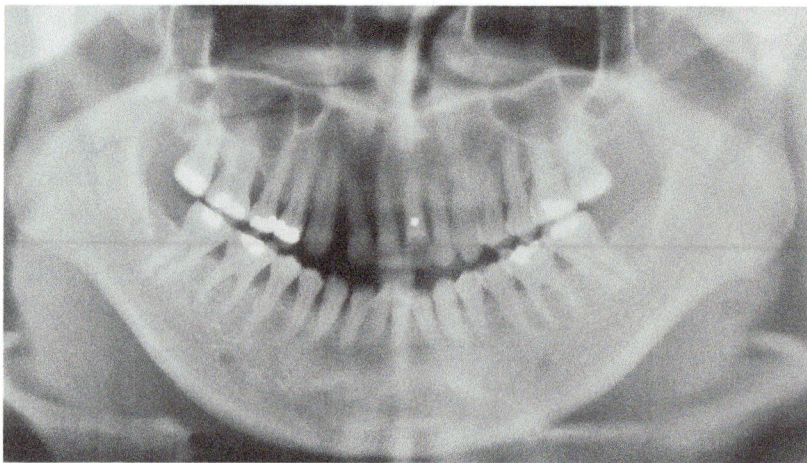

Figure 31–9 Exaggerated smile. Caused by patient's head being tipped forward.

Common Errors During Panoramic Radiography

Quality panoramic radiographs are diagnostic images with good picture clarity and sharpness. A number of errors can occur, however, that will yield poor images. As with all radiographs, retakes should be strenuously avoided. Retakes increase the patient's radiation exposure burden and are not consistent with the ALARA principle.

Common errors include:

- Patient positioning errors
- Film cassette errors
- Exposure and processing errors
- Patient preparation and cooperation errors

Patient Positioning Errors

Proper patient positioning is essential during a panoramic projection. Because panoramic x-ray units have a fixed focal trough, the patient must be perfectly positioned so the dental arches are correctly aligned in the focal trough.

This is especially true in the anterior region, where most machines have a narrower focal trough. Incorrect patient positioning can result in a number of errors:

- If the Frankfort plane is not parallel to the floor, blurry regions, distortions, or other structures superimposed over the radiograph can result. For example, if the Frankfort plane is tipped downward, the radiograph will appear as an exaggerated smile (Figure 31-9). On the other hand, if the Frankfort plane is tipped upward, the radiograph with have an exaggerated "reverse smile."
- If the midsagittal plane is misaligned, the teeth closest to the film appear smaller while the teeth farthest from the film appear magnified.
- If the teeth are positioned either too far forward or too far back from the focal trough, the result is a blurred image. If the patient is positioned too far forward (anterior), the anterior teeth appear too thin, and if the patient is positioned too far back (posterior), the anterior teeth appear overlarge, or fat (Figure 31-10).

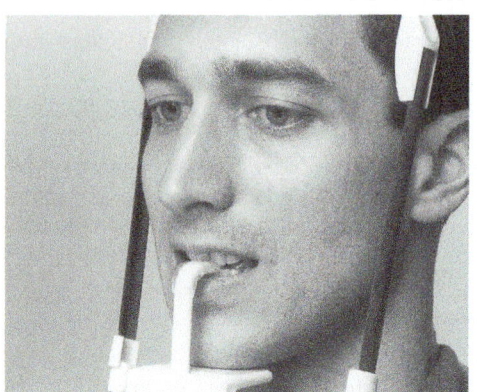 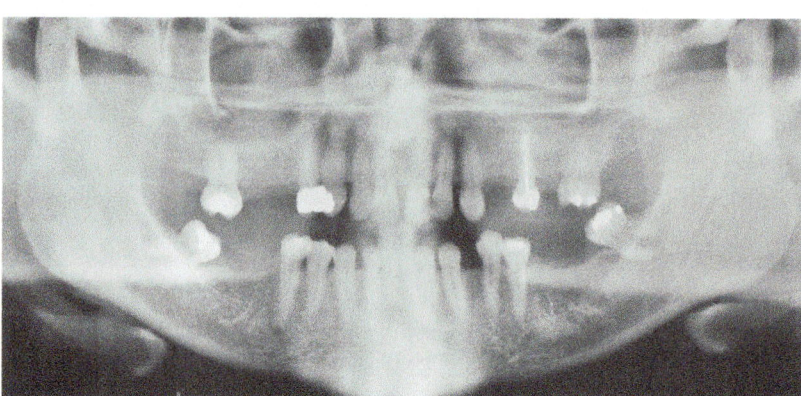

Figure 31-10 Overlarge teeth. Caused by patient positioned too far back.

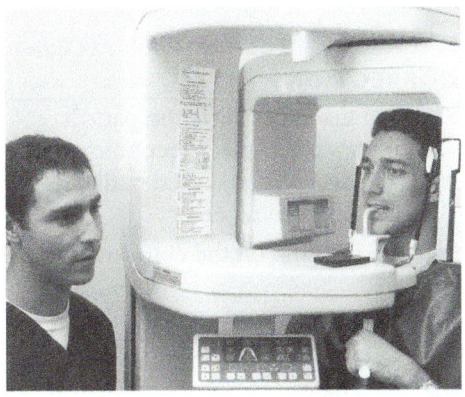
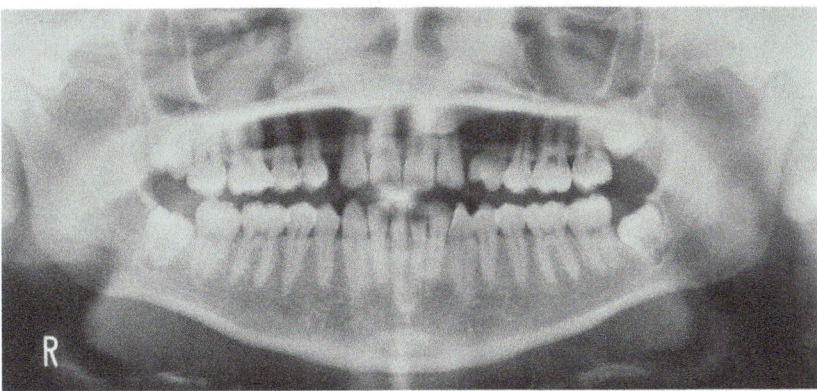

Figure 31-11 **Radiolucent shadows**. Caused by patient's mouth being open and tongue improperly positioned.

- If the patient's lips or tongue are not in the proper positions, radiolucent shadows will obscure parts of the image (Figure 31-11). The lips should be firmly enclosed around the bite block and the tongue should be positioned firmly against the roof of the mouth.
- Any external objects, such as jewelry and lead aprons, should be cleared from the area being visualized.

See Table 31-1 for an analysis of patient positioning errors.

Film Cassette Errors

Three common errors may occur with film and film cassettes:

- The film is not matched to the proper color intensifying screens.
- The film is not oriented correctly in the cassette.
- The cassette is not light-safe, resulting in accidental partial exposure of the film.

TABLE 31-1 Analysis of Panoramic Patient Positioning Errors

ERROR AND CAUSE	IDENTIFYING FEATURES	CORRECTION
Patient too far forward	Narrow blurred anterior teeth with pseudospace Superimposition of spine on ramus Bicuspid overlap bilaterally	Use incisal bite guide Line up incisal edge of teeth with notch Edentulous patients should bite around 5 mm behind notch
Patient too far back	Wide, blurred anterior teeth Ghosting of rami; spread-out turbinates, ears, and nose in image; condyles off lateral edges of film	Use incisal bite guide Line up incisal edge of teeth with notch
Chin tipped too low	Excessive curving of the occlusal plane Loss of image of the roots of the lower anterior teeth Narrowing of the intercondylar distance and loss of head of the condyles at the top of the film	Tip chin down, but ala-tragus line should not exceed -5 to -7 degrees downward Use chin rest
Chin raised too high	Flattening or reverse curvature of occlusal plane Loss of image of the roots of the upper anterior teeth Lengthening of intercondylar distance and loss of head of the condyles at the edges of the film Hard palate shadow wider and superimposed on the apices of the maxillary teeth	Tip chin down -5 to -7 degrees Use chin rest
Head twisted	Unequal right-left magnification, particularly teeth and ramus Severe overlap of contact points and blurring	Line up patient's midline with middle of incisal bite guide Close side guide
Head tilted	Mandible appears tilted on film Unequal distance between mandible and chin rest at a given point on the right and left sides One condyle is higher and larger than the other	Position the chin firmly on both sides of the chin rest Close side guide

TABLE 31-1 Analysis of Panoramic Patient Positioning Errors (*Continued*)

ERROR AND CAUSE	IDENTIFYING FEATURES	CORRECTION
Slumped position	Ghost image of cervical spine superimposed on the anterior region	Stand-up machines: have the patient step forward or place feet on markers All machines: be certain the patient is sitting or standing erect
Chin not on the chin rest	Sinus not visible on the film Top of condyles are cut off Excessive distance between inferior border of the mandible and the lower edge of the film	Position the chin on the chin rest
Bite guide not used	Incisal and occlusal surfaces of the upper and lower teeth overlapped	Use bite guide Compensate for missing anterior teeth with cotton rolls
Tongue not on palate	Relative radiolucency obscuring apices of the maxillary teeth (palatoglossal air space)	Place the tongue firmly against the palate Ask the patient to swallow or suck on his or her tongue
Lips open	Relative radiolucency on the coronal portion of the upper and lower teeth	Close lips
Patient movement	Wavy outline of cortex of the interior border of the mandible Blurring of the image above wavy cortex outline	Ask the patient to hold still and not swallow Explain the function of the machine to avoid startling the patient Be certain the patient's clothing will not interfere
Prostheses	Evidence of prostheses in image Acrylic denture teeth and bases do not show	Remove all complete and partial dentures, eyeglasses, and jewelry

Exposure and Processing Errors

Diagnostic radiographs can be obtained only if the proper settings, including kV and mA, are used. Exposure time is constant on panoramic machines, so this is not an issue. Larger patients with denser tissues will require higher kV to provide enough penetrating power to yield a diagnostic image.

Processing images takes place in the darkroom. See Chapter 32, Film Processing, Mounting, and Evaluation, for a complete discussion.

Patient Cooperation Errors

Patient communication is essential before and during a radiographic exposure. Patients need to understand that there are moving components to a panoramic x-ray unit and that these components will be circling their head during exposure. Additionally, it is imperative that the patient remains still during the length of the exposure, and holds his or her lips and tongue in the correct position. Finally, it is important that the patient remove all objects that might interfere with the image, including jewelry, dental appliances, and even bulky clothing or padded jackets that might interfere with the exposure.

Apply it

During panoramic radiography, patient positioning is essential because the focal trough on most machines is relatively narrow. It is important to properly line up the midsagittal and the Frankfort plane. If the unit has guide lights, this is much easier. During a panoramic exposure:

- The midsagittal plane should be perpendicular to the floor
- The ala-tragus line should be angled slightly down
- The Frankfort plane should be parallel to the floor

See Table 31-2 for an analysis of procedural errors that may occur.

Advantages and Disadvantages of Panoramic Radiography

Panoramic images are the most common type of extraoral image. The main advantages of panoramic radiographs include:

- A wide field of vision at a relatively low radiation exposure. A single panoramic image offers diagnostic quality

TABLE 31-2 Analysis of Panoramic Procedural Errors

ERROR AND CAUSE	IDENTIFYING FEATURES	CORRECTION
Not aligning the machine and/or cassette with the starting point	A portion of the film is blank A portion of the anatomy is lost at the edge of the film	Align the machine and/or cassette with starting point
Cassette resistance	One or several dark vertical bands on the film; these represent areas of overexposure as the cassette is stopped, but radiation continues to be emitted until the end of the cycle	Be certain to remove thickly padded items of clothing In stocky patients with a short neck, the cassette may need to be raised slightly above the ideal position
Paper or lint in screen	Radiopacity of unusual shape and location Foreign object prevents complete exposure of film by fluorescent screen	Periodic inspection and cleaning of the screens
"Fingernail" artifact	Crescent-shaped radiolucency	Avoid rough handling of the film when removing from the box or cassette
Static electricity	Lighting-like radiolucency; dot-like radiolucencies Starburst or other patterns, such as tree-shaped objects	Dry air in the darkroom can be humidified with a humidifier or large bowl of water Avoid rapidly pulling the film from the envelope-type cassettes or full box of film
White-light exposure	A portion of the film appears overexposed	Avoid smoking near film Check other sources of light leaks in the darkroom (i.e., unsafe safelight or display panels on personal electronics [e.g., cell phone or MP3 player]) Check integrity of cassette
Double exposure	Two images on the same film	Always place exposed films in the same location and where they may not be mistaken for unexposed films
Underexposed	Film too light	Increase kV and/or mA depending on the machine Place film between screens, not to one side only Check developer solution
Overexposed	Film too dark	Decrease kV and/or mA depending on the machine
No name	Patient's name or identification number not on the film	Use film imprinter, special labeling tape, or special pen

images of both the maxilla and mandible, with much less overall radiation exposure than a full mouth series. These images tend to be easier for patients to understand.

- Panoramic imaging is relatively easy, with no vertical angulation, and much less time intensive than a full-mouth series.
- Panoramic images are more comfortable and less intrusive for patients, who do not have to worry about uncomfortable film placement, gagging, or multiple exposures. For patients who cannot open their mouths or tolerate intraoral exposures, panoramic projections may be the only option.

The main disadvantages of panoramic radiography include:

- Panoramic images do not yield as much information as intraoral images, and the images are inherently of poorer quality. There is some distortion, magnification, and poor definition present even in well-exposed panoramic exposures.
- Patient positioning in the focal trough is critical.
- Panoramic x-ray units are more expensive than traditional x-ray units.

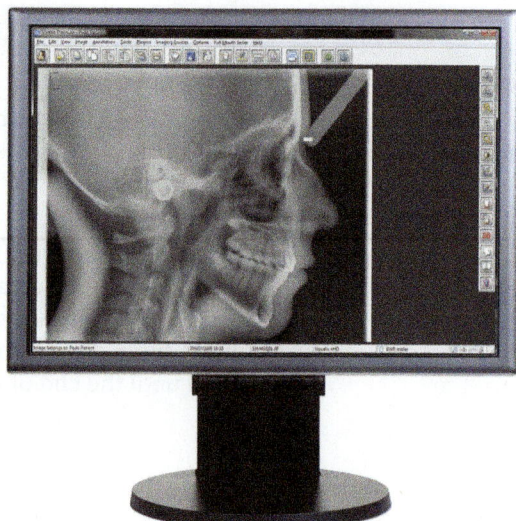

Figure 31–12 Lateral cephalometric (lateral skull) projection.

Other Extraoral Radiographs

Several kinds of extraoral radiographs can be obtained with a traditional dental x-ray unit. These are less common than standard panoramic radiographs and are usually reserved for special situations, such as evaluation by an oral surgeon or for diseases of the bones of the face.

Skull Radiography

Skull radiographs are used to visualize larger areas of the skull, jaws, and bones of the face. Some of these exposures require a device called a **cephalometer** (or cephalostat), which is a head-positioning device. Others do not. Skull radiographs are most commonly used by oral surgeons and orthodontists.

Skull radiographs can be challenging to interpret because of the sheer density of structures in the skull. They often appear overlapping on the final radiographs. Multiple exposures may be required to obtain diagnostic information. There are five basic skull radiograph techniques:

- Lateral cephalometric (lateral skull) projection
- Posteroanterior cephalometric (PA) projection
- Waters radiograph (sinus projection)
- Reverse Towne projection (open mouth projection)
- Submentovertex projection (base projection)

Lateral Cephalometric (Lateral Skull) Projection

Lateral skull projections are used to visualize the entire skull, including the soft tissues of the face. The image is taken from one side, so the sides of the skull are superimposed one upon the other (Figure 31-12). The side nearest to the x-ray tube is magnified slightly.

These projections require the cephalostat. The cephalostat is a large device that is used to position the patient's head parallel to the film and perpendicular to the x-ray beam. It also establishes a standard head position. This is valuable if a series of radiographs are to be taken over time and used for comparison.

These projections are used to visualize the growth and development of the bones of the skull. Dentists use these images to identify fractures, and orthodontists use them to evaluate development and position of the jaws and nearby structures. Additionally, with the use of a special filter, these images are used to obtain a profile of the soft tissues of the face and can be used to evaluate trauma.

Lateral skull projections require use of an 8 × 10 inch film that is positioned in a cassette directly over the patient's shoulder. The patient's head is positioned between the cassette film with the intensifying screens and the x-ray tubehead. The cassette should be parallel to the midsagittal plane of the skull. The central x-ray beam is directed at the acoustic meatus with a fixed vertical angulation of zero degrees.

Posteroanterior Cephalometric (PA) Projection

The posteroanterior cephalometric, or PA, projection, is the companion exposure to the lateral skull radiography. In a PA projection, the x-ray beam passes through the skull from the back (posterior) to the front (anterior), providing a back-to-front view of the entire skull (Figure 31-13).

PA projections are used to evaluate growth in the face, trauma, diseases, and developmental abnormalities. This projection has the advantage that the right and left sides

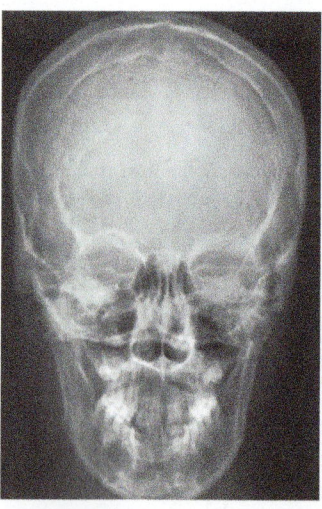

Figure 31–13 Posteroanterior cephalometric (PA) projection.

of the skull are not superimposed over one another, so it is often used in conjunction with lateral skull projections.

PA projections require the use of the cephalostat to position the head relative to the x-ray beam and the film. An 8 × 10 inch film is used with intensifying screens. The film cassette is positioned in front of the patient, so he or she is looking into the film, with the nose and forehead touching the cassette. Vertical angulation is zero degrees, and the central x-ray beam is directed at the external **occipital protuberance** (the large bump near the base of the skull).

The reverse exposure—an anteroposterior projection—is possible, with the central x-ray beam traveling from the anterior (front) to the posterior (back), and the film positioned at the back of the patient's head. However, the PA projection is more common because the facial bones and jaws are nearer to the film and are therefore better visualized. These are the bones of most interest.

Waters Radiograph (Sinus Projection)

Waters radiographs, often called sinus projections, are used to visualize the maxillary sinus area. These images are similar to the PA projections, except they are focused on the middle third of the face, where the sinuses are located.

Patient positioning for a Waters radiograph is similar to a PA, with one notable difference: instead of the patient touching the film cassette with the nose and forehead, the patient touches the cassette with the chin, with the nose slightly (3/4 inch) off the cassette surface. The central x-ray beam is directed through the occipital protuberance.

Reverse Towne Projection (Open Mouth Projection)

Reverse Towne projections are used to visualize the **condylar neck** and **ramus** area. They are called open mouth projections because they are obtained while the patient holds his or her mouth open.

Reverse Towne projections are obtained with the patient facing an 8 × 10 inch film cassette. The patient is positioned with the midsagittal plane perpendicular to the floor and with the mouth wide open. The chin should touch the chest, and the forehead rests against the cassette. The central beam of the x-ray is directed perpendicular to the screen, through the occipital protuberance at the base of the skull.

Submentovertex Projection (Base Projection)

Submentovertex projections are used to visualize the base of the skull and the position of the **condyles** and to evaluate fractures of the **zygomatic arch**, as well as the sphenoid and ethmoid sinuses.

During a submentovertex projection, an 8 × 10 inch film cassette is placed at the top of the head, at the apex of the skull. It is held in place with a holding device. The patient's head and neck should be tipped back as far as possible, as if he or she is craning the neck to look up into the sky or at the ceiling. The midsagittal plane and the Frankfort plane are both positioned perpendicular to the floor.

The central x-ray beam is directed at a perpendicular angle from beneath the mandible through the skull. The exposure factors vary with this exposure, depending on what is being visualized. If the zygomatic arches are of interest, the exposure time is reduced to about one-third the time of a standard submentovertex projection.

Lateral Jaw Radiography

Lateral jaw radiographs are used to visualize the posterior region of the mandible. They are also called *mandibular oblique lateral projections*. These projections are used to visualize impacted molars, fractures, and large areas of pathological concern on the posterior mandible. They are valuable for children, patients who cannot open their mouths, and patients who cannot tolerate intraoral radiographs.

At one time, lateral jaw radiographs were the most common projections obtained with the conventional dental x-ray unit; now, however, they have been largely replaced by panoramic radiography. However, they are still useful when panoramic equipment is not available or when additional information is needed.

During a lateral jaw exposure, the film cassette is placed flat against the cheek on the side of the mandible that is being visualized. It is held in place by the patient, who must place the flat of the palm against the cassette and press slightly. The patient's head should be tilted about 15 degrees toward the side that is being visualized, and the chin is jutted out slightly.

The central x-ray beam is directed toward the first molar from the opposite side of the face, at a perpendicular angle to the film cassette. Different areas of the mandible can be visualized, depending on where the cassette is placed. The film should always be parallel to the long axis of the teeth being visualized, and the central x-ray beam should always be perpendicular to both the long axis and the film.

Temporomandibular Joint Radiography

Temporomandibular joint (TMJ) radiographs are used to evaluate the TMJ (Figure 31-14). This projection is used to diagnose fractures, tumors and pathologies, ankylosis, arthritis, adhesions, and congenital disorders. TMJ projections are called **tomograms**.

A TMJ projection contains information on a number of anatomical structures in the region, including the mandibular condyle, the glenoid fossa, and the articular eminence. Projections are obtained with a 5 × 7 inch film cassette if only one projection is necessary. If multiple projections are necessary, it is possible to fit up to four images on a single 8 × 10 inch piece of film, providing the film cassette is shielded with lead during exposure.

During temporomandibular exposures, the patient is positioned with the head parallel to the cassette and the side to be imaged closest to the cassette. The midsagittal line of the patient's head should be perpendicular to the floor and parallel to the film cassette. The cassette can be resting

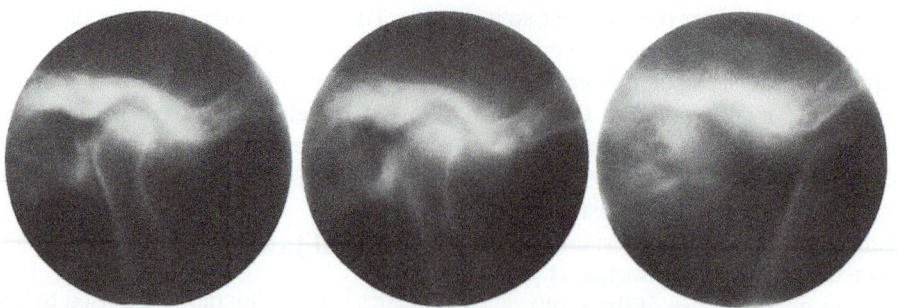

Figure 31–14 Tomographic radiographs of TMJ. From left to right: closed, rest, open.

in place on the patient's shoulder or held in place with positioning devices. The central x-ray beam's point of entry is about 2.5 inch higher than and 1/2 inch in front of the acoustic meatus. Vertical angulation is 20 to 25 degrees.

The major drawback with TMJ radiography is patient movement. Diagnostic images are impossible to obtain if the patient moves during the exposure. Dedicated TMJ radiography machines are available, but they are expensive and relatively rare.

CHECKPOINTS

31-11 List the five basic skull radiograph techniques.

31-12 What area does a lateral jaw radiograph depict?

31-13 What are tomograms?

Other Imaging Systems

Conventional radiography is the oldest and most common imaging modality used in dentistry, but it is not the only tool available. Newer technologies such as **computed tomography** (CT scanning) and **magnetic resonance imaging** (MRI) are also sometimes used.

Computed Tomography

Computed tomography was introduced in the 1970s. It uses ionizing radiation like conventional radiology, but instead of exposing x-ray film to produce radiographs, CT scanners generate highly detailed computer images.

In a CT scanner, patients are surrounded by x-ray detectors or an x-ray beam that moves 360 degrees around the patient. In principle, it is similar to panoramic radiography, except that there are many more sensors in CT scanning. By controlling the rate of rotation, radiographers can isolate very precise layers of tissue or organs in the human body and obtain three-dimensional images of organs at work. CT scans have a wide application in medicine, including skull and head scans of structures in the head and jaws.

In dental practice, a specialized form of CT scanning called *cone-beam imaging* is becoming more popular. This form of CT scanning uses a cone-shaped x-ray beam that rotates around the patient's head, much like panoramic radiographs. During a cone-beam radiograph, the patient lies flat on a table while his or her head is placed into the machine.

Cone-beam radiographs are useful in a number of applications. The machine can be programmed to visualize the TMJ area, dental implant sites, and hard tissues in a variety of planes (Figure 31-15). The resulting images are anatomically accurate.

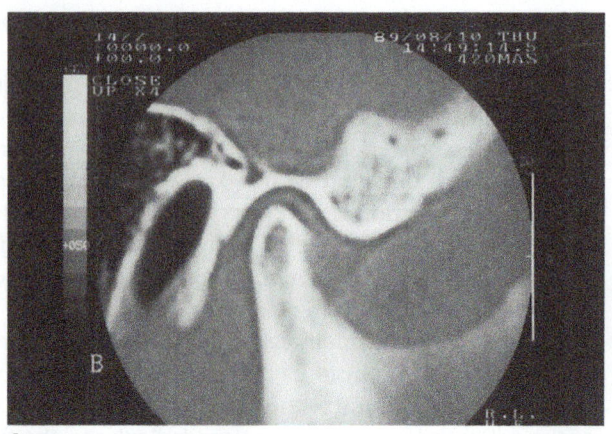

A

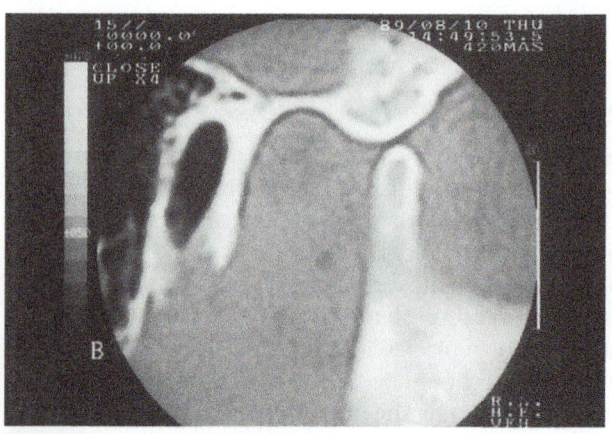

B

Figure 31-15 CT scans of TMJ. (A) Closed. **(B)** Open.

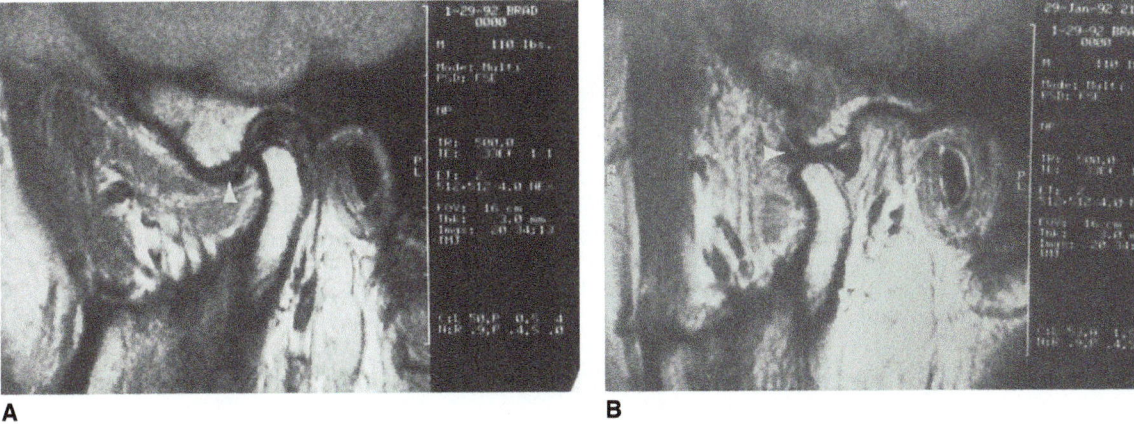

Figure 31-16 **MRI of TMJ.** **(A)** Closed. **(B)** Open.

Advantages of cone-beam imaging include:

- Much less radiation than traditional CT scanning
- Rapid scanning time and enhanced patient cooperation
- Easier-to-interpret, anatomically correct images
- A great degree of flexibility in which area is being imaged
- Digital images that are easily transmitted and stored, similar to digital radiographs

Magnetic Resonance Imaging

Unlike both radiographs and CT scanning, magnetic resonance imaging (MRI) does not rely on ionizing radiation. During an MRI, the patient is placed within a machine that generates a magnetic field. The nuclei of cells react in a predictable way to magnetic fields, and different kinds of cells react differently. By analyzing and measuring the reaction among different cells, the MRI is able to generate a three-dimensional image of internal structures.

Because of the use of strong magnets, all freestanding metal objects must be cleared from the room during an MRI, and patients cannot wear any metal jewelry. Certain implants and other permanent medical devices are contraindications for MRI if they contain metal.

MRIs are particularly good for measuring soft tissues, as opposed to bone. As a result, in dentistry, MRI is used most often to visualize the articular fibrous disk of the TMJ and soft tissue lesions and pathologies (Figure 31-16).

CHECKPOINT

31-14 What form of CT scanning is most often used in dentistry?

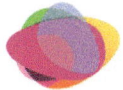

Chapter Highlights

- ◆ Extraoral radiographs are taken with the film positioned outside the patient's mouth. They are used to diagnose large lesions on the skull, TMJ disorders, trauma of the skull and jaws, and impacted teeth, and to evaluate growth and development. They are also useful for patients who are unable to tolerate intraoral radiographs.
- ◆ The most common type of extraoral projection is a panoramic projection, which is taken with a special device that rotates around the patient's head.
- ◆ Useful extraoral projections that can be obtained with a standard x-ray unit include lateral jaw, skull, and temporomandibular radiographs.
- ◆ Cephalometry is a kind of radiograph that uses a cephalometer to hold the patient's head in position during exposure.

- ◆ Extraoral film is larger than intraoral film. There are two varieties—blue and green—which must be matched to corresponding intensifying screens.
- ◆ A completed extraoral film cassette includes the film, two intensifying screens, and the cassette. These must be assembled in a darkroom under safelight conditions.
- ◆ Grids are used to reduce the amount of scatter radiation reaching the patient, but their use requires more primary radiation so they must be carefully considered.
- ◆ Panoramic dental units work by isolating a slice of tissue in a specific region and imaging it. This is accomplished by rotating the film and the x-ray tubehead in opposite directions of one another. The area in focus is called the focal trough.
- ◆ Patient position is critical in panoramic radiography to make sure the dental arches are positioned in the focal trough.

- ✦ Panoramic radiographs are advantageous because they image a large area with relatively little radiation, but disadvantageous because they do not yield as much diagnostic information as intraoral radiographs.
- ✦ Common skull radiographs include lateral skull projection, PA projection, sinus projection, open mouth projection, and base projection.
- ✦ Lateral jaw radiographs visualize the jaws from the side, but have been mostly replaced by panoramic radiographs.

- ✦ Temporomandibular radiographs visualize the region where the mandible is attached to the jaw, or the TMJ.
- ✦ A specialized form of CT scanning called cone-beam imaging is used to visualize hard tissues, implant sites, and disorders in the jaws and skull.
- ✦ MRIs are used in dental practices to visualize soft tissues in the temporomandibular region.

 **Review Questions**

1. What is NOT an advantage of extraoral radiography?
   a. Visualizes larger areas
   b. Is useful for patients who cannot open their mouths
   c. Does not require specialized equipment
   d. Uses less radiation

2. Which components move during a panoramic radiograph?
   a. None
   b. The film
   c. The x-ray tubehead
   d. Both the film and the tubehead

3. Lateral jaw radiographs image which portion of the anatomy?
   a. Anterior portion of mandible
   b. Posterior portion of mandible
   c. Both mandible and maxilla
   d. Posterior portion of maxilla

4. A cephalometer is used to
   a. Hold the head in place during exposure.
   b. Measure bones of the face.
   c. Measure the dental arches.
   d. Collimate the x-ray beam.

5. Screen film works properly only if
   a. Used with the proper intensifying screens.
   b. Protected from light contamination.
   c. Positioned correctly in the cassette.
   d. All of the above.

6. What is the main purpose of a grid?
   a. Helps align the x-ray beam on the patient's skull
   b. Decreases scatter radiation
   c. Helps decrease the amount of primary radiation needed for exposure
   d. Holds the patient's head in place

7. A double-center rotational center on a panoramic unit yields what kind of image?
   a. A single, continuous image
   b. A double exposure
   c. A split image
   d. A digital image

8. What is the ideal vertical angulation for a panoramic projection?
   a. 0
   b. +5
   c. −5
   d. It varies

9. During a panoramic exposure, the Frankfort plane should be
   a. Perpendicular to the ala-tragus line.
   b. Perpendicular to the floor.
   c. Parallel to the floor.
   d. Perpendicular to the primary x-ray beam.

10. In a lateral skull projection, the x-ray beam travels
    a. From the anterior to the posterior of the skull.
    b. From the posterior to the anterior of the skull.
    c. Through the mandibular arch to the apex of the skull.
    d. Through the skull from the side.

11. What is a common problem during temporomandibular exposures?
    a. Wrong exposure factors
    b. Patient movement
    c. Ambient light
    d. Weak signal

Active Learning Exercises

1. Many orthodontic offices use a panoramic, or cephalometric, rather than a periapical full series of x-rays for their patients. What is the difference between the two films? What does each show?

2. Name five placement errors when exposing the panoramic x-ray. What should be done to correct the errors?

3. How is cone-beam technology different from the previous forms of x-ray imaging? In which fields of dentistry would this type of imaging be most useful?

Application Activities

1. Practice assembling a film cassette using exposed film.

2. Practice correctly positioning patients for a panoramic exposure.

3. List and define the various rotational centers of panoramic x-ray units and discuss their importance.

PREPARING FOR CERTIFICATION EXAMS

Review the following topics in this chapter to prepare for the Dental Assisting National Board (DANB) exam:

- **Introduction**

- **Basics of Extraoral Radiography**

- **Equipment Used in Extraoral Radiography**

- **Basics of Panoramic Radiography**

- **Panoramic Equipment**

- **Common Errors During Panoramic Radiography**

- **Other Extraoral Radiographs**

- **Skull Radiography**

chapter 32

Film Processing, Mounting, and Evaluation

CHAPTER OUTLINE

CHAPTER CHECKLIST

On completion of this chapter, students will be able to:

- ☑ Identify the chemicals used in processing radiographs and explain their purpose.
- ☑ Describe how to manually process radiographs.
- ☑ Describe how to automatically process radiographs.
- ☑ Describe how to correctly mount radiographs.
- ☑ Describe the process of interpreting radiographs.
- ☑ Describe how to duplicate and store radiographs.

KEY TERMS

automatic processing – in dental radiography, the use of a machine to transform the latent images on exposed x-ray films to visible images for interpretation and diagnosis, as opposed to manual processing

developer – the first chemical used in the processing of dental films; developer reduces the silver halide on dental films, leaving behind silver specks that correspond to dark areas on the final x-ray image

diagnosis – the practice of identifying diseases, abnormalities, or pathologies based on the information in a radiograph; only dentists are allowed to make diagnoses

duplicating film – special film used in a film duplicator to make exact duplicates of radiographs; duplicate film has emulsion only on one side

film duplicator – a device used to make exact duplicates of radiographs

fixer – the second chemical used in the processing of dental films; fixer solution stops the chemical reaction started by the developer solution and hardens the emulsion to fix the image onto the film

interpretation – the act of reading the information on a radiograph, including anatomical structures, foreign objects, and caries, as distinct from formally diagnosing a patient based on the interpretation of a radiograph

labial mounting – a method of mounting radiographs in which the view is from the front, similar to the perspective of a viewer facing the patient

lingual mounting – a method of mounting radiographs in which the view is from the tongue-side, or back, as if the viewer was located in the back of the patient's throat

manual processing – in dental radiography, the practice of manually transferring exposed dental films from a developer solution to a water bath and then to a fixer solution, under controlled circumstances in terms of time and temperature, to produce diagnostic images

partial image – a processing error resulting from the processing of x-ray film in tanks that are only partially filled

Introduction

Diagnostic radiographs are the result of proper exposure technique, coupled with proper film processing procedures. After exposure, traditional dental film is imprinted with a latent image. Film processing exposes this latent image on the radiographic film, where it is invisible, changing it to a visible image, where a dental professional can interpret it and the resulting permanent image can be stored.

Film processing can be done manually in a darkroom or with an automatic processor. A darkroom is a special room that is designed and used only for film processing. It is light safe, meaning there is no contamination from white light and the lights have special filters that do not affect unexposed film. The darkroom is equipped with the materials, chemicals, and space for proper film exposure.

Film can also be processed in an automatic film processing machine, located either in the darkroom or in the main office area. These machines contain the processing fluids and regulate time and temperature to simplify the processing process. If the automatic unit is equipped with a daylight loader (e.g., a device that allows exposed film to be loaded under white light conditions), then no darkroom is necessary and the film can be processed in a normally lighted area.

No matter how the film is processed, it involves a series of steps that must be followed in order to produce a diagnostic radiograph. This chapter will explain the steps involved in film processing, mounting, and storage, including common mistakes and how to prevent them.

Processing Radiographs

Overview of Film Processing

Successful film processing relies on successful exposure. During a radiograph exposure, dental film is exposed to ionizing radiation, which interacts with emulsion on the film surface. This emulsion is composed of gelatin surrounding silver halide crystals. The silver halide is sensitive to x-ray energy. Crystals that are exposed to x-rays absorb energy. The amount of energy absorbed by the crystals depends on the degree of exposure. The greater the exposure, the more energy is absorbed. The energy pattern stored on the crystals is known as the latent image. The contrast on the final developed radiograph between light areas and dark areas depends on the latent image, with darker areas having absorbed more x-ray energy and lighter areas having absorbed less x-ray energy.

During processing, the film is exposed to processing chemicals in a predictable order for a predictable time. These chemicals include developer and fixer.

Developer

Developer is the first chemical in the process. The developer solution contains two chemicals, hydroquinone and Elon (paradihydroxybenzene).

Developer solutions have a pH above 7, which means they are basic, as opposed to acidic. The developer first softens the gelatin and then interacts with silver halide crystals. In chemical terms, the **developer** *reduces* the silver halide crystals by removing the halide portion of the molecule. What is left behind are silver specks on the film. The higher the energy contained in the silver halide crystals (e.g., the more radiation that reaches the crystals), the more silver that is allowed to precipitate. These areas correspond to the black regions on the final film. They are caused by structures that are radiolucent, or structures through which x-rays easily pass, such as soft tissues and open spaces between teeth. Areas that are more dense, or radiopaque, allow less x-ray energy to get through, so less silver precipitate is created during processing. These are the white areas on the final radiograph.

Time and temperature are critical to the development process. This is a chemical reaction, so it will continue as long as the film is exposed to the developer, and the reaction is accelerated by heat. The so-called time/temperature technique refers to the balance between time in the developer solution and the optimal temperature needed to yield diagnostic radiographs. If film is left in the developer too long, too much silver will be allowed to precipitate and the radiograph will begin to lose contrast between darker and lighter areas. If the film is totally overdeveloped, all the silver will precipitate onto the film and the resulting radiograph will appear totally black.

Besides these two active chemicals, developer solution also contains a preservative (sodium sulfate), an accelerator (sodium carbonate), and a restrainer (potassium bromide). These additives are designed to optimize the function of the developer.

Fixer

After the developer, the film is briefly rinsed in water and then immersed in a fixer solution. The fixer solution contains four ingredients:

- Sodium thiosulfate or ammonium thiosulfate. Commonly called hypo, this is a clearing solution that washes away undeveloped and unexposed silver halide crystals from the gelatin emulsion.
- Sodium sulfate. A preservative that prevents decomposition of the thiosulfate.
- Potassium aluminum sulfate. A hardener that reduces and hardens the gelatin.
- Acetic acid. Maintains the acidic pH level necessary for the other chemicals to work.

Fixer chemicals work to halt the development process, wash away any underexposed or unexposed silver halide, and harden the emulsion.

After the film emerges from the fixer solution, it is washed in running water to remove any trace chemicals and then dried. The finished product can be read and stored as a permanent part of the patient's dental record.

Voice of Experience

I found out firsthand how important it is to replenish old solutions after we had to retake a patient's x-rays because of old solution. Not only did this waste time, it exposed the patient to unnecessary extra radiation. Now we've posted a schedule in the darkroom so everyone will quickly and easily be able to see when the solutions were replenished last.

Manual Processing

Film processing is a chemical reaction that must take place under controlled circumstances. Film processors must make sure that the following variables are optimum to yield diagnostic radiographs:

1. Light conditions
2. Time
3. Temperature

The Darkroom

A darkroom is a dedicated space used for film exposure (Figure 32-1). The darkroom should be located in an out-of-the-way place in the dental office, and it should be used only as a darkroom. It is not a good idea to use the darkroom for storage, as a meeting place, or especially as a place where people eat or drink. After all, the chemicals used in film processing are strong and potentially toxic.

The darkroom should be large enough for one person to work comfortably and safely, usually a minimum of 4 feet × 4 feet. A darkroom must also be light safe. This means no exterior light can sneak into the darkroom around door frames, vents, or electrical outlets. When the safelight is on, it must be the only light in the room. A proper darkroom should also have the following features:

- A safelight (Figure 32-2). Safelights are used when film packets and cassettes are opened, when film is attached to hangers, and during processing. At any one of these stages, exposure to regular white light would ruin the radiographs. A safelight is a low-intensity, long-wavelength light that will not affect x-ray film. Safelights are usually in the red/orange spectrum, although yellow is increasingly common. The safelight should be at least 4 feet away from working areas, although

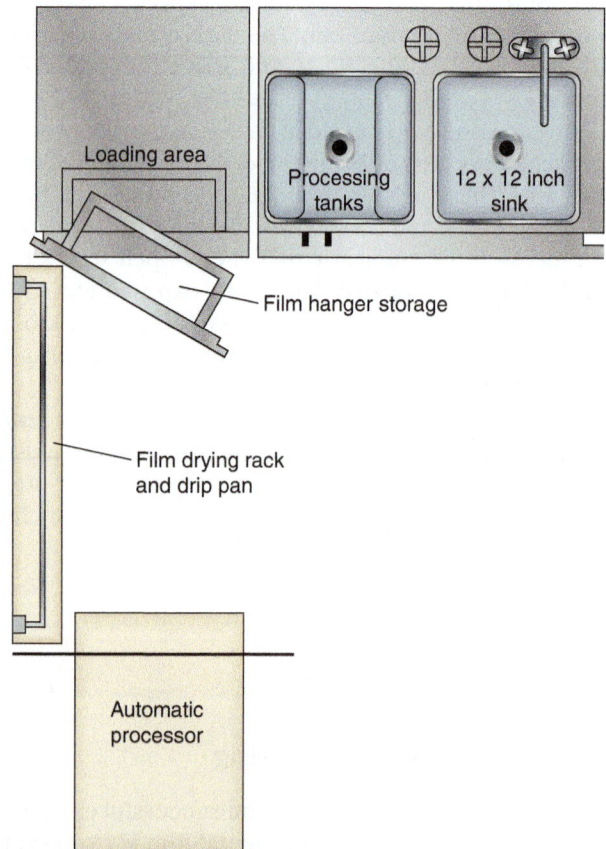

Figure 32–1 Darkroom.

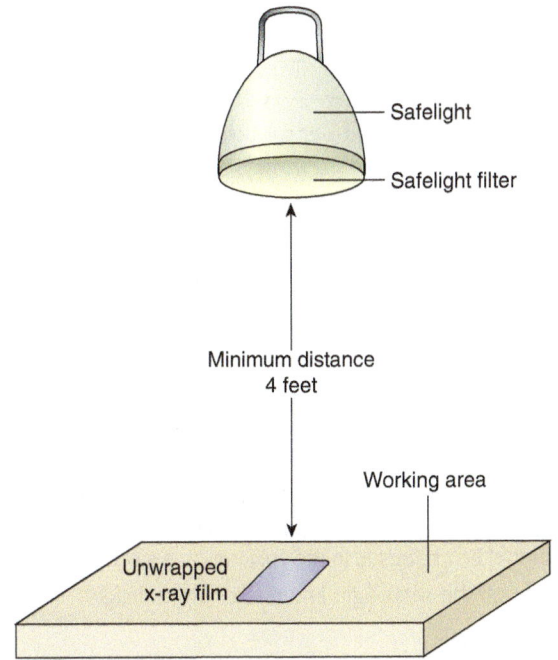

Figure 32–2 **Safelight**. The safelight should be at least 4 feet away from working areas.

low-watt bulbs (e.g., 7.5 watts) may be closer. One important exception, however, occurs with darkrooms that are used to process films taken with intensifying screens. Extraoral screen film might require a special yellow bulb (e.g., Kodak GBX-2 Safelight Filter).

- An overhead white light. The switch for this light should be protected so it cannot accidentally be flipped on or bumped.
- A viewing safelight. This light is used if the film needs to be read while it is still wet, as in the case of an emergency. A viewing safelight is located on the wall above the trays of developer solution. It allows the processor to hold the film up while it is still dripping. Without this light, wet films would have to be held up to the overhead safelight, which means chemicals would drip down on the person holding the film.
- An x-ray view box. This allows for private viewing of the radiographs by the dentist and other dental workers.
- An external warning light. This light should be automatically activated any time safelight conditions are being used in the darkroom. If the warning light is on, no one should open the darkroom door or turn on the overhead white light.
- Sinks for washing equipment.
- Work space, including counter space.
- The processing unit and solutions for manual processing (see the Manual Processing Tanks section later in this chapter).
- A timer.
- Film hangers for transporting films and mounting equipment.

- Film dryer, although automatic units often have dryers built in so if the office relies completely on automatic processing, this may not be necessary.
- Adequate ventilation, to prevent harm from breathing concentrated fumes released by processing solutions.

Manual Processing Tanks

Manual film processing takes place in a special device called a processing tank (Figure 32-3). A typical processing tank contains two removable inserts suspended in a running water bath. Processing tanks are usually built of stainless steel because it does not react with processing chemicals. The insert tanks are usually large enough to hold large 8 × 10 inch extraoral films in a gallon of processing solution.

An overflow valve is built in to control the water level in the master tank, and the unit has a cover that should always be kept in place when the unit is not being used. Fixer and developer solutions lose strength over time because of exposure to oxygen. Using a cover prolongs the life of the solutions.

The two inserts in the processing unit are used to hold developer and fixer solution, respectively. The left insert is often reserved for developer solution, while the right is often reserved for fixer solution. However, to prevent confusion, the sides should still be clearly labeled.

The running water bath between the two insert tanks is used to wash film during processing. This running water bath is also held at a specific temperature so the processing chemicals are always at the correct temperature.

The timer should be located within easy reach and sight of the processing unit, and an accurate thermometer should be affixed to the unit. Correct processing relies on accurate time and temperature, and once the process starts, it should be carried through without interruption.

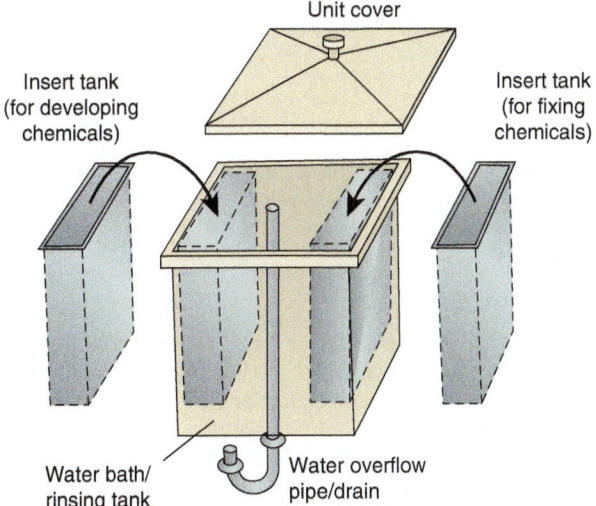

Figure 32–3 **Manual processing tanks**. The two removable insert tanks are large enough to hold 8 × 10 in. films.

Stirring paddles are used to stir the chemicals at the start of the process. Different paddles should always be used for each solution to prevent cross contamination.

Finally, film hangers and drying racks should be close by for use after the films emerge from the final rinse and for use during processing. Intraoral films are transported between the processing solutions in a special film hanger. Film hangers come in various sizes to accommodate the various sizes of dental films. Film hangers can hold up to 20 films. Films should be labeled as soon as practical after processing to prevent confusion.

✔ CHECKPOINTS

32-1 Overdeveloped x-ray film will appear as what?

32-2 What action does fixer solution accomplish?

32-3 What are the two most important variables in manual developing?

32-4 What does *light safe* mean?

Procedure 32-1 Manual X-Ray Film Processing

This procedure details the steps for processing film packets without barriers.

Materials needed (Figure P32-1-1):

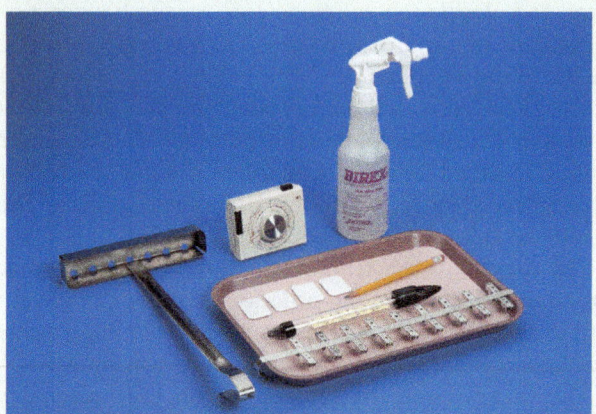

Figure P32-1-1

- Fully equipped darkroom
- Manual processing tanks
- Stirring rods
- Floating thermometer
- Surface barriers or disinfecting solutions for counters
- Exposed films
- Film rack
- Timer
- Pencil
- Film dryer (optional)

1. Lock the darkroom, apply surface barriers or appropriately disinfect surfaces, then locate and label the appropriate film hangers.

2. Open the manual processing unit by removing the cover. Stir the developer and fixer solutions using the stirring rods to ensure an even temperature and chemical concentration throughout the solutions. Do not use the same paddle to stir both solutions as this will contaminate the solutions.

3. Using the floating thermometer, check the temperature of the developer solution and consult the manufacturer's time/temperature chart, which should be located by the solution. The time/temperature chart tells how long a film should be immersed in the solutions at a given temperature.

4. Turn off the white light and turn on the safelight.

5. Wash hands and put on gloves.

6. Open the film packets or cassette. Drop the films onto the work surface without touching them. Discard the contaminated film packets and barrier wraps.

7. Remove gloves. Load the film into the appropriate film hanger, making sure the clips are securely fastened so the films will not fall out during processing.

8. Immerse the film hanger into the developer solution, agitating the hanger to get rid of unwanted air bubbles. Activate the timer.

9. When the timer sounds, remove the film hanger from the developer solution, allowing the excess solution to drain from the film for a few seconds.

10. Immerse the film hanger in the running water bath for 20 to 30 seconds to wash away the developer solution. Agitate the film hanger in the water to make sure as much developer as possible is washed away. Remove the film hanger from the water and allow excess water to drain away.

11. Immerse the film hanger into the fixer solution. Once again, agitate the film hanger in the solution to remove air bubbles and make sure the entire surface of the film is exposed to the solution.

12. Activate the timer for 10 minutes (about twice the developer time). However, it is safe to remove films from the fixer after 3 minutes for a wet reading. After the reading, though, these films should be returned to the fixer solution to complete the process. After the first 3 minutes in the fixer solution, it's no longer necessary to maintain safelight conditions. These films can be safely exposed to white light.

13. When the fixer timer has sounded, remove the film hanger from the solution and let excess solution drain off.

14. Rinse the film hanger in the water bath for at least 20 minutes to remove any excess fixer solution.

15. Place the film hanger in a film dryer or hang them to dry in the darkroom.

16. Mount and label dried films.

Common Errors in Manual Film Processing

Proper processing is necessary to obtain diagnostic radiographs. Errors with processing typically fall into one of the following categories:

- Time and temperature problems
- Contamination of processing chemicals
- Film handling problems
- Light contamination

These may occur individually or several problems may be affecting film. If there is a recurring problem, it is best to work through the possible causes systematically, until the source of the problem is located and can be eliminated. Nondiagnostic images may be fogged, blurred, too light, too dark, clear, or **partial images**, or may contain artifacts and other information that is the result of external factors. In many cases the appearance of the film itself can help diagnose the problem that occurred during processing (Figure 32-4).

See Tables 31-1 to 31-4 for a complete overview of possible processing errors, their effect on film and radiographs, and how to prevent them.

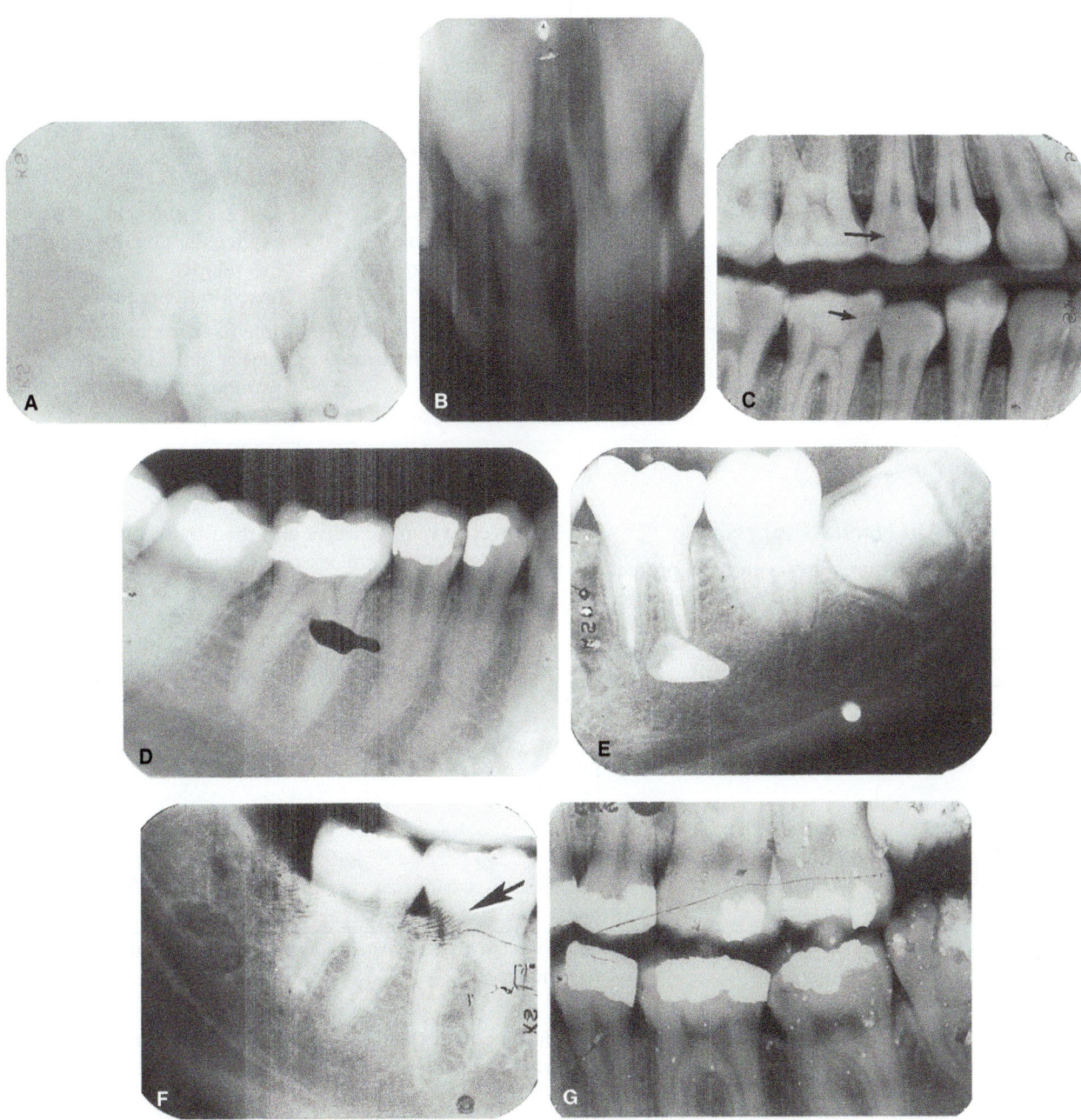

Figure 32–4 Common errors in manual film processing. (**A**) Underdeveloped film is too light. (**B**) Overdeveloped film is too dark. (**C**) Discolored film caused by inadequate rinsing after fixing. (**D**) Black spots caused by developer. (**E**) White spots caused by droplets of fixer. (**F**) Black spot caused by fingerprints. (**G**) White spots caused by air bubbles.

TABLE 32-1 Time and Temperature Problems

FILM APPEARANCE	CAUSE	REASON	PREVENTION
Thin, or light, image (Figure 32-4A)	Underdeveloped	Weak or cold developing solution Insufficient developing time	Replenish/replace developing solution Correct for proper temp/working thermometer Test timer for accuracy
Dense, or dark, image (Figure 32-4B)	Overdeveloped	Excessive developing time Developing solution too hot Concentrated developing solution	Test timer for accuracy Correct for proper temp/working thermometer Replace/replenish developing solution
Wrinkled or cracked image	Reticulation of emulsion	Too great temperature difference between developer (too hot) and water bath (too cold) causes the emulsion to shrink rapidly	Avoid great temperature differences between developer and solutions and water bath
Discolored films (brown) after a period (Figure 32-4C)	Not enough fixer time	Film was not allowed long enough time in fixer bath Film was not rinsed adequately	Make sure film is in fixer for twice the time it was in developer Rinse for 20 minutes
Clear	Emulsion gone entirely	Left in fixer too long or left in running water bath for 24 to 48 hours	Time fixer solution and never leave film hangers in running water bath overnight

Infection Control in Manual Processing

Infection control procedures are critical to protect the health of the dental assistant and the patient. Infection control before and during exposure is covered in Chapter 30, Producing Intraoral Dental Radiographs. This section deals with infection control after the exposure is taken and during processing.

At the end of an exposure series, the exposed film packets should be swiped across a disinfectant-soaked paper towel to remove saliva and then transported in a labeled paper cup to a safe area in the office (e.g., where the film packets will not be exposed to secondary radiation). If disposable plastic film envelopes were used during exposure, the film packets can be safely handed with clean, dry hands or treatment gloves once they have been removed from the envelopes.

Films should be transported to the darkroom where they will be opened and processed under safelight conditions.

TABLE 32-2 Chemical Contamination Problems

FILM APPEARANCE	CAUSE	REASON	PREVENTION
Dark spots (Figure 32-4D)	Developer spots	Film is in contact with developer before processing	Make sure darkroom surfaces are clean and no chemicals are exposed
White spots (Figure 32-4E)	Fixer spots	Film comes into contact with fixer before processing	Make sure darkroom surfaces are clean and no chemicals are exposed
Black spots, fingerprints (Figure 32-4F)	Fluoride contamination	Operator's hands were contaminated with fluoride, which leaves a black stain	Wash hands thoroughly with soap and water before handling radiographs

TABLE 32-3 Film Handling Errors

FILM APPEARANCE	CAUSE	REASON	PREVENTION
White border	Developer cutoff	Low level of developer resulted in a portion of undeveloped film	Make sure film is immersed in developer; add developer solution to insert if necessary
Black border	Fixer cutoff	Low level of fixer resulted in a portion of unfixed film	Make sure film is completely immersed in fixer; add fixer solution to insert if necessary
White lines on film	Scratched film	This occurs when the emulsion is scratched, usually by placing one film hanger in the solution alongside a second hanger; can also be caused by fingernails or any sharp object	Take care never to touch surface of film Discard any broken or damaged film hangers
White spots (Figure 32-4G)	Air bubbles	Air is trapped against the film surface during processing	Agitate film hangers when they are first placed into solutions to shake off air bubbles
Black streaks	Static electricity	Film packets are opened rapidly or before operator has touched a conductive object to discharge static charge on the skin	Touch any conductive object before handling film

As mentioned before, it is safe to handle films that were protected by plastic barrier envelopes with clean, dry hands in the darkroom, but care should still be taken during film handling. In a full-mouth series, for example, all the film packets should be opened and placed in hangers within 2 minutes. Although safelight conditions are designed to prevent damage to film, prolonged, unnecessary exposure of the film to any light increases the risk of damage to the film.

After the film has been placed into the processing tank or automatic film processing unit, aseptic measures should be taken in the darkroom work area. All of the film packets, foil wrappers, cups, and any materials used during transport of the film should be disposed of and the darkroom should be disinfected. Clean all work areas in the darkroom, including anywhere that was touched with gloved hands, such as tables, light switches, and equipment.

TABLE 32-4 Light Problems

FILM APPEARANCE	CAUSE	REASON	PREVENTION
Large black areas	Light leaks	Film is exposed to white light	Never unwrap films in white light Make sure all film packets are factory sealed before using Make sure automatic daylight loaders are sealed and used properly
Grey film, lack of contrast and detail	Fogged film	Leaks in darkroom conditions Improper safelight Contaminated solutions Exposure to secondary radiation Improper film storage or old film Developer too hot	Test for darkroom light tight Check filters and wattage on safelight Do not leave film where it can be exposed to secondary radiation Do not use expired film Store film in cool, dry, protected place Check temperature of developer

Disposing of Processing Solutions

Developer and fixer solutions are strong chemicals that should not be poured down a drain after they are exhausted. In many cities, disposal of these chemicals is regulated by law, and dental offices should check with their local waste management company to make sure they are complying with the law when disposing of used solution.

Automatic Processing

Automatic processing greatly simplifies film processing. An **automatic processing** unit is a machine that contains all of the solutions needed to rapidly process dental radiographs. Automatic processing units are perfect for high-volume practices because they operate much more quickly than **manual processing**. Automatic processing units are capable of going from developer to a dried radiograph in 5 minutes, in contrast to the approximate hour that it takes to manually develop, rinse, fix, wash, and dry a film.

Automatic processing has other advantages also, including:

- Ease of use since time and temperature are automatically controlled inside the unit
- Less space is needed than a fully equipped darkroom
- Less equipment is needed

Although automatic processing has become more popular in recent years, it is not without drawbacks. These include:

- Initial expense of the automatic processing unit
- The potential for equipment malfunction
- The need to replenish chemicals more often because of rapid depletion

Because of the risk of equipment malfunction, many dental offices that rely on automatic processing units also maintain a darkroom as a backup.

Automatic Processing Equipment

A wide variety of automatic processing units are on the market. They vary in size and complexity, as well as in their capabilities. Some automatic processing units handle only intraoral or smaller extraoral films, while others can process any size dental film. Some need to be connected to a plumbing source, while others have their own water source. Still others have a daylight loader that is protected by a light safe baffle so it can be used in white light conditions in a normal office environment.

Nevertheless, all automatic processing units operate on the same basic principle and have similar component systems to move exposed dental film from the beginning to the end of the unit (Figure 32-5). These components include:

- A roller system. Film is moved through the unit on a roller transport belt that carries it between the various

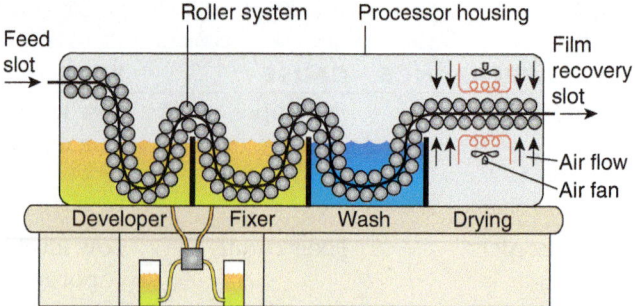

Figure 32–5 Automatic processor. The roller system transports the film through the developer, fixer, wash, and drying cycles.

solutions and dryer compartments of the unit. Rollers are belt- or gear-driven; besides moving film, they also remove excess solution and agitate the solution to eliminate air bubbles.

- Film feed slot. This is located on the outside of the machine. It is where operators insert unwrapped films into the unit. In some units, this is protected by a light safe baffle that allows operators to unwrap films in a protected chamber under safelight conditions.
- Processor housing. This is the "skin" of the unit, covering the unit from end to end in a light-safe condition.
- Developer compartment. This is where the film is immersed in developer solution. Automatic processors use a specially formulated developer solution that works at a higher temperature than traditional developer solution (80°F to 95°F). The high temperatures speed the development process. Manual developer solution should not be used in an automatic developer unit.
- Fixer compartment. This is where the film is immersed in fixer solution. There is no intermediate rinsing step in automatic processing units: film goes straight from the developer to the fixer solution. As with developer solution, the fixer solution used in automatic processing units is specially formulated. Traditional fixer solution should never be used in an automatic processing unit.
- Wash compartment. This compartment holds circulating water, which is used to wash the film after the fixer compartment.
- Drying chamber. Wet film is moved from the wash compartment to the drying compartment, where it is exposed to heat elements and dried.
- Replenisher pump. Some machines have replenisher pumps that automatically keep the developer and fixer solution full. However, this device is not included in all automatic processors; some brands require operator replenishing.
- Film recovery slot. This is where finished, dried radiographs emerge. Processing time is typically 4 to 6 minutes.

Procedure 32-2 **Using an Automatic Film Processor (with a Daylight Loader)**

Materials needed (Figure P32-2-1):

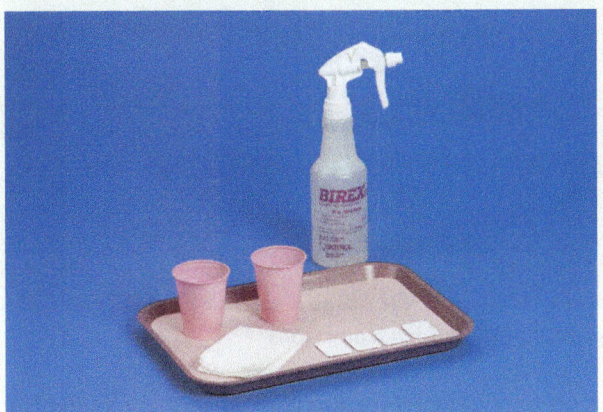

Figure P32-2-1

- Automatic x-ray processor with daylight loader (Air Techniques machine)
- Exposed dental films
- Exam gloves
- Paper towel
- 2 disposable cups/containers
- Disinfectant

1. Turn the unit on and set time and temperature, as indicated by the manufacturer. Some machines will require extended warm-up periods, so make sure the machine is turned on in enough time to warm up before processing the first film packet.
2. Wash and dry your hands.
3. Open the lid of the daylight loader and place a paper towel on the bottom. Place the two disposable cups on the towel. One of these cups should contain the exposed film. Close the lid.
4. Put on gloves and insert hands into the light-safe baffles on the daylight loader (Figure P32-2-2).

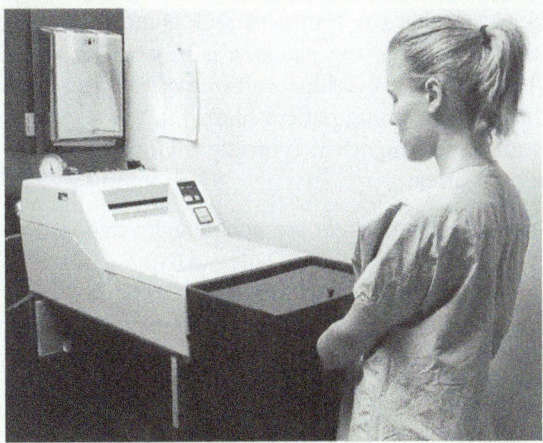

Figure P32-2-2

5. Remove the film from the packet and feed it into the automatic processing unit. Allow the rollers to take the film before releasing it into the unit.
6. Remove the lead foil from the packet and place it into one of the disposable cups. Drop the empty packet onto the paper towel.
7. Allow at least 10 seconds between individual film packets to prevent overlap during processing. Try to alternate films on either side of the film intake slot and make sure films are handled by their edges and fed into the machine straight.
8. After the last film is inserted, remove gloves and place in center of paper towel. Grab the corners of the paper towel and wrap the paper towel over the contaminated film packets and gloves and place into the second disposable cup. Dispose of contaminated waste appropriately, including the cup of lead foil.
9. Retrieve processed and dried radiographs from the film recovery slot at the appropriate time, usually 4 to 6 minutes later.

Maintaining Automatic Processing Units

Automatic processing machines can consistently produce high-quality, diagnostic radiographs in much less time than conventional darkroom processing. However, the units require regular maintenance to work their best.

1. The unit may require daily, weekly, or monthly cleaning, depending on the manufacturer's specifications. Some units may require that a special cleaning film is fed through every day to remove residue from the rollers. Roller assemblies should be removed and cleaned in warm, clean water, per the manufacturer's instructions.
2. Processing solutions should be checked every day (in machines without automatic replenishing pumps). Add new solution as necessary. Never use conventional darkroom processing solutions in an automatic processor.

The solutions used in automatic processors are ultra concentrated and require additional hardeners and other ingredients.

Avoiding Common Errors in Automatic Film Processing

One major advantage of an automatic film processor is the reduced risk for processing errors. A well-maintained machine will monitor the time and temperature automatically, and will not scratch or damage the film packets as they are processed. However, it is essential to check an automatic processing machine before it is used. One of the most common mistakes with automatic processing machines results from not checking the machine before it is used. To check an automatic processor, remove the outer cover before the machine is turned on and make sure the solutions are fresh. The water should be changed daily. After completing this step, turn the machine on and check to see that the transport rack is moving freely. Replace the cover once the machine is in working order. Finally, when using the machine, run one or two test films through before processing patient films.

Common processing errors typically fall into one of the following categories:

- *Light errors.* Film packets are accidentally exposed to white light as they are opened. This can happen in a darkroom or with broken light baffles on a daylight loader.
- *Weak or low processing solutions.* Rigorously follow the manufacturer's instructions regarding processing solutions, and use only the recommended solutions in the machine. Processing solutions may need to be replenished daily or weekly, depending on the workload of the unit.
- *Film loading errors.* Loading too many films at once can lead to overlap. Allow at least 10 seconds before each new film.
- *Poorly maintained machine.* Just as with processing solutions, it is essential to follow the manufacturer's instructions for maintaining and cleaning the automatic processing unit. Rollers should be removed and cleaned on time.

CHECKPOINTS

32-5 During manual processing, a developing solution that is too hot results in what?

32-6 Dark spots on a radiograph indicate what?

32-7 Static electricity causes what during processing?

32-8 Automatic processors typically take how long to produce finished and dried radiographs?

32-9 True or false? The same developer and fixer solutions can be used in automatic and manual processing.

Mounting Radiographs

After processing, dry radiographs should be mounted in holders for better viewing (Figure 32-6). Mounting is typically done as soon as possible after processing. To reduce confusion, radiographs should be labeled with the patient's name and date as soon as possible after drying.

Mounts are available in a variety of sizes and colors to accommodate different sizes of dental film. Mounted radiographs have a number of advantages over loose film:

- Mounted radiographs are easier to read and interpret.
- Mounted radiographs are easier to store.

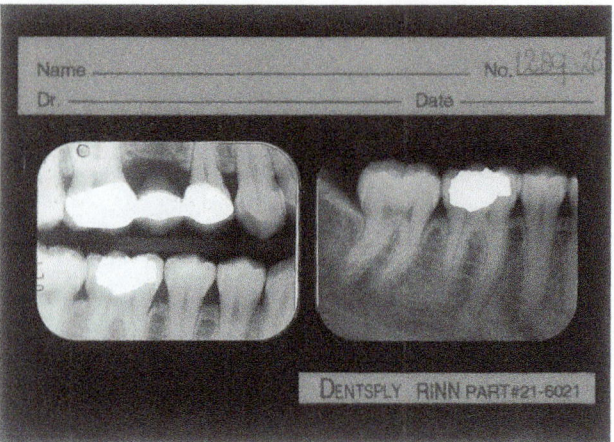

Figure 32–6 Mounted radiographs.

- Correctly mounted radiographs make it easier to distinguish the patient's right and left sides.
- The films are handled less, which decreases the risk of scratches and nicks.
- Film mounts filter out distracting side light, which makes them easier to read.
- Film mounts are easier to label with patient information.

Mounting should always be done on a clean, light-colored surface to protect the films. This makes it easier to see the radiographs when they are laid out on the worktable. During mounting, films are viewed in a view box or illuminator to help guide the operator.

Mounting is generally only performed on intraoral films. Larger extraoral films can be labeled and stored individually. Even single intraoral films benefit from being properly mounted.

Identifying Films

It is helpful to mount all intraoral films, even single images and smaller series. In a larger series, such as a full-mouth series (FMX), mounting them correctly makes it much easier to interpret the radiographs and make accurate diagnoses.

Each dental film is made with a tiny embossed dot on the film itself. This dot is raised on one side and convex on the other, and is used to help orient the film, so that all the films placed into a mount are facing the same way. In a correctly placed intraoral film, the raised side of the dot faces the x-ray beam.

Using the dot as a reference point, there are two methods of mounting radiographs:

- ***Labial mounting.*** Images are mounted with the raised identification dot facing the viewer, or convex. This perspective is most natural for the viewer, since it is the same view as standing directly in front of the mouth and looking at the teeth straight on. The viewer's left is the patient's right, and vice versa. It is also the same

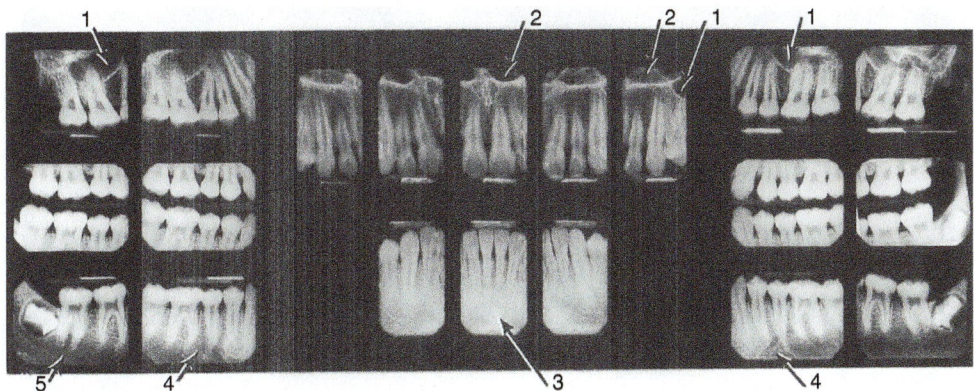

Figure 32–7 Anatomical landmarks for mounting. FMX showing: (1) Maxillary sinuses, (2) Nasal cavities, (3) Genial tubercles, (4) Mental foramen, (5) Mandibular canal.

perspective that is used when the teeth are drawn on most dental or periodontal charts. This method is recommended by the American Dental Association and the American Academy of Oral and Maxillofacial Radiology.

- **Lingual mounting.** Images are mounted with the raised identification dot facing away from the viewer, or concave. This perspective imagines that the viewer is inside the patient's mouth and looking out through the teeth. In this perspective, the viewer's right is also the patient's right. This method is used, but less commonly than labial mounting.

When mounting an FMX that includes both bitewing and periapical exposures, it is helpful to organize all the films on the work surface according to film size, with all the embossed dots facing the same way. During the mounting, teeth should be organized with the dot facing outward. This means the teeth will be depicted from left to right. Bitewing images can be easily distinguished during sorting because they contain both maxillary and mandibular teeth on one film. For more details on how to identify teeth depicted in radiographs, see Anatomical Landmarks below.

Types of Mounts

A variety of mounts and mounting styles are available. Mount colors include clear and black. Most dental offices prefer the black mounts because it enhances the contrast in the radiograph, making it easier to read. Mounts are also available with a number of sizes and spaces for different styles of films. If all the spaces in a particular mount cannot be used, the empty space should be filled with black paper to reduce the amount of light during viewing.

Anatomical Landmarks

An experienced dentist or dental assistant will often be able to immediately identify teeth in radiographs by looking at them. However, novices often use anatomical landmarks on the teeth to help guide them during mounting (Figure 32-7). Ideally, teeth should be mounted following the natural smile line, with the embossed dots facing outward. Anatomical landmarks used to identify radiographs are listed in Table 32-5.

TABLE 32-5 Anatomical Landmarks

REGION	MAXILLARY LANDMARKS	MANDIBULAR LANDMARKS
Incisor	Incisive foramen	Mental ridge
	Median palatine suture	Mental fossa
	Nasal fossa	Lingual foramen
	Nasal septum	Genial tubercles
	Anterior nasal spine	Nutrient canals
Canine	Lateral fossa	
	Inverted Y	
Molar	Coronoid process of mandible	Submandibular fossa
	Hamulus	Mylohyoid ridge
	Maxillary tuberosity	Oblique ridge
	Zygoma	Mandibular canal
	Zygomatic process of maxilla	Mental foramen
	Maxillary sinus	

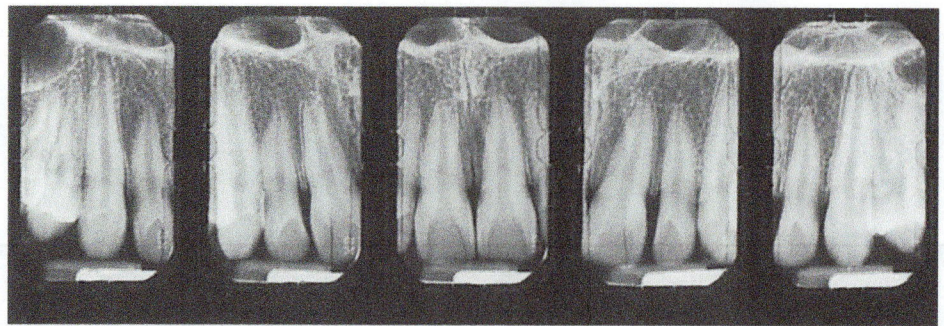

Figure 32–8 Mounted radiographs of maxillary anterior teeth.

The following principles serve as general guidelines:

- Maxillary teeth have larger crowns and longer roots than mandibular teeth.
- Canine teeth have the longest roots.
- Maxillary molars typically have three roots, but the palatal root makes it difficult to visualize all three roots.
- Mandibular molars have two roots with visible bone between them.
- Most roots curve toward the distal.
- Large radiolucent areas of the nasal fossa or maxillary sinus indicate a maxillary radiograph.
- The mandible has a distinctive upward curve in the molar area. Sometimes called the "smile line," this helps orient radiographs.
- Bitewing radiographs should be mounted with the occlusal plane between the mandibular and maxillary teeth (called the curve of Spee) facing upward, toward the distal.

Mounting Techniques

After the mount is selected and the radiographs are sorted, the individual films can be mounted (Figure 32-8). It is best to mount films following a predictable order, much like the film sequence used during exposures. Films of teeth are typically mounted according to their anatomic order. This will reduce errors and alert the operator to any missing or duplicated radiographs.

Films should be securely mounted, and the film mount should be clearly labeled and dated. For more detail on mounting procedures, see Procedure 32-3, Mounting Radiographs below.

Mounting Digital Radiographs

Digital radiography is rapidly changing the practice of radiography, including mounting. Digital radiographs do not need to be processed—they appear on the computer screen almost instantaneously. However, they still need to be viewed, so the same organization principles that apply to mounting apply to digital radiographs.

Digital radiography systems include software for viewing. Operators should be able to "drag and drop" individual images onto virtual mounts for viewing on a computer screen. As with conventional mounting, films of teeth should arranged in anatomic order. Digital mounts can be automatically labeled onscreen with the patient's name, dentist's name, and other information. These should be saved to the patient's electronic record.

Procedure 32-3 Mounting Radiographs

Materials needed (Figure P32-3-1):

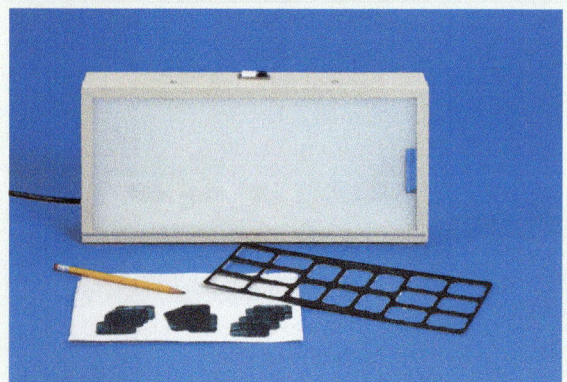

Figure P32-3-1

- Appropriate film mount (cardboard or plastic)
- Pencil
- View box
- Paper towel
- A full-mouth series of radiographs
  1. Prepare the work surface, making sure it is clean and covered with a clean, dry paper towel (to protect the films). Turn on the view box.
  2. Label and date the film mount (Figure P32-3-2).

Procedure 32–3 Mounting Radiographs (Continued)

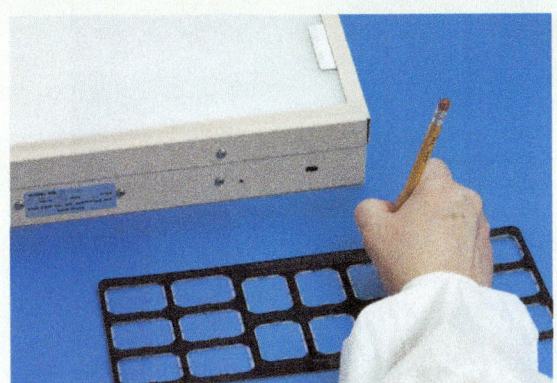

Figure P32-3-2

3. Wash and dry your hands.

4. Handling the radiographs by their edges only, place them onto the paper towel with the embossed identification dot facing up (for labial mounting) (Figure P32-3-3A and B).

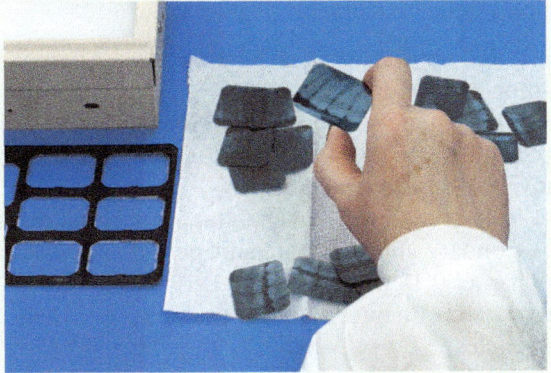

Figure P32-3-3A

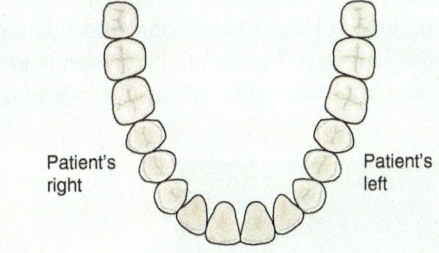

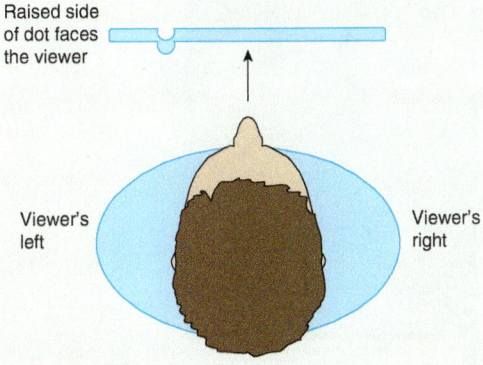

Raised side of dot faces the viewer

Viewer's left

Viewer's right

Figure P32-3-3B. Perspective used for labial mounting.

5. Sort the radiographs into three groups: bitewing, anterior periapical, and posterior periapical. Bitewing radiographs depict the crowns of both the maxillary and mandibular teeth. Anterior radiographs are oriented vertically, with the long axis of the tooth parallel to the long axis of the film. Posterior radiographs are oriented horizontally, with the long axis of the tooth perpendicular to the long axis of the film.

6. Arrange the radiographs on the work surface in anatomic order. Roots usually curve toward the distal, and teeth are typically arranged from the right molars to the left molars. Maxillary and mandibular films can be distinguished through the use of anatomical landmarks. Maxillary teeth are oriented with their roots pointing upward, while mandibular teeth are oriented with their roots pointing downward, as in the mouth.

7. Place the arranged radiographs on the view box in the correct anatomical order (Figure P32-3-4).

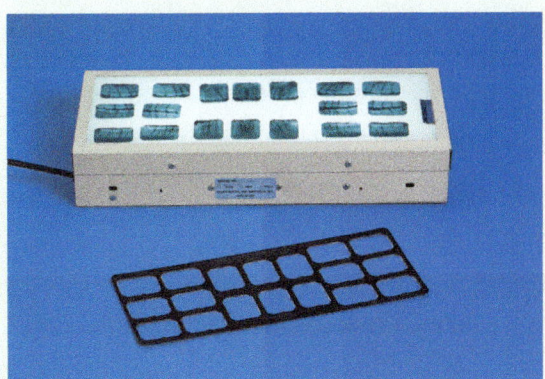

Figure P32-3-4

8. Carefully place each film in the film mount and secure it (Figure P32-3-5). Develop and follow a predictable sequence for every mount. In an FMX, a typical mounting sequence might be:

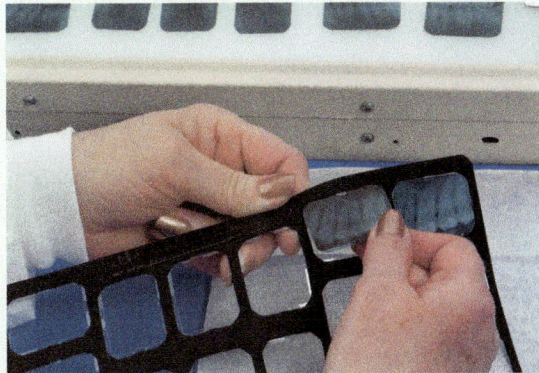

Figure P32-3-5

- Maxillary anterior periapicals
- Mandibular anterior periapicals
- Bitewings

Procedure 32–3 Mounting Radiographs (Continued)

- Maxillary posterior periapicals
- Mandibular posterior periapicals

9. Check your work by verifying that the identification dot is always facing outward (for labial mounting), the films are arranged in anatomic order, all films are mounted securely, and the film mount is properly labeled and dated.

10. Place the mounted radiographs in a view box for viewing and interpretation (Figure P32-3-6).

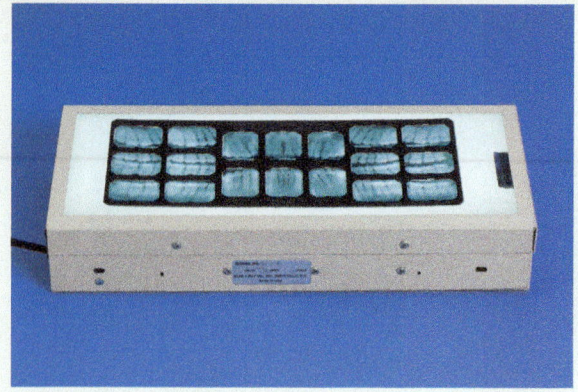

Figure P32-3-6

CHECKPOINTS

32-10 What are the two methods of mounting traditional radiographs?

32-11 How are digital radiographs mounted?

Radiographic Interpretation

Diagnostic radiographs are essential for proper interpretation and diagnosis. Radiographic **interpretation** is the practice of identifying landmarks and anomalies on a radiograph correctly. Any trained dental professional can interpret radiographs, although only dentists can legally diagnose conditions based on dental radiographs. During interpretation, the viewer must be able to identify and distinguish any of the following features that might be present on a dental radiograph (Figure 32-9):

- Normal and abnormal dental anatomy (See Chapter 8, Dentition and Tooth Morphology)
- Restorations, implants, and foreign objects (See Chapter 38, Fixed Prosthodontics, and Chapter 39, Removable Prosthodontics)
- Dental caries (e.g., interproximal, lingual, occlusal, recurrent secondary and rampant) and periodontal disease (See Chapter 9, Dental Caries and Periodontal Disease)
- Trauma (See Chapter 18, Responding to Medical Emergencies)
- Lesions (e.g., cysts, pulp stones, resorption, abscess, fractures, occlusal trauma, etc.) (See Chapter 12, Oral Pathology)

It is important to understand that radiographic interpretation is different from **diagnosis**. Whereas interpretation is identifying landmarks and anomalies present on the radiograph,

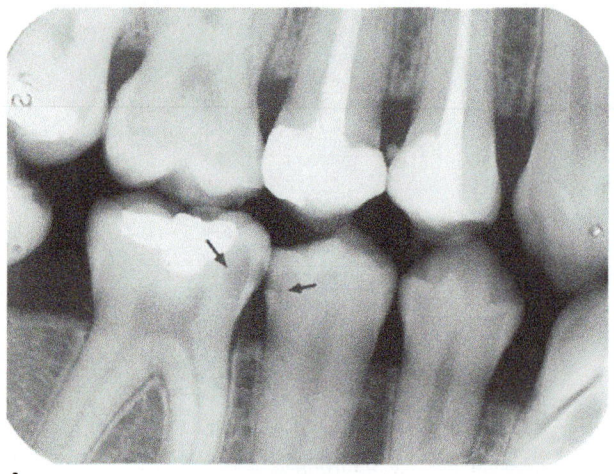

A

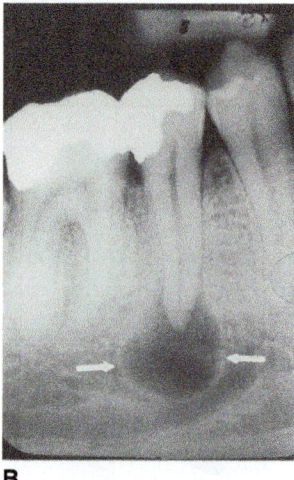

B

Figure 32–9 Radiographic interpretation. (**A**) Dental caries (shown at **arrows**). (**B**) Apical cyst (shown between **arrows**).

diagnosis is the practice of identifying diseases and pathologies based on the information in the radiograph, combined with an expert review of the patient's medical history, dental history, clinical examination, and any lab or clinical tests.

By law, only dentists are allowed to make diagnoses. Dental assistants can help by drawing the dentist's attention to potential abnormalities on the radiograph, but they are not allowed to make diagnoses.

A full discussion of radiographic interpretation is beyond the scope of this text, and beyond the normal job description of most dental assistants. State and local laws governing dental radiography interpretation and diagnosis may vary. Dental assistants should be familiar with the laws in their area.

From the Dentist's Perspective

I run a busy practice, so we are constantly processing and evaluating radiographs in my office. Of course, all of the assistants and hygienists know that I'm the only one who can legally diagnose a condition from a radiograph, but I always appreciate a quick eye from my assistants who take and process x-rays. By drawing my attention to potential problem areas (in private, of course), they allow me more time for direct patient care.

Interpretation in Practice

Dental radiographs are designed to benefit the patient, so ideally, they should be available for interpretation during the patient's normal visit. In practices that rely on traditional darkroom processing, or even automatic processing, dental x-rays should be taken at the beginning of the appointment. During the appointment, radiographs can be processed, dried, and mounted so they are available for interpretation at the end of the appointment. Radiographs are best viewed on a light box in a dim room.

Dental radiographs are also frequently interpreted chairside, where the patient's attention can be directed to the images. Patient input is a valuable part of diagnosis, so having radiographs prepared by the end of an appointment is an invaluable resource for the dentist as he or she evaluates the patient. It is important to note, however, that when patients are viewing radiographs with anybody except the dentist, a potential diagnosis should never be offered. Dental assistants cannot point out caries or any other problem to the patient.

In practices that use digital radiography, processing time is reduced dramatically. The images are available almost instantly on a computer monitor. In this case, it is less pressing to take the radiographs at the beginning of the session.

CHECKPOINTS

32-12 Which member of the dental team is responsible for making diagnoses based on dental radiographs?

32-13 Why should traditional radiographs be taken at the beginning of a patient's appointment?

Duplicating and Storing Radiographs

Radiographs are owned not by the patient but by the dental practice. As such, it is the practice's responsibility to store them safely and to answer any requests for duplication. Radiographs may be duplicated for a number of reasons, including:

- Specialist referral
- Insurance company requests
- Teaching aids
- Legal reasons

Duplications are exact copies of the original radiographs. They can be obtained during exposure by using a two-film packet, or after processing by using a **film duplicator** and **duplicating film** (Figure 32-10). Duplicating film differs from traditional film in that it is only coated on one side with emulsion. A film duplicator is a special device that provides a light source to expose the duplicating film. The light source is typically ultraviolet light. Film duplicators can handle a variety of film sizes.

Film duplication must be done under safelight conditions in a darkroom. The process of duplicating film is simple:

1. Turn the duplicator on, make sure it is clean, and switch to the VIEW function.
2. Remove the radiographs to be duplicated from their mounts and place them on the glass surface of the duplicator. To obtain the best contact between the film and the glass, place the exposed film with the identification dot facing up, so the concave side is down. If the manufacturer of the duplicator has supplied an organizer, use this to organize the radiographs. It will block out extra light.

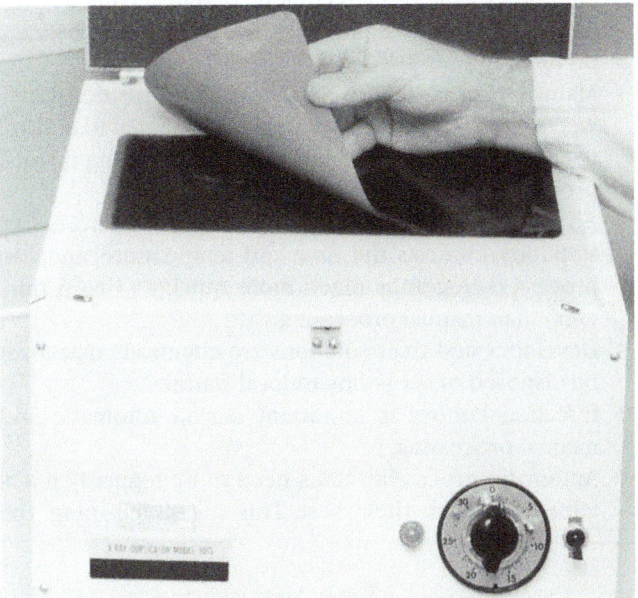

Figure 32-10 Duplication procedure.

3. Turn off the VIEW function to extinguish the view box light. The view box light must be turned off before the box of duplicating film is opened to prevent ruining the unexposed film.

4. Remove an appropriate piece of duplicating film and place it on the films to be duplicated. Note: The emulsion side should face down on duplicators with a light source below the film. The emulsion side is dark in color, while the side without emulsion is shiny. If the light source is above the film, the emulsion side of the duplicating film is placed face up, and the film to be duplicated (the original film) is placed on top of that.

5. Secure the duplicator lid. It is essential to obtain good contact between the duplicating film and the radiographs, so make sure the duplicator's lid is securely latched.

6. Set the desired exposure time, according to the manufacturer's recommendations.

7. Press the exposure button. The longer the duplicating film is exposed to the light source, the lighter it will be. This is the opposite of x-ray film, which becomes darker with prolonged exposure to x-ray radiation.

8. Wait for the indicator light to go off.

9. Remove the duplicator film and process it either manually or with an automatic processor.

10. Place the originals back in their mounts and return to the patient's record.

11. Label and mount the duplicates.

Handling and Storing Radiographs

Radiographs are part of a patient's permanent dental record. Dental radiographs, along with the patient's dental history, should be stored indefinitely. If a patient switches dental practices and requests that records and radiographs be forwarded to the new practice, duplicates of both the dental record and the radiographs should be made. The original copies should never be sent. It is also not advisable to release the copies of dental records and radiographs to the patients themselves. It is better to forward this information straight to the new dental office.

Because they need to last indefinitely, radiographs should be handled and packaged with care. Film should be handled by the edges and care should be taken not to scratch or mar their surfaces. Finished films should be stored in flat envelopes. Under no circumstances should dental films be creased or bent. They should be stored in a cool, dark place, away from visible light.

Digital radiographs should be stored to the appropriate storage device, such as an external hard drive. Permanent radiographs should never be stored on a desktop computer, but should be backed up to a secure drive. Ideally, more than one digital copy should be saved in case of hard-drive failure.

CHECKPOINTS

32-14 Do patients own their radiographs?

32-15 How are duplications of radiographs made?

Chapter Highlights

+ Film processing is the technique of transferring a latent image from exposed radiographic film to a visible image on film.

+ Manual processing involves several steps: developer, water bath, fixer, rinsing, drying. It is essential to control the temperature and timing of solutions during manual processing or the films will be ruined.

+ An automatic processing unit contains all the necessary solutions, controls the time and temperature, and can process radiographs much more quickly (4 to 6 minutes) than manual processing.

+ Developer and fixer solutions are chemicals that must be disposed of according to local statutes.

+ Infection control is important during automatic and manual processing.

+ Automatic processing units need to be regularly maintained to work their best. This means cleaning the machine and replenishing solutions according to the manufacturer's schedule.

+ Dried radiographs should be mounted in special film mounts for viewing and storage. No empty holes should be left in a film mount.

+ Films should be mounted in anatomical order with all the identifying dots facing the same way.

+ Any dental professional with training can interpret a radiograph, but only dentists can diagnose.

+ A film duplicator uses duplicating film to produce an exact copy of a dental radiograph.

+ Dental radiographs belong to the dentist and should be stored indefinitely. Original radiographs should never be sent to outside offices or released to the patient.

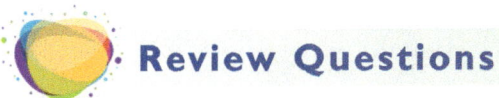
Review Questions

1. Where is the latent image stored in an exposed radiograph?

   a. The front

   b. The back

   c. The gelatin

   d. The silver halide crystals

2. How does temperature affect the development process?

   a. Speeds it up

   b. Slows it down

   c. It depends on whether it is automatic or manual

   d. There is no effect

3. What does the sodium thiosulfate in fixer solution do?

   a. Washes away undeveloped and unexposed silver halide

   b. Preserves the solution

   c. Maintains the pH level

   d. Hardens the gelatin

4. How many light sources are required in every darkroom?

   a. One, a safelight

   b. Two, a safelight and a white light

   c. Three, a safelight, a view box, and a white light

   d. Four, a safelight, a view box, a white light, and a black light

5. About how long do radiographs have to stay in fixer solution?

   a. 17 minutes

   b. Half as long as the developer

   c. 20 minutes

   d. Twice as long as the developer

6. A clear film after processing means what?

   a. Overdeveloped

   b. Too long in the fixer

   c. Exposed to white light

   d. None of the above

7. What do white spots on a film after processing mean?

   a. Too long in the developer

   b. Contact with hands

   c. Fixer solution splattered on the film

   d. Film was defective

8. Which is a disadvantage of automatic processing?

   a. Faster

   b. Less accurate images

   c. Potential radioactive leaks

   d. Expense of the machine

9. How long should you wait between films when feeding them into an automatic unit?

   a. 10 seconds

   b. 30 seconds

   c. 1 minute

   d. 4 to 6 minutes

10. What should you do with extra spaces in a film mount?

    a. Leave them exposed

    b. Cut them away with scissors

    c. Fill them with black paper

    d. Fill them with extra film

11. Who is allowed to interpret radiographs?

    a. Dentists

    b. All trained dental professionals

    c. Hygienists

    d. Dental assistants

12. A labial mount is when

    a. The identifying dot is facing outward on a mount.

    b. The identifying dot is facing inward on a mount.

    c. The films are mounted in anatomical order.

    d. A mount excludes bitewing exposures.

13. How long should radiographs be stored?

    a. 1 year

    b. 7 years

    c. Until the statute of limitations runs out

    d. Indefinitely

Active Learning Exercises

1. What are the differences between manual and automatic dental film processing? What liquids are used in each method and in what order?

2. What are the differences between lingual and labial mounting? Describe your location in viewing the radiographs, including dot placement and other relevant details.

3. How is the process of duplicating films a direct reflection of the professionalism of a dental office? How is duplicating film different from regular film? Describe how to place emulsion on duplicating film.

Application Activity

1. State laws vary regarding what functions a dental assistant is able to perform in the field of dental radiography. Using the Internet or the library, research the laws in your state concerning a dental assistant's scope of practice in the area of radiography. Begin by listing the radiography-related tasks a dental assistant is able to perform in your state. Create a second list that outlines the functions a dental assistant cannot legally perform in your state.

PREPARING FOR CERTIFICATION EXAMS

Review the following topics in this chapter to prepare for the Dental Assisting National Board (DANB) exam:

- **Overview of Film Processing**

- **Manual Processing**

- **Automatic Processing**

- **Mounting Radiographs**

- **Identifying Films**

- **Anatomical Landmarks**

- **Mounting Techniques**

- **Duplicating and Storing Radiographs**

Dental Materials

chapter 33

Dental Cements, Liners, Bases, and Bonding Agents

CHAPTER OUTLINE

CHAPTER CHECKLIST

On completion of this chapter, students will be able to:

- ☑ Describe the important characteristics of dental materials that impact their functioning.
- ☑ Identify the various ways that dental cements are used during procedures.
- ☑ List the general guidelines for mixing dental cement.
- ☑ Describe the main types of dental cements, including their properties, uses, preparation, and placement.
- ☑ Describe the use of etchants, including their properties, uses, and mixing or placement.

- ☑ Describe the use of cavity liners, including their properties, uses, preparation, and placement.
- ☑ Describe the use of cavity varnishes, including their properties, uses, preparation, and placement.
- ☑ Describe the use of cement bases, including their properties, uses, preparation, and placement.
- ☑ Describe the use of bonding agents, including their properties, uses, preparation, and placement.
- ☑ Understand the role of the dental assistant in procedures involving the mixing and placement of dental materials.
- ☑ Explain how to properly remove excess cement after placement of a restoration.

KEY TERMS

acidity – the amount of acid that is present in a substance

adhesion – the joining together of two objects

bonding – the process of using a substance to create adhesion

calcium hydroxide (high-DROK-side) – a dental material used for lining

cavity liner – a dental material used to seal the dentin and to protect the pulp of the tooth being restored

cavity varnish – a dental material used as a liner to create a protective seal over the dentin and pulp of the tooth being restored

cement base – a dental material placed under a restoration to protect the pulp of the tooth being restored; can protect, insulate, and/or sedate the pulp

composite resin – a dental material used for permanent cementing of restorations such as crowns, bridges, inlays, and onlays

corrosion – a breakdown in metal caused by a chemical reaction from metal mixing with water

curing – the process by which dental material sets and hardens

dental flow – changes in the shape of dental materials, such as waxes, due to pressure or force; also called creep

ductility (duk-TIL-uh-tee) – how much a material stretches out or lengthens when under stress

elasticity – the ability of dental material to change shape when force is applied and return to its original shape when force is removed

etchant (ETCH-unt) – acid-based dental material used to improve the bond between a restoration and the tooth

exothermic (ek-so-THER-mik) reaction – a chemical reaction in which heat is released

galvanism (GAL-vuh-nih-zum) – the process by which two metals connect to one another by electric shock when the metals mix with water

glass ionomer (eye-ON-uh-mer) – a dental cement used for permanent cementing of restorations such as crowns, bridges, inlays, onlays, and orthodontic bands and brackets; also used as a base and a permanent liner

hardness – the ability of dental material to resist scratches or marks

luting (LOO-ting) agent – a dental material that is used as an adhesive to hold the tooth and restoration together; also helps create a barrier against microleakage by sealing any gaps between the tooth and restoration

microleakage (my-kroh-LEE-kuj) – leakage of saliva or food particles into the small spaces between the tooth and a restoration

polycarboxylate (pol-ee-kar-BOK-suh-late) – a dental cement used for permanent cementing of restorations such as crowns, bridges, inlays, onlays, and orthodontic bands and brackets; also used for temporary cementing of restorations and as a base

resistance – the degree to which dental material can hold up under force or stress

restoration – a dental material used to restore the health and function of a damaged or missing tooth, such as crowns, bridges, inlays, and onlays

retention – the way in which dental material is held in place

solubility – the degree to which dental material dissolves and breaks apart when it is wet

strain – changes in the shape or function of dental material that are a result of being under stress

stress – the force or pressure applied to dental material

thermal conductivity – the speed at which dental material heats up

thermal expansion – the degree to which dental material expands when heated

tensile strength – the amount of force or pulling dental material is able to resist without tearing or falling out of place

viscosity (vis-KOS-uh-tee) – how well a liquid moves and flows

wettability (wet-uh-BIL-ih-tee) – the degree to which a dental material can be wetted so it can spread across a solid surface

zinc oxide eugenol (YOO-juh-nawl) (ZOE) – a dental cement used for temporary cementing of restorations such as crowns, bridges, inlays, and onlays; also used as a temporary restoration and a base

zinc phosphate (FOS-fate) – a dental cement used for permanent cementing of restorations such as crowns, bridges, inlays, onlays, and orthodontic bands and brackets; also used as a base

Introduction

Dental **restorations** help rebuild the health and function of damaged or missing teeth. Examples of restorations include crowns and bridges. Direct restorations, such as amalgams, are both created and placed inside the mouth. Indirect restorations, such as crowns and bridges, are created outside the mouth and then placed in the mouth. Restorative material, such as dental cement, can be used to create restorations as well as to hold them in place. The selection of the correct material is crucial in determining how well a restoration works. Dental assistants need to know the characteristics and uses of dental materials because they are often involved in preparing, handling, and cleaning up these materials.

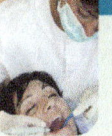

Voice of Experience

Whenever my employer goes to a major dental conference and learns about a new dental material, she purchases it and brings it into the office. Many times, she has handed me new products and asked that I be responsible for teaching the office how to correctly prepare, use, and clean up the product. Those situations always remind me how important it is to read all of the manufacturer's instructions thoroughly before attempting to use the product. Even when I'm not teaching others about a product, I always make sure to sit down and read everything, rather than trying to learn as I go along.

Many dental materials can be used to restore the health of a tooth. Dental professionals must consider several factors in understanding which materials are appropriate for the restoration that needs to be performed.

Adhesion

Adhesion is the joining together of two objects. The process of using a substance to adhere, or join, two objects together is known as **bonding**. Bonding agents, also known as adhesives, are materials used for bonding two objects together. In dentistry, bonding agents often include dental adhesives or cements, which are used for cementing crowns or bridges and for restoring cracked and broken teeth.

Curing

Curing is the process by which dental material hardens or sets. Material that is light-cured requires a special curing light, which is held over the material after it is placed in the oral cavity, causing it to set. Self-cured material does not require an outside light or heat source and instead hardens and sets by itself due to chemical reactions between a catalyst and a base. Dual-cured materials use a combination of light-curing and self-curing.

Flow, Viscosity, Wettability, and Solubility

Some dental materials, such as waxes, change shape when pressure or force is applied to them. This change in shape is called **dental flow**, or creep. Another important feature is the **viscosity** of liquid dental materials. Viscosity describes how easily a liquid moves and flows. Thick liquids flow more slowly, whereas thin liquids flow quickly. Think of the difference between water and honey. Dental materials that are more viscous do not spread over the surface of an object as easily as less viscous liquids. **Wettability** is the degree to which matter can be wetted so that it can be spread across a solid surface. The degree to which matter dissolves and breaks apart when it is wet is called **solubility**. Material that is highly soluble may not work well in some restorations because once it comes into contact with saliva or other liquids, it may break apart.

Elasticity

Elasticity is the ability of dental materials to change shape when force is applied and then return to their original shape when force is removed. Much like a rubber band that stretches when pulled and returns to shape when released, objects with greater elasticity can be shaped and molded easily. But if you have ever stretched a rubber band too far, you know that elasticity has its limits. If the elasticity of an object is tested with too much force, it might not return to its original shape—or it might break altogether. In dentistry, when an impression is made, for example, the material must fit into the interproximal spaces. When the impression is removed, the material must have enough elasticity to stretch enough to be pulled off the teeth, but it is very important that once taken out of the mouth, the material returns to the original impression.

Hardness

The **hardness** of dental material describes how well it can resist scratches or marks. Softer materials are more easily scratched and will wear down more quickly than material with a greater hardness.

Resistance, Stress, Strain, and Ductility

To be effective, dental materials must withstand being subjected to a fair amount of force, such as biting, pushing, or pulling, without breaking. This force or pressure is known as **stress**. The dental material can hold up against force or stress because of **resistance**. Unfortunately, if the material is under too much stress and it does not have enough resistance, changes in the shape or function of the material can occur. This is known as **strain**. In dentistry, when too much stress causes a material to stretch out or lengthen, this is called **ductility**.

Corrosion

Restorative materials that are made of pure metal, such as gold, are at risk for **corrosion**. Corrosion is a chemical process that happens when metal mixes with water, causing the metal to break down and change color. In the mouth, sometimes saliva or bacteria from food can attack the metal in restorations, leading to corrosion.

Galvanism

In addition to corrosion, when metal makes contact with water, an electric flow or shock can occur. If two dissimilar metals contact water, they are connected electrically; this is a process known as **galvanism**. In dentistry, galvanism can occur when saliva causes a new metal restoration to connect electrically with an existing metal restoration, possibly creating a small shock. The same thing can occur, for instance, if a foil gum wrapper is placed in the mouth near a new restoration. The shock is not painful and it usually stops happening after about a week, but it can feel unusual. Explain to patients about galvanism and remind them that this shock is common so that they do not become alarmed or upset.

Thermal Characteristics

Dental materials also have thermal characteristics. The word *thermal* means heat. The speed at which dental material heats up is known as **thermal conductivity**. Materials with higher conductivity heat up quicker, whereas as materials with lower conductivity heat up more slowly. This is important because if materials with greater thermal conductivity come into contact with hot foods and drinks, they can heat up. Heat also causes some materials to expand, a process known as **thermal expansion**. The rate of thermal expansion of a dental material needs to be similar to the thermal expansion of the tooth itself. Otherwise, it can lead to irritation and microleakage can occur.

Retention and Tensile Strength

The way in which dental materials, such as amalgams, are held in place is called **retention**. Retention can be mechanical or chemical. An example of mechanical retention is creating grooves on the surface of a tooth so that a restoration can be held in place. Chemical retention uses chemicals to hold dental materials in place, such as using cements to hold a crown. Similarly, the amount of force or pulling the dental material is able to resist without tearing or falling out of place is known as **tensile strength**. Using dental materials with greater tensile strength is important so that amalgams and other restorations do not fall out of the mouth or tear apart.

Acidity

An acid is a chemical substance that increases the concentration of hydrogen ions when dissolved in water. The amount of acid present in a substance, or its **acidity**, is measured by its pH level. Normally, the mouth has a neutral, or non-acidic, pH. Foods high in acid, such as oranges or lemons, can raise the pH level. Bacteria in the oral cavity also produce acid, which can wear away the tooth enamel and some dental materials. Also, some dental materials may have a certain level of acidity as well. Materials that are high in acidity can cause irritation to the tooth surface, pulp, or gingiva.

> ### Extra Patient Care
> Some dental materials are very toxic and dangerous if handled incorrectly. Always explain the placement procedure to the patient first before placing anything. Be sure to let patients know if a material is hot or cold, as it may cause them sensitivity or irritation. Also be aware of using terms that might make patients feel scared or anxious, such as telling them that you are going to be using "acid" in their mouth.

Microleakage

Saliva or food particles can sometimes leak into small spaces between the tooth and the restoration, a process known as **microleakage**. It is important to know which materials are more likely to cause microleakage because it can result in dental caries and increased tooth sensitivity.

> ### CHECKPOINTS
> **33-1** What is the difference between adhesion and bonding?
>
> **33-2** Why should dental assistants be concerned about microleakage?
>
> **33-3** True or false? The speed at which a dental material heats up is known as thermal expansion.

Dental Cements

Dental cement is a type of restorative adhesive that serves many purposes. The cement typically is made by mixing together small amounts of powder and liquid, which are an acid and a base. Some cements are available in premixed capsules. Even though the dentist will place the cement, dental assistants are responsible for mixing and preparing cements and making sure the mixing equipment is working correctly, is clean, and is stored properly. Preparation, cleaning, and storage all impact whether the cement works as it should, making your role in the restoration process very important.

The American Dental Association classifies dental cements into three categories:

- *Luting agents.* A **luting agent** is an adhesive used to hold the tooth and restoration together. It also helps create a barrier against microleakage by sealing any gaps between the tooth and restorative.
- *Restorative materials.* These cements are used to insulate restorations.
- *Liners or bases.* These cements are used during cavity preparation for the purpose of protecting the pulp from chemicals, bacteria, or other possible injury.

Permanent Cements

Permanent cements are used for long-term restorations that will not be removed, such as bridges, veneers, inlays, and orthodontic appliances. Since permanent restorations will not be removed, it is very important to mix and apply permanent cements carefully.

Temporary Cements

Unlike permanent cements, temporary cements are used for short-term restorative material that will eventually be removed, such as temporary crowns. Sometimes temporary restorations are used to cover and protect the tooth while the permanent restoration is being cast by a dental laboratory technician.

Mixing Techniques

Dental cement is formed by mixing a powder and liquid, which causes a chemical reaction. Many factors can impact whether the dental cement is mixed correctly. One of the most important factors is the cement's consistency. Cement that is too thin or too thick may not work properly. Table 33-1 lists various factors to be aware of when mixing cement.

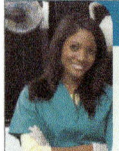

Voice of Experience

Have you heard the saying that big things come in small packages? When I teach dental students how to mix permanent cement, I explain how the $2.00 cement mixed by the dental assistant determines whether the $2,000 crown will stay in the mouth. The strength of the cement depends on how much powder is mixed in while still maintaining the correct consistency. The more powder, the stronger the cement!

Some cements come already mixed in capsules, while others require mixing by hand. The liquid comes in a bottle with a special dispenser-like top that releases the liquid in small drops. When using the dispenser, be sure to hold the dropper vertically and not at an angle.

Follow these general guidelines when mixing dental cements:

- Before mixing, always read the manufacturer's instructions first. Be sure to read *all* of the instructions before you begin rather than reading step-by-step while mixing.

TABLE 33-1	Factors Affecting Cement Mixes
Mixing time	Follow the manufacturer's instructions for the time it takes to mix and use the cement—over- or under-mixing cement can change its consistency, which can reduce its strength.
Temperature	If the environment is humid, the moisture in the air can cause liquids to become drier and powders to become wet.
Amounts of liquid and powder	Using too much powder can make the cement too dry, while using too much liquid can make it runny and thin.

- Mix cements on either a glass mixing slab or a paper mixing pad.
  - If using a glass slab, read the instructions to find out whether the slab should be cool, warm, hot, or cold.
  - The glass slab must always be dry. Water on the slab can make cement too wet or can weaken it altogether.
  - Some cements will require oil-resistant mixing paper, whereas others use standard mixing paper.
- Mix powders and liquids with a mixing spatula.
  - Always make sure the spatula and glass slab are clean before mixing. When using the paper mixing pad, tear off the top sheet if it is not clean.
  - Make sure the cap to the liquid bottle is on tight and that the dispenser is always clean.
  - Do not mix the cement ahead of time; wait until it is needed before mixing. For many types of cement, the liquid evaporates over time, causing unused cement to harden and become unusable.
- Following the manufacturer's instructions, measure the powder and liquid needed for the type and brand of cement being mixed.
  - Always mix for the length of time noted in the instructions. Do not stop mixing just because the cement appears done.
  - Never mix different brands of powders and liquids. Each brand is specially made to react with the powder or liquid of that same brand. Combining brands can result in cement that is weak and ineffective.
- Place the powder on one end of the glass slab or paper mixing pad and the liquid on the opposite end. Use the space in between the two as the mixing area.

CHECKPOINTS

33-4 Name three factors that affect how dental cements will work.

33-5 At what point during a procedure should dental cement be mixed?

Types of Dental Cements

Dental cements can also be classified by the chemicals they contain, including:

- Zinc oxide eugenol
- Zinc phosphate
- Zinc polycarboxylate
- Glass ionomer
- Composite resin cements

Table 33-2 describes the main chemical ingredients of each cement as well as common uses and functions. Table 33-3 provides some guidelines for mixing each type of cement.

TABLE 33-2 Chemical Properties and Functions of Dental Cements

CEMENT	POWDER	LIQUID	USES AND FUNCTIONS
Zinc oxide eugenol	■ Zinc oxide ■ Magnesium oxide ■ Silica	■ Eugenol ■ Acetic acid ■ Zinc acetate ■ Calcium chloride ■ Water	■ Temporary cementing of crowns, bridges, inlays, and onlays ■ Temporary restoration ■ Base (low-strength, sedative) ■ Root canal sealer
Zinc phosphate	■ Zinc oxide ■ Magnesium oxide ■ Silica	■ Phosphoric acid ■ Aluminum phosphate ■ Water	■ Permanent cementing of crowns, bridges, inlays, onlays, and orthodontic bands and brackets ■ Base
Polycarboxylate	■ Zinc oxide	■ Polyacrylic acid ■ Itaconic acid ■ Maleic acid ■ Tartaric acid ■ Water	■ Permanent cementing of crowns, bridges, inlays, onlays, and orthodontic bands and brackets ■ Base (high-strength) ■ Temporary restoration
Glass ionomer	■ Zinc oxide ■ Aluminum oxide ■ Calcium	■ Itaconic acid ■ Tartaric acid ■ Maleic acid ■ Water	■ Permanent cementing of crowns, bridges, inlays, onlays, and orthodontic bands and brackets ■ Base (high-strength, releases fluoride) ■ Liner (low-strength) ■ Root canal sealer ■ Temporary restoration
Composite resin	■ Composite resins vary in their ingredients	■ Composite resins vary in their ingredients	■ Permanent cementing of cast crowns, bridges, inlays, and onlays, resin-bonded bridges, and orthodontic bands

TABLE 33-3 Important Features of Cement Mixing

CEMENT TYPE	FORM	INSTRUMENTS FOR MIXING	CONSISTENCY/APPEARANCE OF MIXED CEMENT
Zinc oxide eugenol	■ Powder and liquid or two pastes ■ Some come in capsule forms	■ Oil-resistant paper mixing pad (for powder/oil) ■ Glass slab (for two pastes)	■ For Type I (temporary), cement should be creamy and drop easily off the end of the spatula ■ For Type II (use as a base), cement should be thick like clay and not drop easily off the end of the spatula; you should be able to roll it into a tacky ball
Zinc phosphate	■ Premixed capsules ■ Powder and liquid	■ Cool glass slab ■ Stainless steel spatula	■ For Type I, cement should be creamy and slightly stringy when hanging from the spatula; cement should spread easily across the glass slab ■ For Type II, cement should be thick like clay, and should not drop easily off the end of the spatula
Polycarboxylate	■ Powder and liquid	■ Nonabsorbent paper mixing pad ■ Glass slab ■ Wide spatula	■ Should be somewhat thick ■ Should be shiny in appearance ■ Becomes "cobweb-like" when overmixed
Glass ionomers	■ Premixed capsules ■ Powder and liquid	■ Nonabsorbent paper mixing pad ■ Glass slab ■ Plastic spatula	■ Very thin and shiny in appearance
Composite resin	■ Powder and liquid (in a syringe-type applicator)	■ Nonabsorbent paper mixing pad	■ Somewhat thin and fluid ■ Chemical properties vary by type of resin used; read the manufacturer's instructions for information on consistency

Zinc Oxide Eugenol

Zinc oxide eugenol (ZOE) comes in two types (Figure 33-1). Type I is used for temporary restorations because it does not have great strength or stability over time. Type II, on the other hand, has special substances added to it that help it remain strong over time, making it useful for permanent restorations. Although ZOE has low acidity, it has a strong odor (resulting from oil of cloves) that some patients may find unpleasant. ZOE has a sedative effect on the dental pulp. Because ZOE contains oil, it cannot be used under a composite restoration; the oil would interfere with the polymerization of the material.

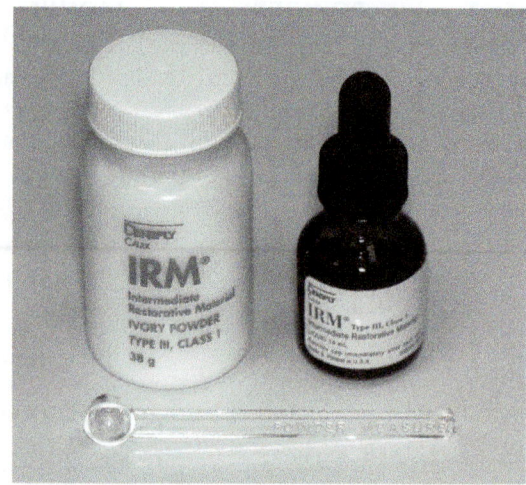

Figure 33–1 Zinc oxide eugenol cement.

Procedure 33–1 Mixing Procedure for Zinc Oxide Eugenol (Powder/Oil Form for Permanent Use)

Materials needed (Figure P33-1-1):

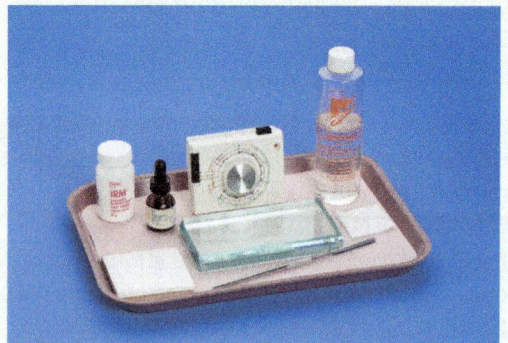

Figure P33-1-1

- Zinc oxide eugenol powder and liquid
- Oil-resistant paper mixing pad or glass slab
- Stainless steel spatula
- Timer
- Cleaning supplies (alcohol or disinfectant)

1. Put on appropriate PPE.
2. Dispense the powder onto the paper or slab according to the manufacturer's instructions. Be sure to replace the cap to the powder container immediately and tightly.
3. Carefully dispense several drops of liquid onto the paper or slab. Place the drops of liquid near the powder but not directly in or right next to the powder (Figure P33-1-2). Cap the liquid immediately and tightly.
4. Using the spatula and following the manufacturer's instructions, mix the powder into the liquid all at once. Use the flat part of the spatula to make sure the powder is spread evenly throughout the liquid.

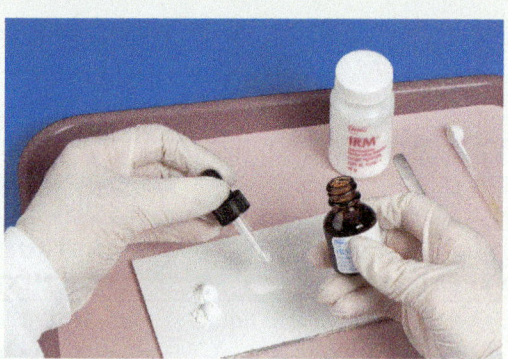

Figure P33-1-2

5. Consulting a timer, mix for 30 seconds.
6. Using the spatula, scrape up all of the mixed cement at once and check for the right consistency (Figure P33-1-3).

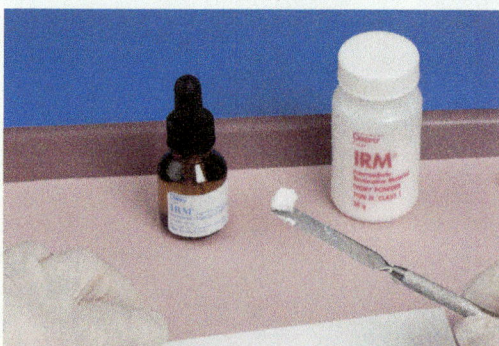

Figure P33-1-3

7. To clean up, tear off the top sheet of paper and fold it in half before throwing it away. This ensures no cement will spill off the paper. Clean any hardened cement off the spatula or glass slab by soaking it in water. Afterward, clean with alcohol or disinfectant.

Procedure 33–2 Mixing Procedure for Zinc Oxide Eugenol (Two Paste Form for Temporary Use)

Materials needed (Figure P33-2-1):

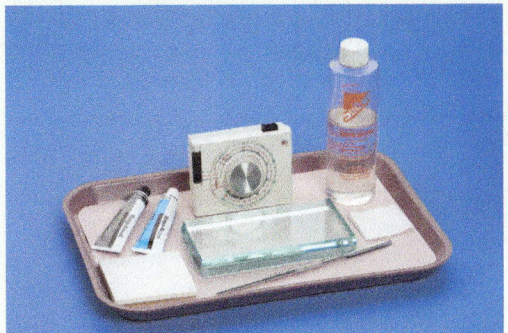

Figure P33-2-1

- Zinc oxide eugenol paste tubes
- Oil-resistant paper mixing pad or glass slab
- Stainless steel spatula
- Timer
- Cleaning supplies

1. Put on appropriate PPE.

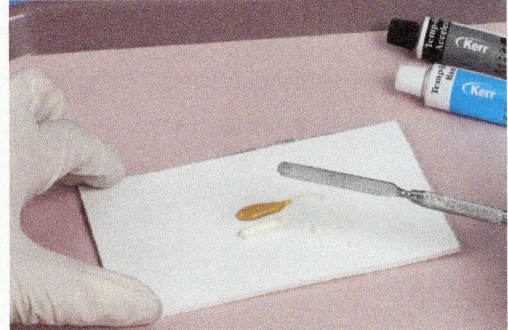

Figure P33-2-2

2. Dispense the pastes onto the paper or slab according to the manufacturer's instructions. Be sure to replace the cap to the paste tubes immediately and tightly (Figure P33-2-2).

3. Using the spatula and following the manufacturer's instructions, mix the pastes together. Use the flat part of the spatula to make sure the pastes are mixed evenly.

4. Consulting a timer, continue mixing for 20 to 30 seconds.

5. Using the spatula, scrape up all of the mixed cement at once and check for the right consistency (Figure P33-2-3).

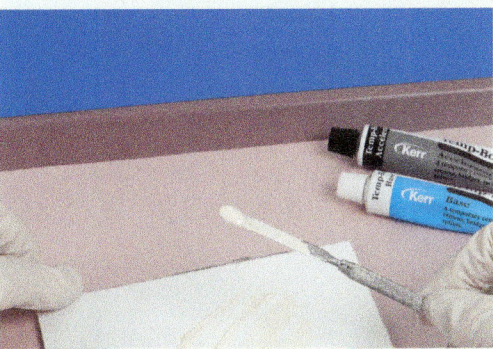

Figure P33-2-3

6. To clean up, tear off the top sheet of paper and fold it in half before throwing it away. This ensures no cement will spill off the paper. Clean any hardened cement off the spatula or glass slab by soaking it in water. Afterward, clean with alcohol or disinfectant.

Zinc Phosphate

Zinc phosphate, an older cement, is available in two types (Figure 33-2). Type I has a fine grain texture, which helps the cement create thin layers needed for permanent restorations. Type II has a medium grain texture and is used as a base to prepare restorations of deep cavities. When used as a base, a subbase, such as ZOE, must be placed underneath zinc phosphate because the phosphoric acid can damage the pulp of the tooth. When mixing zinc phosphate, it is very important to use a cool glass slab—about 68°F. If the slab is too warm, the cement will set too fast and will not work correctly. Also, when mixing, spread the cement over a wide area of the glass slab. Zinc phosphate produces an **exothermic reaction**, meaning it contains chemicals that release heat when mixed. Spreading it allows the cement to cool down before applying.

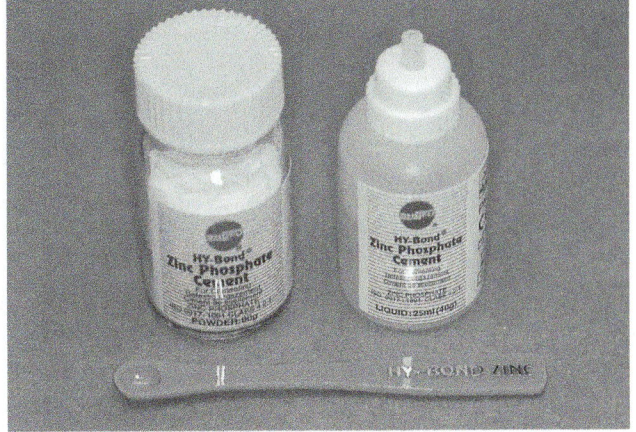

Figure 33–2 Zinc phosphate cement.

Procedure 33-3 Mixing Procedure for Zinc Phosphate

Materials needed (Figure P33-3-1):

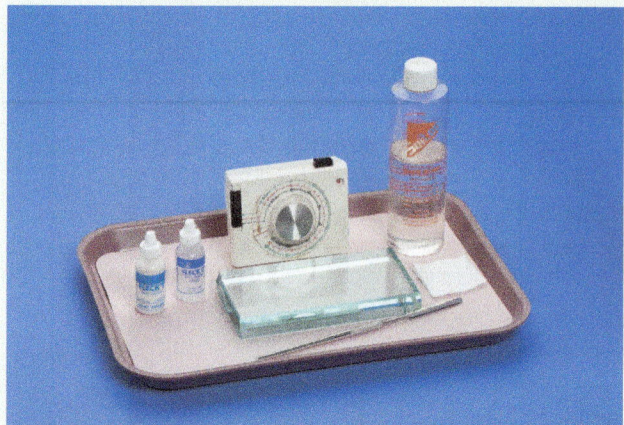

Figure P33-3-1

- Zinc phosphate powder and liquid
- Cool (68°F) glass mixing slab
- Stainless steel spatula
- Timer
- Alcohol wipes and disinfectant

1. Put on appropriate PPE.

2. Measure and dispense the powder onto the glass slab according to the manufacturer's instructions. Replace the cap to the powder container immediately and tightly. Refer to the manufacturer's instructions on how to divide the powder into appropriate increments.

3. Carefully dispense several drops of liquid on the end of the glass slab opposite to the powder (Figure P33-3-2). Cap the liquid immediately and tightly.

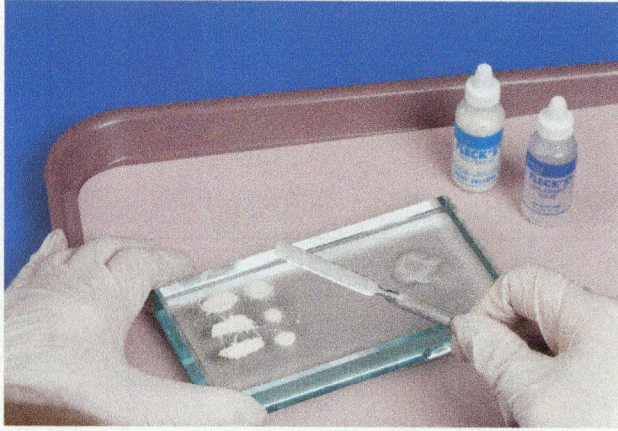

Figure P33-3-2

4. Using the spatula and following the manufacturer's instructions, mix one increment of the powder into the liquid. Use the flat part of the spatula to spread the cement over a wide area of the glass slab so it can cool (Figure P33-3-3). Spreading the cement in a figure-eight motion helps it cool faster.

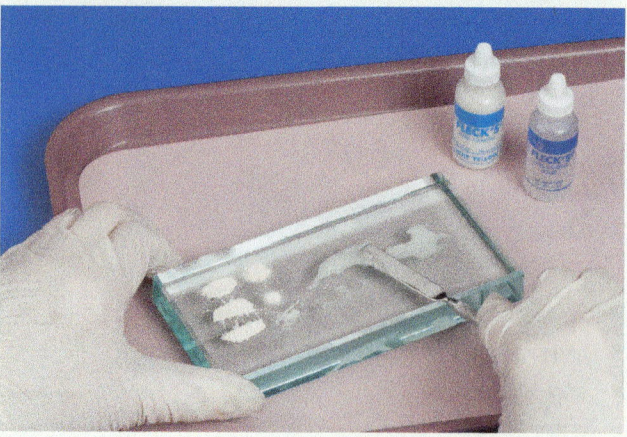

Figure P33-3-3

5. Consulting a timer, continue mixing the material for the length of time recommended in the manufacturer's instructions.

6. Using the spatula, scrape up all of the mixed cement at once and check for the right consistency (Figure P33-3-4).

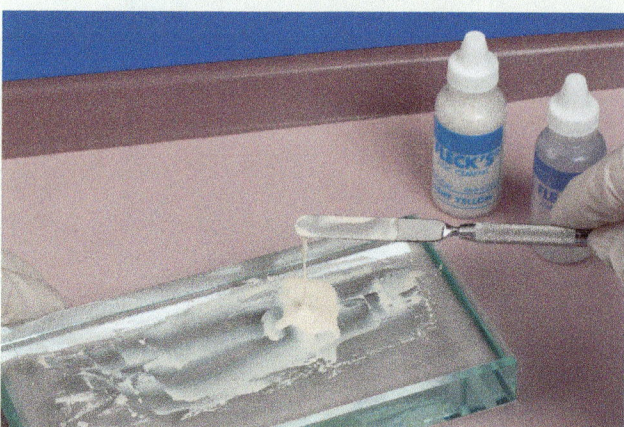

Figure P33-3-4

7. Clean up cement immediately using an alcohol wipe. Afterwards, clean the glass slab with a disinfectant.

Polycarboxylate

Polycarboxylate is a permanent cement used for casts and stainless steel crowns (Figure 33-3). It is also used as a base for amalgams and as a restoration. Polycarboxylate contains a liquid that evaporates quickly, which makes the cement thicken easily. For this reason, it must be used quickly and cannot sit on the slab for long. Polycarboxylate does not irritate the pulp of the tooth like zinc phosphate. However, the pH level of polycarboxylate rises as it sets, making it become highly acidic. This is another reason why it must be applied quickly. Polycarboxylate has low solubility, but when mixed with lactic acid, which is an acid that occurs naturally in the body, it becomes very soluble. For example, individuals with excess dental plaque also have excess lactic acid in their mouth, which can cause polycarboxylate to break down.

Glass Ionomer

Glass ionomer cement is the most commonly used type of cement. It serves many functions and comes in three types. Type I is for cementing metal restorations. Type II is used as a

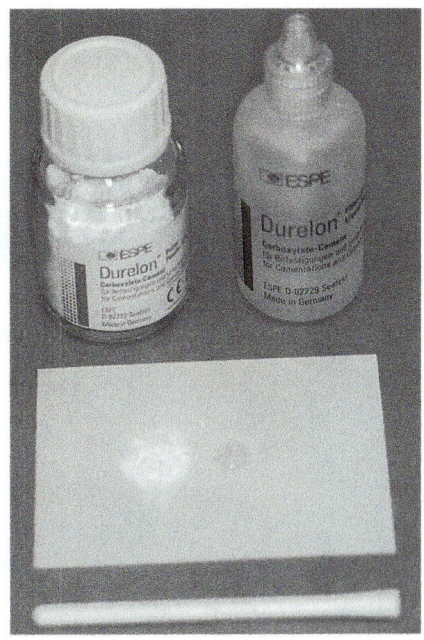

Figure 33–3 Polycarboxylate cement.

Procedure 33-4 Mixing Procedure for Polycarboxylate

Materials needed (Figure P33-4-1):

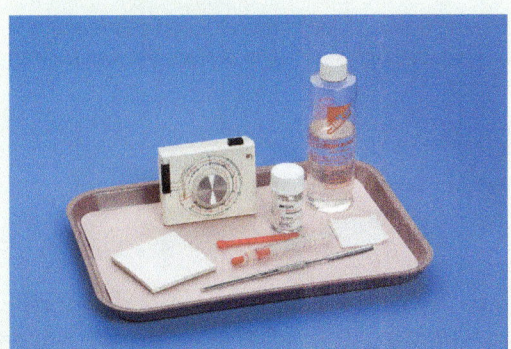

Figure P33-4-1

- Polycarboxylate powder and liquid (in syringe-type applicator)
- Paper mixing pad
- Stainless steel spatula
- Timer
- Alcohol wipes

1. Put on appropriate PPE.
2. Gently shake the powder and dispense onto the paper according to the manufacturer's instructions. Replace the cap to the powder container immediately and tightly.
3. Carefully dispense several drops of liquid onto the paper. Place the drops of liquid near the powder but not directly in or right next to the powder. Cap the liquid immediately and tightly.

4. Using the spatula and following the manufacturer's instructions, mix the powder into the liquid. Use the flat part of the spatula to make sure the powder is spread evenly throughout the liquid.
5. Consulting a timer, continue mixing the material for 30 seconds.
6. Using the spatula, scrape up all of the mixed cement at once and check for the right consistency. To determine the correct consistency, place the flat side of the spatula on the cement and lift the spatula up. The cement should follow the spatula up about 1 inch before it breaks away (Figure P33-4-2).

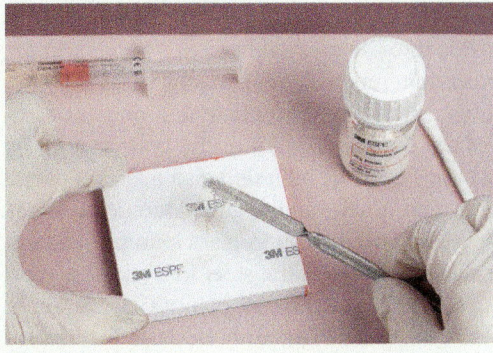

Figure P33-4-2

7. To clean up, tear off the top sheet of paper and fold it in half before throwing it away. Soak the spatula in a solution that is 10% sodium hydroxide. Afterward, clean the spatula with alcohol.

Procedure 33-5 Mixing Procedure for Glass Ionomer Cement

Materials needed (Figure P33-5-1):

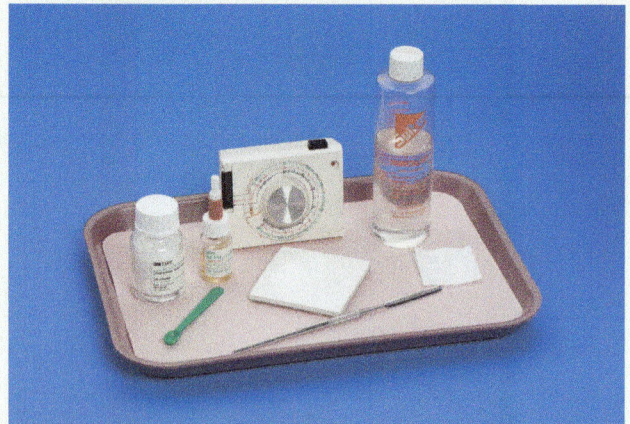

Figure P33-5-1

- Glass ionomer powder and liquid
- Paper mixing pad or cool, glass mixing slab
- Plastic spatula
- Timer
- Alcohol wipes

1. Put on appropriate PPE.
2. Dispense the powder onto the paper or slab according to the manufacturer's instructions. Replace the cap to the powder container immediately and tightly.
3. Carefully dispense several drops of liquid onto the pad or slab. Place the drops of liquid near the powder but not directly in or right next to the powder. Cap the liquid immediately and tightly.

4. Using the spatula and following the manufacturer's instructions, mix the powder into the liquid. Use the flat part of the spatula to make sure the powder is spread evenly throughout the liquid.
5. Consulting a timer, continue mixing for the amount of time noted in the manufacturer's instructions.
6. Using the spatula, scrape up all of the mixed cement at once and check for the right consistency (Figure P33-5-2).

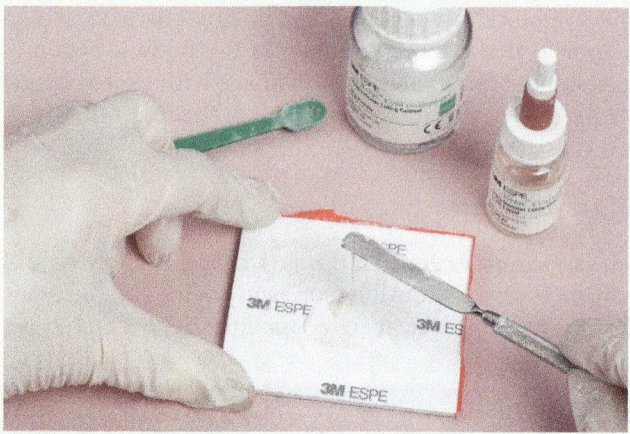

Figure P33-5-2

7. To clean up, tear off the top sheet of paper and fold it in half before throwing it away. Clean any hardened cement off the spatula or glass slab by soaking in water. Afterward, clean with alcohol.

---

restorative material, especially for areas of the tooth near the gingiva. Type III is used as a liner and bonding agent. Glass ionomer cement helps fight caries by slowly releasing a small amount of fluoride into the tooth. It has low solubility in the mouth and strong adherence to wet surfaces. Glass ionomer cement is stronger than zinc phosphate and does not irritate the pulp of the tooth, making it useful both as a luting agent and as a base. Its strong adhesion also makes it useful in cementing crowns. When mixing glass ionomer cement, use a plastic spatula. The particles in glass ionomer cement are hard and will wear away at the steel in a stainless steel spatula, causing the cement to change colors. Glass ionomer cement needs to be applied right away because it sets very quickly. Once it becomes rubbery, it should not be used.

Composite Resin Cement

Composite resin cements have many purposes, including cementing ceramic or resin inlays and onlays, ceramic veneers, orthodontic bands and brackets, and metal castings. Composite resin cements have no solubility in the mouth, but can irritate the pulp. Unlike some other types of dental cement, composite resin cements can only be used on a tooth or restoration that is clean, dry, and prepared beforehand with an etchant and bonding system. They usually come in a powder and liquid or in a syringe-like applicator. Composite resin cement should be mixed on a paper pad and should be mixed rapidly.

Check Your Ethics

As a dental assistant, a dentist asks you to permanently cement a crown. You are aware that this is not a legally allowed function for dental assistants to perform in your state. What should you do?

CHECKPOINTS

33-6 What is required before placing zinc phosphate cement on the tooth?

33-7 What is the most commonly used dental cement today?

Procedure 33–6 Mixing Procedure for Composite Resin Cement

Materials needed (Figure P33-6-1):

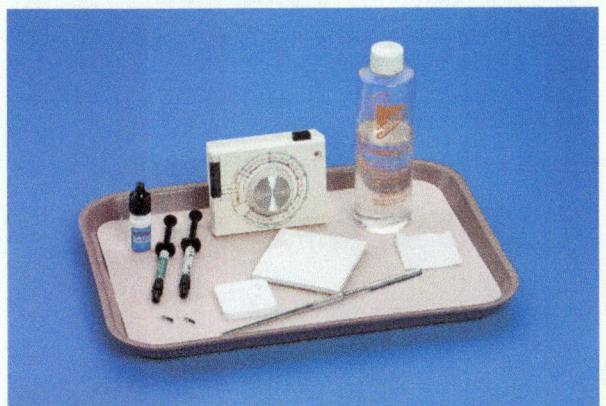

Figure P33-6-1

- Composite resin cement powder and liquid (in syringe-like applicator)
- Paper mixing pad
- Stainless steel spatula
- Timer
- Alcohol wipes or orange solvent
1. Put on appropriate PPE.
2. Dispense equal parts of powder and liquid onto opposite ends of the mixing pad.

3. Consulting a timer, mix the powder into the liquid for 10 seconds.
4. Using the spatula, scrape up all of the mixed cement at once and check for the right consistency (Figure P33-6-2).

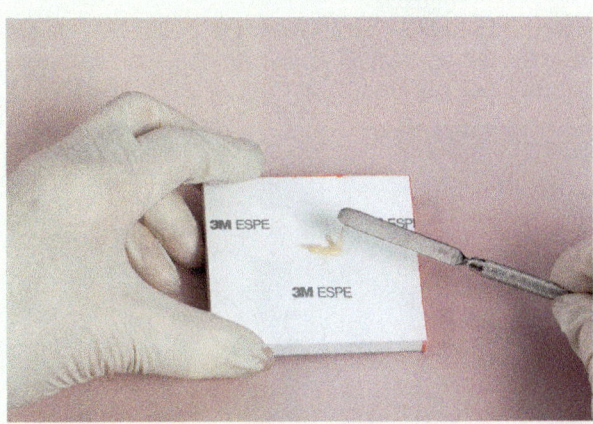

Figure P33-6-2

5. To clean up, tear off the top sheet of paper and fold it in half before throwing it away. This ensures no cement will spill off the paper. Clean any hardened cement off the spatula by wiping it with alcohol or orange solvent.

Etchants

Etching is a process that improves the bond between two objects. Dental professionals use **etchants** for strengthening the bond between restorations and the tooth's enamel and dentin. Etchants are acid-based, to roughen the surface of the tooth or restoration to which they are applied, making adhesion easier and stronger. Most etchants today contain about 30 to 40% phosphoric acid, while others may contain 10% maleic acid or other acids. Etchants come in both liquid and gel form. Many etchants are available on the market and they have different manufacturers' instructions; be sure to read all instructions before using.

CHECKPOINT
33-8 What is the purpose of using an etchant?

Procedure 33–7 Placing Procedure for Etchants

Some states allow qualified dental assistants to place etchants; in other states the dental assistant assists the dentist during this procedure. Check the regulations governing your state for more information about the specific duties dental assistants are allowed to perform.

Materials needed (Figure P33-7-1):

- Acid etchant solution with applicator or syringe or microbrush
- Cotton rolls
- Air-water syringe
- HVE or suction

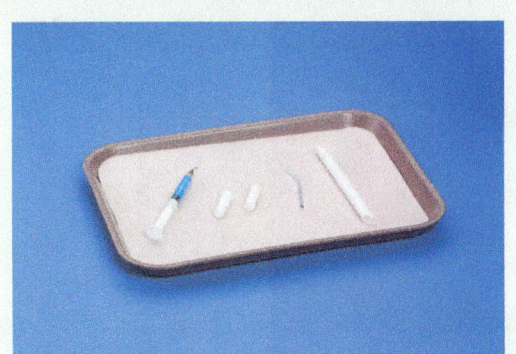

Figure P33-7-1

Procedure 33-7 Placing Procedure for Etchants (Continued)

1. Put on appropriate PPE.
2. Use a cotton roll(s) to isolate the etched tooth from other teeth and soft tissues.
3. Clean and dry the tooth's surface.
4. Prepare and pass the etchant to the dentist. The dentist applies the etchant according to the manufacturer's instructions using the applicator or syringe (Figure P33-7-2).

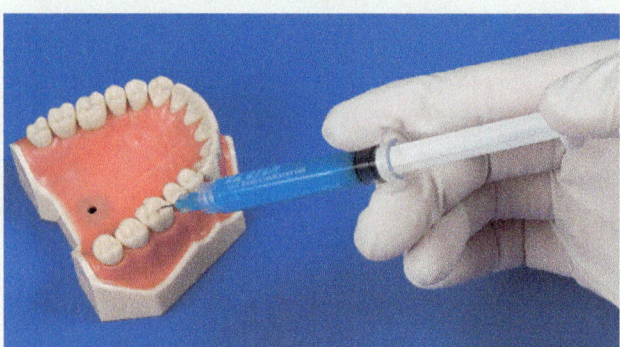

Figure P33-7-2

5. Use the air-water syringe to rinse and dry the etched tooth for 15 to 30 seconds.

6. The surface of the etched tooth should appear frosty white (Figure P33-7-3). If it does not appear this way, contamination has occurred and the process must be done again. Be sure not to allow any saliva or other liquid to touch the etched tooth. Keeping the surface of the tooth clean and dry is very important.

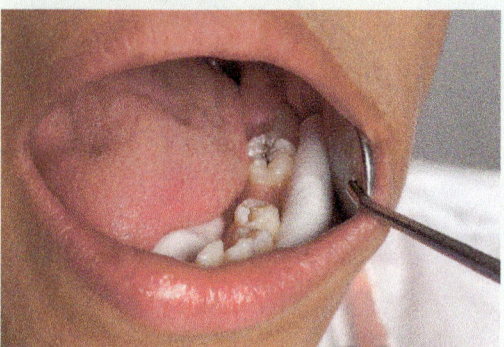

Figure P33-7-3

Cavity Liners

Cavity liners, also called dental liners, are used to seal the dentin and to protect the pulp of the tooth being restored. They include glass ionomer cement, described earlier, as well as calcium hydroxide. **Calcium hydroxide** is thin and low in strength, but it does provide some protection for the pulp and helps restore the health of the dentin. Calcium hydroxide can be used with all types of restorations and is especially helpful for deep cavities. Cavity liners come in two pastes called a base and a catalyst, as well as a single application as a light-cured system. Dycal is an example of a commonly used calcium hydroxide liner.

Procedure 33-8 Mixing Procedure for Cavity Liner (Calcium Hydroxide Catalyst and Base Pastes)

Materials needed (Figure P33-8-1):

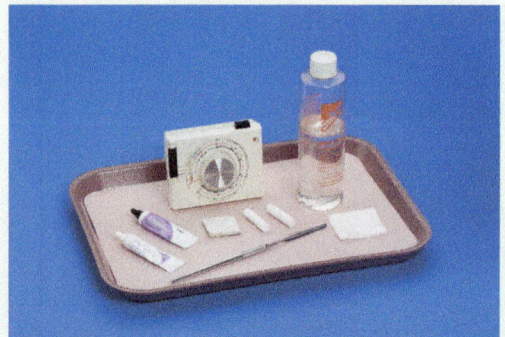

Figure P33-8-I

- Calcium hydroxide catalyst and base paste tubes
- Calcium hydroxide applicator
- Paper mixing pad
- Stainless steel spatula
- Cotton roll
- Timer
- Alcohol wipes

1. Put on appropriate PPE.
2. Gently dispense equal amounts of the catalyst and base onto opposite ends of the paper pad. Replace the caps to the tubes immediately and tightly.

Procedure 33-8 Mixing Procedure for Cavity Liner (Calcium Hydroxide Catalyst and Base Pastes) (Continued)

3. Using the spatula and following the manufacturer's instructions, mix the pastes together. Consulting a timer, continue mixing for 10 to 15 seconds (Figure P33-8-2).

4. To clean up, tear off the top sheet of paper and fold it in half before throwing it away. Clean any hardened material off the spatula with alcohol.

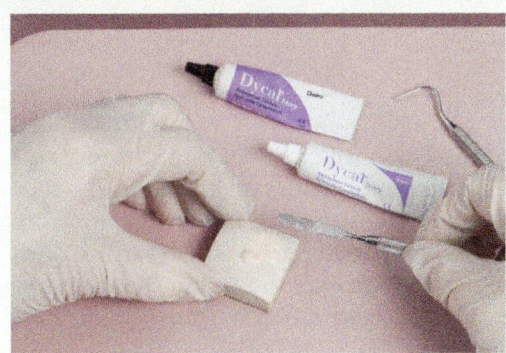

Figure P33-8-2

Procedure 33-9 Placing Procedure for Cavity Liner (Light-Cured Application)

Some states allow qualified dental assistants to place cavity liners; in other states the dental assistant assists the dentist during this procedure. Check the regulations governing your state for more information about the specific duties dental assistants are allowed to perform.

Materials needed (Figure P33-9-1):

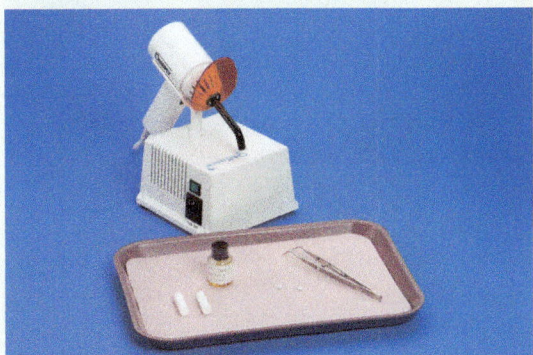

Figure P33-9-1

- Cavity liner light-cured system
- Curing light
- Liner applicator
- Cotton rolls

1. Put on appropriate PPE.

2. Transfer the explorer and mirror. The dentist uses the dental explorer and mirror to examine the cavity and determine where the liner will be placed.

3. Use a cotton roll(s) to isolate the treated tooth from the other teeth and soft tissues.

4. Transfer the cavity liner to the dentist. Light-cured liners typically do not have to be mixed.

5. Using the applicator, the dentist applies the liner directly to the preparation area, beginning with the deepest part of the preparation area and applying the liner in a thin layer (Figure P33-9-2).

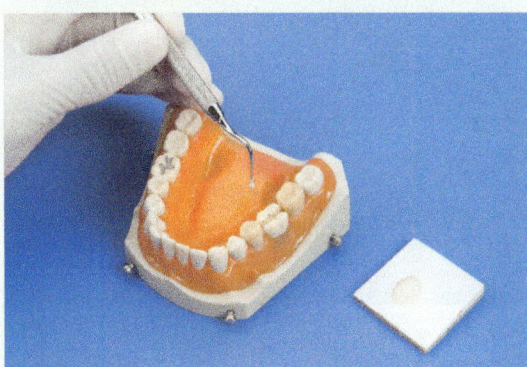

Figure P33-9-2

6. The dentist holds the curing light over the area for 10 to 20 seconds to harden the liner.

7. Transfer the mirror and explorer to the dentist for examination of the placement of the material. After the liner has cured, the dentist examines it to make sure it covers the deepest portion of the cavity preparation. If it does not, the dentist applies a second layer, making sure to reach the deepest areas.

8. Clean up supplies and equipment.

Cavity Varnishes

Cavity varnishes (also called dental varnishes) are sealants that are placed on top of the cavity liner and underneath the restoration. Cavity varnishes are liquid resins that contain ether or chloroform. When the varnish dries, it creates a protective seal over the dentin and pulp that helps reduce microleakage. Cavity varnishes cannot be used under composite restorations because the varnish may interfere with the composite polymerization.

One specific type of varnish is fluoride varnish. Fluoride varnishes release fluoride into the dentin and enamel of the tooth, helping to strengthen it. They are also used on children to provide ongoing protection after a cavity has been treated. Some dentists do not use cavity varnishes because they feel that, because they are so thin, they break down too easily. Others, however, argue that cavity varnishes are very useful.

Procedure 33-10 Placing Procedure for Cavity Varnishes

Some states allow qualified dental assistants to place cavity liners; in other states the dental assistant assists the dentist during this procedure. Check the regulations governing your state for more information about the specific duties dental assistants are allowed to perform.

Materials needed (Figure P33-10-1):

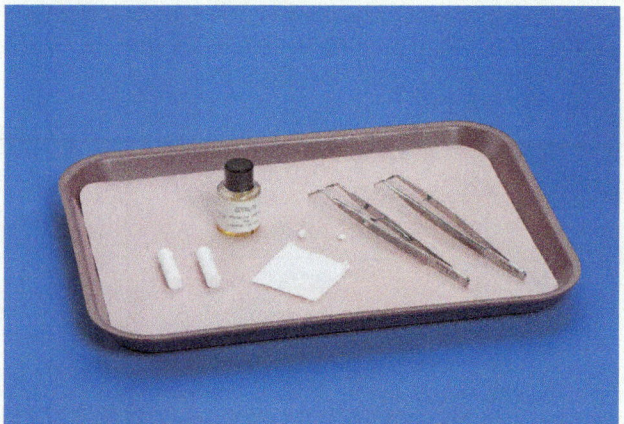

Figure P33-10-1

- Dental varnish and solvent
- Two college pliers
- Cotton pellets and roll or microbrush
- Cleaning supplies

1. Put on appropriate PPE.
2. Transfer the dental explorer and mirror to the dentist. The dentist uses the dental explorer and mirror to examine the cavity and determine where the varnish will be placed.
3. Use the cotton roll to isolate the treated tooth from the other teeth.
4. Open the bottle of varnish.

5. Holding the cotton pellet with one of the pliers—not the fingers—dip the pellet into the varnish. Replace the cap to the varnish immediately and tightly. If the cap is not replaced tightly, the liquid in the varnish can evaporate, causing it to become too sticky for use.
6. Transfer the pliers and cotton pellet to the dentist.
7. The dentist applies a thin layer of varnish to the walls and margins of the cavity preparation (Figure P33-10-2).

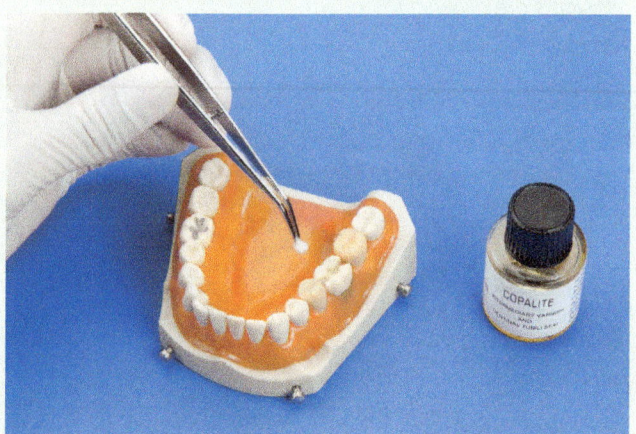

Figure P33-10-2

8. When first layer is dry, repeat the process of dipping the pellet into the varnish, using the second set of pliers and a new cotton pellet. (Make sure to use the second set of pliers and a new cotton pellet to avoid any contamination from the first application.) Replace the cap to the varnish immediately and tightly.
9. Transfer the pliers and cotton pellet to the dentist.
10. The dentist applies a second layer of varnish.
11. Throw away the cotton pellets and clean the pliers with solvent before sterilizing.

Cement Bases

Like cavity liners and cavity varnishes, **cement bases** are placed under the restoration to protect the pulp. There are three types of cement bases, grouped according to the way in which they affect the pulp:

- *Protective* bases are used to shield the pulp prior to placing the restoration.
- *Sedative* bases are used to treat pulp that has been damaged by dental caries or infection.
- *Insulating* bases protect the pulp from sudden changes in temperature that naturally occur within a tooth.

Many of the cements described earlier serve one or more of these functions. For instance, ZOE is insulating and protective, but because of its soothing oil, it is also a sedative base. Zinc phosphate is used as an insulating base because it heats up at the same rate as the dentin, allowing it to keep the pulp from becoming too hot or too cool. Polycarboxylate can be used both as a protective base and as an insulating base.

CHECKPOINT

33-11 What are the three groups of cement bases?

Procedure 33-11 Mixing and Placing Procedure for Cement Base

Some states allow qualified dental assistants to place cement bases; in other states the dental assistant assists the dentist during this procedure. Check the regulations governing your state for more information about the specific duties dental assistants are allowed to perform.

Materials needed (Figure P33-11-1):

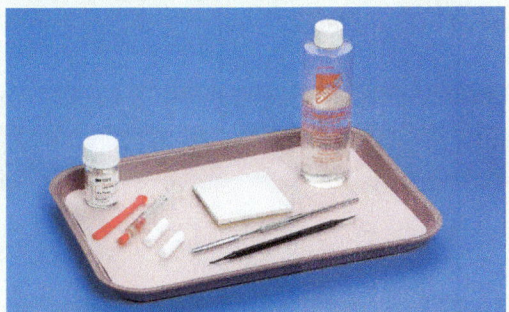

Figure P33-11-1

- Cement base materials (powder and liquid) (ZOP, ZOE, or polycarboxylate)
- Paper mixing pad
- Stainless steel spatula
- Plastic filling instrument
- Timer
- Cleaning supplies

1. Put on appropriate PPE.
2. Transfer the dental explorer and mirror so the operator can examine the prepared tooth and determine where the base will be placed.
3. Gently mix the cement materials on the paper pad, as described in the manufacturer's instructions. Replace the caps to the cement containers immediately and tightly.
4. The cement should be the consistency of putty. Using the spatula, divide the cement into two halves and roll each half into a ball.
5. Use the plastic filling instrument to pick up one of the balls of cement (Figure P33-11-2). If the base material sticks to the instrument, you can dip the end of the instrument in

some extra powder before picking up the base and placing it in the preparation (like placing flour on a rolling pin before rolling out dough).

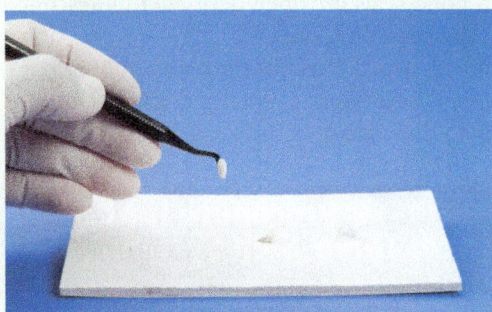

Figure P33-11-2

6. Transfer the plastic filling instrument to the operator.
7. The operator covers the entire floor of the preparation area with the cement but leaves enough room for the restoration to be placed (Figure P33-11-3). If needed, both halves of the cement can be used. The base should be approximately 1 mm thick.

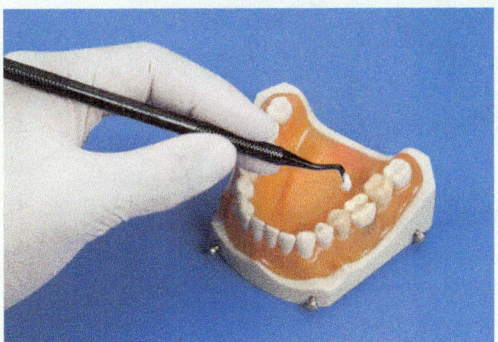

Figure P33-11-3

8. To clean up, tear off the top sheet from the paper pad and fold it in half before throwing it away. This ensures no cement will spill off the paper. Clean any cement off the spatula by wiping it clean with a wet gauze pad before the cement hardens. Hardened cement can be removed with alcohol. Afterward, prepare the spatula for sterilization.

Bonding Agents

Dental bonding is important for ensuring that restoration materials adhere strongly and correctly. Bonding is used for all types of restorations, including crowns, bridges, inlays, and onlays. The two types of bonding are dentin bonding and enamel bonding.

Bonding to the dentin first requires removal of the smear layer, which is a thin film of fluids and particles that forms over the dentin when a cavity is prepared. During cavity preparation, thousands of tiny dentinal tubules are cut, leaving numerous openings that allow bacteria and moisture to leak into the pulp. This can damage the pulp and cause pain, although some moisture must remain in order to keep the pulp from drying out. The smear layer provides a shield that keeps moisture in and keeps bacteria and other particles out. The smear layer is commonly called "nature's Band-Aid." During dentin bonding, an etchant is used to remove the protective smear layer, and the dentin bond seals the open dentinal tubules, once again keeping the pulp protected.

Enamel bonding, which is used for placement of bridges, resin veneers, and orthodontic brackets, uses agents to adhere directly to the enamel of the tooth. Prior to placing an enamel bonding agent, etchants are used to create a rough surface. This allows for greater adhesion and retention of the restorative material to the enamel.

Bonding agents can be self-curing, light-cured, or dual-curing. Some are premixed in applicators while others require mixing together two liquids.

Although a variety of bonding systems are available, each system typically includes three basic processes: etching, priming, and bonding. The systems differ in the techniques used to achieve these results. Some systems use separate steps for each process; others combine two or more processes in a single application. Three types of bonding systems are commonly available:

- One-step system (also called a "self-etching" system or "all-in-one" system): This method combines etching, priming, and bonding in a single step.
- Two-step system: These systems combine in one step the etching and priming process or the priming and bonding processes.
- Three-step system: This method uses a separate application for each step in the process.

Because the methods can differ significantly, be sure to read all the manufacturer's instructions before preparing a bonding agent.

Procedure 33–12 Procedure for Preparing and Applying Bonding Agent (Light-Cured, Three-Step System)

Materials needed (Figure P33-12-1):

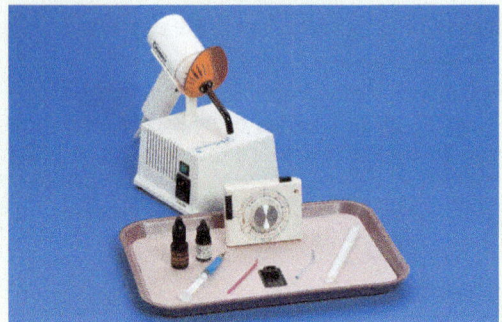

Figure P33-12-1

- Bonding agent
- Etchant
- Primer (if both enamel and dentin are involved)
- Bonding agent applicator
- Air-water syringe
- Curing light
- Timer

1. Put on appropriate PPE.
2. Transfer the dental explorer and mirror so the dentist can examine the cavity and determine where the bonding agent will be placed.

3. Prepare and pass the etchant. The dentist applies the etchant according to the manufacturer's instructions.
4. Use the air-water syringe to rinse and dry the etched tooth for 15 to 30 seconds. Be sure the tooth is dry and has a frosty white appearance.
5. If the restoration involves the enamel and the dentin, the dentist applies a primer.
6. The dentist applies the bonding agent according to the manufacturer's instructions (Figure P33-12-2).

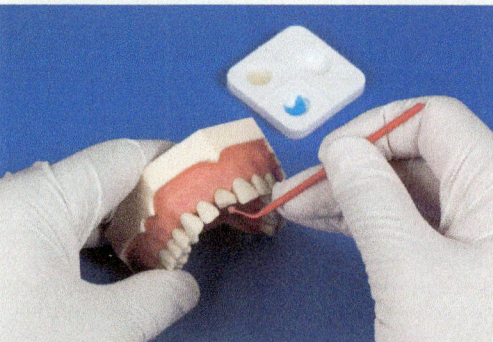

Figure P33-12-2

7. After the bonding agent is applied, the curing light is placed over the preparation area to harden the bond.
8. To clean up, dispose of the bonding applicator tip.

✔ **CHECKPOINT**

33-12 What type of bonding is used for placement of bridges?

✔ **CHECKPOINT**

33-13 What instrument is typically used to remove excess cement?

Cement Removal

After a restoration is cemented and placed in the mouth, the patient will bite down on a cotton roll to make sure the restoration is securely set. At this time, some extra cement typically leaks out from under the edge of the restoration and onto the tooth and gingiva. This cement must be removed or else it can cause irritation and pain. The dental explorer is used to remove the excess cement from the edge of the tooth, and dental floss can be used to remove cement from between teeth.

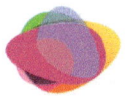

From the Dentist's Perspective

The field of dentistry is always growing, and what we know about dental materials seems to change each year. I appreciate working with a dental assistant who reads the dental journals and stays on top of the latest research. Attending courses and lectures is part of keeping up with the field. This helps our office offer the latest and most effective services to our patients. Not only does this make the dental assistant a valuable addition to my practice, it also makes him or her worthy of raises!

Chapter Highlights

- Understanding the properties of dental material includes understanding which material should be used in a restoration and which features can impact whether it works correctly.
- Dental cements serve many purposes, including acting as a luting agent, a restoration, and a base or liner.
- Dental cements are made by hand-mixing powder and liquid. Several factors can impact whether the cement is mixed properly, including the mixing time, temperature of the environment, and the amount of powder and liquid used.
- When mixing cement, always read the full manufacturer's instructions first. Follow all instructions and never mix different brands of powder and liquid.
- Types of dental cement include zinc oxide eugenol, zinc phosphate, polycarboxylate, glass ionomer, and composite resin.
- Zinc eugenol comes in two types and is used for both temporary and permanent cementing. It has low acidity and contains an oil that can soothe against irritation.
- Zinc phosphate comes in two types. It can be used for permanent cementing and as a base. Because it contains acid that can irritate the pulp, a subbase must be applied underneath it. Because zinc phosphate contains chemicals that release heat when mixed, it must be spread over a wide area of the mixing slab so it can cool prior to placement.
- Polycarboxylate is used for permanent cementing and as a base. It does not irritate the pulp, but it becomes more acidic and thickens as it sets.

- The most commonly used cement is glass ionomer cement, which comes in three types and is used for a variety of functions. Glass ionomer does not irritate the pulp, is high in strength, and helps release fluoride to fight dental caries.
- Composite resin cements can be used for cementing ceramic or resin inlays and onlays, ceramic veneers, orthodontic bands and brackets, and metal castings. This material can only be used on clean, dry teeth. An etchant and bonding system must be applied before placing composite resin cements.
- Dental etchants are acid-based materials that roughen the surface of a tooth or restoration, making adhesion easier and stronger.
- Cavity liners seal and protect the dentin and pulp prior to restoration. Glass ionomer cement and calcium hydroxide are two common cavity liners.
- Cavity varnishes, also known as dental varnishes, seal and protect the cavity liner.
- Cement bases are placed underneath restorations to protect the pulp, sedate pulp that has been damaged, and insulate the pulp from temperature changes.
- Bonding agents ensure that restorations are strongly and properly adhered to the tooth. They can be applied to the dentin of the tooth or to the enamel. Before a bonding agent is placed, an etchant must be used to roughen the surface of the tooth or restoration.

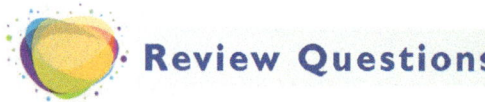

Review Questions

1. The degree to which a dental material can withstand stress is known as

   a. Resistance.

   b. Strain.

   c. Elasticity.

   d. Ductility.

2. Dental material that is high in solubility is

   a. More likely to break apart in water.

   b. Less likely to break apart in water.

   c. More easily spreadable when wet.

   d. Made up of a higher water content.

3. When mixing dental cement

   a. Always use a glass mixing slab.

   b. Make sure the mixing slab is dry and clean.

   c. Use the dispenser to drop the liquid into the powder.

   d. Read the directions as you mix the cement.

4. Which of the following provides the strongest protection of the pulp as a base?

   a. Calcium hydroxide

   b. Type I zinc oxide eugenol

   c. Polycarboxylate

   d. Zinc phosphate

5. Which of the following types of dental cement should have a thick, clay-like consistency?

   a. Type I zinc oxide eugenol

   b. Type II zinc oxide eugenol

   c. Type I zinc phosphate

   d. Calcium hydroxide

6. Which two types of dental cement can irritate the pulp of the tooth?

   a. Zinc phosphate and polycarboxylate

   b. Zinc phosphate and zinc oxide eugenol

   c. Zinc phosphate and composite resin

   d. Polycarboxylate and composite resin

7. Before placement of zinc phosphate, its exothermic reaction must be reduced by

   a. Adding water to the cement

   b. Letting the mixed cement sit for 24 hours

   c. Spreading the cement over a wide area of the mixing slab

   d. Placing the slab in the freezer prior to mixing

8. Because of its high acidity, a protective base must be applied before placing which cement?

   a. Phosphoric acid etchant

   b. Zinc oxide eugenol

   c. Glass ionomer

   d. Zinc phosphate

9. What is an added benefit (or benefits) of glass ionomer cement?

   a. It helps fight dental caries.

   b. It is stronger than zinc phosphate but does not irritate the pulp.

   c. Neither A nor B.

   d. Both A and B.

10. How is placement of composite resin different from placement of other dental cements?

    a. Composite resin must be spread across a wide area of the mixing slab to reduce its heat.

    b. Composite resin must be placed on top of another cement base due to its high acidity.

    c. Composite resin must be preceded by placement of an etchant and bonding agent.

    d. Composite resin must be placed on a glass slab that is 68°F in temperature.

11. Which types of cement can be used as cavity liners?

    a. Glass ionomer and calcium hydroxide

    b. Zinc oxide eugenol and calcium hydroxide

    c. Composite resin and glass ionomer

    d. Glass ionomer and polycarboxylate

12. Which cement base has insulating, protective, and sedative properties?

    a. Polycarboxylate

    b. Zinc phosphate

    c. Zinc oxide eugenol

    d. Glass ionomer

Active Learning Exercises

1. Name seven unique characteristics that make dental materials especially useful in dentistry. What precautions should be taken when using a glass slab to mix certain materials? How might this affect the material?

2. How does using a liner and a varnish during restorative procedures help protect the tooth pulp? What role does each material play in the protection of the tooth?

3. Why is fluoride becoming increasingly used in dental materials? Name at least two types of materials in which fluoride is found.

Application Activities

1. Fold a piece of paper in half. In one column, list the common characteristics of dental materials discussed in this chapter. In the other column, for each characteristic, provide an example of a type of dental material that demonstrates a high or low level of that feature.

2. Imagine you are in the office mixing cement. You quickly realize that your mixture is too wet. Write a paragraph describing what you would do. Should you keep adding more powder? Should you ask someone for help? Should you start over? Would you tell your supervisor about your mistake? Why or why not? Consider what problems may occur if you make a mistake in mixing cement and do not correct that mistake before the material is placed in the patient's mouth.

PREPARING FOR CERTIFICATION EXAMS

Review the following topics in this chapter to prepare for the Dental Assisting National Board (DANB) exam:

- **Introduction**
- **Dental Cements**
- **Mixing Techniques**
- **Glass Ionomer**
- **Etchants**
- **Cavity Liners**
- **Cavity Varnishes**
- **Cement Bases**
- **Bonding Agents**
- **Cement Removal**

Dental Materials

CHAPTER OUTLINE

CHAPTER CHECKLIST

On completion of this chapter, students will be able to:

- ☑ Identify the four classes of amalgam.
- ☑ Describe the properties, uses, preparation, and placement of amalgam.
- ☑ List some guidelines for safely working with mercury.
- ☑ Describe the main types of composite materials, including their properties, uses, preparation, and placement.
- ☑ Describe the characteristics and uses of glass ionomers and compomers.
- ☑ Describe the main types of temporary materials, including their properties, uses, preparation, and placement.
- ☑ Understand the role of the dental assistant in procedures involving common restorative materials.

KEY TERMS

alloy (AL-oi) – a combination of two or more metals

amalgam (uh-MAL-gum) – a restorative dental material composed of an alloy mixed with mercury, primarily of two types: silver-tin alloy, containing small amounts of copper, zinc, and perhaps other metal, and a second type containing more copper by weight; amalgams are used in restoring teeth and making dies

amalgamator (uh-MAL-guh-may-tur) – a device for combining mercury with a metal or an alloy to form a new alloy; also used for some newer dental materials that come prepared in a premeasured capsule

bonding agent – a material used to obtain a strong seal between the tooth surface and a restoration material

intermediate restorative material (IRM) – reinforced zinc oxide eugenol; a dental material used to create provisional restorations, as well as liners, bases, and cements, and to create impressions; IRM restorations can only last for about a year in the oral cavity

pestle (PES-ul) – rodlike instrument with one rounded and weighted extremity, used for mixing substances; in restorative dentistry, pestles are included within amalgam capsules to combine alloy and mercury during amalgamation

polymerization (pol-ih-mer-uh-ZAY-shun) – a process by which composite material hardens

trituration (trit-you-RAY-shun) – mixing dental amalgam with a mortar and pestle or with a mechanical device

triturator (trit-you-RATE-ur) – a device used to triturate; another term for an amalgamator

Introduction

Dental materials are central to modern dentistry. Dental amalgam has been used for decades for restorations in posterior teeth, and recently, newer materials have been developed that more closely mimic the look of a natural tooth and address lingering safety concerns associated with amalgam. These new materials include composites and glass ionomers.

Dental assistants have a critical role in restoration processes. Although the functions they are authorized to perform vary from state to state, all dental assistants should remain current on dental restoration materials and procedures.

This chapter discusses direct restoration materials, or materials that are placed and formed in the patient's tooth cavity. Indirect restorations, or those that are shaped outside of the patient's mouth, are discussed in the next chapter.

Amalgam

Dental **amalgam** is one of the oldest and most common materials used in restorations. It is inexpensive and easy to work with. Originally, amalgam was made by combining powdered silver with mercury to form a workable metal compound. This compound was placed into the tooth cavity before it hardened, then carved to fit the existing tooth anatomy. After hardening in place, the amalgam becomes a permanent part of the tooth.

Today, amalgam fillings are not made entirely from silver but are composed of an **alloy** of copper, zinc, and tin. The underlying process, however, is still the same: powdered metals are mixed with liquid mercury into a paste and used to restore tooth structure. In recent years, extensive public safety concerns have arisen about the use of mercury in dentistry, and dental assistants should be fully informed about the safety profile of mercury, as well as trained in using it. Guidelines for safely using mercury are discussed in a later section.

Indications and Contraindications for Amalgam

Amalgam is often used in posterior restorations because of its strength and long-term impact resistance. It is indicated in the following situations:

- Primary and permanent teeth
- Posterior teeth
- Severe tooth destruction
- Poor moisture control
- Poor patient oral hygiene
- As a foundation for cast restorations
- When an economical restoration is needed

Amalgam, however, should not be used in restorations in anterior teeth that are visible or when a large restoration is needed and cost is not a factor.

Classes of Amalgam

Amalgam is classified several ways, depending on which types of metal alloy are used with the mercury, the alloy's particle shape, and in what proportions (Table 34-1). The following metals are used in various combinations:

- *Silver.* The main constituent of amalgam, silver provides strength, increases expansion of the alloy, and hardens quickly.
- *Tin.* Tin helps the mercury blend with the component metals.
- *Copper.* Copper increases the strength of the amalgam and resists corrosion. Amalgam is classed by how much copper it contains: *high-copper amalgam* and *low-copper amalgam*. These differ not only in the proportion of copper, but also in the shape of the copper particles in the alloy: spherical (round) or irregular (lathe-cut). High-copper alloys are valuable because they are easier to work with and fit to the tooth cavity. Low-copper alloys contain only lathe-cut particles, while high-copper amalgam can contain lathe-cut, spherical, or mixed particles.
- *Zinc.* Very small amounts of zinc are sometimes used in amalgam to reduce oxidation or discoloration of the restoration.

The proportion of the various alloys changes the properties of the resulting amalgam. Amalgam (like all restoration materials) is evaluated on the following properties:

- *Contraction and expansion.* Amalgam can contract or expand in the tooth depending on temperature changes. This might occur, for example, when a person eats ice cream while sipping hot chocolate. The temperature extremes can cause the dental material to pull away from the tooth, creating a tiny fissure. This can result in microleakage or faulty restorations. Microleakage can increase the patient's risk for sensitivity and recurring decay.

TABLE 34-1 Amalgam Properties		
METAL	**PROPORTION**	**CLASSIFICATION**
Silver	52–70%	High copper
	68–72%	Low copper
Tin	15–30%	High copper
	21–37%	Low copper
Copper	11–29%	High copper
	2–9%	Low copper
Zinc	0–1%	High and low copper

- *Tarnish and corrosion*. Metal products that come into contact with oxygen can oxidize, or become tarnished and corroded. Amalgam is designed so that proper polishing can reduce tarnishing.
- *Flow and creep*. Dental restoration materials must be supple enough to work with during the restoration procedure, but then solid enough to remain in place for the long term. Amalgam creeps, or moves, very slightly in the restoration over time due to the occlusal stress placed on it.
- *Adhesion*. The restorative material must form a permanent, tight bond with the healthy tooth material during the restoration. Adhesives are often used during restorations to improve adhesion between the tooth and the restoration material. Using an adhesive also lowers the risk of microleakage.

Mercury-to-Alloy Ratio

In addition to the right proportion of various alloys, the ratio between mercury and alloy is very important. Amalgam is usually mixed with a 1:1 ratio of mercury and alloy. This is known as the *Eames technique*.

In modern dentistry, however, amalgam typically comes prepacked in capsules. Dental assistants do not usually have to measure mercury and alloy in proportion.

Preparing Amalgam

The type of amalgam chosen depends on the situation and the type of restoration. For safety reasons, amalgam is delivered to dental offices in capsules (Figure 34-1). Each capsule is sealed and designed for a single use. Inside the capsule, the metal alloy is separated from the liquid mercury by a thin membrane. Capsules also contain a tiny **pestle,** which is used during mixing to achieve the desired consistency.

Amalgam capsules are available in three sizes; the term *spill* is often used to indicate the amount of amalgam in each capsule:

- 400 mg (single spill). These are designed for small or single-surface restorations.
- 600 mg (double spill). These are designed for medium-size restorations.
- 800 mg (triple spill). These are designed for large restorations.

Multiple capsules might be required during a restoration procedure, depending on the size of the restoration.

To prepare amalgam, the mercury and alloy have to be thoroughly mixed. This process is called **trituration**, or amalgamation. This is accomplished with a special machine known as an **amalgamator** or **triturator** (Figure 34-2).

These machines somewhat resemble the paint mixers used in hardware stores. They are designed to vibrate the capsule for the appropriate time and at the appropriate speed to thoroughly mix the mercury and alloy and create usable amalgam. Carefully follow the manufacturer's instructions for the specific kind of amalgam you are using. If the mixing time of the amalgam is too short, it may be difficult to remove from the capsule and have a soupy texture. If it is mixed too long, it may harden.

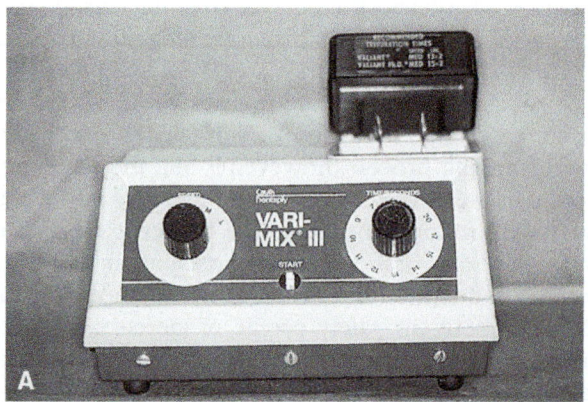
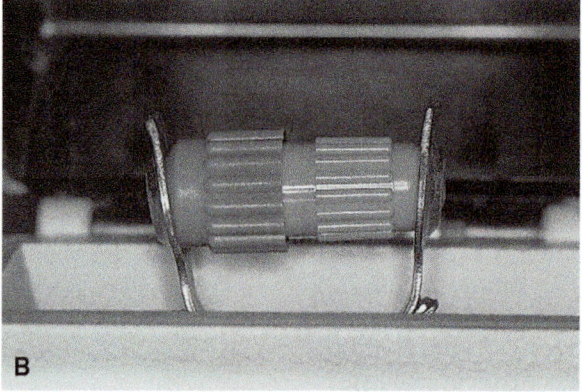

Figure 34–2 Amalgamation. (A) Amalgamator. **(B)** Amalgam capsule in place ready to be triturated.

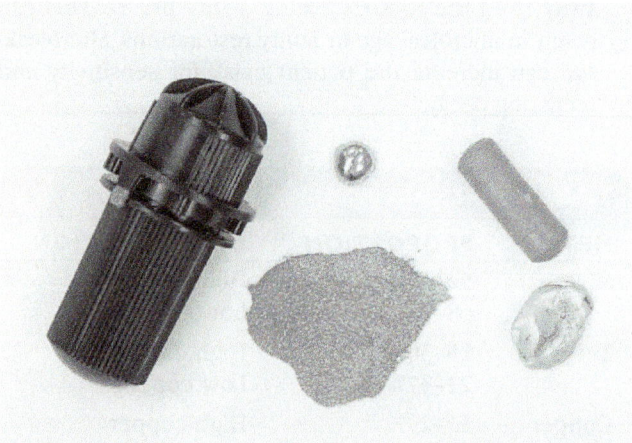

Figure 34–1 Dental amalgam. Starting at the left and moving clockwise: capsule, liquid mercury, pestle, freshly mixed amalgam, and powdered amalgam alloy.

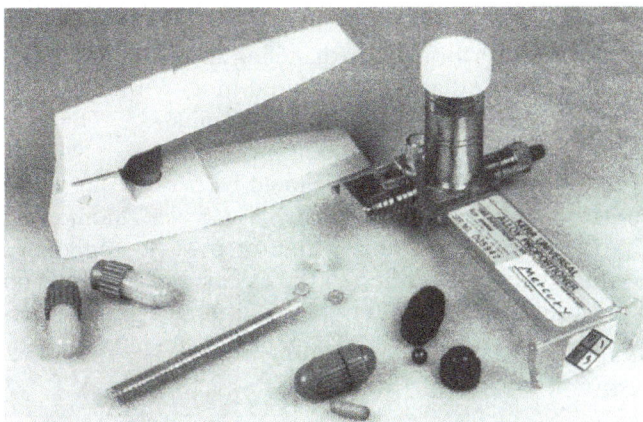

Figure 34–3 **Activator**. Activator is shown at the top left. Other materials shown include amalgam capsules with pestles, individual alloy pellets, and mercury dispenser.

Before using the amalgamator, however, the capsule must first be placed into an activator (Figure 34-3). This is a simple device that is used to break the membrane inside the capsule, allowing for the mixture of mercury and alloy. Activators are designed to protect and contain the capsule to prevent the escape of any mercury vapor. Not all capsules need activators; check the manufacturer's instructions. Many companies now make self-activating capsules.

Using Amalgam

After it emerges from the amalgamator, the finished capsule is opened, the pestle is removed, and the amalgam is ready to be loaded into the amalgam carrier (Figure 34-4). Properly mixed amalgam should be pliable and workable. Some states allow dental assistants to load amalgam into the carrier, while others do not. In either case, it is still important to understand the steps that are involved between amalgamation and condensing.

Which end of the amalgam carrier should be loaded first depends somewhat on the dentist's preference. Amalgam carriers have a small and a large end. Some dentists prefer the small end to be filled first, allowing them to condense small amounts of amalgam into the crevices of the cavity before filling the bulk of the cavity.

The following steps are involved with filling the cavity:

■ *Condensing*. The process of transferring amalgam from the amalgam carrier into the cavity is called condensing. Dentists use hand instruments, such as a condenser or a plugger, to condense the amalgam into the cavity preparation. During condensing, it is vital that the amalgam is securely packed into the small crevices and cracks in the cavity. For this reason, some dentists prefer using small amounts of amalgam at first, followed by larger quantities. In many states, an expanded functions dental assistant can place and condense amalgam. Refer to your state's dental practice act to determine if qualified dental assistants are allowed to perform these procedures.

■ *Carving and finishing*. This process involves carving back amalgam to fit the natural contours of the patient's tooth. This is accomplished with the use of hand-carving instruments and burnishers. In some states, expanded functions dental assistants can perform carving of a final restoration, both amalgams and composites.

In some cases, a **bonding agent** might be used before condensing begins. Bonding agents are special compounds that increase the adhesion between the amalgam and the tooth. Bonding agents typically are made from resin. Their use is covered in greater depth in Chapter 33, Dental Cements, Liners, Bases, and Bonding Agents.

Using Mercury Safely

Mercury is regulated as a hazardous material, and its use in dentistry is carefully monitored. In some countries, the

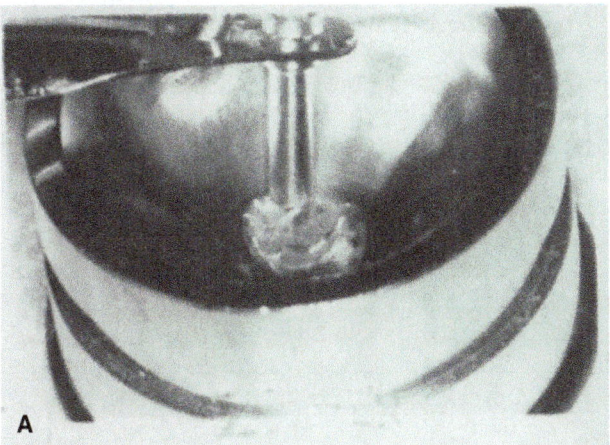

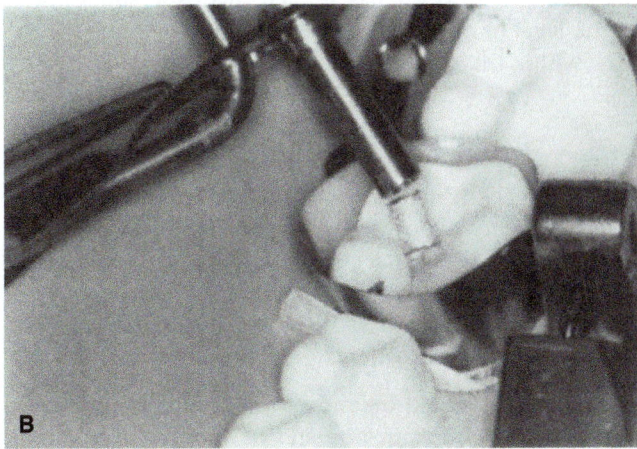

Figure 34–4 **Using amalgam**. (**A**) An amalgam carrier being forced into an amalgam mass in an amalgam well. (**B**) Amalgam being dispensed into the prepared area.

use of amalgam in minors may be prohibited, while in other countries, amalgam is banned entirely because of its mercury content. In response to these concerns, a number of dental offices in the United States have opted not to use mercury and are amalgam-free.

It is important to note, however, that the American Dental Association does not consider mercury to be dangerous in the dental office when properly used and disposed of. Nevertheless, because dental personnel are at risk for exposure to mercury, it is imperative to practice mercury hygiene perfectly.

Sources of Mercury Contamination

Mercury is a unique metal because it is liquid at room temperature, and it has a very low vaporization point. Mercury vapors are easily absorbed through the skin and mucus membranes and can contribute to a number of diseases and cause birth defects in children. Mercury may also contaminate groundwater supplies. Mercury exposure is cumulative: it is stored in the fat tissues in the body for a very long time, so mercury exposure builds up over time until toxic levels are reached.

In the dental office, mercury exposure can occur through a number of avenues:

- Vapors escaped from capsules during amalgamation
- Vapors released during burnishing and polishing
- Vapors released during transfer of amalgam
- Vapors released from storage of open capsules
- Direct physical contact with amalgam
- Small particles of amalgam that collect on surfaces in the treatment room, especially carpets, and then are sent airborne during cleaning
- Amalgam scraps

Some patients might also express a concern about mercury outgassing. This is the tendency of amalgam restorations to release very small levels of mercury over a long period of time in the patient's mouth. The American Dental Association, however, has studied this issue and found that the level of mercury exposure created by outgassing is well within the safe limits.

Mercury Hygiene

All dental offices need to practice comprehensive mercury hygiene. Mercury exposure risk is actually higher among dental personnel—who regularly work with mercury—than among the patients who receive restorations. The following guidelines are designed to protect dental professionals as well as their patients.

1. Dental staff should be aware of all potential sources of mercury contamination and be thoroughly versed in local and Environmental Protection Agency (EPA) regulations for mercury handling and disposal.
2. Proper ventilation is required in all working areas, and air conditioning filters should be changed regularly.
3. The office environment should be periodically monitored for atmospheric mercury levels. Monitoring is also necessary after a spill or possible contamination event. According to the Occupational Safety and Health Administration (OSHA), the currently acceptable mercury limit is 50 mg/cubic meter in any 8-hour work shift over a 40-hour week.
4. Floors in working areas should be easy to clean and nonabsorbent. Carpet is not recommended in dental offices as it absorbs mercury that can be released during vacuuming.
5. Bulk mercury should not be used; all dental offices should switch to precapsulated amalgam.
6. Amalgamators should be equipped with a protective cover so that the capsule is completely covered during amalgamation. This helps prevent mercury vapors from escaping faulty capsules.
7. Avoid any direct contact with mercury or freshly mixed amalgam. If contact occurs, wash the affected skin with soap and water and rinse under running water.
8. Re-cap capsules after amalgamation and dispose of them according to local ordinances.
9. Store mercury and amalgam scraps according to local and EPA regulations The material should be stored in a designated and clearly labeled container. Use only qualified mercury disposal companies to recycle old amalgam.
10. Use a high-volume evacuator and water spray when cutting old amalgam or polishing a new restoration. Masks should be worn.
11. Immediately clean up spilled mercury with trap bottles, tape, or fresh amalgam. Commercial clean-up kits are available and may be part of the standard safety equipment. Do not vacuum spilled mercury.
12. Wear appropriate PPE, such as gloves, a mask, and protective eyewear, when working with mercury, and remove these items before leaving the office.

CHECKPOINTS

34-1 What are the main components of amalgam?

34-2 What are the two main types of amalgam? How do they differ?

34-3 Describe an amalgam capsule, including its internal components.

34-4 In what forms is mercury dangerous?

Procedure 34–1 Mixing and Transferring Amalgam

Materials needed (Figure P34-1-1):

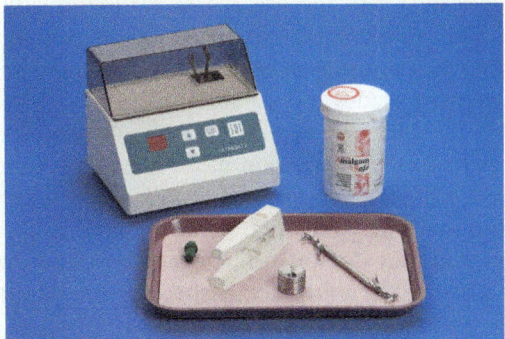

Figure P34-1-1

- Amalgam capsule
- Capsule activator
- Amalgamator
- Amalgam well
- Amalgam carrier
- Amalgam condenser
- Scrap amalgam container

1. Put on appropriate PPE.
2. Set the amalgamator for the proper time and speed as directed by the amalgam manufacturer.
3. Activate the capsule with the activator. This requires crushing or twisting the capsule to pierce the internal membrane and allow the alloy and mercury to mix. Remember, not all capsules need to be activated before use; check the manufacturer's instructions.
4. Put the capsule into the amalgamator (Figure P34-1-2).

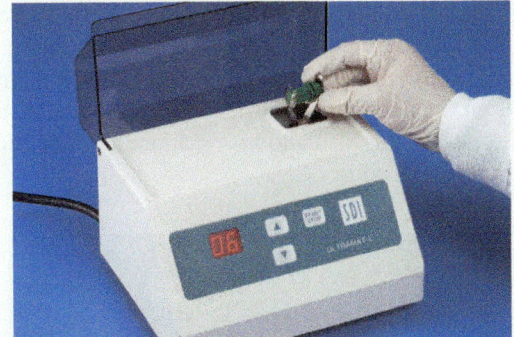

Figure P34-1-2

5. Close the cover and activate the amalgamator. Continue to hold the cover closed throughout the entire activation.
6. Remove the capsule after the amalgamator is done.
7. Twist open the capsule and empty the freshly mixed amalgam into the amalgam well. Do not touch freshly mixed amalgam (Figure P34-1-3).

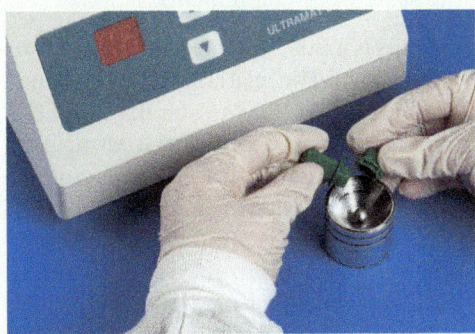

Figure P34-1-3

8. Reassemble the capsule and set it aside for proper disposal later.
9. Load the amalgam into the carrier. Some dentists prefer the small side to be filled first; others prefer the large side to be filled first.
10. Transfer the carrier to the dentist and get ready to transfer a condenser next.
11. Repeat the process of loading and transfer until the amalgam is condensed and the restoration is filled to the dentist's satisfaction. As the amalgam begins to harden, it will be more difficult to load into the carrier.
12. Clean up the work area and dispose of the used capsule.
13. Store any unused or scrap amalgam in a sealed container. (Scrap amalgam containers are available from dental supply companies.)

Composite Materials

Composite resins are becoming a material of choice for dental restorations. These materials are naturally colored and do not have the mercury concerns associated with amalgam. At one time, composites were used only for anterior applications, but new materials and technologies have created composites that can be safely used in posterior applications as well.

As research continues into composites, glass ionomers, resins, and porcelain materials, they will likely continue to displace amalgam as the dental material of choice. Current composites are designed to last for long periods of time in the oral cavity, withstand occlusal pressure, and be worked to fit the existing tooth anatomy. Composites are usually self-curing or cured with special lights, or a combination of both. Unlike amalgam, they do not need to be amalgamated but often come in syringes or single-use applicators. In some cases, composites are radiopaque, which makes it possible to identify them on dental radiographs.

Properties of Composites

Although there are a number of composites on the market, they all include the same basic components:

- *Organic matrix*. This is a fluid-like substance that forms the basis of composites. The material used in dental composites is called *dimethacrylate*, or BIS-GMA. BIS-GMA, however, is not strong enough by itself to form a long-lasting dental restoration, so it must be complemented with fillers and coupling agents.
- *Fillers*. Fillers are inorganic compounds that provide structure to the composite resin. They can constitute more than 80% of any composite. Common fillers include quartz, silica, glass, and lithium aluminum silicate. Composites are classified by the size of the filler particles because this affects their strength, wear-resistance, and tone and color. The different classes of composites are listed in the next section.
- *Coupling agents*. Coupling agents are used to bond the filler to the organic matrix. Compounds used as coupling agents include *organosilanes*.
- *Pigments*. These are used to provide natural color to the composite so it matches the nearby tooth surfaces.

Classes of Composites

Composites are classed by the particle size and type of the filler compound. Because fillers are the largest percentage of composites, the nature of the filler determines the properties of the composite. Types of composites include:

- *Macrofilled composites* have the largest particle size, with particles ranging from 1 to 3 microns. These were used more extensively in the 1960s and 1970s and are still used in Class IV restorations. Macrofill composites are stronger than other composites, but do not polish to the same degree as other composites.
- *Microfilled composites* have smaller particle sizes, ranging from 0.01 to 0.1 microns. These are used in both Class III and Class IV restorations, as well as veneers and diastema closures. Microfill composites are cured with UV light and can be polished to a high sheen, making them more aesthetically pleasing.
- *Hybrid composites* contain both large and small particles, usually including more than one type of filler (e.g., glass and silica). These newer composites have the best properties of both macrofilled and microfilled composites: they can be polished to a high sheen and feature the strength needed for posterior as well as anterior applications.

In addition to these classifications, composites are also identified as *flowable composites* and *packable composites*.

Flowable composites have a low viscosity and can be used in tight spaces. They are typically applied with a syringe directly into the cavity preparation. A dentist might use a flowable composite in narrow cavities with irregular contours, for sealing pits and fissures, or for lining larger restorations. Flowable composites are generally not very strong, but they can be used in very small spaces and come in a wide variety of shades.

Packable composites are stronger and less viscous than flowable composites. They contain more filler by volume and are used to fill larger restorations and in areas where strength is required. They are often built up in the restoration in layers, and they do not shrink as much as flowable composites. Their major drawback is they are not supple enough to work in very tight, narrow areas.

Using Composites

Composites differ from amalgam in several important ways.

First, shade matching is extremely important during composite restoration. If the shade is incorrect, patients will see the mismatched composite after the restoration. Composite manufacturers have designed shade matching systems (Figure 34-5) to guide the dental team and make sure the composite matches the patient's natural enamel color.

Cavity preparation is also different when using composites. Before composite application, cavities are often prepared with an etchant. After etching, the tooth appearance will be dull, and the preparation will be ready for the bonding agent (if one is being used). Bonding agents help ensure that the composite tightly binds to the tooth and forms a lasting restoration.

During placement, composites are often applied in thin layers and light cured between layers. To make this process easier, manufacturers have developed single-paste, lightproof syringes that can be used directly in the oral cavity (Figure 34-6). After each layer is applied, it is light cured, and then the next layer is applied. Besides forming a stronger restoration, this also allows for adjustment of the shade during the procedure.

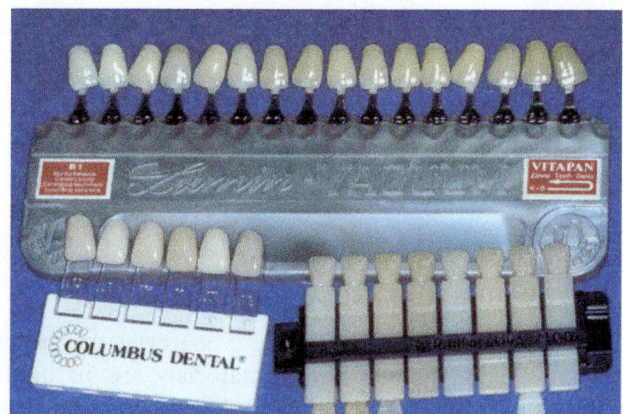

Figure 34–5 Shade matching. Photo shows several shade guides including a Vita shade guide.

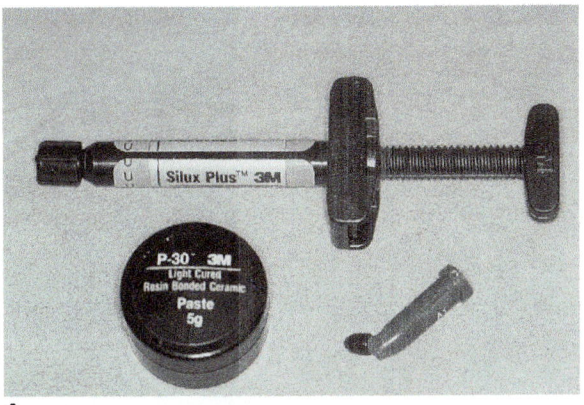

A

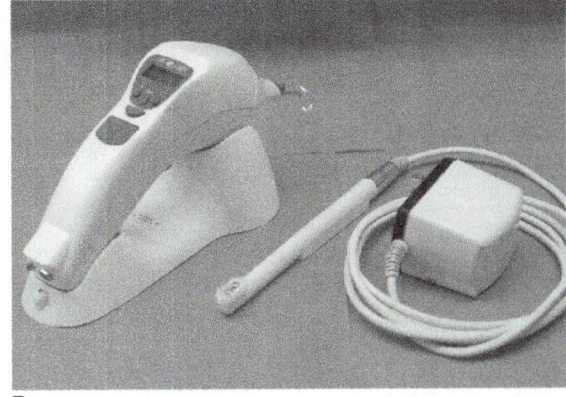

B

Figure 34–6 Using composites. (**A**) Light-cure composites are supplied as a jar, screw-type syringe, and compule (unit dose). (**B**) Light-emitting diode curing lights.

After the final layer is in place, it is light cured one last time, and then polished. Light-cured composites are cured with a blue light that *polymerizes* the material. (**Polymerization** is the process by which composite material hardens.) The exact length of curing depends on the composite used; follow the manufacturer's instructions. Darker composite colors require a longer curing time.

The restoration process varies depending on the composite used and the nature of the restoration. In some cases, for example, a cavity liner or base might be applied before the etchant to protect the tooth pulp. The manufacturer should provide instructions in the composite kit for etching, bonding, and curing.

Finishing a Composite Restoration

Composites differ from amalgam in another important way: they cannot be shaped using hand-cutting instruments. Unlike amalgam, which gradually hardens and allows the dentist to carve away excess amalgam by hand, composites instantly cure as they are polymerized.

In place of hand-cutting instruments, composite restorations are finished with finishing burs and abrasive materials. Although this procedure will be performed by the dentist, the dental assistant is responsible for preparing, assembling, and transferring the necessary instruments during the procedure. Instruments that might be required during a composite restoration include diamond burs, finishing burs, various discs, finishing strips, and polishing paste.

CHECKPOINTS

34-5 Name the components of a typical composite.

34-6 What is a hybrid composite?

34-7 What is the purpose of acid etching?

Procedure 34–2 Mixing and Transferring Composite Restoration Materials

Composite restoration materials can be mixed by dental assistants, and in some states, an expanded function dental assistant may place and condense the material into a cavity preparation.

Materials needed (Figure P34-2-1):

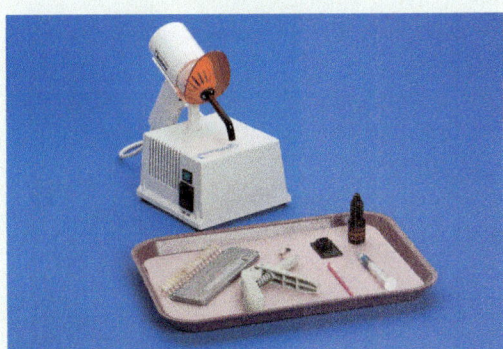

Figure P34-2-1

- Shade guide
- Composite materials
- Composite syringe if a capsular type being used
- Microbrushes
- Composite well to hold etch and bonding agent
- Etch
- Bonding agent
- Curing light

1. Put on appropriate PPE.
2. Select the shade guide and match the composite materials against the patient's teeth. Make sure both the shade guide and the patient's teeth are wet. When matching the shade, use natural lighting because fluorescent lighting can change the appearance of colors. Involve the patient in the decision on the shade. Make a note of the shade (Figure P34-2-2).

Procedure 34–2 Mixing and Transferring Composite Restoration Materials (Continued)

3. Assist the dentist in the correct sequence of applying the etch and bond material. If needed, light cure the material.

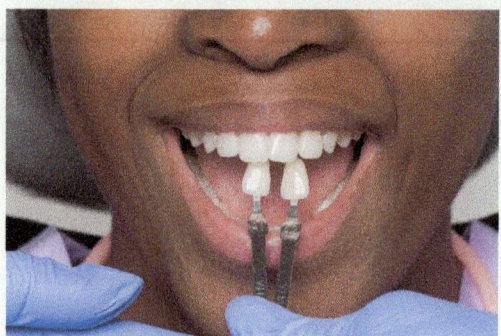

Figure P34-2-2

4. Prepare the composite. Composite materials are usually packaged in syringes or capsules that are ready for use; some self-curing composites need to be mixed before use. Many composites are sold in single-use syringes, which can be used to apply the material.

5. Transfer the composite to the dentist (Figure P34-2-3). The dentist applies the composite directly to the prepared cavity in layers.

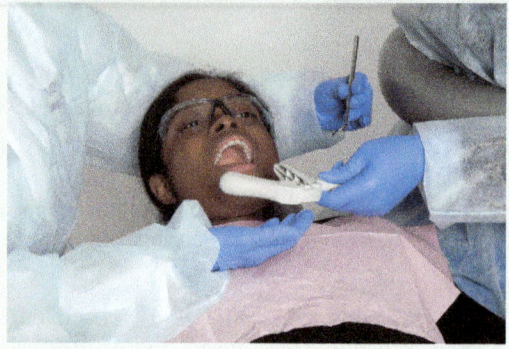

Figure P34-2-3

6. If light curing is needed, the composite is cured after every layer is added.

Glass Ionomers

Glass ionomers are specialized materials with a wide range of applications. They can be used for restorations that are not subject to stress, such as Class V restorations or root surfaces (Figure 34-7). They are also used on primary teeth and as preparation materials during composite restorations.

Glass ionomers differ from amalgam and composite because they chemically bond with the tooth surface, which means less preparation is needed of the tooth surface. Most importantly, however, glass ionomers can release fluoride to prevent further decay.

Research into the development of stronger glass ionomers continues. Newer hybrids, called *resin-modified ionomers,* include resin with the original material. This makes the material stronger and more aesthetically pleasing. These newer ionomers can be auto cured or light cured. Another form of ionomer includes the addition of a spherical silver-tin alloy with glass ionomer. These metal-reinforced ionomers have improved workability and setting time, as well as fluoride release and erosion resistance. They are used for repair of restorations, core buildups, and as a base.

Glass ionomers are similar to some composites in their preparation and applications. They can be supplied as a powder and liquid that must be mixed before application,

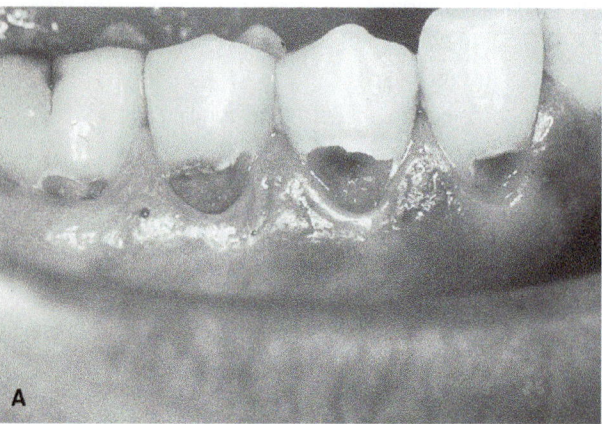
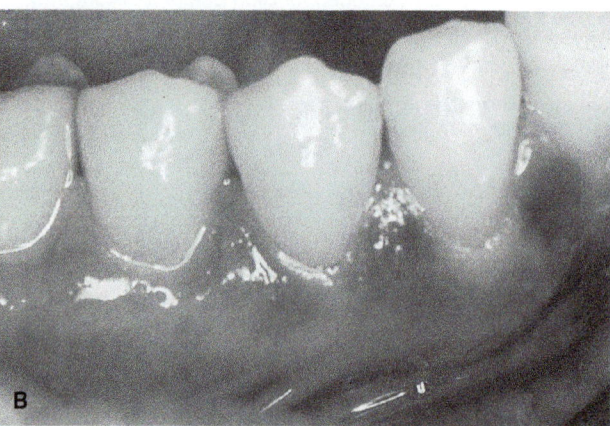

Figure 34–7 Glass ionomers. (**A**) Several Class V carious lesions. (**B**) Light-cured glass ionomer restorations. (Courtesy of GC America, Inc.)

or they are supplied in premixed application tubes or capsules. Follow the manufacturer's instructions for tooth preparation, ionomer preparation, and application.

Compomers

Compomers are hybrid materials that combine glass ionomers and composites. They are light cured like composites, but can release fluoride like ionomers. No etchant is needed during tooth preparation, but a primer/adhesive is required to form a solid bond with the tooth material.

CHECKPOINT

34-8 What type of restorations are glass ionomers typically used for?

Temporary Materials

Temporary restorations are used in emergency situations or when a tooth is waiting for a permanent restoration. A number of materials and techniques are used for temporary restorations that are unique to temporary restorations. Because these are not permanent restorations, in many states with expanded dental assistant functions, they can be performed by dental assistants.

Temporary restorations may be used to:

- Prevent shifting of teeth until a permanent restoration is placed
- Maintain tooth function and aesthetics for the short-term
- Allow time for a proper diagnosis

Intermediate Restorative Materials

Intermediate restorations are used when a short-term restoration is needed. For example, a dentist might request an intermediate restoration if primary teeth are affected during an emergency or during a caries management program.

Intermediate restorations are typically performed using a material called **intermediate restorative material**, or IRM. IRM is made from reinforced *zinc oxide eugenol*. The material has a mild sedative property and can be enhanced through the addition of fillers. It is also used for a liner, base, and cement, as well as an impression material.

IRM is available as premixed capsules that are triturated like amalgam, or as liquid and powders that must be mixed before application. These materials typically do not last more than a year, but this is plenty of time for a provisional restoration.

Procedure 34-3 Using Intermediate Restorative Material (IRM)

Some states allow qualified dental assistants to perform this procedure; in other states the dental assistant assists the dentist during the procedure. Check the regulations governing your state for more information about the specific duties dental assistants are allowed to perform.

This procedure gives steps for mixing powder/liquid IRM. Some IRM is sold in capsules that are triturated.

Materials needed (Figure P34-3-1):

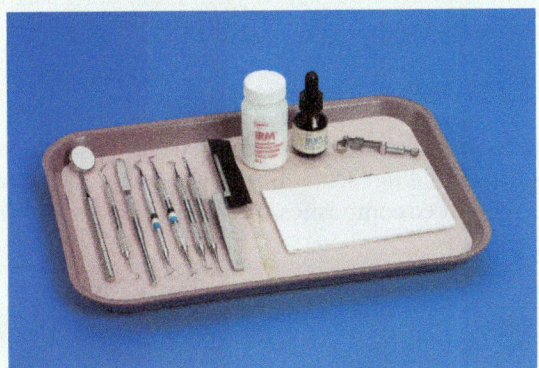

Figure P34-3-1

- Intermediate restorative material
- Paper mixing pad or glass slab
- Spatula
- Mirror
- Plastic instrument
- Condenser
- Explorer
- Cotton Pliers
- Articulation paper
- Hollenback carver
- Cleoid-discoid carver
- Matrix band
- Matrix band retainer
- Wedges

1. Put on appropriate PPE.
2. Assemble the matrix band and retainer for the designated tooth. Transfer the assembled retainer to the dentist, followed by the correct number of wedges.
3. Dispense the powder and liquid onto the paper or slab according to the manufacturer's instructions. Mound the powder and make a well, then dispense the correct amount of liquid into the well. The ratio of liquid to powder is determined by the manufacturer (Figure P34-3-2).
4. Mix the two materials together with a spatula until stiff.
5. Work the mixture on the pad, smoothing it repeatedly with the spatula until it is smooth and workable. Work quickly: you have only a minute before it starts to set.

Procedure 34-3 **Using Intermediate Restorative Material (IRM) (Continued)**

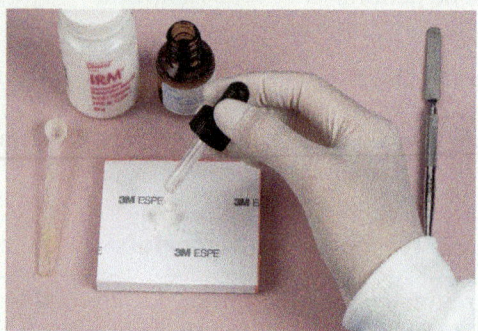

Figure P34-3-2

6. Using the plastic instrument, transfer the IRM to the dentist (Figure P34-3-3).

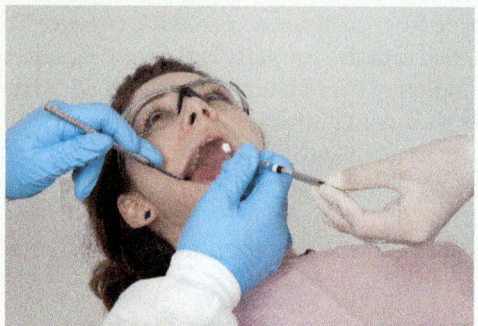

Figure P34-3-3

7. The dentist loads the IRM into the restoration, condensing after each increment with the small end of a condenser and continuing the process until the restoration is overfilled.

8. Transfer the explorer to the dentist. The dentist uses an explorer to carve away excess IRM from the proximal box and matrix band.

9. Retrieve the explorer and pass the cleoid-discoid carver to the dentist. The dentist uses the cleoid-discoid carver to remove excess material from the occlusal surface. The restoration material should now be contained within the margin of the final restoration, and the matrix system can be removed.

10. Retrieve the cleoid-discoid carver and transfer the Hollenback carver to the dentist. The dentist carves the IRM back to the normal anatomy of the tooth with the cleoid-discoid carver.

11. The dentist removes excess IRM from the interproximal space with the Hollenback carver. The interproximal area should be clear, with no overhangs.

12. Use articulation paper to check the occlusal contact. Ask the patient to gently bite down on the paper.

13. The dentist adjusts the restoration with the final carving.

Provisional Crowns

Provisional crowns are acrylic, aluminum, or stainless steel crowns that are cemented into place with temporary cement (Figure 34-8). These temporary crowns can usually be carved, but they are strong enough to withstand occlusal pressure and carry the patient over until a permanent restoration can be placed.

Acrylic crowns are formed on the tooth during preparation. To make one, a matrix is filled with mixed acrylic and then placed on the tooth. After a predetermined period of time, it should be removed from the tooth and exposed to air and then replaced. This allows the chemical heat generated by the acrylic bonding agent to disperse so the patient is not injured. This place-and-remove procedure should be repeated until the proper contour has been achieved and the crown is ready for placement. The acrylic crown is then trimmed with a laboratory bur and final adjustments are made. Acrylic crowns are fixed in place with temporary cement.

Temporary crowns are a cost-effective solution until permanent crowns can be placed. Their main drawback is a lower aesthetic value.

Other Provisional Materials

Composites are also sometimes used as provisional restorations, including self-curing, light-cured, or glass ionomer–reinforced composites. These are usually supplied

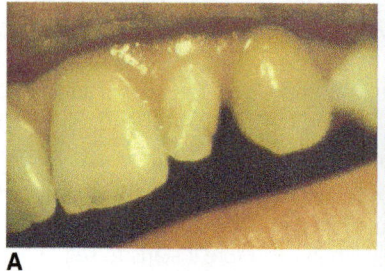
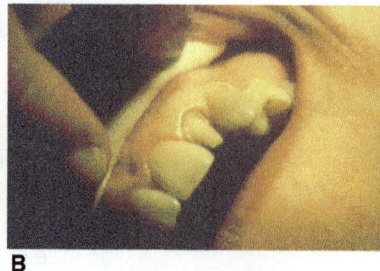
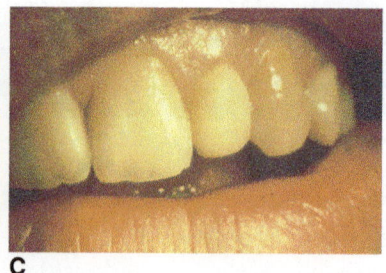

A   B   C

Figure 34–8 Provisional crowns. (**A**) Preoperative peg-shaped lateral incisor. (**B**) Crown preparation. (**C**) Temporary crown in place.

in a gun-style applicator that can be applied directly to the restoration (Figure 34-9). They do not generate heat like acrylic resins and are less irritating to the oral cavity. However, some of these materials are prone to discoloration, and there is some evidence of plaque adherence.

During the application, they are injected directly into the restoration and can be carved as they set. Final curing is accomplished either through light or through the material curing on its own.

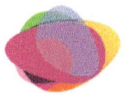 **CHECKPOINT**
34-9 How long can intermediate restorations typically last?

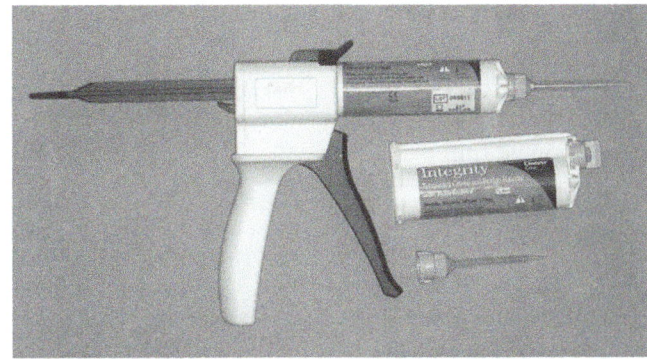

Figure 34–9 Gun-style applicator. For provisional composite restorations.

Chapter Highlights

+ Amalgam restorations are made from the combination of mercury and a metal alloy or element, including silver, copper, zinc, and tin.
+ Amalgam fillings cannot be color-matched to the tooth and are used on posterior teeth, as well as in situations with poor moisture control or extensive damage, or when patient oral hygiene is a concern.
+ High copper amalgam has a higher percentage of copper than low copper amalgam; high copper amalgams are easier to work with.
+ The typical ratio of mercury to alloy is 1:1.
+ Amalgam comes in capsules that contain mercury and alloy separated by a thin membrane. To prepare them, they are first activated and then mixed in an amalgamator.
+ Mercury is a highly toxic chemical: all dental offices that use amalgam need a comprehensive mercury hygiene plan, including contamination protection procedures.

+ Composites are replacing amalgam as their quality and strength improves. These materials can be color-matched to existing teeth.
+ Composites are made from the combination of an organic matrix (BIS-GMA) with fillers, coupling agents, and pigments.
+ Composites are classified by the size of the filler particles. Newer hybrid composites have both large (macro) and small (micro) particles.
+ Composites are either auto cured or light cured. They are usually applied in thin layers and cured between layers.
+ Composites require the use of acid etchants and bonding agents to form a good bond between the tooth and the restoration.
+ Glass ionomers are made from glass and resins; their main advantage is the ability to release fluoride after the restoration is complete.
+ Intermediate restorative material (IRM) is used to create provisional restorations.

Review Questions

1. What is the main alloy constituent of the typical amalgam?
   a. Silver
   b. Tin
   c. Copper
   d. Zinc

2. Which is not a typical application for amalgam?
   a. Posterior tooth
   b. Patient with poor oral hygiene
   c. Anterior tooth
   d. Primary tooth

3. What is the Eames technique?
   a. The process of forming an amalgam
   b. A method of combining composites
   c. A method of condensing glass ionomer
   d. The ratio of mercury to alloy in amalgam

4. In capsulated amalgam, what is the pestle for?
   a. To protect against mercury contamination
   b. To mix the amalgam and alloy
   c. To keep the alloy and mercury separated
   d. To pulverize the alloy before mixing

5. Which of the following is not a common size for amalgam capsules?
   a. Complete spill
   b. Single spill
   c. Double spill
   d. Triple spill

6. If a mercury spill occurs
   a. Quickly vacuum it up.
   b. Close the office and call a detox service.
   c. Use a spill kit, tape, or trap bottle to clean it up.
   d. Destroy all exposed clothing and fabrics.

7. What is the main constituent of the typical composite?
   a. BIS-GMA
   b. Filler
   c. Coupling agent
   d. Pigment

8. How are composites cured?
   a. Air cured
   b. Auto cured
   c. Light cured
   d. Either auto cured or light cured, depending on the composite

9. What are the three classes of composites?
   a. Ionomers, compomers, composites
   b. Microfill, macrofill, hybrid
   c. Cosmetic, structural, restorative
   d. Posterior, anterior, hybrid

10. What differentiates flowable composites from packable composites?
    a. Cost
    b. Aesthetics
    c. Time to cure
    d. Viscosity

11. What is acid etching?
    a. The process of mixing composite bases with acids before use
    b. Preparing a tooth cavity with acid
    c. Cleaning and polishing a composite restoration
    d. Removing a faulty composite restoration

12. Which instruments are used to finish composite restorations?
    a. Finishing burs and abrasive materials
    b. High-speed cutting disks
    c. Hand-cutting instruments
    d. Laser etchers

13. What is the main advantage of glass ionomers?
    a. Strength
    b. Versatility
    c. Ability to release fluoride
    d. Aesthetics

Active Learning Exercises

1. Imagine that you have recently begun working in a dental office and have just completed an amalgam restoration. The dentist throws the remaining amalgam scrap in the trash can and says, "It's only a little. It's no big deal." Why is the dentist wrong? How should you handle this situation? What is your professional obligation?

2. If a patient is having financial problems and simply cannot afford a permanent restoration at this time, what specific material could be used for a temporary restoration that would withstand a longer duration in the mouth? How is this material different from other temporary materials?

Application Activities

1. Visit the website of the EPA and review the guidelines for mercury releases and spills (www.epa.gov/mercury/spills). Write a detailed description of a scenario in which mercury is spilled in a dental office and outline the step-by-step procedures you would follow to safely clean up the spill.

PREPARING FOR CERTIFICATION EXAMS

Review the following topics in this chapter to prepare for the Dental Assisting National Board (DANB) exam:

- **Introduction**
- **Preparing Amalgam**
- **Composite Materials**
- **Glass Ionomers**
- **Temporary Materials**
- **Intermediate Restorative Materials**

chapter 35

Laboratory Materials and Techniques

CHAPTER OUTLINE

CHAPTER CHECKLIST

Upon completion of this chapter, students will be able to:

- ☑ Describe the safety precautions necessary in a dental laboratory.
- ☑ Identify typical laboratory supplies and equipment and explain the purpose of each.
- ☑ Explain the use of a casting, including examples of the various types and the materials used to create them.
- ☑ Identify substances commonly used to obtain dental impressions and describe the purpose of each.
- ☑ Describe the purpose and procedure for making custom impression trays.
- ☑ Explain the role of the dental assistant in procedures for obtaining patient impressions.
- ☑ Identify types of dental wax and describe the purpose of each.
- ☑ Identify types of gypsum products and describe their purpose in dentistry.
- ☑ Describe the role of the dental assistant in pouring and trimming patient study models.

KEY TERMS

alginate (AL-juh-nate) – an irreversible hydrocolloid material used to obtain impressions of teeth and soft tissues

articulator (ar-TIK-yoo-lay-ter) – device built to resemble the temporomandibular joint and human jaw to which casts of the mandibular and maxillary arches may be attached

base metal – metal, such as iron, tin, and zinc, known for its hardness

cast – a positive reproduction of the patient's mouth; three-dimensional representation of the teeth and other tissues of the oral cavity; also called a model

casting – indirect restoration formed by pouring molten material into a previously obtained mold

ceramic casting – restoration made of clay-like material topped by a metallic glaze

distortion – a change in the dimensions of an impression that has already set; also changes that occur during removal of an impression from a patient's mouth

custom tray – an impression tray specially constructed for an individual patient

elastomeric – having a rubbery elastic quality

gypsum (JIP-sum) – a form of calcium sulfate used in dental plasters, investments, and stone

imbibition (im-buh-BISH-un) – changes in a set alginate impression due to swelling or additional moisture

impression tray – a metal or plastic tray used in obtaining impressions

impression – an imprint or negative reproduction/likeness of the teeth or other tissues of the oral cavity

indirect restoration – a restoration, such as a crown, that is created outside the patient's mouth

investment material – material used to envelope or cover an object during laboratory procedures, such as soldering, curing, or casting

lathe (LAYTHE), dental – an appliance fitted with attachments for grinding, cutting, and polishing dental materials and appliances

model trimmer – appliance used to trim away excess plaster or dental stone from models or casts

noble metal – metal such as gold, palladium, or platinum, known for resistance to tarnish and etching

plaster – a type of gypsum containing calcium sulfate hemihydrate and porous crystals that is used to make dental casts

polysulfide (pol-ee-SUL-fide) – synthetic elastic material used to make elastomeric dental impressions

porcelain – a commonly used dental ceramic

polyether (pol-ee-EH-thur) – material used to make elastomeric impressions for crowns and bridges

sandblaster – small hand-held instrument used to roughen smooth surfaces for better adhesion

silicone – material used in dentistry to make elastomeric impressions

spatula, mixing – a flat blade used for mixing plaster and other dental materials

spatula, wax – a double-ended flat blade used to shape wax

stock tray – a prefabricated impression tray intended to fit a wide variety of patients

syneresis (sih-NER-uh-sis) – changes in a set alginate impression due to dryness and loss of moisture resulting in shrinkage

vacuum former – an appliance used to warm plastic and construct custom trays

vibrator – a platform used to agitate mixes

work pan – a plastic tray used to hold ongoing laboratory work

Introduction

A dental assistant trained in dental laboratory materials and techniques is a valuable addition to the dental care team. Dental offices typically include a laboratory area separate from the patient treatment area. The laboratory area is furnished with a countertop to provide work space and cabinets for storage of laboratory supplies and equipment (Figure 35-1). Only dental assistants and other trained members of the dental team use the resources of the dental laboratory. The laboratory tasks you may perform as a dental assistant are essential to patient education and appropriate treatment. In the dental laboratory you might:

- Pour preliminary impressions
- Trim and finish diagnostic models

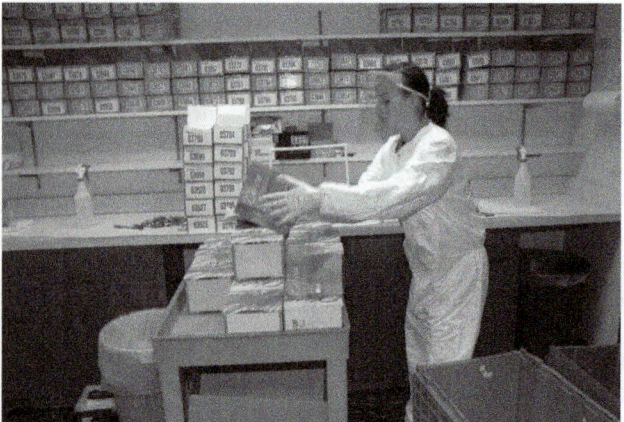

Figure 35–1 Dental office laboratory. (Photograph courtesy of Olson Dental Company, Inc., Clinton Township, MI.)

- Prepare custom impression trays
- Polish certain restorations

Pouring, trimming, and polishing diagnostic models are important tasks for patient education. A model is a **cast**, or three-dimensional representation and positive reproduction, of the teeth and other tissues of the oral cavity. Dentists use diagnostic models when presenting treatment plans to patients. A properly poured, trimmed, and polished model allows a patient to understand potential treatments, as well as any individual concerns or problems, more fully.

Tasks and procedures that cannot be completed in the office dental laboratory are accomplished in a commercial dental laboratory.

CHECKPOINT
35-1 What is another name for a dental model?

Laboratory Safety

Safety is an extremely important consideration in a dental laboratory. Safety concerns fall into the following general categories:

- Following infection control procedures
- Operating equipment according to the manufacturer's instructions
- Handling chemicals and other potentially harmful materials correctly
- Preventing and extinguishing fires
- Reporting any accidents to the dentist promptly

Personal Safety

Safe operating procedures begin with you. Take the following personal precautions whenever you work in a dental laboratory:

- Do not eat, drink, or smoke in the laboratory
- Wear personal protective equipment as instructed
- Keep your hair pulled back and away from materials and equipment
- Keep cosmetics or other personal care items out of the area

Physical Safety

Follow these guidelines when operating electrical equipment or other laboratory instruments at high temperatures:

- Keep a fire extinguisher nearby
- Plan a fire escape route
- Keep all equipment in good working order
- Do not operate faulty equipment in need of repair; report any faulty equipment immediately to the dentist
- Follow manufacturer guidelines for equipment use
- In laboratories equipped with a natural gas line, make sure to turn the gas supply completely *on* before operating equipment and completely *off* when finished
- Ensure that the laboratory has an adequate ventilation system

Chemical Safety

Exercise caution when handling materials in the dental laboratory. Many chemicals or substances used there are:

- Toxic—poisonous
- Corrosive—damaging to the skin, eyes, nose, clothing, or other surfaces
- Carcinogenic—capable of causing cancer

Familiarize yourself with the material safety data sheets provided by chemical manufacturers, and perform all laboratory procedures as instructed. These measures will help ensure that you do not inhale or swallow dangerous substances or contact them in ways that allow absorption into your skin and eyes. Plan how you will respond should a chemical accident occur. Familiarize yourself with the location of the eyewash station. Regularly check the station to ensure it is in good working order. Do the same with spill kits. Make sure all dental personnel know the location of the kits and how to use them.

Biohazards and Infection Control

Remember that impressions and other items brought into the laboratory from the patient treatment area can contain potentially infectious bodily fluids, such as blood and saliva. Avoid cross-contamination and exercise infection control measures in the laboratory as you would in the treatment area. Disinfect the laboratory area and any contaminated items or equipment after each use.

Laboratory Supplies and Equipment

Laboratory Supplies

In addition to the workbenches and counters in the typical dental laboratory, wall-mounted storage cabinets may be used to hold bulk supplies of the following materials:

- Stone, for mixing with water and creating models. Stone may be laboratory stone, used to create sturdier diagnostic casts or study models; orthodontic stone, used to create models for orthodontic diagnosis and treatment; die stone, used to create positive replicas of teeth or especially strong models or casts; or high-strength, high-expansion die stone, an especially strong stone mix requiring less water for preparation.
- **Plaster**, for mixing with water and creating models. Plaster may be impression plaster, used mainly for mounting casts on articulators, or laboratory plaster, used primarily to create diagnostic casts or study models. Plaster models are weaker than stone models.
- **Investment materials**, for covering prostheses or restorations during curing, soldering, or casting procedures.

A typical dental laboratory also has the following supplies:

- Plastic **work pans** marked with individual patient names to hold laboratory work in progress. In some dental laboratories, these work pans are color-coded to indicate the nature of ongoing work.
- Rubber bowls for use in both the treatment and laboratory areas of a dental practice. In the treatment area, they are used for the mixing of alginate, and in the laboratory, for mixing plaster or stone.

Spatulas used in a dental laboratory differ in shape and style depending on their use (Figure 35-2).

- **Wax spatulas** are double-ended instruments used for waxing a pattern or for working with wax for dentures.
- **Mixing spatulas** are used to mix materials such as alginate, stone, or plaster. Their size and sturdiness depend on the nature of the material being mixed.

Dental assistants are often in charge of keeping dental offices stocked with necessary materials and supplies.

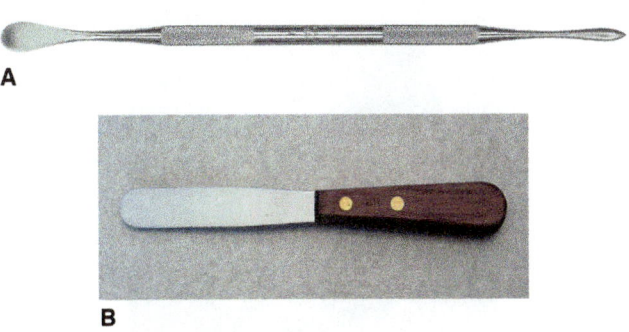

A

B

Figure 35–2 Spatulas. (**A**) Wax spatula. (**B**) Mixing spatula.

When ordering supplies and stocking shelves, ensure that an adequate supply of plaster, stone, trays, mixing bowls, and spatulas remains available for ongoing work in your dental practice.

CHECKPOINT

35-2 Mixing spatulas and bowls are used to mix which materials in the dental laboratory?

Laboratory Equipment

Heat Sources

Dental laboratories use heat sources to heat wax and other substances. A propane or butane torch is typically used for this purpose. In laboratories equipped with a natural gas line, a rubber hose will run from the gas outlet to a Bunsen burner that is used as a heat source.

Model Trimmers

A **model trimmer** is used to trim stone or plaster models (Figure 35-3). It is equipped with a wheel for grinding away stone or excess plaster. Do not allow stone or plaster to build up between trimmings. The wheel must be kept clean for maximum effectiveness. A stream of water runs continuously across the wheel to cut down on dust and make cutting and trimming easier. The water runs into a sink where a plaster trap catches bits of plaster and grindings before they can block the drain. Be sure to wear safety goggles when operating a model trimmer. A splash shield should also be in place to prevent splatter on the operator.

Dental Lathes

A **dental lathe** is used to trim and polish custom impression trays, dentures, and some restorations. The lathe has a protective plastic see-through shield that is lowered over the work area. A revolving threaded extension runs from each end of the motor. Attachments, such as grinding wheels, are placed on these extensions. Sterilize any previously used attachments before the next use.

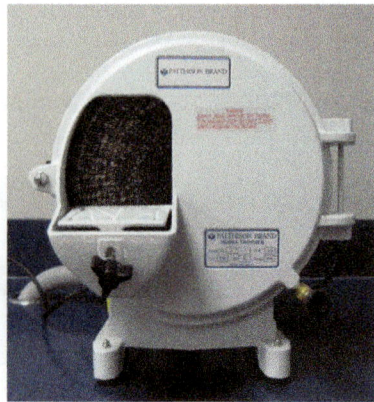

Figure 35–3 Model trimmer.

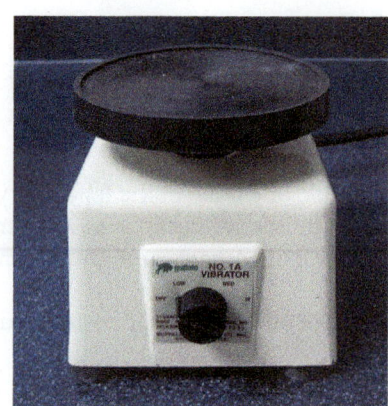

Figure 35–4 Vibrator.

Laboratory Handpieces

Low-speed laboratory handpieces are used for a variety of tasks, including trimming custom impression trays, trimming and contouring temporary crowns, and trimming and relining removable partial plates and dentures, as well as trimming and contouring orthodontic appliances. The low-speed handpiece is sometimes called a straight handpiece because of its straight-line design. Low-speed handpieces come in standard-length and short designs. The rotating portion of the handpiece, the bur, can operate with a forward or backward motion. A straight attachment, also known as a sleeve, is attached to the handpiece to adapt it for common laboratory procedures. Laboratory burs are used in the lab handpiece. Like restorative burs, these burs are cleaned and sterilized after use.

Vibrators

A dental laboratory **vibrator** is a canister-like appliance topped by a flat working surface (Figure 35-4). Bowls or work trays containing mixes and other work in progress are placed on top and vibrated. Vibrators remove air from plaster and stone mixes and help material flow more smoothly when a diagnostic model is poured. The flat top of the vibrator is often lined with a disposable cover to help keep it clean. Many vibrators have variable speeds.

Vacuum Formers

A **vacuum former** (Figure 35-5) is an electrical appliance used to construct custom trays for bleaching, mouth guards, and positioners for orthodontics. The upper portion of the vacuum former heats and softens a sheet of thermoplastic resin. Holes along the work surface allow the vacuum to pull and shape the warmed plastic around a mold.

Articulators

An **articulator** is a device built to resemble the temporomandibular joint and human jaw (Figure 35-6). When individual patient casts of the mandibular and maxillary arches are attached to an articulator, their motion and the individual patient's bite may be examined closely. Some articulators mimic only the up and down motion of the jaws. Others also mimic side-to-side motion. The observations and

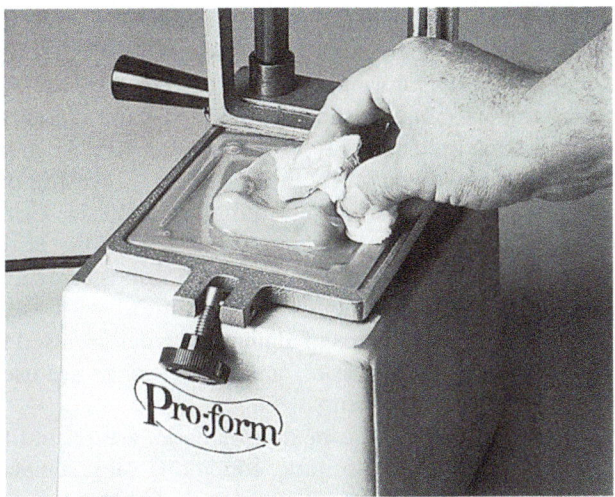

Figure 35–5 **Vacuum former**.(Courtesy of DR Dental Resources, Inc.)

measurements done with an articulator help the dentist diagnose problems, plan dental appliances, and create restorations for individual patients. You may help mount individual patient models onto the articulator. Models should be trimmed so that they fit onto the articulator easily.

Sandblasters

A **sandblaster** is a small hand-held instrument used to roughen surfaces for better adhesion. The sandblaster sprays sand at a high rate of speed, creating small pits on acrylic, metal, or porcelain surfaces of dental restorations. Ensure that proper ventilation is used while operating a sandblaster.

> **CHECKPOINT**
> **35-3** Which dental laboratory device mimics the motions of the human jaw?

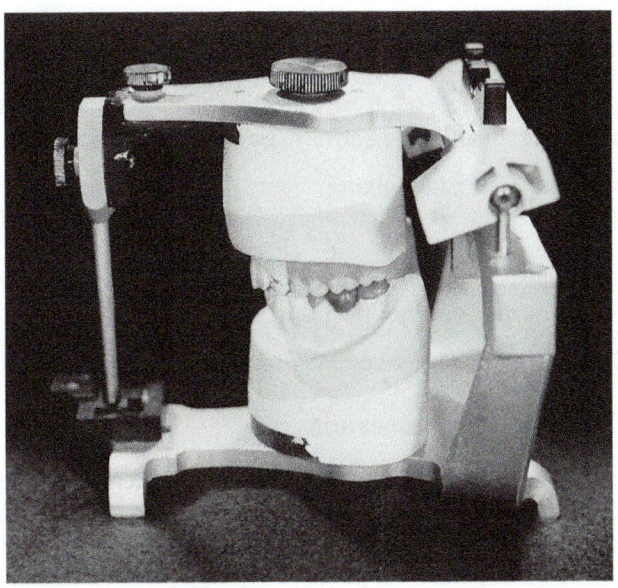

Figure 35–6 Articulator.

Castings

Castings are one type of **indirect restoration**. Indirect restorations are created outside the patient's mouth and then placed in position by the dentist and dental team. **Castings** are replicas of teeth or parts of teeth formed by pouring molten material into a previously formed mold. They may be made of gold-metal alloys, ceramic, or porcelain. A porcelain crown is an example of a casting. Castings usually are ordered by the dentist but produced in full-scale dental laboratories outside of the dental practice. Dental offices with a high volume of indirect restorations may have a full-scale dental laboratory on site.

Castings involve a series of procedures that begins with obtaining an impression of the tooth to be restored, waxing a pattern, investing the pattern, casting the restoration, and finishing and polishing the casting. The final step in an indirect restoration is the bonding or cementing in place of the finished casting by the dentist and dental team.

Gold-Noble Metal Alloys

Gold-noble metal alloys combine **noble metals**, such as gold, palladium, or platinum, with **base metals**, such as iron, tin, and zinc. Noble metals are known for their resistance to tarnish and corrosion, while less-valuable base metals are known for their hardness and resistance to wear. Gold alloys combine these characteristics into durable and reliable castings.

Gold alloys are classified according to their composition and resulting hardness. There are four different types:

- The softest alloy, the Type I, contains 83% noble metals. It is suitable for restorations that will receive only mild stress, such as inlays.
- Type II alloys contain 78% noble metals. Their medium hardness makes them suitable for inlays and some posterior bridge abutments.
- Hard Type III alloys contain 77% noble metals. They are suitable for inlays, three-quarter crowns, full crowns, and both posterior and anterior bridge abutments.
- Type IV alloys contain 75% noble metals. Classified as extra hard, they are suitable for crowns, bridges, and some partial dentures.

Ceramic Castings

Ceramic castings are fashioned from clay-like materials and covered with a metallic glaze to ensure durability.

Porcelain is a commonly used dental ceramic that in its finished form resembles natural tooth enamel. Its natural appearance and color make it a popular choice for veneers. When used to create crowns, porcelain or other ceramics are frequently used in combination with metal to provide increased durability. The ceramic is fused to a metal backing and the casting is glazed and fired to produce an extremely smooth, natural-looking surface. See Chapter 38, Fixed Prosthodontics, for more information about the use of porcelain in indirect restorations.

✔ **CHECKPOINT**

35-4 The hardest gold alloys, Type IV, contain what percentage of noble metals?

Impression Materials and Techniques

Impressions are negative reproductions of the patient's mandibular and maxillary arches. "Negative" means that each tooth in the arch forms a space in the impression material into which another type of material can be poured to form a "positive" model or study cast of the patient's teeth. Impressions are the first step in creating restorations such as bridges and crowns.

The accuracy of study casts and models varies with the type of impression material was used to create them. A dentist will instruct the dental assistant on what type of impression to obtain depending on the accuracy required.

Alginate

Hydrocolloid is the material most commonly used to obtain an impression. Irreversible hydrocolloid is typically known as **alginate**. The term *irreversible* simply means that the alginate cannot be returned to its original powdery state once it is mixed with water into a gel. Alginate provides sufficient accuracy for most study casts and primary models, but is not the material associated with greatest accuracy. It is typically used to make models for orthodontic appliances, mouth guards, bleach trays, temporary restorations, and custom trays.

The dental assistant mixes additional materials, including calcium sulfate (which may already be included in the alginate mix) and water, into the alginate to form the gel that is used to obtain impressions. Retardants can also be added to the gel to ensure that it will not harden too quickly before being placed in the patient's mouth. Alginate offers many advantages as an impression material:

- Its rapid setting ability and mild taste enhance patient comfort
- It may be used to obtain impressions of both teeth and soft tissues
- It is economical and easy to use

Alginate is available in fast-set and regular-set types. Each has a specific working time (the amount of time you have between mixing the material and loading it into the tray) and setting time (the amount of time from the start of mixing until the material has set in the patient's mouth). Fast-set alginate requires a faster mixing time and will set up in the patient's mouth at a faster rate. This type of alginate is recommended for fidgety children or patients with strong gag reflexes.

The fast setting time makes this type of alginate suitable for use by more experienced dental assistants. Regular-set alginate gives the operator more time to mix the alginate, load the material into the tray, and seat it in the patient's mouth.

The setting time of any type of alginate material can be sped up or slowed down by increasing or decreasing the temperature of the water used to mix the material. Using warmer water results in the material setting up faster (decreasing the setting time), while the opposite occurs with cold water (increasing the setting time).

On average, two scoops of alginate powder are used to take a mandibular impression, and three scoops are used for a maxillary impression.

Alginate's most significant disadvantages are related to its vulnerability to atmospheric conditions. Most alginate impressions must be filled ("poured up") within 1 hour of being obtained. If the impression is stored unfilled for a longer period of time, it may change in size slightly due to the loss or gain of additional moisture. Stored in a dry environment, the impression may shrink (**syneresis**); stored in a humid environment, the material may swell (**imbibition**).

Another disadvantage of alginate is the possibility of tearing or **distortion** as the impression is removed from the patient's mouth. Distortion refers to any stretching or changes in dimension.

Dental Facts

Before alginates were introduced in dentistry, the impression material of choice was agar hydrocolloid. It originated from a by-product of ocean waste and seaweed found off the coast of Japan. The availability of agar hydrocolloid was cut off abruptly with the outbreak of war with Japan in World War II. Scientists responded by inventing a synthetic product, alginate, to take its place.

Innovation is a constant in modern dentistry. Although not yet widely used, some newer alginate products offer advantages over established product lines. New products may offer the following advantages:

- Require no hand mixing
- Be dispensed from specially designed automatic dispensers
- Produce impressions that remain stable for longer periods of time and can be "poured up" when convenient.

These benefits may save time in a busy practice.

Elastomeric Materials

Elastomeric materials are used to obtain dental impressions when accuracy of the impression is of great importance. Once elastomeric materials have set, their rubbery elastic quality makes it possible to remove them from the patient's mouth without any tearing or distortion.

Elastomeric materials contain both a base ingredient and a catalyst. You add the catalyst to the base as you prepare the impression material. Elastomeric materials are self-curing. Adding the catalyst to the base sets in motion chemical changes that change the base into its necessary consistency.

Elastomeric bases come packaged as paste in a tube or cartridge, or as putty in a jar. The catalyst, sometimes called an *accelerant*, is also packaged as paste in a tube or cartridge, or as liquid in a bottle. Elastomeric materials come in three forms: light-bodied, regular, and heavy-bodied.

Light-bodied elastomeric materials are sometimes referred to as *syringe-type* or *wash-type* materials. Light-bodied materials are injected into the mouth to flow into and around details of teeth and increase the accuracy of the resulting impression.

Regular-bodied elastomeric materials may also be referred to as *tray-type* materials. They are not applied with a syringe, but rather prepared in a tray. Because they are heavier than light-bodied materials, the pressure they exert forces the light-bodied material already in place to flow as closely as possible around prepared teeth, thereby increasing the accuracy of the impression. Heavy-bodied materials are used in this manner also.

✔ **CHECKPOINTS**

35-5 The process by which an alginate impression loses moisture and shrinks in a dry environment is known as what?

35-6 When mixing elastomeric materials, what is added to the base?

35-7 Light-bodied elastomeric materials are sometimes applied to the patient's mouth with what?

Elastomeric materials are also classified according to their chemical composition.

Polysulfide

Sometimes referred to as "rubber base," **polysulfide** has longer working and setting times than other elastomeric impression materials. It has a long history of use in dentistry, but its disadvantages include a strong odor, along with the potential for staining clothing. Polysulfide impressions are not particularly stiff, allowing for ease and flexibility during removal from the patient's mouth.

Silicone

Silicone is easy to mix from a paste and liquid catalyst. Silicone has no odor and does not stain clothing. In addition, impressions made from silicone maintain their dimensions well.

Polyether

Both the base and the catalyst of **polyether** are supplied as pastes. Polyether can prove to be particularly stiff and difficult to manipulate. For this reason, thinners are added to the base and catalyst once they are mixed.

Impression Trays

Once impression material has been mixed and prepared, it is transferred into an **impression tray** to be inserted into the patient's mouth to obtain the impression. Impression trays come in two general categories:

- Ready-made **stock trays**, which may be ordered and kept on hand, are available in a wide range of sizes and styles to fit a variety of patients. When ordering supplies for the dental practice, make sure a sufficient number of styles and sizes are always available.
- **Custom trays**, which are sometimes constructed by dental assistants and dental laboratory technicians, are specially designed and fabricated to fit a particular patient's mouth. Custom trays may be necessary in situations where a stock tray would not allow adequate space for the amount of impression material needed or where an excess of material would compromise the accuracy of the impression. Custom trays follow a model provided by a preliminary impression of the patient's teeth and soft tissues.

Any stock or custom impression tray you use must be:

- *Sturdy* enough to reliably hold sufficient impression material
- *Spacious* and *adaptable* enough to allow a uniform thickness of impression material throughout the arch
- *Adaptable* enough to hold the impression material as close as possible to the teeth
- *Strong* enough not to break as you remove it from the patient's mouth
- *Rigid* enough not to warp the impression as you remove it from the patient's mouth

Selecting a proper tray from among a supply of stock trays requires trying several before choosing one that causes the patient as little discomfort as possible (Figure 35-7). A properly fitting stock tray should also extend beyond the patient's teeth in the following directions:

- Slightly beyond, or in front of, the facial surface of the teeth
- Approximately 2 to 3 mm beyond the last molar or tuberous area of the arch in the back of the mouth
- Below the arch enough to allow approximately 2 to 3 mm of impression material between the tray and the incisal or occlusal surfaces of the teeth

Not all stock trays cover the entire arch.

- *Full-arch* trays cover the entire maxillary or mandibular arch
- *Quadrant* trays cover half of an arch
- *Section* trays cover the anterior portion of an arch

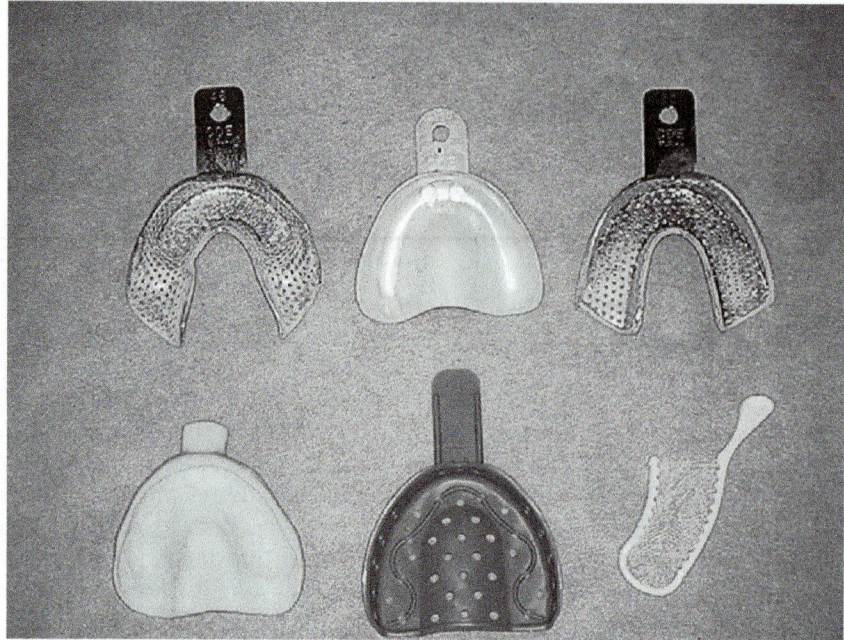

Figure 35–7 **Impression trays**. From upper left, moving clockwise: metal perforated tray for partially edentulous impressions, solid metal tray for edentulous impressions, metal tray for dentulous impressions, bite registration tray, plastic tray for dentulous impressions, and a custom tray.

The surface of an impression tray affects how its contents are held in place. Some trays are perforated with holes through which the impression material oozes and locks the material in the tray solidly in place. Trays without perforations require an adhesive to be sprayed or painted along their smooth surface to hold the impression material securely in place. Adhesives should be sprayed onto a smooth tray at least 15 minutes before an impression is taken to allow for adequate drying time. Elastomeric impression materials require adhesives that match the material. Silicone adhesives are used with silicone materials; polyether materials require vinyl polysiloxane (VPS) adhesives.

Though stock trays are intended to fit a wide variety of patients, they can be adapted to fit special circumstances. Utility wax can be added along the border of the tray to lengthen it or to increase its depth. Wax can also be added to the stock tray's palate area to accommodate a patient with an unusually high palate. Thermoplastic materials, as well, are increasingly being used to adapt stock trays for special circumstances.

Custom Impression Trays

Custom trays are made by a dental assistant in a dental office laboratory or by a laboratory technician in an outside laboratory. Specially designed for individual patients and their needs, custom trays must meet all the requirements of stock trays, but are specifically intended to allow accurate impressions of any irregular areas in the patient's mouth (see Figure 35-7, lower right). Like stock trays, custom trays may be either perforated or smooth.

CHECKPOINTS

35-8 Which elastomeric impression material is sometimes referred to as "rubber base"?

35-9 A stock tray that covers half of a maxillary or mandibular arch is what type of tray?

35-10 Which type of impression tray does not require an adhesive spray?

35-11 Impression trays designed and built to fit one particular patient are called what?

Several types of materials may be used to construct a custom impression tray. It may be made of self-curing or light-cured acrylic resin, a vacuum resin, or a thermoplastic material. These materials are composed of different ingredients, but also are distinguished by their curing method.

Curing is also known as *polymerization*. It occurs when chemical and physical processes cause a plastic to change from a pliable to a rigid state. Custom trays begin as pliable plastic so that they may be contoured to fit individual patient models. They must then harden to provide the rigidity and sturdiness required of impression trays. The process of hardening them is known as curing. Custom trays may be cured in one of four ways:

- Self-cured
- Light-cured
- Vacuum formed
- Thermoplastic, or cured by warm water

Self-Cured

Most custom trays are created out of self-curing acrylic resin. Like some elastomeric impression materials, acrylic resin uses a powder base and a liquid catalyst for self-curing. Self-curing materials go through several stages before the curing process is complete. In the initial stage the newly mixed material is sticky but can still be pulled apart, leaving strands hanging. In the second stage the material is sturdy enough to be handled and rolled into a ball. At this point it is contoured onto the model of an individual patient's teeth and soft tissues. At the third stage the material exudes heat as it hardens and continues to set. When the heat has subsided and the material can no longer be manipulated or shaped, the curing has reached its final stage. Custom trays made from self-curing acrylic resin should be allowed to sit for 24 hours before they are used to obtain an impression. During this time the tray becomes dimensionally stable and ready for patient use.

The major disadvantage of self-curing acrylic resin is the precaution required when handling the liquid catalyst (monomer methylmethacrylate). Its vapors are highly flammable and hazardous when inhaled in large quantities. It also can irritate unprotected skin. Dental assistants or other members of the dental team who are pregnant should remain aware of exposure to vapors, which can drift from the laboratory into other areas of the dental office.

Light-Cured

Use of light-cured acrylic resin requires a small oven-like appliance in which the premixed material is shaped to a patient model and then exposed to and cured by a special light. Dental assistants and laboratory technicians can exercise greater control over light-cured materials than self-curing materials. You can initiate the process when convenient and quickly obtain a dimensionally stable product for use. In addition, light-cured acrylic resin lacks monomer methylmethacrylate, the irritating and highly volatile catalyst needed for self-curing.

Vacuum-Formed

Vacuum-forming units also utilize heat in the curing process. In another oven-like appliance, a sheet of premixed heavy plastic resin is heated to softness. It is then draped over the patient model while vacuum pressure pulls and shapes the plastic to the model.

Thermoplastic

Warm water enables prepackaged thermoplastic beads and buttons to become a plastic soft and pliable enough to be shaped to the patient model. This process is relatively simple and requires no mixing or polymerization. It is also free of harmful fumes and chemicals. When soft, thermoplastic material appears clear and becomes increasingly opaque as it hardens. Thermoplastic has a variety of uses in a dental practice, including customizing stock trays.

CHECKPOINTS

35-12 The chemical and physical process that changes a plastic from a pliable to a rigid state is known as what?

35-13 Which custom tray material can release harmful vapors as you are working with it in the laboratory?

35-14 Thermoplastic beads and buttons become soft and pliable in what medium?

Extra Patient Care

Consider patient comfort when obtaining an impression. Ask whether the patient would like to apply a lip balm or lubricant for greater comfort. Patients' lips and mouths are stretched very wide during an impression procedure. Lip lubricant can provide welcome comfort. Keep it handy. Second, some impression materials may stain clothing. Do not just use a bib while obtaining an impression. Cover the entire front of the patient's body with a large vinyl drape.

Procedure 35-1 Mixing Alginate and Preparing for Impression

Materials needed (Figure P35-1-1):

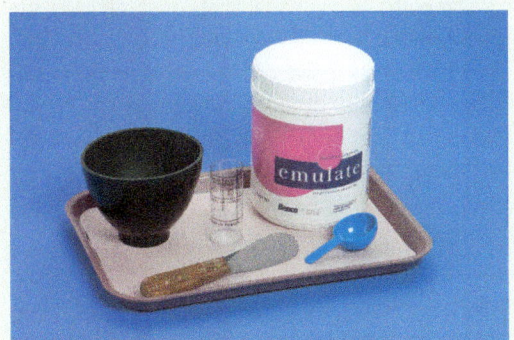

Figure P35-1-1

- Alginate
- Powder measuring cup
- Water measuring cup
- Medium-sized rubber bowl
- Wide-blade spatula

1. Put on appropriate PPE.
2. Using the water measuring cup, measure out and place the appropriate amount of room-temperature water into the rubber bowl.
3. Shake the alginate can gently to "fluff up" the contents. Remove the lid carefully.
4. Measure the alginate into the powder measuring cup.

Procedure 35-1 Mixing Alginate and Preparing for Impression (Continued)

5. Add the appropriate amount of powder to the water in the rubber bowl.

6. Mix with the spatula to moisten.

7. Continue to mix until the mixture appears smooth and creamy (Figure P35-1-2).

8. Spread the mixed alginate around the sides of the rubber bowl.

9. Finally, gather the fully mixed alginate into one mass in the bowl.

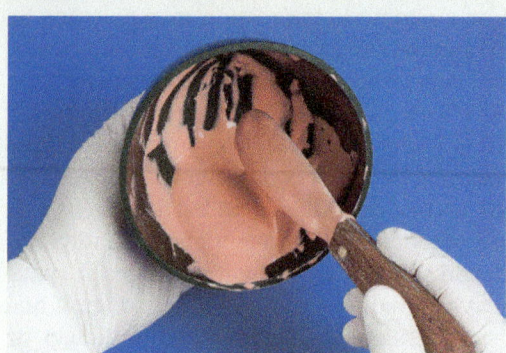

Figure P35-1-2

Procedure 35-2 Obtaining an Alginate Impression

Some states allow qualified dental assistants to perform this procedure; in other states the dental assistant assists the dentist during the procedure. Check the regulations governing your state for more information about the specific duties dental assistants are allowed to perform.

Materials needed (Figure P35-2-1):

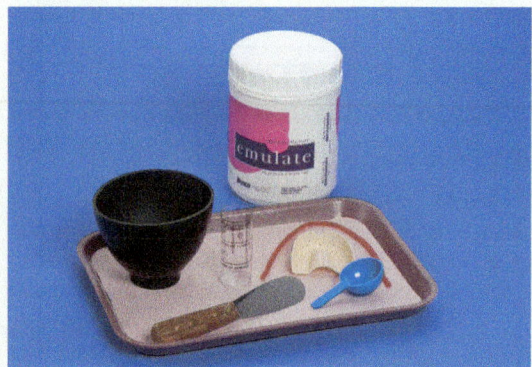

Figure P35-2-1

- Mixed alginate in rubber bowl
- Wide-blade spatula
- Sterile impression tray
- Tray adhesive (if using a nonperforated tray)
- Utility wax for extending tray if necessary

Loading the Impression Tray

1. Put on appropriate PPE.

2. Gather the alginate material from the bowl.

3. Fill one side of the mandibular impression tray at a time. Fill the tray from the lingual aspect.

4. Fill the entire maxillary impression tray at once and move the bulk of the alginate material toward the anterior area of the tray (Figure P35-2-2).

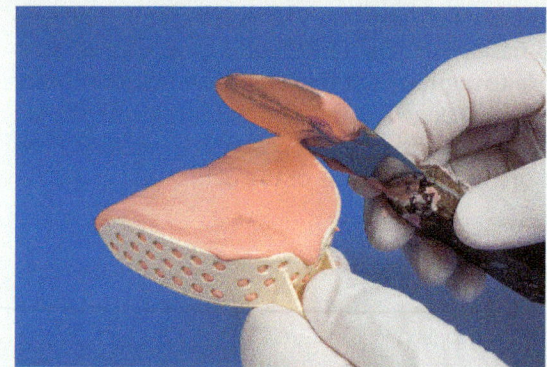

Figure P35-2-2

5. Press the alginate material down into the base of the tray.

6. Moisten your fingertip with water.

7. Smooth the surface of the alginate material with the moistened fingertip.

Seating the Impression Tray

Mandibular Arch

1. Have the patient rinse with water or mouth rinse to remove debris.

2. The dentist smooths additional alginate material over the occlusal surfaces of the mandibular arch.

3. While pulling back on the patient's cheek, the dentist inserts the tray sideways into the patient's mouth.

4. The dentist centers the impression tray over the patient's central and lateral incisors.

5. The dentist presses down on the tray, beginning with the posterior border.

6. Ask the patient to raise the tongue to the roof of the mouth and relax it.

7. The dentist presses down on the anterior portion of the tray (Figure P35-2-3).

Procedure 35-2 Obtaining an Alginate Impression (Continued)

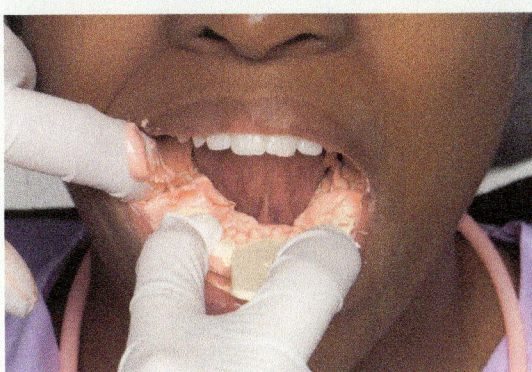

Figure P35-2-3

8. The dentist lifts the patient's lip around the tray.

9. Observe the alginate material around the sides of the tray to determine when it has set.

Maxillary Arch

1. Have the patient rinse with water or mouth rinse to remove debris.

2. The dentist smooths additional alginate material over the occlusal surfaces of the maxillary arch.

3. The dentist stands behind the patient so that it will be easier to center the tray and keep the patient's head from moving.

4. While pulling back on the patient's cheek, the dentist inserts the tray sideways into the patient's mouth.

5. The dentist centers the tray over the patient's central and lateral incisors.

6. The dentist presses up on the tray, beginning with the posterior border.

7. The dentist gently lifts up the patient's lips while seating the anterior portion of the tray.

8. The dentist checks for and wipes away any excess alginate material.

9. The dentist holds the tray firmly in place while the alginate material sets (Figure P35-2-4).

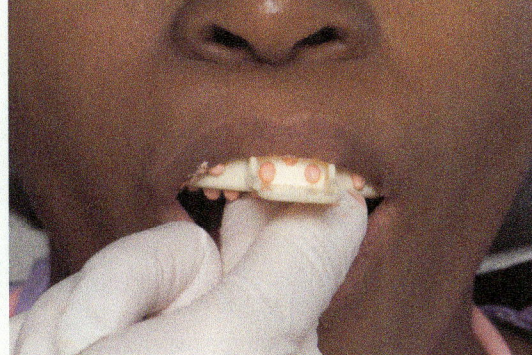

Figure P35-2-4

Removing the Impression Tray

Mandibular Arch

1. The dentist gently runs his or her fingers around the patient's cheeks and lips to loosen the tray's grip on the peripheral tissues.

2. The dentist positions one hand in the patient's mouth to shield the maxillary arch.

3. The dentist gently but firmly pulls up on the handle of the tray to loosen its seal around the teeth.

4. The dentist snaps up the tray as the seal loosens (Figure P35-2-5).

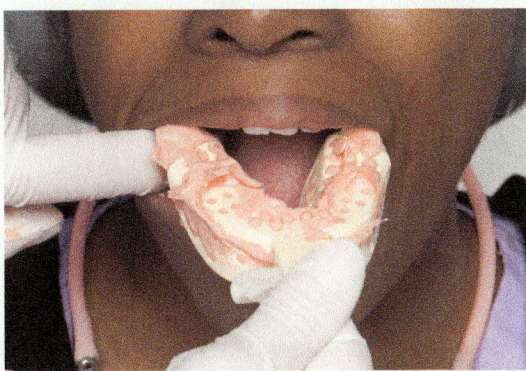

Figure P35-2-5

5. Have the patient rinse with water to remove excess alginate material from the teeth and soft tissues.

Maxillary Arch

1. The dentist gently runs his or her fingers around the sides of the tray to loosen its grip on the peripheral tissues.

2. The dentist positions one hand in the patient's mouth to shield the mandibular arch.

3. The dentist gently but firmly pulls down on the tray to loosen its seal around the teeth.

4. The dentist snaps the tray down as the seal loosens (Figure P35-2-6).

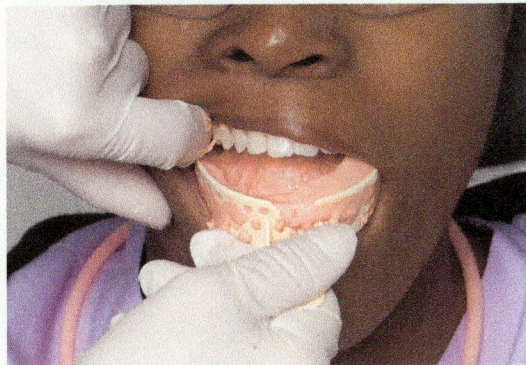

Figure P35-2-6

5. Have the patient rinse with water to remove excess alginate material from the teeth and soft tissues.

Procedure 35-2 Obtaining an Alginate Impression (Continued)

Evaluating the Impression for Accuracy

1. Ensure that the impression is free of tears and holes (Figure P35-2-7).

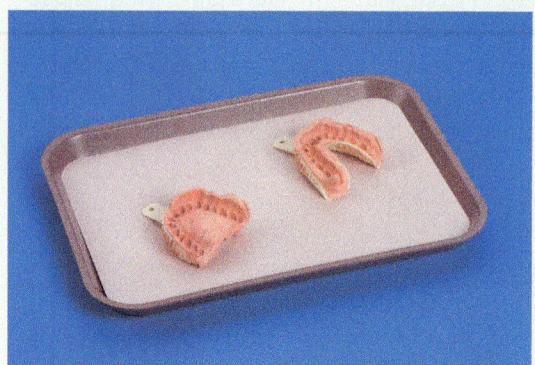

Figure P35-2-7

2. Ensure that it provides sharp detail of all teeth and soft tissues.

3. When reviewing a mandibular impression, ensure that it shows such important anatomical details as the tongue space, lingual frenum, mylohyoid ridge, and retromolar area.

4. When reviewing a maxillary impression, ensure that it shows such important anatomical details as the hard palate and tuberosities.

Care of Impressions

1. Gently rinse away saliva and any other fluids under cold running tap water.

2. Spray the impression with a disinfectant approved for the purpose.

3. In the case of any delay before "pouring up" the impression, wrap it in a moistened paper towel and store it in a covered container, such as a plastic bag or box.

Procedure 35-3 Making a Polysulfide Impression

Some states allow qualified dental assistants to perform this procedure; in other states the dental assistant assists the dentist during the procedure. Check the regulations governing your state for more information about the specific duties dental assistants are allowed to perform.

Materials needed (Figure P35-3-1):

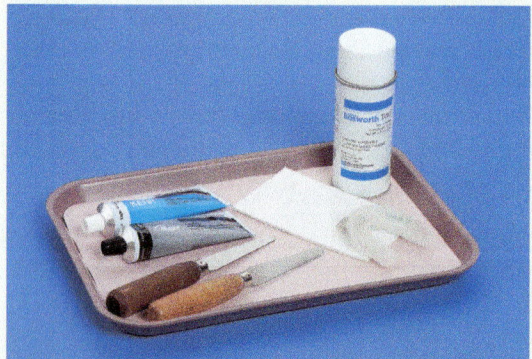

Figure P35-3-1

- Two rigid laboratory spatulas
- Tube of polysulfide base
- Tube of polysulfide catalyst
- Paper mixing pad
- Custom tray coated with appropriate adhesive

Mixing the Material

1. Put on appropriate PPE.

2. Dispense the base and catalyst onto the paper mixing pad. Always dispense equal lengths, *not* equal amounts (Figure P35-3-2). Avoid contaminating the material with glove powder.

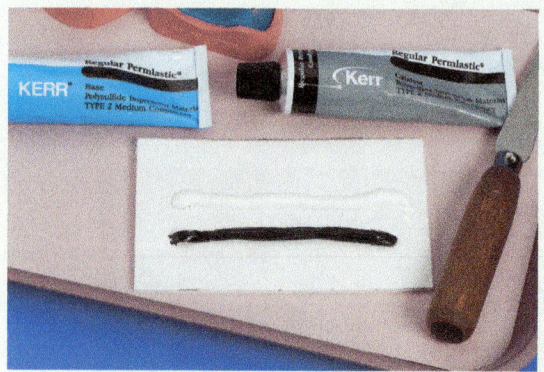

Figure P35-3-2

3. Leave enough space in between the materials to prevent premature mixing and polymerization.

4. When ready, use the spatula to mix the materials.

5. Transfer the newly mixed material to a fresh surface of the pad.

Procedure 35-3 Making a Polysulfide Impression (Continued)

6. Continue mixing with the spatula for 45 to 60 seconds until the mixture is a single color (homogenous) without any visible streaks (Figure P35-3-3).

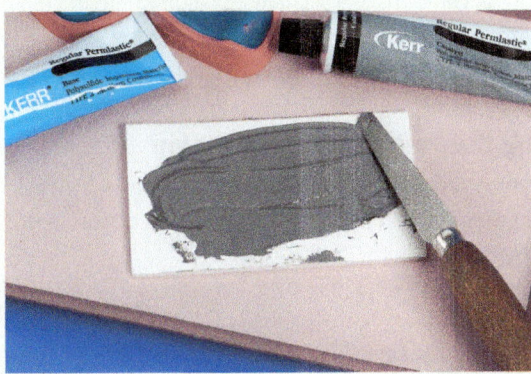

Figure P35-3-3

7. Using one stroke with the tip of the spatula, load the thoroughly mixed material onto the custom tray. Spread the material as broadly and evenly as possible onto the tray (Figure P35-3-4).

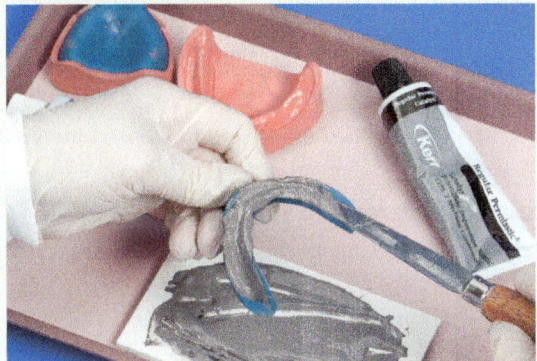

Figure P35-3-4

Obtaining the Impression

1. The dentist addresses any patient questions or concerns.
2. While pulling back on the patient's cheek, the dentist inserts the tray sideways into the patient's mouth.
3. The dentist centers the tray over the patient's central and lateral incisors.
4. The dentist presses firmly up on the maxillary tray or down on the mandibular tray, beginning with the posterior border.
5. The tray is held in place for the 6 to 10 minutes required for a polysulfide impression.

Removing the Impression Tray

1. The dentist gently runs his or her fingers around the sides of the tray to loosen its grip on the peripheral tissues.
2. The dentist positions one hand in the patient's mouth to shield the opposing arch.
3. The dentist gently but firmly pulls down on the maxillary tray and up on the mandibular tray to loosen its seal around the teeth.
4. The dentist snaps the tray up or down to loosen the seal further.
5. Have the patient rinse with water to clean the teeth and soft tissues.

Evaluating the Impression for Accuracy

1. Ensure that the impression provides sharp detail of all teeth and soft tissues (Figure P35-3-5).

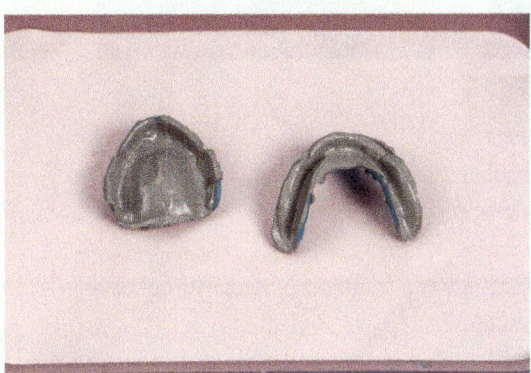

Figure P35-3-5

2. When reviewing a mandibular impression, ensure that it shows such important anatomical details as the tongue space, lingual frenum, mylohyoid ridge, and retromolar area.
3. When reviewing a maxillary impression, ensure that it shows such important anatomical details as the hard palate and tuberosities.

Care of Impressions

1. Gently rinse away saliva and any other fluids under cold running tap water.
2. Spray the impression with a disinfectant approved for the purpose.

Procedure 35–4 Making a Final (Silicone) Impression

Some states allow qualified dental assistants to perform this procedure; in other states the dental assistant assists the dentist during the procedure. Check the regulations governing your state for more information about the specific duties dental assistants are allowed to perform.

Materials needed (Figure P35-4-1):

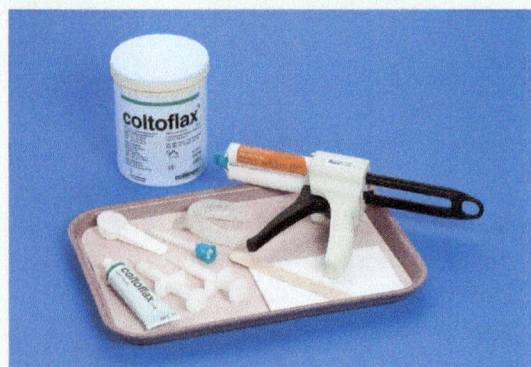

Figure P35-4-1

- Putty base material
- Putty or liquid catalyst material
- Paper mixing pad
- Spatula
- Stock or other tray painted with appropriate adhesive
- Plastic sheet
- Extruder gun with mixing tip and intraoral delivery tip
- Injection syringe
- Cartridges of light-body impression material

Preparing Preliminary Impression Material

1. Put on appropriate PPE.
2. Measure the base and catalyst onto the paper mixing pad according to the manufacturer's instructions.
3. Knead the mixture with a spatula or your hands for approximately 30 seconds until the mixture is a single color throughout without any visible streaks (Figure P35-4-2).

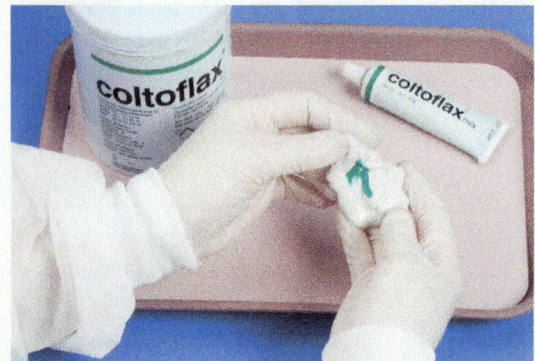

Figure P35-4-2

4. Form the properly blended material into a patty.
5. Load the material onto a prepared impression tray.
6. Use your finger to make a slight indentation where the teeth will appear.
7. Place the plastic spacer sheet on top of the tray. This will allow space for additional injectable impression material later.

Obtaining the Preliminary Impression

1. The dentist addresses any patient questions or concerns.
2. While pulling back on the patient's cheek, the dentist inserts the tray sideways into the patient's mouth.
3. The dentist centers the tray over the patient's central and lateral incisors.
4. The dentist pushes gently up on the maxillary tray or down on the mandibular tray.
5. Allow 3 minutes for the impression material to set.

Removing the Preliminary Impression

1. The dentist gently runs his or her fingers around the sides of the tray to loosen its grip on peripheral tissues.
2. The dentist positions one hand in the patient's mouth to shield the opposing arch.
3. The dentist gently but firmly pulls down on a maxillary tray and up on a mandibular tray to loosen its seal around the teeth.
4. The dentist snaps the tray up or down to loosen the seal further.

Evaluating the Impression for Accuracy

1. Ensure that the impression provides ample detail of all teeth and soft tissues (Figure P35-4-3).

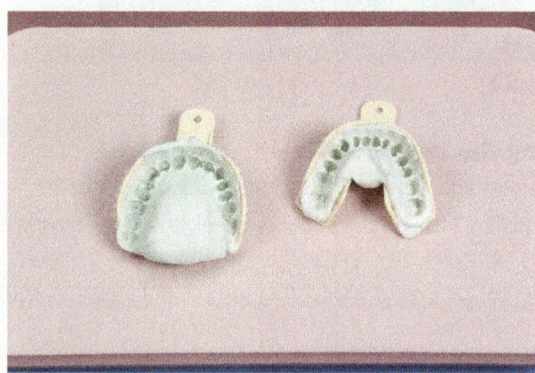

Figure P35-4-3

2. Ensure that a mandibular impression shows such important anatomical details as the tongue space, lingual frenum, mylohyoid ridge, and retromolar area.
3. Ensure that a maxillary impression shows such important anatomical details as the hard palate and tuberosities.
4. Lay the impression aside to set further.

Procedure 35-4 Making a Final (Silicone) Impression (Continued)

5. Rinse the impression to remove potentially infectious materials and disinfect prior to manipulation to avoid cross contamination.

Obtaining the Final Silicone Impression

Injectable light-body impression material is used to obtain a final silicone impression.

1. Load the extruder gun with injectable material according to the manufacturer's instructions.

2. Use the mixing tip to load material into a prepared tray or into the preliminary impression obtained earlier (Figure P35-4-4).

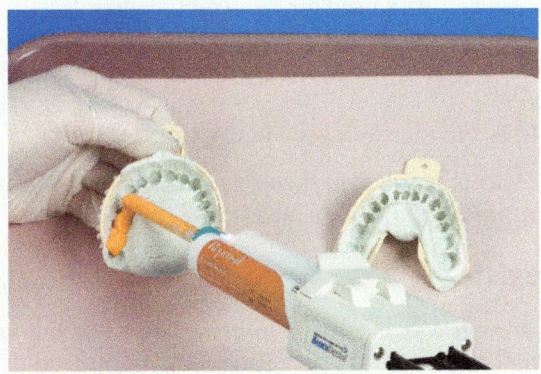

Figure P35-4-4

3. When finished, wipe excess light-body material off mixing tip.

4. Transfer the prepared tray to the dentist. The dentist inserts the tray into the patient's mouth.

5. Assist as needed while the dentist uses a syringe to inject additional material around the prepared tooth.

6. The tray is held in place for 3 to 5 minutes while the material sets.

Removing the Final Silicone Impression

1. The dentist gently runs his or her fingers around the sides of the tray to loosen its grip on peripheral tissues.

2. The dentist positions one hand in the patient's mouth to shield the opposing arch.

3. The dentist gently but firmly pulls down on a maxillary tray and up on a mandibular tray to loosen its seal around the teeth.

4. The dentist snaps the tray up or down to loosen the seal further.

5. The dentist removes the tray from the patient's mouth.

6. Rinse the tray under cool running water.

7. Let the tray air dry.

8. Disinfect the tray according to the material manufacturer's instructions.

Dental Waxes

Waxes have been used in dentistry for more than two hundred years. Dental waxes are made from a variety of natural and synthetic materials. Beeswax, fatty acids, fats, gum, and oils are among the natural products from which dental waxes are derived. Dental waxes can take several different forms depending on their purpose (Figure 35-8). Uniform color is important, as is the ability to provide consistent results.

Waxes used in dentistry are classified into three broad categories:

- Pattern waxes
- Impression waxes
- Processing waxes

Utility Wax

Utility wax, also known as periphery or bending wax, is a soft, pliable processing wax used to extend the borders of an impression tray or cover bothersome metal in orthodontic appliances. Utility wax is packaged as sticks, strips, or ropes, and consists of beeswax, petrolatum, and similar soft waxes (see Figure 35-8).

Sticky Wax

Packaged as brittle sticks or blocks (see Figure 35-8), sticky wax becomes tacky or sticky when heated. As its name suggests, sticky wax adheres well to surfaces such as gypsum, metal, and porcelain, and is used to join objects together until they can be repaired. Sticky wax is also used to form wax patterns. Beeswax and resin are its chief ingredients.

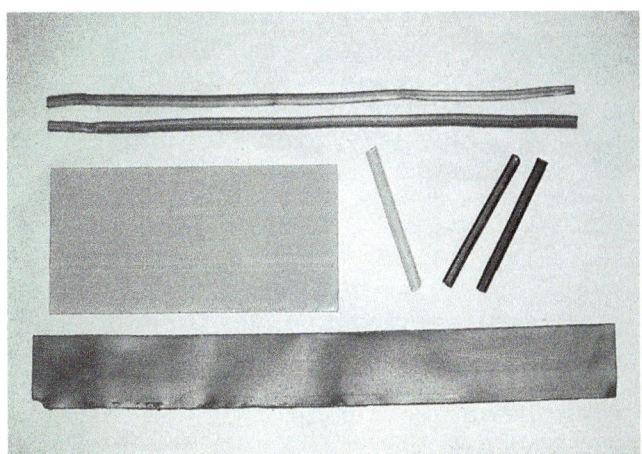

Figure 35-8 Dental waxes. Rope wax (*top*), baseplate wax (*middle left*), sticky wax (*middle center*), inlay wax (*middle right*), and boxing wax (*bottom*).

Boxing Wax

The purpose of boxing wax is suggested by its name. Boxing wax is a processing wax used to frame a preliminary impression when it is poured up. This produces a cleaner, more even model that does not require as much trimming.

Boxing wax is available in long, narrow strips, approximately 1 to 1½ inch wide and 12 to 18 inch long (see Figure 35-8).

Casting Wax

The purpose of casting wax may also be guessed by its name. Regular casting wax is a pattern wax used to create molds for indirect porcelain or metal restorations of single teeth, as well as for fixed bridges and metal portions of a partial denture.

Inlay casting wax has a variety of purposes and is classified into several different types.

- Type A is a hard wax used by dental laboratory technicians to create the pattern of an indirect restoration onto a patient model.
- Type B is a medium wax used to wax patterns of direct restorations in the mouth.
- Type C is a soft wax used by technicians during the creation of indirect restorations in a dental laboratory.

Inlay casting wax may be made from paraffin wax, carnauba wax, beeswax, and resin. Regular casting wax is made up of paraffin, beeswax, ceresin, and resins. Both types of casting wax are supplied in sheets of varying thickness (see Figure 35-8).

Baseplate Wax

Baseplate wax is a pattern wax used in the creation of dentures, including for recording the occlusal rims of teeth for the initial arch form, for setting denture teeth, and for creating a denture wax-up (trial denture). Like casting wax, baseplate wax is classified into three different types. Because its consistency is affected by room temperature, three classifications relate to its use in various climates.

- Type I is a soft wax used for constructing dentures.
- Type II is of medium hardness and is used in moderate climates. It is most often used to create baseplates for dentures.
- Type III is a harder wax used in tropical climates.

Baseplate wax is supplied in sheets and made up of paraffin or ceresin, beeswax, and carnauba wax (see Figure 35-8).

Bite Registration Wax

Bite registration wax is a soft impression wax that is softened further under warm water. Patients bite down on the wax to record an imprint of the teeth. Bite wafers are thin sheets of bite registration wax held in place by a horseshoe-shaped ring placed between the patient's maxillary and mandibular arches.

Procedure 35-5 Taking a Wax Bite Registration

Some states allow qualified dental assistants to perform this procedure; in other states the dental assistant assists the dentist during the procedure. Check the regulations governing your state for more information about the specific duties dental assistants are allowed to perform.

Materials needed (Figure P35-5-1):

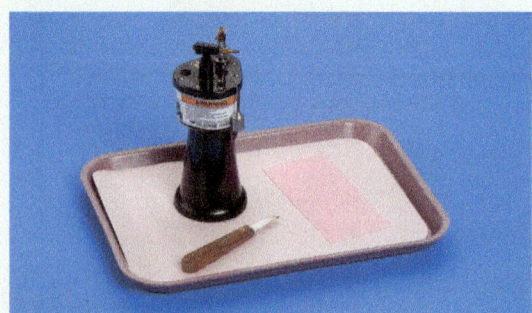

Figure P35-5-1

- Baseplate wax
- Laboratory knife
- Rubber bowl with warm water or a Bunsen burner

Obtaining the Bite Registration

1. Put on appropriate PPE.
2. Explain the procedural steps to the patient and reassure the patient that the wax will be warm, not hot.
3. Address any additional patient questions or concerns.
4. Ask the patient to open and close the mouth several times, observing the patient's normal pattern for doing so.
5. Have the patient rinse with water or mouth rinse to remove debris.
6. Place the cold wax over the occlusal and incisal surfaces of the patient's teeth to determine whether it is of sufficient length to cover all the teeth.
7. If the wax is long enough to prove uncomfortable, use a laboratory knife to trim away extra length.
8. Use a heat source, such as warm water, a Bunsen burner, or a torch, to soften the wax.
9. Place the softened wax against the occlusal and incisal surfaces of the teeth.
10. Instruct the patient to bite gently and naturally into the softened wax (Figure P35-5-2).

Procedure 35-5 Taking a Wax Bite Registration (Continued)

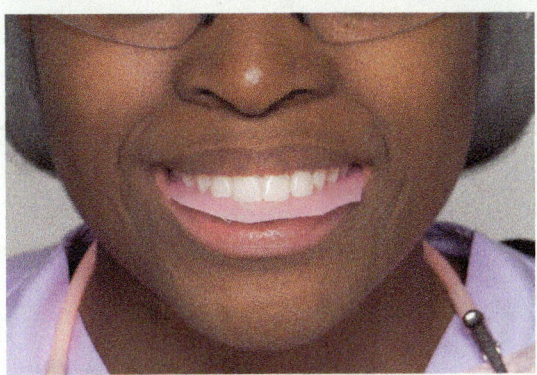

Figure P35-5-2

11. Allow the wax to cool and harden for approximately 1 to 2 minutes before removing it from the patient's mouth.

Removing the Bite Registration

1. Remove the bite registration carefully to avoid causing distortion.

2. Rinse the impression to remove potentially infectious materials and disinfect prior to manipulation to avoid cross contamination (Figure P35-5-3).

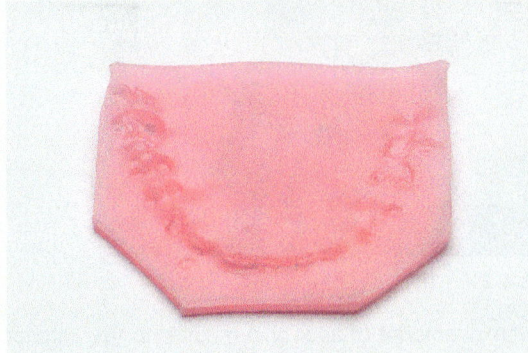

Figure P35-5-3

3. Write the patient's name on a tag and attach it to the container used to store the bite registration.

Procedure 35-6 Taking a Polyvinylsiloxane (PVS) Bite Registration

Some states allow qualified dental assistants to perform this procedure; in other states the dental assistant assists the dentist during the procedure. Check the regulations governing your state for more information about the specific duties dental assistants are allowed to perform.

Materials needed (Figure P35-6-1):

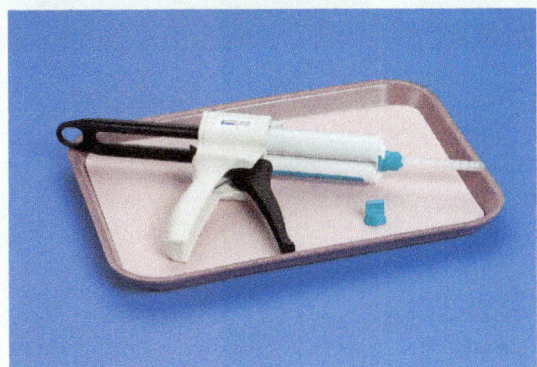

Figure P35-6-1

- Plunger unit containing tubes of vinyl polysiloxane base and catalyst
- Mixing cartridge, dispenser, and disposable tips

Precautions

Observe the following precautions when working with PVS bite registrations:

1. Do not contaminate PVS bite material with latex or sulfur-containing gloves. This includes touching the patient's teeth with a latex-gloved hand prior to the procedure. Use vinyl or other nonlatex gloves. Do not use certain hand soaps or lotions that can interfere with the setting action.

2. Make sure the material is at room temperature.

3. Block out any severe undercuts.

Preparing the Patient

1. Put on appropriate PPE.

2. Explain the procedural steps to the patient.

3. Reassure the patient that the material used will be room temperature and not excessively hot or cold.

4. Address any patient questions or concerns.

5. Ask the patient to open and close the mouth several times while observing the patient's normal pattern for doing so.

6. Have the patient rinse with water or mouth rinse to remove debris.

Obtaining the Bite Registration

1. Follow the manufacturer's instructions to release the base and catalyst from the plunger unit into mixing the cartridge and dispenser.

2. Use the dispenser to extrude the material directly onto the occlusal surface of the patient's mandibular arch (Figure P35-6-2).

Procedure 35-6 Taking a Polyvinylsiloxane (PVS) Bite Registration (Continued)

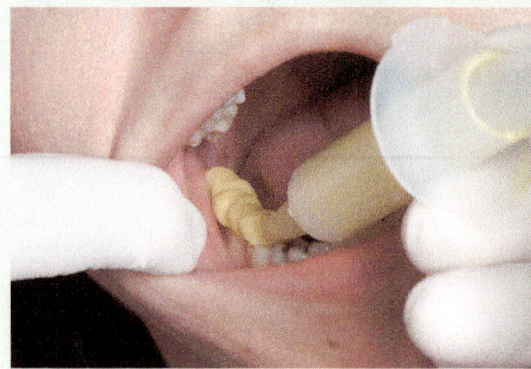

Figure P35-6-2

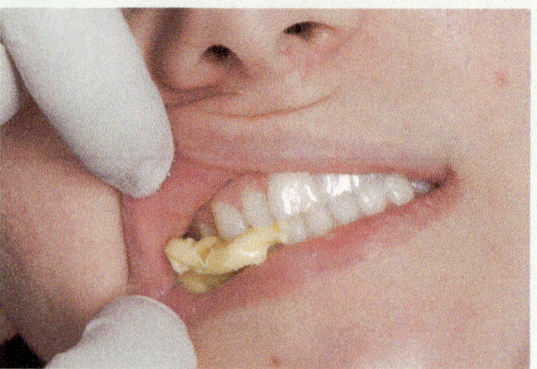

Figure P35-6-3

3. Add a small amount of additional material to the anterior teeth of the maxillary arch.

4. Squeeze the dispenser trigger evenly using moderate pressure. A layer of material approximately 5 mm thick is usually sufficient.

5. Do not take longer than 30 seconds to dispense the material.

6. When finished, wipe away any excess from the dispenser tip.

7. Leave the tip in place or remove and replace with original cap. Replace the tip before next use.

8. Instruct the patient to bite down gently but firmly in a normal manner (Figure P35-6-3).

9. Wait for approximately 1 minute while the material sets.

Removing the Bite Registration

1. Ask the patient to open his or her mouth.

2. Carefully release the bite registration from the teeth.

3. Check for residual material in any undercuts.

4. Rinse the bite registration under cold running water.

5. Allow the registration to air dry.

6. Disinfect the registration with standard disinfecting solution or spray.

7. Store the registration away from direct sunlight.

8. Unset material may be removed from clothing with a manufacturer-provided cleaning solvent or isopropyl alcohol, or by dry cleaning.

Procedure 35-7 Fabricating a Self-Curing Acrylic Custom Tray

Materials needed (Figure P35-7-1):

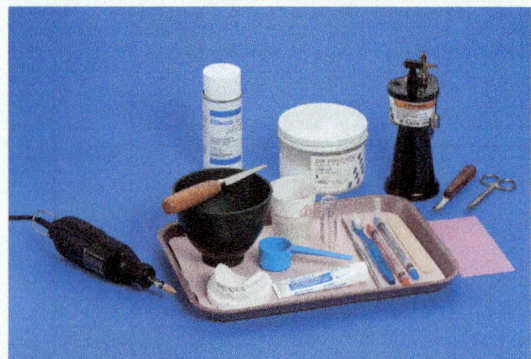

Figure P35-7-1

- Diagnostic patient model of maxillary or mandibular arch
- Black or red/blue pencil
- Tray resin

- Water measuring cup
- Powder measuring cup
- Baseplate wax
- Separating medium with brush
- Mixing container
- Laboratory knife and scissors
- Laboratory spatula
- Tongue blade
- Wax spatula #7
- Warm water or laboratory torch
- Petroleum jelly
- Glass jar with lid or wax-lined paper cup
- Appropriate tray adhesive
- Acrylic bur or similar rotary instrument
- Old toothbrush

Procedure 35–7 Fabricating a Self-Curing Acrylic Custom Tray (Continued)

Preparing the Model

1. Put on appropriate PPE.

2. Fill any undercuts on the patient diagnostic cast.

3. Use a pencil to outline the outer margin of the tray onto the diagnostic cast (Figure P35-7-2).

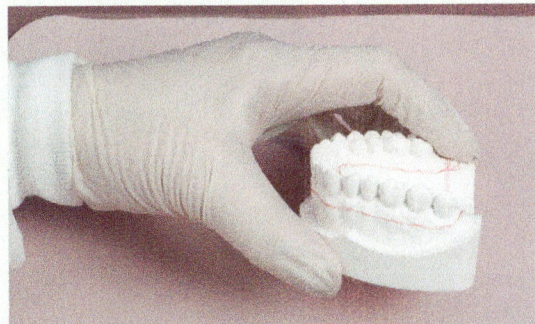

Figure P35-7-2

4. Place the baseplate wax spacer onto the model.

5. Use heat to soften the wax and seal the spacer to the model.

6. Use a laboratory knife and an angle cut to trim the spacer to fit the outline.

7. Cut appropriate stops into the spacer to allow for the impression material.

8. Paint the spacer and the surrounding area with separating medium.

Mixing the Resin

Mixing acrylic resin according to manufacturer's instructions is essential. Fumes from the mixture are toxic and, in the absence of adequate precaution, can drift throughout the dental office. When working with acrylic resin, use a ventilation system, if available.

1. Measure the monomer and polymer into a wax-lined paper mixing cup.

2. Add an equal part water.

3. Stir the mixture with a tongue blade until uniformly mixed.

4. Allow the mixture to go through polymerization for 2 to 3 minutes.

5. Some manufacturers recommend covering the mixing cup during this time.

Contouring the Custom Tray

1. After initial polymerization, the material is ready for contouring when it is no longer sticky. Spread petroleum jelly over the palms of your hands and gather the material into a ball.

2. Use your fingers to knead the material further.

3. Set aside a small amount of material to construct a handle for the tray.

4. Divide the remaining material into a "patty" for the maxillary arch or a "roll" for the mandibular arch.

5. For the maxillary arch, place a patty of material over the maxillary cast to cover the wax spacer and extend 1 to 2 mm beyond it.

6. For the mandibular arch, place a roll of material over the mandibular cast and extend it 1 to 2 mm beyond the wax spacer.

7. Take the material set aside for a handle and shape it to fit.

8. Place a drop of the monomer liquid onto both the handle tip and the midline area of the tray where you will place it.

9. Extend the handle directly outward for a patient with existing teeth. For a patient without existing teeth, extend the handle up and then outward.

10. Press the handle to the custom tray until the handle is firmly affixed. (Figure P35-7-3)

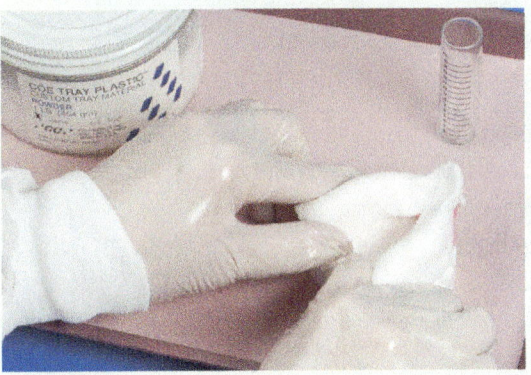

Figure P35-7-3

Finishing the Custom Tray

1. Wait 8 to 10 minutes before removing the tray from the model cast and taking out the baseplate wax spacer.

2. Use hot running water, a wax spatula, and an old toothbrush to remove any remaining wax from the finished tray.

3. Wait a minimum of 30 minutes for the acrylic to finally set.

4. Trim the edges of the tray with an acrylic bur or similar instrument. Do not trim the inside of the tray (Figure P35-7-4).

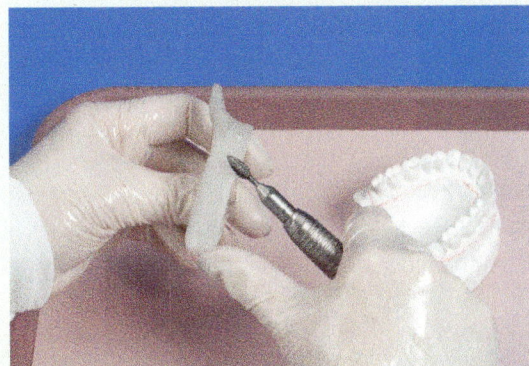

Figure P35-7-4

5. Clean and disinfect the tray according to the manufacturer's instructions.

6. Write the patient's name on the tray.

7. Apply appropriate adhesive provided by the manufacturer along the inside and edges of the tray.

Procedure 35–8 Fabricating a Light-Cured Resin Custom Tray

Materials needed (Figure P35-8-1):

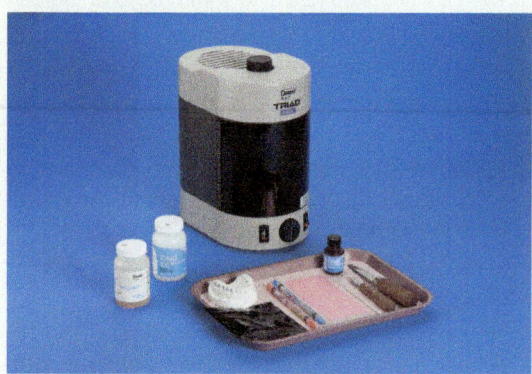

Figure P35-8-1

- Patient diagnostic model
- Light-curing system
- Black or red/blue pencil
- Tray material
- Baseplate wax
- Separating medium with brush
- Laboratory knife
- Barrier coating
- Spatula

Preparing the Diagnostic Model

1. Put on appropriate PPE.
2. Use a pencil to outline the tray border onto model.
3. Paint the model with separating medium.
4. Place the baseplate wax spacer onto the model.
5. Use heat to soften the wax and seal the spacer to the model.
6. Use a laboratory knife and an angle cut to trim the spacer to fit the outline.
7. Cut appropriate stops into the spacer to allow for the impression material.
8. Paint the spacer and the surrounding area with the separating medium.
9. Lay a precut sheet of tray material onto the model.
10. Adapt and contour the material to fit the maxillary or mandibular model (Figure P35-8-2).
11. Push the material through the "occlusal stop" areas to facilitate contact with occlusal surfaces.
12. Trim excess tray material away with laboratory knife.

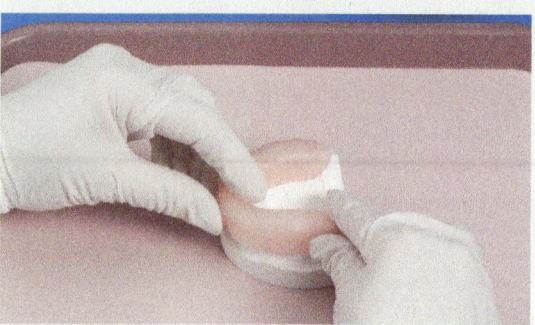

Figure P35-8-2

13. Use the excess material to form a handle for the tray (Figure P35-8-3).

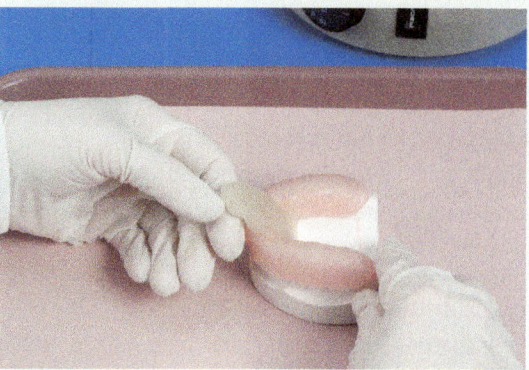

Figure P35-8-3

Preparing the Light-Curing Tray

1. Place the patient model with the tray material into the light-curing unit (Figure P35-8-4).

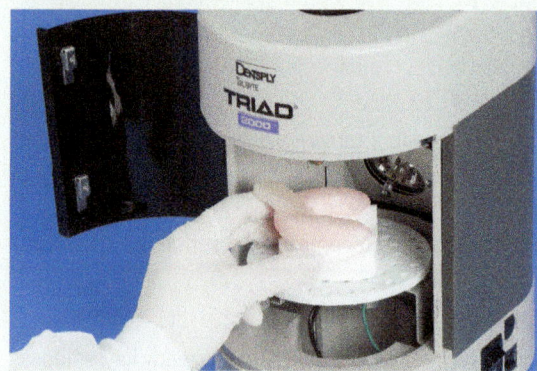

Figure P35-8-4

2. Leave it in the unit for 2 minutes to cure.
3. Remove it from the unit and rinse under cool running water.
4. Separate the model from the newly cured tray (Figure P35-8-5).

Procedure 35-8 Fabricating a Light-Cured Resin Custom Tray (Continued)

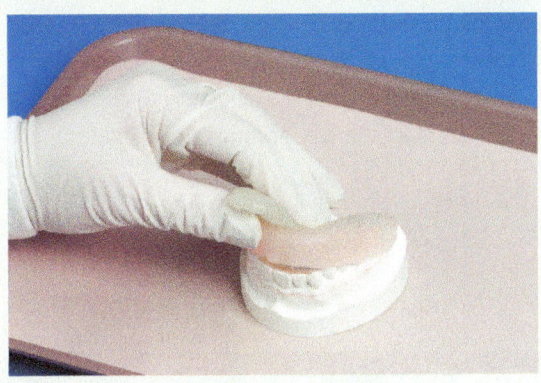

Figure P35-8-5

5. Using a wax spatula, gently remove the spacer wax from the tray.
6. Use hot water to remove any remaining wax from the interior of the tray.
7. Trim the borders of the tray with an acrylic bur.
8. If desired, use a thin acrylic bur to create perforations in the tray.
9. Clean and disinfect the tray according to the manufacturer's instructions.

Procedure 35-9 Fabricating a Vacuum-Formed Acrylic Resin Custom Tray

Materials needed (Figure P35-9-1):

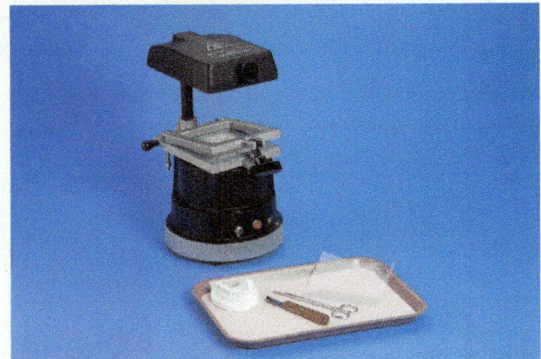

Figure P35-9-1

- Diagnostic patient cast of maxillary or mandibular arch
- Laboratory knife and scissors
- Vacuum former
- Acrylic custom tray sheet
- Bunsen burner
- Baseplate wax (if necessary)

Preparing the Cast

Soak the cast in warm water for up to 30 minutes before beginning procedure. Doing so eliminates small air bubbles that can otherwise rise to the surface during the remainder of the procedure and compromise the accuracy of the custom tray.

1. Put on appropriate PPE.
2. Place a spacer onto the cast, if necessary.
3. Mark the desired outline of the tray onto the cast.

Creating the Tray

1. Place the cast onto the platform of the vacuum-forming unit.
2. Select an appropriate acrylic resin sheet.
3. Place the sheet between the unit's heater frame and gasket frame.
4. Tighten the anterior knob of the unit to secure the material in place.
5. Confirm the position of the heating element above the acrylic sheet.
6. Turn on the heating element.
7. Carefully observe the acrylic sheet as it heats.
8. When the acrylic sheet has begun to "droop" approximately 1 inch, lower the frame containing it over the cast (Figure P35-9-2).

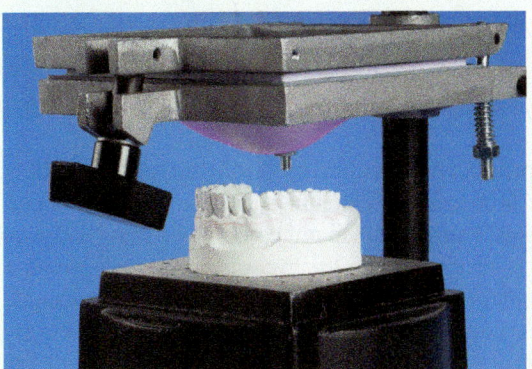

Figure P35-9-2

Procedure 35–9 **Fabricating a Vacuum-Formed Acrylic Resin Custom Tray (Continued)**

9. Turn on the vacuum forming unit once the sheet is positioned over the cast.

10. Turn off the heating element.

11. Allow the vacuum to form for 1 to 2 minutes.

Finishing the Tray

1. After the acrylic material has cooled, remove it from the vacuum forming unit.

2. Separate the new custom tray from the cast.

3. Use laboratory scissors to trim away excess material.

4. Affix a handle to the tray using a laboratory torch.

5. Clean and disinfect the tray according to manufacturer's instructions.

6. Write the patient's name on it.

Procedure 35–10 **Fabricating a Thermal Bead Custom Tray**

Materials needed:

- A cup of hot water (155°F to 185°F)
- Prepackaged thermal beads with measuring cup
- Patient diagnostic model
- Spacer material, if needed
- Laboratory handpiece and burs
- Laboratory torch
- Thermal plastic molding sticks

Preparing the Tray

1. Put on appropriate PPE.

2. Measure the manufacturer recommended amount of hydroplastic beads into a cup of hot water.

3. Wait 1 minute while the beads form a soft putty-like material.

4. Remove the material from the cup and knead briefly.

5. Apply the manufacturer's provided spacer material, if necessary.

6. Contour the material onto the patient diagnostic model.

Finishing the Tray

1. The material will harden after 5 minutes in the open air. If necessary, the material will harden instantly under cold running water.

2. Remove the material from the patient diagnostic model.

3. Trim away excess material or overextensions with laboratory handpiece and acrylic burs.

4. Warm and soften with a laboratory torch if other adjustments are necessary.

CHECKPOINT

35-15 Which dental wax is typically used to create a wax bite registration?

- Laboratory stone
- Orthodontic stone
- Die stone
- High-strength die stone

Gypsum Materials

Gypsum products are widely used to make dental models. **Gypsum** is a form of calcium sulfate, a naturally occurring mineral. During the manufacturing process most of the water is removed from the gypsum to create a powder-like substance. All dental gypsum products are packaged in a plastic bag or container to prevent contamination by unwanted moisture. Adding water back into the powder in the dental laboratory results in gypsum impression materials, sometimes referred to as "plaster of Paris." Dentistry typically uses six types of gypsum products, which vary by strength, durability, uses, setting time, and powder-to-water ratio.

- Impression plaster
- Model plaster

Powder-to-Water Ratio

Gypsum products are characterized by the size of crystals in the powder and by how much water must be added to create the intended products. This "recipe" for gypsum products is called the powder-to-water ratio, or P/W ratio. It determines how strong and durable the resulting product will be. Gypsum products requiring more water in their preparation are significantly weaker than those requiring less. The P/W ratios and other characteristics of the six main types of gypsum products used in dentistry are shown in Table 35-1.

Note that measurements of water and powder must be exact. If too much water is used, the mix will be thin and runny. If too little water is used, the powder and water will not mix sufficiently or properly. As with alginate, the temperature of the water influences the setting time of the gypsum product.

TABLE 35-1 Gypsum Products

GYPSUM TYPE	NAME	P/W RATIO	COLOR	USES
Type I	Impression plaster (rarely used today)	100 g to 60 mL	White	Mounting casts onto articulator; repairing casts
Type II	Model plaster	100 g to 50 mL	White	Preliminary impressions and study models
Type III	Laboratory stone	100 g to 30 mL	Yellow	Articulating models for partial and full dentures
Type IV	Die stone	100 g to 24 mL	White Variety of colors	Dies for bridges, crowns, and indirect restorations
Type V	High-strength die stone	100 g to 18–22 mL	White Variety of colors	Strongest gypsum available
No type	Orthodontic stone (mix of model plaster and laboratory stone)	100 g to 40 mL	White	Orthodontic treatment and diagnosis

Procedure 35-11 Mixing Gypsum for Models

Materials needed (Figure P35-11-1):

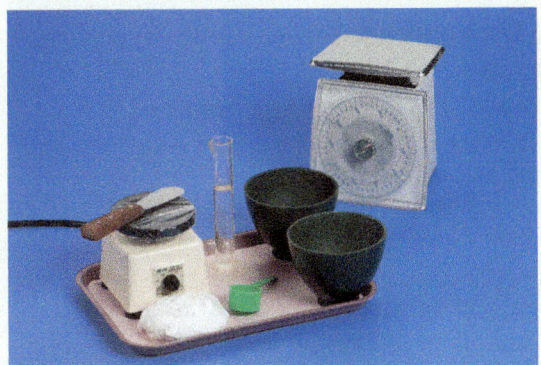

Figure P35-11-1

- Sturdy metal laboratory spatula
- Two rubber mixing bowls
- Laboratory scale
- Gypsum
- Powder measuring cup
- Room temperature water
- Liquid measuring cup
- Laboratory vibrator with disposable cover on platform

Mixing the Plaster

1. Put on appropriate PPE.
2. Measure the indicated amount of water into a rubber mixing bowl.
3. Set a second bowl onto the laboratory scale and set the scale to zero (Figure P35-11-2).

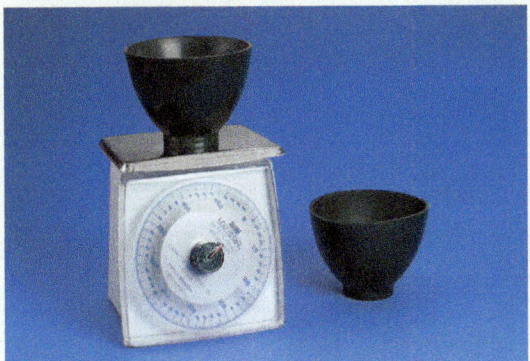

Figure P35-11-2

4. Measure 100 g of gypsum into the second bowl.
5. Remove the bowl from the scale and add the powder to the water in the first mixing bowl.
6. Wait several seconds for the powder to dissolve.
7. Mix the material together slowly with a spatula for approximately 1 minute.

Procedure 35–11 Mixing Plaster for Models (Continued)

8. Lift the bowl to the vibrator platform and set the unit on slow-to-medium speed (Figure P35-11-3).

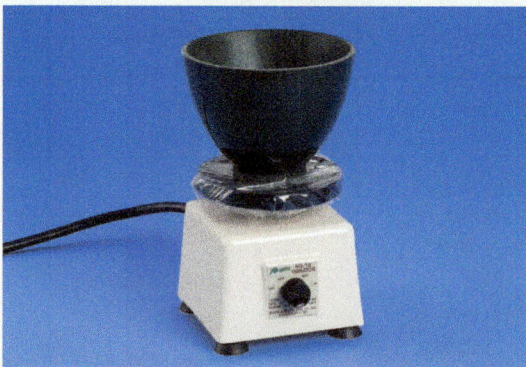

Figure P35-11-3

9. Rotate the bowl slowly on the platform for approximately 2 minutes.

10. The gypsum is ready when it appears smooth and creamy (Figure P35-11-4).

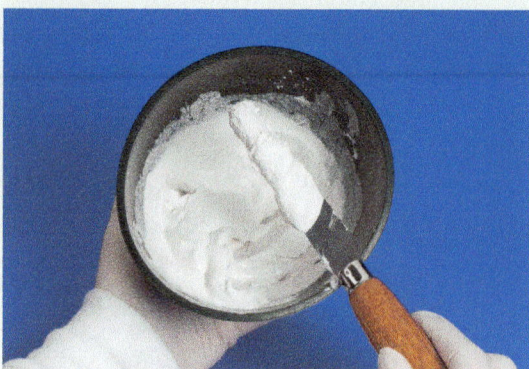

Figure P35-11-4

11. Test the mixture by holding a spoonful on the end of the spatula. An adequately mixed plaster with correct powder-to-water ratio will remain in place on the spatula.

Procedure 35–12 Pouring the Anatomic Portion of a Study Model

Pouring the anatomical portion of a study model is the first step in what is known as the "two-step" pour. The second step, described in the next procedure, Pouring the Base of a Study Model, will form the base of the model.

Materials needed (Figure P35-12-1):

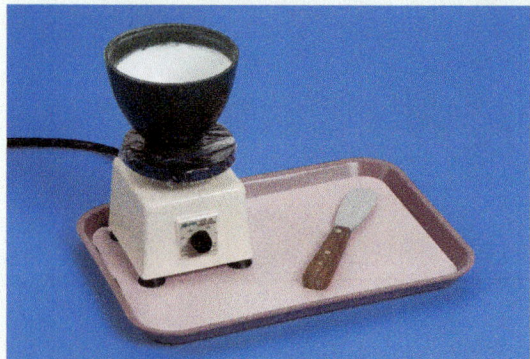

Figure P35-12-1

- Sturdy metal laboratory spatula
- Mixed dental plaster or stone
- Laboratory vibrator with disposable cover on platform

Pouring the Impression

1. Put on appropriate PPE.
2. Turn the vibrator to low or medium speed.
3. Set the impression tray on the vibrator platform and hold the impression by its handle.
4. Take a small amount of prepared plaster and add it to one end of the arch.
5. Watch as the vibration helps the plaster or stone flow smoothly into and fill the negative spaces of the impression.
6. As plaster continues to flow toward impressions of the anterior teeth, continue to add small amounts of plaster to the impression (Figure P35-12-2).

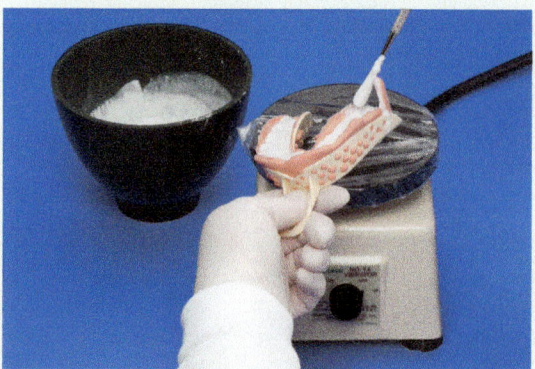

Figure P35-12-2

Procedure 35–12 Pouring the Anatomic Portion of a Study Model (Continued)

7. Rotate the impression as it sits on the vibrator platform.

8. Continue adding material until the plaster has filled in anatomical details and flows out of the opposite end of the impression (Figure P35-12-3).

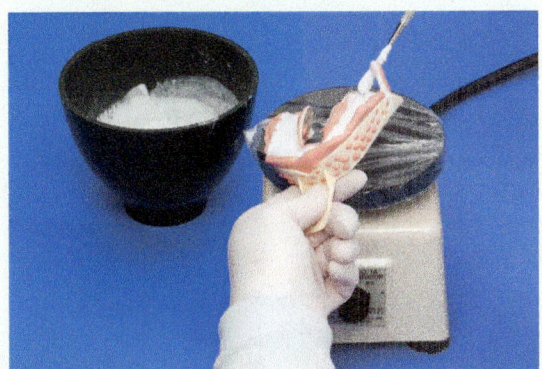

Figure P35-12-3

9. Remove the impression from the vibrator platform.

10. Add larger amounts of plaster to completely fill the impression (Figure P35-12-4).

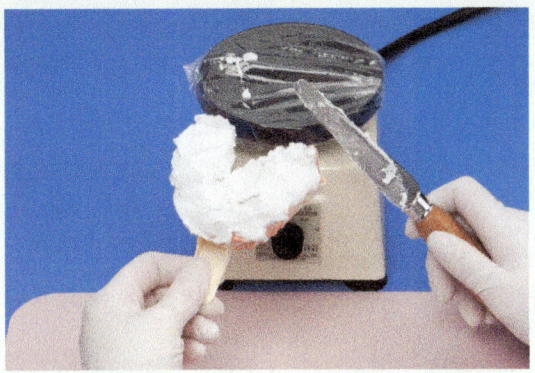

Figure P35-12-4

11. Return the plaster-filled impression to the vibrator platform and allow it to vibrate slightly.

12. Remove the filled impression from the vibrator platform and allow it to set for 5 to 10 minutes.

13. If you will be adding additional plaster to form a base for the model, leave blobs of plaster material in place along the top of the impression.

Procedure 35–13 Pouring the Base of a Study Model

Materials needed (Figure P35-13-1):

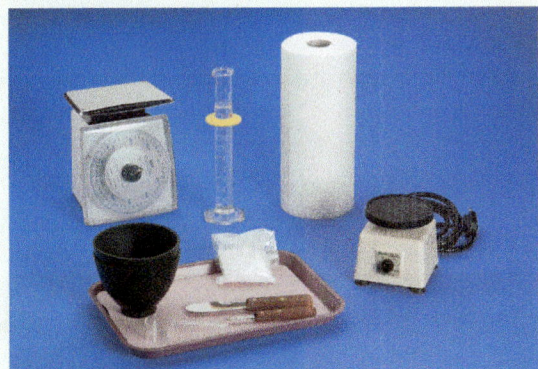

Figure P35-13-1

- Sturdy metal laboratory spatula
- Two rubber mixing bowls
- Laboratory vibrator with disposable cover on platform
- Paper towels
- Plaster or stone powder
- Powder measuring cup
- Room temperature water
- Liquid measuring cup
- Laboratory knife

Preparing for the Second Pour

1. Put on appropriate PPE.

2. Wipe the rubber bowls and laboratory spatula clean of previous plaster mix.

3. Wash and dry the bowls and spatula.

4. Measure *slightly less* than the indicated amount of water into the first rubber mixing bowl.

5. Set the second bowl onto a laboratory scale and set the scale to zero.

6. Measure 100 g of plaster or stone into the second bowl.

7. Remove the bowl from the scale and add the powder to the water in the first mixing bowl.

8. Wait several seconds for the powder to dissolve.

9. Mix the material together slowly with the spatula for approximately 1 minute.

10. Lift the bowl to the vibrator platform and set the unit on slow-to-medium speed.

11. Rotate the bowl slowly on the platform for approximately 2 minutes.

12. The mix is ready when it appears smooth and creamy.

13. Test the mixture by holding a spoonful on the end of a spatula. An adequately mixed plaster with correct powder-to-water ratio will remain in place on the spatula.

14. This mix will appear *thicker* than the plaster mixed to form the anatomical portion of the model.

Procedure 35-13 **Pouring the Base of a Study Model (Continued)**

Pouring to Form the Base

1. Gather the mixed plaster or stone onto a glass slab or paper towel.

2. Do not allow the material to spread out.

3. Turn the anatomical portion of the impression upside down onto the base.

4. Hold the tray and impression steady, with the tray handle parallel to the glass slab or paper towel.

5. Using a spatula, combine the impression and base by filling in any voids.

6. Wipe excess material away from the tray margins.

7. Allow the model to set for 40 to 60 minutes (Figure P35-13-2).

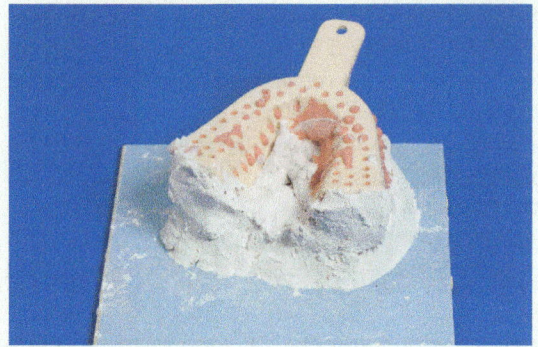

Figure P35-13-2

Removing the Plaster Model from the Impression

1. Use a laboratory knife to remove any excess material from the margins of the tray.

2. Hold the handle of the impression tray and lift the tray upward.

3. If the tray does not lift off immediately, examine it for areas of sticking plaster or stone.

4. If necessary, remove the sticking plaster or stone.

5. Do not wiggle the tray from side-to-side or lift it sideways in an attempt to dislodge it.

6. Continue lifting straight upward until tray is lifted free of the model. (Figure P35-13-3)

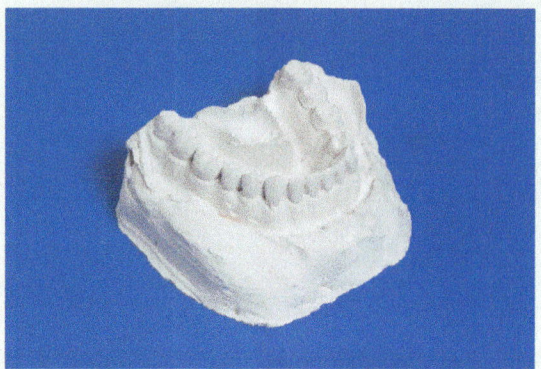

Figure P35-13-3

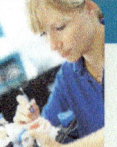

Voice of Experience

When removing an impression, have a 4 × 8 inch ceramic tile ready. Inverting the model onto the tile's smooth surface will allow an easy separation. Rinse the model under cool running water, and it will immediately slide off the tile for separation.

CHECKPOINT

35-16 Identify the six types of gypsum products commonly used in dentistry.

Procedure 35-14 **Trimming, Finishing, and Polishing Study Models**

Materials needed (Figure P35-14-1):

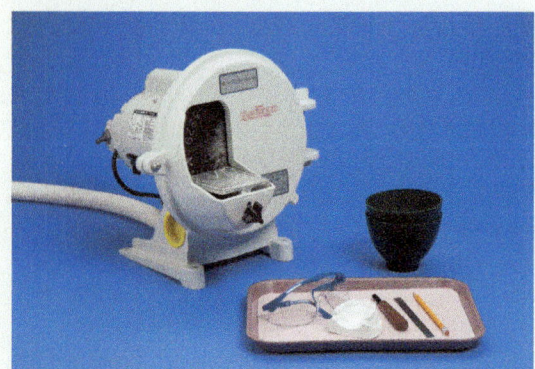

Figure P35-14-1

- Poured and set study models
- Safety goggles
- Model trimmer
- Two mixing bowls
- Laboratory knife
- Pencil
- Ruler
- Spray gloss

Prepare for Trimming

1. Put on appropriate PPE.

2. Dampen dry models by soaking in a bowl of warm water for 5 minutes.

Procedure 35-14 Trimming, Finishing, and Polishing Study Models (Continued)

3. Put on safety goggles.
4. Turn on the model trimmer.
5. Confirm that an adequate amount of water is running over the grinding wheel.

Trimming the Maxillary Arch Model

1. Lay the maxillary model onto the counter top with the anatomical impression side facing down.
2. Draw a line around the model 1¼ inch up from the bottom (Figure P35-14-2).

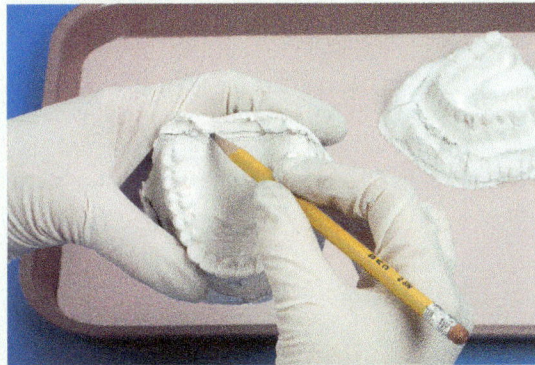

Figure P35-14-2

3. Hold the model firmly against the trimmer.
4. Keep the heels of your hands on the countertop and your fingers away from the wheel.
5. Trim the model base down to the previously drawn line (Figure P35-14-3).

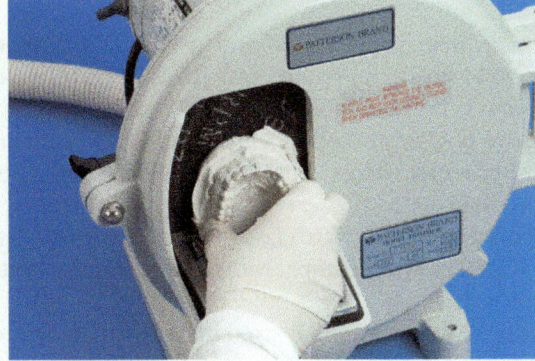

Figure P35-14-3

6. Draw another line ¼ inch behind the arch's maxillary tuberosities.
7. Trim the posterior portion of the model to this line.
8. Draw a third line down the center of the model's occlusal ridges.

9. Measure ¼ inch toward the model's outer edge and draw another line.
10. Trim the model's side to this line, using care not to trim away the mucobuccal fold.
11. Draw a line down the center of the occlusal ridge on the opposite side of the model.
12. Measure ¼ inch toward the model's outer edge and draw another line.
13. Trim the model's remaining side to this line, using care not to trim away the mucobuccal fold.
14. Draw a line at each of the model's heels that is perpendicular to the canine tooth on that side.
15. Trim each heel of the model to that line.
16. Finally, on the occlusal surface of the model, draw an angled line on each side from the canine teeth to the midline (Figure P35-14-4).

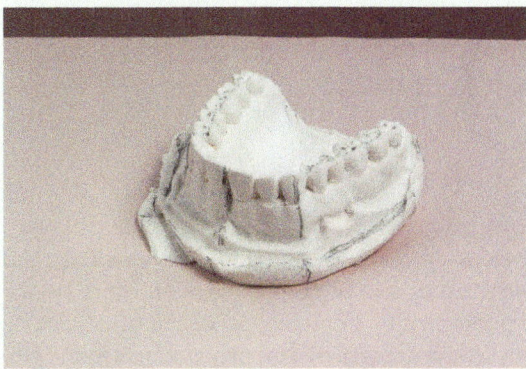

Figure P35-14-4

17. Trim the front of the model to this line.
18. Take care not to trim away protruding teeth.

Trimming the Mandibular Arch Model

Use the trimmed maxillary arch as a model for trimming the mandibular arch.

1. Join the mandibular and maxillary arches in correct occlusion.
2. Trim the posterior portion of the mandibular arch until it is even with the maxillary model.
3. Place the maxillary base on the countertop and measure 3 inch from the top surface.
4. Draw a line around the base of the mandibular arch at this point.
5. Trim the mandibular base to the line drawn.
6. Trim the lateral cuts on the mandibular base to match those on the maxillary base.

Procedure 35-14 Trimming, Finishing, and Polishing Study Models (Continued)

7. Trim the mandibular heel cuts to match those on the maxillary arch.

8. Trim and round out the anterior of the mandibular arch from right canine to left canine.

9. Confirm that the maxillary and mandibular arches can remain in correct occlusion.

Finishing the Study Models

1. Fill voids in either arch with a slurry of newly mixed plaster.

2. Use a laboratory knife to trim away beads of excess plaster.

Polishing the Study Models

1. Spray the models with gloss.

2. Buff the surface with dry cloth (Figure P35-14-5).

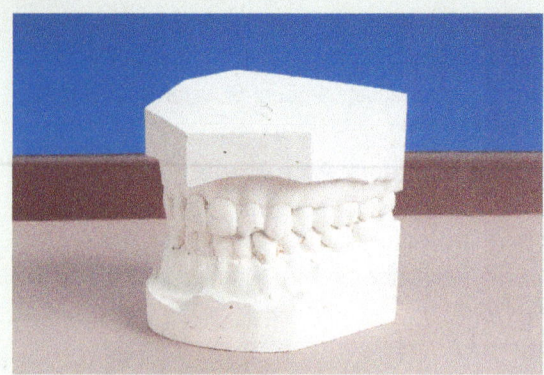

Figure P35-14-5

3. Label both the mandibular and maxillary arches with the patient's name and the date of the model.

4. In an orthodontic practice, include a pediatric patient's age.

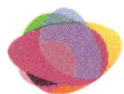 ## Chapter Highlights

◆ Dental offices typically include a laboratory area. Tasks and procedures that cannot be completed in the office laboratory are performed by a commercial dental laboratory.

◆ Common tasks a dental assistant may perform in the laboratory include pouring preliminary impressions, trimming and finishing diagnostic models, preparing custom impression trays, and polishing certain restorations.

◆ Safety is of primary importance in the dental laboratory. Following infection control procedures, operating equipment according to manufacturer's instructions, handling chemicals correctly, preventing and extinguishing fires, and reporting any accidents to the dentist promptly are all essential.

◆ A dental office laboratory typically is furnished with countertops and cabinets, as well as wall-mounted covered bins holding bulk supplies. Typical laboratory equipment includes heat sources, model trimmers, dental lathes, and laboratory handpieces. More specialized equipment includes the laboratory vibrator, the vacuum former, and the articulator.

◆ Impressions are the first step in creating patient casts. The accuracy of study casts and models varies with the type of impression used to create them. A dentist instructs the dental assistant on what type of impression to obtain depending on the accuracy required.

◆ Hydrocolloid is most commonly used to obtain an impression. Alginate provides sufficient accuracy for most study casts and primary models but does not have the greatest accuracy.

◆ Elastomeric impression materials are preferred when accuracy of the impression is especially important. Elastomeric materials include polysulfide, silicone, and polyether.

◆ Impression material is mixed and prepared and then transferred into an impression tray that is inserted into the patient's mouth to obtain the impression.

◆ Curing, or polymerization, occurs when chemical and physical processes cause a plastic to change from a pliable to a rigid state.

◆ Waxes used in dentistry are classified in three broad categories: pattern waxes, impression waxes, and processing waxes.

◆ Gypsum products are widely used in dentistry to create dental models. Six types of plaster are commonly available, varying by strength, durability, uses, setting time, and powder-to-water ratio. These are impression plaster, model plaster, laboratory stone, orthodontic stone, die stone, and high-strength die stone.

◆ Gypsum products differ according to the size of crystals in the powder and how much water is added. This recipe for gypsum products is called the powder-to-water ratio, or P/W ratio. Gypsum products requiring more water in their preparation are significantly weaker than those requiring less.

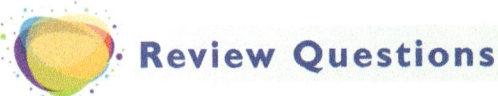

Review Questions

1. Dental models are poured using which of the following materials?

   a. Stone or plaster

   b. Thermoplastic

   c. Wax

   d. Alginate

2. A dental laboratory vibrator is used to remove air bubbles from

   a. Alginate impressions.

   b. Custom trays.

   c. Self-curing resins.

   d. Stone and plaster mixes.

3. Gold in a gold-noble alloy provides castings with which of the following characteristics?

   a. Enhanced appearance

   b. Durability

   c. Resistance to corrosion and tarnish

   d. Patient comfort

4. A dentist may ask for an impression made from an elastomeric material when

   a. Accurate detail is not needed.

   b. Accurate detail is essential.

   c. Setting time needs to be short.

   d. The impression will not be "poured up" immediately.

5. With what materials might stock trays be adjusted to fit a particular patient better?

   a. Plaster or stone

   b. Polysulfide or sulfide

   c. Dental wax or thermoplastic

   d. "Rubber base" or acrylic resin

6. The sheet of acrylic resin used to create a vacuum-formed custom tray is softened by which of the following means?

   a. Warm water

   b. Heat source

   c. Vibration

   d. Polymerization

7. Which of the following is *not* required when constructing custom trays out of thermoplastic beads?

   a. Hot tap water

   b. Polymerization

   c. Accurate patient model

   d. Laboratory torch

8. Inform a patient of what to expect during an impression procedure by discussing which of the following?

   a. The impression material's taste, temperature, and setting time

   b. Side effects of the material

   c. The purpose of the procedure

   d. What the poured model will look like

9. Dental waxes are classified by which of the following purposes?

   a. Bite registration and extension waxes

   b. Impression, pattern, and processing waxes

   c. Tray and boxing waxes

   d. Casting and inlay waxes

10. The strength of gypsum products used in dentistry is determined by the size of crystals in the gypsum powder and by the

    a. Powder-to-water ratio.

    b. Purpose for which the gypsum is intended.

    c. Polymerization process used.

    d. Quality of the natural gypsum from which the material was manufactured.

Active Learning Exercises

1. What is the purpose of the vacuum former? What steps need to be taken to prepare the model?

2. Describe the differences in function between a bite registration and an articulator.

3. Imagine that upon removing an impression from a patient's mouth, you realize the patient has moved and you become concerned that the impression may be compromised. How can this be avoided?

Application Activities

1. Using the Internet or the library, research new alginate materials that can be used to obtain impressions. Select one new material and write a paragraph or two describing the product, outlining its benefits and drawbacks.

2. Practice describing the alginate impression process for patients. Pretend that you are preparing to obtain an alginate impression for a patient, and develop a basic overview that outlines what a patient should expect during the process.

PREPARING FOR CERTIFICATION EXAMS

Review the following topics in this chapter to prepare for the Dental Assisting National Board (DANB) exam:

- **Introduction**
- **Biohazards and Infection Control**
- **Impression Materials and Techniques**
- **Alginate**
- **Elastomeric Materials**
- **Impression Trays**
- **Dental Waxes**
- **Utility Wax**
- **Sticky Wax**
- **Boxing Wax**
- **Casting Wax**
- **Baseplate Wax**
- **Bite Registration Wax**
- **Gypsum Materials**

part IX

Assisting in Dental Procedures

Assisting in Restorations

CHAPTER OUTLINE

CHAPTER CHECKLIST

On completion of this chapter, students will be able to:

- ☑ Identify and use the terminology used to describe cavity preparation.
- ☑ Describe the steps involved in preparing a site for restoration.
- ☑ Describe the various permanent restoration procedures outlined in the chapter.
- ☑ Describe the various matrix systems outlined in the chapter.
- ☑ Explain the role of the dental assistant during common restoration procedures.
- ☑ Identify situations in which an intermediate restoration is appropriate.

KEY TERMS

axial (AK-see-ul) wall – the internal wall of a cavity running parallel to the tooth's long axis

cavity wall – the internal surface of the restoration

cavosurface (kay-voh-SUR-fus) margin – the intersection between the cavity and the healthy surface of a tooth

convenience form – alterations in the shape of a cavity preparation to allow removal of decay and to enable proper instrumentation for cavity preparation and insertion of a dental restoration

dentinal (DEN-tun-ul) wall – an external wall that includes dentin

enamel wall – an external wall that includes enamel

external wall – the surface of the cavity that extends to the tooth surface; usually identified by its location, such as medial, distal, lingual, facial, and gingival

gingival (jin-JIH-vul) wall – the internal wall nearest the gingiva, running perpendicular to the long axis of the tooth

internal wall – the wall of the cavity that does not extend to the tooth surface

line angle – in a cavity preparation, the angle formed when two walls or surfaces intersect

outline form – the shape of the tooth surface area included within the cavosurface margins of a cavity preparation of a dental restoration

point angle – the junction of three surfaces

pulpal (PUL-pul) wall – the internal wall that runs perpendicular to the long axis of the tooth, usually covering the tooth pulp; also called the floor or pulpal floor

resistance form – the shape given to a cavity preparation that enables a dental restoration to withstand masticatory forces

retention form – the shape of a cavity preparation that prevents displacement of a dental restoration by lateral or tipping forces as well as masticatory forces

Introduction

Dental restorations are a foundation of modern dentistry. As opposed to aesthetic dentistry, which is concerned with the appearance of the teeth, restorative dentistry's aim is to restore teeth to the original state by replacing diseased and decayed matter with the appropriate dental materials.

Dental assistants play a very important role in restorative dentistry. Your job as a dental assistant might include helping to take dental radiographs and setting up for procedures, controlling moisture and transferring instruments, mixing and preparing materials, and maintaining proper infection control to protect the patient and the dental staff.

Even though only dentists can diagnose conditions that require a restoration, dental assistants still need to be familiar with the procedures and materials used during restorations. Dental assistants do well to anticipate the dentist's and patient's needs, making the procedure faster, more efficient, and smoother for everyone involved.

Cultural Diversity

Among some cultures and faiths, such as Muslim, the addition to or removal of any part of the body, including teeth, is forbidden unless because of a defect. Conversely, in some cultures, patients adorn or replace their teeth with gold or jewels as a sign of their status and wealth. Knowing how to convincingly explain the need for a tooth extraction or restoration to one patient and respecting another's choice for adornment is essential. This kind of cultural sensitivity can help you help the patient make educated decisions about oral health.

Cavity Preparation

A number of conditions might require a permanent restoration, including:

- Recurring caries
- Old or broken restorations
- Worn down tooth structure

Once the dentist has diagnosed one of these conditions, the patient will likely be scheduled for a restorative procedure. Restorations range in complexity from relatively simple single-surface restorations to more complicated multisurface restorations.

Before the restoration can be performed, the cavity site must be prepared. Cavity preparation is performed by the dentist and requires specialized knowledge about the anatomy and structure of the tooth. This includes knowing the unique properties of the tooth enamel, the dentin, the tooth pulp, and the tooth crown. Any or all of these might be affected by the restoration, so the dentist will have to take all of these factors into account during preparation.

Preparation Terminology

A number of terms are used to describe the tooth anatomy and the resulting preparation. These terms describe the walls, lines, and angles that are formed as the dentist cuts away diseased tooth structure or old restorative material and creates a space for a new preparation. They include:

- **Cavity wall**: The internal surface of the restoration space
- **Internal wall**: A cavity wall that does not extend all the way to the external tooth surface
- **External wall**: The surface that extends to the external tooth surface; these are used as descriptors based on their location, such as medial, distal, lingual, facial, and gingival
- **Axial wall**: An internal wall that runs parallel to the long surface of the tooth
- **Pulpal wall**: An internal wall that runs perpendicular to the long axis of the tooth, usually covering the tooth pulp; also called the floor or pulpal floor
- **Gingival wall**: An internal wall nearest the gingiva, running perpendicular to the long axis of the tooth
- **Enamel wall**: An external wall area that includes enamel
- **Dentinal wall**: An external wall area that includes dentin

The planes of these walls form lines. Where two or more lines meet, angles are formed. The following terms are used to describe the angles formed during restorative dentistry (Figure 36-1):

- **Line angle**: An angle formed by the intersection of two tooth surfaces, or walls. Line angles are described by combining the names of the two walls that intersect. For example, the line angle formed by the intersection of the lingual wall and the pulpal wall would be identified as the *lingopulpal angle*. It is important to understand and correctly use these terms as they describe the properties of the cavity preparation.

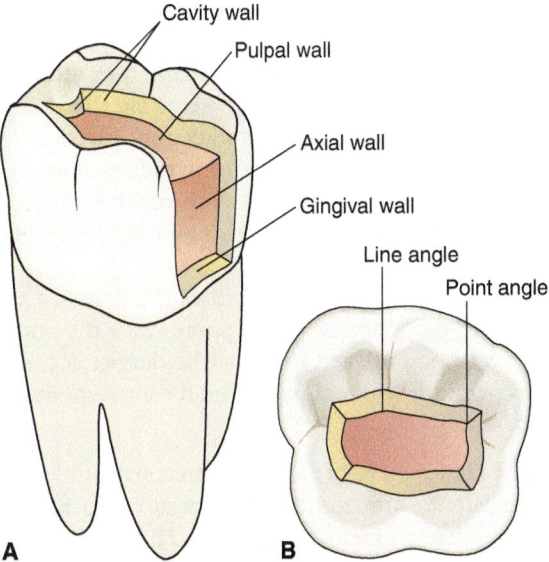

Figure 36–1 **Preparation terminology. A.** Tooth preparation walls. **B.** Tooth preparation angles.

■ **Point angle**: Points are formed when three or more tooth surfaces, or walls, intersect. They are also named according to the walls that form the angle, so the point angle formed by the intersection of the distal, lingual, and pulpal walls is called the *distolinguipulpal angle*.

Finally, the **cavosurface margin** is the intersection between the preparation surface and the normal, healthy tooth surface. It is very important for this area to be properly prepared. A loose cavosurface margin can result in leakages into the restoration, which can ruin the restoration. In some cases, the cavosurface margin will be slightly beveled to allow for a better restoration.

Planning for the Preparation

The actual preparation is performed by the dentist using a variety of instruments. You must be familiar with the necessary instruments and be prepared to transfer them to the dentist as needed. Dental instruments and instrument transfer are covered more completely in Chapter 26, Dental Instruments and Equipment.

To prepare a tooth for restoration, the dentist must remove all of the diseased tooth structure and any old restorative material in the cavity, leaving behind enough tooth to anchor the new restoration. To do this, the dentist follows a number of steps and takes into account specific factors that will ensure success.

These factors include:

■ **Outline form**. The shape and form of the cavity preparation, which is determined by the extent of healthy tooth material, the type of restorative material, and the necessary structures to bind the restorative material.
■ **Resistance form**. The internal shape of the restoration, taking into account the placement of the restoration and the stresses it will be subject to.
■ **Retention form**. The internal shape and structure of the restoration as it relates to securing the restoration in place. This can take into account physical elements, such as slightly undercutting the restoration to form an overhang, and other structures that might be necessary to help lock the restoration in place, such as fissures.
■ **Convenience form**. This describes the dentist's ease of access to the working area. In some cases, the outline form has to be enlarged to allow the dentist access to the preparation with enough room for instrumentation and materials.

Once these factors have been taken into consideration, the dentist is ready to prepare the actual restoration. Steps in the final preparation include (Figure 36-2):

■ Removing the tooth structure, old restorative material, or decay

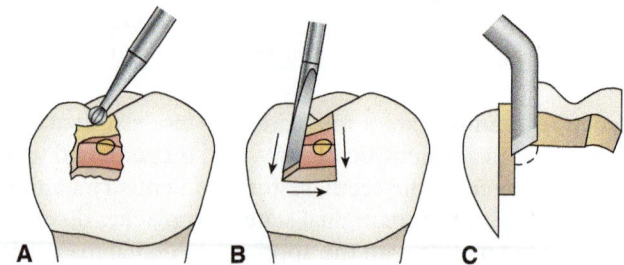

Figure 36–2 Steps of cavity preparation. (**A**) Open the cavity. (**B**) Outline the cavity. (**C**) Refine and finish the cavity.

■ Creating an optimal space for the restoration, which might include making retention notches, grooves, and other structures for restoration retention. In some cases, retention pins might be required
■ Cleaning the cavity to remove debris
■ Preparing the cavity if necessary through the addition of liners, cements, bases, and other materials
■ Maintaining moisture control with a rubber dam, cotton rolls, or other methods

✓ CHECKPOINTS

36-1 Where is the axial wall in a cavity preparation?

36-2 What is a point angle and how is it distinguished from a line angle?

36-3 Name the four forms that dentists consider while planning a restoration.

Restoration Procedures

Dental restorations are classified to make identification and discussion easier. Dental assistants must be familiar with the differences between the various types of restorations, including the instrumentation used in each procedure, the materials required, and the dentist's and patient's needs during the procedure.

Your role as the dental assistant depends in part on the specific legal requirements and regulations of your state. In states with expanded functions dental assistants, qualified dental assistants may be allowed to perform more complex tasks, such as placing bases, liners, and varnishes, or creating temporary restorations. In states without this function, the dental assistant helps the dentist perform these tasks.

Permanent Restorations

Permanent restorations range in complexity from simple and conservative to multisurface. Black's Classification of Cavities is a standard method of classifying the pattern and extent of decay (see Chapter 20, Oral Diagnosis and Treatment Planning). Before the procedure begins, the dentist diagnoses the cavity, plans the procedure, administers the anesthetic, and prepares the tooth for restoration.

Class I Restorations

Class I restorations are the simplest form of restorations. These lesions are located in the pits and fissures of teeth, without extending into the tooth's inner anatomy (Figure 36-3). Class I restorations typically occur in the following teeth:

- Premolars and molars, including the occlusal surfaces, buccal pits and fissures, and lingual pits and fissures. These areas can be very difficult to effectively clean, allowing for locally limited decay.
- Maxillary anterior teeth, including the lingual pits. These lesions are most often located near the cingulum.

Tooth preparation for a Class I restoration is typically simple. The dentist needs only remove the local decay on the pit, fissure, or groove where it is located. This is often done with a bur, which is used to create a shallow, smooth

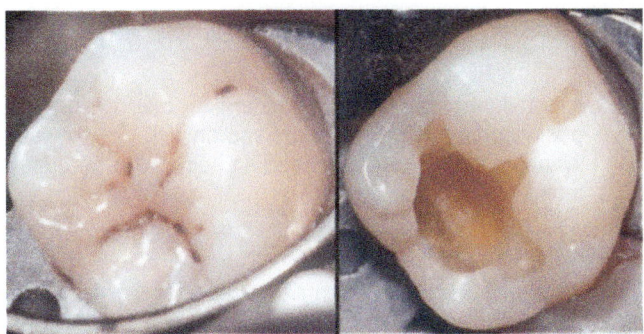

Figure 36–3 Class I lesion. Before (*left*) and after (*right*) preparation.

indentation in the enamel. Care is taken not to create angles that would complicate the restoration.

For a restoration on an occlusal surface, the dentist may use articulating paper before opening up the enamel to gauge how the occlusal surfaces meet. Ultimately, the goal is to restore the occlusal surfaces to a natural contour.

Procedure 36–1 Assisting with a Class I Restoration

Materials needed (Figure P36-1-1):

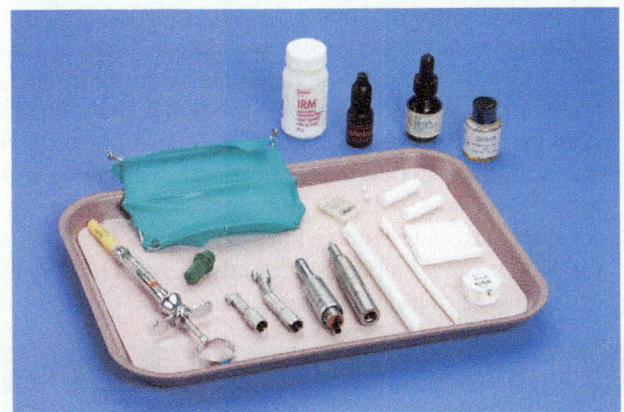

Figure P36-1-1

- Restorative tray setup
- Local anesthetic setup
- Dental dam setup
- High-volume evacuator (HVE)
- High-speed handpiece
- Low-speed handpiece
- Saliva ejector
- Burs, assorted
- Cotton pellets
- Cotton rolls
- Gauze (2 × 2-inch)
- Dental liners, bases, bonding agents, sealers

- Permanent restorative material (composite or amalgam)
- Dental floss

Tooth Preparation

1. Put on appropriate PPE.
2. Transfer the mouth mirror and explorer to the dentist for the initial examination of the tooth (Figure P36-1-2).

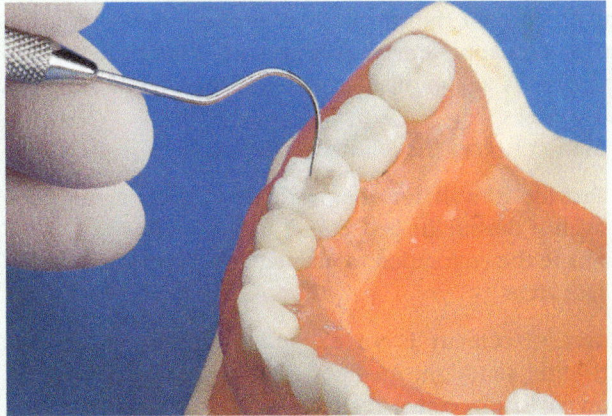

Figure P36-1-2

3. Where necessary, assist in the administration of anesthetic.
4. Apply moisture control and isolation measures, such as cotton rolls. In some cases, a dental dam may be used.

Cavity Preparation

1. Transfer the mouth mirror and high-speed handpiece with the appropriate cutting instrument to the dentist. For Class I restorations, burs are commonly used.

Procedure 36-1 Assisting with a Class I Restoration (Continued)

2. Assist during the tooth preparation by making sure the operating field is well lit, clean, and dry. Use the air-water syringe and HVE to apply water and air and, if necessary, retract the patient's tissues.

Placing Dental Materials

1. Prepare the necessary dental materials for transfer to the dentist. These materials might include bases, liners, or sealers, depending on the restoration and the dentist's preferences.

2. If necessary, assist with etching and bonding by transferring instruments and materials in the proper sequence.

3. Prepare the amalgam, if necessary, with the amalgamator, according to the manufacturer's instructions.

4. Prepare the composite, if necessary, according to the manufacturer's instructions.

Placing Restorative Materials

1. If using amalgam, transfer the amalgam to the dentist in the amalgam carrier, followed by a condenser for amalgam condensing.

2. Transfer the amalgam carrier and condensing instruments as needed until the restoration is filled.

3. Transfer burnishers as needed after the amalgam is filled.

4. If using composite, transfer the composite to the dentist as needed and prepare to transfer the curing light as necessary.

Finishing the Restoration

1. If using amalgam, transfer carvers as needed.

2. If using composite, transfer the high-speed handpiece and finishing burs as needed.

3. Use the HVE throughout the procedure to remove pieces of debris.

Checking for Proper Occlusion

1. After the restoration is placed, remove cotton rolls or other isolation devices and check the occlusal surfaces with articulating paper.

2. Transfer the high-speed handpiece and/or finishing burs to the dentist to adjust the occlusal surface.

3. Clean the new restoration with a cotton pellet or roll.

Matrix Systems with Class II, III, and IV Restorations

Class I restorations are the simplest and require the least amount of special instrumentation and set-up. Class II, III, and IV restorations are more complicated. These preparations sometimes require removal of one or more interproximal surfaces, which means there is no external wall to contain the restoration. In these cases, an artificial wall must be temporarily created during the restoration. This is accomplished through the use of matrices and wedges.

Matrices serve the following purposes:

1. Provide a wall for the restorative material to push against during the procedure

2. Shape the restoration to maintain proper proximal contact areas

Matrix placement is an expanded function. In states with this function, qualified dental assistants may be allowed to place matrices. In other states, dental assistants can assemble the matrix and assist the dentist during placement.

A matrix system includes the following components:

- *Retainer*. Retainers are secured to the tooth during a procedure to hold everything in place. Several types of retainers are available. The most common type, a Tofflemire retainer, is a metal device that firmly holds the band in place during posterior restorations.

- *Band*. The band is a narrow strip of stainless steel shaped into a circle and fitted around the tooth being restored. The band is held firmly in place by the retainer

and wedges. In anterior restorations, clear plastic strips are used without retainers.

- *Wedges*. Wedges are typically made from wood or plastic. They are used in Class II, III, and IV restorations to maintain the integrity of the restoration wall at the gingival margin. This prevents small amounts of restorative material from seeping out beneath the band and creating an overhang, which is potentially damaging to the sensitive gingival tissue and the restoration. In addition, the wedge must be placed properly to avoid impinging upon the restoration, called cupping.

Voice of Experience

When I first heard of matrices, the concept sounded a little confusing—but not anymore. Using a Tofflemire matrix can seem complicated at first, but practicing on a model or with the matrix alone can help you better understand how to use the device. Now that I've learned how to correctly assemble and place all different kinds of matrices, it allows us to provide faster, more efficient care for the patients in our office. The dentist's time is better spent elsewhere. This is why we now provide intensive training for all new dental assistants on assembling and placing matrices.

Posterior Matrix Systems (Tofflemire Matrix Systems)

Posterior restorations typically use the Tofflemire matrix system, which includes a metal retainer, thin stainless steel bands, and wedges (Figure 36-4). Also known as the universal matrix system, the Tofflemire is the most common matrix used in restorative dentistry.

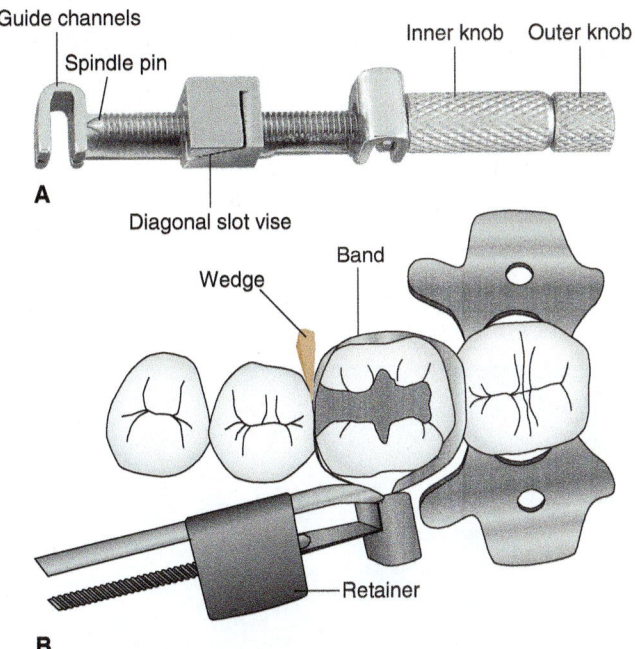

Figure 36–4 **Tofflemire system.** (**A**) Retainer. (**B**) Tofflemire system shown in place.

To place a Tofflemire matrix, the retainer is usually placed from the buccal side of the tooth, while the wedges are firmly inserted into the interproximal space from the lingual side.

Before placing the matrix, the band must first be selected and contoured. Contouring the band will make it more malleable and easier to place on the tooth. Bands are specially shaped so they fit the planned restoration. When the ends of the band are brought together, they form a circle with varying sizes, or circumferences. The smaller circumference edge always faces toward the gingiva, while the larger circumference edge always faces toward the occlusal surface.

After the band has been bent into shape, it is inserted into the diagonal slots on the retainer and positioned with the guide channels, and then it is screwed into place with the spindle pin. Once this is completed, the size of the loop can be adjusted using the inner knob on the retainer.

After the band has been properly adjusted, the retainer can be fastened to the tooth. The retainer handle is positioned so that it extends outside of the oral cavity. The band should extend approximately 1 mm below the gingival margin of the restoration and should not exceed the occlusal surface of the tooth by more than 2 mm.

Wedges are often positioned after the band is placed. Wedges are inserted firmly with cotton pliers or no. 110 pliers. Considerations include:

- The wedge must be tall enough to apply pressure across the face of the restoration, from the gingival and apical walls. Wedges come in four main sizes: small, slim, large, and wide base.
- The wedge should slightly separate the teeth.

Procedure 36–2 Assembling a Tofflemire Matrix System

Materials needed (Figure P36-2-1):

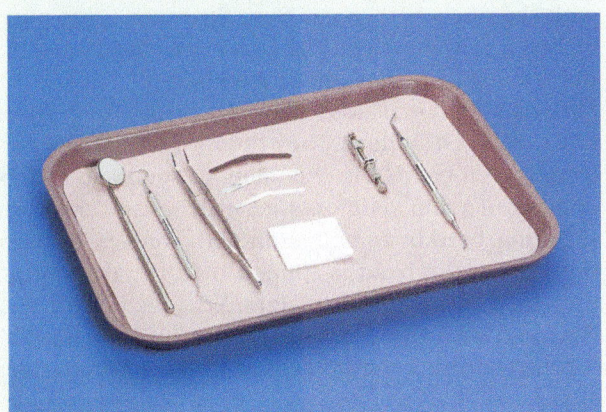

Figure P36-2-1

- Basic setup
- Universal retainer
- Matrix bands
- Paper pad
- Ball burnisher

1. Determine the size of the band to be used during the preparation. This is dictated by the outline of the cavity, including the tooth size and the depth of the preparation.

2. Contour the band by placing it on a piece of paper and rubbing its center with a burnisher (Figure P36-2-2). This creates a thin area where the interproximal contacts are located.

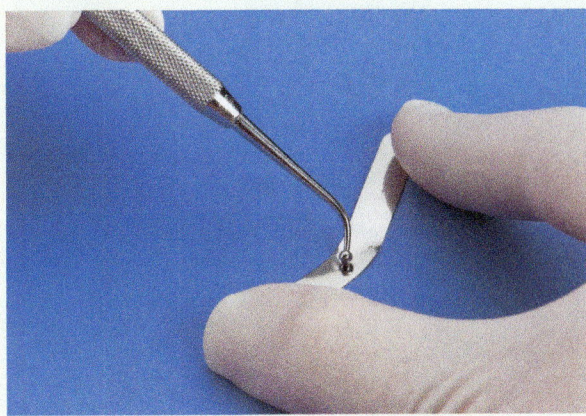

Figure P36-2-2

Procedure 36–2 Assembling a Tofflemire Matrix System (Continued)

3. Prepare the retainer handle. Hold the retainer with the diagonal slots and guide channels facing you (Figure P36-2-3).

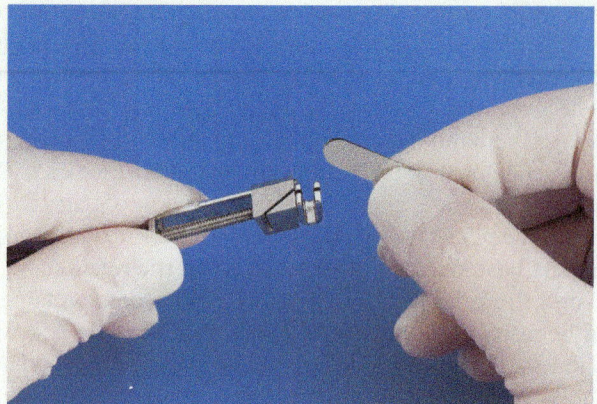

Figure P36-2-3

4. Turn the outer knob counterclockwise until the tip of the spindle becomes visible, away from the diagonal slots.

5. Turn the inner knob until the vise on the end is within a quarter inch of the guide slots.

6. Holding the band, gently bend it into a circle or teardrop shape. Pay attention to the circumferences: the smaller circumference is the gingival edge; the larger circumference is the occlusal edge. Do not crease the band.

7. Holding the band with the gingival edge facing up, slide the occlusal edge into the diagonal on the vise. The loop should be facing the guide slots.

8. Slide the band into the guide channels. The orientation of the matrix band depends on the direction of the restoration.

9. Once the band is placed in the guide channels, turn the outer knob until the spindle tip firmly grips the band in place in the vise slot (Figure P36-2-4).

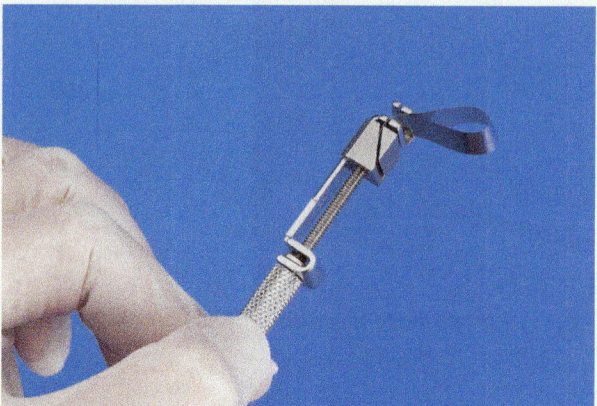

Figure P36-2-4

Alternative Posterior Matrix Systems

Although the Tofflemire matrix is the most common, other matrix systems are available for posterior applications (Figure 36-5). These include:

- *AutoMatrix System*. The AutoMatrix system relies on preformed bands that do not require a retainer to hold them in place. The bands, available in a variety of sizes, come with an autolock loop that is fixed in place with a wrench included with the system. Wedges are still used as needed. After the procedure, the band is loosened with the wrench, then cut from the tooth using pliers included in the system. The bands are disposable, but the wrench and pliers can be sterilized.

- *Palodent System*. Palodent systems can also be used in Class II restorations. They do not require retainers or universal bands. The Palodent, or sectional matrix, consists of a thin, stainless-steel matrix band and a tension ring, used in combination with wedges. To place the matrix, the band is slipped over the restoration, then held in place with wedges. Next the tension ring is placed with the prongs between the band and the wedge to form a secure margin in the interproximal space.

- *T-band System*. The T-band is used for primary teeth, which are too small to accommodate the universal band and retainer system. T-bands are made from pliable copper with a U-shaped retainer system. To assemble the T-band, the copper is bent into an oval to accommodate the restoration. One end of the band is slipped through the U-shaped retainer, which is bent into position to firmly hold the band's shape. The band is then placed over the tooth and the restoration can continue.

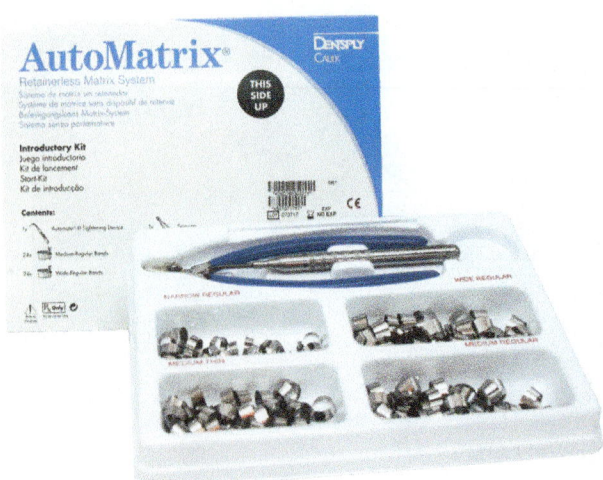

Figure 36–5 AutoMatrix system.

■ *Spot-Welded Bands.* Spot-welded bands are custom-fitted bands made from stainless steel. Like T-bands, these are often used on primary teeth. To assemble a spot-welded band, the stainless steel is formed to fit the restoration with no. 110 pliers. The band is then removed from the mouth, making sure it retains its form, and then spot-welded with a special piece of equipment into a solid band. The bands are disposed of after the procedure.

Anterior Matrix Systems

Posterior matrix systems such as the Tofflemire system are designed to be used with amalgam. However, these are inappropriate for anterior restorations, which are typically made from composites for aesthetic purposes. Instead of the universal system, the most common matrix systems used in anterior applications are plastic strip matrices (Figure 36-6).

Plastic strip matrices are made from clear plastic, which allows for light-curing of the composite material. Also, the material does not harm the composites, which can be scratched or otherwise deformed by the stainless steel bands used in the universal system. These systems are used in Class III or Class IV anterior restorations where the proximal wall is absent. No retainer is required, but they are held in place with wedges.

To place a plastic matrix system, the band is first slightly contoured so it follows the natural curvature of the anterior teeth. This is accomplished by rubbing the band over the rounded handle of a mouth mirror or cotton pliers until it begins to curve slightly.

The matrix is then placed between teeth before etching and priming to protect the nearby teeth from the etchants. The composite material is placed within the plastic band, which aids in shaping the restoration. Light-curing takes place with the matrix band still in place, as the clear plastic allows light to penetrate the band.

Class II Restorations

A Class II restoration is similar to a Class I restoration, except the decay extends into the proximal surfaces of molars and premolars (Figure 36-7). Class II restorations involve at least two surfaces, and can involve three or more surfaces, making them more complex than Class I restorations.

As with a Class I restoration, a number of factors influence the tooth's preparation. Because reaching the proximal surfaces can be difficult, the dentist might choose to involve the occlusal surface of the tooth. If the decay extends into the dentin, it may involve the use of additional retention and, possibly, bonding materials to help secure the restoration. Either amalgam or composite can be used, depending on the situation. If additional strength is called for, the dentist might use an amalgam restoration.

Matrix systems are required with Class II restorations because of the removal of one or both proximal tooth surfaces.

From the Dentist's Perspective

We're lucky in our state to have expanded functions dental assistants. This has allowed me to provide better service by relying on dental assistants to select and place the appropriate matrix without needing any oversight. I don't even need to be in the room! It's such a great feeling to walk into the treatment room and find the patient completely ready, with a matrix in place and proper isolation and moisture control measures already taken.

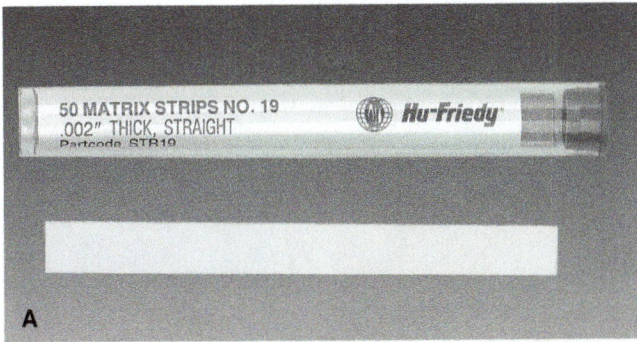
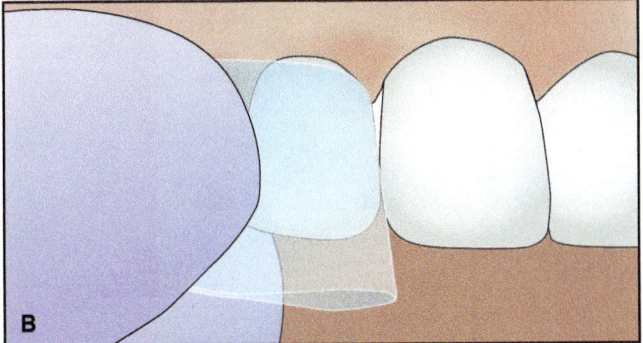

Figure 36-6 Plastic matrix system. (A) Plastic strips. (B) Placed around tooth.

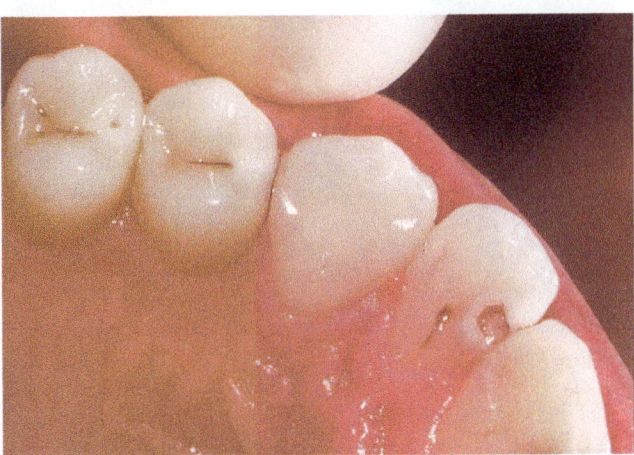

Figure 36-7 Class II and III lesions. Premolars have Class II lesions. The lateral has a Class III lesion.

Procedure 36–3 **Placing a Matrix Band for a Class II Restoration**

Some states allow qualified dental assistants to perform this procedure; in other states the dental assistant assists the dentist during the procedure. Check the regulations governing your state for more information about the specific duties dental assistants are allowed to perform.

Materials needed (Figure P36-3-1):

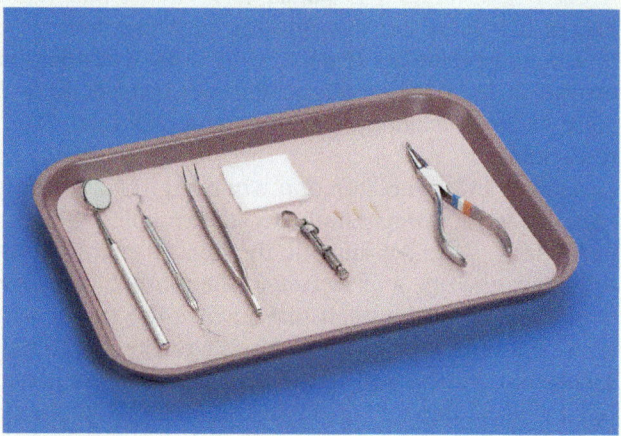

Figure P36-3-1

- Basic setup
- Prepared matrix band
- Prepared retainer
- No. 110 pliers
- Wedge, for each proximal space involved

1. Put on appropriate PPE.
2. Prepare the band. During placement in the retainer, the band may have become misshapen or smaller. Use the handle of a mouth mirror to open the band, and if necessary, adjust the size of the band with the inner knob on the retainer (Figure P36-3-2).

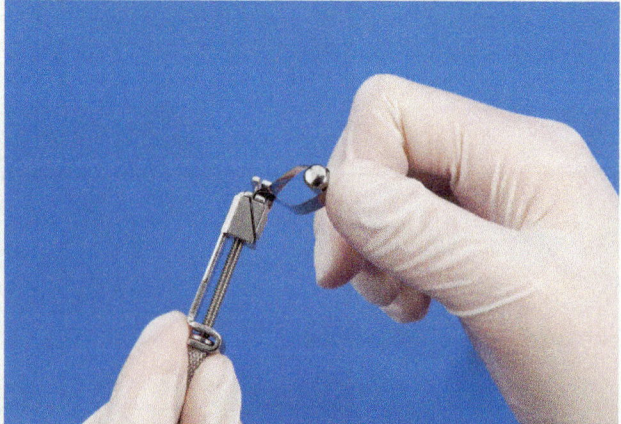

Figure P36-3-2

3. Transfer the retainer to the dentist.
4. The dentist inserts the retainer into the oral cavity, parallel to the buccal surface, sliding the open band down over the

occlusal surface of the tooth. The band should extend 1.0 to 1.5 mm above the occlusal plane (Figure P36-3-3).

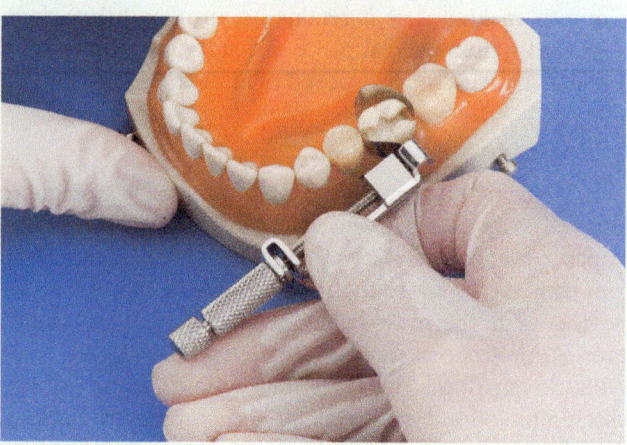

Figure P36-3-3

5. Holding the band securely in place so it does not slide up and off the tooth, the dentist adjusts the inner knob until the band has tightened around the tooth.
6. Transfer an explorer to the dentist when needed.
7. Using the explorer, the dentist makes sure the band is adapted to the tooth surface and there is no material or tissue between the band and the tooth.
8. Transfer the burnisher to the dentist. The dentist contours the band slightly with a burnisher at the contact area. It should be slightly concave.
9. Transfer a wedge to the dentist.
10. The dentist slides the wedge into the interproximal space with the wide, flat side of the wedge toward the gingival tissue. Wedges should be inserted wherever preparations are being placed (Figure P36-3-4).

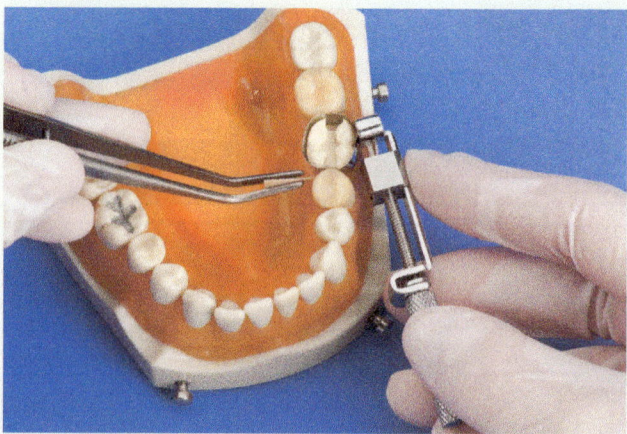

Figure P36-3-4

11. The dentist double checks to make sure the seal at the gingival area is secure.
12. The dentist can now proceed with the restoration.

Procedure 36–4 **Assisting with a Class II Restoration**

Materials needed (Figure P36-4-1):

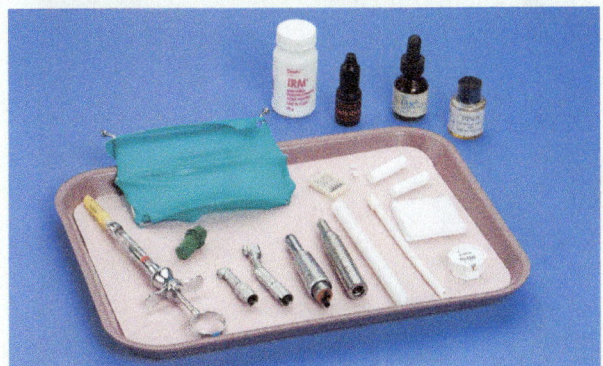

Figure P36-4-1

- Restorative tray
- Local anesthetic setup
- Dental dam setup
- High-volume evacuator (HVE) tip
- High-speed handpiece
- Low-speed handpiece
- Saliva ejector
- Burs, assorted
- Matrix setup
- Wedges
- Cotton pellets
- Cotton rolls
- Gauze (2 × 2-inch)
- Dental liners, bases, bonding agents, sealers
- Premeasured amalgam capsules
- Composite material
- Composite shade guide
- Curing light
- Amalgamator
- Dental floss

Tooth Preparation

1. Put on appropriate PPE.
2. Transfer the mouth mirror and explorer to the dentist for examining the tooth.
3. Assist in the administration of anesthetic.
4. Apply moisture control and isolation measures, such as cotton rolls. In some cases, a dental dam may be used.

Preparing the Restoration

1. Transfer the mouth mirror and the high-speed handpiece to the dentist, with the appropriate bur. Typically, cutting burs are used to remove diseased tissue and tooth matter.
2. During tooth preparation, keep the operating field clean and well lit using the HVE and air-water syringe and by adjusting the dental light. Supply retraction as necessary.

Preparing Dental Materials

1. After the tooth preparation is complete, evaluate with the dentist what materials are needed. If a base, liner, or sealer will be required, prepare the material according to the manufacturer's instructions.
2. Transfer materials to the dentist in the proper sequence.
3. Transfer the assembled matrix band and wedges.
4. If bonding is required, prepare the bonding material and transfer it to the dentist.
5. If amalgam is being used, prepare the amalgam according to the manufacturer's instructions.
6. If composite is being used, prepare the composite according to the manufacturer's instructions.

Placing Dental Materials

1. If amalgam is being used, triturate the amalgam, empty the mixture into the amalgam well and fill the amalgam carrier. Many dentists prefer to condense the amalgam in small batches, so fill the small end of the amalgam well with amalgam and transfer (Figure P36-4-2).

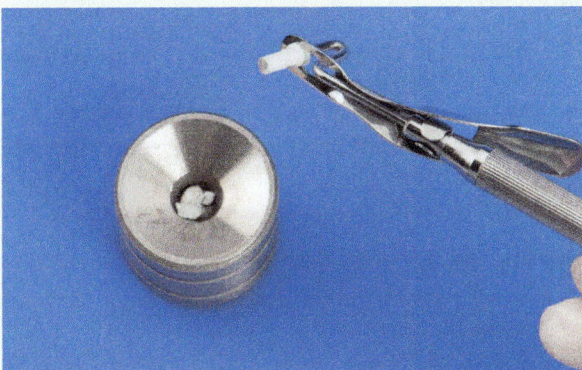

Figure P36-4-2

2. Transfer the amalgam carrier, followed by the condenser. Repeat filling the condenser and transferring the amalgam until the condensing is complete.
3. After the condensing is complete and the restoration is slightly overfilled (Figure P36-4-3), transfer the burnisher.

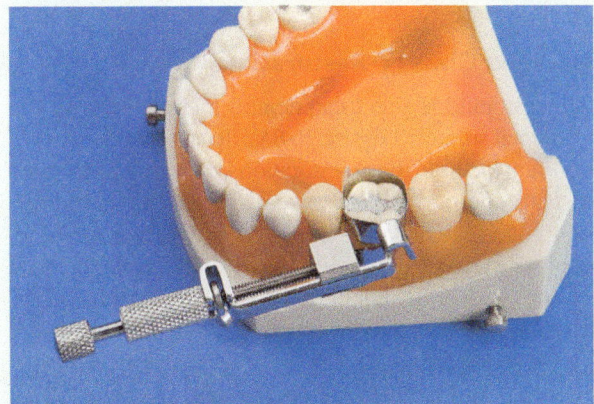

Figure P36-4-3

Procedure 36-4 **Assisting with a Class II Restoration (Continued)**

4. If composite is being used, prepare to transfer the composite in increments, alternating with the curing light between each increment.

Carving and Finishing the Restoration

1. If amalgam is being used, transfer carvers as needed until the initial carving is complete (Figure P36-4-4).

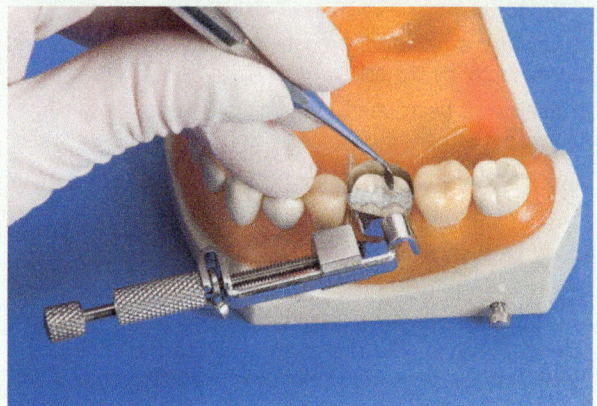

Figure P36-4-4

2. The dentist will remove the matrix after initial carving is complete and then proceed with final carving.

3. If composite is being used, the dentist will remove the matrix first, and then you will transfer the high-speed handpiece with the appropriate finishing burs.

4. Assist with the HVE to keep the field free from debris.

Adjusting the Occlusal Surface

1. Remove all moisture control devices, including cotton rolls and dental dam. Rinse and dry the area.

2. Use articulating paper to check the occlusal contact. Insert the paper between the jaws and ask the patient to gently bite down on the paper (Figure P36-4-5A). High points will appear as dark blue marks on the tooth (Figure P36-4-5B).

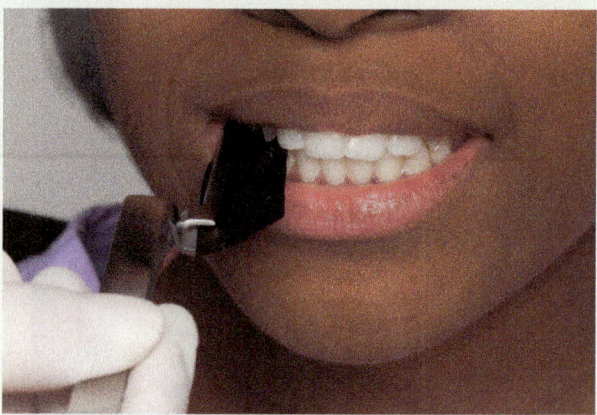

Figure P36-4-5A

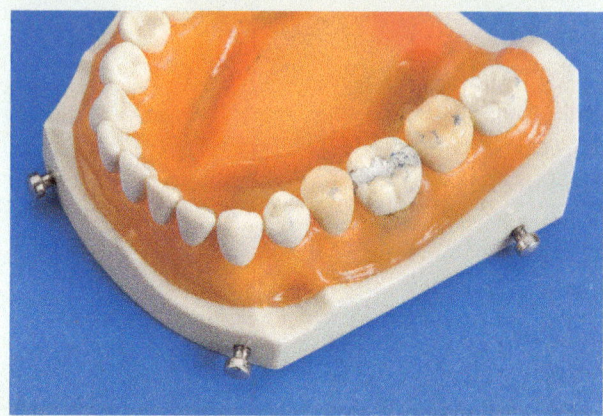

Figure P36-4-5B

3. Transfer finishing burs and carvers as necessary while the dentist removes any high spots and adjusts the occlusion.

4. Clean the newly finished restoration with a damp cotton pellet or ball.

Class III and Class IV Restorations

Class III restorations affect canine and incisor teeth on the interproximal surfaces (Figure 36-8A). Because aesthetics are an important factor in these restorations, they are usually completed with composite restorative materials that have been carefully color-matched to the patient's tooth color. Additionally, dentists may enter the tooth from the lingual side, thus preventing more involvement of the facial tooth surface. Plastic strip matrices are often used with Class III restorations.

A chief concern with Class III restorations is moisture control and isolation. Dental dams are very useful during these restorations to help retract the gingival tissue and keep the area drier. Finally, during the color matching, it is important to make sure the colors are matched appropriately, so use natural lighting with the composite shade chart.

Like Class III lesions, Class IV lesions also affect anterior teeth including the canines and incisors. The difference, however, is that Class IV lesions involve a larger surface area and include the incisal edge and interproximal surfaces (Figure 36-8B). Matrices are also necessary for Class IV restorations.

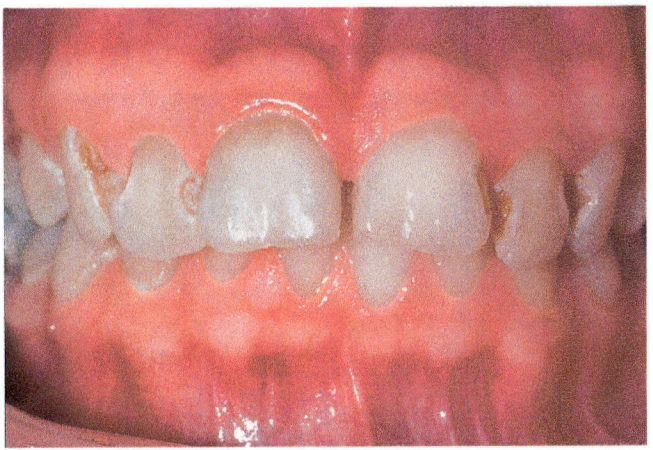

A

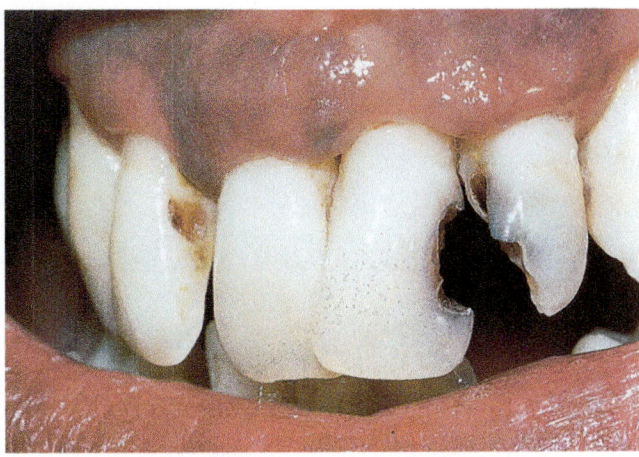

B

Figure 36–8 Class III and IV lesions. (A) Class III lesions on centrals, laterals, and canines. (B) Class IV lesions on mesial of lateral incisor.

Procedure 36-5 Assisting with a Class III or Class IV Restoration

Materials needed (Figure P36-5-1):

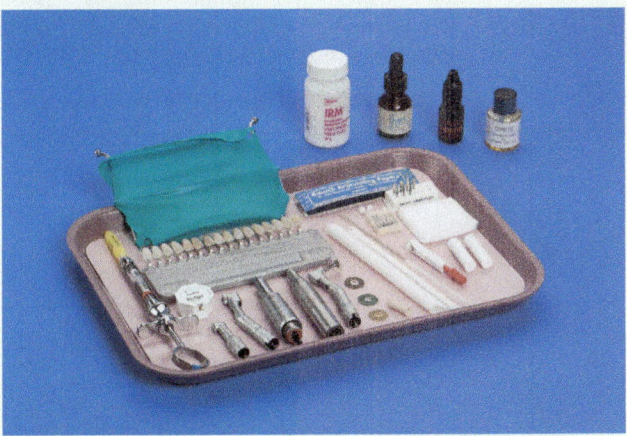

Figure P36-5-1

- Restorative tray
- Composite shade guide
- Local anesthetic setup
- Dental dam setup
- High-volume evacuator (HVE) tip
- High-speed handpiece
- Low-speed handpiece
- Mylar matrix setup
- Saliva ejector
- Burs, assorted
- Cotton pellets
- Cotton rolls

- Gauze (2 × 2-inch)
- Dental liners, bases, bonding agents, sealers
- Composite material
- Curing light with protective shield
- Finishing burs and diamonds
- Dental floss
- Articulating paper
- Polishing kit (disk and mandrel)
- Polishing paste

Tooth Preparation

1. Put on appropriate PPE.
2. Transfer the mouth mirror and explorer to the dentist for examining the tooth.
3. Assist in the administration of anesthetic.
4. Assist with shade selection for composite restoration material.
5. Apply moisture control and isolation measures, such as cotton rolls. In some cases, a dental dam may be used.

Preparing the Restoration

1. Transfer the mouth mirror and the high-speed handpiece to the dentist, along with hand-cutting instruments as needed.
2. During the tooth preparation, keep the operating field clean and well lit using the HVE and air-water syringe and by adjusting the dental light. Supply retraction as necessary.

Etching, Bonding, and Placing Composite

1. Assist in the placement of the plastic strip matrix with wedges if necessary (Figure P36-5-2).

Procedure 36-5 **Assisting with a Class III or Class IV Restoration (Continued)**

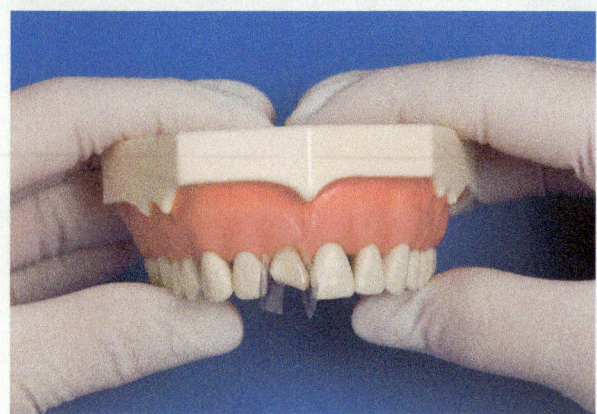

Figure P36-5-2

2. Prepare and assist in the application of the etch, primer, and bonding resins according to the manufacturer's instructions.

3. Prepare the composite material according to the manufacturer's instructions, including dispensing onto a paper pad for application and using a composite syringe (Figure P36-5-3).

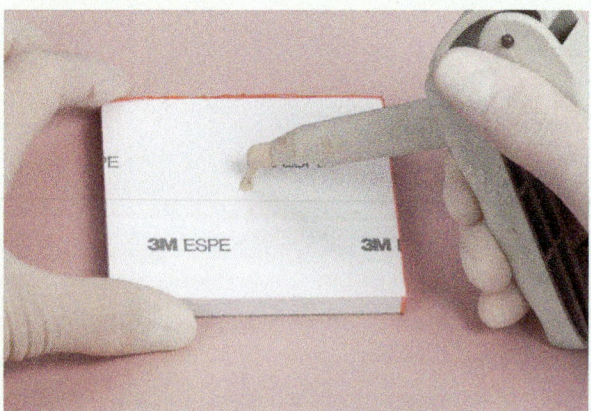

Figure P36-5-3

4. Transfer the composite material to the dentist with a composite instrument (Figure P36-5-4). The dentist will place the composite material for the restoration (Figure P36-5-5).

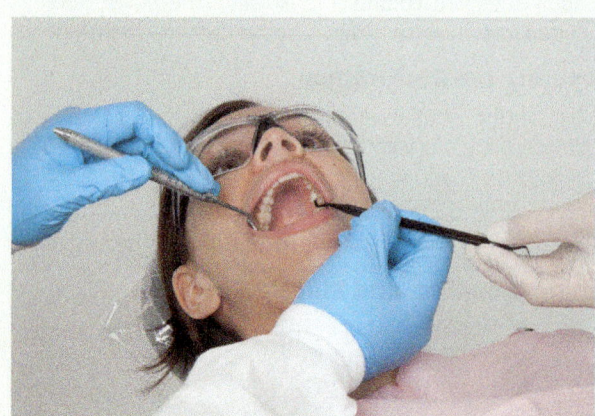

Figure P36-5-4

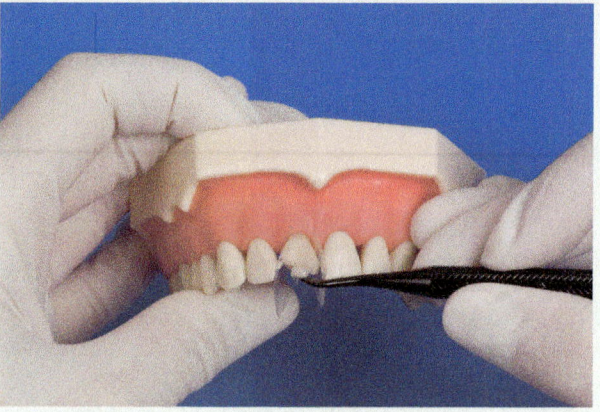

Figure P36-5-5

5. Assist during light-curing by making sure the matrix remains in place.

Finishing

1. After the composite is light-cured, the dentist will remove the plastic strip matrix and wedge, if a wedge was used.

2. Transfer finishing instruments, including the high-speed handpiece with finishing burs or diamonds, as needed while the dentist contours the restoration (Figure P36-5-6).

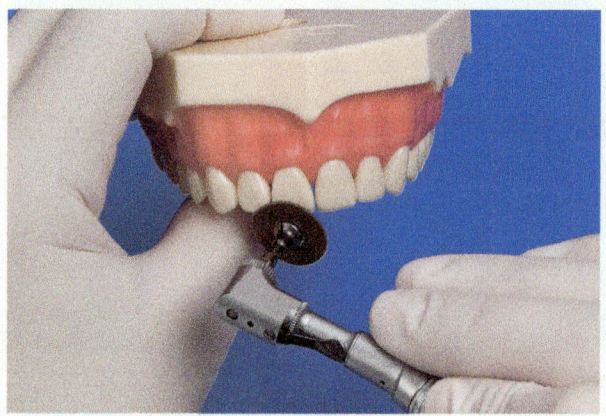

Figure P36-5-6

3. Transfer finishing strips or other materials and instruments as needed.

4. Remove moisture control measures and check the occlusion with articulating paper.

5. Transfer any polishing instruments as the dentist finishes the restoration.

Class V Restorations

A Class V lesion is a smooth-surface lesion that occurs in the gingival third of any tooth, either on the facial or lingual surface (Figure 36-9). Like Class I restorations, these are fairly uncomplicated restorations that require removal of the lesion without any angles in the target area. Typically, composites are used to repair Class V restorations for aesthetic purposes, but in some cases, composite may be inappropriate so amalgam must be used.

During a Class V restoration, moisture control and gingival retraction is essential. Because these lesions are located in the immediate vicinity of the gingival margin, excess moisture is a persistent issue. Dental dams are usually used, and in some cases, cervical clamps or gingival retraction cords are needed to achieve proper gingival retraction.

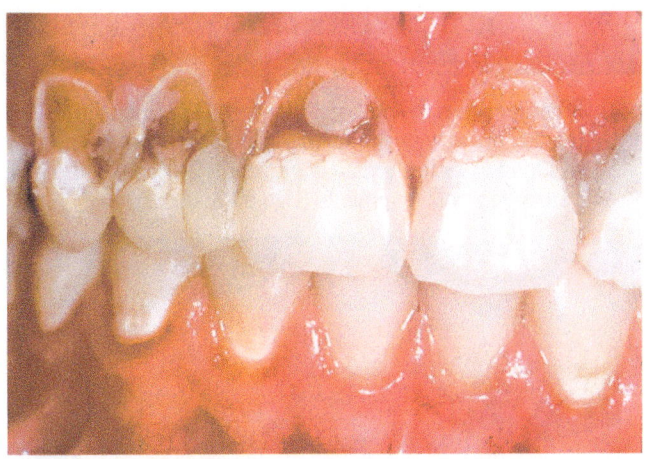

Figure 36–9 Class V lesions on maxillary anteriors.

Procedure 36–6 Assisting with a Class V Restoration

Materials needed (Figure P36-6-1):

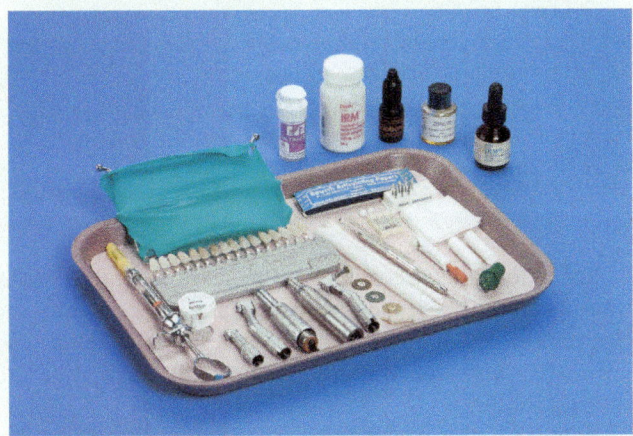

Figure P36-6-1

- Restorative tray
- Local anesthetic setup
- Dental dam setup (cervical clamp)
- Retraction cord and packer
- High-volume evacuator (HVE) tip
- High-speed handpiece
- Low-speed handpiece
- Saliva ejector
- Burs, assorted
- Cotton pellets
- Cotton rolls
- Gauze (2 × 2-inch)
- Dental liners, bases, bonding agents, sealers
- Permanent restorative material (composite or amalgam)
- Dental floss

Tooth Preparation

1. Put on appropriate PPE.
2. Transfer the mouth mirror and explorer to the dentist for examining the tooth.
3. Assist in the administration of anesthetic.
4. Apply moisture control and isolation measures, such as cotton rolls. A dental dam may be used.

Preparing the Restoration

1. Transfer the mouth mirror and the high-speed handpiece to the dentist.
2. During removal, keep the operating field clean and well lit using the HVE and air-water syringe and by adjusting the dental light. Supply retraction as necessary.

Preparing Dental Materials

1. Mix and prepare any materials such as bases, liners, or sealers as required.
2. Once the tooth preparation is completed, assist with the application of a bonding system, if necessary.
3. If amalgam is being used, prepare the amalgam by amalgamating the capsule according to the manufacturer's instructions.
4. If composite is being used, prepare the composite according to the manufacturer's instructions.

Placing Dental Materials

1. If amalgam is being used, transfer the amalgam in increments to the dentist using the small end of the amalgam carrier. Transfer the condenser as needed.
2. Continue transferring amalgam and condenser until the cavity is slightly overfilled.
3. Transfer the burnisher to the dentist for burnishing.

Procedure 36–6 **Assisting with a Class V Restoration (Continued)**

4. If composite is being used, transfer the composite to the dentist, along with the curing light as needed. Composite is added in increments (Figure P36-6-2A) and light-curing occurs between increments (Figure P36-6-2B).

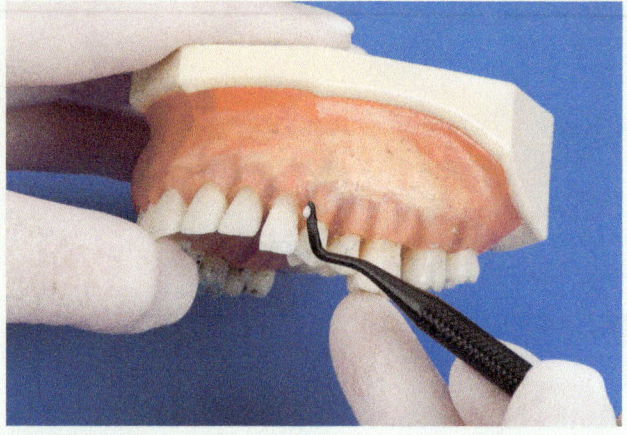

Figure P36-6-2A

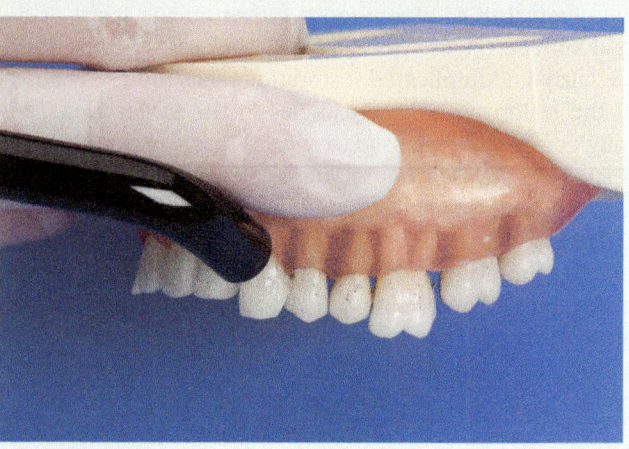

Figure P36-6-2B

Finishing the restoration

1. If amalgam is being used, transfer the carver to the dentist for initial carving.
2. If composite is being used, transfer the high-speed handpiece with the appropriate finishing bur.
3. Throughout the final steps, keep the operating field clear with the high-volume evacuator.

Use of Retention Pins

Retention pins are used when a lesion extends too deeply into the tooth or compromises the structure of the remaining tooth such that retention grooves and bonding agents would not be strong enough to secure the restoration in place (Figure 36-10). Typically, one retention pin is required for each missing cusp.

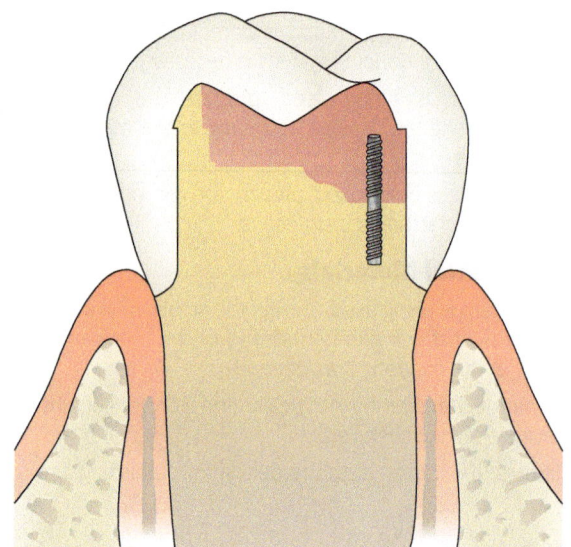

Figure 36–10 Retention pin in place in restoration.

Retention pins are small pins that are anchored firmly into the healthy remaining tooth and extend into the restoration. Much like the use of steel bars in reinforced concrete, they supply additional strength and stability to the restoration.

Retention pins are available in different sizes. However, even the largest retention pins are very small. It is essential to place a retention pin only after a dental dam is in place to prevent accidentally dropping a pin into the patient's throat.

Temporary and Intermediate Restorations

Temporary restorations are used when a permanent restoration is not possible, for any number of reasons. Temporary restorations might be prescribed if:

1. The patient cannot yet afford a permanent restoration
2. The permanent restoration cannot be placed yet due to ongoing work
3. The health of the remaining tooth is in question.

Temporary restorations are usually made from a material called intermediate restorative material (IRM). IRM and other dental materials are covered more thoroughly in Chapter 34, Dental Materials. Typically, temporary restorations are designed to last for up to one year. Beyond that, the integrity of the restoration might be compromised.

Placing temporary restorations is an expanded function. In states with expanded functions dental assistants, a qualified dental assistant can place temporary restorations. In states without this function, dental assistants can help the dentist place the temporary restoration.

CHECKPOINTS

36-4 Define a Class I lesion.

36-5 What is the most common form of matrix system and when is it used?

36-6 Which matrix system is commonly used for anterior restorations?

36-7 Which class of lesion occurs in the gingival third of a tooth?

Procedure 36-7 Assisting with an Intermediate Restoration

Some states allow qualified dental assistants to perform this procedure; in other states the dental assistant assists the dentist during the procedure. Check the regulations governing your state for more information about the specific duties dental assistants are allowed to perform.

Materials needed (Figure P36-7-1):

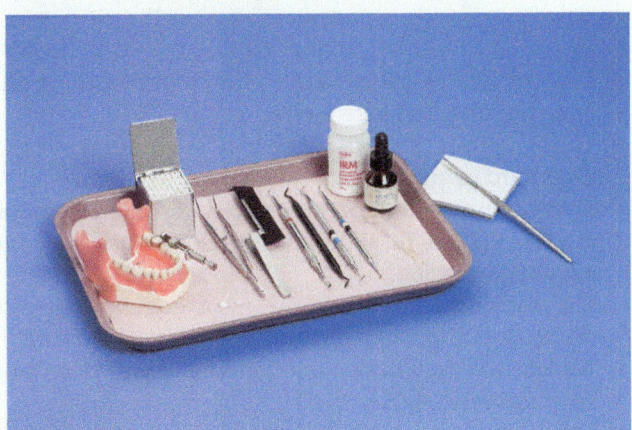

Figure P36-7-1

- Tofflemire matrix retainer (for Class II)
- Matrix band system (for Classes II, III, and IV)
- Wedge (for Classes II, III, and IV)
- Intermediate restorative material (IRM) setup (material, spatula, treated pad)
- Condenser
- Discoid-cleoid carver
- Plastic instrument
- Hollenback carver
- Cotton pellet
- Cotton rolls
- Articulating paper
- Mixing pad

1. Put on appropriate PPE.
2. Prepare the tooth preparation, making sure it is clean, dry, and isolated using either cotton rolls or a dental dam.
3. The dentist plans the restoration, making an outline of the planned preparation.
4. If the restoration includes a proximal wall, the appropriate matrix and wedge system is placed.
5. Prepare the IRM to the proper consistency according to the manufacturer's instructions.
6. Transfer the IRM to the dentist with a plastic instrument for placement into the restoration.
7. The dentist condenses the IRM in the cavity in increments, beginning in the interproximal box if there is one, continuing to condense until the cavity is slightly overfilled (Figure P36-7-2).

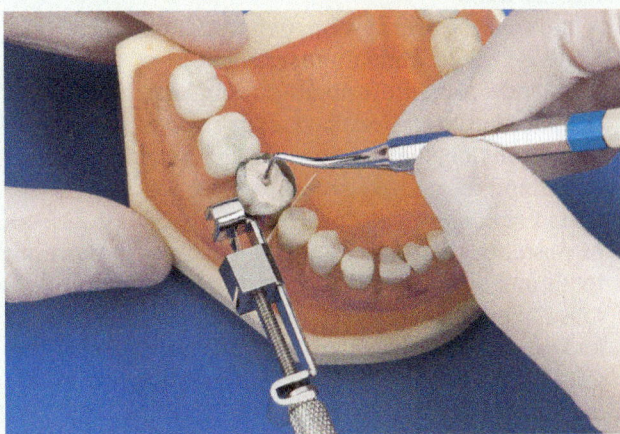

Figure P36-7-2

8. After the tooth is filled, retrieve the plastic instrument from the dentist and transfer an explorer. Before the IRM hardens, the dentist removes any excess material from the matrix band with an explorer, clearing the proximal box and marginal ridge.
9. Pass the discoid-cleoid carver to the dentist. The dentist carves away any excess material from the occlusal surface with a discoid-cleoid carver (Figure P36-7-3).

Procedure 36–7 Assisting with an Intermediate Restoration (Continued)

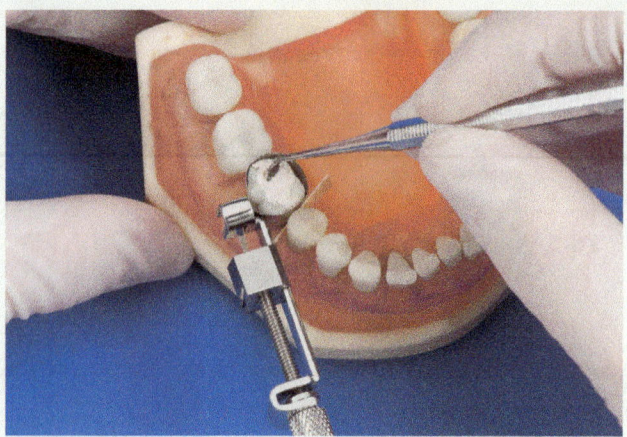

Figure P36-7-3

10. The dentist removes the matrix.

11. The dentist finishes carving with the discoid-cleoid carver, retaining the natural anatomy of the tooth.

12. Provide the dentist with the Hollenback carver. The dentist clears the interproximal area with a Hollenback carver, making sure to clear away any overhangs.

13. The dentist will remove the wedge if one was placed.

14. Use articulating paper to check the patient's occlusion. Ask the patient to gently bite down on the articulating paper. Dark areas signal high points.

15. The dentist finishes the final carving to restore the natural occlusion, then cleans the restoration with a wet cotton pellet or swab.

16. Provide the patient with postoperative instructions for the temporary filling.

 **Chapter Highlights**

✦ Dental assistants play a crucial role in restorative dentistry by preparing materials, transferring equipment, maintaining isolation and moisture control, and, in some cases, performing simple tasks.

✦ Restorations are described according to the anatomy they affect, such as the external wall, pulpal wall, and enamel wall.

✦ A line angle is formed when two walls intersect; a point angle is formed when three walls intersect.

✦ The dentist plans the restoration using a number of forms that take into consideration factors such as the shape of the restoration, the steps involved in creating the restoration, and the access to the area to be restored.

✦ Class I restorations are located on the occlusal surfaces of posterior teeth, buccal and lingual pits of posterior teeth, and lingual pits of maxillary anterior teeth.

✦ Class II lesions involve the proximal surfaces of molars and premolars and may involved two or more surfaces.

✦ Class III lesions affect canine and incisor teeth on the interproximal surfaces.

✦ Class IV lesions affect canine and incisor teeth on the interproximal and incisal edge.

✦ Class V lesions affect the surface of the tooth at the gingival third of any tooth.

✦ Matrices are used to provide a form for the restoration in Class II, Class III, and Class IV lesions when an external wall is missing.

✦ The Tofflemire matrix is the most common type of matrix. It comprises a retainer and band.

✦ Wedges are used in conjunction with matrices to help keep the band stable.

✦ Alternative matrix systems include the AutoMatrix, Palodent system, T-band, and spot-welded systems.

✦ Anterior matrix systems are made from plastic strips that can be used with light-curing systems for composite restorations.

✦ Retention pins are used when the restoration needs additional support; these tiny screws are anchored in healthy tooth tissue and extend into the restoration.

 **Review Questions**

1. Which describes the pulpal wall?

   a. An external wall that includes enamel

   b. An internal wall running parallel to the long surface of the tooth

   c. An internal wall running perpendicular to the long surface of the tooth

   d. None of the above

2. What is the cavosurface margin?

   a. The occlusal surface of the tooth

   b. The gingival margin

   c. The region where the cavity intersects with healthy external tooth

   d. The inner wall of the cavity restoration

3. Which form describes the occasional need to extend a restoration to allow for access?

   a. Outline form

   b. Resistance form

   c. Retention form

   d. Convenience form

4. Which best describes Class I restorations?

   a. Uncomplicated surface lesions

   b. Multisurface lesions

   c. Anterior lesions

   d. Interproximal lesions

5. What is purpose of a matrix?

   a. To aid in removal of diseased tissue

   b. To assist in isolation

   c. To prevent debris and help moisture control

   d. To provide form to a restoration

6. What is the retainer's purpose?

   a. Hold the dental material in place

   b. Hold the band in place

   c. Help adjust tooth alignment

   d. None of the above

7. What is the inner knob of a universal retainer used for?

   a. Apply pressure to the tooth during restoration

   b. Release the band after restoration

   c. Adjust the diameter of the band

   d. Apply pressure to the spindle

8. Which describes a Class II lesion?

   a. Can involve more than one surface

   b. Affects molars and premolars

   c. Affects posterior teeth

   d. All of the above

9. Which describes a Class III lesion?

   a. Affects only anterior teeth

   b. Affects the incisal edge of anterior teeth

   c. Affects the interproximal surface of anterior teeth

   d. Affects both anterior and posterior teeth

10. What type of matrix is used with a Class IV restoration?

    a. AutoMatrix

    b. T-band

    c. Strip matrix

    d. Universal matrix

11. Which describes a Class V lesion?

    a. Multisurface, involving anterior teeth

    b. Affecting the gingival margin of any tooth

    c. Affecting the gingival margin of anterior teeth only

    d. Affecting the occlusal surface of any tooth

12. How long do temporary restorations typically last?

    a. 1 month

    b. 6 months

    c. 12 months

    d. 18 months

Active Learning Exercises

1. What is the purpose of a matrix system? Can anyone place a matrix band on a patient? Why or why not?

2. What is the purpose of contouring the matrix band?

Application Activities

1. Practice assembling a Tofflemire matrix and inserting a band.

2. Practice using the proper terminology to describe line and point angles.

PREPARING FOR CERTIFICATION EXAMS

Review the following topics in this chapter to prepare for the Dental Assisting National Board (DANB) exam:

- **Restoration Procedures**
- **Permanent Restorations**
- **Temporary and Intermediate Restorations**

Expanded Clinical Functions

CHAPTER CHECKLIST

On completion of this chapter, students will be able to:

- ☑ Describe the differences between indirect and direct supervision.
- ☑ Describe the skills needed for working as an operator in allowed dental procedures.
- ☑ Understand the role of the dental assistant in the various expanded function procedures outlined in the chapter.

KEY TERMS

direct supervision – supervision provided by a dentist who has diagnosed and authorized the condition to be treated, remains on the premises while the procedure is being performed, and approves the work performed before the patient is dismissed

general supervision – supervision provided by a dentist who has diagnosed and authorized the condition to be treated but is not necessarily on the premises while the procedure is being performed

indirect supervision – supervision provided by a dentist who has diagnosed and authorized the condition to be treated and remains on the premises while the procedure is being performed

Introduction

Successful operation of a dental office requires that patients move smoothly in and out for their procedures and that each member of the office staff, from administrative staff to the dentist, operates as part of a team.

In some states, dental assistants are allowed to act as operators in some procedures, assuming they have the proper licensing and training. This helps the dental office function more smoothly and expands the role of the dental assistant in terms of patient care. These functions are known as expanded functions, and states with these rules are known as expanded functions dental assistant (EFDA) states.

As the name implies, EFDAs can perform specific procedures that might otherwise be performed only by the dentist. This usually requires written certification that the dental assistant has completed additional training and passed any required examinations. State regulations vary; refer to your state's dental practice act for details. Qualified EFDAs are a great resource for dentists, who can delegate many time-consuming but important patient procedures, thereby making the whole office function more efficiently.

This chapter describes the role of an EFDA and lists specific procedures often performed by EFDAs. Some of these procedures are described elsewhere in this text with the dental assistant in the role of assisting the dentist as operator; here the dental assistant is the operator.

From the Dentist's Perspective

As a general dentist, I've enjoyed having EFDAs in the office. Well-trained EFDAs will come to you if they are concerned that something might be done improperly or if they need help. They're an excellent boon to the practice and have allowed me to see more patients in a streamlined manner. This permits me to spend more one-on-one time with all my patients … something that I love to do!

The Dental Practice Act

The role of the EFDA is covered by the dental practice act in each state. This act lays out specific procedures and responsibilities, including the need for supervision, of the EFDA. There are two forms of supervision:

- **Indirect supervision.** The dentist is in the office, but not necessarily in the same treatment room as the dental assistant during the procedure. The dentist is available to evaluate and assess the EFDA's work and in case of emergencies.
- **Direct supervision.** The dentist is in the same treatment area as the EFDA.

No matter the situation, the dentist is ultimately responsible for everything that happens in the dental office, even if the dentist is not in the same treatment room during a procedure.

Check Your Ethics

EFDAs can help a dental practice run more smoothly—but it is important to remember this is a tightly controlled job description and that both the dentist and you can be held responsible for any unapproved procedures you perform (although only the dentist will likely be legally liable). If a dentist asks you to do something that falls outside the scope of the dental practice act in your state, how should you respond?

Working as an Operator

The transition from assistant to operator requires rethinking the way you approach a procedure. When you are acting as an operator, performing expanded functions requires the following skills:

- *Correct instrumentation.* This means understanding the proper use of instruments such as the explorer or the mouth mirror. EFDAs often work alone, without the benefit of four-handed dentistry, so it is important to learn how to position the mouth mirror correctly, for example.
- *Proper hand position.* Reducing strain and stress on your hand during longer procedures is important. EFDAs should know how to establish a fulcrum, or stabilize hand position, during the procedure. A good fulcrum allows the operator to rest his or her hand while grasping and using the instrument. This often means resting fingers against the teeth (an intraoral fulcrum) or the patient's chin or cheek (an extraoral fulcrum).
- *Knowledge of tooth anatomy.* The EFDA must have a thorough understanding of the dental anatomy, including tooth structure, contour, position, and the relationships among these. This is covered in depth in Chapter 8, Dentition and Tooth Morphology.
- *Knowledge of the procedure.* EFDAs need to understand the instrumentation, materials, and methods used in the particular procedure. Also, if the EFDA procedure is performed before another procedure, the EFDA should be aware of the final goals of the following procedure to better help the dentist accomplish the ultimate goal.

CHECKPOINT
37-1 What is a fulcrum?

Applying Dental Sealants

Pit and fissure sealants are used to prevent caries from developing in the pits and fissures of posterior teeth. Sealants are most commonly used on pediatric patients, although they may in some cases be used on adults. The decision to place sealants is made by the dentist, but in certain states, the actual placement is an EFDA function. Procedure 37-1 describes how to place sealants. For more information on dental sealants, see Chapter 10, Prevention of Caries and Periodontal Disease and Chapter 43, Pediatric Dentistry.

Moisture control and tooth isolation are essential during sealant placement. The most common reason for sealant failure is poor moisture control. To some degree, the method and timing of moisture control—before or after polishing, dry angles or not—depends on the operator. The most efficient moisture control usually occurs with the use of a dental dam. Specific instructions on placing dental dams can be found in Chapter 27, Moisture Control and Isolation, and later in this chapter in Procedure 37-2: Placing a Dental Dam.

✔ CHECKPOINT

37-2 What is the most common reason for sealant failure?

Procedure 37–1 Applying Pit and Fissure Sealants

Materials needed (Figure P37-1-1):

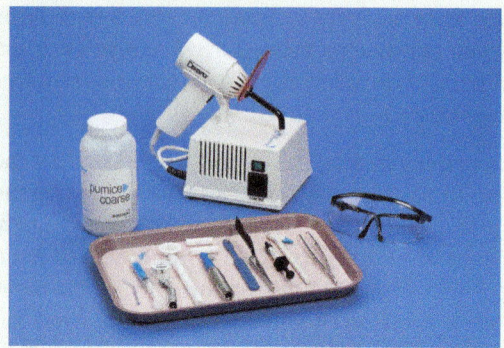

Figure P37-1-1

- Protective eyewear for patient and operator
- Dental dam, dry angles, or cotton rolls
- Basic setup
- Cotton tip applicator
- Sealant material
- Etching agent, gel or liquid
- Pumice and water
- Prophy brush
- Prophy angle
- Applicator device or syringe
- High-volume evacuator (HVE)
- Saliva ejector
- Air-water syringe
- Curing light with appropriate shield
- Articulating paper and holder
- Low-speed dental handpiece
- Round white stone, latch type
- Materials for occlusal adjustments, when filled resin product is used
- Dental floss

1. Put on appropriate PPE, including protective eyewear for yourself and the patient.
2. Prepare the teeth with pumice and water. Do not use standard tooth polish, which may contain fluoride, flavors, and oils that can interfere with the sealant. Air polishers may also be used. If a sodium bicarbonate polisher is used, cleanse the teeth with hydrogen peroxide after cleaning to neutralize the sodium bicarbonate, and then thoroughly rinse the teeth with water.
3. Check the fissures with an explorer to make sure they are clear, then rinse and dry again with the air-water syringe.
4. Isolate and dry the teeth using a dental dam, cotton rolls, and/or dry angles (Figure P37-1-2).

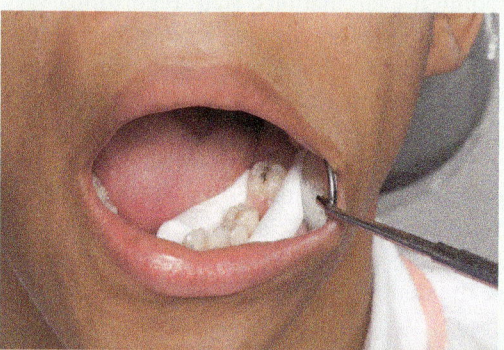

Figure P37-1-2

5. Apply the etchant, following the manufacturer's directions, extending the margin of the etched area just beyond the margin of the area to be sealed (Figure P37-1-3). Etch between 15 and 30 seconds for permanent dentition, depending on the product, or between 50 and 60 seconds for primary dentition, but not for more than 60 seconds in either circumstance.

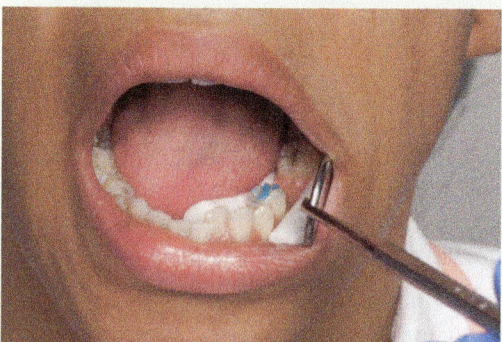

Figure P37-1-3

6. Use the evacuator to remove any excess etchant and then rinse the area to completely remove all the etchant. Suction away water immediately.
7. Dry the tooth again, and replace the cotton rolls, if used. Properly etched areas will be a frosty white (Figure P37-1-4).

Procedure 37-1 Applying Pit and Fissure Sealants (Continued)

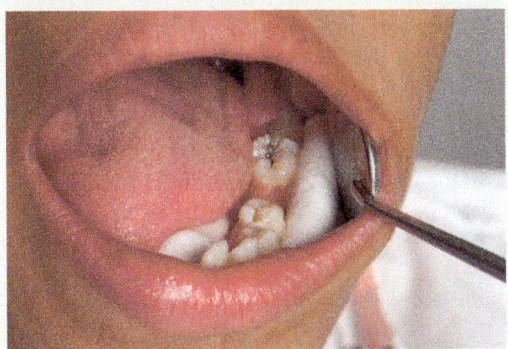

Figure P37-1-4

8. Apply the sealant according to the manufacturer's directions (Figure P37-1-5). Do not let sealant flow beyond the etched areas. Check the sealed areas with an excavator to make sure the tooth is completely sealed. If there are gaps in coverage, apply more sealant as long as no saliva has contacted the area. If saliva has contacted the unsealed area, it must be etched again before sealing.

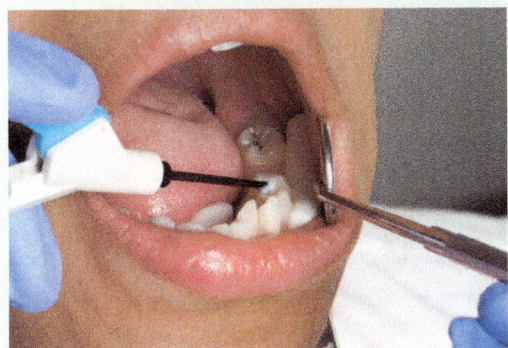

Figure P37-1-5

9. Cure the sealant if necessary, according to the manufacturer's instructions.

10. Check the sealant again with an explorer, and fill in any gaps in coverage.

11. Remove the moisture control devices and check the interproximal areas with dental floss to make sure that no extra sealant is obstructing the space.

12. Wipe the hardened sealant with a cotton applicator to remove the haze (Figure P37-1-6).

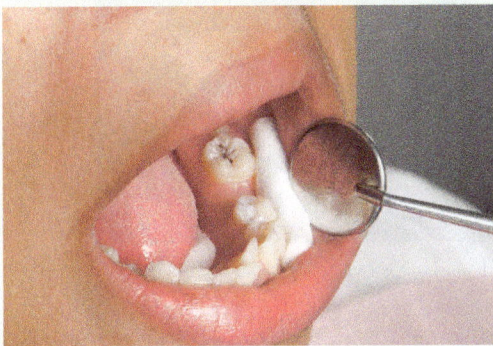

Figure P37-1-6

13. Check the patient's occlusion using the articulating paper. Inform the dentist of any adjustments needed.

14. Document the procedure in the patient's record and provide the patient with postoperative instructions.

Placing a Dental Dam

Dental dams are used in isolation and moisture control. Although they take a few minutes to place successfully, they offer the most complete isolation and moisture control, and they protect patients from swallowing debris generated during the procedure. Several types of dental dams are available, and the best choice depends on the patient and the application. Dental dams can be used with almost any patient, including pediatric patients and patients missing teeth.

Dental dam systems consist of several components, including:

- *Latex and nonlatex dental dam material.* Dental dam sheets are available in a variety of sizes and weights.
- *Frames.* These are plastic or metal devices that hold the dam in place.
- *Dental dam punch.* Punches are used to punch appropriately sized holes in the dental dam prior to placement.
- *Dental dam clamps.* Metal clamps are fastened to teeth near the target tooth and used to hold the dental dam in place during the procedure.

With practice, placing a dental dam should take less than 5 minutes and can be done solo, without any assistance. The following procedure covers placement of a dental dam on an adult patient. The procedure for pediatric dental dams and Quickdams varies slightly. Dental dams should be placed after the anesthetic has been administered by a dentist.

For more information on dental dams, see Chapter 27, Moisture Control and Isolation.

✔ CHECKPOINT
37-3 How long should it take to place a dental dam?

Procedure 37-2 Placing a Dental Dam

There are several variations in dental dam placement, and placing pediatric dental dams is also slightly different. This general procedure is meant to cover the basics, but details might vary among different offices.

Materials needed (Figure P37-2-1):

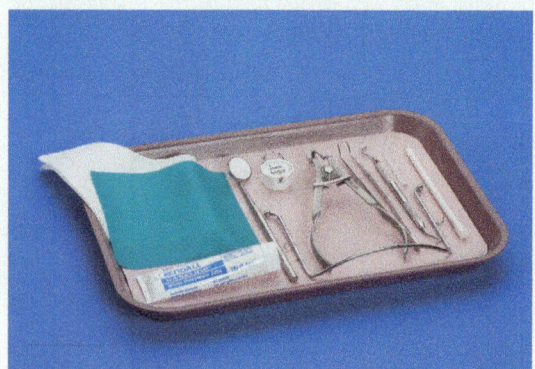

Figure P37-2-1

- Prepared dental dam
- Lip lubricant
- Cotton tip applicator
- Mouth mirror
- Dental floss
- Dental dam lubricant
- Dental dam clamp (winged or wingless)
- Dental dam frame (Young frame)
- Dental dam forceps
- Cotton pliers
- Dental dam stabilization cord (if needed)
- Plastic instrument or beavertail burnisher
- Dental napkin
- Spoon excavator (if needed)
- Plastic instrument or beavertail burnisher
- Air-water syringe
- Saliva ejector

1. Put on appropriate PPE.
2. Before placement of the dam on a patient, and after the anesthetic has taken effect, apply lubricant to the patient's lips using a cotton swab.
3. Use a mouth mirror to examine the site where the dental dam will be placed. Make sure the site is free from plaque and debris. Floss all contacts and make note of tight contacts for later.
4. Prepare the dental dam. If using latex dam material, the powdered side of the dam goes toward the patient's face. There is no powder on latex-free dam material. Mark the dental dam for the appropriate teeth, then punch the keyhole and the holes for individual teeth. Each hole should be separated by a slight ligature that will be eased into the interproximal space.

5. Select an appropriate clamp. The clamp should be the right size to fit securely at the cementoenamel junction (CEJ) of the anchor tooth.
6. Tie a safety line of dental floss to the clamp by doubling it and running it through one anchor hole, across the bow, and through the next anchor hole. Use a long enough piece of floss that it can be strung through the dental dam and attached to the dam frame (Figure P37-2-2).

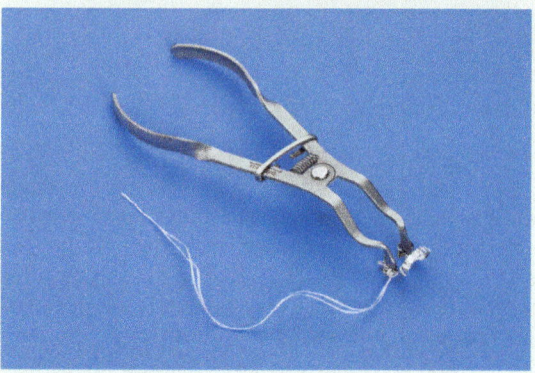

Figure P37-2-2

7. Grip the clamp with the forceps by inserting the forceps beaks into the clamp and using gentle pressure to spread the beaks of the forceps. If the dental dam is already in place, insert the forceps through the dental dam material. Use the sliding bar to hold the forceps open. If the clamp and dental dam are being placed simultaneously, slide the key hole over the bow at this time.
8. Place the clamp by sliding it over the anchor tooth. Begin with the lingual side of the clamp, which allows for better visibility, and then place the buccal side. Gently rotate the clamp to slide it into position. The clamp should not pinch gingival tissue but should be firmly placed at the CEJ (Figure P37-2-3). During placement, hold an index finger over the clamp so it does not spring off and potentially injure you or the patient.

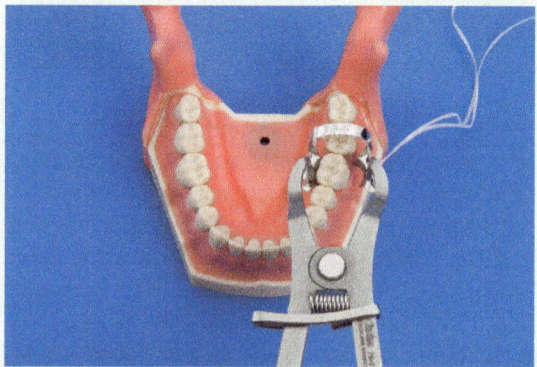

Figure P37-2-3

9. Confirm with the patient frequently that there is no discomfort. The patient should only experience pressure.
10. Gently release the forceps and remove the beaks from the anchor holes.

Procedure 37–2 **Placing a Dental Dam (Continued)**

11. If you have not already placed the dental dam, slide the key hole over the bow of the placed clamp.

12. Retrieve the dental floss ligature with cotton pliers and slide it through the dental dam.

13. Secure the dental dam to the opposite tooth (typically the opposite canine), using either a double loop of dental floss, a small slit of dental dam material, or dental dam stabilization cord (Figure P37-2-4).

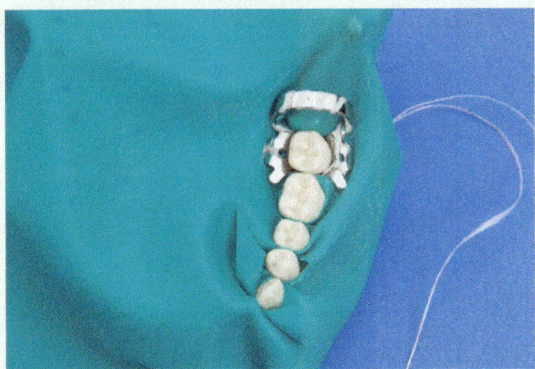

Figure P37-2-4

14. Place the dental napkin around the patient's oral cavity and slide the frame into position. Hook the dental dam material on the frame to hold it steady. Frames can be placed over or under the dental dam material (Figure P37-2-5).

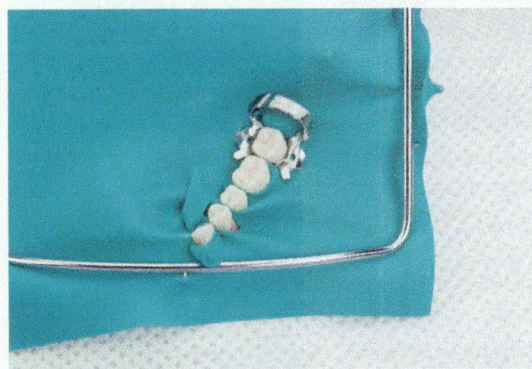

Figure P37-2-5

15. Using your fingers and dental floss, work the remaining teeth to be isolated through the punched holes in the dental dam material. Work the dental dam ligature in between the tooth contacts, using floss if necessary to ensure that the dental

dam is located below the contacts (Figure P37-2-6). This increases the isolation and moisture control.

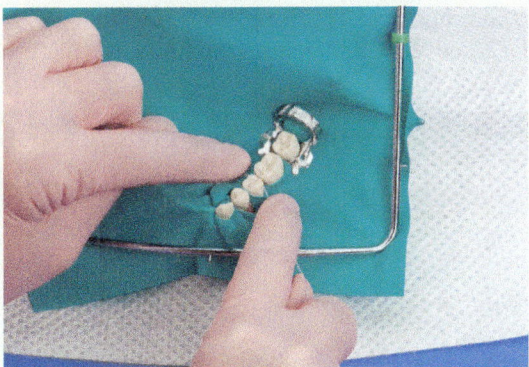

Figure P37-2-6

16. After the dental dam is placed, invert (or tuck) the material. To do this, gently stretch the dental dam, causing the fabric to bend toward the sulcus as it is released. If this does not work, a hand instrument such as a spoon excavator can be used to tuck the dental dam under, along with a stream of air from the air-water syringe.

17. Use the air-water syringe to dry the isolated teeth (Figure P37-2-7).

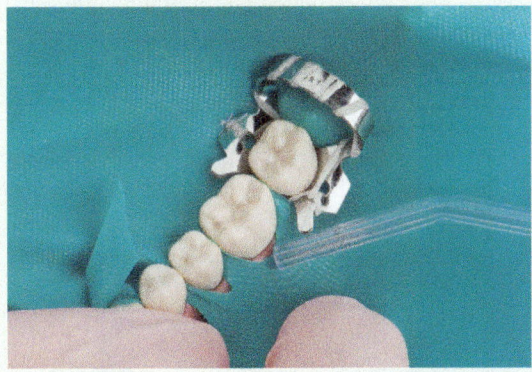

Figure P37-2-7

18. Place a saliva ejector and/or bite block for patient comfort. If the patient is having trouble breathing through the nose, cut a small hole in the dental dam to facilitate breathing.

19. Confirm the dental dam is well placed, with all the edges inverted and secure.

Placing a Matrix Band and Wedge for Restorations

Matrix systems are used with Class II, III, and IV restorations, when the restoration involves a missing interproximal surface. In these cases, there is no external wall to hold the dental material in place during the restoration, so the dental team must use a matrix to provide a temporary wall and help shape the restoration.

Matrix systems include the Tofflemire matrix (also called universal matrix), which is the most common, AutoMatrix systems, Palodent systems, T-bands, and spot-welded bands for posterior teeth, and plastic strip matrices for anterior teeth. These matrices are covered in greater depth in Chapter 36, Assisting in Restorations.

The choice of matrix system depends on the location of the repair, the extent of the repair, and operator preference. In anterior teeth, where amalgam is usually avoided, plastic strip matrices are typically used because they can be used in conjunction with composite. For posterior restorations, the most common matrix system is the Tofflemire system. Procedure 37-3 covers placement of the Tofflemire matrix.

CHECKPOINT
37-4 What is the purpose of using a matrix system during a restoration procedure?

Procedure 37-3 Placing a Matrix Band and Wedge (Tofflemire Matrix) for Restorations

Materials needed:

- Basic setup
- Universal retainer
- Matrix bands
- Paper pad
- Ball burnisher
- Locking cotton pliers
- Wedge for each proximal space involved

1. Put on appropriate PPE.
2. Select the appropriate sized band for the restoration and contour the band by rubbing it with the handle of the burnisher. The band should be thinned slightly and slightly concave to allow proper placement in the interproximal contacts.
3. Place the band into the retainer handle.
4. Before placing the band on the tooth, confirm that it is still shaped properly. If the band has become misshapen, open it with the handle of a mouth mirror and, if necessary, adjust the size of the band with the inner knob on the retainer (Figure P37-3-1).

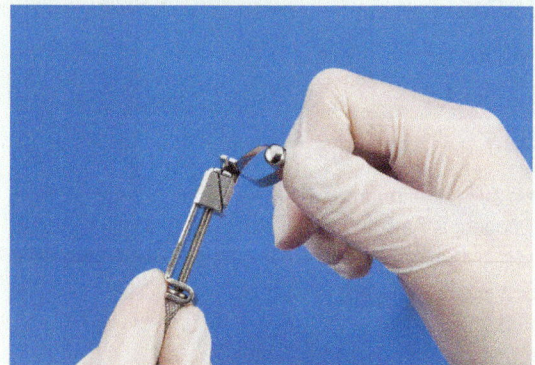

Figure P37-3-1

5. Insert the retainer into the oral cavity, parallel to the buccal surface. Slide the open band down over the occlusal surface of the tooth, making sure that the band extends 1.0 to 1.5 mm above the occlusal plane (Figure P37-3-2).

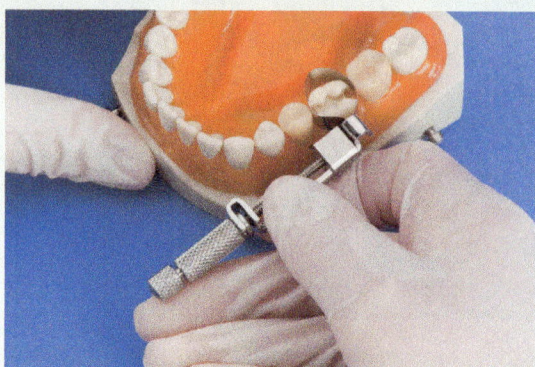

Figure P37-3-2

6. Holding the band securely in place so it does not slide up and off the tooth, adjust the inner knob until the band has tightened around the tooth.
7. Using an explorer, make sure the band is adapted to the tooth surface and there is no material or tissue between the band and the tooth. This prevents aggravation to gingival tissue and leakage of restorative material.
8. Contour the band slightly with a burnisher at the contact area. It should be slightly concave.
9. Select a wedge and slide it into the interproximal space with the wide, flat side of the wedge toward the gingival tissue (Figure P37-3-3). Wedges should be inserted wherever preparations are being placed.

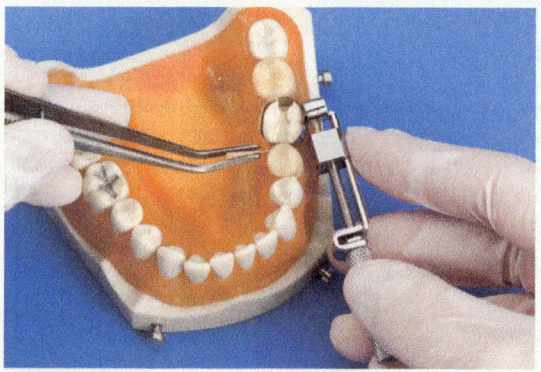

Figure P37-3-3

10. Double check to make sure the seal at the gingival area is secure.
11. The dentist can now proceed with the restoration.

Placing Cements, Bases, and Liners

Dental materials such as cements, bases, and liners are used to prepare and strengthen restorations. Liners and bases are typically used to protect the sensitive tooth pulp. A number of products are available, and the indications and procedures for each may vary slightly based on the manufacturer's recommendations and the type of restoration. For example, amalgam restorations require different materials from composite restorations. Common cements, bases, and liners include calcium hydroxide, zinc oxide eugenol, glass ionomer, zinc phosphate, and polycarboxylate.

Dental cements, bases, and liners are covered in greater depth in Chapter 33, Dental Cements, Liners, Bases, and Bonding Agents. The following procedure covers placement of a cement base.

Procedure 37-4 Placing a Dental Cement Base

Materials needed (Figure P37-4-1):

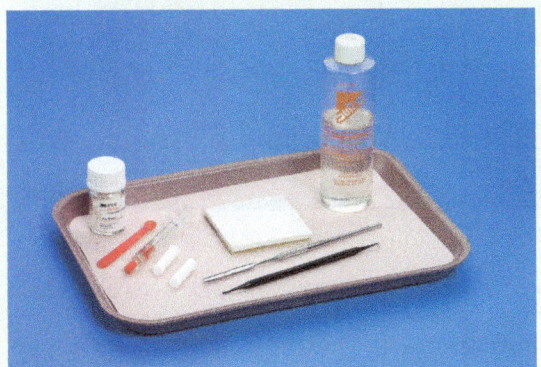

Figure P37-4-1

- Basic setup
- Cement base materials (powder and liquid) (ZOP, ZOE, or polycarboxylate)
- Paper mixing pad or chilled glass slab (for zinc phosphate cement)
- Stainless steel cement spatula
- Plastic filling instrument
- Timer
- Cleaning supplies

1. Put on appropriate PPE.
2. Use the dental explorer and mirror to examine the prepared tooth and determine where the base will be placed.
3. Gently mix the cement materials on the paper pad or glass slab, as described in the manufacturer's instructions. Replace the caps to the cement containers immediately and tightly.
4. The cement should be the consistency of putty. Using the spatula, divide the cement into two halves and roll each half into a ball.
5. Use the plastic filling instrument to pick up one of the balls of cement (Figure P37-4-2). If the base material sticks to the instrument, you can dip the end of the instrument in some extra powder before picking up the base and placing it in the preparation (like placing flour on a rolling pin before rolling out dough).

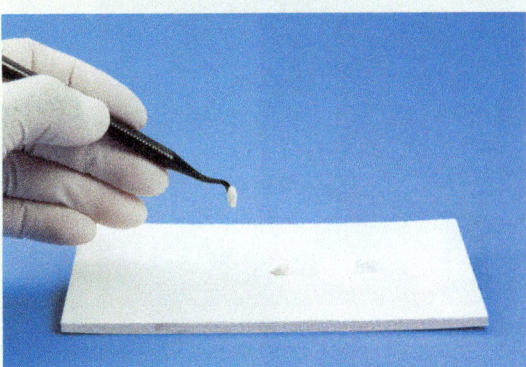

Figure P37-4-2

6. Cover the entire floor of the preparation area with the cement but leave enough room for the restoration to be placed (Figure P37-4-3). If needed, both halves of the cement can be used. The base should be approximately 1 mm thick.

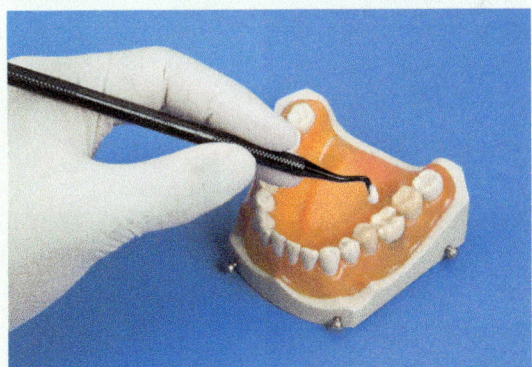

Figure P37-4-3

7. To clean up, tear off the top sheet from the paper pad and fold it in half before throwing it away. Clean any cement off the spatula by wiping it clean with a wet gauze pad before the cement hardens. Hardened cement can be removed with alcohol. Afterward, prepare the spatula for sterilization.

CHECKPOINT

37-5 How thick should the base be when placed in the preparation area?

Performing Intermediate Restorations

Intermediate restorations serve as temporary restorations. There are a number of reasons an intermediate restoration might be performed, including financial issues or to

---

Procedure 37-5 Creating an Intermediate Restoration

Materials needed (Figure P37-5-1):

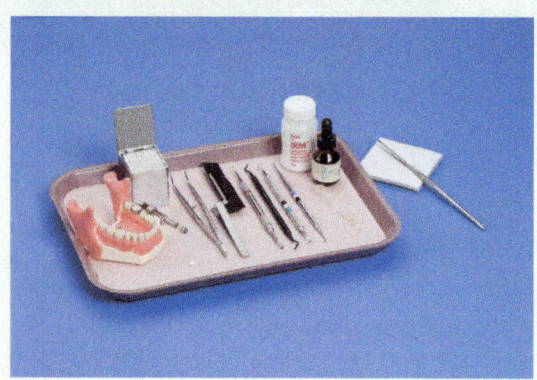

Figure P37-5-1

- Tofflemire matrix retainer (for Class II)
- Matrix band system (for Classes II, III, and IV)
- Wedge (for Classes II, III, and IV)
- Intermediate restorative material (IRM) setup (material, spatula, treated pad)
- Condenser
- Basic setup
- Discoid-cleoid carver
- Plastic instrument
- Hollenback carver
- Cotton pellet
- Cotton rolls
- Articulating paper
- Mixing pad

1. Put on appropriate PPE.
2. Prepare the tooth preparation, making sure it is clean, dry, and isolated using either cotton rolls or a dental dam.
3. Plan the restoration, making an outline of the planned preparation.
4. If the restoration includes a proximal wall, place the appropriate matrix and wedge system.
5. Prepare the IRM to the proper consistency according to the manufacturer's instructions.
6. Condense the IRM in the preparation in increments, beginning in the interproximal box if there is one, continuing to condense until the cavity is slightly overfilled (Figure P37-5-2).

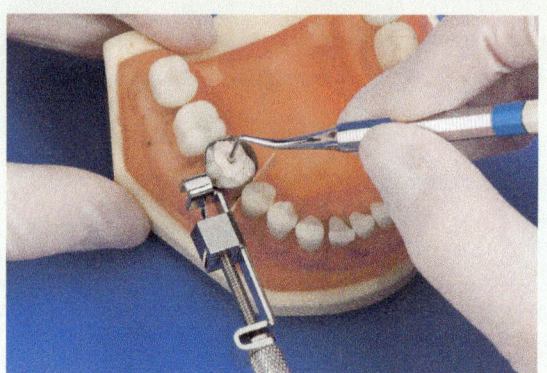

Figure P37-5-2

7. Before the IRM hardens, remove any excess material from the matrix band with an explorer, clearing the proximal box and marginal ridge.
8. Carve away any excess material from the occlusal surface with a discoid-cleoid carver.
9. Remove the matrix.
10. Finish carving with the discoid-cleoid carver, retaining the natural anatomy of the tooth (Figure P37-5-3).

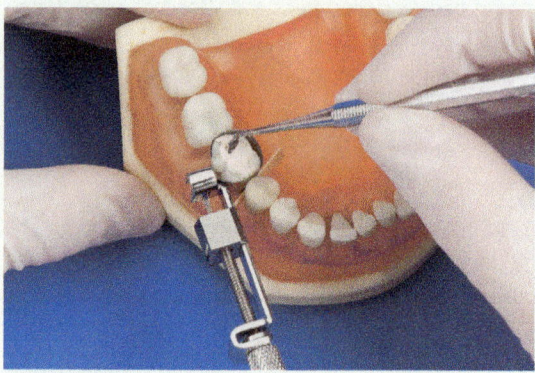

Figure P37-5-3

11. Clear the interproximal area with a Hollenback carver, making sure to clear away any overhangs.
12. Remove the wedge if one was placed.
13. Use articulating paper to check the patient's occlusion. Ask the patient to gently bite down on the articulating paper. Dark areas signal high points.
14. Finish the final carving to restore the natural occlusion, then clean the restoration with a wet cotton pellet or swab.

provide structure while the dentist completes a long-term treatment program.

Intermediate restorations use intermediate restorative material (IRM). Generally, they do not last longer than a year. For more information on intermediate restorations, see Chapter 36, Assisting in Restorations.

✔ CHECKPOINT

37-6 What does the abbreviation IRM stand for?

Performing Tooth Whitening

Tooth whitening has rapidly become one of the most popular procedures in dental offices today. A number of tooth-whitening products are available, both over-the-counter (OTC) and through the dental office. OTC products often use the same ingredients as dental preparations, but in lesser concentrations. It is important to communicate with patients regarding their expectations. They may need to be made aware that only a few shades of brightness can realistically be accomplished and that intrinsic stains cannot be treated with this method.

Tooth whitening offered through a dental office falls into two categories: in-office procedures and at-home procedures. In-office bleaching includes internal bleaching, which is performed during the course of a root canal. This procedure must be performed by a dentist. Other whitening procedures are expanded functions.

In-office tooth whitening systems involve an application of bleaching materials for a specified amount of time. This procedure can be performed in a relatively short period of time, with excellent results. Some products can be applied with a special tray that is custom fitted to the patient's teeth. Others are brushed onto the tooth surface. Some materials are light-cured with a special light wand, while others must be continuously washed away and reapplied every 10 minutes

during the procedure. The choice of which whitener to use is a matter of personal choice for each dental office.

For more information on tooth whitening, including at-home procedures, see Chapter 46, Cosmetic Dentistry.

✔ CHECKPOINT

37-7 What should be communicated to patients before a tooth whitening procedure?

Performing Coronal Polishing

Coronal polishing is a largely cosmetic procedure used to remove stains and discoloration from the coronal surfaces of teeth. It does, however, have some therapeutic benefit as it reduces the presence of small grooves where caries might form.

Coronal polishing differs from a routine dental prophylaxis cleaning in that it only polishes the visible surfaces of the teeth. The coronal polish is not designed to remove calculus, plaque deposits, or debris. Instead, a coronal polish is designed only to remove stains and discoloration.

Coronal polishing can be accomplished with either air-powder polishing, rubber cup polishing, or bristle brush polishing. Of these, rubber cup polishing is more common. This procedure relies on the use of a mildly abrasive agent that is applied with a rubber polishing cup that gently scrubs the tooth surface clean.

For more information on tooth stains and polishing, including the procedures for performing rubber cup polishing, see Chapter 44, Coronal Polishing.

✔ CHECKPOINT

37-8 What does a coronal polishing procedure remove from the teeth?

Procedure 37-6 In-Office Tooth Whitening

Materials needed:

- Protective eyewear for patient and operator
- Basic setup
- Protective gel or dental dam
- Tooth whitener product (components will vary by product)
- Low-speed handpiece
- Prophylaxis polishing cup
- Fluoride prophy paste
- Light or laser source if used to enhance the application

1. Take "before" photos of the patient's teeth and explain the procedure.
2. Put on appropriate PPE.

3. Isolate the teeth. This can be accomplished with a protective gel or with a dental dam (which provides the best isolation).
4. Polish the crowns of the teeth to be whitened.
5. Apply the whitener following the manufacturer's instructions, light-curing it if appropriate. Multiple applications may be necessary.
6. Rinse the teeth and then remove the dental dam. Rinse and cleanse again to remove any leftover whitening gel and protective gel.
7. Polish the newly whitened teeth with a resin polishing cup or a fluoride prophy paste.
8. Examine the teeth and discuss the procedure's outcome with the patient. The full bleaching affect may take several days to become apparent, and the teeth may be sensitive for the first few days.

Performing Gingival Retraction

Gingival retraction is performed whenever it is necessary to create accurate impressions that extend below the gingival surface (or in certain Class V restorations).

Gingival retraction may be accomplished by use of gingival retraction cord or by surgical retraction. Use of gingival retraction cord is the most common and, in some states, can be performed by a qualified EFDA. Surgical gingival retraction is performed only by a dentist.

Gingival retraction cord is designed to temporarily widen the sulcus after the preparation is complete but before the final impression is taken. There are two types of gingival retraction cord:

- *Impregnated.* This type of cord has been impregnated with a special solution that causes temporary retraction of the gingival tissue.
- *Nonimpregnated.* This type of cord does not contain any chemical solution and must be placed by force.

Cords are available in different thicknesses, and as plain, twisted, or braided. The exact choice of cord depends on the situation and what is best for the patient and operator. For more information about gingival retraction, see Chapter 38, Fixed Prosthodontics.

Procedure 37–7 Gingival Retraction Cord Placement

Materials needed (Figure P37-7-1):

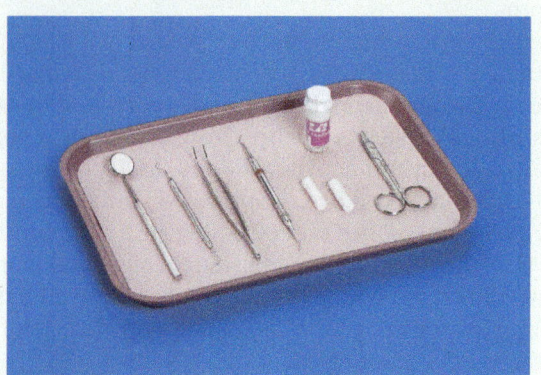

Figure P37-7-1

- Basic setup
- Cotton pliers
- Scissors
- Air-water syringe
- Cotton rolls
- Cord packing instrument
- Gingival retraction cord

1. Put on appropriate PPE.
2. Rinse and dry the target teeth with the air-water syringe, then isolate the quadrant with cotton rolls.
3. Cut a length of cord about 1 inch in length. The cord should be long enough to circle the tooth in question, with enough left over to allow for manipulation.
4. Form the cord into a loop with cotton pliers.
5. Slip the looped cord over the target tooth and slide the loop over the sulcus (Figure P37-7-2).

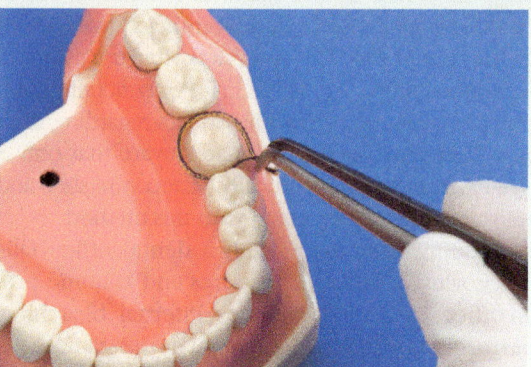

Figure P37-7-2

6. Using a blunt cord packing instrument, work the cord clockwise gently into the sulcus. Keep the ends of the cord on the facial aspect. To pack the cord, gently rock the cord packing instrument and move around the tooth (Figure P37-7-3).

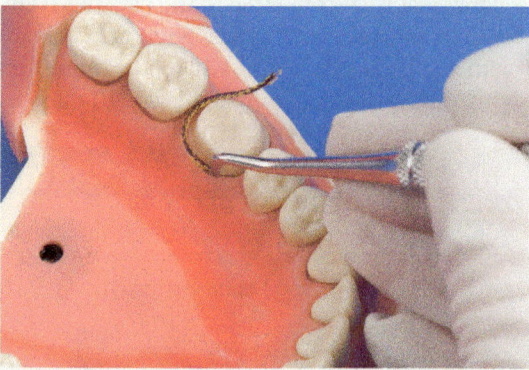

Figure P37-7-3

7. Overlap the ends of the cord when the loop is fully packed. Alternatively, leave a little tail sticking out for easier removal.
8. Leave the cord in place for at least 5 minutes. During this time, the patient should remain still and the area should remain dry. If a nonimpregnated cord is used, the wait time may be as long as 15 minutes.
9. At the end of the desired time, remove the cord in a counterclockwise direction using the cotton pliers.
10. The impression material should be placed immediately after.

37-9 When is gingival retraction necessary?

Performing Provisional Coverage Procedures

A provisional coverage is a temporary covering that is put in place during placement of a permanent prosthetic. Provisional coverings, including crowns and bridges, protect the prepared tooth and maintain its function between the time the final impression is taken and the permanent prosthetic is cemented in place. This period may last from several days to a few weeks. Provisional coverings also prevent adjacent teeth from shifting and maintain the margins of the prepared tooth.

There are several types of provisional coverings, including custom provisionals, which are created specifically for each patient, and prefabricated crowns. Custom provisionals provide better coverage and protection, but they are more time consuming and expensive to create.

For more information about provisional covers, see Chapter 38, Fixed Prosthodontics.

37-10 What is the purpose of a provisional coverage?

Procedure 37–8 Fabricating and Placing a Provisional Crown

This procedure covers the creation of a provisional crown. The steps are similar for provisional bridges, which are also formed from alginate impressions and cemented in place with provisional cement.

Materials needed (Figure P37-8-1):

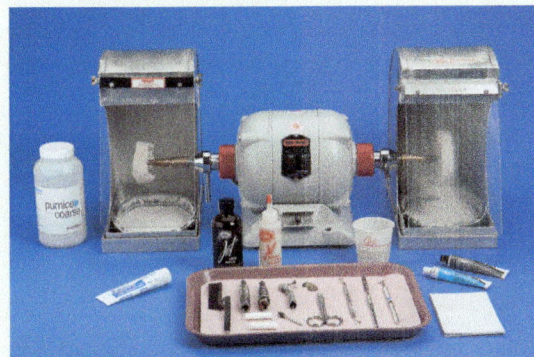

Figure P37-8-1

- Basic setup
- Spoon excavator
- Alginate impression, obtained before preparation of teeth
- Separating medium
- Cotton rolls
- Self-curing acrylic resin, liquid and powder
- Spatula, small cement type
- Dappen dish
- Scissors
- Laboratory knife, optional
- Burnisher, ball or "beaver tail"
- Straight handpiece and mandrel
- Acrylic burs
- Finishing burs, diamond, or discs

- Pumice
- Articulating paper
- Lathe and sterile white rag wheel
- Provisional cementation setup

1. Put on appropriate PPE.
2. Inspect and prepare the alginate impression. This includes making sure it is free from defects in the area of the provisional crown. You should also disinfect it and moisten it, then set it aside until it is needed.
3. Maintain moisture control and isolation of the prepared tooth using cotton rolls.
4. Prepare the site with petroleum jelly, which will help the provisional crown separate from the mold.
5. Retrieve the alginate impression and dry it in preparation for loading with the resin.
6. Prepare the liquid monomer in a dappen dish. Mix it according to the manufacturer's instructions and add the proper shade of self-curing powder.
7. Blend the monomer with a spatula (Figure P37-8-2), then set it aside until it forms a doughy mass.

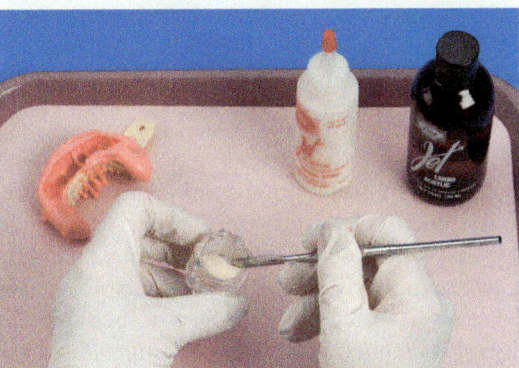

Figure P37-8-2

Procedure 37–8 Fabricating and Placing a Provisional Crown (Continued)

8. Load the resin into the prepared impression (Figure P37-8-3), and then place the impression onto the patient's prepared tooth.

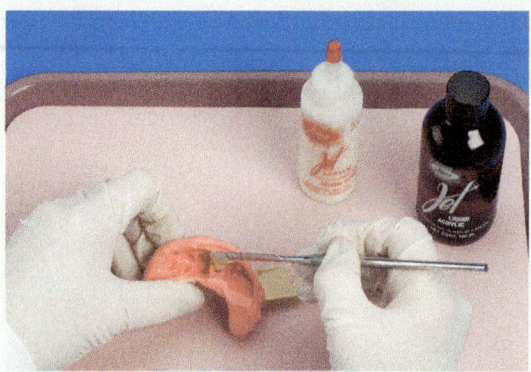

Figure P37-8-3

9. Let the resin set for about 3 minutes, then gently lift the impression tray away and remove it from the patient's oral cavity.

10. Remove the provisional crown from the impression and place it on the patient's prepared tooth.

11. Mark the provisional crown with a pencil (Figure P37-8-4A), then trim it to within 1 mm of the gingiva with an acrylic bur or stone (Figure P37-8-4B).

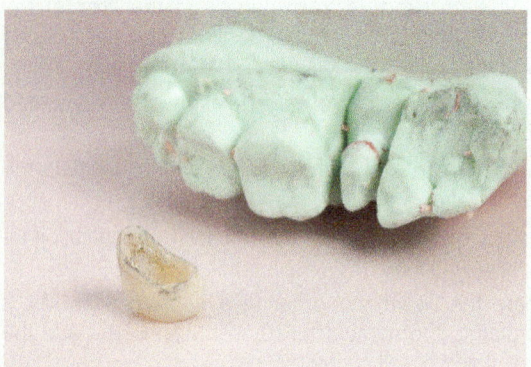

Figure P37-8-4A

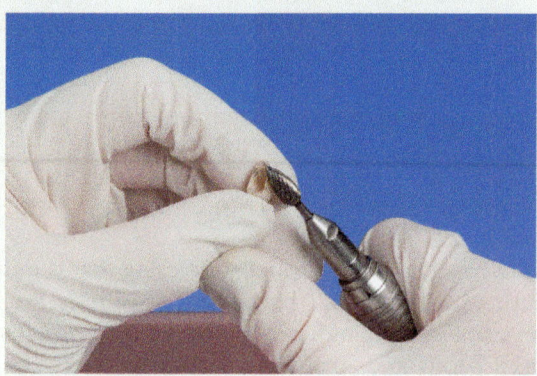

Figure P37-8-4B

12. Adjust the fit and occlusion, removing it and further trimming with an acrylic bur as needed.

13. Polish the provisional crown in the laboratory with the sterile white rag wheel and pumice stone. Always wear eye protection during this procedure.

14. Cement the provisional crown in place with a provisional cement, then check the occlusion with articulating paper. If further trimming is necessary, the dentist can perform it with an acrylic bur.

Removing Sutures

Sutures are used to control bleeding and promote healing after tissue has been cut during a procedure or through a trauma. Several types of sutures are available, including absorbable and nonabsorbable sutures. Absorbable sutures do not need removal—they are naturally absorbed into the body over a period of time. Nonabsorbable sutures, however, must be removed during a follow-up appointment. Nonabsorbable sutures are typically made from silk, polyester, or nylon. Suture removal is typically performed 5 to 7 days after they are placed. The timing and process of removal depends on the rate of healing and the type of suture used.

CHECKPOINT
37-11 When are nonabsorbable sutures typically removed?

Procedure 37–9 **Removing Sutures**

Materials needed (Figure P37-9-1):

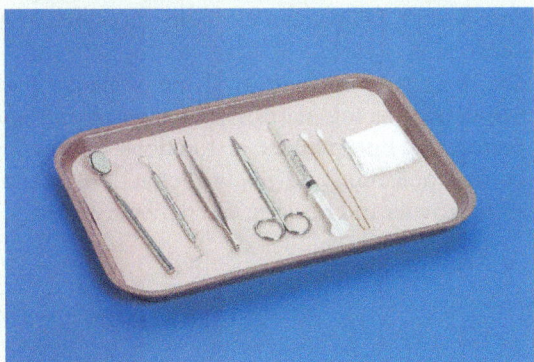

Figure P37-9-1

- Basic setup
- Cotton pliers
- Suture scissors
- Cotton-tipped applicator
- Antiseptic solution
- Sterile cotton gauze
- Sterile saline

1. The site is inspected by the oral surgeon or dentist to make sure healing is satisfactory.
2. Put on appropriate PPE.
3. Refer to the patient's chart to determine how many sutures must be removed.
4. Swab the site with an antiseptic to cleanse the area and remove debris.
5. Using cotton pliers, grasp the suture and pull it gently away from the tissue to expose the knot (Figure P37-9-2).

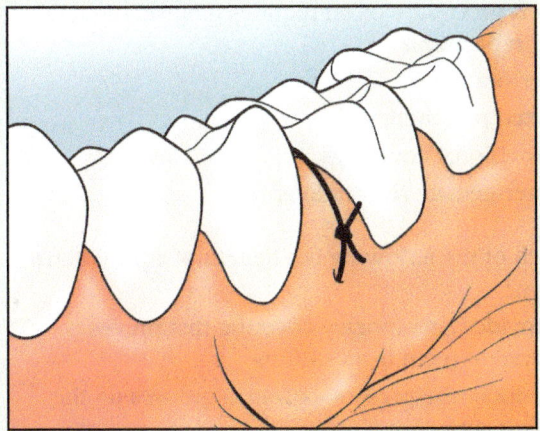

Figure P37-9-2

6. Using suture scissors, cut the sutures near the tissue. Be careful not to cut the tissue, but to slide the blade under the sutures and then snip (Figure P37-9-3).

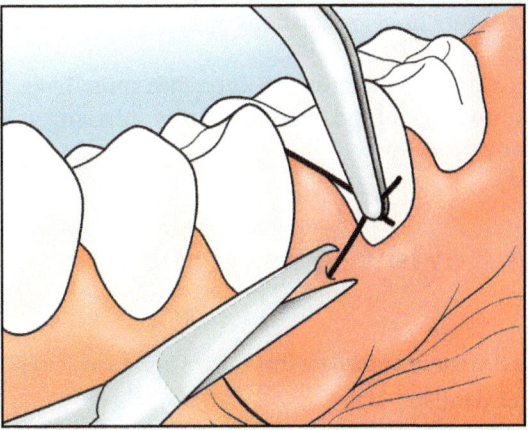

Figure P37-9-3

7. Use cotton pliers to gently grasp the suture by the knot and slide it through the tissue (Figure P37-9-4).

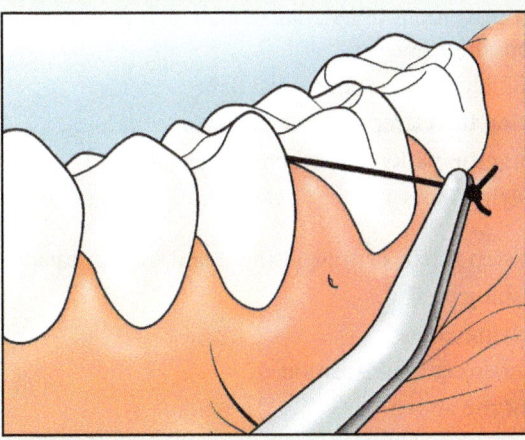

Figure P37-9-4

8. Prevent bleeding with gentle pressure applied with a compress. Swab bleeding areas with antiseptic to prevent infection.
9. Count during suture removal to make sure the number of sutures you remove corresponds to the number of sutures placed according to the patient's record.
10. Rinse the entire surgical site with sterile saline.

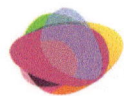

Chapter Highlights

✦ Expanded functions dental assistants receive special training that allows them to perform certain tasks by themselves, under supervision of the dentist.

✦ Expanded functions regulations vary from state to state.

✦ EFDAs act as the operator and therefore must have a sound knowledge of the instrumentation, anatomy, and goal of any procedure.

✦ Dentists are ultimately liable for anything that happens in the office, but EFDAs can be held accountable as employees.

✦ Expanded functions include applying sealants; placing dental dams; placing matrices; placing cements and bases; performing intermediate restorations, tooth whitening, coronal polishing, and gingival retraction; creating provisional crowns and bridges; and removing sutures.

Review Questions

1. What is the name of the law that covers EFDAs in states?
   a. Better dentistry act
   b. Dental practice act
   c. Dental assistant assistance act
   d. Responsible dentist act

2. During placement of a dental dam, which function is prohibited for EFDAs?
   a. Punching holes in the dental dam
   b. Placing the clamps on the patient's teeth
   c. Giving the patient anesthetic
   d. Applying frames

3. Which step is part of applying a pit and fissure sealant?
   a. Polishing teeth
   b. Applying etchant
   c. Maintaining total isolation
   d. All of the above

4. Name the matrix system that EFDAs cannot legally place, even in states that allow EFDAs.
   a. Tofflemire
   b. Strip
   c. Palodent
   d. None of the above

5. Which of the following is a component of a basic matrix system?
   a. Retainer
   b. Bur
   c. Explorer
   d. Curet

6. During placement of an intermediate restoration, which material is used most frequently?
   a. Amalgam
   b. Glass ionomer

   c. IRM
   d. Composite

7. EFDAs can legally perform which type of tooth whitening?
   a. At-home
   b. In-office
   c. Neither
   d. Both

8. Coronal polishing is performed with which instrument?
   a. Low-speed handpiece
   b. High-speed handpiece
   c. White rag polisher
   d. Buffing stone

9. Which procedure often requires gingival retraction as a preparation?
   a. Restorations
   b. Fixed prosthetics
   c. Provisional coverings
   d. Intermediate restorations

10. Which of the following is a benefit of a provisional crown?
    a. Provides a temporary covering that prevents adjacent teeth from shifting
    b. Reduces the presence of small grooves on the tooth surface
    c. Prevents exogenous stains from developing
    d. Eliminates the need for a permanent prosthetic

Active Learning Exercise

1. Imagine that a patient presents to the office for removal of a periodontal dressing. Describe the removal process if sutures have been used under the dressing.

Application Activities

1. Practice establishing an intraoral fulcrum using a mouth mirror.

2. Research online to find your specific state practice act. Describe the EFDA duties that are permissible in your state.

3. In comparison to over-the-counter and at-home treatment regimes, explain the advantages that a patient may expect by having tooth whitening performed in the dental office.

PREPARING FOR CERTIFICATION EXAMS

Review the following topics in this chapter to prepare for the Dental Assisting National Board (DANB) exam:

- **Applying Dental Sealants**
- **Placing a Dental Dam**
- **Placing a Matrix Band and Wedge for Restorations**
- **Performing Tooth Whitening**
- **Performing Coronal Polishing**
- **Removing Sutures**

Fixed Prosthodontics

CHAPTER OUTLINE

CHAPTER CHECKLIST

On completion of this chapter, students will be able to:

- ☑ Describe the types of fixed prostheses, including general appearance and function.
- ☑ Identify the materials used in the construction of various fixed prostheses.
- ☑ Identify fabricating techniques for various fixed prostheses.
- ☑ Explain the use of dental implants, including examples of types of implants and their functions.
- ☑ Identify retention techniques used to place prostheses.
- ☑ Describe the procedures for selecting, fabricating, and placing crowns, veneers, and bridges, including retention techniques and gingival retraction.
- ☑ Understand the role of the dental assistant during common prosthodontic procedures.
- ☑ Discuss the role of provisional coverages, as well as their placement.
- ☑ Describe important aspects of patient education and home care for patients receiving fixed prostheses.

KEY TERMS

bridge – a restoration used to replace one or more missing teeth

computer-aided design/computer-aided manufacture (CAD/CAM) – a special method of fabricating prosthodontic restorations using a computerized system

core buildup – a retention technique that provides support for a crown and helps restore the natural shape of the tooth; involves using amalgam or composites to replace damaged or missing parts of a tooth prior to crown placement

endosteal (en-DOS-tee-ul) implant – an implant that is inserted directly into the alveolar bone of the maxillary or mandibular jawbone

fabrication – in dentistry, the ways in which restorations are manufactured and assembled

fixed bridge – a fixed, nonremovable prosthesis used to fill the gap where one or more teeth are missing

fixed prosthesis – a prosthodontic restoration that cannot be removed from the oral cavity; includes crowns, inlays, onlays, bridges, and veneers

gingival retraction – the process of pulling the gingival tissue away from the tooth so that the entire area of the tooth surface can be molded for an accurate impression

gold alloy – a combination of gold with silver, copper, zinc, or other elements, which creates a restorative material that is hard and durable

Maryland bridge – a bridge that has small, metal, wing-like extensions that are bonded to the lingual surface of the anterior teeth

pontic (PON-tik) – an artificial tooth that serves as a substitute for a missing tooth (or teeth)

prosthodontics (pros-thuh-DON-tiks) – an area of dentistry focused on restorations that replace missing or broken teeth or parts of the tooth

provisional coverage – a temporary prosthesis, such as a crown or bridge, that is placed while a permanent prosthesis is being fabricated

retention pin – a nail-like device placed into the dentin of the tooth and placed underneath a core buildup for strength

retention technique – a technique used to make sure a prosthesis stays in place

retraction cord – used to move gingival tissue either by hand or by chemicals in the cord

subperiosteal (sub-per-ee-OS-tee-ul) implant – an implant that is inserted into the gingival tissue but sits on top of the jawbone

Introduction

Prosthodontics is an area of dentistry that focuses on restorations that replace missing teeth or parts of a tooth. Many prosthodontic procedures are performed by general dentists; others require the specialization of a prosthodontist. In either case, working with prosthodontics requires additional training after dental school.

The dental assistant's role in prosthodontics is to prepare for appointments, assist during procedures, take measurements, and record other information necessary for the creation of prostheses. The dental assistant plays an important role in educating patients and may also perform some laboratory procedures.

Overview of Fixed Prosthodontics

Fixed prostheses are prostheses that cannot be removed from the oral cavity. Indirect prostheses are restorations that cannot be created directly in the oral cavity (such as crowns), while direct restorations are made and applied directly in the oral cavity (such as inlays). Impressions, or molds, are usually taken of the patient's oral cavity, and the fixed prosthesis is made either in the dental office or in a dental laboratory. Fixed prostheses are generally classified in two ways:

- The way in which they restore a tooth's structure
- The material from which they are made

Both types of fixed prostheses are used not only to help the teeth function properly but to improve the overall appearance and stability of the remaining natural teeth. Examples of fixed prostheses include crowns, inlays, onlays, bridges, and veneers.

Indications and Contraindications

Patients who are to receive a fixed prosthesis need to have healthy gingival tissue and surrounding teeth as solid support for the restoration. Radiographs and impressions are often used to determine the health of the patient's oral cavity to ensure the prosthesis can be well-supported. Prosthesis recipients also need to be in generally good health overall so that the oral cavity will heal well after the prosthesis is placed. Patients who might not receive a fixed prosthesis include:

- Patients with severe gingival disease or other oral problems that would prevent the prosthesis from being supported
- Patients with bleeding disorders
- Patients with significant health problems that might reduce healing, such as cancer patients who are undergoing radiation or chemotherapy
- Patients who will not or cannot maintain the health of their prosthesis, including cleaning the prosthesis properly and attending appointments as needed

CHECKPOINTS

38-1 What are fixed prostheses?

38-2 Identify some contraindications for fixed prostheses.

Types of Fixed Prostheses

Crowns

Crowns act as caps for teeth that are decayed or broken. They are used to restore damaged teeth that have a large part of the tooth structure missing. A full crown is placed

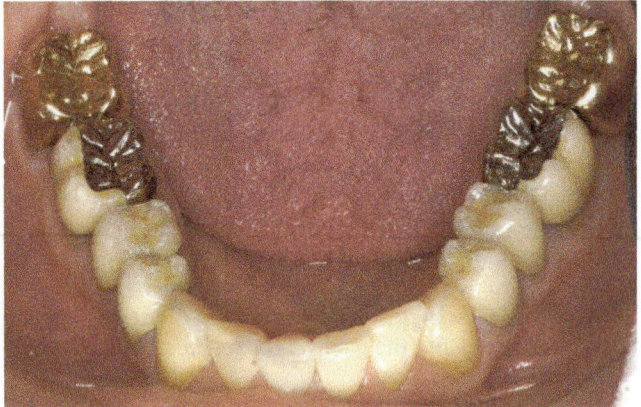

Figure 38–1 Full and partial crowns.

on a tooth that needs to be completely covered and held together. A ¾ crown, however, may cover much of the cusp surface, but it does not completely cover the entire cusp. Figure 38-1 shows full and partial crowns.

Inlays and Onlays

Inlays are restorations that are placed inside the cusps of the teeth. They replace small to medium-sized portions of the damaged tooth structure and allow a crown to be placed correctly. They are most commonly used to restore grooves or pits as well as to repair the posterior side of the tooth surface. Like inlays, onlays (or overlays) replace the structure of the tooth but are used when a much larger portion of the tooth structure needs to be replaced. Onlays not only sit inside the cusp but cover the surface ridges of the cusp as well. Both can be made of plastic/resin, porcelain, or gold and are cemented with permanent cement (Figure 38-2).

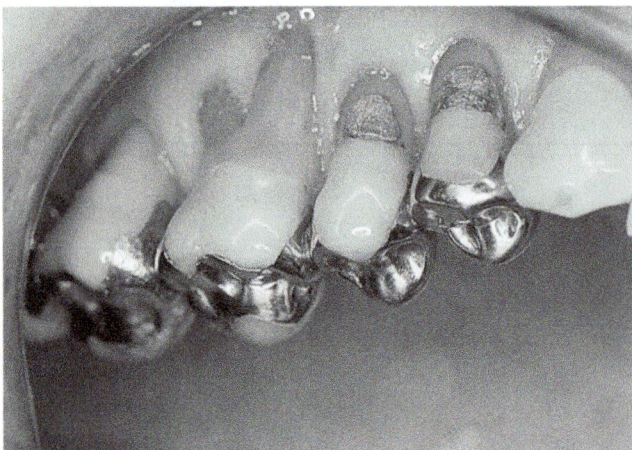

Figure 38–2 **Inlays and onlays.** Tooth no. 3 is restored with an inlay. Tooth no. 4 is restored with an inlay/onlay combination. Tooth no. 5 is restored with an onlay.

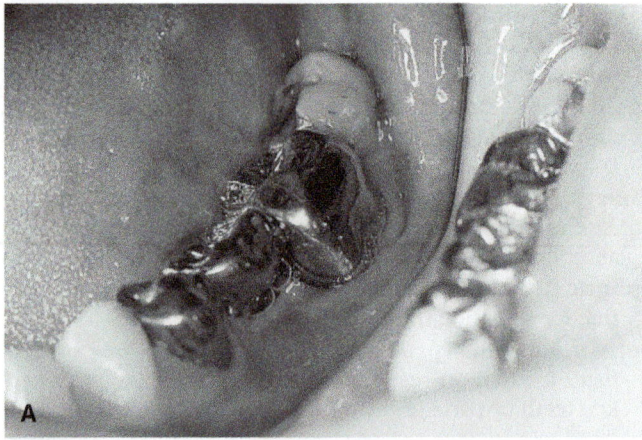

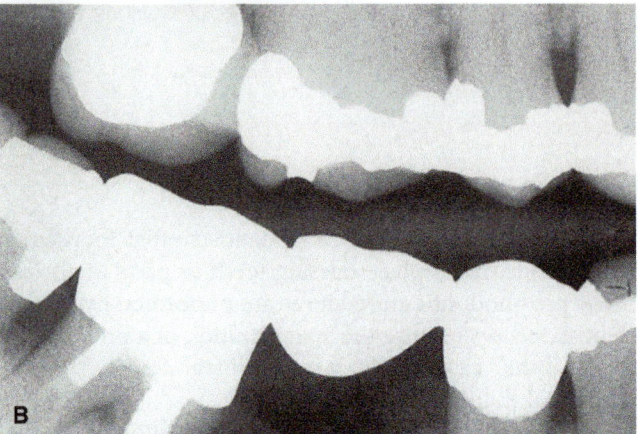

Figure 38–3 **A gold bridge.** (**A**) Photograph and (**B**) radiograph.

Fixed Bridges

Another type of fixed prosthesis is a bridge, which functions exactly like its name sounds. A **bridge** (Figure 38-3) is used to fill the space where a tooth is missing. Bridges include artificial teeth called **pontics**, which fill the space where a missing tooth once was. The supporting teeth located next to the pontic are called abutments. Abutment teeth may be fitted with crowns, inlays, or onlays to provide extra support for the pontic. A fixed bridge may be used to replace one tooth or several missing teeth.

Veneers

Much like the shell of a hard-boiled egg, a veneer is a thin layer of material that protects another material. A veneer is placed on the outer surface of the tooth to improve its appearance, such as treating darkened or yellowed teeth, or to repair a tooth's abnormalities, such as crooked or misshapen teeth. Veneers can be bonded or cemented with permanent cement.

✔ **CHECKPOINT**
38-3 Why might a patient want a veneer?

Materials

Numerous materials are used to create fixed prostheses. The material chosen can affect how well the restoration functions and stays in place. Different materials are used for different types of prostheses.

Gold Alloys

Gold alloys are among the most commonly used materials for prosthetic restorations such as inlays, onlays, and crowns. An alloy is a combination of two or more metals. Some restoratives use gold alloys rather than pure gold, which is too soft. **Gold alloys** combine gold with silver, copper, zinc, or other elements to create a material that is hard and durable. Gold alloys, however, are generally used to improve the health and functioning of a tooth, not to improve its appearance.

Porcelain

Porcelain is a ceramic material that is often used in prosthodontics to improve the appearance of teeth, such as when a tooth is discolored or misshapen. Although porcelain effectively makes teeth appear healthier and more natural-looking, as a material it is not very strong and does not resist fracturing as well as other materials. This is why porcelain is generally used in making veneers, not inlays, onlays, or crowns.

Porcelain-fused-to-metal (PFM) crowns, which combine the strength of metal and the aesthetic benefit of porcelain, are often used in restorations. An underlying metal substructure provides strength and stability while the porcelain covering on the outer surfaces provides a pleasing appearance. This is one of the most commonly used combinations for bridges and crowns. In certain cosmetic cases, or in cases of metal allergy, all-ceramic crowns might be used.

Composites

Restoratives made of composites are becoming more popular as laboratory techniques have improved their strength and durability. Composites are tooth-colored resins made from the mineral quartz. Their natural-looking appearance makes them a popular alternative for patients who do not like the appearance of metal restorations or amalgams. Composites are frequently used for inlays, onlays, and crowns. At present, composites

generally fracture and wear at a greater rate than metal restorations, but the materials are constantly improving.

✔ **CHECKPOINT**
38-4 What is the benefit of a porcelain-fused-to-metal crown?

Fabrication

Dental **fabrication** refers to the ways in which restorations are manufactured and assembled. Dental assistants play several important roles in fabricating prostheses, including preparing the equipment and materials, educating patients, assisting the dentist in preparing and placing the materials, and, in some states, performing some procedures, such as making impressions of the patient's oral cavity.

Dental Laboratory

In a dental laboratory, technicians fabricate prostheses using materials such as waxes, plastics, alloys, and porcelain. The fabrication techniques include the following:

- Creating dental casts, which are then used to fabricate the restorations
- Making replications of a prepared tooth
- Creating full or partial dentures or fixed bridges for missing teeth
- Finishing and polishing crowns

CAD/CAM Systems

Special dentistry computers are being used today to help fabricate restorations. Such systems use a computer to both design and manufacture the restoration and are therefore known as **computer-aided design/computer-aided manufacture (CAD/CAM)** systems (Figure 38-4). These systems are used largely with porcelain materials and allow dentists to create and place nonmetal restorations in a single appointment. In addition, physical molds and impressions do not need to be taken, as the CAD/CAM systems can create impressions using special light-based lasers, called optics. This makes the procedure easier and more pleasant for the patient. Because these systems are computerized, they allow dentists to fabricate the restorations more accurately. However, being all porcelain, these restorations have a higher fracture rate than traditional crowns or bridges.

✔ **CHECKPOINT**
38-5 In the CAD/CAM systems, what is used to create impressions?

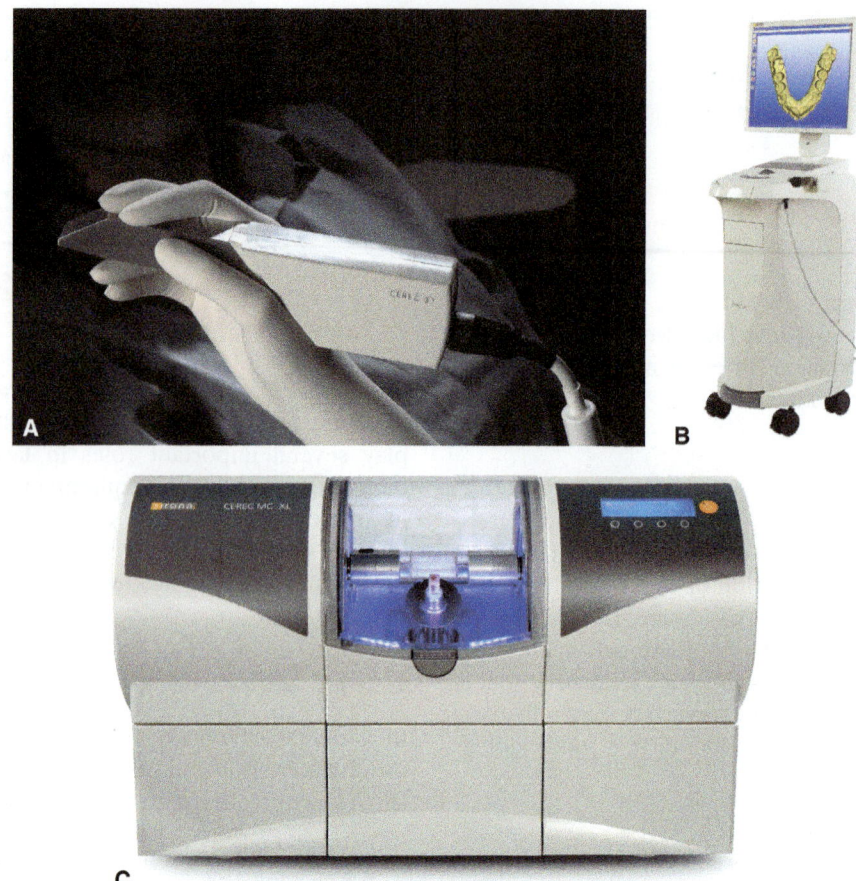

Figure 38–4 **CAD/CAM system.** **(A)** Intraoral digital scanning device. **(B)** CAD component to design a virtual model of the restoration. **(C)** CAM component to fabricate the restoration from a ceramic or composite resin block.

Retention Techniques

Patients who require a fixed prosthesis usually have damaged or weakened tooth structures. As a result, **retention techniques** are used to make sure the restoration stays in place and that the underlying tooth structure is strong enough to support the restoration. Several different methods can be used to ensure that restorations are correctly placed and remain in place.

Dental Implants

When a patient's oral health is so poor that the remaining teeth cannot provide enough support for a prosthesis, dental implants (Figure 38-5) can provide additional support for restorations. Implants are placed directly into the bone or gingival tissue. Over the following 6 months the bone slowly grows around the implant, helping to provide stability. A crown, bridge, or other restoration can then be attached to the implant.

Indications and Contraindications

Patients with missing teeth and who have healthy jaw bone structure are considered good candidates for dental

implants. Also, patients who receive dental implants should have healthy gingival tissue that is free of disease or inflammation. Dental professionals who specialize in the tissues and bone of the oral cavity, called periodontists, examine the patient to determine whether the oral cavity is healthy enough to support an implant.

Types of Implants

Implants can be fixed, or cemented in place, and can also be removable. Removable implants, including overdentures and copings, are discussed in Chapter 39, Removable Prosthodontics. Fixed implants are classified in the following categories:

- **Endosteal implants** are implants that are inserted directly into the alveolar bone of the mandibular or maxillary jawbone. These are the most common types and usually come in the form of screws or cylinders. They can be used to replace one or more missing teeth and are useful for patients who need bridges but who do not have strong enough supporting teeth to act as abutments.
- **Subperiosteal implants** are inserted into the gingival tissue but sit on top of the jawbone. The implants protrude through the gingival tissue, where the restoration can be securely attached. These are ideal for patients who do not have adequate bone to support endosteal implants.

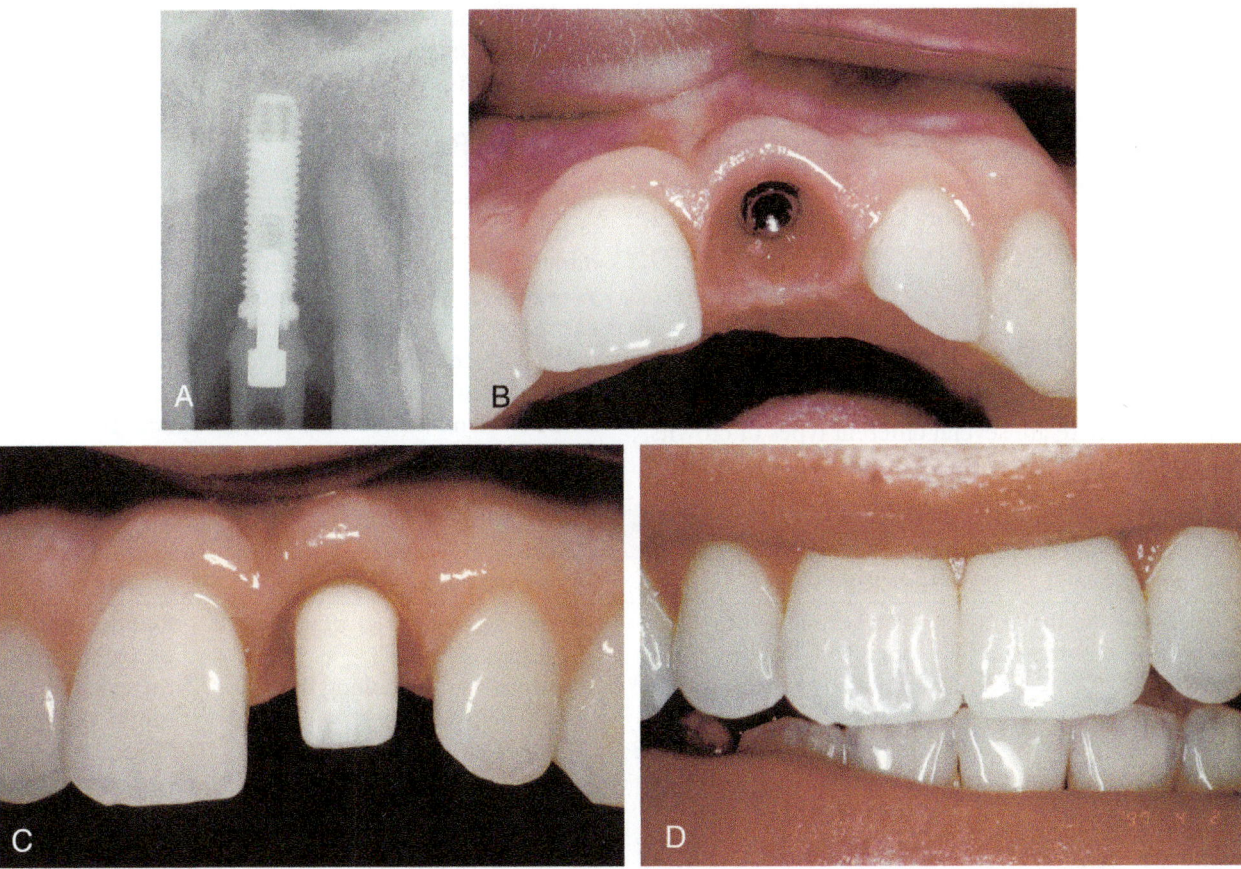

Figure 38–5 Implant restored with a crown. (**A**) Radiograph of the implant, abutment, and abutment screw. (**B**) Photograph of implant. (**C**) Esthetic abutment and cylinder. (**D**) Crown. (Courtesy of Dr. Roger A. Lawton, Olympia, WA, and Nobel Biocare, Yorba Linda, CA.)

- Transosteal implants are implants that pass through the full thickness of the jaw bone. Because of the invasive nature of this type of implant, it is rarely used in modern dentistry, although it may be used as a last resort in cases involving severe resorption of the mandibular ridge.
- Mini-implants are a newer form of implant that is popular for orthodontic movements and to support overdentures. The tiny implants are inserted directly into the bone and the restoration is attached immediately, without any waiting period for the bone to fuse with the implant.

Implants can be used for prostheses that replace one missing tooth, several missing teeth, or an entire set of teeth.

Core Buildups

For especially damaged teeth that require a crown, a **core buildup** is often performed. The core buildup provides support for the crown and helps restore the natural shape of the tooth. A root canal is first performed to remove infected or necrotic pulp tissue and any remaining decay. The core buildup, usually made from amalgam or composite resin, replaces the missing tooth material and strengthens the remaining parts of the tooth to ensure the crown will stay in place. A weak tooth that does not receive a core buildup before placement of a crown may develop a tooth fracture and possibly lead to loss of the tooth.

Post and Core

The post and core procedure may be necessary when placing a restoration on a tooth that is weakened due to root canal. In this procedure, a metal post is placed inside the tooth canal about two-thirds of the way down the canal, allowing the remaining one-third to remain sealed with the gutta percha, and secured using dental cement. Then, a core buildup can be performed to prepare for placement of the restoration.

Retention Pins

To provide even more support for a core buildup, the dentist may use a device called a **retention pin**. The pin is anchored into the dentin of the tooth and placed underneath the core buildup. Retention pins are also used in live teeth, without root canals, to help support large amalgam or composite restorations.

CHECKPOINT
38-6 List the four types of fixed implants.

Crown Procedures

Crowns help restore the function of a damaged tooth. Depending on the type of crown selected, they can also improve the appearance of a misshapen or discolored tooth. Because crowns are fabricated in a dental laboratory, placement of a provisional crown is usually necessary until the permanent crown is available.

Selection and Preparation

The crown procedure begins by determining which type of crown to use. There are several different types of crowns, each with their own benefits and weaknesses (Table 38-1). The dentist examines the patient's oral cavity and decides which type is most appropriate.

Gingival Retraction

Before a crown can be placed, an impression of the tooth is made. To accomplish this, the area of the tooth just under the gingival tissue must be exposed. **Gingival retraction** is the process of pulling the gingival tissue away from the tooth so that the entire area of the tooth surface can be molded for an accurate impression. A **retraction cord** may be used to move the gingival tissue by hand (called mechanical retraction), or the cord

TABLE 38-1 Types and Features of Dental Crowns

TYPE OF CROWN	DESCRIPTION	STRENGTHS	WEAKNESSES
Porcelain-fused-to-metal crowns or ceramometal crowns	■ Metal crowns with porcelain veneers attached to them ■ Very popular because they not only help restore the function of the tooth, but the veneer helps restore the appearance of the tooth	■ Strong, resist fracturing and discoloration ■ More natural looking than all-metal crowns	■ Require more preparation for the existing tooth ■ Porcelain is fragile and can break easily ■ Not as natural looking as ceramic
All-ceramic, all-porcelain, and all-resin crowns	■ Made entirely of ceramic, porcelain, or resin; no metal is used	■ Ceramic and porcelain are the most natural-looking crowns ■ Useful for front teeth ■ All-resin crowns tend to be less expensive	■ Not as durable or tough as metal crowns ■ Not useful for posterior teeth due to excessive pressure from biting and chewing
Full gold crowns	■ Made completely from gold alloy ■ Covers the entire anatomic portion of the tooth	■ Durable ■ Last longer than non-metal crowns ■ Can hold up under the pressure of biting and chewing, making them suitable for placement on posterior teeth	■ Less natural-looking than ceramic
Three-quarter gold crowns	■ Also known as onlays ■ Cover approximately ¾ of the tooth	■ Durable ■ Can hold up under the pressure of biting and chewing, making them suitable for placement on posterior teeth	■ Less natural-looking than ceramic

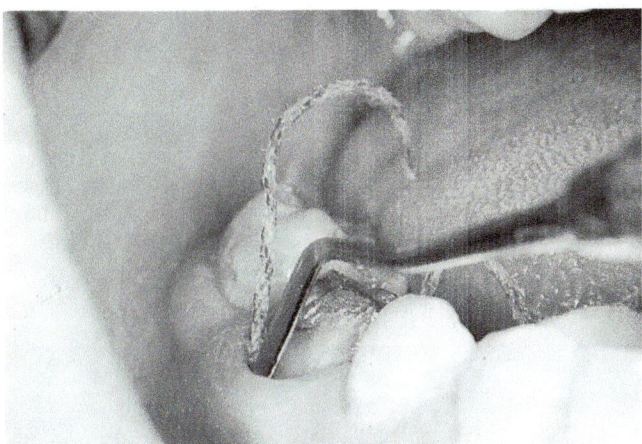

Figure 38–6 Gingival retraction cord.

may contain a chemical (vasoconstrictor) that causes the gingival tissue to shrink (called chemical retraction), revealing the underlying area of the tooth (Figure 38-6). Surgical retraction is sometimes used when a patient's gingival tissue is overgrown and covers an unusually large surface area of the tooth.

Table 38-2 outlines different types of retraction cords. The type of cord used may depend on factors such as the patient's medical history or the dentist's personal preference. Remember to ask patients about their medical history before using a retraction cord. If the patient has a history of heart problems or excessive bleeding, special solutions can be applied to the cord beforehand to reduce bleeding.

TABLE 38-2 Types of Gingival Retraction Cords	
Untwisted cord	■ Also known as a plain cord ■ Must be twisted before placement
Twisted or braided cord	■ Can be placed directly without additional twisting
Impregnated cord	■ Uses chemicals that cause the gingival tissue to shrink ■ Contains 10% aluminum chloride to reduce bleeding
Non-impregnated cord	■ Does not contain any chemicals ■ Gingival tissue is pulled away from the tooth by force ■ Also called mechanical retraction

Retraction cords are placed using a packing instrument. The rounded end of the packing instrument pushes the cord into the gingival tissue firmly; care must be taken not to press so firmly that the tissue is damaged. Once the tissue is pulled away from the tooth, the cord is quickly removed, and the impression is taken immediately. See Chapter 37, Expanded Clinical Functions, for a detailed description of the procedure for placing gingival retraction cord.

Provisional Coverage

After the impression has been made, a temporary cover—called a **provisional coverage**—is placed over the tooth or, in some cases, where a tooth or teeth are missing. A provisional coverage performs several functions:

- Provides protection for the outside areas of the tooth
- Helps reduce sensitivity and increase patient comfort while waiting for the permanent restoration to be fabricated
- Keeps nearby teeth from shifting before the final restoration can be placed
- Maintains the overall appearance and function of the tooth

Provisional coverages typically stay in the patient's oral cavity for a short time, generally from several days to a few weeks, until the final cementing of the permanent restoration. Because they are temporary restorations, they are cemented using temporary, lower-strength cements, such as zinc oxide eugenol.

Materials and Fabrication

Provisional coverages are commonly custom fabricated. A prefabricated type of provisional coverage is also available in many different sizes and materials. For example, prefabricated crowns include:

- Polymer crowns that are filled with a composite resin to cement the crown to the tooth
- Polycarbonate crowns that can be customized for anterior teeth
- Stainless steel crowns that are strong and used mostly for posterior teeth

In states with expanded functions dental assistants (EFDAs), qualified dental assistants can fabricate and place a provisional crown. In other states dental assistants help as the dentist places the restoration. The steps are similar for provisional bridges, which are also formed from alginate impressions and cemented in place with provisional cement. See Procedure 37-8 in Chapter 37, Expanded Clinical Functions, for this procedure for an EFDA.

Procedure 38–1 **Fabricating and Placing a Provisional Crown**

This procedure is described for dental assistants who are assisting the dentist with the creation and placement of a provisional crown.

Materials needed (Figure P38-1-1):

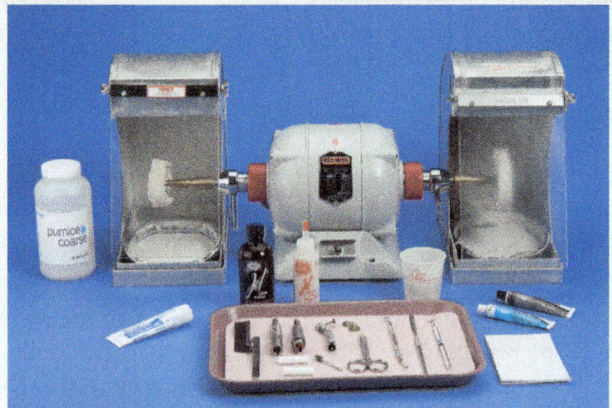

Figure P38-1-1

- Basic setup
- Spoon excavator
- Alginate impression, obtained before preparation of teeth
- Separating medium
- Cotton rolls
- Self-curing acrylic resin, liquid and powder
- Spatula, small cement type
- Dappen dish
- Scissors
- Laboratory knife, optional
- Burnisher, ball or "beaver tail"
- Straight handpiece and mandrel
- Acrylic burs
- Finishing burs, diamond, or discs
- Pumice
- Articulating paper
- Lathe and sterile white rag wheel
- Provisional cementation setup

1. Put on appropriate PPE.
2. Inspect and prepare the alginate impression. This includes making sure it is free from defects in the area of the provisional crown. Disinfect and moisten it, then set it aside until it is needed.
3. Maintain moisture control and isolation of the prepared tooth using cotton rolls.
4. Prepare the site with petroleum jelly, which will help the provisional crown separate from the mold.

5. Retrieve the alginate impression and dry it in preparation for loading with the resin.
6. Prepare the liquid monomer in a dappen dish. Mix it according to the manufacturer's instructions and add the proper shade of self-curing powder.
7. Blend the monomer with a spatula (Figure P38-1-2), then set it aside until it forms a doughy mass.

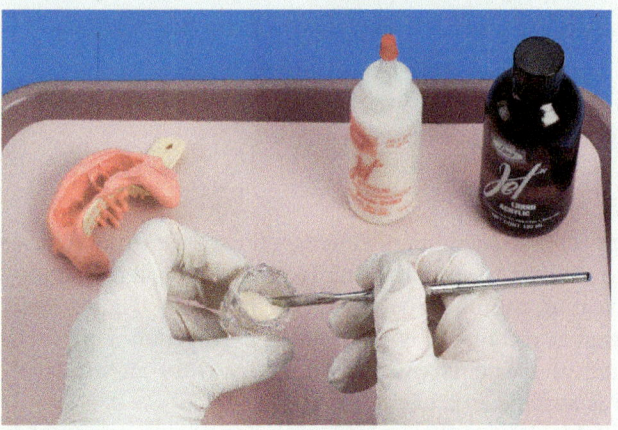

Figure P38-1-2

8. Load the resin into the prepared impression (Figure P38-1-3) and transfer the impression to the dentist.

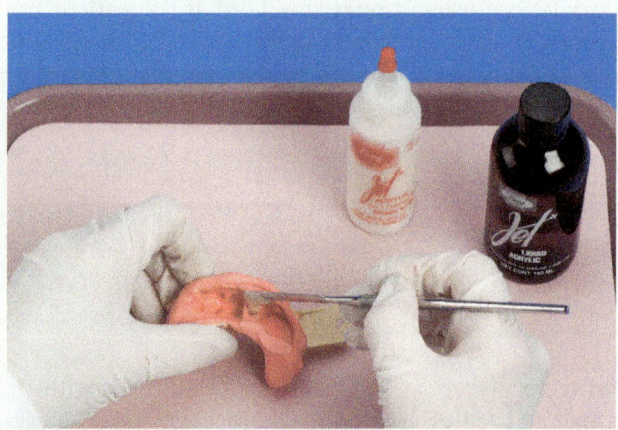

Figure P38-1-3

9. The dentist places the impression onto the patient's prepared tooth.
10. The resin sets for about 3 minutes. The dentist then gently lifts the impression tray away from the patient's oral cavity.
11. The dentist removes the provisional cover from the impression and places it on the patient's prepared tooth.
12. The dentist marks the provisional crown with a pencil (Figure P38-1-4), then trims it to within 1 mm of the gingiva with an acrylic bur or stone.

Procedure 38–1 Fabricating and Placing a Provisional Crown (Continued)

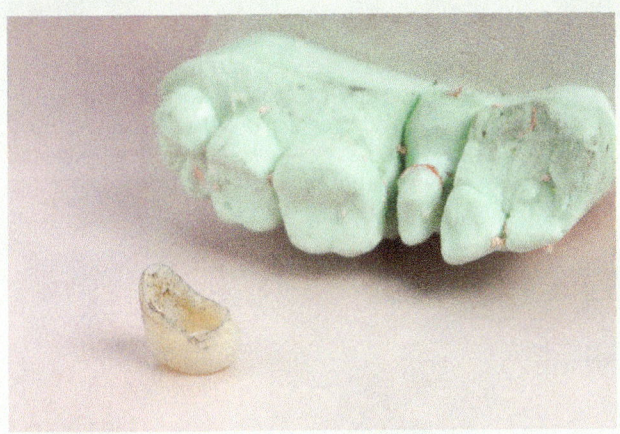

Figure P38-1-4

13. The dentist adjusts the fit and occlusion, removing it and further trimming with an acrylic bur as needed.

14. Polish the provisional crown in the laboratory with the sterile white rag wheel and pumice stone. Always wear eye protection during this procedure.

15. The dentist cements the provisional crown in place with a provisional cement.

16. Check the occlusion with articulating paper. If further trimming is necessary, the dentist can perform it with an acrylic bur.

Assisting in Crown Procedures

Placement of a crown usually occurs in several stages. If a porcelain crown is being used, be sure to select the right shade by examining the patient's surrounding teeth. The crown must also be selected to fit the general shape and height of the tooth, although the dentist will reduce the size of the tooth so that the crown will fit properly. If excessive decay or damage is present, the dentist will apply any necessary retention aids, including core buildups or retention pins. Follow the steps for gingival retention and take an impression so that the crown can be accurately shaped to the tooth. The impression is then sent to a dental laboratory, where the crown is fabricated. This process takes approximately 2 weeks, except with CAD/CAM procedures. During this time, a provisional crown can be placed to help the patient eat, speak, and function normally. When the permanent crown is ready for placement, the provisional coverage is removed and saved in case it is needed later, such as if the permanent crown has to be removed and refabricated. When the permanent crown is ready, the dentist secures it in place with a bonding agent.

Procedure 38–2 Permanent Crown Placement (After Removal of the Provisional Coverage)

Materials needed (Figure P38-2-1):

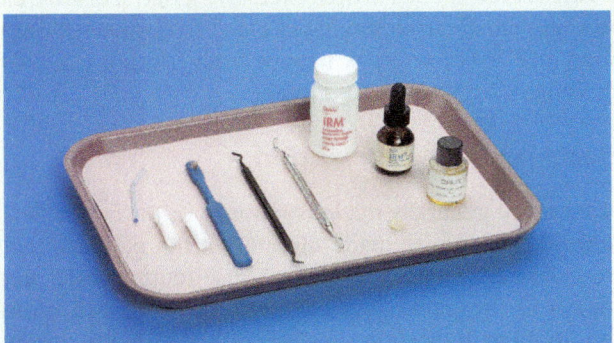

Figure P38-2-1

- Air-water syringe
- Saliva ejector
- HVE
- Basic setup
- Cotton rolls
- Bite stick
- Plastic filling instrument
- Cavity varnish or liner (optional)
- Permanent luting cement
- Scaler or explorer
- Custom fabricated crown
- Floss

1. Put on appropriate PPE.

2. The dentist cleans away any excess cement left after removing the temporary crown.

3. Rinse and dry the tooth with the air-water syringe and surround it with cotton rolls to keep it isolated from nearby teeth.

4. Transfer the crown to the dentist. The dentist places the crown on the patient's tooth to make sure it fits properly. A bite stick can be used to make sure it fits securely. If the cast crown fits, the dentist may proceed. If not, the crown is returned to the dental laboratory to be adjusted.

Procedure 38-2 Permanent Crown Placement (After Removal of the Provisional Coverage) (Continued)

5. The dentist uses a cavity varnish or liner on the prepared tooth before applying the permanent crown.

6. Mix the permanent cement according to the manufacturer's instructions.

7. Transfer the cement to the dentist.

8. The dentist puts the cement inside the crown as well as directly on the prepared tooth using the plastic filling instrument.

9. The dentist places the crown on the tooth and asks the patient to bite down hard to ensure the crown is secure. The patient can bite on the bite stick to help (Figure P38-2-2). Insert the saliva ejector to aid in keeping the field dry.

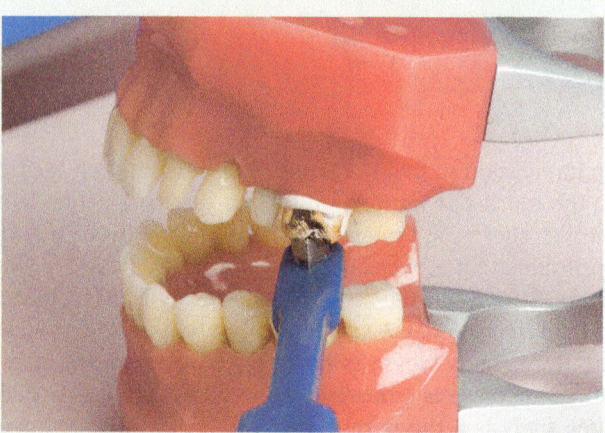

Figure P38-2-2

10. After the cement has hardened, remove the cotton rolls and transfer the scaler or explorer to the dentist. The dentist uses the scaler or explorer to carefully remove any excess cement that has leaked outside the edges of the crown, being careful not to scratch or displace the crown (Figure P38-2-3).

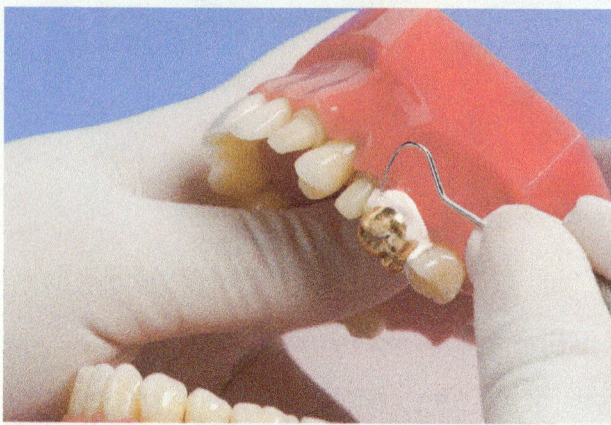

Figure P38-2-3

11. Tie a knot in the dental floss and floss the teeth to remove excess cement from the interproximal areas.

12. Advise patients to not eat for at least 30 to 60 minutes and to avoid hard foods or very chewy or sticky foods for the first 24 hours.

CHECKPOINTS

38-7 What is gingival retraction?

38-8 Why should you ask about the patient's medical history before using a gingival retraction cord?

38-9 What are some benefits of using all-porcelain crowns? What are some of the disadvantages?

Veneers

Veneers are helpful not only for restoring the function of teeth but for improving their appearance as well. Veneers have become increasingly popular.

Indications and Contraindications

Patients who receive veneers usually have stained or discolored teeth; teeth that are crooked or oddly shaped; or a diastema (Figure 38-7). Patients who are not good candidates for veneers include individuals at high risk for dental caries and those who are not likely to maintain the health of their teeth. Further, excessive gingival disease can prevent veneers from staying in place. Extensive malocclusions may also prevent a patient from being a candidate for veneers.

Materials and Fabrication

Veneers are generally made from resin or porcelain. Resin veneers that can be made directly on the patient's teeth are called direct resin veneers. These require little preparation of the patient's tooth and can be placed in one appointment. Indirect resin veneers, however, require two appointments—one to prepare the tooth and a second to place the veneer. The veneer is fabricated in an outside laboratory. Resin veneers are considered weaker and less durable than porcelain veneers. Porcelain veneers are tough and have a very natural-looking appearance, making them ideal for treating teeth that are stained or discolored. Like indirect resin veneers, porcelain veneers require two appointments for preparation and placement.

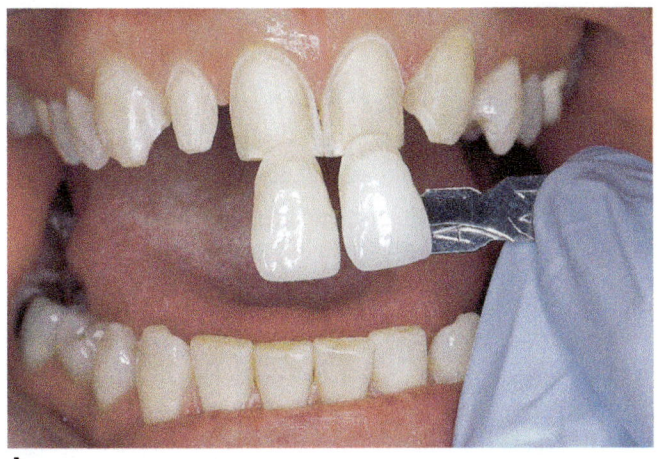 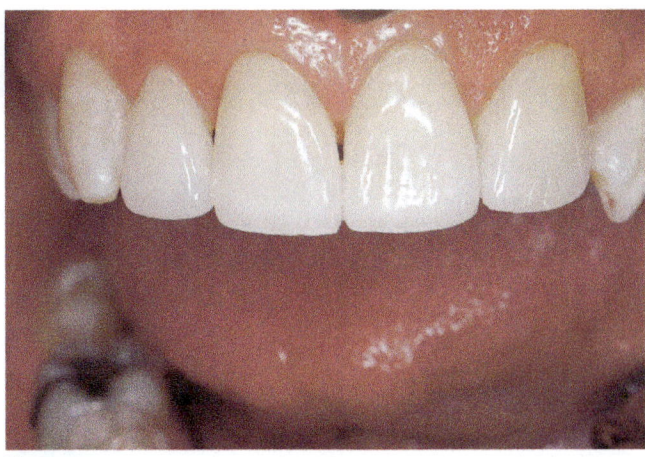

A **B**

Figure 38–7 Veneers. (**A**) Teeth prepared for indirect veneers. (**B**) Veneers cemented in place. (Courtesy of Ultradent Products, Inc.)

Procedure 38-3 Assisting with Cementing of Porcelain Veneers (After Fabrication)

Dental assistant duties in this procedure can vary greatly depending on the preference of the dentist and the regulations of each state.

Materials needed (Figure P38-3-1):

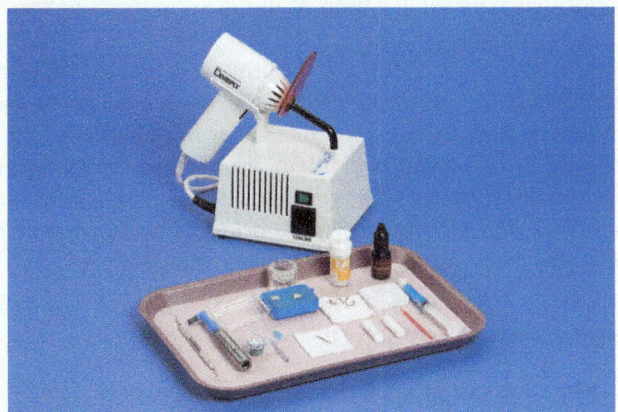

Figure P38-3-I

- Protective eyewear for the patient
- Air-water syringe
- Cotton rolls
- Basic setup
- Fabricated veneer
- Retraction cord
- Etchant and applicator
- Light-cured bonding agent
- Curing light
- Finishing diamonds or burs (if needed)

- Rubber wheels and cusp for polishing
- Polishing paste
- Pumice
- HVE
- Saliva ejector
- Floss

1. Put on appropriate PPE.
2. Measure the tooth to determine the size of the veneer. Once a veneer is selected, try it on for size. Be very careful—veneers are fragile.
3. Once the fit is determined, the dentist uses an etchant to clean and dry the inside of the veneer (Figure P38-3-2).

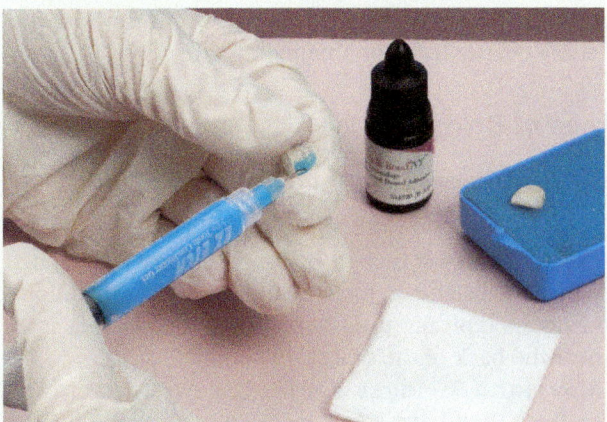

Figure P38-3-2

4. The dentist places light-cured bonding agent in the veneer (Figure P38-3-3). The veneer is held in a light-protected area until ready to be placed on the prepared tooth.

Procedure 38–3 Assisting with Cementing of Porcelain Veneers (After Fabrication) (Continued)

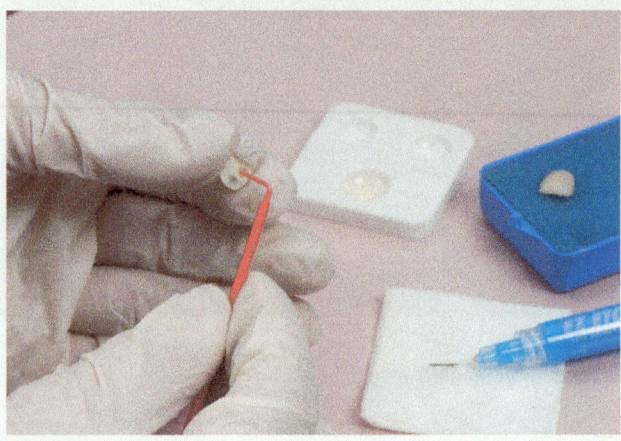

Figure P38-3-3

5. The dentist prepares the tooth for bonding with a retraction cord and cleans the surface of the tooth thoroughly.
6. Make sure the tooth is dry and free of all moisture using the air-water syringe. Use cotton rolls to isolate the tooth.
7. The dentist etches the surface of the tooth being bonded, following the manufacturer's instructions on the etching agent.
8. The dentist applies an adhesive to the tooth and places the veneer on the tooth.
9. The veneer is light-cured in place and the dentist removes any excess cement with the explorer.
10. If needed, the dentist uses a handpiece, with finishing diamonds or burs, to ensure the margins of the veneer are clean and even.
11. The dentist polishes the veneers with polishing paste, rubber wheels, and cusp.

CHECKPOINT

38-10 What materials are commonly used to create veneers?

Bridges

Fixed bridges are made of a metal framework and one or more pontics that act as artificial replacements for missing teeth. The bridge stays in place due to support provided by nearby teeth, or abutment teeth.

Types of Bridges

There are three main types of fixed bridges:

- Traditional crown-and-bridges (see Figure 38-3) are exactly as they sound—a bridge with crowns attached, which are placed on the abutment teeth. The traditional bridge is typically used when teeth are missing in or near the back of the oral cavity.
- **Maryland bridges** are bridges without crowns. Instead, they have small, metal, wing-like extensions that are bonded to the lingual surfaces of the abutment teeth. Maryland bridges are also known as resin-bonded bridges. This bridge is typically used when teeth are missing in the anterior portion of the oral cavity.
- Cantilever bridges are used when abutment teeth are present only on one side of the missing tooth or teeth.

Selection and Preparation

The type of bridge selected by the dentist depends on many factors, such as the location of the missing tooth or teeth, whether nearby abutment teeth are present, and whether the neighboring teeth are healthy enough to support the bridge. To prepare a bridge, the dentist prepares the abutment teeth to make them smaller in size to allow the crowns to be placed over them. Impressions of the teeth are taken, which serve as a model for fabricating the bridge, pontic(s), and crowns. While the bridge is being fabricated in a dental laboratory, a provisional coverage is used.

Provisional Coverage

A temporary bridge allows patients to maintain the function of their teeth while their permanent bridge is being fabricated, which usually takes 2 to 3 weeks. Provisional bridges are usually fabricated with acrylics, composites, or self-curing resins, which become doughy once set and are easily molded to fill the space of missing teeth. Prior to preparing the provisional, an impression of the patient's existing teeth and arch is made. This impression is used as a mold for creating the provisional. After the provisional material is shaped and set, it is placed back in the patient's oral cavity to finish setting.

Materials and Fabrication

Traditional bridges are usually made from porcelain fused to metal or ceramics. Maryland bridges are typically made from resin and metal. Fabrication takes place in a dental laboratory. Bridges can be fabricated either by being molded from a cast or by using a CAD/CAM system.

Procedure 38-4 **Fabricating and Cementing a Provisional Bridge**

Some states allow qualified dental assistants to perform this procedure; in other states the dental assistant assists the dentist during the procedure. Check the regulations governing your state for more information about the specific duties dental assistants are allowed to perform.

Materials needed (Figure P38-4-1):

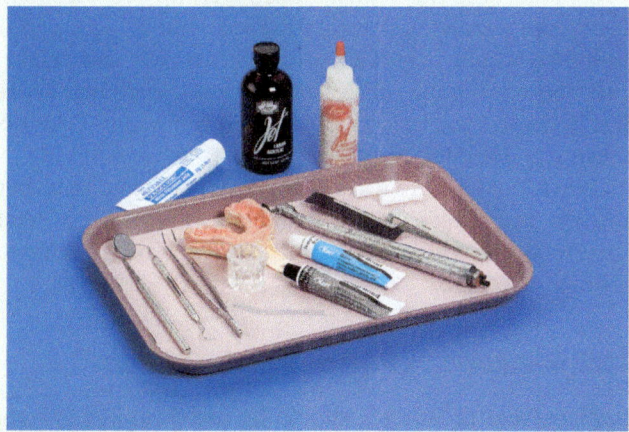

Figure P38-4-1

- Basic setup
- Air-water syringe
- Cotton rolls
- Petroleum jelly or other lubricant
- Alginate impression
- Self-curing acrylic resin
- Cement spatula
- Mixing pad
- Temporary cement
- Finishing diamonds or burs
- Acrylic burs
- Lathe
- Rag wheel
- Pumice
- Saliva ejector
- HVE
- Crown and bridge scissors
- Slow speed handpiece
- Articulating paper
- High speed handpiece
- Mandrels
- Floss

1. Put on appropriate PPE.
2. An impression of the teeth and arch is made before the teeth are prepared. Be sure the impression is clean and keep it slightly moist until it is needed later.
3. Clean and dry the teeth using an air-water syringe, and isolate the teeth with a cotton roll. Apply a light layer of petroleum jelly to the teeth so the provisional bridge can be easily removed.
4. Place the liquid monomer in the mixing area according to the manufacturer's instructions.
5. Quickly add the self-curing powder and mix immediately with a spatula. Cover the mixture immediately and let it sit 1 to 2 minutes, until it looks glossy and dough-like.
6. Unwrap the initial impression and dry off any moisture. Place the resin mixture directly into the impression.
7. The dentist places the impression into the patient's oral cavity.
8. The resin sets for approximately 3 minutes, and the dentist removes the impression from the patient's oral cavity.
9. Carefully remove the provisional bridge from the impression. Cut any flash with the crown and bridge scissors.
10. The dentist places the provisional bridge back in the patient's oral cavity to avoid any further shrinking while it continues to set.
11. Using a pencil, the dentist marks the border where the provisional bridge meets the gingival tissue to identify where excess material needs to be trimmed. After the provisional bridge is completely set and is removed from the patient's oral cavity, the dentist trims within 1 millimeter of the border.
12. The dentist checks the provisional bridge for cleanliness and to make sure the size fits in the patient's oral cavity. Using temporary cement, such as zinc oxide eugenol, the dentist cements the provisional bridge in the patient's oral cavity (Figure P38-4-2).

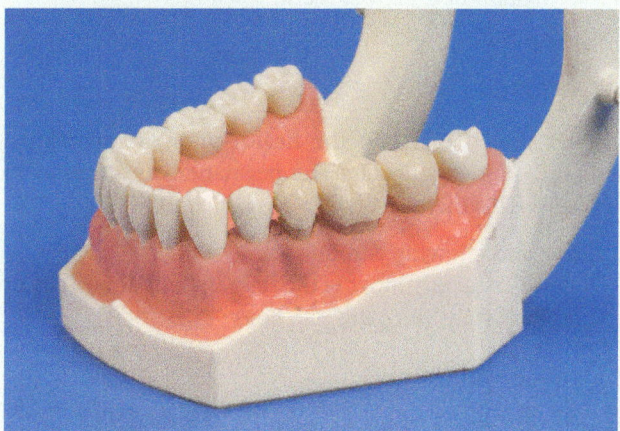

Figure P38-4-2

Assisting in Bridge Procedures

Dental assistants serve several key functions throughout the bridge fabrication and cementing procedures. Providing and maintaining suction is important to keep the prepared area clean and dry; otherwise, the provisional material may not set properly or stay cemented in place. Placement and removal of the gingival cord allows an accurate impression to be taken, which helps ensure the provisional is fabricated to the correct size. Further, as a dental assistant, you may assist with fabricating the provisional bridge by mixing the composite or resin material. Dental assistants also are responsible for mixing the zinc oxide eugenol that is used to temporarily cement the provisional in place. Be sure to follow the instructions carefully on the cement packaging. Excess cement can be removed using an explorer or scaler.

CHECKPOINTS

38-11 What are the three main types of bridges?

38-12 What are some of the purposes of a provisional coverage?

Patient Education and Home Care

It is vital that patients understand how to properly care for their prostheses. Good oral hygiene is the most important factor affecting how long a prosthesis will last. Without proper care, these restorations may not work properly or may break altogether. Encourage patients to take the same time and care to maintain the health of their restorations as they would their natural teeth.

Provisional Coverage

Patients should maintain the health of their provisional coverage while waiting for the permanent restoration to be placed. This includes:

- Biting and chewing carefully
- Flossing by gently moving the floss up and down, rather than forcefully "popping" the floss

- Brushing regularly, including after meals
- Avoiding eating or chewing on the side of the oral cavity with the provisional coverage, as much as possible
- Avoiding sticky foods, such as caramel, toffee, or chewing gum
- Avoiding foods that require lots of hard chewing or crunching, such as raw carrots

If a provisional coverage becomes loose or falls out, the patient must call the dentist immediately for a replacement. If not, the permanent restoration may not fit or function properly, which may lead to having to refit and refabricate the restoration. Make sure patients understand that just because a provisional coverage is temporary does not mean it is not important.

Provisional coverages are more likely to stain than permanent prostheses. Advise patients to avoid or cut back their intake of wine, coffee, or tea while wearing their provisional coverage.

Maintenance of Fixed Prosthodontics

Implants and prostheses should be cared for just as natural teeth, including flossing and brushing after every meal. A special toothbrush made especially for implants and bridges can be used to clean the abutments. A brush with an angled handle can be used to clean underneath the abutments. Supply patients with a floss threader or a special type of floss that has a stiff end to help with proper flossing of the area between the prosthesis and the gingiva. Patients should also schedule regular check-ups every 6 months to ensure the restoration still fits and functions as it should. In addition to checking the patient's prosthesis during these appointments, the dentist checks the health and stability of the jaw, gingival tissue, and existing teeth as well.

Just as with provisional coverages, if a permanent crown or bridge chips or falls out, patients should immediately contact the dental office. Chipped, broken, loose, or dislodged restorations can allow bacteria to leak in and cause dental caries or infection around implant-supported crowns and bridges.

CHECKPOINT

38-13 What is the most important factor affecting how long a prosthesis lasts?

Chapter Highlights

- Fixed prostheses are permanent restorations that cannot be removed from the oral cavity and are used to replace missing or broken teeth or parts of a tooth. Common fixed prostheses include crowns, bridges, inlays, onlays, and veneers.

- Crowns are like caps for teeth that are broken or decayed. They may partially or completely cover a tooth.
- Bridges are used to fill the space where a tooth is missing. The artificial tooth that fills that space is known as

a pontic. The surrounding teeth that support the bridge in place are known as abutment teeth.

♦ Veneers help restore the natural color of discolored teeth, as well as restoring the natural shape of teeth that are broken or crooked or have large gaps between them.

♦ Materials such as gold alloys, porcelain, or resin composites can be used to fabricate the prosthesis. They can be fabricated in a dentist's office or outside the office in a dental laboratory. Computerized systems are frequently used to help fabricate fixed prostheses accurately.

♦ Retention techniques ensure the fixed prosthesis stays in place. Common techniques include implants, which are inserted directly into the jaw bone, core buildups, and retention pins.

♦ Crowns can be fabricated from several different materials. Metal alloy crowns tend to be more durable, but are less natural-looking. Ceramic, porcelain, and resin-based crowns have a more desirable appearance but are more prone to breakage.

♦ When placing a crown, gingival retraction is performed to expose the area of the tooth that normally is hidden by the gingival tissue. This allows an accurate impression of the tooth to be taken, which is then used to fabricate a crown that is correctly shaped.

♦ Fixed prostheses that are fabricated in a dental laboratory may take up to 4 weeks to complete. During that time, provisional coverages are used as temporary prostheses.

♦ There are three main types of bridges (traditional, cantilever, and Maryland). Traditional bridges are attached to surrounding teeth by a crown, while Maryland bridges attach using a wing-like structure that is bonded to the back of the abutment teeth. Cantilever bridges are used when there are abutment teeth only on one side of the pontic.

♦ One of the most important factors in determining the lifespan of a fixed prosthetic is oral hygiene. Patient education is important to ensure that patients take care of their restoration and report any problems immediately.

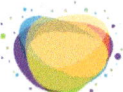 ## Review Questions

1. Fixed prostheses
   a. Are always fabricated in a laboratory.
   b. Are permanently cemented.
   c. Include inlays, onlays, and amalgams.
   d. Are usually made of gold alloys.

2. What type of prosthetic is typically used to repair misshapen teeth in the anterior portion of the oral cavity?
   a. Ceramic crown
   b. Ceramic veneer
   c. Porcelain bridge
   d. Implant

3. What type of crown is generally best for teeth in the posterior portion of the oral cavity?
   a. Porcelain-fused-to-metal crown
   b. All-ceramic crown
   c. Composite resin crown
   d. Three-quarters gold crown

4. Mechanical retraction cords
   a. Do not contain chemicals.
   b. Are generally used when a patient's gingival tissue is excessively overgrown.
   c. Can only be used on patients with heart conditions or bleeding disorders.
   d. Are also known as impregnated retraction cords.

5. A provisional coverage
   a. Is usually removed after a few days.
   b. Is temporary, and therefore not placed using any type of cement or bonding agent.
   c. Is only used when a patient is receiving a crown.
   d. Is to be cared for in the same ways that patients should care for their natural teeth.

6. When replacing a missing tooth in the front of the oral cavity, which bridge is most likely to be used?
   a. Cantilever
   b. Traditional
   c. Maryland
   d. Any of the above

7. What factor has the largest influence on the lifespan of a fixed prosthesis?
   a. The material it is made from
   b. The experience of the dentist in placing fixed prostheses
   c. The oral hygiene of the patient in caring for the prosthesis
   d. The age of the patient

Active Learning Exercises

1. Explain the differences between an inlay and an onlay. What is the difference between this type of restoration and a full crown?

2. Many patients will choose to have tooth-colored restorations in all areas of their mouth. Why would a porcelain occlusal surface on a posterior crown not be an appropriate choice for a patient who has a severe bruxism problem?

3. Postoperative instruction regarding the home care of a dental bridge is very important in the daily care process for the patient. Take a trip to your local supermarket or pharmacy. Identify all of the self-care aids available for cleaning under a dental bridge. What are the differences in prices?

Application Activities

1. Using crowns provided by your instructor, examine the different types of crowns for differences and similarities. Do the surfaces appear natural looking? How do they feel? Suppose a patient asked you about the difference between metal and nonmetal crowns. What would you tell the patient?

2. A patient comes in to receive her permanent crown. Upon examination, you see that the provisional is broken. The patient says that it broke a few days ago but that she did not want to bother coming in since her appointment was only a few days away and the provisional was just temporary anyway. How do you respond? What important information do you need to tell the patient about the impact of her failing to call the dentist's office when her provisional broke? How might this impact the procedure for placement of the permanent crown?

PREPARING FOR CERTIFICATION EXAMS

Review the following topics in this chapter to prepare for the Dental Assisting National Board (DANB) exam:

- **Dental Laboratory**

- **Dental Implants**

- **Crown Procedures**

- **Selection and Preparation**

- **Materials and Fabrication**

- **Assisting in Crown Procedures**

- **Bridges**

- **Selection and Preparation**

- **Materials and Fabrication**

- **Assisting in Bridge Procedures**

Removable Prosthodontics

CHAPTER OUTLINE

CHAPTER CHECKLIST

On completion of this chapter, students will be able to:

- ☑ Identify the two types of removable prostheses, including general appearance and function.
- ☑ Describe the typical treatment plan for a patient considering a removable prosthesis.
- ☑ Describe the use of an overdenture.
- ☑ Describe the use of a partial denture, including indications and contraindications, components, and appointment sequencing.
- ☑ Understand the role of the dental assistant during procedures for final impressions, wax denture try-in, and placement of a partial denture.
- ☑ Describe the use of a full denture, including indications and contraindications, components, and appointment sequencing.
- ☑ Understand the role of the dental assistant during procedures for final impressions and placement of a full denture.
- ☑ Describe the use of an immediate denture, including indications and contraindications, components, and appointment sequencing.
- ☑ Describe the process of denture relining.
- ☑ Explain how to receive dentures for repairs.
- ☑ Describe important aspects of patient education and home care for patients receiving removable prostheses.

KEY TERMS

abutment (uh-BUT-munt) – a tooth or implant used for the support or retention of a fixed or removable prosthesis

baseplate – the rigid acrylic resin structure that serves as the base of a denture, used to fit a full denture

flange (FLANJ) – the part of a denture that extends from the cervical margin to the border of the prosthesis

full denture – a prosthesis that replaces all the teeth in a single dental arch; also called a complete denture

immediate denture – a removable dental prosthesis fabricated for placement immediately after the removal of a natural tooth or teeth

overdenture – a removable prosthesis that rests on one or more remaining natural teeth, tooth roots, or dental implants

partial denture – a removable prosthesis used to replace one or more missing teeth

post dam – the seal at the posterior area of a maxillary denture that secures it in place; also called the posterior palatal seal

rebasing (re-BAY-sing) – a procedure in which the denture base is replaced

relining – a procedure in which the tissue side of the denture base receives a new lining to improve fit and comfort

rest – a metal projection that is part of the framework of a removable partial denture and which comes into contact with the occlusal or lingual surface of the abutment teeth and aids in the support of the pontic tooth

retainer – a clasp that comes into contact with abutment teeth and prevents a partial denture from moving

Introduction

Dental appliances that replace missing teeth and tissues and that can be taken out of the oral cavity by the patient are referred to as removable prostheses. Unlike fixed prostheses, these devices can be easily removed for cleaning, maintenance, and adjustment. Understanding the various types of removable prostheses available to patients helps the dental assistant play a valuable role in the treatment process.

Functions you may perform include assisting with the initial consultation, impressions, try-in, and placement of removable prostheses. You should also understand the procedures involved in denture repair and maintenance. In addition, you may provide patients with instructions for oral hygiene and denture care.

Overview of Removable Prosthodontics

The two primary types of removable prosthodontics are partial dentures and full dentures. A **partial denture**, often referred to simply as a "partial," is a substitute for a missing tooth (or teeth) and is held in place by the remaining teeth and tissues. A **full denture** (or complete denture) is a substitute for all the teeth in an arch and is supported by the oral tissues and mucosa, alveolar ridges, and hard palate.

Removable prostheses serve various purposes, including providing the ability to chew food and speak well. Another purpose is to improve aesthetics.

Indications and Contraindications

Most patients are suitable candidates for removable prostheses. General good health is important for fitting, tolerating, and maintaining a removable prosthesis. Factors that may affect a patient's suitability include:

- An unhealthy bone structure, which may not be able to support removable prostheses
- A resorbed alveolar ridge, which can cause the prosthesis to irritate the mucosa and negatively affect chewing
- Tori, or abnormal bone growths, which may have to be removed to create the right fit for the prosthesis (Figure 39-1)
- Diabetes or another physical condition that makes the tissues in the oral cavity intolerant of the pressures of the prosthesis
- Poor nutrition that negatively affects tissue health and, ultimately, the ability to comfortably wear a prosthesis
- A mental health condition or mental disability that affects the ability to keep the device in place and maintain oral hygiene
- Weak facial muscle tone, including paralysis
- Extreme facial tics or contortions that may dislodge a prosthesis

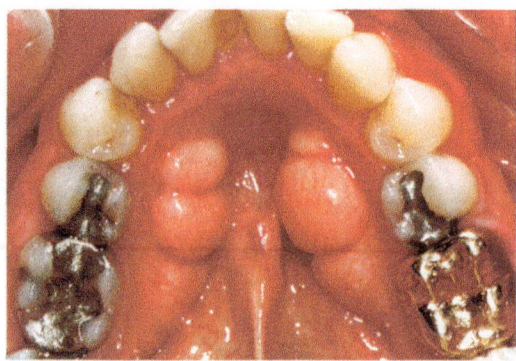

Figure 39–1 Mandibular tori.

- Mouth breathing, which may affect the ability to keep the device in place
- Chronic teeth clenching or grinding that affects any remaining natural teeth and the prosthesis
- Inadequate flow of saliva that may make the fit and comfort of a prosthesis difficult
- Oral mucosa conditions that may negatively affect prosthesis comfort or cause irritation

The Treatment Plan

When a removable prosthesis is considered, the initial appointment typically includes an examination, along with a thorough medical history; radiographic films; photographs of the full face, frontal view, profile view, and close-up; and preliminary impressions.

At a subsequent consultative appointment, the dentist explains the proposed treatment plan to the patient. The dental assistant usually prepares materials and visual aids, including photographs of the patient's face and models of the patient's oral cavity; radiographs; and appropriate booklets, videos, photographs, and models.

Important considerations for the patient include the cost estimate, insurance coverage, and other financial information. Ideally, the dental office will have contacted the insurance company in advance so that the patient can be informed about financial responsibilities at this appointment.

Also important to the patient are time considerations such as the number and duration of appointments. This information can be prepared in advance and presented to the patient. Once the patient agrees to a treatment plan and financial matters are settled, this series of appointments can be scheduled.

Use of Implants and Overdentures

A dentist may save parts of a patient's original teeth—most often, the canine teeth—or place implants in the patient's dental arch to provide a base to which full dentures can attach for support. (See Chapter 38, Fixed Prosthodontics, for a discussion of the types of implants available.)

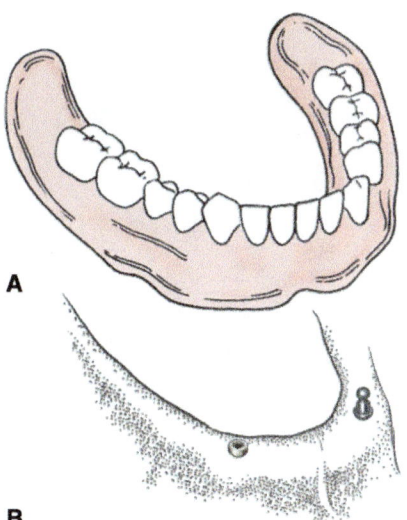

Figure 39–2 Overdenture. (**A**) Mandibular complete denture. (**B**) Examples of two types of implant abutments.

This is called an **overdenture**, and it can significantly improve the stability of a denture, similar to how natural teeth are anchored (Figure 39-2). An overdenture may also be used in cases when bone shrinks or absorbs and makes a denture less stable. These patients may not have a sufficient alveolar ridge to support a denture without an overdenture.

When the patient's retained teeth are used for support, they are treated and prepared with posts and cores or prefabricated attachments. The part of the denture that faces the tissue is made with an attachment for the retained tooth or implant.

Patients who have this type of procedure must be particularly attentive to controlling plaque in the area around implants and retained teeth. Uncontrolled plaque can lead to bone loss.

✓ CHECKPOINT
39-1 What is an overdenture?

Partial Dentures

Indications and Contraindications

Removable partial dentures are suitable for patients seeking a replacement for several teeth in the same quadrant or in both quadrants of the same arch (Figure 39-3). In some cases, this denture is used instead of a fixed bridge. A removable partial denture also may be suitable for a pediatric patient who is missing teeth.

If a patient has chronically poor oral hygiene causing a severe periodontal condition or rampant caries, he or she may not be a good candidate for a removable partial denture. This type of denture requires natural teeth in the arch and adequate alveolar bone and mucosa for support. Patients who lack these characteristics may not be good candidates.

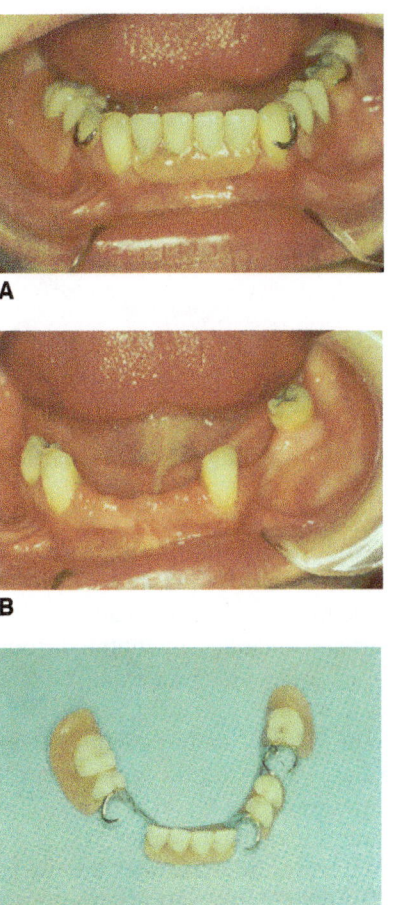

Figure 39–3 Removable partial denture. (**A**) Denture in place. (**B**) Mouth without denture in place. (**C**) Removable partial denture.

Components and Fabrication

Partial dentures are created for each individual patient, depending on his or her needs. The skeleton of a typical partial denture consists of a stable metal framework made of chrome cobalt (Figures 39-4 and 39-5). Connecting metal bars link the parts of the denture and provide support for the remaining natural teeth. In a maxillary partial denture, the palatal connector serves this purpose. Its counterpart in a mandibular partial denture is the lingual connector. Other minor connectors link these major connectors to the base, clasps, and other components of the framework.

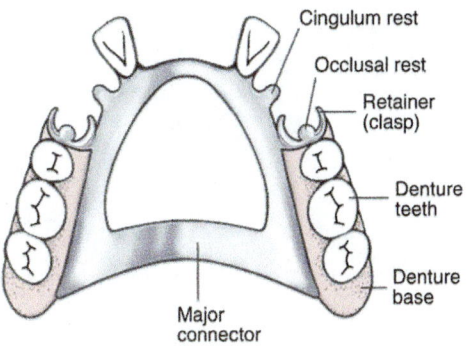

Figure 39–4 Components of a removable partial denture.

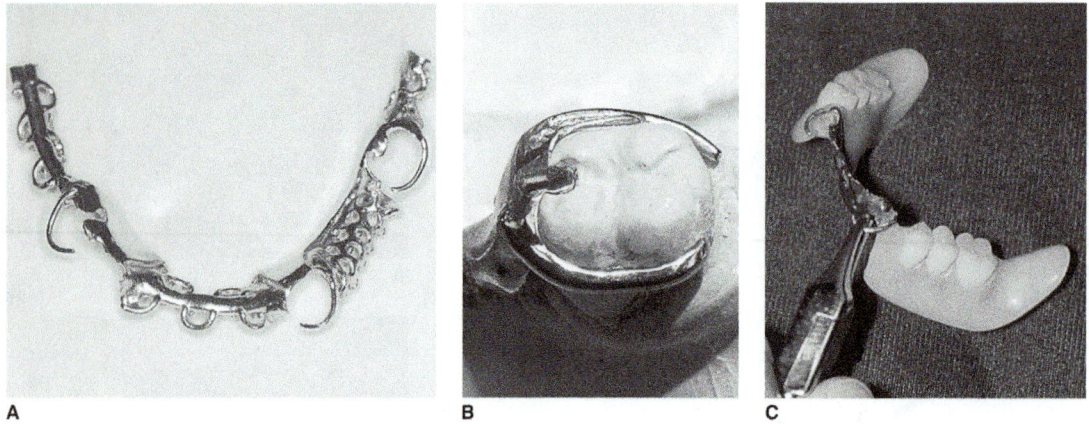

A   B   C

Figure 39–5 Components of a partial denture. (**A**) Framework. (**B**) Clasp. (**C**) Denture base with clasp being adjusted.

The framework engages with **abutment** teeth with a clasp assembly, also called a **retainer**. The retainer helps to secure the denture in place. Typically, a circumferential-type clasp partially encircles an abutment tooth. Another type of clasp, a bar-type, extends from the gingiva to the occlusal surface.

For aesthetic reasons, some patients opt for a design in which no clasps show on the faces of visible teeth. In these dentures, the clasps fit on the lingual surface and may extend onto the occlusal surface.

Another adjunct to the framework are the **rests**, metal projections that come into contact with the natural teeth to position the denture in the oral cavity. Rests may be positioned on occlusal or lingual surfaces to help distribute the load of the denture to several teeth.

The base of the partial denture is usually made of plastic acrylic resin. The base holds the artificial teeth, called pontics, and rests on the oral mucosa. Base material is available in shades to match most patients. A flexible, lightweight material is available for improved comfort. To fit a partial denture made of flexible material, the device is immersed in hot tap water and then fitted in the patient's oral cavity.

Pontics are made of acrylic, porcelain, or plastic resin and are available in a variety of sizes, shapes, and shades to suit the patient's appearance (Figure 39-6). Acrylic teeth have the advantage of not making a clicking sound during chewing. However, acrylic teeth are more prone to staining. Porcelain teeth last longer but are more prone to breakage. Many patients opt for acrylic teeth in one arch, with natural or porcelain teeth in the opposing arch, which can minimize the clicking sound associated with porcelain teeth.

Appointment Sequencing

The first appointment to prepare a patient for a partial denture focuses on information gathering, including health and dental history, radiographs, and photographs (intraoral and extraoral). Oral prophylaxis may also be performed. At this appointment, preliminary impressions are taken for the dental laboratory to make custom trays for the final impression.

The second appointment focuses on preparing the oral cavity for the dentures. The dentist selects the type of rest that will be used, which determines how abutment teeth will be prepared. An abutment tooth may need a slight modification, including modifying a restoration, to receive the rest or another attachment. The patient's bite and occlusal registration are taken, and the shade and mold of the artificial teeth are determined. This appointment also involves taking final impressions with an elastomeric material.

At the third appointment, a model of the denture is tried on the patient. This "try-in" involves a cast framework of the prosthesis with the teeth set in wax. Consulting with the patient, the dentist checks the fit, function, comfort, and appearance of the teeth. Any changes made are noted, and the disinfected prosthesis is sent to the dental laboratory with the prescription.

The patient receives the partial denture in a 20- to 30-minute subsequent appointment.

The patient is scheduled to return for a fifth appointment several days later. At this 10- to 20-minute checkup, the dentist removes the denture, examines the mucosa for pressure and sore areas, and makes any minor adjustments. The patient is instructed to return several months later for another checkup, including an assessment of the patient's oral hygiene with the prosthesis.

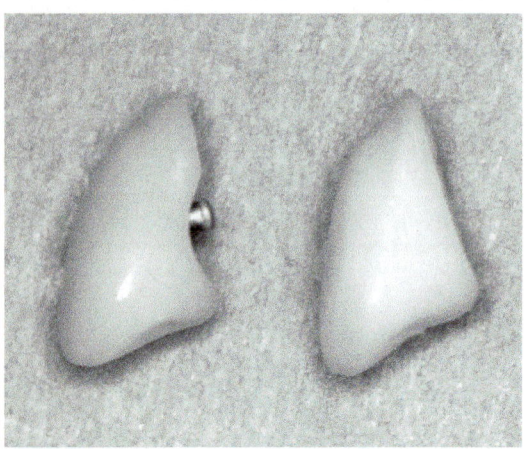

Figure 39–6 Pontics. (*Left*) Porcelain. (*Right*) Acrylic.

Procedure 39–1 Assisting with a Final Impression for a Partial Denture

Materials needed (Figure P39-1-1):

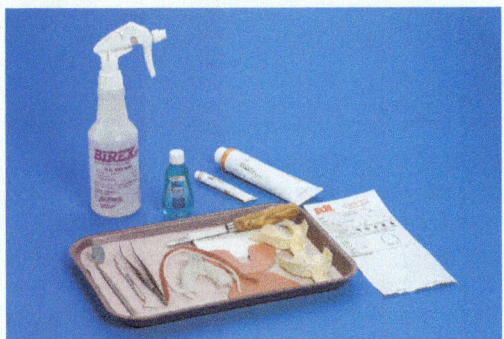

Figure P39-1-1

- Basic setup, including mouth mirror, explorer, and cotton pliers
- Mouthwash
- Custom impression tray created for the patient or a stock tray
- Contouring wax and impression materials (spatula and mixing pad or dispensing gun and tips)
- Laboratory prescription form
- Disinfectant
- Wax or silicone bite registration materials
- Container for the impressions and bite registration
- Tooth shade and mold guides

1. Put on appropriate PPE.
2. Seat and drape the patient and explain what will happen during the procedure.
3. The dentist places the impression tray in the patient's oral cavity and uses contouring wax as needed to improve the fit. Then the dentist paints an adhesive on the inside of the tray.
4. Prepare the final impression material according to the manufacturer's instructions and load the impression tray.
5. The dentist places the impression tray in the patient's oral cavity.
6. When the impression is taken, the dentist gives you the final impression for disinfecting (Figure P39-1-2).

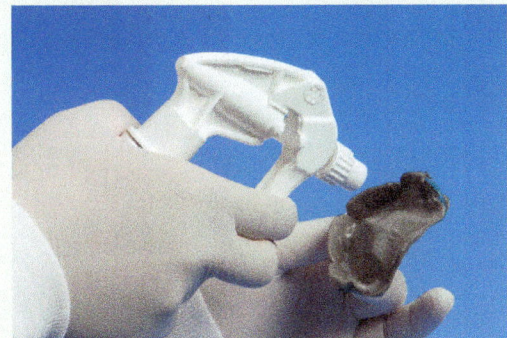

Figure P39-1-2

7. Prepare materials for taking the bite registration. This includes softening the wax in warm water (Figure P39-1-3A) and preparing it for placement in the patient's oral cavity. If not using wax, mix the impression materials on a paper pad and put them on a quadrant tray (Figure P39-1-3B).

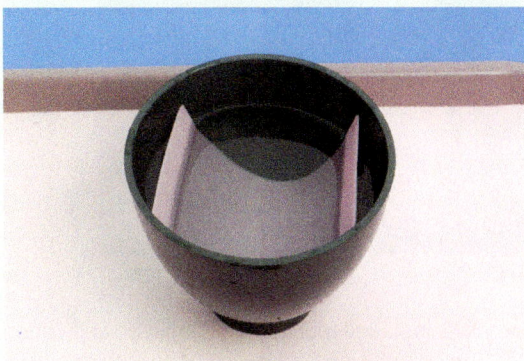

Figure P39-1-3A

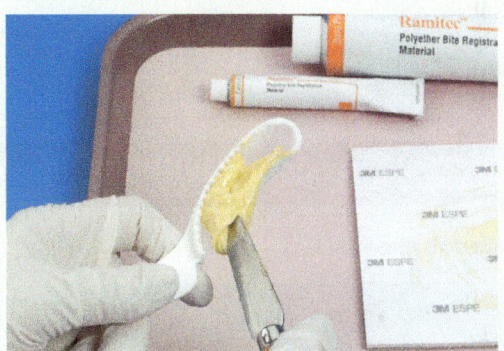

Figure P39-1-3B

8. The dentist takes the bite impression. After these materials have set, the dentist will give you the bite impression for disinfecting.
9. The dentist uses a moistened shade guide under natural light to check the shade of the artificial teeth.
10. Help check the shade and record the information in the patient's chart and on the laboratory prescription.
11. The dentist reviews the prescription and provides final details about the construction of the denture.
12. Document the procedure in the patient's record and provide the patient with postprocedure instructions.

Procedure 39–2 **Assisting with a Wax Denture Try-In**

Materials needed (Figure P39-2-1):

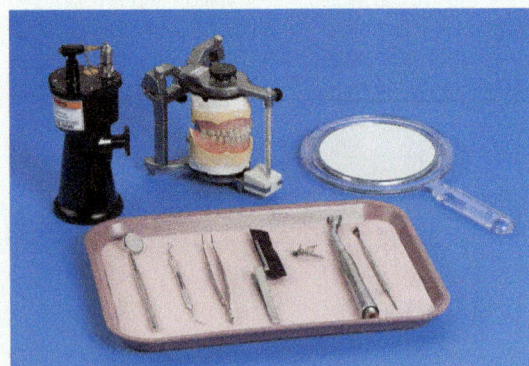

Figure P39-2-1

- Basic tray setup, including mouth mirror, explorer, and cotton pliers
- Hand mirror
- Articulating paper and forceps

- Adjusting instruments (wax spatula and heat source)
- Low-speed handpiece with burs, discs, and stones
- The patient's full denture

1. Put on appropriate PPE.
2. Disinfect the denture and rinse it in water in preparation for the patient.
3. The dentist places the denture in the patient's oral cavity and makes any necessary adjustments.
4. Be prepared to provide the dentist with the warmed spatula as needed for adjustments that involve the base of the denture. You also provide the dentist with articulating paper for occlusion evaluation and the handpiece and accessories for occlusion adjustments.
5. When the denture is in place, provide the patient with a hand mirror to view the denture.
6. When the denture is removed, disinfect it and prepare it for the laboratory.
7. Document the procedure in the patient's record and provide the patient with postprocedure instructions.

Procedure 39–3 **Assisting with the Placement of a Partial Denture**

Materials needed (Figure P39-3-1):

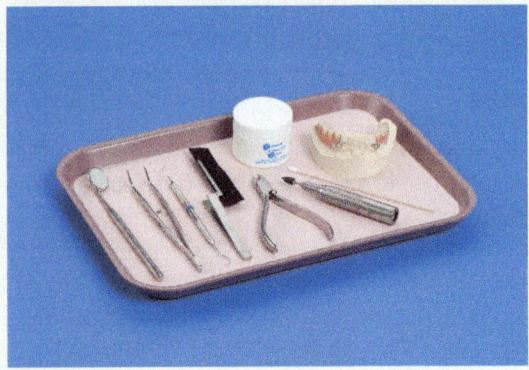

Figure P39-3-1

- Basic tray setup, including mouth mirror, explorer, and cotton pliers
- Articulating paper and forceps
- Pressure indicator paste
- Low-speed handpiece and acrylic and finishing burs
- Three-pronged pliers
- The patient's partial denture

1. Put on appropriate PPE.
2. Disinfect the denture and rinse it in water in preparation for placement.

3. Seat the patient and explain what will happen during the procedure.
4. The dentist positions the new denture in the oral cavity.
5. To assist the dentist in checking the occlusion, place articulating paper on the occlusal surface of the mandibular teeth. Instruct the patient to make a chewing motion.
6. The dentist checks the occlusion and reduces the denture as necessary with a bur.
7. The dentist checks for pressure points that may cause discomfort. Assist by placing pressure indicator paste on the tissue surface of the denture (Figure P39-3-2).

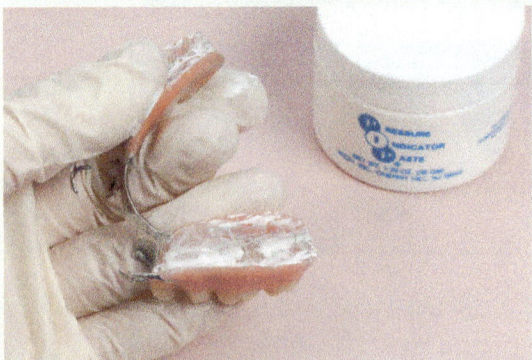

Figure P39-3-2

Procedure 39–3 Assisting with the Placement of a Partial Denture (Continued)

8. The dentist places the denture in the patient's oral cavity and checks for pressure points, making adjustments as necessary.

9. The dentist checks the tension of retainers on the abutment teeth. Have the pliers ready for the dentist to adjust tension.

10. The denture is removed for polishing on the laboratory lathe.

11. Scrub the denture with soap and water, disinfect and rinse it, and return it to the patient.

12. Provide the patient with instructions on how to place and remove the denture and how to care for it.

13. Document the procedure in the patient's record.

CHECKPOINTS

39-2 What is the term for the major connecting metal bar in the maxillary partial denture?

39-3 What is the term for the major connecting metal bar in the mandibular partial denture?

39-4 What is the term for the clasp assembly that links abutment teeth to the framework?

39-5 What is the term for the metal projections attached to the framework that come into contact with natural teeth to position the denture in the oral cavity?

Full Dentures

Indications and Contraindications

Full dentures are appropriate for patients who have no remaining natural teeth or poorly maintained or supported natural teeth and who wish to have their chewing function restored and a more pleasing appearance (Figure 39-7).

It is generally desirable for denture patients to be in good overall health. Often, poor health is evident in the oral cavity.

Patients need good muscle coordination to keep a denture in place and healthy oral tissues to support it. Dentures rely on oral mucosa and alveolar ridges for support, but the prosthesis also can stress these tissues. Therefore, denture patients should ideally have healthy mucosa and alveolar ridges. Patients who are losing or gaining substantial amounts of weight also may not be ideal candidates for a full denture because the weight change can affect the prosthesis fit.

It takes time, patience, and understanding to adjust to dentures. Patients who know what to expect and are prepared generally have a better experience. As the dental assistant you have an important role in helping to educate and prepare the patient.

From the Dentist's Perspective

Patients who need dentures can be very self-conscious, especially after any remaining natural teeth are extracted. No people feel like they look their best toothless. This can make patients feel very vulnerable. I really value a dental assistant who understands this and has a manner that puts patients at ease. A professional, compassionate assistant makes patients feel special and unique. One assistant told me she tries to picture each denture patient as her grandmother, whom she loves very much. That feeling of hers translated to patients as respect and comfort. That's invaluable to have in a practice.

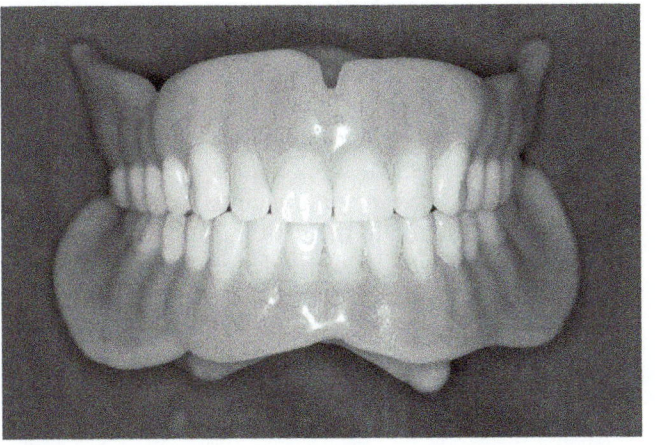

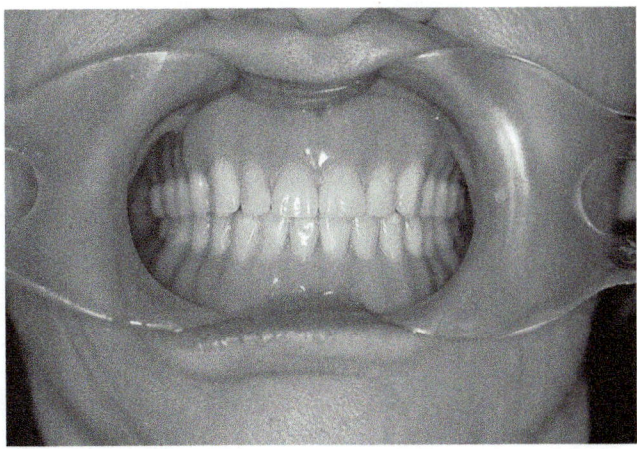

A   B

Figure 39–7 Completed dentures. (**A**) From laboratory. (**B**) In place.

Components and Fabrication

A full denture includes a base, usually made of plastic acrylic resin, which rests on the oral mucosa and to which the pontics are attached. Sometimes the base is reinforced with metal mesh for extra support.

The base extends over the mucosa from the cervical margin to the denture border. This part is called the **flange**. In the mandibular denture, it extends over the residual ridge and attached mucosa, to the oblique and mylohyoid ridges, and over the genial tubercles and retromolar pads. In the maxillary denture, the flange extends past the residual ridge and the attached mucosa to the tuberosities and the junction of the hard and soft palates.

A maxillary denture has a base that encompasses the entire hard palate. The suction seal occurs where the tissues and posterior border of the denture meet. This seal—called the **post dam**, or posterior palatal—is essential to keep the maxillary denture in place. From one buccal space in the back of the palate behind the maxillary tuberosity to the opposite buccal space, the post dam goes across the posterior part of the prosthesis.

Keeping a mandibular denture in place can be more challenging because it does not have the large suction area of a maxillary denture. In addition, tongue movement can negatively affect suction. The alveolar ridge plays a key role in keeping this prosthesis in place because suction can occur between the denture and tissue that covers the ridge.

You should be able to describe the various surfaces of the denture (Figure 39-8). The surface that rests on the residual ridge and adjacent tissues is called the impression surface. A patient may place an adhesive material on the impression surface before inserting the denture. This adhesive is removed from the denture and from tissues in the oral cavity during daily cleaning. Sometimes the impression surface is lined with a material such as a temporary soft liner, tissue conditioner, or permanent soft silicone liner that is not to be removed by the patient.

The outer-facing surface of the denture is referred to as a polished surface and is fabricated to resemble natural tissues. This surface extends over the retromolar pad on the mandible or over the maxillary tuberosity area on the maxilla.

The area where the denture makes contact with the corresponding surface of the opposing denture or natural teeth is called the occlusal surface.

A denture arch features 14 pontics in anterior and posterior sets—two central incisors, two laterals, two cuspids, four bicuspids, and four molars, respectively. As in a partial denture, the pontics are made of acrylic, porcelain, or plastic resin in sizes, shapes, and shades to suit the patient's appearance. Acrylic pontics have the advantage of not making a clicking sound during chewing. However, acrylic pontics are more prone to staining. Porcelain pontics last longer but are more prone to breakage. Porcelain against porcelain in opposing arches can wear down the pontics. Many patients, therefore, opt for acrylic pontics in one arch, with natural or porcelain pontics in the opposing arch. Acrylic pontics are bonded into the denture base, whereas porcelain pontics require mechanical fastening with pins or holes.

When the dentist makes adjustments to acrylic pontics in a denture, they can be polished in the office. Porcelain pontics must go to the laboratory for refinishing.

Appointment Sequencing

If a full denture patient has remaining natural teeth, these need to be extracted first. A period of 4 to 6 months of healing usually is necessary before the denture can be created. Many patients opt for an immediate denture rather than be without teeth for that long. In this case, the remaining natural posterior teeth are extracted, and the patient is fitted with an immediate denture (see Immediate Dentures section later in this chapter). The anterior teeth are extracted and the alveolar bone is shaped when the immediate denture is ready. An immediate denture ensures that the patient is never without teeth, which is an important aesthetic and functional consideration. Immediate dentures often require subsequent relining in a period of a few months once the bone has healed; some patients may even need a new prosthesis.

The information-gathering appointment for a full denture, like that for a partial denture, includes obtaining a medical and dental history and completing a comprehensive oral examination, including tissues and ridges. Photographs, radiographs, and impressions are taken. Patients also are asked to provide photographs to help ensure the denture is well suited to their natural appearance. During this process, you will help the dentist prepare a patient-friendly diagnosis, treatment plan, and financial estimate. Some dentists prefer to gather the necessary information and records in an initial appointment and present the treatment plan in a subsequent appointment.

Once the plan has been agreed upon, construction of the patient's denture begins with an alginate impression poured in plaster or stone. Custom acrylic trays are created

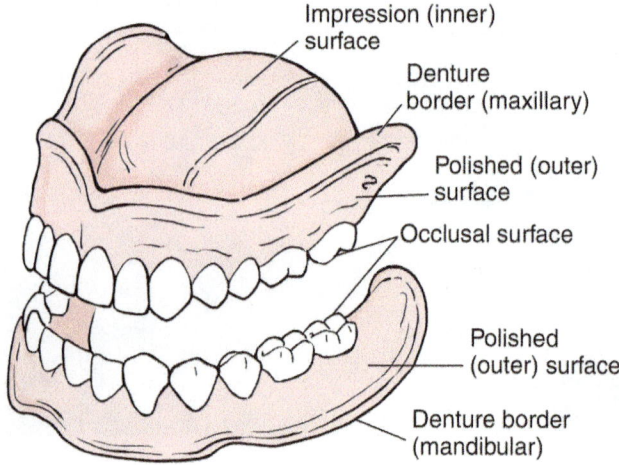

Impression (inner) surface

Denture border (maxillary)

Polished (outer) surface

Occlusal surface

Polished (outer) surface

Denture border (mandibular)

Figure 39-8 Denture surfaces.

from these models. If the patient has an immediate denture, the trays account for the presence of anterior teeth.

Next, final impressions are taken in the dental office. This appointment should not occur until the patient has healed after having the posterior teeth removed and the alveolar bone has been contoured.

After final impressions are taken, they are sent to the dental laboratory, where a stone master cast is produced (Figure 39-9A). This is used to make an acrylic resin **baseplate**, which serves as a makeshift base for the denture. Several layers of wax are affixed to the baseplate, comprising the bite rim and representing where teeth normally would be (Figure 39-9B).

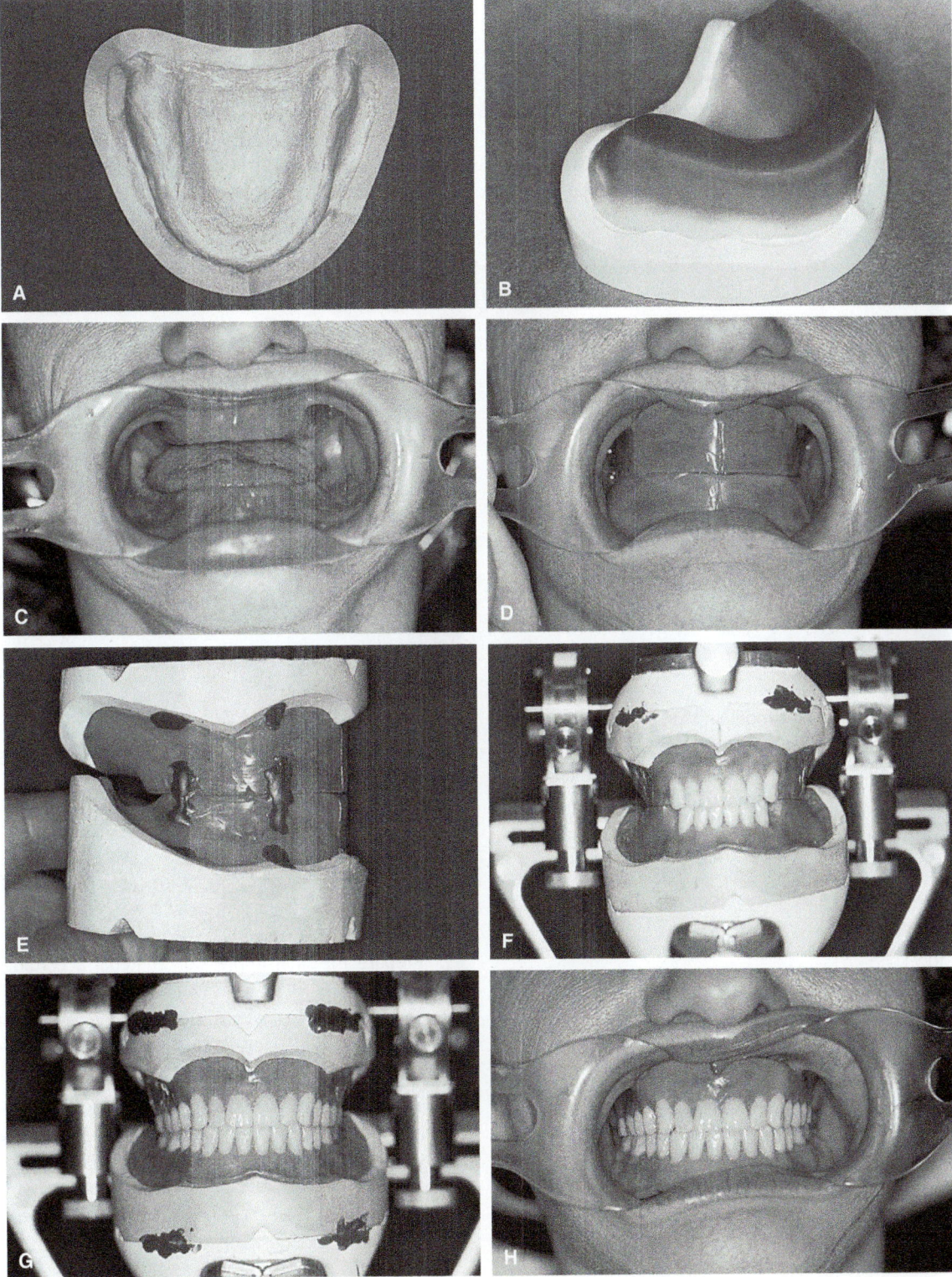

Figure 39–9 Steps in the construction of a denture. See text for description. Note that the plastic cheek retractors in **C**, **D**, and **H** are to aid in photography and are not typically used during the dental procedure.

The bite rim helps determine the vertical dimension for the denture—the distance between the upper and lower jaws.

Another patient appointment is scheduled to allow the dentist to further customize the denture. The dentist places the baseplates and bite rims in the patient's oral cavity and adjusts them as needed to ensure a natural lip drape and the appropriate amount of tooth and gingival tissue showing (Figure 39-9C). The dentist also determines the centric occlusion, protrusion, retrusion, and lateral excursion, which guide the laboratory technician in making a wax denture that duplicates the patient's normal jaw motions (Figure 39-9D, E). The shade, mold, and material of the teeth for the denture are also determined.

The laboratory then prepares a try-in denture, with pontics mounted in the bite rim and adjusted by the dentist (Figure 39-9F, G). The patient returns to the dental office for a try-in appointment. The entire dental team works closely together to ensure the patient is happy with the denture before its construction is finalized.

The laboratory finalizes the denture by replacing the try-in denture with one with an acrylic resin base and pontics. The patient returns to the dental office for placement of the denture (Figure 39-9H).

Another appointment is scheduled 2 to 3 days after placement of the denture to allow the dentist to evaluate the fit, checking for pressure spots or tenderness in the oral cavity. Minor adjustments can be made at this time. Additional appointments are scheduled as needed until both the patient and the dentist are satisfied that the denture is functioning properly.

Procedure 39–4 Assisting with a Final Impression for a Full Denture

Materials needed (Figure P39-4-1):

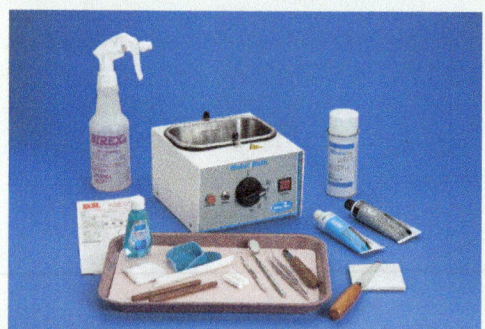

Figure P39-4-1

- Basic tray setup, including a mouth mirror, explorer, and cotton pliers
- High-volume evacuator (HVE) and air-water syringe tips
- Cotton rolls and gauze
- Mouthwash
- The patient's custom trays
- Compound wax and a Bunsen burner
- Water heater
- Laboratory knife
- Impression materials (spatulas, mixing pads, or dispensing gun and tips)
- Laboratory prescription form
- Disinfectant
- Container for the impressions and bite registration.

1. Put on appropriate PPE.
2. Before the dentist begins making impressions, have the patient rinse the oral cavity with mouthwash and explain what will happen during the appointment.

3. The dentist inserts the custom tray into the patient's oral cavity and checks the fit. The tray is then removed.
4. Heat the impression compound. The water heater can be used to temper the compound after it has been heated.
5. The dentist positions the impression compound in the borders of the tray (Figure P39-4-2).

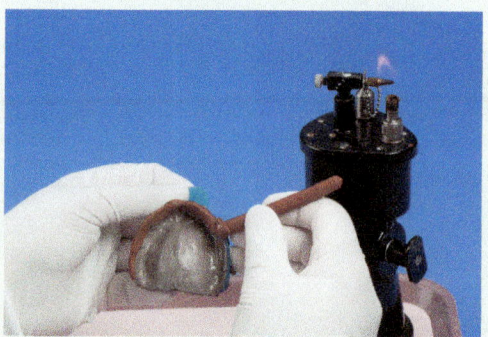

Figure P39-4-2

6. When cool, the dentist places the tray in the patient's oral cavity for border molding, a process used to define the edges of the denture. The tray is again removed from the patient's oral cavity.
7. Prepare the final impression material according to the manufacturer's instructions and load the impression tray.
8. The dentist places the impression tray in the patient's oral cavity.
9. When the material has set, the tray is removed and the oral cavity rinsed.
10. The process is repeated with the other arch.
11. Once the final impressions are taken, the dentist gives you the final impressions for disinfecting. Prepare the impressions and prescription for the laboratory.
12. Document the procedure in the patient's record and provide the patient with postprocedure instructions.

Procedure 39–5 Assisting with the Placement of a Full Denture

Materials needed (Figure P39-5-1):

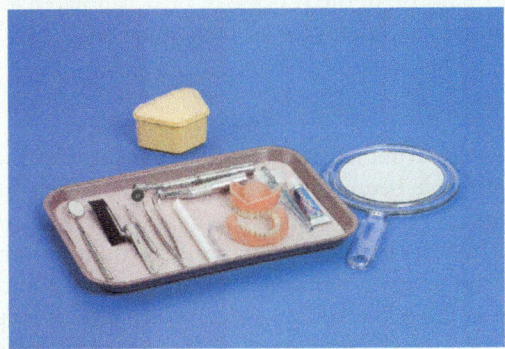

Figure P39-5-1

- Basic tray setup, including mouth mirror, explorer, and cotton pliers
- High-volume evacuator (HVE) and air-water syringe tips
- Hand mirror
- Articulating forceps and paper
- High-speed and low-speed handpieces and accompanying burs and discs
- The patient's dentures from the laboratory
- Take-home materials and hygiene aids

1. Put on appropriate PPE.
2. Seat the patient and place any dental appliances in containers. Explain what will happen during the procedure.
3. The dentist places the denture in the patient's oral cavity. A patient who is receiving an immediate denture has it placed after the remaining extractions.
4. The dentist gives the patient time to adjust the denture and then examines the denture to ensure it appears natural and checks the occlusion with articulating paper.
5. The denture is removed from the oral cavity for adjustments with burs and discs. If the denture requires laboratory polishing, disinfect the denture before it is returned to the patient's oral cavity.
6. The dentist instructs the patient to move his or her mouth in different positions and performs various functions to check how well the denture stays in place.
7. Ensure that the patient knows how to remove and replace the denture and care for it at home. Give the patient take-home materials and hygiene aids.
8. Document the procedure in the patient's record. Before dismissing the patient, make sure he or she knows to call with any problems or questions. Schedule an appointment for a few days later for a recheck.

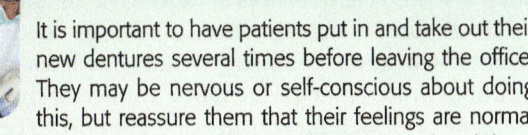

Voice of Experience

It is important to have patients put in and take out their new dentures several times before leaving the office. They may be nervous or self-conscious about doing this, but reassure them that their feelings are normal and urge them to take their time. They will feel more relaxed if you act as if you have all the time in the world and do not rush them. Provide a mirror if that will help them. Demonstrate how to clean the dentures and have them actually do it over the sink in the treatment room. Go through the entire process and fill the sink with water or line it with a towel to show them every step they should take at home. This experience helps to embed a visual image in their mind and will serve them well in caring for their dentures at home.

From the Dentist's Perspective

I always compliment my patients on how nice their new dentures look. I think this is important because teeth play a vital role in appearance, and patients who have been without teeth may be particularly sensitive about appearance.

We strive as a team to select and fit dentures that are comfortable and appealing looking. I appreciate it when the dental assistant also tells patients how natural, beautiful, or flattering the new dentures look. Little references to photographs the patient provided to show us how their natural teeth looked can make a big difference in boosting patients' self-image. One assistant said, "Mrs. Hamilton, you look just like you did in the 25th anniversary picture you showed us. With your new dentures, you'll look just as beautiful for your 50th anniversary pictures next month." The patient just beamed when she heard that. Remembering details like that and mentioning them to patients goes a long way toward satisfying patients and providing excellent care.

39-6 What is the part of the base of a full denture that extends over the mucosa from the cervical margin to the border of the denture?

39-7 What is the name for the suction seal of a maxillary denture base?

39-8 Why is it more difficult to keep a mandibular denture in place?

39-9 How many pontics are in a full denture arch?

39-10 What is affixed to the baseplate to represent where pontics would be to help the dentist determine the vertical dimension for the denture?

Immediate Dentures

When a patient waiting for the construction of a full denture has posterior teeth extracted but the anterior teeth remain, construction of an **immediate denture** can begin upon healing of the hard and soft tissues. Although an immediate denture generally needs relining or replacement within 3 to 6 months, it allows the patient to avoid being without teeth. In addition to aesthetic benefits, an immediate denture makes speaking and eating easier.

After the immediate denture is constructed, the anterior teeth can be extracted and the denture put in place. This denture has an additional benefit of compressing and protecting the post-extraction area.

An immediate denture is appropriate for only 3 to 6 months because the alveolar ridge typically undergoes changes during the healing process. At that time, the denture must be relined or replaced with a full denture.

Indications and Contraindications

Because an immediate denture must be relined or replaced, the patient should be aware of the additional expense. Most patients who are in the process of being prepared for a full denture are candidates for an immediate denture.

Fabrication

The wax setup for an immediate denture takes place after the posterior teeth have been extracted, the alveolar bone contoured, and tissues healed. At this point, the anterior teeth are still in place. The process of taking impressions requires consideration of the patient's bite and jaw configuration. Photographs taken in the office and provided by the patient help ensure that the manufactured denture looks natural. Based on the impressions, the immediate denture is manufactured. The laboratory also makes a surgical template—a clear plastic impression tray—of the anterior area. This template guides the oral surgeon in further contouring the alveolar ridge.

39-11 Which teeth are still in place when a patient is fitted for an immediate denture?

39-12 What benefit, besides function and aesthetics, does an immediate denture provide?

Denture Relining

Patients who have dentures should have an annual exam to check for fit and the health of oral tissues. Some patients will need **relining**, which involves placing a layer of denture resin on the tissue surface of the denture, to ensure a better fit and greater comfort. The dentist takes an impression, using the patient's existing denture, then allows an elastomeric impression material to flow into the tissue side of the denture. The dentist guides the

---

Procedure 39-6 Assisting with the Placement of an Immediate Denture

Materials needed:
- Basic tray setup, including mouth mirror, explorer, and cotton pliers
- Articulating paper and forceps
- Pressure indicator paste
- Low-speed handpiece and acrylic and finishing burs
- The patient's immediate denture

1. Put on appropriate PPE.
2. Disinfect the denture and rinse it in water in preparation for placement.

3. When the denture is ready for placement, the anterior teeth are extracted, the alveolar ridge contoured, and the denture positioned.
4. Document the procedure in the patient's record. Instruct the patient how to care for the denture and maintain good oral hygiene at home. Remind the patient that the denture should be worn at all times except when it is removed for cleaning.
5. Arrange for the patient to return the next day and on subsequent days for a checkup, including irrigation with an antiseptic, until healing is underway and sutures are removed. This time period is usually 2 to 3 days after surgery.

patient in a process to mold the denture lining until the impression is set. The dentist removes the denture from the oral cavity for disinfection and relining, usually by a laboratory technician.

After relining is complete, the denture should be disinfected again and checked for fit and comfort by the dentist.

Another procedure, **rebasing**, involves replacing the base material of a denture.

One of these procedures may be required when a denture is loose or ill-fitting or when changes have occurred in the patient's tissue.

✓ CHECKPOINT

39-13 How often should patients with dentures be checked by a dentist?

Denture Repairs

Some denture repairs can be performed in the dental office while others require laboratory repair.

When a patient brings in a denture for repair, first disinfect the denture to prevent cross-contamination. Provide the patient with a disposable cup to place the denture in. Then, wearing appropriate PPE, rinse the prosthesis under slowly running water; avoid splashing. Place the denture in a denture cleaning solution in an isolated bag in an ultrasonic cleaner.

Some denture repairs require patients to see the dentist, and others simply involve a drop off and return later to pick up the repaired denture. In most cases, the dentist needs to see patients whose dentures have been repaired to ensure the fit is satisfactory.

> ### Extra Patient Care
>
> When a patient brings in a damaged denture for repair, assess how the damage occurred without making the patient feel guilty. Assure the patient that these things happen to many denture patients. Then say that you would like to do your 10-minute denture care refresher course. Walk through the steps of denture care, from preparing the area to cleaning and storing the denture to performing other oral hygiene. Watch for signs that the patient might need help in a particular area, and involve the spouse or another family member in this process if appropriate. Provide take-home supplies and written materials and reassure the patient that no question is too small to call the office about.
>
> Most people become a little lax with routines over time, and a friendly, gentle refresher in denture care might remind the patient about steps he or she has forgotten and help to prevent the need for future repairs.

✓ CHECKPOINT

39-14 What should you always do when a patient gives you dentures for repair?

Patient Education

Maintenance and Home Care

Like all dental patients, those who have dentures should be instructed to practice good oral hygiene. This practice is particularly important for patients who have dentures.

Being fitted with dentures is a big step for most patients. They may not recall every aspect of instructions given in the dental office. You can help by providing written instructions to take home. Patients should be instructed to care for their dentures by storing unworn dentures in water or in a moist, airtight container at night during sleep.

Remind patients to remove their dentures after eating to brush or rinse, reminding them also that regular toothpaste is too abrasive for use on dentures. During cleaning, patients should hold their dentures over a sink partially filled with cool water or lined with a towel, in case the dentures are dropped. They should avoid soaking dentures in hot water or strong solutions. They should use a different toothbrush for their dentures from that used for their natural teeth because the clasps and metal parts of a prosthesis can wear out a toothbrush, making it ineffective for use on natural teeth. Patients also should not use an electric toothbrush on dentures. Special toothbrushes and pastes are available for brushing dentures (Figure 39-10).

Remind patients to brush and floss abutment teeth and supportive structures, and rinse oral tissues at least once a day with their dentures removed. The health of underlying tissues can be negatively affected by a removable denture because biofilm tends to accumulate more readily. Controlling this biofilm is a key factor in preserving the health of abutment teeth for a removable partial denture.

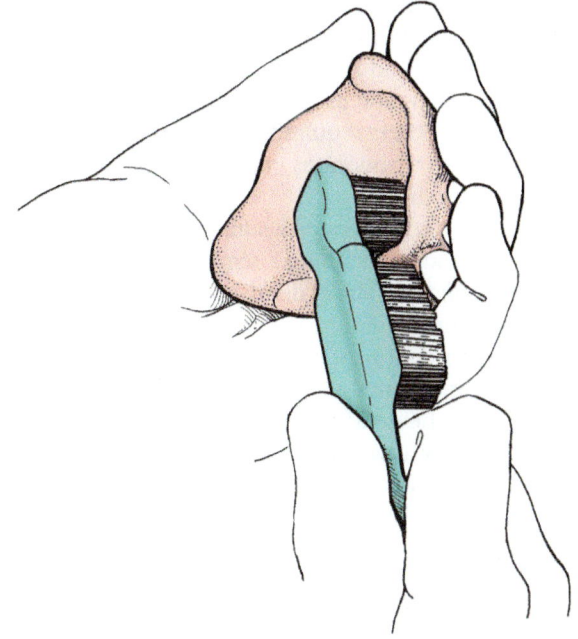

Figure 39-10 Denture brush.

Patients also should be advised not to attempt to adjust their dentures but instead to see their dentist with any problems.

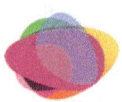

Voice of Experience

Assemble a kit of brushes, pastes, adhesives, and other materials used to care for dentures. Many people are visual learners and will remember what you show them better than what you say to them. If you recommend several brands of cleaning pastes, for example, have a tube of each to show patients. This visual reminder will help them when they are purchasing their own materials.

To reinforce that patients should not submerge a denture in hot water, obtain a denture that has been damaged by this process and show it to patients as you explain why this is not a good idea. Do the same to demonstrate why some pastes are too harsh or abrasive to a denture. Show a denture that has been damaged in this way.

Any examples you can show patients of both "do" and "do not" behaviors will help to reinforce your important instruction. This denture care kit will become an invaluable aide in your patient instruction.

Extra Patient Care

For many patients, the information provided about caring for dentures can be overwhelming. For this reason, walking the patient through each step of denture care while he or she is in the office will help the patient retain the information. Pretend that the patient is getting ready for bed at night and go through the process of preparing for denture care, cleaning and storing the denture, and performing other oral hygiene. Show each instrument or material the patient should use, and provide a take-home kit. You may want to first model each step and then ask the patient to do it.

In addition to this "show-and-tell" method of teaching, provide the patient with take-home written materials that outline everything you have taught. Sit down with the patient and walk through the materials, encouraging him or her to call the office with any questions.

This process of both demonstrating and providing materials that reinforce your messages will help to ensure maximum retention of important information.

CHECKPOINT

39-15 Should you advise a patient to use a regular toothbrush and paste on dentures?

Chapter Highlights

- Removable prostheses are dental appliances that replace missing teeth and tissues and can be taken out of the oral cavity at will.
- Partial dentures substitute for a missing tooth or teeth in the same arch and are held in place by the remaining teeth and tissues.
- A full (or complete) set of dentures substitutes for all the teeth and is supported by the oral tissues and mucosa, alveolar ridges, and hard palate.
- Many prosthodontic procedures are performed by general dentists; others require the specialization of a prosthodontist. Prosthodontics requires additional training after dental school.
- The patient's good general health is important for fitting, tolerating, and maintaining a removable prosthesis.
- Patients' concerns about dentures will include financial worries, time required for the series of appointments, adjusting to dentures, and being without teeth while healing from natural teeth extraction and during construction of the denture.
- A dentist may save parts of a patient's original teeth or place implants in the dental arch to provide a supportive base for full dentures. This is called an overdenture, and it can significantly improve the stability of dentures.
- The metal framework of a partial denture clasps onto abutment teeth to secure the denture in place.

- A laboratory prescription for a denture provides an exact blueprint for construction of the prosthesis and includes precise impressions and information about the patient's bite and occlusal registration and the shade and mold of the artificial teeth.
- Appointments for a partial denture include information gathering and preliminary impressions, oral cavity preparation and final impressions, wax try-in, and delivery of the denture.
- The base of a full maxillary denture encompasses the entire hard palate—a relatively large area for suction to keep the denture in place. A mandibular denture, on the other hand, lacks this large area for suction and works best when natural teeth or implants help to provide support.
- A full denture arch features 14 pontics in anterior and posterior sets—two cuspids, two laterals, two central incisors, four bicuspids, and four molars, respectively.
- If a full denture patient has remaining natural teeth, these need to be extracted, and the healing takes 3 to 6 months. Many patients opt for an immediate denture rather than be without teeth for that long.
- Appointments for a full denture include information gathering, alginate impressions to create custom trays, final impressions, bite rim and try-in, and delivery of the denture.
- Dental assistants play a key role in educating patients about the care of dentures and the importance of good oral hygiene with dentures.

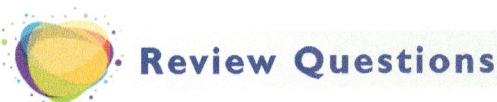

Review Questions

1. Why is an immediate denture only appropriate for 3 to 6 months?

   a. The materials used to create an immediate denture will break down after that time.

   b. Biofilm will build up in the underlying tissue and make the denture unwearable.

   c. The tissues in the oral cavity undergo changes during the healing process, making denture adjustment or replacement necessary.

   d. The abutment teeth are unable to support a denture for longer than 6 months.

2. Which of these is *not* a possible barrier to a patient being a good candidate for dentures?

   a. Tori

   b. Great fluctuations in weight

   c. Facial paralysis

   d. Heavy saliva flow

3. Which of a patient's original teeth are most often saved to serve as a base to which to attach a full denture?

   a. Third molars

   b. Buccal

   c. Bottom

   d. Canine

4. From what material is the metal framework of a partial denture made?

   a. Chrome cobalt

   b. Platinum

   c. Porcelain

   d. Nickel

5. Which of the following patients would not be a good candidate for a partial denture?

   a. An individual missing several teeth in the same quadrant

   b. A pediatric patient

   c. An individual with rampant caries

   d. An older patient

6. Pontics in a denture can be made from all of these except which one?

   a. Plastic resin

   b. Cobalt

   c. Acrylic

   d. Porcelain

7. At the final impressions appointment for a partial denture, which of these is done?

   a. Bite and occlusal registration taken

   b. Shade and mold of pontics determined

   c. Abutment teeth modified

   d. All of the above

8. Which of these is used to evaluate occlusion?

   a. Ink

   b. Paste

   c. Articulating paper

   d. Laboratory prescription

9. How long must a patient being fit for a full denture heal after natural teeth are extracted before receiving the denture?

   a. 4 to 6 days

   b. 4 to 6 weeks

   c. 4 to 6 months

   d. There is no wait; they can receive the full denture right away

10. If a patient wanting a full denture opts for an immediate denture, how long after the extraction of the teeth can the immediate denture be placed?

    a. Immediately

    b. A week later

    c. A month later

    d. A full denture patient cannot have an immediate denture

Active Learning Exercises

1. What is the best explanation you can provide to a patient who does not understand the differences between immediate and final dentures? How would you respond if that patient insisted on getting only the immediate denture?

2. Imagine that a patient tells you she keeps her denture in her mouth 24 hours a day and refuses to take it out. What advice or options can you give the patient?

Application Activities

1. Write a paragraph or two describing a patient who would benefit from the choice of porcelain dentures. What specific characteristics of the patient's condition would make porcelain the best choice? What benefits of porcelain would make it the best choice?

2. Pretend that one of your patients is having a hard time adjusting to her new set of full dentures. What would you say to make her more comfortable? Write a paragraph describing some strategies and advice you could share with the patient.

PREPARING FOR CERTIFICATION EXAMS

Review the following topics in this chapter to prepare for the Dental Assisting National Board (DANB) exam:

- **Partial Dentures**
- **Assisting with a Final Impression**
- **Assisting with a Wax Denture Try-In**
- **Assisting with the Placement of a Partial Denture**
- **Full Dentures**
- **Assisting with a Final Impression**
- **Assisting with the Placement of a Full Denture**
- **Patient Education**
- **Maintenance and Home Care**

chapter 40

Endodontics

CHAPTER OUTLINE

CHAPTER CHECKLIST

On completion of this chapter, students will be able to:

- ☑ Describe the purpose of endodontic dentistry and the various conditions it treats.
- ☑ Describe the methods used to diagnose pulpal disease, including possible outcomes of diagnostic testing.
- ☑ Identify the instruments, equipment, and materials used in endodontic treatment.
- ☑ Describe the procedure for root canal therapy, including preparation for therapy and post-therapy care.
- ☑ Describe the types of pulpal therapies and the purpose of each.
- ☑ Understand the role of the dental assistant in providing support during common endodontic procedures.
- ☑ Describe the types of endodontic procedures available when root canal therapy fails.

KEY TERMS

apex (A-peks) finder – an electronic device that helps determine the length of the root of the tooth by measuring the distance to the tooth apex; also called an apex locator

apexification (a-pek-sih-fih-KAY-shun) – placement of a paste to aid a root in closing; placed after an apicoectomy

apexogenesis (a-pek-suh-JEN-eh-sis) – a procedure used to close an open tooth apex

apical curettage (AP-ih-kul kyur-ih-TAZH) – removal of apical tissue

apical periodontitis (per-ee-oh-don-TIE-tis) – inflammation of the periapical tissue

apicoectomy (ap-ih-koh-EK-tuh-mee) – a surgical procedure that removes a small amount of the root apex, usually 1 to 3 mm

endodontics (en-doh-DON-tiks) – a branch of dentistry that deals with the functions of and problems with the tooth pulp and surrounding tissues

gutta percha (GUT-uh PUR-chuh) – a rubber-like substance used to fill a root canal; available in the form of cones, called gutta percha points

hemisection (heh-mee-SEK-shun) – a procedure in which half of the entire tooth is removed

irrigant – water-based solution used to disinfect the canal system by killing bacteria and dissolving the pulp tissue

obturation – obstruction or occlusion

paper point – used to dry a root canal before it is filled

percussion test – tapping the tooth with the handle of a dental mirror to determine whether pulpal damage is present

periapical (per-ee-AP-ih-kul) abscess – breakdown of the periapical tissue caused by a build up of purulent material and fluids in the tissue

periapical area – the area of the gingiva at the apex of the tooth

pulp – the soft inner core of the tooth that contains the tooth's nerves and blood vessel

pulp cap – placement of a cement base underneath a restoration in order to provide extra protection of the pulp

pulp necrosis (neh-KROH-sis) – death of the tooth's pulp

pulpectomy (pul-PEK-tuh-mee) – removal of all pulp from both the crown and the root canal

pulpotomy (pul-POT-uh-mee) – removal of pulp from the crown of the tooth but not from the root canal

transillumination (tranz-ih-LOO-muh-NAY-shun) testing – pulpal testing using a fiber optic light to look for cracks or other signs of bacteria leakage that could cause pulp necrosis

Introduction

Endodontics is a branch of dentistry that addresses the functions of and problems with the tooth pulp and surrounding tissues. The **pulp** is the soft inner core of the tooth that contains the tooth's nerves and blood vessels (Figure 40-1). It runs from the crown of the tooth down to the bottom of the tooth's root. An endodontist is a dentist who is specially trained to provide endodontic therapy, also known as root canal therapy.

As a dental assistant you should be familiar with the techniques used to diagnose endodontic problems and the various treatment options available, including surgical procedures. You should understand the steps involved in root canal therapy and know how to assist during a root canal procedure.

Pulpal Disease and Damage

Different types of pulpal disease include:

- *Irreversible pulpitis:* Inflammation of the pulp that cannot be healed by medication alone. In this case, the tooth is usually sensitive to cold or heat and causes the patient significant pain. Treatment for irreversible pulpitis involves root canal therapy or removal of the tooth.

- *Reversible pulpitis:* Inflammation of the pulp that can be healed. In this case, inflammation is usually caused by dental caries or damage to the tooth itself. Treatment for reversible pulpitis involves removing or treating the cause of the inflammation and applying medication to allow the pulp to heal.

- *Pulp necrosis:* Death of the pulp tissue. When the pulp has been overwhelmed by bacteria or disease, the pulp tissue in the root canal slowly dies. As it dies, bacteria and byproducts from the dead tissue can cause nearby tissue surrounding the tooth to become inflamed and infected.

If left untreated, damage to the pulp can spread to the apex. If this happens, the gingival tissue at the apex, called the **periapical area**, can become infected as well. As with pulpal diseases, there are different types of periapical diseases, with different causes and treatments. These include:

- **Apical periodontitis**: Inflammation of the periapical tissue. This can usually be treated by removing the cause of the inflammation, such as a cyst. Patients with this disease usually report pain, and the inflamed area may be red and swollen in appearance. A dentist diagnoses apical periodontitis through radiography of the inflamed area (Figure 40-2).

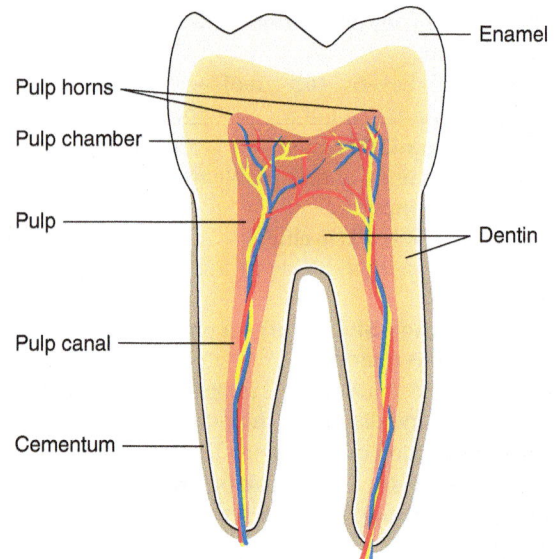

Figure 40-1 Anatomy of the tooth.

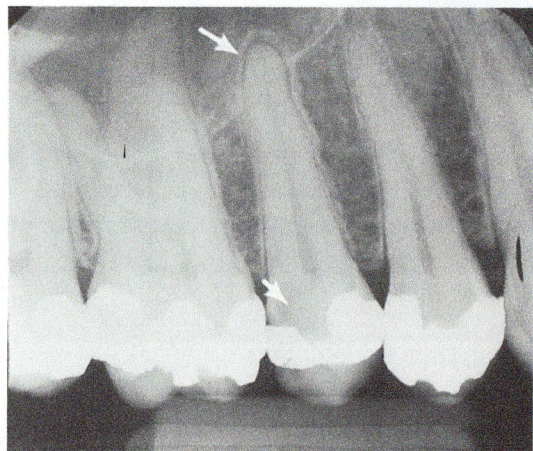

Figure 40-2 Apical periodontitis. Upper second premolar has large, recurrent caries on distal surface. The tooth gave abnormal responses to pulp testing, elicited spontaneous pain, and was painful to percussion. The pulp was severely inflamed.

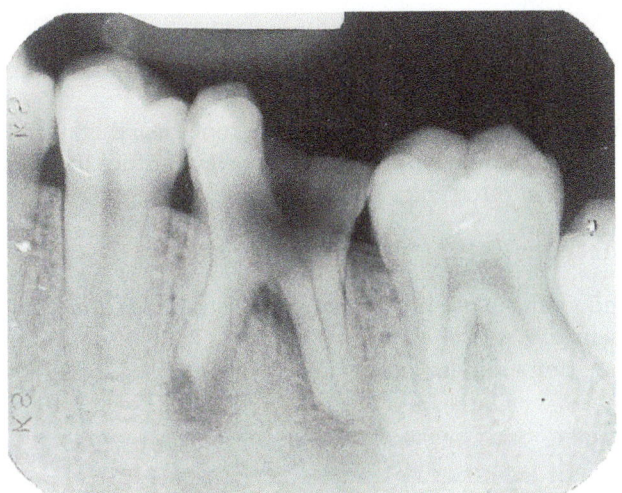

Figure 40–3 Periapical abscess. Radiograph shows caries, chronic periapical inflammation, and an abscess of the first molar.

- **Periapical abscess:** Breakdown of the periapical tissue caused by a build-up of purulent material and fluids in the tissue (Figure 40-3). Patients usually report feeling pain in the periapical region, and the area may be red and swollen in appearance. Periapical abscesses are treated by cleaning out the purulent material and fluids, removing the diseased tissue, and performing root canal therapy.

✓ CHECKPOINT
40-1 Why might a patient need to visit an endodontic dentist?

Endodontic Diagnosis

Endodontic diagnosis helps the dentist determine the type of pulp or apical disease present and which tooth, if any, may require treatment. Dental professionals make the diagnosis in different ways. Determining the right diagnosis also helps the dentist determine whether root canal therapy can restore the tooth's health and function, or whether the tooth is too damaged to treat. In addition to reviewing a patient's dental and medical history, diagnosing endodontic disease begins with an examination of the patient's teeth and gingiva.

Palpation

Palpation is a common way to determine the health of the tooth. The endodontist gently applies pressure to the gingival tissue near the tooth in question. Swelling, sensitivity, or pain can indicate inflammation. Additional areas are palpated for comparison.

Percussion

Percussion tests involve tapping the tooth with the handle of a dental mirror. If the patient cannot feel the tapping in the tooth, the pulp is likely dead. If the pulp is inflamed, the patient generally reports feeling pain upon percussion.

Thermal Testing

Thermal pulp testing uses extreme temperatures to see how the pulp reacts. If the pulp reacts to extreme cold, it can indicate early stages of inflammation. The reaction to cold should disappear once the cold stimulus is removed. If the pulp continues to react, however, that can indicate more advanced inflammation. If applying a hot stimulus causes pain, and application of cold further provides relief, the inflammation is likely advanced. If the pulp does not respond to heat or cold, it likely is dead and cannot be healed.

Electric Testing

Electric pulp testing is performed using a tester called a vitalometer (Figure 40-4). Several teeth are tested with an electric current to determine whether pulp necrosis has occurred and if the pulp can be treated. Care must be taken when using this machine to prevent false readings.

Radiography

Dental radiographs allow the dentist to examine the health of the pulp, the root canal space, and the bone, and to detect possible dental caries. In some instances, pulp damage may not be seen on the radiograph, in which case other tests, such as thermal testing, may be necessary.

Transillumination Testing

Transillumination testing uses a fiber optic light to look for cracks or other signs of bacteria leakage that could cause pulp necrosis. The fiber optic light is used to compare the color of the tooth in question to other teeth. Dark discolorations often mean that pulp necrosis has occurred.

✓ CHECKPOINT
40-2 How are endodontic problems diagnosed?

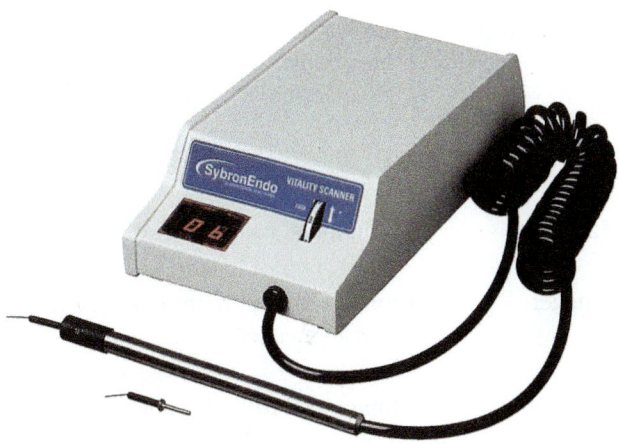

Figure 40–4 Vitalometer.

Treatment Planning

After a diagnosis is made and the dentist determines that root canal therapy is needed, the treatment plan is developed. This includes describing the procedure to the patient, answering any questions, and asking the patient to sign a consent form. Brochures or videos can be helpful for patients with many questions or who seem overly nervous about the procedure.

Root Canal Therapy

When damage to the pulp is severe, root canal therapy may be needed to save the tooth and prevent further infection. Treatment often takes place in two or three appointments.

Instruments

Endodontists use a wide range of instruments and equipment to perform root canal therapy (Table 40-1). A common tray setup for a root canal is shown in Figure 40-5.

TABLE 40-1 Common Endodontic Instruments

INSTRUMENT	DESCRIPTION	FUNCTION
Barbed broach	A long rod made of wire that contains small, sharp barbs or extensions; the handles come in different colors according to the size of the broach	The broach is placed in the pulpal canal, and as it is removed, the barbs scrape away excess tissue
File	A long, twisted rod that comes in different widths and lengths; the handles come in different colors according to the size of the rod; some files are flexible and bend easily to fit into small spaces	The file is used to scrape and clean the pulpal canal of excess tissue; also used to remove dead tissue from the canal
Reamer	A long twisted rod, shaped much like a file; the handles come in different colors according to the size of the reamer	The reamer is used to clean and remove tissue from the pulpal canal
Gates-Glidden	A long metal rod with an oval-shaped tip; they come in different sizes according to the thickness of the canal	The Gates-Glidden cleans the upper area of the canal
Peeso reamer	Shaped much like the Gates-Glidden, but instead of an oval-shaped tip, it has a pointed tip; Peeso reamers come in different sizes depending on the width of the reamer	The Peeso reamer is used to make the inside of the canal even and straight for placement of a post
Lentulo spiral	A long flexible wire that is twisted into a spiral shape	The Lentulo spiral is used to apply root canal sealer
Endodontic spoon excavator	A long metal rod with two ends curved into the shape of a spoon	The endodontic spoon excavator is used to remove material, such as caries or cement, from deep within the pulpal canal
Endodontic explorer	A long metal rod with curved, pointed ends	The endodontic explorer helps the dentist find the canal opening
Rubber stop	A circular rubber disc that slides onto reamers and files; comes in different colors and has holes already punched in the center	A rubber stop is placed onto a file or reamer to mark the length of the root canal; placement is determined by holding the file or reamer up to a radiograph of the canal and sliding the rubber stop to be in line with the edge of the cusp
Spreader	A long metal rod with two pointed ends	A spreader is used to apply a material called gutta percha into the canal
Plugger	A long metal rod with two flat ends shaped much like a spreader	A plugger is used to pack excess filling material to create extra space in the canal for additional gutta percha to be applied
Glick no. 1	A long metal rod with one flat end and one pointed end	A Glick no. 1 instrument is for both packing and removing excess gutta percha

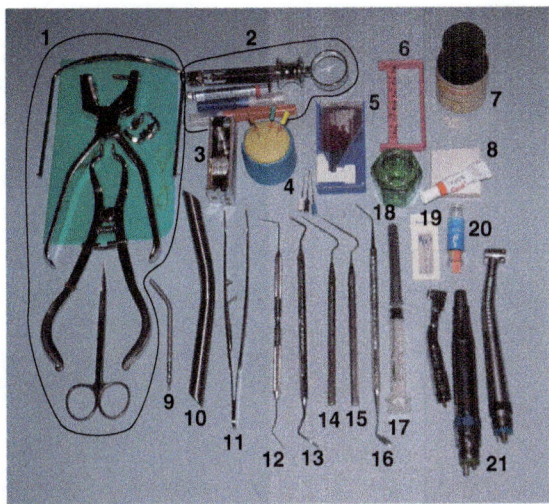

Figure 40–5 Tray setup for root canal. (**1**) Dental dam setup. (**2**) Local anesthesia set-up. (**3**) File gauge. (**4**) Files. (**5**) Stops. (**6**) Burs. (**7**) Intracanal medications. (**8**) Temporary filling material. (**9**) Air/water syringe tip. (**10**) Oral evacuator tip. (**11**) Cotton pliers. (**12**) Endo explorer. (**13**) Endo excavator. (**14**) Endo spreader. (**15**) Endo plugger. (**16**) Endo plastic instrument. (**17**) Irrigating syringe. (**18**) Irrigating solution. (**19**) Paper points. (**20**) Gutta percha points. (**21**) Handpieces (high and low speed).

Equipment

Modern technology has allowed dental professionals to improve root canal therapy, including the following:

- An **apex finder**, also called an apex locator, is an electronic device that helps determine the length of the root of the tooth by measuring the distance to the tooth apex (Figure 40-6). Its digital screen displays an image showing when the endodontic file is nearing the apex. Other apex finders make a sound signal as the file gets closer to the apex.
- Heating units perform several functions, including automatically warming gutta percha for easier placement and performing heat tests to diagnose possible endodontic disease.
- Endodontic handpieces attached to low-speed hand instruments are used to apply endodontic materi-

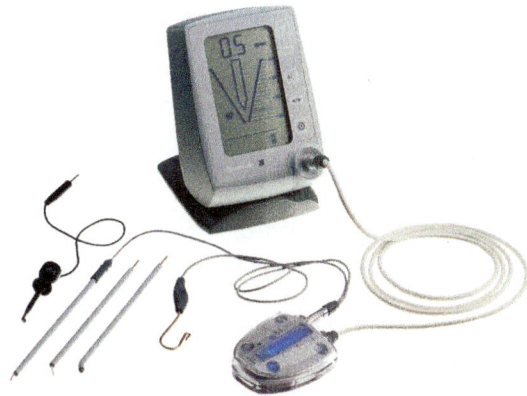

Figure 40–6 Apex finder.

als correctly and evenly. They also aid in cleaning and preparing the root canal for treatment.

- Ultrasonic units perform a variety of endodontic tasks, such as preparing root canal posts, cleaning cement or debris from canals, placing or removing crowns, preparing the root canal for therapy, and acting as a spreader. Special tips are used for different functions.
- Benders are used to bend endodontic instruments, including reamers, files, pluggers, and spreaders, to match the shape of the canal.

Materials

Dental assistants use many different materials to prepare for and assist in root canal therapy. **Irrigants** are water-based solutions used to disinfect the canal system by killing bacteria and dissolving the pulp tissue. Irrigants also flush out debris and keep the canal from becoming overly dry. Common irrigants include sodium hypochlorite, parachlorophenol, chlorhexidine, and sterile saline. Irrigants are injected into the canal with a syringe and needle, and removed with suction. A **paper point** is then used to dry the canal before it is filled.

Once the canal space is prepared and shaped, filling material is applied. The filling material, called **gutta percha**, is a rubber-like substance that is made mostly from zinc oxide. It is available in the form of cones, called gutta percha points. Since it is rubbery in texture, gutta percha is very flexible and easily molded into the canal space. It softens and becomes even more flexible when heated. To make the gutta percha especially soft, you may heat it with a solvent before placing into the canal space. Gutta percha is used in combination with an endodontic sealer, which coats the canal space and fills any gaps between the canal pulp and the gutta percha. The root canal sealer, which is a type of dental cement, is typically made from resin, glass ionomer, zinc oxide eugenol, or calcium hydroxide. Sealers can come in either paste or powder and liquid form. Finally, disinfectants are used to keep the root canal clean throughout the procedure.

Preparation

Before root canal therapy begins, the endodontist decides whether to use anesthesia and, if so, which type. If the nerves inside the pulp are no longer alive, anesthesia may not be needed. Additionally, after the pulp has been removed during the root canal procedure, anesthesia may not be needed during follow-up appointments. When anesthesia is used, the anesthetic is usually injected into the surrounding tissues with a syringe. Sometimes anesthetic agents may be taken in pill form or inhaled as a gas.

Before accessing the root, the area being treated must be isolated using a dental dam. For the canal to be properly reshaped and filled during the procedure, the endodontist must know the canal's length. You may aid in preparation by taking a radiograph of the tooth and placing rubber stops on the endodontic files and reamers for the correct filling of the canal.

Root Canal Procedures

Root canal therapy involves several steps. Generally, treatment involves removal of damaged pulp, reshaping the root canal, filling and sealing the canal, and placement of a permanent restorative, such as a crown.

A root canal involves the following steps:

1. The dentist makes an opening in the tooth's crown to expose the pulp.
2. Damaged pulp (or areas of **obturation**) is removed and the root canal is cleaned.
3. The root canal is reshaped so that it is larger and can be irrigated to flush out the bacteria.
4. The root canal is sealed with a cotton pellet and a restoration material. Depending upon the extent of the infection and the preference of the dentist, a temporary restoration is often used at this step, to allow more time to treat the infection. In such cases a follow-up appointment is scheduled to complete the procedure.
5. At the final appointment, the temporary restoration is removed, and the root canal is cleaned and filled with gutta percha and root canal sealer.
6. A permanent crown and a post and core can be placed over the tooth.

Be sure to educate patients on what to expect after root canal therapy. Some tenderness of the tooth is normal, and patients should avoid chewing, biting, or putting pressure on the treated tooth in the days immediately following therapy. Patients should also avoid crunchy foods as well as foods and beverages that are extremely hot or cold. If pain or swelling occurs, the patient should call the office immediately. If a permanent restoration was not placed, the patient needs to schedule an appointment for this. After root canal therapy, patients should visit the endodontist at 3 to 6 months to determine the effectiveness of the treatment.

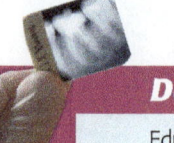

Dental Facts

Educating (and comforting) your patient is especially important with root canal therapy. According to the American Association of Endodontists, more people are afraid of getting a root canal than speaking in public or going on a job interview!

Root Canal Retreatment

If there is enough healthy tooth structure remaining after the root canal therapy, the opening of the tooth crown by which the pulp was accessed can be restored using a composite or amalgam material. Since a tooth undergoing endodontic treatment often has significant weakening from decay, the tooth structure is restored with a crown. After root canal therapy, a post and core is placed to provide support for a prosthetic crown.

Procedure 40–1 Assisting with Root Canal Therapy

Dental assistant duties in root canal therapy can vary greatly depending on the preference of the dentist and state regulations. Typical duties may include taking radiographs and preparing gutta percha cones by dipping them in sealant before transferring to the dentist for placement.

Materials needed (Figure P40-1-1):

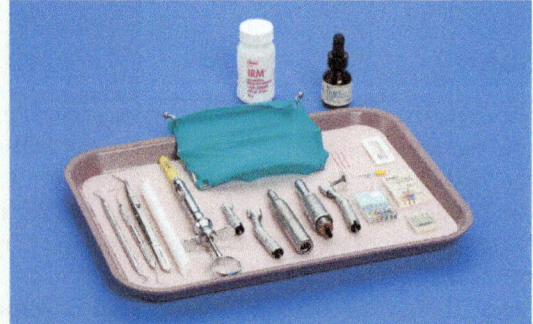

Figure P40-1-1

- Local anesthetic agent setup (optional)
- Dental dam setup
- Handpiece (high-speed) with burs (at dentist's discretion)
- Handpiece (low-speed) with latch attachment
- Irrigating syringe (5-6 mL with 27-gauge needle)
- Irrigating solution
- Broaches and Hedstrom/K-type files of assorted lengths/sizes
- Rubber instrument stops
- Lentulo spiral
- Paper points
- Gutta percha points
- Spoon excavator
- Endodontic explorer
- Endodontic sealer supplies
- Glick no. 1
- Locking cotton pliers
- High-volume evacuator (HVE) tip
- Temporary and/or final restorative material and instruments

1. Put on appropriate PPE.
2. In the first appointment, anesthesia is used to numb the tooth and gingiva. After the first appointment, the dentist decides if anesthesia is needed.
3. Isolate the tooth being treated by assisting with preparation and placement of a dental dam. Clean the area to be treated with disinfectant and a cotton swab.
4. The dentist uses a handpiece to create an opening in the crown of the tooth (Figure P40-1-2).

Procedure 40-1 Assisting with Root Canal Therapy (Continued)

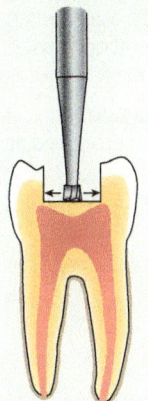

Figure P40-1-2

5. Once the root canals are located, an endodontic spoon excavator is used by the dentist to remove decayed pulp (Figure P40-1-3).

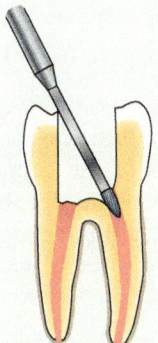

Figure P40-1-3

6. The dentist cleans the canals and an irrigating solution is used.

7. Using the radiograph for guidance, rubber stoppers are placed on the files and reamers the dentist will use to mark the length of the root canals (Figure P40-1-4).

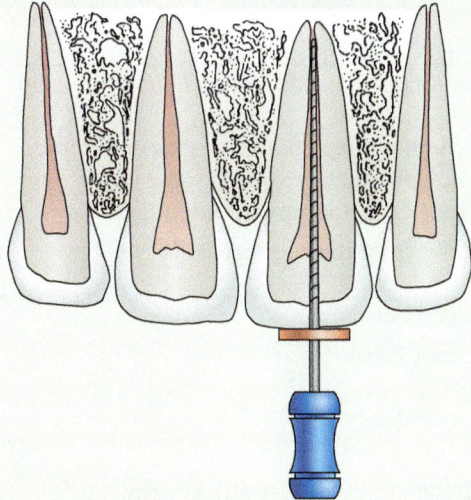

Figure P40-1-4

8. The dentist uses a series of files to reshape and enlarge the root canals (Figure P40-1-5). During the reshaping process, the root canal should be continually rinsed to keep it free from shavings. Paper points may be used to dry the canals after rinsing. This routinely marks the end of the first appointment, depending on the preferences and judgment of the dentist. For example, a dentist may choose to utilize temporary restoratives at this stage to allow time to treat a more extensive infection.

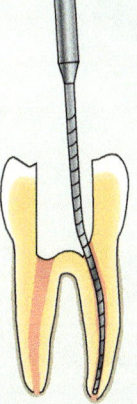

Figure P40-1-5

9. If a follow-up appointment is appropriate, at the next appointment, the dentist removes any temporary restoratives placed previously.

10. The dentist prepares to permanently fill the root canals with gutta percha. The dentist selects the gutta percha cone and tests it for fit before filling the root canal.

11. The root canal sealer is mixed, and the dentist places it using a Lentulo spiral or a gutta percha cone that has been dipped in sealer (Figure P40-1-6).

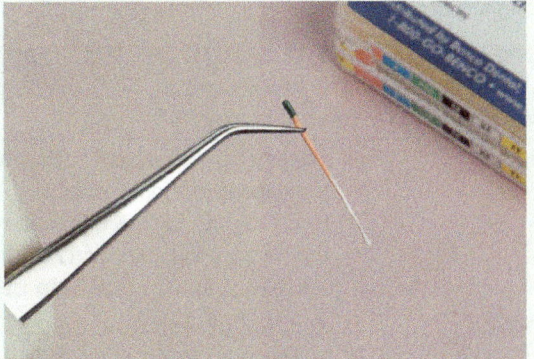

Figure P40-1-6

12. The dentist places gutta percha cones in the canals, one at a time. After placing a cone, the dentist uses the spreader to create space for the next cone and continues placing gutta percha cones until the root canal is filled.

13. A radiograph is taken to confirm the root canal is filled correctly (Figure P40-1-7).

Procedure 40–1 Assisting with Root Canal Therapy (Continued)

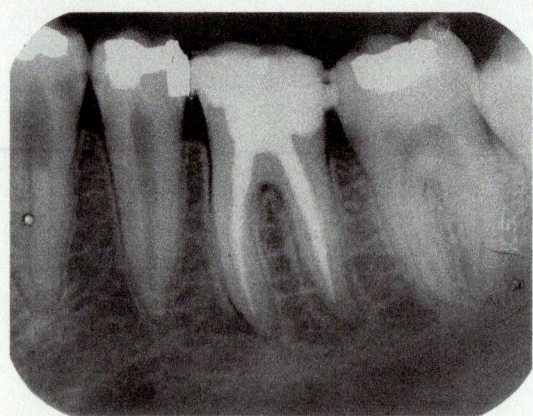

Figure P40-1-7

14. The dentist seals the crown of the tooth with a temporary or permanent restoration. If a temporary restoration is used, this marks the end of the second appointment.
15. During a final appointment, a temporary restoration is removed and a permanent restoration is cemented in place.

CHECKPOINTS

40-3 Which instrument is used to apply root sealer?

40-4 What material is used to fill the canal space during a root canal procedure?

40-5 Why are radiographs needed in preparation for root canal therapy?

Pulpal Therapies

Although root canal therapy is the most common endodontic treatment, other treatment options are typically used when the pulp of the tooth is damaged but not to the extent that root canal therapy is needed. These pulp treatments are described in Table 40-2.

Pulpotomy

A pulpotomy is a frequently performed procedure designed to completely remove the coronal portion of the dental pulp, while maintaining the healthy pulp tissue deeper in the tooth canals. This procedure is indicated in certain emergencies, for vital primary teeth, and for teeth with deep carious lesions.

CHECKPOINT

40-6 What is the difference between a pulpotomy and a pulpectomy?

TABLE 40-2 Types of Pulp Therapies

THERAPY	DESCRIPTION
Pulp cap	■ Placement of a cement base underneath a restoration to provide extra protection for the pulp ■ Used for deep tooth decay ■ Indirect pulp caps are placed when decay is deep but not deep enough to expose the pulp ■ Direct pulp caps are placed when decay is deep enough to have exposed some of the pulp ■ Use of a pulp cap may help prevent the need for root canal therapy in the future
Pulpotomy	■ Removal of pulp from the crown of the tooth but not from the root canal ■ Typically performed on pediatric patients ■ Used when an infection or tooth damage causes deep decay
Pulpectomy	■ Removal of all pulp from both the crown and the root canal ■ Usually performed on pediatric patients ■ Used when an infection or tooth damage causes deep decay
Apexogenesis	■ A procedure to close an open tooth apex ■ Used for teeth that have some damage to the pulp but are otherwise still healthy ■ Used in combination with a pulp cap or pulpotomy ■ Usually performed on pediatric patients

Procedure 40-2 Assisting with Pulpotomy of a Primary Tooth

Dental assistant duties in pulpal therapy vary greatly depending on the dentist's preferences and state regulations.

Materials needed (Figure P40-2-1):

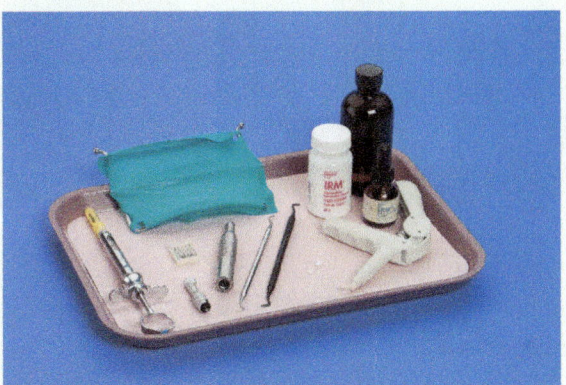

Figure P40-2-1

- Local anesthetic agent setup
- Dental dam setup
- Low-speed handpiece
- Round burs
- Spoon excavators (various sizes)
- Sterile cotton pellets
- Formocresol
- Zinc oxide eugenol (ZOE) base
- Final restorative material (and instruments for placement)

1. Put on appropriate PPE.
2. Anesthesia is used to numb the tooth and gingiva.
3. Isolate the tooth being treated by assisting with preparation and placement of the dental dam. Clean the area to be treated with disinfectant and a cotton swab.
4. The dentist exposes the pulp chamber using a round bur in the low-speed handpiece (Figure P40-2-2).

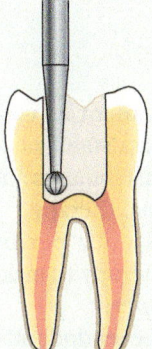

Figure P40-2-2

5. Transfer a spoon excavator to the dentist for removal of pulp tissue in the coronal chamber.

6. To control bleeding, transfer to the dentist a sterile cotton pellet moistened with formocresol for placement in the pulp chamber (Figure P40-2-3A and B).

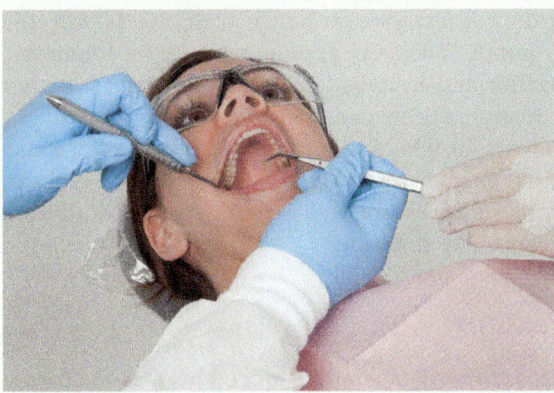

Figure P40-2-3A

Sterile cotton pellet moistened with formocresol

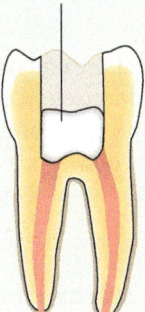

Figure P40-2-3B

7. After approximately 5 minutes, once bleeding has been controlled, the dentist uses ZOE base with a drop of formocresol added to fill the pulp chamber (Figure P40-2-4).

ZOE base

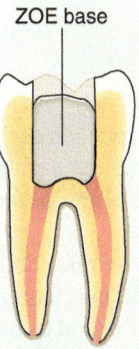

Figure P40-2-4

8. The dentist places the final restorative material.
9. Document procedure in the patient's record and provide the patient with postprocedure instructions.

Surgical Endodontics

Root canal therapy is successful in 90% to 95% of all cases but may fail, usually due to infection, inflammation, or damage to the root canal. Patients with failed root canal therapy do not always experience pain; this is why the 3 to 6 month follow-up appointment is so important. A radiograph and examination usually indicate whether further treatment is needed.

In patients for whom root canal therapy was not a success, endodontic surgery may be needed. Several types of endodontic surgeries can help save the treated tooth from further damage or removal.

Apicoectomy

An **apicoectomy** is a surgical procedure that removes a small amount of the root apex, usually 1 to 3 millimeters. Depending on whether the tissue around the root is infected, an **apical curettage**, or removal of tissue, may take place.

Root End Filling

During an apicoectomy, a filling is placed to seal the end of the root. This process is called root end filling, or retrograde restoration. Different materials, including gutta percha and composites, may be used to fill the end of the root.

Root Amputation

When root damage is severe, an endodontist may have to remove one or more of the roots of a multi-root tooth, a procedure called root amputation. At least one root must be left for the tooth to continue to be healthy.

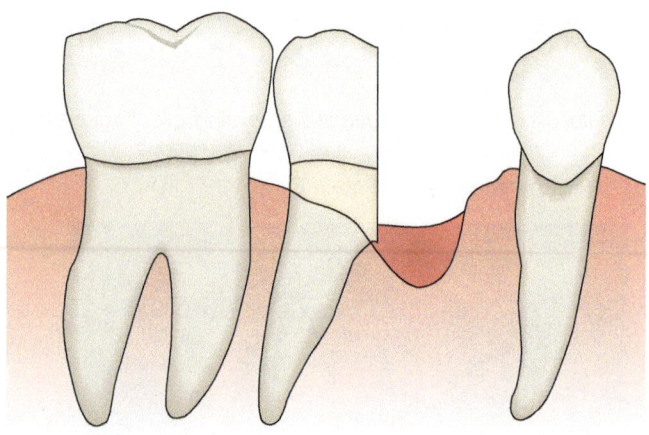

Figure 40–7 Hemisection.

Hemisection

An option for heavily decayed mandibular molars with two roots is a **hemisection** (Figure 40-7). In this procedure, the overlying crown and one root of the tooth are surgically removed ("hemi" means half). Once the damaged half of the tooth is removed, a bridge may be fabricated to help the remaining healthy tooth function normally.

Apexification

Following an apicoectomy, the endodontist may help the root close by placing a special paste in a procedure called **apexification**. The paste is usually made from calcium hydroxide.

CHECKPOINT
40-7 How successful is root canal therapy?

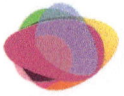

Chapter Highlights

✦ Endodontics is a branch of dentistry that specializes in treating problems with the tooth's pulp, including pulp infection, pulp necrosis, and inflammation of the periapical tissue.

✦ A variety of techniques are used to diagnose endodontic problems, including palpating the tooth, percussion tests, thermal and electric testing, radiographs, and transillumination testing.

✦ Pulpal therapy may include placement of pulp caps and removal of pulp from the crown and/or root canal.

✦ Root canal therapy is the most common endodontic treatment and frequently takes place in two or three appointments. It involves removal of damaged pulp, reshaping and cleansing of the root canal, filling and sealing the canals, and placement of a restoration.

✦ Special endodontic instruments and equipment are used during the root canal procedure. Dental assistants need to be knowledgeable about the various instruments and equipment and their function in root canal therapy.

✦ Materials such as irrigants, paper points, gutta percha, and sealants are used during root canal therapy to make sure the canal is clean, dry, and filled properly.

✦ Before root canal therapy can occur, the endodontist decides whether anesthesia is needed. The tooth to be treated must be isolated, and a radiograph is taken to determine the length of the root canal.

✦ Although root canal therapy is highly effective, it may be unsuccessful if infection, inflammation, or damage to the root canal occurs. In such cases, a variety of surgical procedures may help save the tooth.

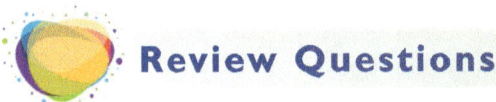 **Review Questions**

1. If a patient cannot feel tapping during percussion testing,
   a. The tooth is likely healthy.
   b. The tooth is likely infected.
   c. The tooth is likely dead.
   d. None of the above.

2. Which type of pulpal therapy involves removal of pulpal tissue from the crown and root?
   a. Root canal therapy.
   b. Pulpectomy.
   c. Pulpotomy.
   d. Hemisection.

3. Rubber stops may be used to mark the length of the root canal, which is helpful when using
   a. Endodontic files.
   b. Endodontic spreaders.
   c. Endodontic excavators.
   d. Barbed broaches.

4. During root canal therapy
   a. Anesthesia is not necessary since the nerves in the damaged pulp are dead.
   b. The root canal is filled with zinc oxide eugenol.
   c. Both A and B.
   d. None of the above.

5. How often does root canal therapy fail?
   a. About 50% of cases
   b. About 20 to 25% of cases
   c. About 5 to 10% of cases
   d. Less than 5% of cases

6. After an unsuccessful root canal treatment, a patient returns to the endodontist, who determines that one of the damaged roots must be removed. This is known as
   a. Root amputation.
   b. Root curettage.
   c. Apioectomy.
   d. Apexification.

7. After completion of a root canal procedure, the patient should have a follow-up appointment
   a. Within 6 weeks.
   b. In 3 to 6 months.
   c. In a year.
   d. Only if experiencing pain.

8. Which of the following terms refers to a surgical procedure that removes a small amount of the root apex?
   a. Apexogenesis
   b. Apex finder
   c. Apicoectomy
   d. Hemisection

Active Learning Exercises

1. What are the differences among a file, a reamer, and a broach? What are the visual differences? In what order would they be used?

2. What does the term *obturation* mean? What instruments would be used to complete this procedure?

3. Imagine that a patient presents with an extreme toothache and undergoes a pulpotomy. How is this different than a pulpectomy? What are the indications for performing pulpotomy rather than a pulpectomy?

Application Activities

1. Using the instruments and equipment your instructor provides, practice identifying each instrument and its use. Which instruments are similar in appearance and might be easily confused? For each item, describe your role as a dental assistant in using, preparing, and cleaning the instruments and equipment.

2. It is not unusual for patients to feel nervous or scared about undergoing root canal therapy. How can you make sure you educate your patient without frightening him or her? What are some things you can say to comfort patients? Suppose a patient who had root canal therapy in the past complains of having had a bad experience. How would you handle this situation? What might you say to reassure the patient?

PREPARING FOR CERTIFICATION EXAMS

Review the following topics in this chapter to prepare for the Dental Assisting National Board (DANB) exam:

- **Pulpal Disease and Damage**
- **Endodontic Diagnosis**
- **Electric Testing**
- **Root Canal Therapy**
- **Root Canal Procedures**
- **Pulpal Therapies**

Periodontics

CHAPTER OUTLINE

CHAPTER CHECKLIST

On completion of this chapter, students will be able to:

- ☑ Describe the steps of a periodontal examination.
- ☑ Identify and describe the various instruments used in periodontal examinations and procedures.
- ☑ Identify nonsurgical periodontal procedures and describe when each is appropriate.
- ☑ Explain the role of the dental assistant when providing support during nonsurgical periodontal procedures.
- ☑ Identify surgical periodontal procedures and describe when each is appropriate.
- ☑ Explain the role of the dental assistant when providing support during surgical periodontal procedures.
- ☑ Describe how to prepare, place, and remove a periodontal dressing.

KEY TERMS

bone grafting – adding bone or bone substitute to an area

curette (kyu-RET) – instrument used to perform gingival curettage; also used to remove calculus from the teeth, mainly subgingival calculus

débridement (day-BREDE-mahnt) – a procedure that involves scaling and ultrasonic instrumentation of the root surfaces of the teeth to attain healthy gingival tissue

frenectomy (fruh-NEK-tuh-mee) – surgical removal of the frenum

gingival curettage – procedure to remove inflamed tissue and debris from the gingival lining of a periodontal pocket

gingival grafting – taking tissue from one area and replacing it where gingival tissue is missing

gingivectomy (jin-juh-VEK-tuh-mee) – surgical removal of diseased gingival tissue

gingivoplasty (jin-juh-voh-PLAS-tee) – surgical reshaping and contouring of gingival tissues

ostectomy (os-TEK-tuh-mee) – removing bone

osteoplasty (OS-tee-oh-plas-tee) – contouring and shaping bone

planing – procedure to smooth tooth surfaces by removing calculus and necrotic cementum that may be embedded in the root surface; this procedure is rarely performed in modern dentistry

pocket marker – tweezer-like dental instrument used to perforate gingival tissue with small markings, indicating locations for incisions

scaling – type of tooth surface débridement that removes plaque, calculus, and stains

Introduction

Periodontics is the branch of dentistry that focuses on the prevention, diagnosis, and treatment of diseases affecting the tissues that surround the teeth and attach them to the alveolar bone. A dentist who specializes in this field is known as a *periodontist*. To become a periodontist, an individual must complete an accredited dental program and go on to receive 3 or more years of advanced training in the study and treatment of periodontal diseases.

Various periodontal diseases affect the gingival tissues, periodontal connective tissues, and alveolar bone. These diseases can be classified into two major categories: gingivitis and periodontitis. *Gingivitis* is a bacterial infection that is characterized by inflammation of the gingival tissue, typically as a result of bacterial plaque. It results in reversible damage to the gingival tissue. Left untreated, gingivitis may lead to periodontitis, a bacterial infection of all parts of the periodontium. *Periodontitis* results in irreversible destruction to the tissues of the periodontium and can lead to tooth loss.

This chapter focuses on the instruments and procedures used in the treatment of periodontal disease. For a detailed look at the types, causes, and symptoms of periodontal disease, see Chapter 9, Dental Caries and Periodontal Disease. For information about methods used to prevent periodontal disease, see Chapter 10, Prevention of Caries and Periodontal Disease.

Periodontal Examination

Medical and Dental History

As with any dental examination, the dental team should take a current dental and medical history of a periodontal patient, including a medication history. A review of the patient's medical history and additional information gathering, if necessary, can help the dental team determine if the patient has any medical conditions that may affect dental treatment. Studying a patient's family health history can also indicate whether a patient has a genetic predisposition to a particular illness. A patient with a systemic illness may have lowered resistance to infection, which increases the severity of periodontal disease. Diseases such as diabetes, human immunodeficiency virus (HIV), and acquired immunodeficiency syndrome (AIDS) are among the diseases that can lower resistance.

Diagnostic Techniques

The dentist's or dental hygienist's visual inspection of the patient's gingival tissues, teeth, and oral cavity is an integral part of any examination and can provide clues about the patient's health, hygiene, and habits.

During the periodontal examination, the dentist or dental hygienist checks the teeth for mobility. Teeth normally have some mobility, but too much can indicate periodontal disease.

The dentist or dental hygienist also checks for plaque and calculus buildup and assesses gingival health, bone levels, and periodontal pockets. Because healthy gingival tissue does not bleed, gingival health and the extent of inflammation are indicated by the amount of bleeding that occurs when the gingival tissue is gently probed.

Periodontal probing is a technique used to determine epithelial attachment lost to periodontal disease. The dentist or dental hygienist uses a probe to measure pocket depth around individual teeth (Figure 41-1). The probe, which is tapered and rounded, is inserted into the gingival sulcus until it meets resistance. Six measurements are taken for each tooth—three facial sites and three lingual sites. Periodontal probes measure the depth of periodontal pockets in millimeters, with a normal sulcus depth

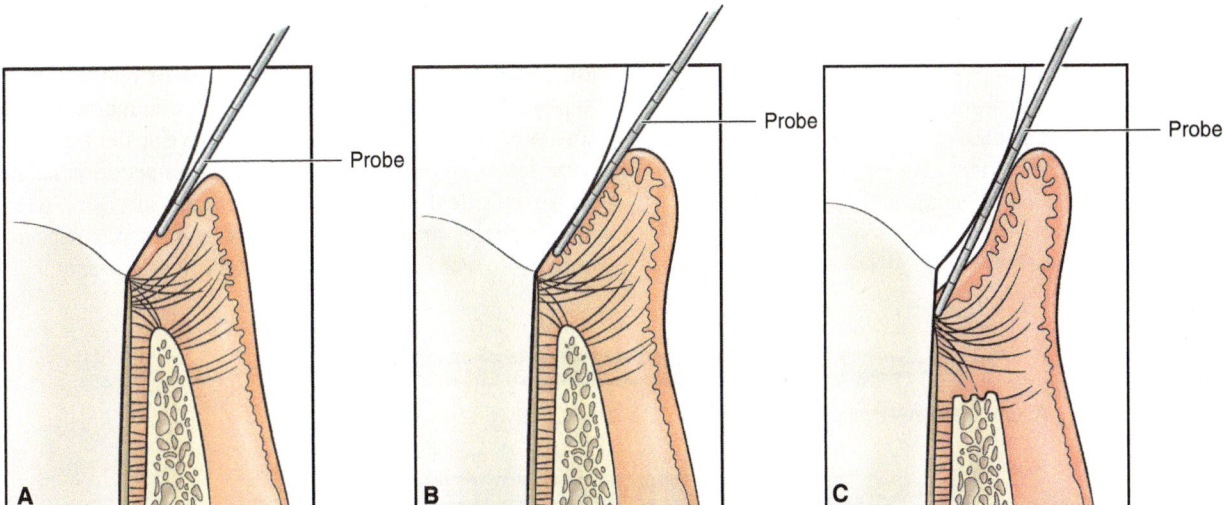

Figure 41-1 **Periodontal probing.** The dentist or dental hygienist uses a probe to measure pocket depth around individual teeth. **(A)** Minimal inflammation of tissues. **(B)** Moderate inflammation. **(C)** Severe inflammation.

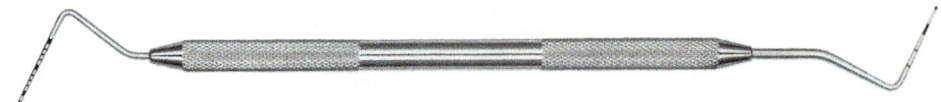

Figure 41–2 Periodontal explorer.

measuring 3 mm or less. If the sulcus depth is greater than 3 mm, it is considered a periodontal pocket. Periodontal pockets can be difficult to keep clean and can harbor bacteria and debris. Untreated, bacteria in periodontal pockets will multiply, which may eventually lead to tooth loss. The level of the gingival margin is also assessed. A periodontal probe is used to measure the level of the free gingival margin in relationship to the cementoenamel junction (CEJ) and mucogingival junction. Attachment loss is recorded in the patient's chart.

The dentist also checks the patient's occlusal adjustment. If the patient's bite is putting pressure on particular areas, it can cause trauma and can lead to tooth mobility, bone destruction, and pain. The dentist can adjust the patient's bite to ensure equally distributed occlusal force.

Radiography is another important part of the examination. Periodontal disease results in recession of the alveolar bone. Bitewing radiographs, in particular, help to show bone height at the surface of the root.

Voice of Experience

You can help the patient understand what the dentist is measuring during periodontal probing. More importantly, you can counsel the patient on ways to prevent pockets from worsening. And at subsequent appointments in which pocket depth is measured, you can praise the patient when efforts have halted or improved damage and offer continued encouragement to practice the self-care regimen required for good oral health.

CHECKPOINTS

41-1 How many measurements per tooth does the dentist or dental hygienist take when documenting periodontal pockets?

41-2 What is the normal sulcus depth measured with a periodontal probe?

Periodontal Instruments

Examination Instruments

Periodontal probes are used during the examination to measure periodontal pockets, bleeding, and recession. Probes are calibrated in millimeters and may be indented or color-coded to indicate increments. Also available is a computerized probe system that records the information during measurement.

A periodontal explorer (Figure 41-2) helps to identify calculus deposits, root surface irregularities, and abnormalities in restoration margins. Because they are used to reach the base of pockets and furcations, explorers used in periodontics generally are longer than those used in general dental practice. They are also finer and thinner for working around root surfaces, and the working end is typically more curved for exploring all tooth surface angles.

Scalers and Curettes

A periodontal scaler is a sharp instrument used to remove calculus deposits from the teeth. Scalers are available in various shapes and angles (Figure 41-3). One type is a sickle scaler, appropriate for removing supragingival calculus. It has a long, straight shank, a curved blade, and two cutting edges. A chisel scaler is used on anterior teeth and features a slightly curved blade and a beveled cutting edge. A hoe scaler is used to remove heavy deposits from the buccal and lingual surfaces of posterior teeth. It has a beveled, sharp cutting edge and a bent blade.

An ultrasonic scaler is a handheld device that uses rapid vibration to remove calculus and other hard deposits from the surface of the teeth. It is also used to remove orthodontic cement and overhanging margins of restorations. Two types of ultrasonic scalers are available: magnetostrictive and piezoelectrical. A magnetostrictive scaler has a tip that vibrates at 18,000 to 45,000 cycles per second and moves in an elliptical pattern. A piezoelectrical scaler has a tip that vibrates at 25,000 to 50,000 cycles per second and moves forward and backward in a linear pattern.

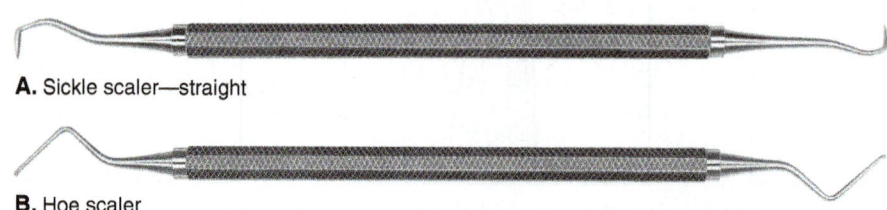

A. Sickle scaler—straight

B. Hoe scaler

Figure 41–3 Scalers. (A) Sickle scaler—straight. **(B)** Hoe scaler.

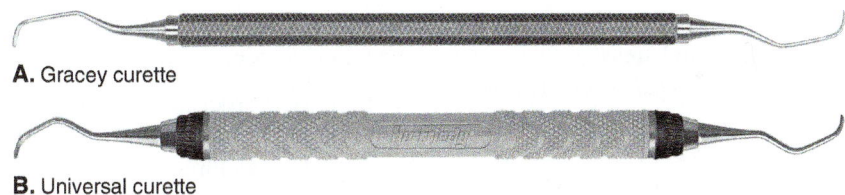

A. Gracey curette

B. Universal curette

Figure 41–4 **Curettes.** (**A**) Gracey curette. (**B**) Universal curette.

The scaler sprays water from its tip that flushes out debris and aids in keeping the ultrasonic tip cool. The dental assistant (DA) has an important role when using the high-volume evacuator (HVE) to prevent contamination with this aerosol spray. This is particularly important with patients who have a communicable disease that could be transmitted via contaminated spray.

The ultrasonic scaler should not be used on patients who are particularly vulnerable to infection, such as those who have had an organ transplant or who are having chemotherapy and those who have a respiratory condition, such as asthma or emphysema. Other patients for whom this scaler may be contraindicated include those who have a cardiac pacemaker and those who have difficulty swallowing.

Additionally, some restorations, dental implants, and dental conditions may make the ultrasonic scaler a less-than-ideal choice. For example, if a patient has demineralized areas, the scaler could negatively affect any remineralization.

Because the tissues of pediatric patients are sensitive to ultrasonic vibrations, the ultrasonic scaler should not be used on patients who have primary or new permanent teeth.

Files featuring various blade shapes and angles are used in a pulling motion to break up heavy calculus. They also may be used for the removal of overhanging margins of restorations.

Another commonly used instrument is the **curette**, which is used to remove subgingival calculus, smooth root surfaces, and remove soft tissue lining periodontal pockets. Two basic types are the universal curette, which is designed for use throughout the mouth, and the Gracey curette, which is designed for site-specific use (Figure 41-4). The working end of a curette is similar to that of a scaler, but the end of the curette is rounded, not pointed.

Surgical Instruments

Surgical knives are commonly used in periodontal procedures to remove gingival or soft tissue (Figure 41-5). Kirkland knives have kidney-shaped blades. Orban knives

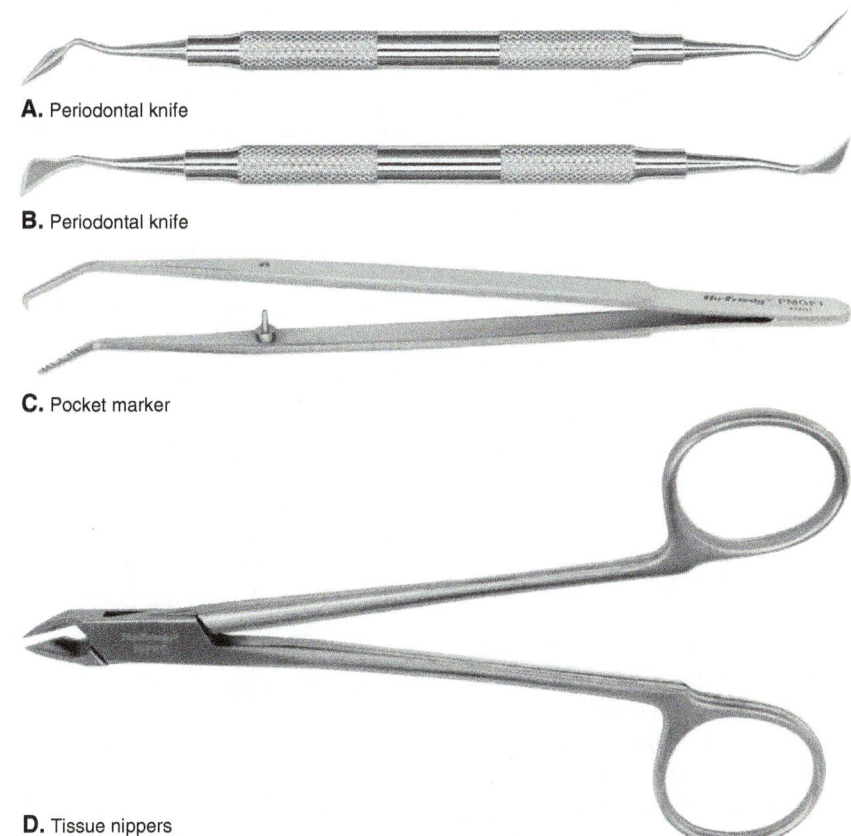

A. Periodontal knife

B. Periodontal knife

C. Pocket marker

D. Tissue nippers

Figure 41–5 **Surgical instruments.** (**A, B**) Periodontal knives. (**C**) Pocket marker. (**D**) Tissue nippers.

are shaped like spears, feature two cutting edges, and are used to remove tissue from interdental areas.

The periotome is an instrument used to cut the periodontal ligament fibers prior to an atraumatic extraction or in preparation for an implant. The blades are sharp, thin, and flexible, and the instruments are available in various designs.

The **pocket marker** has a straight side and a tip bent at a right angle. The straight side is placed in the periodontal pocket. When the two sides are pushed together in a tweezer-like fashion, the other side—the bent, sharp side—perforates the gingival tissue with small markings. These indicate the location for an incision.

The periosteal elevator is used by the dentist to detach gingival tissue from around the cervix of the tooth. Typically, this instrument has a long, tapered end and a round blade end.

Scissors are used during periodontal procedures to trim tissue. The blades may be straight or curved, with smooth or serrated edges.

Tissue forceps are used to pull back and hold tissue in place, typically during oral surgery (see Chapter 42, Oral and Maxillofacial Surgery).

It is important to keep periodontal instruments appropriately sharp so they perform at their peak. Instruments can be sharpened either by hand using sharpening stones or by using a mechanical sharpener; both techniques require practice.

✓ **CHECKPOINTS**

41-3 What instrument is used to measure the depth of periodontal pockets?

41-4 What is the pocket marker used for?

Periodontal Equipment

When performing periodontal surgery, a dentist may use an electrosurgical unit that uses a high-frequency electrical current to make precise cuts. The dentist uses foot pedals to operate the equipment, which includes a probe with cutting tips, a plate placed behind the patient's back, and a control box. During this type of procedure, the DA uses the HVE to remove debris.

Laser technology may also be used in periodontal treatment. A laser produces a narrow beam of light with a single wavelength that can produce intense energy. The beam can be used to remove soft tissue or make incisions in the oral cavity. One benefit of using lasers in dentistry is that laser incisions produce very little bleeding, thus allowing

a clearer view of the surgical area for the dentist. Additional benefits include:

- Increased precision in cutting
- Reduced trauma to healthy tissue
- Reduced swelling and discomfort
- Reduced risk of infection
- Reduced procedure time for increased convenience and comfort of the patient
- Reduced need for anesthesia

Among the periodontal procedures for which laser technology can be used are crown lengthening surgeries, implant exposure, tissue fusion, removal of tumors and lesions, sulcular debridement, laser curettage, gingivectomy, gingivoplasty, frenectomy, and ulcer treatment.

A dentist who uses a laser in practice must be trained in its use. When a laser is in use, members of the dental team and the patient must wear protective eyewear.

✓ **CHECKPOINT**

41-5 How can laser technology result in a clearer view of the surgical area?

Nonsurgical Periodontal Procedures

Removing calculus, soft deposits, plaque, and stains from supragingival and unattached subgingival tooth surfaces are common nonsurgical treatments for patients who have periodontal diseases.

Scaling and Polishing

A dentist or dental hygienist performs **débridement** to help restore tissues to health by removing deposits from the teeth and bacteria from periodontal pockets. Débridement generally requires a local anesthetic. One type of débridement is **scaling**, which removes supragingival and subgingival plaque and calculus from the teeth. Devices employed in this procedure can include ultrasonic instruments and hand instruments, such as scalers and curettes.

Coronal surfaces of the teeth are often polished after scaling (see Chapter 44, Coronal Polishing).

Root Planing

Root **planing** is a technique designed to remove any remaining calculus that may be embedded in the root surface. Following the process used for scaling, the cementum

Procedure 41-1 Assisting with Scaling and Polishing

Materials needed (Figure P41-1-1):

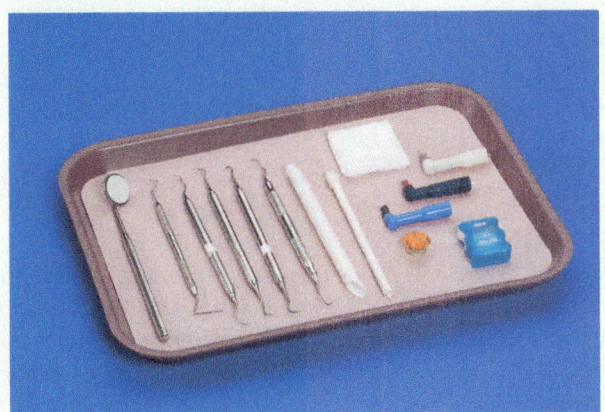

Figure P41-1-1

- Mouth mirror
- Explorer
- Probe
- Scalers and curettes
- Gauze
- Cotton pliers
- Dental floss and tape
- Prophy angle with rubber cups and brushes
- Prophy paste
- High-volume evacuator (HVE)
- Saliva ejector

1. Put on appropriate personal protective equipment (PPE).
2. Retract the patient's lips, tongue, and cheeks to provide the dentist or dental hygienist with access and visibility during the procedure.
3. The operator uses scalers and curettes to remove calculus from the teeth (Figure P41-1-2A). An ultrasonic scaler also may be used for this procedure (Figure P41-1-2B).

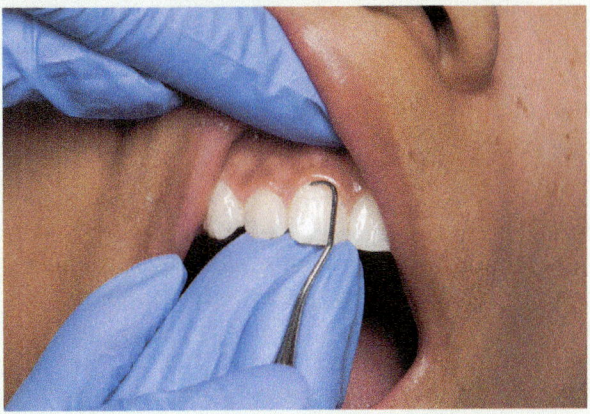

Figure P41-1-2A

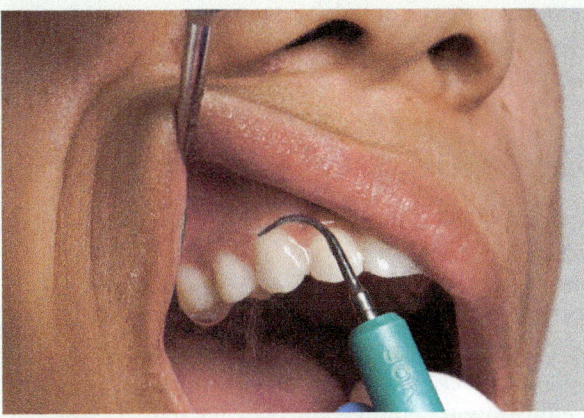

Figure P41-1-2B

4. Throughout the procedure, assist with the transfer of instruments and use the HVE to remove excess saliva, fluids, and debris.
5. The operator polishes the crown portion of the teeth using a rubber cup and prophy paste.
6. Finally, the operator cleans the interproximal areas with dental floss and tape to remove any remaining debris.
7. Make a note of the procedure in the patient's record and provide the patient with self-care instructions.

covering the root surfaces is smoothed, or planed, making it more difficult for plaque to adhere to the surfaces. This technique is now seldom performed because it is now known that planing is not necessary for removing calculus on most root surfaces.

Gingival Curettage

In addition to treating the surfaces of the tooth, **gingival curettage** may be performed on the soft tissue lining the periodontal pocket. Gingival curettage is a procedure in which the gingival lining of the periodontal pocket is removed with a curette. The goal is to remove all inflamed tissue and eliminate bacteria and debris.

Occlusal Adjustment

An uneven, unequal bite can cause trauma that affects the health of the periodontium, including tooth mobility, bone destruction, and joint pain. The dentist may elect to adjust an unequal bite to better distribute occlusal forces over the patient's teeth. Instruments used in this process include articulating paper, stones, and burs.

Use of Antibiotics in Periodontal Procedures

Because of their antibacterial properties, antibiotics, especially tetracycline, can be used to combat periodontitis, often in combination with surgical and nonsurgical procedures. A dentist may prescribe an antibiotic oral medication or mouth rinse or may apply an antibiotic directly into the patient's periodontal pockets. Often, this latter method is used when the patient's condition does not respond to other methods or if the patient cannot take systemic medications. A directly applied antibiotic can be in the form of a fiber, an injected gel, or a dissolvable chip. The dissolvable chip contains chlorhexidine, an antimicrobial agent.

Patient Education

Review proper oral hygiene practices with each patient, including brushing and flossing techniques. Note any problem areas and recommend techniques and instruments that can help with the patient's unique challenges, including cleaning large interdental spaces and around dental appliances. Maintain a kit of models and supplies to demonstrate techniques for patients and to show particular devices to patients. Be sure to record your oral hygiene instructions and product recommendations in the patient's chart.

If the patient has had a procedure that requires tissue healing, advise the patient to avoid alcoholic beverages and spicy or citrus foods that could impair recovery. Another impediment to healing is smoking. Patients who smoke should be cautioned that smoking impedes healing.

Voice of Experience

Generally speaking, you are not going to be the impetus for a patient to quit smoking, although you can inform the patient about available tobacco cessation programs. You should, however, emphasize to the patient the importance of not smoking while healing from a periodontal procedure. Patients who smoke already know that smoking is not a healthy choice, and they will quit smoking only when they decide the time is right. Instead of lecturing patients about the negative effects of smoking, suggest instead that they refrain from smoking for a specific time period while healing. Explain how smoking impedes recovery. If given a reasonable number of days to either not smoke or simply cut back on smoking, the patient may see the request as more achievable and may be more likely to comply.

CHECKPOINTS
41-6 What is the form of debridement that removes plaque, calculus, and stains from tooth surfaces?

41-7 What procedure removes inflamed tissue and debris from the gingival lining of a periodontal pocket?

Surgical Periodontal Procedures

Nonsurgical treatment is generally the first course of action to stop periodontal disease. When that fails, surgery may be recommended. Periodontal surgery provides the dental professional with greater access to the root surfaces for scaling.

Gingivectomy

Gingivectomy is the surgical removal of diseased gingival tissue (Figure 41-6). This procedure is appropriate when periodontal pocket depth is too great and fibrous tissue is present. Removal of the pocket improves the patient's access to the area for better cleaning. Gingivectomy may also be performed on patients with gingival hyperplasia, an overgrowth of gingival tissue due to medications such as Dilantin.

The dentist marks the gingival tissue using pocket markers, and uses knives and scissors to remove the tissue. Lasers also may be used for this procedure. With the pocket size reduced, the patient can more easily perform adequate self-care.

Gingivoplasty

Gingivoplasty is surgical reshaping and contouring of gingival tissues and is appropriate when periodontal pocket depth is too great and fibrous tissue is present. Patients who have gingivectomy also often have gingivoplasty.

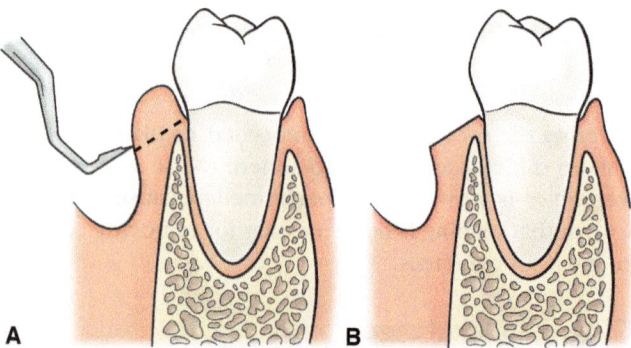

Figure 41–6 Gingivectomy. (A) A gingivectomy knife is used to incise excess gingival tissue. **(B)** Removing the excess tissue creates a more natural level and contour of the gingiva on the tooth surface.

Procedure 41-2 Assisting with Gingivectomy

Materials needed (Figure P41-2-1):

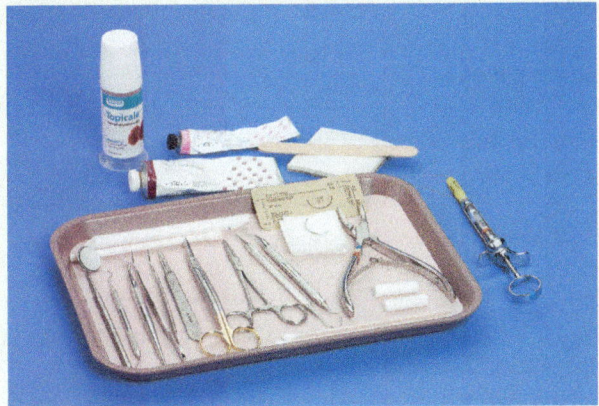

Figure P41-2-1

- Mouth mirror
- Explorer
- Cotton pliers
- Periodontal probe
- Cottons rolls and gauze sponges
- HVE and saliva ejector
- Pocket markers
- Periodontal knives
- Scalpel
- Blades
- Burs

- Scalers and curettes
- Soft tissue rongeurs
- Surgical scissors
- Hemostat
- Sutures
- Needle holder
- Anesthetic supplies
- Periodontal dressing supplies

1. Put on appropriate PPE.
2. The dentist administers anesthetic and examines the patient's periodontium with a probe, marking pocket depths with pocket markers. Be prepared to transfer instruments as needed and to retract the patient's cheeks, lips, and tongue.
3. Using a knife or scalpel, the dentist incises the marked gingiva (see Figure 41-6A). Evacuate the area and provide instruments to the dentist as needed.
4. The dentist uses interdental knives, scissors, rongeurs, and burs to remove interproximal tissue and tissue tags (see Figure 41-6B). Use gauze to clean instruments as needed.
5. The dentist next scales the root surfaces. Provide instruments and evacuation of the surgical area.
6. If sutures are used, prepare the suture materials and pass them to the dentist.
7. Prepare the periodontal dressing for placement.
8. Once the dressing is in place, gently clean the patient's face.
9. Make a note of the procedure in the patient's record and provide the patient with self-care instructions.

To contour tissue, knives, burs, curettes, and surgical scissors are used. The gingival margin is thinned and given a natural-looking, attractive edge.

Periodontal Flap Surgery

Periodontal flap, or incisional, surgery is the surgical separation of the gingiva from underlying tissue (Figure 41-7). It is performed instead of gingivectomy or gingivoplasty. Tissue is not removed but is pushed aside to allow the dentist to scale the exposed root surfaces or recontour underlying bone.

Mucogingival Surgery

Mucogingival surgery, also called *periodontal plastic surgery*, is considered reconstructive surgery on oral cavity tissues. Common types of mucogingival surgery are gingival grafting and frenectomy.

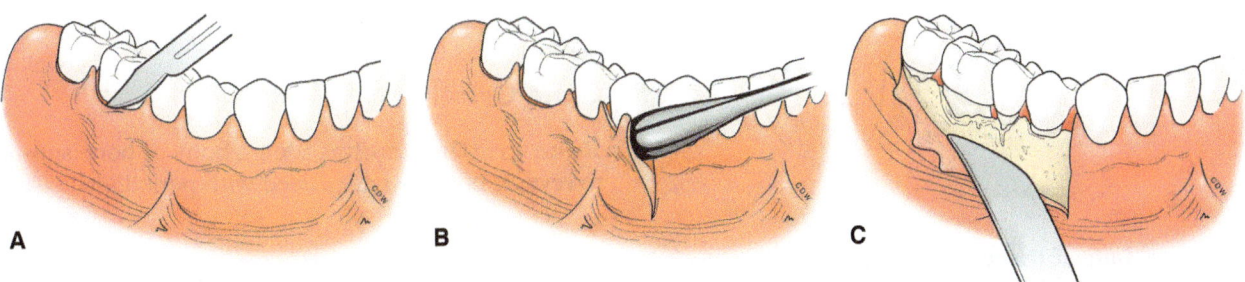

Figure 41-7 Periodontal flap surgery. (A) An incision is made to allow for separation of the soft tissue from the roots and alveolar bone. **(B)** The soft tissue flap is elevated. **(C)** The tooth roots and alveolar bone contours can be visualized.

Gingival Grafting

Gingival grafting involves taking tissue from one area and placing it where gingival tissue is missing. In one type, the graft is taken from an adjacent tooth or area. In another type, tissue for the graft is taken from the patient's palate and placed at the graft site. The flap helps supply nutrients to the grafted tissue during healing.

Frenectomy

A **frenectomy** is a procedure to surgically remove a frenum, a small flap of tissue attaching the lip, cheek, or tongue to the gingiva. A labial frenectomy involves the removal of the frenum connecting the inside of the lip to the gingival tissue. The procedure is typically performed to close a gap between the front teeth or to improve the fit of dentures. A lingual frenectomy is performed on patients who are tongue-tied.

Guided Tissue Regeneration

Guided tissue regeneration is a surgical procedure that uses barrier membranes to direct the growth of new soft tissue where a periodontal defect exists (Figure 41-8).

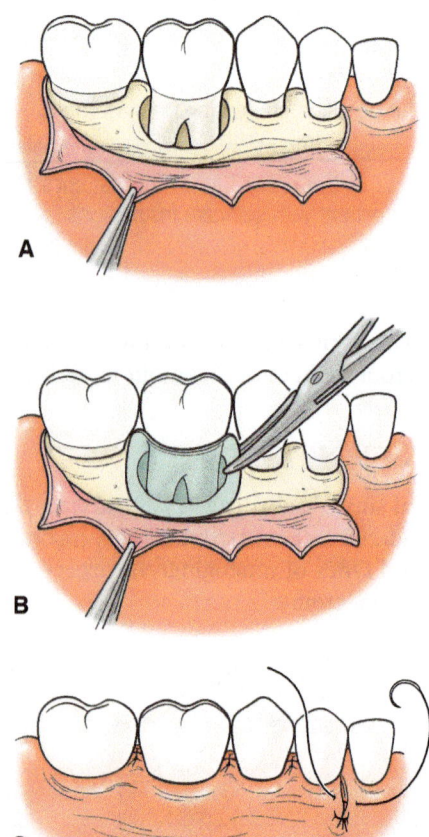

Figure 41–8 Guided tissue generation. (A) Flap is incised and elevated prior to débridement of the osseous defect and tooth root. (B) A barrier is trimmed to size and sutured into place. (C) Flap is sutured into place covering the barrier material.

Cells that can help to grow new cementum, periodontal ligament, and alveolar bone produce these tissues in the surgical site. This requires that gingival tissue from the flap be kept free from the site in order for this growth to occur.

CHECKPOINTS

41-8 What is the surgical removal of diseased gingival tissue performed when periodontal pocket depth is too great and fibrous tissue is present?

41-9 What is the surgical reshaping and contouring of gingival tissues?

41-10 What procedure involves taking tissue from one area and replacing it where gingival tissue is missing?

Osseous Surgical Procedures

When periodontitis or another condition causes a defect in the alveolar bone supporting the teeth, osseous surgery may be necessary. Osseous surgery may involve reshaping, removing, or enhancing the bone to improve periodontal health.

Osteoplasty

An **osteoplasty** is a surgical procedure in which the alveolar bone is contoured and shaped; in some cases, additional bone or bone material is added through grafting. The procedure involves incising the soft tissue to expose the bone and shaping the bone with a bur or a bone chisel to eliminate periodontal pockets and restore normal contours in the bone.

Ostectomy

An **ostectomy** involves removing a portion of the alveolar bone. In this surgical procedure, bone is removed with a bur or a bone chisel to eliminate periodontal pockets and establish normal gingival contours.

Bone Grafting

Bone grafting involves adding bone or bone substitute to reverse bone loss associated with periodontal disease.

CHECKPOINT

41-11 Of osteoplasty and ostectomy, which one involves removal of bone?

Procedure 41-3 Assisting with Osseous Surgery

Materials needed (Figure P41-3-1):

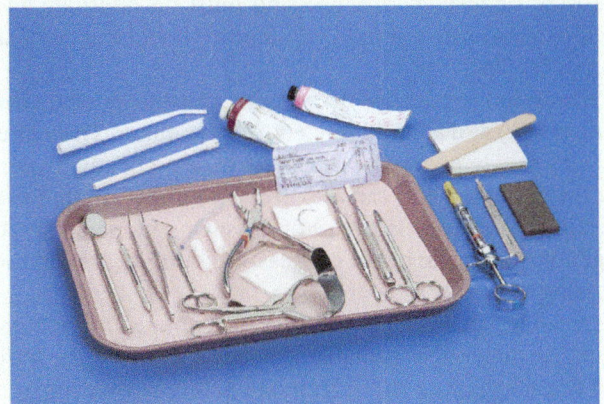

Figure P41-3-1

- Mouth mirror
- Explorer
- Cotton pliers
- Periodontal probe
- Cotton rolls and gauze sponges
- Sterile saline solution
- Saliva ejector
- HVE
- Air-water syringe tip
- Surgical aspirating tip
- Scalpel and blades
- Periodontal knives
- Tissue retractor
- Periosteal elevator
- Burs and stones
- Rongeurs, chisels, and files
- Scalers and curettes
- Scissors
- Suture materials
- Periodontal dressing materials
- Anesthesia supplies

1. Put on appropriate PPE.
2. The dentist administers anesthetic, and incises and retracts the patient's soft tissue.
3. Help maintain ease of visibility and access for the dentist.
4. The dentist removes or reshapes the bone (Figure P41-3-2A and B).

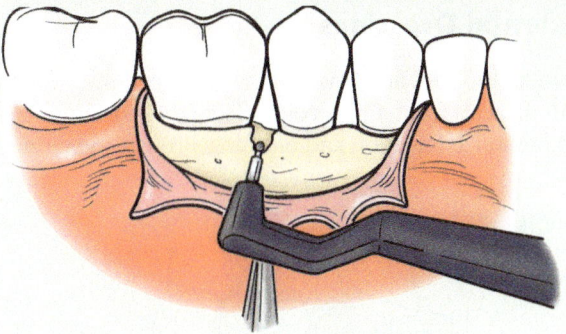

Figure P41-3-2A

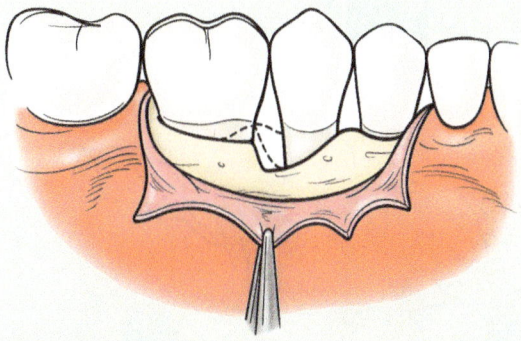

Figure P41-3-2B

5. The dentist removes calculus with scalers and curettes.
6. Throughout the process, rinse the patient's mouth as necessary and transfer instruments as needed for shaping and contouring.
7. Prepare the suture materials and pass them to the dentist (Figure P41-3-3).

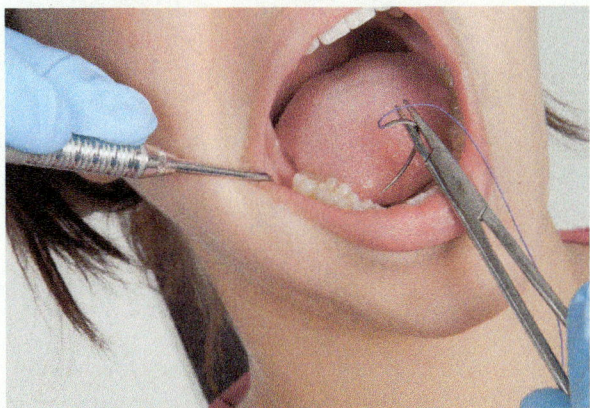

Figure P41-3-3

8. Prepare the periodontal dressing for placement.
9. Once the dressing is in place, gently clean the patient's face.
10. Document the procedure in the patient's record and provide the patient with self-care instructions.

Postsurgical Procedures

Periodontal Dressings

Periodontal dressings are bandages that protect tissues while the patient heals from a procedure (Figure 41-9). Dressings help to minimize infection and bleeding, protect the tissues

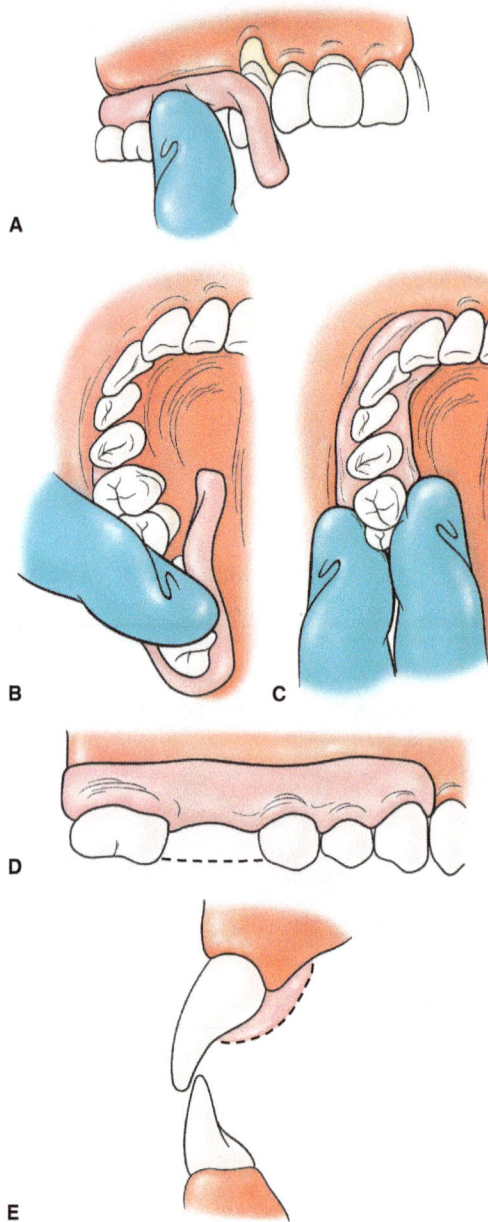

Figure 41–9 Periodontal dressing. (**A**) Dressing is pressed into interdental spaces with gentle finger pressure on the facial. (**B**) Dressing is looped around the most distal tooth and pressed into the interdental spaces on the palatal. (**C**) Gentle finger pressure is used to join the dressing on the facial and palatal aspects. (**D**) Dressing can be bridged across edentulous areas. (**E**) Dressing amount should be minimal to avoid contact of dressing with the teeth in the opposite arch.

during chewing, help to hold flaps in place, protect the surgical site from irritation, and help support teeth.

A dressing should adhere to the teeth and adjacent tissues and provide stability and flexibility without becoming distorted or displaced. A dressing must be nontoxic and nonirritating, and it should be smooth to resist accumulation of biofilm.

A zinc oxide eugenol dressing is available as a powder (zinc oxide) and a liquid (eugenol) to be mixed. This material sets slowly, giving the dental team some flexibility during the application. It can also be mixed ahead of time and stored for later use. Be aware of possible patient allergy to eugenol, which can cause redness and burning around the dressing.

Dressings that do not contain eugenol are more common. The material is available in tubes containing the base and the accelerator. These materials set more quickly.

Also available are light-cured and gelatin-based dressing materials. Light-cured dressing comes in syringes and can be placed directly on the surgical area, then shaped and cured. Gelatin-based dressings dissolve after 1 to 2 days.

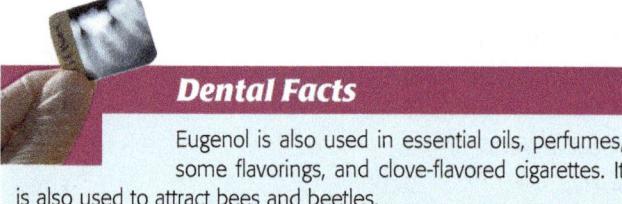

Dental Facts

Eugenol is also used in essential oils, perfumes, some flavorings, and clove-flavored cigarettes. It is also used to attract bees and beetles.

Patient Education

You have an important role in helping ensure that the patient understands and follows postsurgical instructions. Patients who receive thorough instruction in self-care are more likely to understand *why* the procedures should be followed, which makes them more likely to comply.

If a patient has a dressing following a surgical procedure, explain that the dressing protects the surgical wound and that it should remain in place until the next appointment. For the first few hours after it is placed, the dressing will be setting, or becoming hard, and should not be disturbed. That means the patient should not eat foods that require chewing, should drink only cool liquids, and should try to rest quietly. Some slight bleeding may occur during the first few hours. Until anesthesia wears off, the patient should also be careful to not bite his or her lips or cheeks. If pain persists after the anesthesia wears off, the patient should take any prescribed medication or use ice packs or cold compresses, if advised, to reduce swelling.

Advise the patient not to disturb the dressing or try to clean under it. Small pieces of the dressing may break off. If large pieces break off, the patient should contact the dentist. Not including the day the dressing is placed,

Procedure 41-4 **Preparing and Placing a Periodontal Dressing**

Some states allow qualified dental assistants to perform this procedure; in other states the dental assistant assists the dentist during the procedure. Check the regulations governing your state for more information about the specific duties dental assistants are allowed to perform with additional training.

Materials needed (Figure P41-4-1):

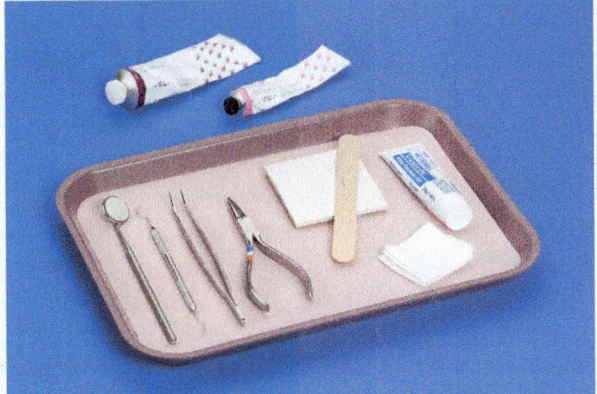

Figure P41-4-1

- Mouth mirror
- Explorer
- Cotton pliers
- Gauze sponges
- Dressing materials
- Paper pad
- Tongue blade
- Lubricant
- Contouring instrument

1. Put on appropriate PPE.
2. Apply a lubricant on the patient's lips.

3. Mix dressing materials in equal parts with a tongue blade on a paper pad until the material is no longer tacky.
4. Place lubricant on your gloved fingers for easier handling.
5. With your hands, mold the dressing into two thin strips a little longer than needed.
6. Mold a hook shape on one end of one strip, and wrap it around the distal surface of the most posterior tooth.
7. Then mold the strip on the facial surface, pressing the material into interproximal spaces. Apply the second strip in the same way on the lingual surface (Figure P41-4-2).

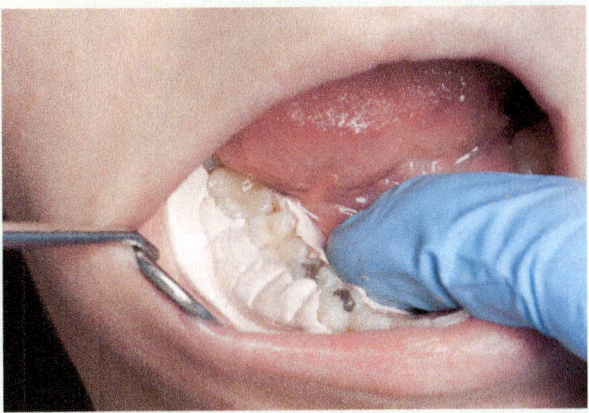

Figure P41-4-2

8. Join the strips at the distal surface of the last tooth at each end.
9. Ask the patient how the pack feels and make sure it does not interfere with occlusion, tongue movement, or frenum attachments.
10. Contour and trim any overextended areas of the dressing.
11. Document the procedure in the patient's record and provide the patient with self-care instructions.

Procedure 41-5 **Removing a Periodontal Dressing**

Some states allow qualified dental assistants to perform this procedure; in other states the dental assistant assists the dentist during the procedure. Check the regulations governing your state for more information about the specific duties dental assistants are allowed to perform with additional training.

Materials needed (Figure P41-5-1):

- Mouth mirror
- Explorer
- Cotton pliers
- Spoon excavator
- Suture scissors
- Floss
- Saliva ejector

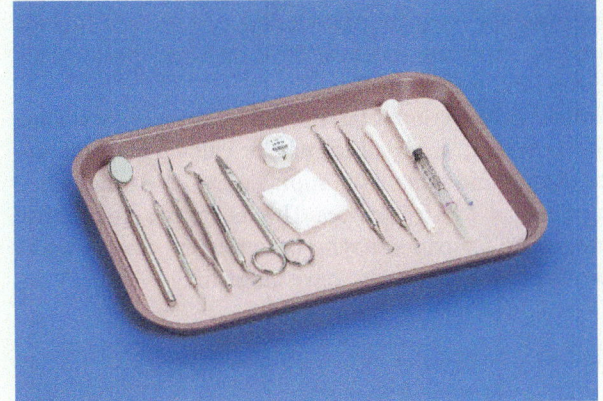

Figure P41-5-1

Procedure 41-5 Removing a Periodontal Dressing (Continued)

- Air-water syringe tip
- Gauze sponges
- Tissue
1. Put on appropriate PPE.
2. Use a spoon excavator to remove the dressing, taking care not to cause trauma to the surgical site (Figure P41-5-2).
3. If sutures have been used, cut the sutures with the suture scissors.
4. Gently remove the sutures.
5. Use scalers and floss to remove any stray particles.
6. Irrigate the area to remove any remaining debris.
7. Document the procedure in the patient's record and provide the patient with self-care instructions.

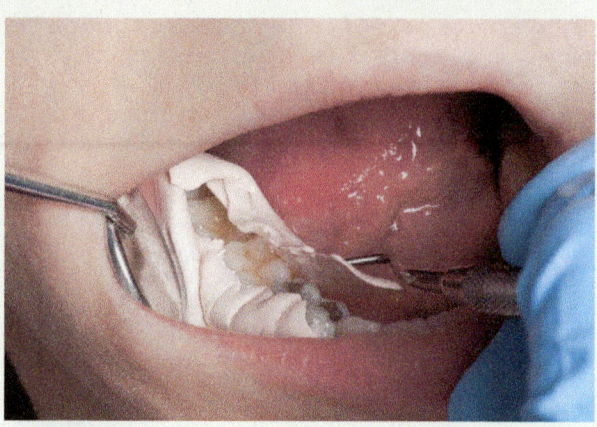

Figure P41-5-2

the patient should rinse with a saline solution twice a day after tooth brushing. Normal tooth brushing in non-treated areas should continue as well as light brushing of the dressing material surface with a soft brush and water.

A healthy diet will aid healing. The patient should avoid highly seasoned foods and spicy, hot, sticky, crunchy, and coarse foods. Too much chewing can hamper healing, so patients should avoid foods that require considerable chewing and should chew only on the untreated side of the mouth.

Smoking or using other tobacco products is never advisable but should especially be avoided after any periodontal procedure. Tobacco use delays healing, and the heat and smoke irritate the gingiva. If it is not realistic that a patient will cease all tobacco use, urge the patient to reduce use as much as possible until healing occurs.

CHECKPOINT
41-12 Which are more common—periodontal dressings that do or do not contain eugenol?

Chapter Highlights

- The two major categories of periodontal disease are gingivitis and periodontitis.
- During a periodontal exam, the dentist checks for plaque and calculus buildup, assesses gingival health and bone levels, and measures pocket depth.
- Instruments used in periodontal procedures include probes, explorers, scalers, files, curettes, periotomes, knives, and pocket markers.
- Nonsurgical periodontal procedures, such as scaling and polishing, are used to remove calculus, soft deposits, plaque, and stains from supragingival and unattached subgingival tooth surfaces. This is both a preventive procedure for patients who have healthy gingiva and a treatment for those who have gingivitis.

- When nonsurgical treatment fails, surgical periodontal procedures may be used. Surgical procedures include gingivectomy, gingivoplasty, periodontal flap surgery, and mucogingival surgery.
- When periodontitis causes a defect in the bone, osseous surgery may be necessary to reshape, enhance, or remove the bone.
- Periodontal dressings protect tissues while the patient heals from a procedure. Dressings help to minimize infection and bleeding, protect the tissues during chewing, help to hold flaps in place, protect the surgical site from irritation, and support teeth.

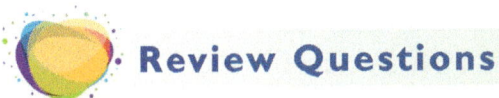

Review Questions

1. When performing periodontal probing, the dentist inserts the probe into the sulcus until what occurs?

   a. Bleeding

   b. Resistance

   c. A depth of 3 mm is indicated on the probe

   d. The patient expresses discomfort

2. Which type of scaler is used to remove heavy deposits from the buccal and lingual surfaces of posterior teeth?

   a. Hoe

   b. Kirkland

   c. Chisel

   d. Sickle

3. An ultrasonic scaler may be contraindicated for which of these patient groups?

   a. Pediatric patients

   b. Patients who have a cardiac pacemaker

   c. Patients who have difficulty swallowing

   d. All of the above

4. Which of the following is *not* a function of the curette?

   a. Measuring depth of periodontal pockets

   b. Removing subgingival calculus

   c. Smoothing root surfaces

   d. Removing soft tissue lining periodontal pockets

5. One benefit of using a laser in a procedure is

   a. Lower cost to the patient.

   b. Less training is required for dental office staff.

   c. Lasers are less expensive than traditional instruments.

   d. Reduced trauma to healthy tissue.

6. Which of the following procedures involves reshaping and contouring of gingival tissue?

   a. Ostectomy

   b. Osteoplasty

   c. Gingivoplasty

   d. Gingivectomy

7. A normal sulcus depth measures

   a. 3 mm or less.

   b. 4 mm.

   c. 5 mm.

   d. 6 mm or more.

8. Which of the following instruments is used to cut the periodontal ligament fibers?

   a. Periotome

   b. Pocket marker

   c. Gracey curette

   d. Orban knife

9. Which of the following is not an osseous surgical procedure?

   a. Osteoplasty

   b. Ostectomy

   c. Bone grafting

   d. Frenectomy

10. A periodontal dressing is used to

    a. Correct occlusal adjustment.

    b. Restore gingival health.

    c. Protect a surgical site from irritation.

    d. Minimize tooth decay.

Active Learning Exercises

1. There are two types of periodontal dressings: eugenol- and non–eugenol-based dressings. What are the differences between the two regarding mixing, manipulation, and storage of the materials?

2. Surgical procedures can be quite invasive. What are some important postoperative instructions the patient should be given after undergoing osseous surgery?

3. Lasers are being used more frequently for periodontal surgeries. What are some advantages of using the laser as opposed to a traditional scalpel? What could be some drawbacks to using a laser?

Application Activities

1. Create a detailed plan to educate patients about proper postsurgical self-care methods. Be sure to include information explaining why each step is necessary.

2. A patient is scheduled to come in for her first periodontal examination. Prepare a basic overview of the examination that you could use to explain to the patient what she should expect during the procedure.

PREPARING FOR CERTIFICATION EXAMS

Review the following topics in this chapter to prepare for the Dental Assisting National Board (DANB) exam:

- **Introduction**
- **Diagnostic Techniques**
- **Nonsurgical Periodontal Procedures**
- **Scaling and Polishing**
- **Postsurgical Procedures**
- **Periodontal Dressings**

chapter 42

Oral and Maxillofacial Surgery

CHAPTER OUTLINE

CHAPTER CHECKLIST

On completion of this chapter, students will be able to:

☑ Identify conditions that commonly require oral surgery.

☑ Identify the members of an oral surgery team and describe their responsibilities.

☑ Identify and describe the two common settings for oral surgery.

☑ Identify and describe the various instruments used in oral surgery.

☑ Explain the sterilization and infection control procedures used during oral surgery.

☑ Identify common surgical procedures and describe when each is appropriate.

☑ Understand the role of the dental assistant in providing support during common oral surgery procedures.

KEY TERMS

alveolitis (al-vee-oh-LIE-tis) – inflammation of a tooth socket

alveoplasty (al-vee-oh-PLAS-tee) – surgical preparation of the alveolar ridges for the reception of dentures; reshaping and smoothing of socket margins after extraction of teeth

crepitus (KREP-uh-tis) – the sound or sensation of grating or clicking

hemostat (HEE-moh-stat) – a locking, pliers-like instrument used during surgical procedures to hold tissue and objects

impacted tooth – a tooth that has been prevented from erupting normally

osseointegration (os-ee-oh-in-tuh-GRAY-shun) – apparent direct attachment or connection of osseous tissue to an inert alloplastic material without intervening connective tissue, as with dental implants

periosteal (per-ee-OS-tee-ul) elevator – a surgical instrument used to separate the attached periosteum from the underlying alveolar bone

retractor – an instrument for holding oral tissues away from the operating field or holding back structures adjacent to the operating field

surgical asepsis (a-SEP-sis) – procedures used to ensure a sterile environment in the operating area

tinnitus (TIN-ih-tus) – a ringing in the ears

Introduction

Oral and maxillofacial surgery involves the diagnosis and treatment of diseases and malformations that occur in the oral cavity, face, jaws, and neck. Oral and maxillofacial surgeons treat a wide array of conditions, including malformations, diseases, and injuries.

Although all dentists receive training in oral surgery in dental school, oral surgeons receive further training in specialized surgical techniques. Dentists generally refer to oral surgeons those patients who need surgical care that goes beyond their own experience or training.

Just as in dental offices, surgical dental assistants (DAs) are an important part of the oral surgeon's team. They help prepare patients, make the office run more efficiently, and assist the surgeon during procedures. In some states, expanded functions allow surgical DAs with additional training to take a more direct role in procedures.

Overview of Oral and Maxillofacial Surgery

Oral and maxillofacial surgeons are dentists who have received specialized training in oral surgery techniques. Their additional schooling includes training in pain management and anesthesia, oral and facial anatomy, and surgical techniques. Patients are typically referred to oral surgeons by dentists to deal with more complex cases or procedures that cannot be managed in the dental office.

Indications for Surgery

There is some overlap between dentists and oral surgeons. Some dentists perform complex procedures in their offices, whereas others are more likely to send patients to an oral surgeon.

Conditions that are routinely referred for oral surgery include:

- Tooth extraction for decayed, impacted, or nonvital teeth
- Ankylosis
- Surgery to contour and smooth the alveolar ridge before placing a prosthesis
- Procedures related to orthodontic treatment, including tooth extraction
- Cyst removal
- Tumor removal
- Removal of shattered roots or root fragments
- Surgical biopsies for suspected malignancies
- Treatment of trauma, such as fractures to the maxilla or mandible

- Cosmetic surgeries
- Surgery involving the temporomandibular joint
- Reconstructive oral surgery
- Surgeries for cleft lip and palate
- Surgeries on salivary glands
- Oral implants

In many cases, the oral surgeon is part of an overall treatment team. For example, correction of cleft palates and cleft lips might include oral surgeons, plastic surgeons, and rehabilitative specialists.

The Oral Surgical Team

The oral surgical team is similar to a dental team. The team consists of the lead operator, in this case the oral surgeon, as well as office support staff and DAs. The main difference is the addition of a nurse anesthetist or, if the surgeon's office is in a hospital or a busy practice, the services of an anesthesiologist.

Oral Surgeon

The oral and maxillofacial surgeon is the lead operator in surgical procedures. These professionals have finished dental school and received up to 6 years of additional training in surgical techniques. Oral surgeons are board certified by the American Board of Oral and Maxillofacial Surgeons. Many oral surgeons also go on to receive a medical license.

Oral surgeons can operate in their own offices, which are equipped with all the instruments needed to perform most oral surgeries. Some oral surgeons perform more complex or challenging oral surgery in local hospitals.

Surgical Dental Assistant

The surgical DA is a specialized DA who has received training in surgical techniques, oral anatomy, and surgical asepsis. Like an assistant in a dental office, surgical DAs also help with patient communication, record maintenance, and maintaining infection control procedures before, during, and after surgery.

Although exact roles vary from office to office, surgical DAs may perform any of the following tasks:

- Instrument transfer, which may include six-handed dentistry, using two DAs: one DA transfers instruments to the oral surgeon while the other acts as an assistant to the first assistant
- Patient monitoring and assessment, including monitoring vital signs before and during the surgery
- Sterilization of the treatment area and instruments
- Preparation of the treatment room, including maintaining infection control procedures
- Maintenance of surgical asepsis, which requires an advanced level of infection control to protect the patient and the operating team

- Stabilization and positioning of the patient
- Postoperative patient care, including assisting the patient during recovery and giving postsurgical instructions for wound care
- Suture removal, which is an expanded function and is allowed in some states after completion of additional training
- Exposing preoperative and postoperative radiographs when necessary

Training for surgical DAs can be obtained through schools that offer special courses.

Nurse Anesthetist or Anesthesiologist

One of the main differences between the office of a dentist and that of an oral surgeon is the presence of a professional to handle anesthesia. During oral surgery, different degrees of anesthesia are required, from local pain relief to general anesthesia that must be performed and continuously monitored by an anesthesiologist or nurse anesthetist.

The choice of nurse anesthetist or anesthesiologist depends on the procedure and the location. Nurse anesthetists often work in oral surgeon's offices, whereas anesthesiologists usually work in hospitals and are not part of the oral surgeon's staff but are hired on a per-case basis.

Administering and monitoring anesthesia are specialized skills that require constant attention to the patient's vital signs and training in anesthetic techniques and materials. It is very important that, prior to receiving anesthesia, patients clearly communicate any possible risks, including previous adverse reactions to anesthesia, allergies of any kind, and any additional medications or illicit drugs they might be taking.

Office Staff and Receptionist

As in a dental office, the oral surgeon's office is staffed by a receptionist to greet patients and office support personnel who handle the business aspects of the practice. This might include an office manager to run the office as well as other professionals who deal with insurance claims, request and process dental radiographs from referring offices, and manage the patient's files and records.

The Oral Surgical Setting

Oral surgery usually takes place in a private office or a hospital operating room. The choice of location depends on many factors, including the oral surgeon, the complexity of the surgery, and the available facilities. Neither setting is automatically preferable over the other, as long as the chosen facility has all the equipment and instruments required for a successful surgery.

Private Practices

Most oral surgeons operate from private practices that are equipped with the supplies and treatment areas necessary to complete most oral surgeries. These offices might resemble a dental office, with the addition of a surgical suite and recovery areas.

The surgical suite is similar to that in a hospital, although it is typically smaller and only equipped for oral surgeries. An oral surgeon's surgical suite is equipped with the treatment chair or table, instrumentation, patient monitoring equipment, pain control units, and mobile trays.

Oral surgery practices usually include a recovery area for patients recovering from anesthesia. These special areas are separate from the treatment room and may include a reclining chair or bed so the patient can relax and recover after the procedure. This is also where the surgical DA gives postoperative instructions and dispenses prescriptions for pain medicines and other medications.

Hospital Operating Room

For some cases, oral surgeons might work from operating rooms in local hospitals. These are usually more complicated cases that require the services of an anesthesiologist and, sometimes, access to equipment that is not available in the private office. To gain access to a hospital operating room, the oral surgeon has to be granted privileges from the hospital administration. Operating privileges are based on the surgeon's training, competency, and experience.

Operating rooms are typically larger than the surgical suite in private practices. They include overhead lighting, operating tables and mobile trays, patient monitoring equipment, anesthesiology equipment, and surgical equipment. Operating rooms are also large enough to allow standing room for multiple professionals, including surgeons, an anesthesiologist, and assistants.

CHECKPOINTS

42-1 Name some reasons a patient might be referred for oral surgery.

42-2 How is a surgical dental assistant different from a traditional dental assistant?

42-3 What is one major difference between oral surgery and dentistry?

42-4 When might an oral surgery take place in a hospital?

Oral Surgery Instruments

Oral surgeons work with specialized equipment. Surgical equipment is designed to cut away bone and tissue and perform many tasks involved with complicated oral surgeries, such as loosening and removing teeth from sockets. Surgical DAs must be familiar with all the instruments used in oral surgery. Assistants are often responsible for setting up the treatment room, including setting up the instrumentation trays for surgeries.

Oral surgery instruments are made from either stainless steel or disposable plastic. Stainless steel and plastic instruments are classified as critical instruments and must be sterilized between uses and packaged in sterile coverings that are opened only during the actual procedure. For more information on sterilization techniques, see Chapter 14, Disease and Infection Control.

Dental Facts

The basic instrumentation used in oral surgery has changed very little over the years. The first extraction instrument was called a "turn key" and looks very similar to a T-handled elevator today. Early examples can still be seen in the Smithsonian Institutes and the Dental Museum at the University of Maryland at Baltimore.

Mouth Props

Mouth props made from rubber, hard plastic, or silicone are used to keep the patient's mouth open during longer procedures or when patients are under anesthesia and cannot hold open their own mouths (Figure 42-1). They are inserted into the oral cavity on the opposite side of the planned procedure and slid into the appropriate position to hold the mouth open. Basic mouth props include bite blocks, which are made from rubber or plastic and inserted between the patient's jaws. Some devices are equipped with dental floss safety ligatures in case the device is accidentally aspirated.

One common type of mouth prop is known as the *Molt mouth gag*. This device features a hinged beak that is inserted into the patient's mouth in the closed position. When the operator gently squeezes the handle, the beak of the device opens, thus opening the patient's jaws. It can be locked into position for the duration of the procedure.

Retractors

Retractors are used to hold the patient's lips, tongue, and soft tissues out of the way during a procedure. Tissue damage during procedures delays recovery and poses a danger of infection. Retractors come in several forms, depending on their function (Figure 42-2):

- *Cheek retractors*. Cheek retractors are curved or shaped pieces of plastic or metal that are inserted in the patient's oral cavity and used to gently pull the patient's cheek away.
- *Tongue retractors*. Tongue retractors are made from metal or plastic and shaped like spoons or long blades. They are used to hold the tongue away from the operating site, usually by inserting the tongue retractor between the tongue and lingual surface of the tooth and gently pulling the tongue back and away.

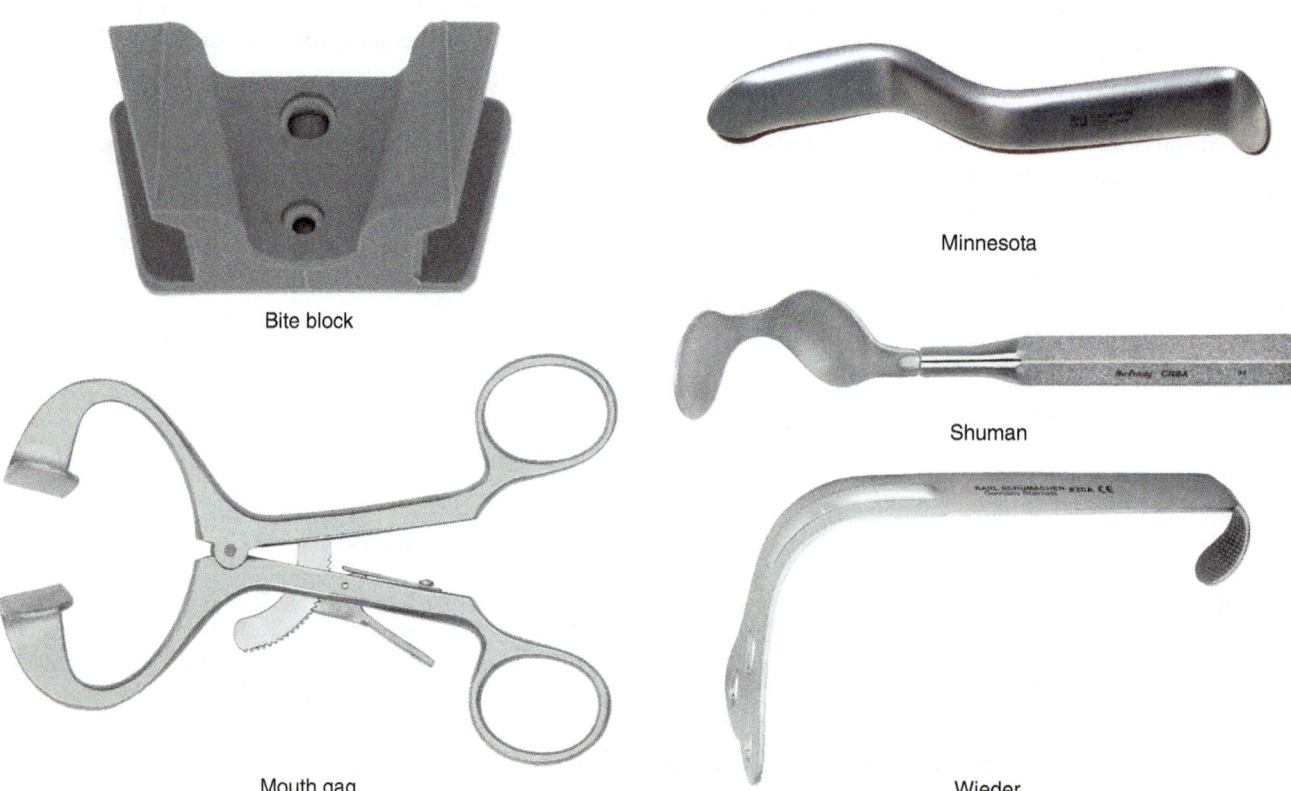

Bite block

Mouth gag

Minnesota

Shuman

Wieder

Figure 42–1 Mouth props.

Figure 42–2 Tongue and cheek retractors.

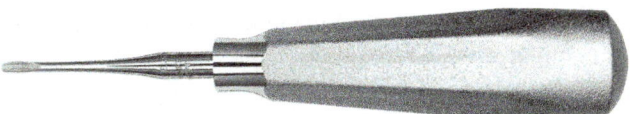

Figure 42–5 Straight elevator.

and the gingival tissue at the tooth cervix, then rocking gently to separate the tissue.

Straight Elevators

Straight elevators are used during extractions to loosen teeth from the periodontal ligament, as well as to remove teeth, roots, and root fragments. Elevators are available in a number of different configurations and styles, depending on the manufacturer (Figure 42-5). They are single-ended instruments that are designed so the oral surgeon can maintain a firm grip on the tooth and exert significant pressure during the extraction. Some of the common designs include:

- *Potts elevators*. Potts elevators feature a T-handle that provides a strong grip. Their working ends are angled.
- *Cryers elevators*. Cryers elevators have bulbous handles that fit into the palm. Their working ends are flat, angled blades. They are designated for the right or left side of the mouth.
- *Apical elevators*. Apical elevators are similar to straight elevators, but have an angled working end with a narrow blade that is useful for removing retained roots and root fragments.

Root Tip Picks

Root tip picks are a specialized type of elevator with a narrow, sharper working end that may be straight or angled (Figure 42-6). These instruments are used to remove retained root tips or root fragments. Root tip picks are usually paired left or right. They are not built to withstand the same pressures that are applied to larger elevators.

Forceps

Forceps are used to extract a tooth from its socket after the application of elevators to loosen the tooth. A variety of sizes and shapes are available, depending on the procedure and the operator's preference.

Like pliers, forceps are hinged instruments that end in a pair of beaks. The beaks may be smooth or serrated to grasp the tooth. Similarly, their handles might be situated

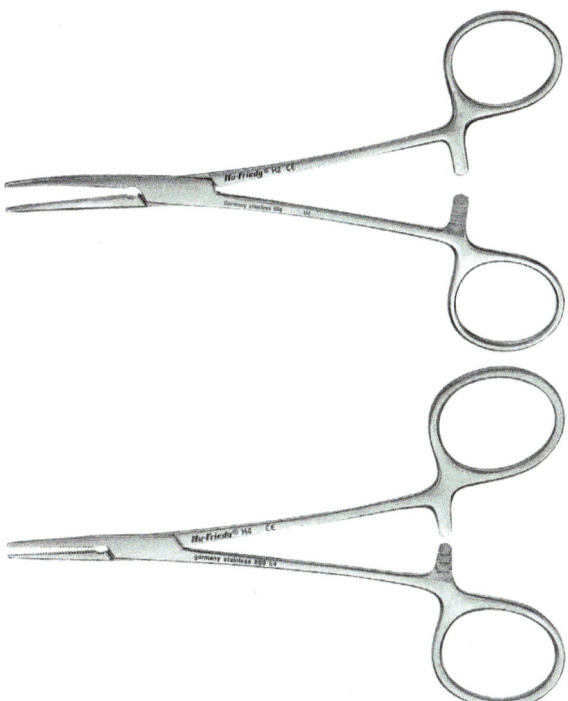

Figure 42–3 Hemostats.

- *Tissue retractors*. Tissue retractors are shaped like forceps or pliers. They are used to pull smaller pieces of tissue away from the operating field and usually have tiny teeth or gripping pads on their working ends.

Hemostats

Hemostats are all-purpose surgical instruments that are used to hold items, much like electrician's pliers (Figure 42-3). Hemostats can be used to grasp bone or tooth fragments and retract and remove tissue. They are also used to clamp off small blood vessels and feature a locking mechanism that can hold them in place once they are clamped shut. Hemostats do not have sharpened beaks but have long and narrow jaws with gentle serrations for improved holding power. Hemostats are available with both straight and curved ends.

Periosteal Elevators

Periosteal elevators are all-purpose instruments included on most oral surgery trays (Figure 42-4). These instruments are available in a variety of configurations, but most include either a long, flat blade or a rounded end. They can be single ended or double ended.

These instruments are most often used to separate the tooth from the gingival tissue prior to grasping the tooth with surgical forceps during an extraction. This is accomplished by working the flat blade between the tooth wall

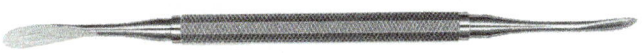

Figure 42–4 Periosteal elevator.

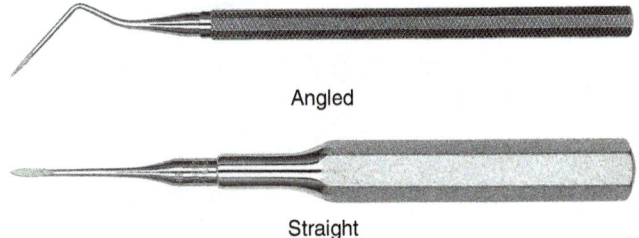

Angled

Straight

Figure 42–6 Root tip picks.

on a horizontal or vertical plane in relation to the beaks, depending on their function. Some forceps have finger rings or hooks on their handles to make them easier to grasp and hold during extractions.

Forceps are classified by which teeth they are designed to remove or where they are designed to operate in the mouth. One way to easily identify forceps is by their manufacturer's number and letter. Names often include an "R" or "L," for right or left. This indicates which side of the mouth they are used on. They are also labeled by number; for example, forceps #88L is designed for use on the left maxillary first and second molars. Some forceps also have descriptive names, such as the cowhorn forceps, which is used to extract the mandibular first and second molars. Some forceps are designed to be used in pedodontics; these tend to have shorter handles. These forceps are identified by an "S" after the designated forceps number.

Forceps can also be identified by how they are shaped. Depending on the orientation of the beaks and the handle, they may be intended for use in the:

- Right or left quadrant
- Maxillary and mandibular arches
- Anterior or posterior

If the beaks point upward, the forceps are designed to be used on the maxillary arch. If the beaks point toward the sides, they are designed to be used on the mandibular arch.

TABLE 42-1 Forceps	
NAME/NO.	USE
#222	Mandibular third molars
#15	Mandibular first and second molars
#23 (cow horns)	Mandibular first and second molars
#151	Mandibular incisors, cuspids, and roots
#210	Maxillary third molars
#88R/L	Maxillary first and second molars, right or left side
#53R/L	Maxillary first and second molars, right or left side
#150	Maxillary incisors, cuspids, bicuspids, and roots

If the beaks touch together, they are designed to be used on anterior teeth. If there is a space between the beaks, they are designed to be used on a posterior or larger tooth.

Universal forceps are designed for use in any quadrant. Refer to Table 42-1 and Figure 42-7 for a listing of specific forceps.

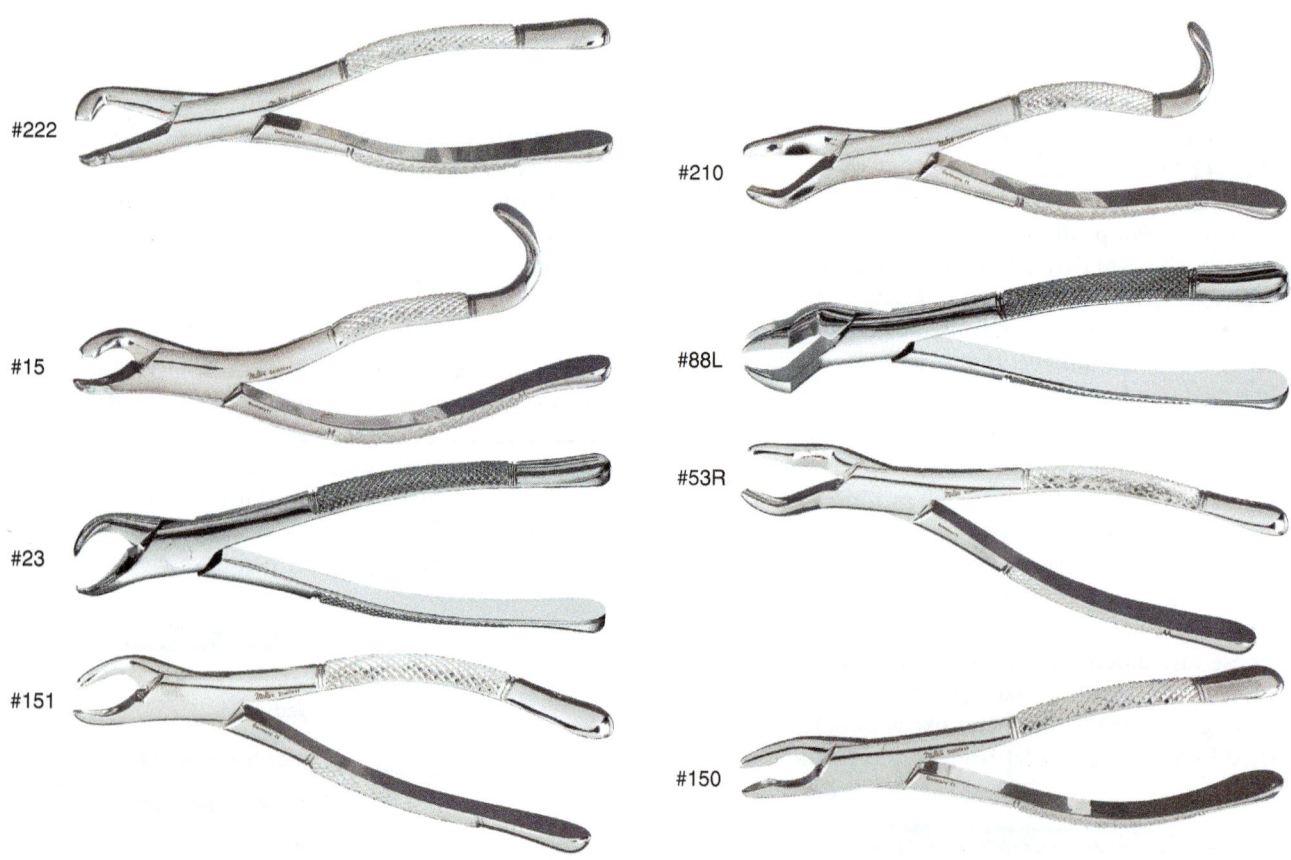

Figure 42–7 Forceps.

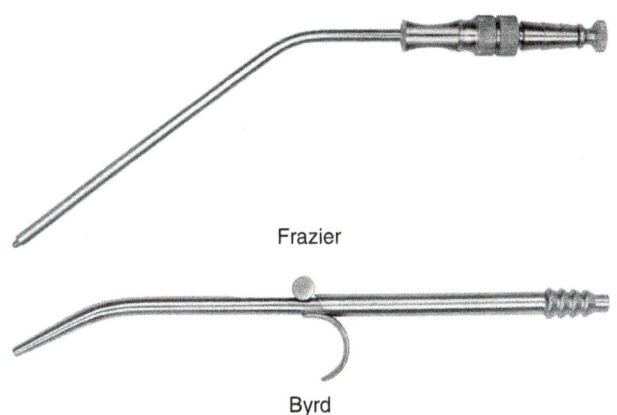

Frazier

Byrd

Figure 42–8 Aspirating tips.

Aspirating Tips

Aspirating tips are long, slender tubes that are used to remove blood and debris from a surgical site (Figure 42-8). They can be made of metal or plastic. Plastic aspirating tips are often disposable, whereas metal aspirating tips must be sterilized. Use of a surgical aspirating tip during oral surgery prevents an extracted tooth from being evacuated into the suction system. If this were to happen, the operator would not have the chance to review the extracted tooth to determine if all root structures were intact after removal.

Scalpels

Scalpels are surgical knives used to excise soft tissue. They are exceptionally sharp to cause the least amount of trauma to the patient and allow the surgeon maximum control when making an incision. Scalpels feature two components: the handle and the blade. Each is available in different styles and sizes (Figure 42-9). Handles are typically made from metal and are designed to be used with disposable blades. The most common handle style is the Bard Parker, which is a flat metal handle that features a metric ruler on the side. Disposable blades are available in various sizes, usually identified by number. Disposable plastic handles are also available; these can be used with disposable metal blades. All disposable scalpels must be discarded into a sharps container. As a general rule, when a scalpel is used, sutures will be required.

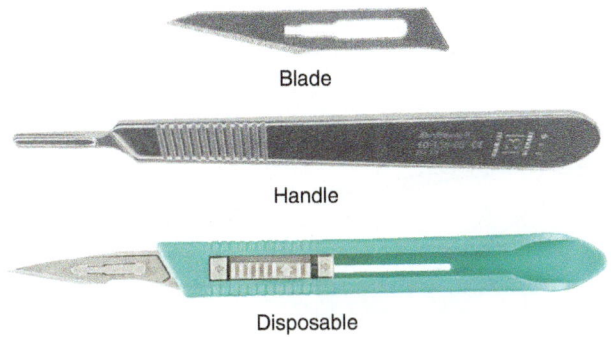

Blade

Handle

Disposable

Figure 42–9 Scalpels.

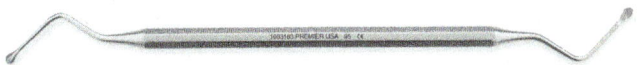

Figure 42–10 Curette.

Surgical Curettes

A surgical curette is a double-ended instrument with a curved or straight shank and spoon-shaped working end (Figure 42-10). They are used to débride and curette the interior of a tooth socket after an extraction to remove diseased tissue and abscesses.

Surgical Scissors

Surgical scissors are very sharp scissors used to cut soft tissues or remove sutures (Figure 42-11). They are made from metal and must be sterilized between uses. In order to maintain their cutting edge, surgical scissors should only be used for their intended purpose.

Rongeurs

Rongeurs somewhat resemble forceps, except they have sharp, cutting edges on the beaks and a spring in the handle, similar to nail clippers. The beaks may be side cutting or front cutting, depending on the design (Figure 42-12). Rongeurs are used during extractions to trim the alveolar bone or to trim away sharp points along the edentulous ridge. A simple extraction does not require the use of a rongeur, which is most commonly used during a multiple extraction procedure.

Bone Files

Bone files are used to smooth and shape the alveolar bone during an extraction, after the ridge has been roughly

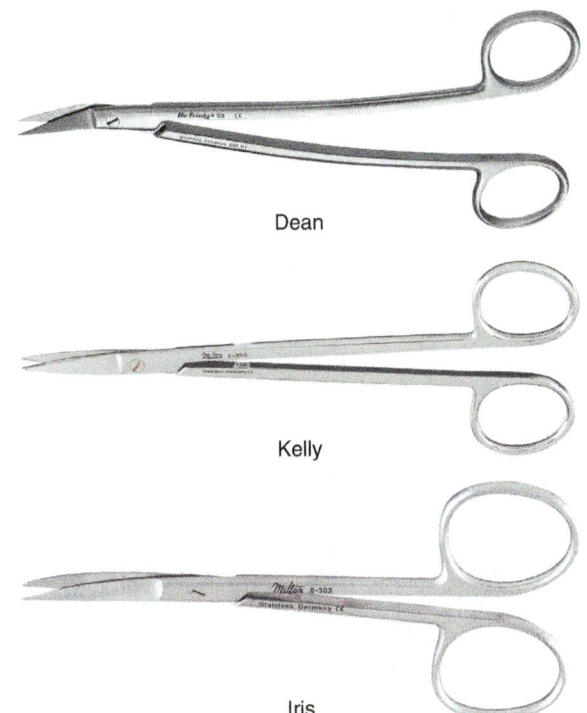

Dean

Kelly

Iris

Figure 42–11 Surgical scissors.

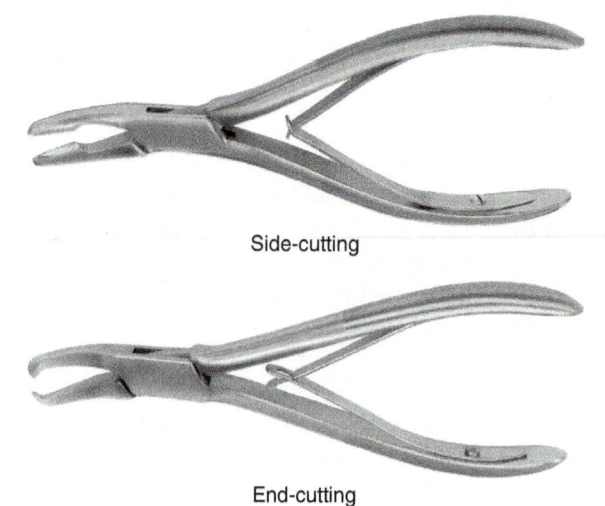

Side-cutting

End-cutting

Figure 42–12 Rongeurs.

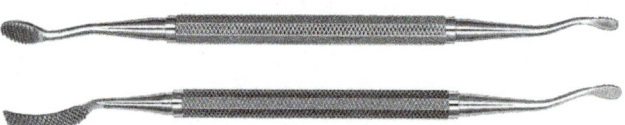

Figure 42–13 Bone files.

contoured with the rongeurs. They are available in a number of sizes, shapes, and roughness (Figure 42-13) and are used with a push-and-pull motion.

Surgical Handpiece

A surgical handpiece is a power instrument that is designed for use with surgical burs in oral surgery (Figure 42-14A).

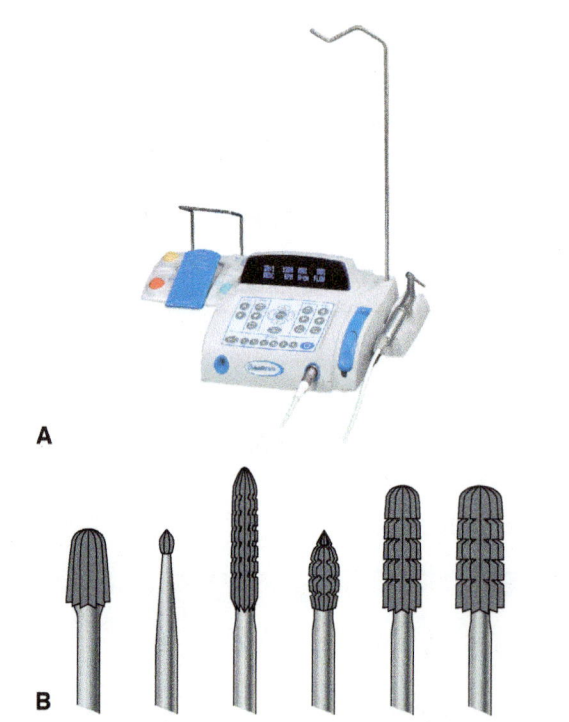

A

B

Figure 42–14 Surgical handpiece and burs. (A) Surgical handpiece. **(B)** Surgical burs.

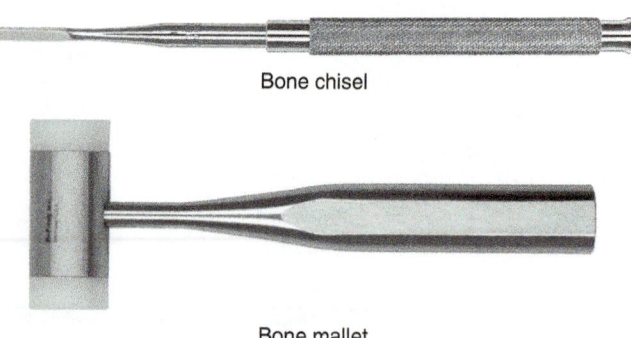

Bone chisel

Bone mallet

Figure 42–15 Bone chisel and mallet.

Like a dental handpiece, this device must be sterilized and prepared for use in a sterile surgical environment.

Surgical Burs

Surgical burs are used with surgical handpieces (Figure 42-14B). They are used during extractions to split crowns or roots, as well as remove pieces of bone.

Bone Chisels and Mallets

Bone chisels and mallets are hand instruments used to shape and contour, or remove, bone during extractions (Figure 42-15). Chisels can be single or double beveled. Single-beveled chisels are often used to shape or contour bone, whereas double-beveled mallets are used to break teeth into smaller pieces for easier extraction.

Chisels can be used by hand, but if the bone is hard or dense, the surgeon might require a mallet to apply extra force. To use a mallet, the head of the chisel is held in place, and the mallet is gently tapped against the chisel handle.

Needle Holders

Needle holders are used during suturing to hold the suture needle while sutures are placed. They are similar in shape and structure to hemostats, with grooved beaks that are either bent or straight and handles that lock into place during the procedure (Figure 42-16). One difference is that needle holders' beaks are shorter.

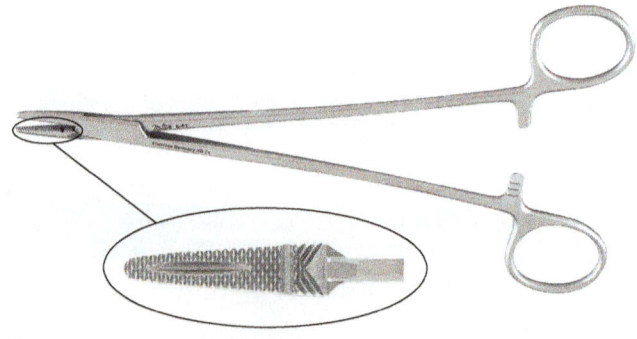

Figure 42–16 Needle holder.

Surgical Asepsis

Surgical asepsis refers to the procedures used to ensure a sterile environment in the operating area. Infection control is a critical part of all dentistry, but the need for stringent asepsis is heightened during oral surgery because of the direct exposure to bodily fluids and tissue during invasive procedures.

Surgical asepsis begins before the patient enters the office, with proper sterilization of surgical equipment and office personnel. The treatment area must also be prepared with barrier measures, such as draping and plastic covering. All of these measures reinforce and support one another—a breach anywhere in the chain of infection control results in potential contamination for any exposed instruments or people. If any breach occurs, new measures should be taken. Additionally, if a prepared treatment room is left alone for more than 1 hour before use, it should be considered contaminated and new infection control measures taken.

This section covers sterilization and infection control as they relate to oral surgery; for a broader, more detailed treatment of infection control concepts, see Chapter 14, Disease and Infection Control.

The Sterile Field

A sterile field is an area considered free of microorganisms, such as the area where surgical instruments are held during a surgery or the area around a patient who has been prepped for surgery. Equipment setups should only be brought into the surgical field in sterilized packages and opened immediately preceding the surgery (Procedure 42-1).

Handwashing is an essential part of any infection control program. In oral surgery, washing the hands and forearms before a procedure is known as "scrubbing in" (Procedure 42-2). This is essentially a more thorough form of handwashing that should be performed before surgical gloves are donned for the procedure. For more information on handwashing, including Centers for Disease Control and Prevention Guidelines on Hand Hygiene, see Chapter 14, Disease and Infection Control.

The use of gloves is mandatory in all oral surgeries (Procedure 42-3). The U.S. Food and Drug Administration identifies two types of treatment gloves: examination gloves (nonsterile) and surgical gloves (sterile). Only surgical gloves should be used. Surgical gloves are designed to fit either the right or left hand specifically. For more information on gloving, see Chapter 14, Disease and Infection Control.

Procedure 42-1 Preparing and Maintaining a Sterile Field for Instruments

Materials needed (Figure P42-1-1):

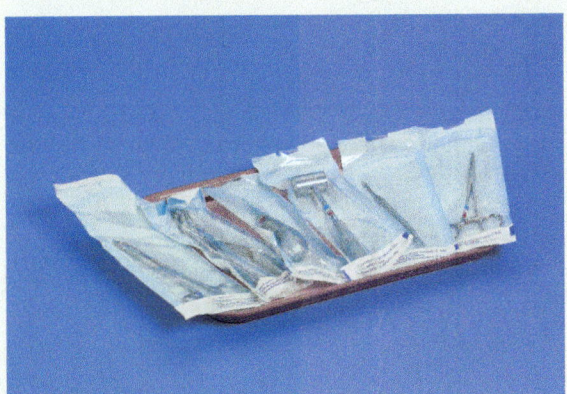

Figure P42-1-1

- Sterile surgical pack
- Mobile treatment tray

1. Handle setups only after hands are thoroughly washed and dried.
2. Place the wrapped, sterile surgical pack on the mobile tray, which has been positioned behind the patient chair in the treatment area.
3. Position the sterile packaging so the wrapping will open away from you.

4. Open the wrapping so the sterile field is facing upward (Figure P42-1-2).

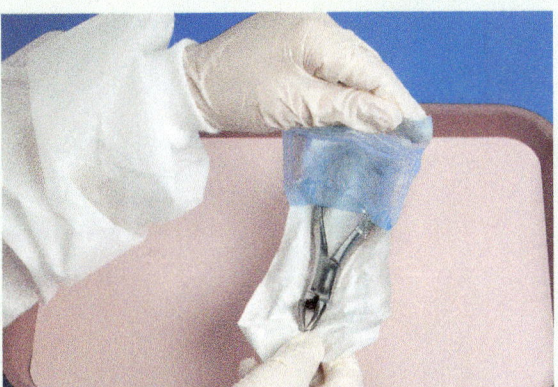

Figure P42-1-2

5. Using the wrapping, gently shake the contents of the package out onto the mobile tray. Do not touch the contents with your bare hands, but let them slide out while you handle only the wrapping paper.
6. Add any additional items to the mobile treatment tray, such as instrumentation and sutures.

Procedure 42-2 **Surgical Scrub**

The first surgical scrub of the day should be 10 minutes in length, and subsequent scrubs should be 3–5 minutes.

Materials needed:

- Orange stick
- Antimicrobial soap
- Sterile surgical brush
- Sterile towel
- Sterile operating gown

1. Make sure your eyes, face, and hair are covered with appropriate personal protective equipment (PPE) before performing a scrub to prevent contamination. Remove all jewelry.

2. Use an orange stick to scrub under your nails under running water (Figure P42-2-1). After you are done, discard the stick and rinse your hands. Do not touch any part of the sink or faucets with your hands.

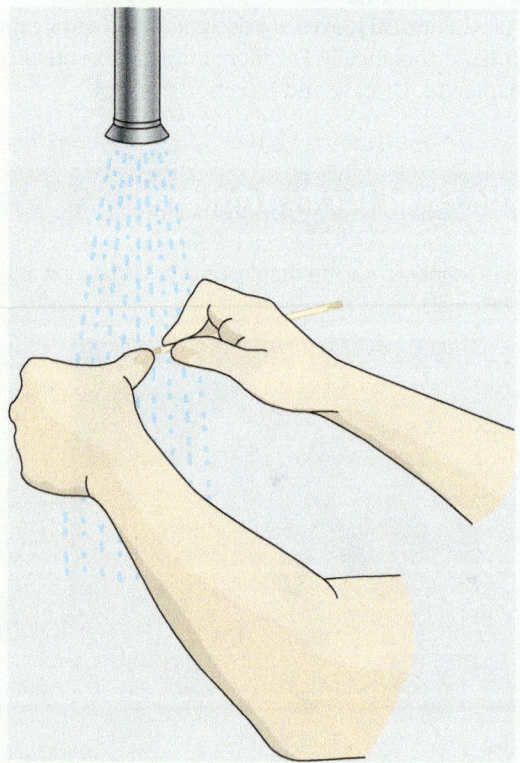

Figure P42-2-1

3. Moisten your hands and forearms up to your elbows in running water, then dispense a small amount (5 mL) of an approved antimicrobial soap into your hands. Lather vigorously with strong rubbing motions.

4. Scrub your hands and forearms with the sterile surgical brush for one-half of the allotted scrub time (5 minutes for the first scrub of the day and 1.5 to 2.5 minutes for each subsequent scrub) (Figure P42-2-2).

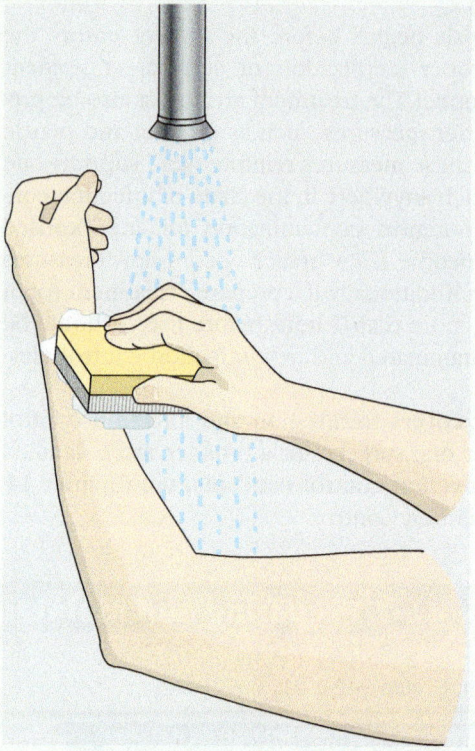

Figure P42-2-2

5. Rinse off the soap residue. When rinsing, hold your hands up so the water runs from your fingertips down to your elbows to prevent any possible contamination of your hands with dirty water.

6. Repeat the scrub with more soap and the surgical brush for the remaining time and rinse again.

7. Dry your hands with a sterile towel.

8. Hold your hands above waist level to don a sterile operating gown.

9. Proceed to gloving.

Procedure 42–3 Surgical Gloving

Materials needed (Figure P42-3-1):

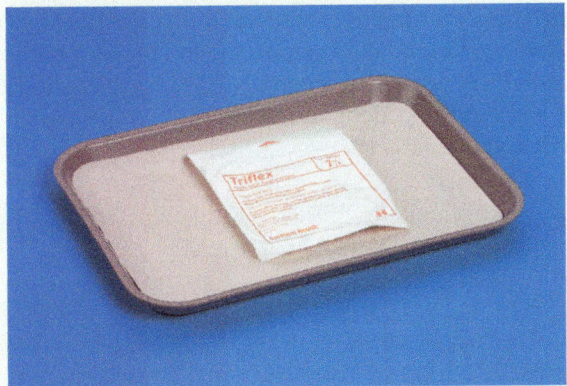

Figure P42-3-1

- Surgical gloves (package already opened)

1. Remove a glove from an open package of surgical gloves, touching only the cuff of the glove itself. Do not handle the container, which may be contaminated.

2. Glove your dominant hand by pulling the glove over your hand, touching only the folded cuff. You should come into direct contact only with material on the inside of the glove, not the outside. Unroll the cuff.

3. Using your gloved hand, pick up the sterile second glove, being careful to touch only the cuff of the second glove.

4. Slide the second glove over your nondominant hand and unroll the cuff.

Other Surgical Personal Protective Equipment

PPE is a standard part of maintaining asepsis during oral surgery. In addition to gloves, surgical PPE includes gowns, face masks, face shields, protective eyewear, and surgical hats. These items are designed to prevent both the patient and the wearer from contamination with bodily fluids by supplying a physical barrier. PPE should be worn in any surgical situation to protect the eyes, nasal passages, mouth, and any exposed skin. See Chapter 14, Disease and Infection Control, for a detailed discussion of the various types of PPE.

The Surgical Dental Assistant's Role

Surgical DAs have a wide range of roles in the oral surgery practice. Their involvement begins long before the patient sits in the treatment chair and ends well after the surgery is over. In some states with expanded functions dental assistant (EFDA) laws, surgical DAs with additional training are allowed to take an even more direct role in procedures, including suture removal and other necessary tasks. EFDA rules vary by state.

Voice of Experience

Oral surgery may seem routine to me, but it can be scary and unknown for patients, who often dread oral surgery as some kind of "worst-case visit" to the dentist. I try to remind myself when I'm dealing with nervous patients how I'd feel if I was parachuting from an airplane: I'd sure appreciate a little extra support from the group leader. Sometimes all it takes is a gentle, reassuring touch on the shoulder to really let patients know I'm there for them.

Before the Procedure

Surgical DAs are often responsible for much of the presurgery preparation. They may be asked to confirm that the patient's dental records and radiographs are available and current and follow up with the patient's dentist and physician to see if there are any concerns. Similarly, they may work with prosthetics labs and other vendors to make sure everything needed for the procedure is in place.

Finally, surgical DAs are typically responsible for the surgical tray set-up. The exact composition of the tray set-up depends on the procedure and operator, so it is essential to understand the nature of the surgery and the surgeon's preferences while assembling the set-up.

Immediately before the surgery, the DA prepares the treatment room to establish surgical asepsis. This includes placing barriers over equipment and making sure the surgical set-up is readily available, along with oxygen, pain control measures, and any emergency equipment that might be unique to the surgery. As noted previously, sterile surgical set-ups should not be opened until immediately before the surgery.

Surgical DAs also usually work directly with patients as they enter the office for their surgery. This means updating the medical history and obtaining new lab reports (if there are any) as well as following up on dietary and medication recommendations. Take care to ensure that the patient has followed preoperative instructions to reduce the risk of complications.

Just before the surgery is to begin, the surgical DA helps the patient into the treatment chair, takes vital signs, and drapes the patient in preparation for anesthesia.

During the Procedure

The role of the surgical DA during surgery depends on the individual's training and whether the state allows EFDA roles. DAs may be called upon to help administer local anesthetic, nitrous oxide, and intravenous medications.

Once the surgery is underway, the DA helps with instrument transfer, retraction, and moisture control. During complex surgeries, two or more assistants might be required. Surgical DAs may also be expected to monitor the patient's vital signs, including heart rate and the amount of oxygen in the blood.

Finally, assistants are sometimes called upon to stabilize and hold the patient during surgeries, including holding the patient's head or mandible if necessary.

From the Dentist's Perspective

Experienced dental surgical assistants are crucial to my success. In complicated cases, it's not unusual to have three assistants in the treatment area during the surgery: one transfers instruments, one assists with suctioning and keeping a clear operating field, and one monitors vital signs and secures the patient's head. When every member of the team works well together, we can provide excellent patient care and achieve great results.

After the Surgery

Surgical DAs typically remain with a patient while the patient recovers from anesthesia and becomes able to leave the treatment area or office. Many offices have recovery rooms for this purpose, and a surgical DA might sit with the patient in the recovery room.

During this time, the assistant gives postoperative care and medication instructions, based on the surgeon's recommendations. It is important to clearly explain issues like medication schedules and wound care. The assistant also updates the patient's medical record with a record of the surgery and any prescriptions, and then schedules any necessary follow-up visits.

Finally, the assistant breaks down the treatment room, disposes of any waste, and begins the sterilization procedures for instruments used in the surgery.

CHECKPOINTS

42-5 Describe uses for the following instruments: elevators and root tip picks.

42-6 How are forceps classified?

42-7 What are rongeurs used for?

42-8 How long can you leave an open surgical packet unattended before it can no longer be considered sterile?

Surgical Procedures

Surgical DAs help with a wide range of procedures. Although the oral surgeon is ultimately responsible for the procedure's outcome, it is important for the assistant to understand the procedure in order to explain the surgery and its goals to the patient and to anticipate the surgeon's needs during the surgery.

Extra Patient Care

When patients show up for their surgery, they are often nervous and may be distracted. After the surgery is over, they might still be feeling the effects of anesthesia and dealing with uncomfortable bandages and gauze pads in the mouth. Naturally, you can understand why they might not catch all of your pre- and postoperative instructions. But these instructions are very important, so it is a good idea to print out the patients' instructions and hand them the sheet. Later, when they are calm and clear-headed, they will appreciate it!

Simple Tooth Extraction

Simple, or routine, tooth extraction involves removing primary or permanent teeth that have erupted into the oral cavity. These procedures require forceps to firmly grasp the tooth to be removed and additional instrumentation. Although sutures are often not required, this is a surgery. See Procedure 42-4 for the steps involved in assisting with a simple tooth extraction.

Alveoplasty

An **alveoplasty** is performed in conjunction with multiple tooth extractions. Although the process is the same for single or multiple extractions, the end result is different. Multiple extractions are typically performed when the patient requires implants or a partial or full denture. After the extractions, the alveolar ridge must be contoured and smoothed to accommodate the new appliance. Thus, this procedure is called an *alveoplasty*.

Procedure 42-5 outlines the steps involved in assisting with an alveoplasty.

Check Your Ethics

During the course of an oral surgery, a patient under general anesthesia mumbles a potentially embarrassing personal detail—a fairly common occurrence when people are under anesthesia. Later, the patient asks if she said anything unusual under anesthesia. What should you do?

Procedure 42–4 **Simple Tooth Extraction**

Materials needed (Figure P42-4-1):

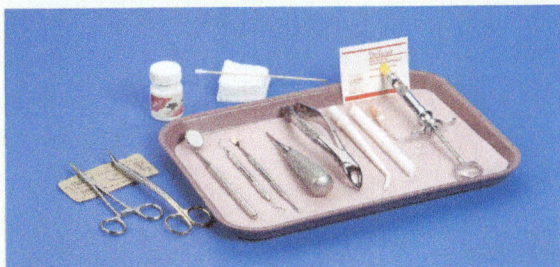

Figure P42-4-1

- Anesthetic supplies
- Mouth mirror
- Explorer
- Periosteal elevator
- Straight elevator
- Forceps
- Surgical curette
- Retraction instrument
- Sterile gauze pad
- High-volume evacuator (HVE)
- Surgical aspirator tip
- Suture supplies

1. Put on appropriate PPE.
2. Prepare the patient for the surgery and for administration of a local anesthetic. During this step, the surgeon examines the patient with a mouth mirror and explorer, then applies a topical anesthetic, followed by the injection of a local anesthetic (Figure P42-4-2).

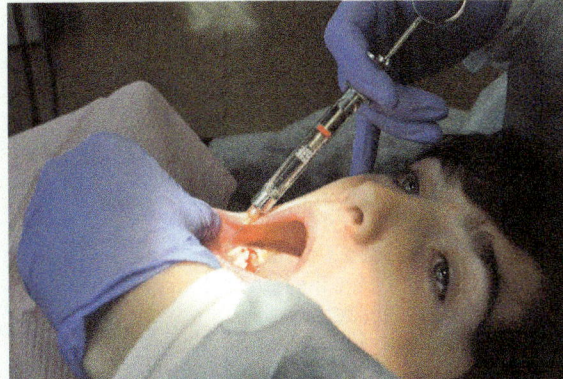

Figure P42-4-2

3. Transfer the elevator to the surgeon, who loosens the gingival tissue around the tooth cervix. During the loosening, the assistant should be ready with gauze to remove blood and debris from the instruments and make sure the light is adjusted. Use the HVE and sterile water to keep the operating field clean and free of blood and debris.
4. Transfer the forceps to the surgeon, who firmly grasps the tooth and luxates it, moving it in the socket to loosen it in the

alveolar bone (Figure P42-4-3). If the tooth does not easily slide from the socket, the surgeon might require the elevator again, followed by another round with the forceps. These instruments should be ready for transfer until the tooth is removed. You may also assist with tissue retraction.

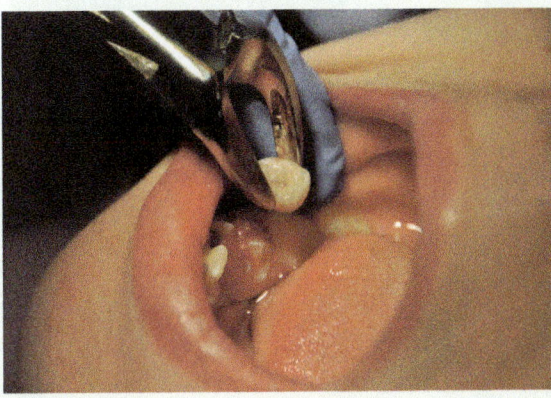

Figure P42-4-3

5. After the tooth is removed, the surgeon examines it for fractured roots. Aspirator tips are used to débride and clean the empty tooth socket of debris, granulated tissue, and cysts.
6. Fold several pieces of gauze to make a firm pad and place it in the empty socket to stop bleeding (Figure P42-4-4). Instruct the patient to gently bite down on the gauze.

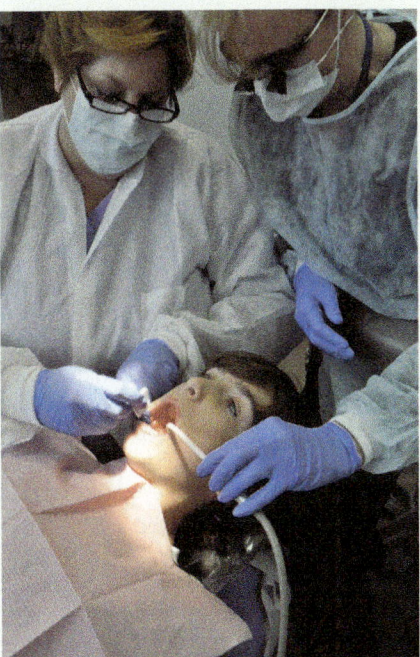

Figure P42-4-4

7. If sutures are necessary, the surgeon places them after bleeding subsides.
8. Return the patient to a sitting position and prepare for recovery. Document the procedure in the patient's record and provide the patient with self-care instructions.

Procedure 42–5 Assisting with Multiple Extractions and Alveoplasty

Materials needed (Figure P42-5-1):

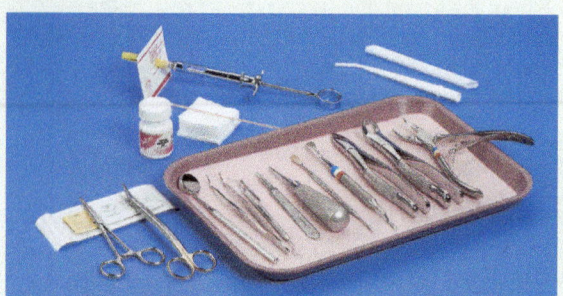

Figure P42-5-1

- Anesthetic supplies
- Mouth mirror
- Explorer
- Periosteal and straight elevators
- Forceps
- Surgical curette
- Scalpel
- Rongeurs
- Surgical chisel and mallet
- Scalpel and blade
- Surgical bur
- Bone file
- Mouth and cheek retractors
- Mouth prop
- Hemostat
- Aspirating syringe and sterile saline
- Surgical suction tip
- Surgical aspirator tip
- Sterile gauze pad or sponges
- Plastic stent (if needed)
- Suture supplies

1. Put on appropriate PPE.
2. Prepare the patient for the surgery and for administration of anesthetic. During this step, the surgeon examines the patient with a mouth mirror and explorer. The surgeon then introduces an intravenous line and administers the general anesthetic until the proper sedation is achieved.
3. Transfer the elevator to the surgeon, who loosens the gingival tissue around the tooth cervix. During the loosening, the assistant should be ready with gauze to remove blood and debris from the instruments and make sure the light is adjusted. Use the HVE and sterile water to keep the operating field clean and free of blood and debris.
4. Transfer the forceps to the surgeon, who firmly grasps the tooth and luxates it, moving it in the socket to loosen it in the alveolar bone (Figure P42-5-2). If the tooth does not easily slide from the socket, the surgeon might require the elevator again, followed by another round with the forceps. These instruments should be ready for transfer until the tooth is removed. You may also assist with tissue retraction.

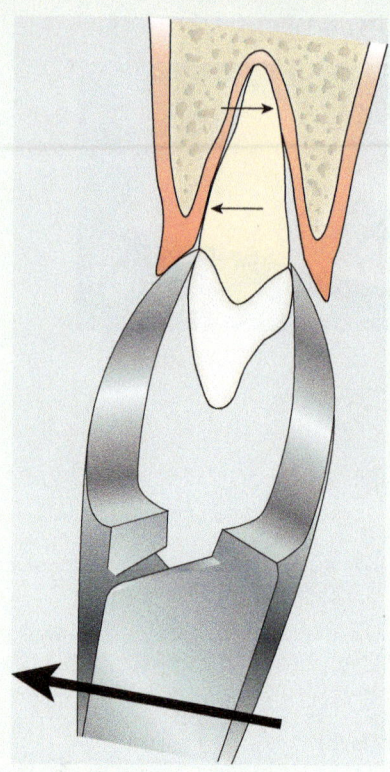

Figure P42-5-2

5. Repeat steps 3 and 4 until all necessary teeth have been removed.
6. After the extractions, transfer the scalpel to the surgeon. The surgeon makes an incision through the gingival tissue on the lingual and buccal sides and retracts the tissue with the periosteal elevator to expose the alveolar bone. During this procedure, keep the area free from debris and blood. Additionally, you may be called upon to retract the tissue with forceps.
7. Transfer the rongeurs and/or surgical bur to the surgeon for contouring the alveolar ridge. During the contouring process, use sterile gauze, the HVE, and sterile water to keep the operating field clean and free of blood and debris.
8. After the bone has been contoured, transfer the bone file. The surgeon uses this to make the alveolar ridge conform to the shape of the appliance. If a denture is to be placed, the surgeon uses a plastic stent, or a clear plastic model of the denture, to make sure the bone is correctly shaped. This might involve several attempts to fit the stent, so keep the stent clean between filing.
9. Once the surgeon is satisfied with the alveolar ridge, the tissue flaps are put back in place and sutured. The surgeon then sutures the multiple extraction sites closed.
10. Prepare a sterile gauze packet or sponges to be placed over the surgical wound immediately after the sutures are completed.
11. Return the patient to a sitting position and prepare for recovery. Document the procedure in the patient's record, provide postoperative instructions, and schedule follow-up visits. Be sure to give clear instructions about pain medications and oral care.

Extraction of Impacted Teeth

Impacted teeth are those that have not yet erupted. These types of extractions are known as *complex extractions*, as opposed to *simple extractions*, because they require additional skills. Impacted teeth may be impacted in the soft tissue (a *soft tissue impaction*) or in the bone (a *hard tissue impaction*). The exact approach to the extraction, and the instruments required, depend on each unique case. Many factors can influence an impacted tooth extraction, such as tooth direction, whether it is a hard or soft impaction, surrounding structures, depth of the impacted tooth, and others.

The most common impacted teeth to be removed are the third molars, which patients sometimes call the *wisdom teeth*. Third-molar extractions can be performed in one or multiple appointments. For steps on assisting with an impacted tooth extraction, see Procedure 42-6.

Procedure 42-6 Assisting with Extraction of Impacted Teeth

Materials needed (Figure P42-6-1):

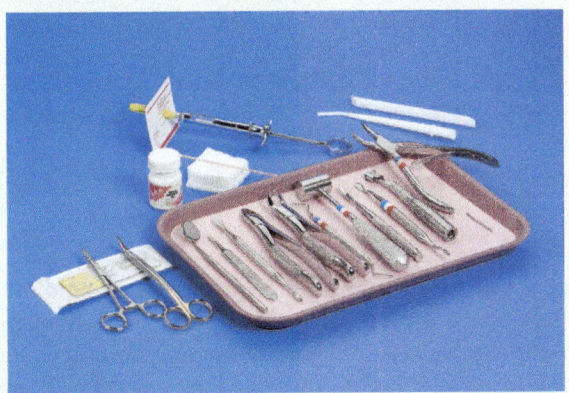

Figure P42-6-1

- Anesthetic supplies
- Mouth mirror
- Scalpel
- Periosteal elevator
- Forceps
- Curettes
- Rongeurs
- Bone file
- Suture supplies
- Sterile gauze pad
- High-volume evacuator (HVE)
- Surgical chisel and mallet or low-speed handpiece and surgical bur

1. Put on appropriate PPE.
2. Assist the surgeon with anesthesia. The choice of general anesthesia or local anesthesia depends on the case, the surgeon's preference, and the patient's preference.
3. Transfer the scalpel to the surgeon for the first incision. This incision is made through the gingival tissue and periosteum along the alveolar ridge (Figure P42-6-2). During this incision, use the HVE to keep the field clear of blood and debris.

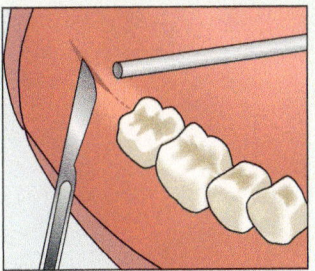

Figure P42-6-2

4. Transfer the periosteal elevator to the surgeon for tissue retraction from the alveolar bone (Figure P42-6-3). After the tissue is retracted, keep the tissue flap retracted and maintain a field clear of debris, blood, and saliva.

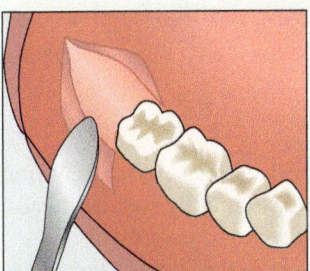

Figure P42-6-3

5. Transfer a surgical chisel and mallet or low-speed handpiece and surgical bur to the surgeon to break up the tooth. As the tooth is exposed and prepared for extraction, continue to evacuate and maintain a clear field (Figure P42-6-4). In some cases, nearby teeth might have to be sectioned to gain access to the impacted tooth.

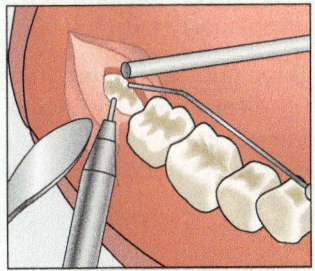

Figure P42-6-4

Procedure 42-6 Assisting with Extraction of Impacted Teeth (Continued)

6. Transfer the forceps or elevators for the extraction of the tooth or tooth pieces (Figure P42-6-5). As the surgeon removes the tooth or tooth pieces, they are placed on a tray and examined to ensure that all tooth fragments have been removed.

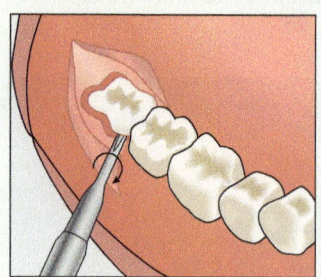

Figure P42-6-5

7. After the tooth is completely removed, curettes are used to remove the tooth follicle. The surgeon may also require rongeurs or the bone file to contour the bone socket. Afterward, the socket is débrided and then irrigated with sterile water and evacuated to ensure it is completely free of fragments.

8. Once the socket is free of any possible infectious agents, the tissue flap is replaced and the surgeon places sutures. During this process, you can assist by placing the sutures in the needle holder and retracting the cheeks.

9. When suturing is complete, return the patient to a sitting position and prepare for recovery. Provide the patient with gauze and ice packs as well as postoperative instructions for wound care and pain control. Document the procedure in the patient's record. Schedule an appointment for suture removal, if necessary. When the patient is ready to leave, assist him or her to their escort.

CHECKPOINTS

42-9 Give an example of a simple extraction.

42-10 Give an example of a complex extraction.

Dental Implants

Dental implants are used to replace missing teeth. When placed correctly, dental implants are highly successful and provide both function and aesthetics to patients.

During dental implant surgery, the native teeth are removed and a titanium screw or frame is implanted into the bone. Through a process known as **osseointegration**, the titanium fuses with the bone over time and provides a stable base for prosthesis. Implants can be fashioned for fixed or removable prosthetics, depending on the situation. They can be used with crowns, bridges, full dentures, or partial dentures.

Implant surgery is generally very successful, although a number of factors might cause implants to fail, including:

- The load on the prosthetic is too great. Implants with a great deal of pressure, such as those in posterior teeth, are more likely to fail than anterior implants.
- The implant does not integrate with the bone (lack of osseointegration).
- The site becomes infected.
- The implant breaks or fractures.
- The mandible is damaged during implant surgery.
- The maxillary sinus or nasal cavity is damaged during surgery.

Despite these risks, however, implant surgery is commonly a very attractive option for patients who are committed to the process, understand and follow the directions, and seek a long-term solution. In some cases, if there is not enough bone to place an implant, bone grafting may be necessary before the implant is placed.

Types of Implants

Subperiosteal and endosteal implants are the most common types of implants. A third type, the mini-implant, is becoming increasingly popular. A fourth type, the transosteal implant, is available but used only rarely in extreme cases involving severe resorption of the mandibular ridge. For a complete discussion of dental implants, see Chapter 38, Fixed Prosthodontics, and Chapter 39, Removable Prosthodontics.

Phases of Treatment

Dental implants can be placed in either one or two surgeries, depending on the implant, the patient, and the surgeon's recommendation. After the surgeries are completed, the restoration is finished with the prosthesis. Successful implant surgery requires a team of oral professionals, including a dentist (who typically refers the patient to an oral surgeon); the oral surgeon; and, frequently, a periodontist.

The surgical phase may include:

- One surgery. In the single-surgery approach, the implants are placed into the bone during the surgery and the rods or abutments extend through the gingival tissue. The abutments are capped after the surgery with healing caps, and the prosthesis is not placed. As a result, there is no load on the implants during the healing and integration process, which can take from 3 to 6 months.

- Two surgeries. In the two-surgery approach, the tissue is opened during the first surgery and the implant is placed. However, the abutment or rods do not extend through the gingival tissue, which is sutured back into place after the surgery is completed. After 3 to 6 months healing and integration time, the patient is scheduled for another surgery. During the second surgery, the tissue is opened back up and the surgeon checks the stability of the implants. If they are stable, then abutments or rods are placed that extend through the gingival tissue and are used to support the prosthesis. Temporary dentures can be worn during the interval.

After the surgeries are performed and the caps or abutments are placed, the patient is ready for the prosthetic phase. During this phase, impressions for the prosthesis are taken; the prosthesis is fabricated; and, finally, the prosthesis is placed.

Postoperative care and instructions are essential for successful implant surgery.

Procedure 42–7 Assisting with Dental Implant Surgery

This procedure describes the two-surgery procedure (Figure P42-7-1). The one-procedure surgery is similar, without the follow-up surgery.

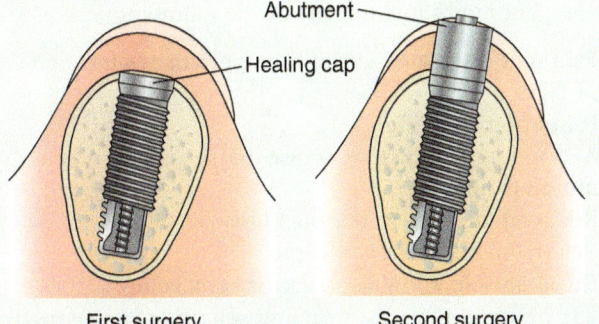

First surgery   Second surgery

Figure P42-7-1

Materials needed:

- Anesthetic supplies
- Surgical template (stent)
- Scalpel
- High-volume evacuator (HVE)
- Periosteal elevator
- Spiral burs
- Implant with healing caps
- Mallet or ratchet wrench
- Electrosurgical loop
- Contra-angle screwdriver
- Sterile saline solution
- Hydrogen peroxide
- Sterile cotton pellet
- Sterile gauze pad

1. Put on appropriate PPE.
2. Prepare the patient for the surgery and assist the surgeon with anesthesia.
3. Assist with placement of the surgical template (stent) in the patient's oral cavity. The tissue is marked through the template.
4. Transfer the scalpel to the surgeon, who makes an incision into the soft tissue and exposes the ridge of bone. During incisions, transfer the scalpel and keep the operating field clear of blood.
5. Transfer a periosteal elevator, which is used to separate the tissues and fully expose the bone.
6. Transfer spiral burs as necessary while the surgeon prepares to place the implant. Several burs might be necessary to obtain the correct size. During this process, irrigate the surgical site with sterile saline solution.
7. The surgeon places the implant. During placement, transfer both the implant and the mallet or ratchet wrench to the surgeon.
8. Once the implant is placed, transfer the healing cap and a contra-angle screwdriver. The healing cap is left exposed in the mouth.
9. Return the patient to a sitting position and prepare for recovery. Document the procedure in the patient's record and provide the patient with postoperative instructions.

Second Surgery

1. Put on appropriate PPE.
2. Prepare the patient for the surgery and assist the surgeon with anesthesia.
3. Assist with the placement of the template over the implants. The tissue is marked where the implants are located under the tissue.
4. Remove the template and assist the surgeon as the tissue is excised with an electrosurgical loop to expose the healing cap. During excision, maintain the surgical field.
5. Prepare to receive the healing caps in a gauze pad after they are removed.
6. Clean the inside of the implant with hydrogen peroxide on a sterile cotton pellet. Transfer the cotton pellet to the surgeon.
7. Transfer the implant to the surgeon, who places it so it protrudes slightly from the mucosa.
8. Prepare sutures and transfer to the surgeon so the gingiva can be sutured around the implant.
9. Return the patient to a sitting position and prepare for recovery. Document the procedure in the patient's record and provide the patient with postoperative instructions.

Biopsy Procedures

A biopsy is a procedure for removing a tissue sample for diagnostic purposes. Biopsy tissue samples are examined to detect a malignant (cancerous) or benign (noncancerous) growth. Three forms of biopsy are used most often in oral surgery: incisional, excisional, and exfoliative.

Incisional Biopsy

An incisional biopsy occurs when the surgeon removes a small slice of tissue from a relatively large lesion. Incisional biopsies are performed only on lesions that are at least 1 cm in size and are located in areas where removal might affect functionality or aesthetics. This slice of tissue is compared to a sample of normal tissue. If the tissue is malignant, then treatment may include complete surgical removal of the lesion, chemotherapy, and radiation therapy.

Excisional Biopsy

An excisional biopsy is one in which the surgeon completely removes the suspected lesion, along with some normal tissue for comparison. Excisional biopsies are performed for lesions that are smaller than 1 cm and not located in areas that would affect functionality or aesthetics. The tissue is examined after removal to detect malignancies.

Exfoliative Biopsy

An exfoliative biopsy is an alternative to excisional biopsies. In this procedure, a sample of cells is obtained from a suspected lesion. This sample can be obtained with a brush, which is rubbed against the lesion, or with other instruments. Once the cells are collected, they are examined by a pathologist to detect malignancies. This form of biopsy is just as effective for certain kinds of lesions as an excisional biopsy but is less invasive.

Biopsy Results

Ideally, the biopsy will return a conclusive result, indicating that the lesion is either nonmalignant or malignant. Treatment depends on the result. In some cases, nonmalignant lesions are left alone, or they might be removed to prevent progression into a malignancy. Certain forms of skin cancer form precancerous lesions that, over time, can become more dangerous. A malignancy requires immediate intervention from a qualified health professional. Oral cancers are covered more completely in Chapter 12, Oral Pathology.

Temporomandibular Joint Dysfunction

The temporomandibular joint (TMJ) is located in the region where the mandible attaches to the bones of the skull (refer back to Figure 6-11 in Chapter 6, Head and Neck Anatomy).

It comprises the bones, muscles, and joints that enable free movement of the mandible and related jaw structures (see Chapter 6, Head and Neck Anatomy). A healthy TMJ makes mastication and speech possible.

Causes and Symptoms of TMJ Dysfunction

Any condition that affects the TMJ can result in serious problems, because patients who cannot effectively chew or swallow risk compromising their overall health through poor nutrition. Any number of conditions can affect the TMJ, including:

- Trauma to the jaw
- Bruxism (clenching and grinding of the teeth)
- Jaw clenching
- Misalignment of the teeth
- Osteoarthritis or other systemic diseases

Signs and symptoms vary, depending on the severity of the disease, but might include any of the following:

- Pain that originates in the jaw and radiates into the ear or face
- Pain upon chewing
- A popping or clicking noise or sensation when the mouth is opened
- Reduced mobility in the mandible
- Recurring headaches or earaches
- Facial muscle, shoulder, back, or neck aches
- **Tinnitus** in the ear (a ringing sensation) or **crepitus** (the sound or sensation of grating or clicking)
- Trismus, spasms affecting the muscles of the jaw
- Fremitus, a vibration in the teeth caused by trauma from occlusal contact

Diagnosing TMJD

Patients who complain of any of these symptoms should be tested for temporomandibular joint dysfunction (TMJD). In many cases, the patient may be unaware of habits that led to the TMJD, such as nighttime bruxism. In other cases, the symptoms may be caused by another medical condition unrelated to the TMJD (differential diagnosis). As with all oral diseases, it is very important to have an updated medical and dental history.

Steps to diagnose TMJD include:

1. Physical examination. During the examination, the dentist asks the patient to open and close the mouth, and the dentist palpates the jaw muscles and bones while listening closely for any sounds. Additionally, the patient is asked to open the mouth as wide as possible to test for range of motion.
2. Diagnostic tests. Tests such as magnetic resonance imaging and computed tomography scans may reveal structural abnormalities that might be causing symptoms.

3. Casts. Models may be taken of the patient's teeth (dental casts) to reveal problems with the patient's bite and occlusion.

Treating TMJD

Treatment of TMJD depends on the severity of the symptoms and the patient's long-term outlook. Even seemingly benign TMJD caused by bruxism, for instance, might warrant preventive treatment to prevent more serious problems later. In many cases, the dentist or surgeon tries the least invasive treatments first. If the patient does not respond, then more invasive treatments may be considered.

TMJD treatments include:

- Jaw resting exercises
- Heat and cold packs
- Medical treatment, including pain relief, muscle relaxers, and other medications
- Biofeedback treatment
- Stress relief
- Physical therapy
- Massage
- Ultrasound
- Splints
- Orthodontic treatment
- Steroid injections to reduce inflammation
- Arthrocentesis, or rinsing of the joint with injections
- Arthroscopic surgery using tiny, minimally invasive instruments to access the joint
- Open surgery to repair severe damage to the soft tissue and joint

Suture Placement and Treatment

Sutures are a common feature of many oral surgeries. They are used to hold tissue in place while it heals. Sutures are always placed by the oral surgeon, and the type of suture used depends on the situation. Absorbable sutures are absorbed into the body over time. Nonabsorbable sutures, however, need to be removed after healing has taken place. Suture removal is typically performed by the oral surgeon or the dental hygienist, but in states with EFDA rules, they may be removed by qualified DAs who have completed additional training and licensing requirements.

DAs have a number of roles to play during suture placement, including:

- Preparing the sutures
- Counting the number of sutures along with the surgeon
- Observing placement
- Updating the patient's record
- Providing postoperative instructions

Types of Sutures

Sutures are placed in repetitive patterns to hold the tissue in place, then secured with simple square knots. The DA should know how the sutures were placed and how many. The following patterns are commonly used (Figure 42-17).

Simple Suture

This is the most common and versatile suture pattern. A simple suture is a loop through two flaps of tissue that is tied off to hold them together (Figure 42-17A).

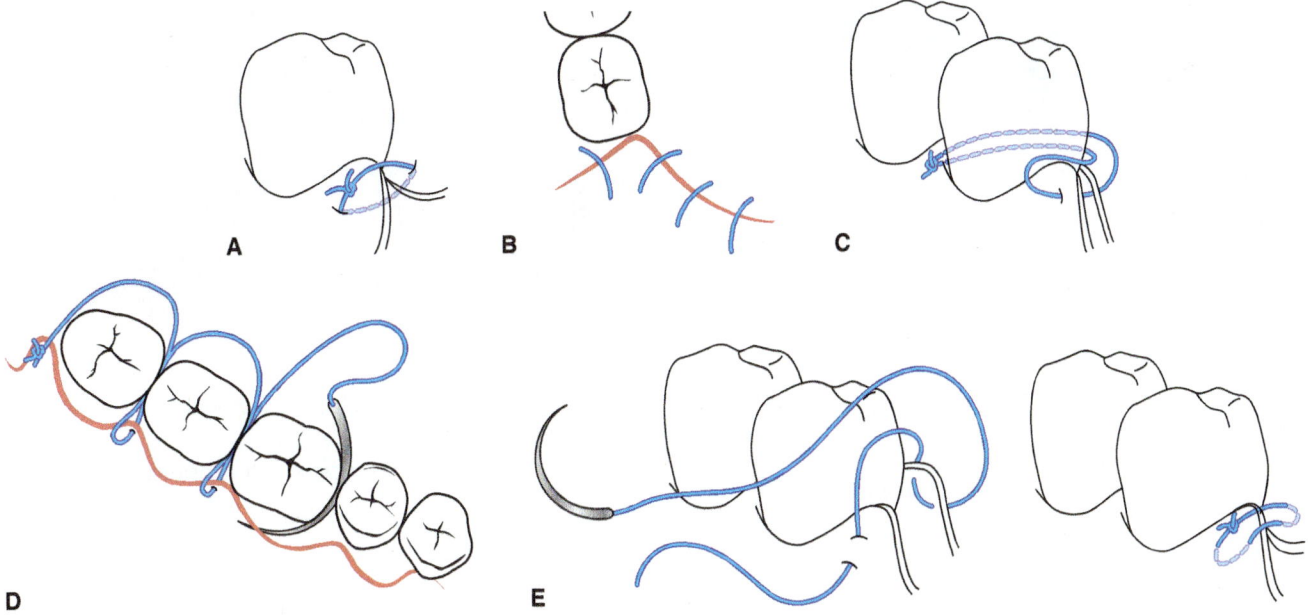

Figure 42–17 Suturing techniques. (**A**) Simple sutures. (**B**) Continuous simple sutures. (**C**) Simple sling suture. (**D**) Continuous sling suture. (**E**) Mattress suture.

Continuous Simple Suture

A continuous simple suture is a series of simple sutures placed in a row along the seams of an incision (Figure 42-17B). It resembles the stitching placed in hems. The number of sutures depends on the length of the wound. Both ends are tied off with a square knot.

Simple Sling Suture

A simple sling suture is used to join interproximal flaps. The suture is placed by first inserting the needle through the tissue on the facial surface of the tooth, continuing through the interproximal space, then wrapping the suture around the tooth to the far side, where it is inserted through both sides of a tissue flap and brought back around, through the interproximal space, and tied off (Figure 42-17C).

Continuous Sling Suture

The continuous sling is used when a larger flap of tissue needs to be secured. Like the simple sling, the needle is first passed through the gingival tissue and then the suture is passed through the interproximal space, looped around the tooth, and brought back to the open tissue. After securing the tissue flap in place, the suture passes back through the interproximal space, and is then looped around to the next interproximal space, where the pattern repeats itself until the flap is sutured (Figure 42-17D). The suture is secured at both ends with knots.

Mattress Suture (Horizontal and Vertical)

Mattress sutures are also used to hold tissue flaps in place. They are created by passing the suture through the tissue surface and emerging again from the same surface, then looping the suture to the other side of the tissue flap and repeating the procedure (Figure 42-17E). The ends of the suture are held in place by tying it off where the first suture was placed. Horizontal mattress sutures are placed when the initial suture is horizontal, while vertical sutures are created by placing a vertical suture in the first tissue flap.

Procedure 42–8 Assisting with Suture Placement

Materials needed (Figure P42-8-1):

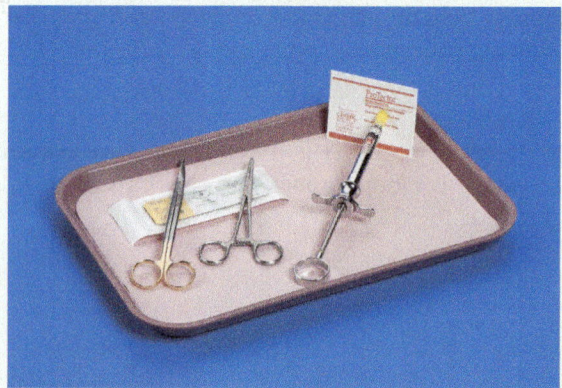

Figure P42-8-1

- Suture supplies
- Needle holder
- Suture scissors

1. Put on appropriate PPE.
2. Prepare for suture placement by removing sterile suture material from its packaging.
3. Using a needle holder, hold the needle in the upper third, away from the sharp point.
4. Transfer the needle holder to the surgeon when it is needed. During the transfer, hold the needle holder by the hinge and transfer it handle first.

5. Provide tissue retraction during placement of the sutures. Observe the number and placement of sutures.
6. After the sutures are tied, cut the ends of the sutures with suture scissors, if required. Do not snip sutures flush to the tissue, but leave a 2 to 3 mm end.
7. When the sutures are finished (Figure P42-8-2), accept the suture material from the surgeon and place on the treatment tray.

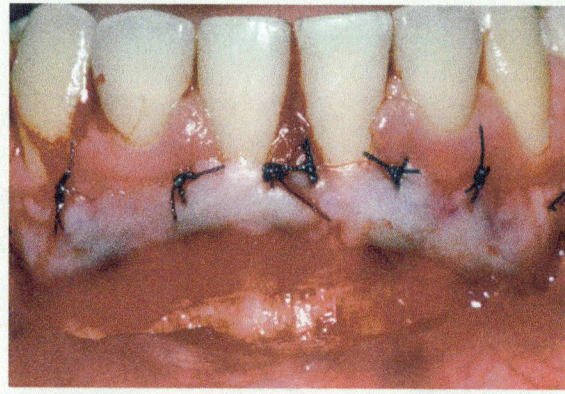

Figure P42-8-2

8. Record the number and placement of sutures in the patient's record.
9. Provide the patient with postoperative instructions.

Procedure 42-9 Assisting with Suture Removal

In some states, dental assistants are allowed to perform suture removal as an expanded function after meeting additional training and licensing requirements (see Procedure 37-9 in Chapter 37, Expanded Clinical Functions). This procedure covers assisting with suture removal. Sutures are ready for removal when the wound site has healed (Figure P42-9-1).

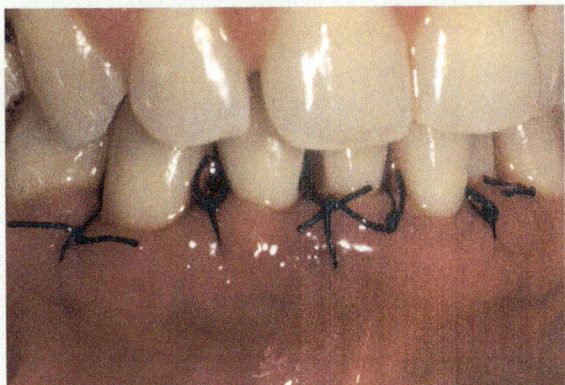

Figure P42-9-1

Materials needed (Figure P42-9-2):

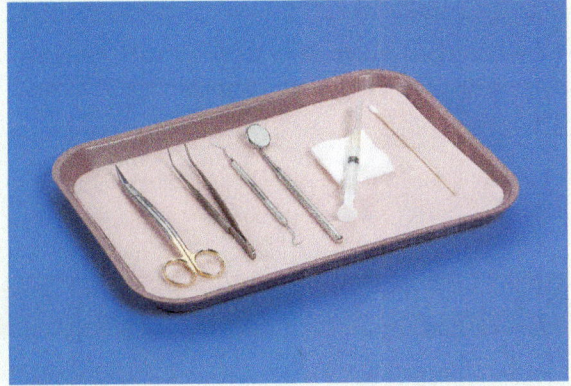

Figure P42-9-2

- Basic setup tray
- Cotton pliers
- Suture scissors
- Cotton-tipped applicator
- Antiseptic solution
- Sterile cotton gauze

1. Put on appropriate PPE.
2. Transfer a cotton-tipped applicator that has been dipped in an antiseptic solution to the surgeon who swabs the site with an antiseptic to cleanse the area and remove debris.
3. Transfer the cotton pliers to the surgeon to lift away the suture and expose the knot.
4. Transfer suture scissors to the surgeon to cut the sutures.
5. Retract tissues as necessary to provide a well-lit working area.
6. Accept removed sutures for placement on a gauze sponge; this helps keep track of how many sutures have been removed. Count the number of sutures removed and compare it to the dental record to make sure all sutures are removed.
7. Make a note of the procedure in the patient's record and provide the patient with postoperative instructions.

Care After Suture Removal

Sutures are typically removed 5 to 7 days after placement. During removal, the site may bleed slightly. Apply pressure with a gauze pad to stop the bleeding. Heavier bleeding may require intervention from the surgeon.

After the sutures are removed, inspect the patient's oral cavity to make sure it is free from debris, bleeding, or lesions. Also, check the number of sutures removed against the dental record to make sure there are no sutures remaining in the patient's mouth. The patient should be advised to eat only soft foods and rinse with saltwater for a few days after suture removal. A follow-up appointment should not be necessary. After the patient is dismissed, update the patient's record with the number of sutures removed and any notes from the procedure.

Postsurgical Care and Complications

Bleeding and Swelling

After oral surgery, some bleeding or oozing (even from freshly sutured surgical wounds) and swelling is expected. Bleeding can be controlled with cotton or gauze pads, and swelling can be controlled with cold packs placed on the swollen tissues. Cold packs should be applied in 20-minute cycles during the first 24 hours after the surgery. After the initial 24 hours, switch to a gentle heating pad. Pain relief is usually given in the form of medication, depending on the nature of the surgery. Patients should be instructed to take any prescribed pain medication before the anesthetic wears off.

Normal swelling and light bleeding are not considered complications of oral surgery, but rather side effects. However, bleeding that cannot be stopped or extreme pain could signal a possible complication. These conditions should be examined by an oral surgeon or dentist to see if further treatment is warranted.

Patients should also be advised to continue with their oral care regiment after surgery, including brushing and flossing. The surgical site can be avoided until it is completely healed.

Finally, patients should be advised to avoid strenuous physical activity, chewing on hard or tough foods, sucking on straws or hard candy, smoking, chewing gum, or operating any types of machinery or vehicles while under the influence of pain medications. They should also avoid vigorously rinsing the mouth for at least 48 hours.

Alveolitis

After an extraction, a blood clot forms over the empty socket as part of the normal healing process. The blood clot is the first step in refilling the empty socket with bone. In the normal healing process, the blood clot is replaced with granulated tissue, connective tissue that forms on the wound during the early stages of healing. As healing progresses, this tissue is replaced by healthy tissue and finally bone.

If a clot fails to form or is dislodged, a condition called **alveolitis** (dry socket) may occur. Alveolitis usually manifests itself within 2 to 4 days of surgery and is extremely painful. Signs and symptoms include sharp pain radiating up and down the head and neck, halitosis, exposed bone, and a bad taste in the mouth. The most common site for alveolitis is the third molar. Alveolitis is a dental emergency that requires immediate attention.

There are a number of possible causes for alveolitis, including:

- Lack of blood supply to the affected socket
- Infection within the socket that prevents blood from flowing in
- Trauma to the socket
- Dislodging of the clot, sometimes by the patient's tongue, smoking, drinking through a straw, spitting, or rinsing

Assisting in treatment for alveolitis is covered in Procedure 42-10.

✓ CHECKPOINTS

42-11 How long does it typically take for implants to heal and fuse with bone?

42-12 What are the three forms of biopsy most often used in oral surgery?

42-13 If a structural abnormality is suspected as the cause of temperomandibular joint dysfunction, what diagnostic tests may be prescribed?

42-14 What is done if slight bleeding occurs after oral surgery?

Procedure 42-10 Assisting with the Treatment of Alveolitis

Materials needed (Figure P42-10-1):

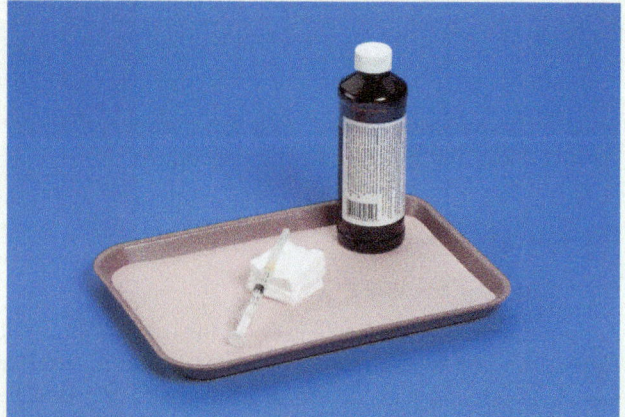

Figure P42-10-1

- Syringe
- Saline solution
- Iodoform gauze

1. Put on appropriate PPE.
2. Prepare a syringe filled with warm saline solution. Transfer the syringe to the surgeon.
3. The surgeon irrigates the empty socket with the warm saline solution to remove any accumulated debris.
4. Cut a narrow strip of iodoform gauze to fit the socket. Iodoform gauze contains a topical antiseptic that helps reduce infection. Transfer the gauze to the surgeon.
5. The surgeon gently packs the gauze into the socket. The gauze takes the place of the normal blood clot, soothing the socket and preventing food and microbes from gaining access to the socket.
6. Make a note of the procedure in the patient's record and provide the patient with self-care instructions. A follow-up appointment is set for 1 to 2 days to change the dressing and repeat the procedure. This is repeated until the socket begins to heal normally.

Chapter Highlights

✦ Oral surgery is performed by specialized oral surgeons, who have completed up to 6 years of additional training after dental school.

✦ Surgical dental assistants have also received training in assisting with oral surgery; in states with expanded functions dental assistants, they can perform some basic procedures after additional training.

✦ Indications for surgery include extractions, biopsies and tumor removal, trauma, cosmetic surgeries, reconstructive surgeries, temperomandibular joint dysfunction, and orthodontic surgeries.

✦ Oral surgery can be performed with local anesthetic or general anesthesia administered by a nurse anesthetist or anesthesiologist, depending on the surgery.

✦ Oral surgery instruments are designed to retract tissue and remove and shape bone and tissue. Surgical dental assistants need a thorough understanding of the various instrumentation and how to assemble sterile surgical set-ups.

✦ The chain of surgical asepsis refers to all the steps that are required to maintain a sterile operating environment, including personal preparation, instrumentation, and treatment area preparation.

✦ Simple tooth extractions are performed to remove one tooth.

✦ Alveoplasty is performed to shape the alveolar ridge after multiple extractions and in preparation for dentures or an appliance.

✦ Impacted teeth are those that have not erupted; the most commonly removed impacted teeth are the third molars.

✦ Dental implants are fastened directly to the bone to hold appliances in place and can be used with bridges, crowns, and dentures.

✦ Biopsies are performed to remove and assess lesions for malignancies.

✦ Temporomandibular joint (TMJ) dysfunction has a number of causes, and treatments range from medication to appliances to surgery.

✦ Sutures are placed by surgeons but may be removed by expanded functions dental assistants.

✦ Some bleeding and swelling is normal after surgery, but severe pain or bleeding that cannot be controlled should be evaluated by a dentist or surgeon.

✦ Alveolitis occurs when there is no blood clot in the socket after a tooth extraction; it is extremely painful and needs to be treated.

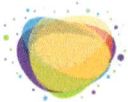

Review Questions

1. Which task may be performed by expanded functions dental assistants?

   a. Suture placement

   b. Extractions

   c. Suture removal

   d. None of the above

2. What are elevators used for?

   a. Tongue retraction

   b. Cheek retraction

   c. Tooth extraction

   d. Reflecting tissue

3. Which teeth are universal forceps used to extract?

   a. Posterior molars

   b. Incisors

   c. Mandibular teeth

   d. All of the above

4. What does the "R" stand for in #88R forceps?

   a. Reflecting

   b. Radiopaque

   c. Right

   d. Retained

5. When are bone chisels used?

   a. To shape teeth

   b. To reflect tissue

   c. To contour bone

   d. To loosen teeth

6. How long should you wash your hands in each step of a surgical scrub?

   a. 5 min.

   b. 7 min.

   c. 9 min.

   d. 12 min.

7. During a simple tooth extraction, how many teeth are typically removed?

    a. 1

    b. 2

    c. 3

    d. 4

8. Which teeth are most likely to be removed because they are impacted?

    a. Old, dull teeth

    b. Third molars

    c. Primary teeth

    d. Teeth affected by trauma

9. Which is the implant used most often for patients whose dentures have failed?

    a. Subperiosteal

    b. Endosteal

    c. Mini

    d. None of the above

10. What is the purpose of the second surgery during implant surgery?

    a. To place titanium rods in the bone

    b. To place abutments on the rods

    c. To test the appliance

    d. To permanently place the appliance

11. During an excisional biopsy

    a. The whole lesion is removed for evaluation.

    b. A tissue sample is removed for evaluation.

    c. A scraping is removed for evaluation.

    d. None of the above.

12. Alveolitis is treated by

    a. Pain control and time.

    b. Gentle rinsing of the empty socket.

    c. Packing the empty socket with treated gauze.

    d. Bone grafts.

Active Learning Exercises

1. Identify the three main types of retractors and explain their uses in oral surgery.

2. What is the purpose of surgical aspirating tips during a surgical procedure? The suction tips come in various widths. For what reasons might different widths be needed? In what procedure might both a slender and a wider tube be used and why?

3. Although routine extractions use a basic surgical armamentarium setup, what additional instruments or materials would be necessary for extracting impacted teeth? How are these procedures different?

Application Activities

1. Demonstrate how to open a surgical set-up without compromising asepsis.

2. Demonstrate how to count and identify sutures; also demonstrate suture removal on a cotton roll.

3. Develop a handout for your oral surgery patients with preoperative and postoperative instructions. Be specific and complete.

PREPARING FOR CERTIFICATION EXAMS

Review the following topics in this chapter to prepare for the Dental Assisting National Board (DANB) exam:

- **The Surgical Dental Assistant's Role**
- **Surgical Procedures**
- **Simple Tooth Extraction**
- **Extraction of Impacted Teeth**
- **Suture Placement and Treatment**
- **Postsurgical Care and Complications**

chapter 43

Pediatric Dentistry

CHAPTER OUTLINE

Introduction
The Pediatric Dental Office
The Role of the Pediatric Dental Assistant
Characteristics of Pediatric Patients
    Childhood Stages of Development
    Patients with Special Needs
Pediatric Behavior Management
    The Frankl Scale
    Behavior Management Techniques

Pediatric Treatments
    Medical and Dental History
    The Examination
    Preventive Dentistry
    Pit and Fissure Sealants
    Restorative Procedures
    Endodontic Procedures
    Prosthodontic Procedures
    Treatment of Dental Trauma
Child Abuse and Reporting Laws

Procedures
    43-1   **Assisting with Application of Pit and Fissure Sealants**
    43-2   **Assisting with Stainless Steel Crown Placement**

CHAPTER CHECKLIST

On completion of this chapter, students will be able to:

- ☑ Identify the features unique to a pediatric dental office and describe their purpose.
- ☑ Describe the role of the pediatric dental assistant.
- ☑ Describe the characteristics of pediatric patients, including stages of childhood development.
- ☑ Identify the ratings on the Frankl scale.
- ☑ Describe common behavior management techniques.
- ☑ Describe common preventive and restorative pediatric treatments.
- ☑ Explain the role of the dental assistant in providing support during pediatric procedures.
- ☑ Describe how to treat dental trauma.
- ☑ Explain child abuse reporting requirements.

KEY TERMS

festooned (fes-TOONDE) – a crown or other restoration sculpted to follow the natural contours of gingival tissue

papoose board – a type of restraint made from a still board and Velcro straps that restrains a pediatric patient's arms and legs

stainless steel crowns – crowns made from stainless steel used for pediatric restorations

Introduction

Pediatric dentistry is the branch of dentistry focused on dental care for children and some adult patients with special needs. This is specialized dentistry that requires knowledge of the physical and emotional development of children. Pediatric dentists are intimately involved with growth and jaw development; caries prevention; and restoration of primary, mixed, and permanent teeth, as well as treatment of dental trauma.

Patients are referred to pediatric dentists by other dentists, family physicians, and other specialists. Pediatric dentists are a very important first step for children and their families because good oral hygiene habits and impressions of dentistry formed in childhood are likely to last a lifetime. Thus, pediatric dentists and dental assistants often spend significant time dealing with young patients who might be afraid or intimidated by the dental visit.

Additionally, pediatric dentists, dental hygienists, and dental assistants have special training to adapt adult procedures to the specialized circumstances sometimes presented by pediatric patients or adults with special needs. This chapter covers the main points of pediatric dentistry as a specialty, with a special focus on how pediatric dental assistants can improve the dental experience for children and the occasional adult with special needs who might be referred to a pediatric dentist.

The Pediatric Dental Office

Pediatric dental offices usually are designed to encourage and keep patients cheerful. The office decor is typically child-friendly, with bright colors and themes that children find interesting and comforting. Some offices are themed, with waiting areas that are painted to resemble aquariums, outer space, or even movie sets.

The reception areas in a pediatric dental office are filled with objects to keep children occupied while they wait. Coloring books, reading books, televisions, games, and even video game consoles are all regular features of pediatric dental offices.

The treatment area of the pediatric dental office is also frequently designed to comfort the child. Many pediatric dental offices are designed with "open bays," so the treatment areas are visible to each other. Many children benefit from seeing other children receiving dental care, and this may encourage children to be brave together.

Pediatric treatment areas also frequently include distractions to keep children occupied during treatment. This might include headphones with music, televisions playing movies or cartoons, or even hand-held games at treatment chairs that children can use with the dentist's or dental assistant's permission.

Some pediatric dental offices are also equipped with a "quiet room." Children who become unmanageable may be escorted to the quiet room until they bring themselves back under control, in the company of their parent or guardian. This prevents them from upsetting other children in the treatment area.

The general cheerfulness of the pediatric office frequently extends to the uniforms worn by staff and other little touches. The idea is to render the office more friendly and less medical, to put children at ease.

CHECKPOINT
43-1 How is the decor in a pediatric dental office different from that in a general dental practice?

The Role of the Pediatric Dental Assistant

The pediatric dental office is staffed with many of the same positions found in a general dental practice. The office is headed by a dentist who specializes in pediatric patients, along with dental hygienists, dental assistants, and office staff.

Pediatric dental assistants receive the same training as other dental assistants, which can vary from state to state. Some states allow expanded functions dental assistants, who have additional training and are legally allowed to perform some pediatric procedures that would otherwise be performed by the dentist or hygienist. Pediatric dental assistants must be thoroughly versed in pediatric tooth development, as well as the age and emotional development of the children they see in the office.

Pediatric dental assistants should also enjoy working with children and their families. In many offices, the pediatric dental assistant is the first dental professional the child sees, and the assistant leads the child to the treatment area and acclimates him or her to the treatment chair. When the assistant is in charge of the child, he or she should be able to establish an easy connection and keep the child under control.

Finally, a pediatric dental assistant should be able to answer questions about procedures for both children and their guardians. This means being able to describe to children and adults procedures such as restorations, polishing and sealing, and treatment for trauma.

From the Dentist's Perspective

A pediatric dental assistant is a special kind of person! In our office, like many offices, the dental assistants are more than just medical professionals—they're also the child's voice and advocate. Our dental assistants show children to their chairs and sit with them during procedures, helping soothe them and talk them through what can be scary for many kids.

CHECKPOINT
43-2 What specialized knowledge should a pediatric dental assistant have?

Characteristics of Pediatric Patients

Children are not "little adults" when it comes to medical and dental treatment of any kind. Aside from the fact that children have unique dental needs, they are also at different places along the developmental spectrum. It is important to recognize where a particular child patient is in his or her emotional, mental, and physical development in order to anticipate how best to provide appropriate patient care.

Although broad generalities can be drawn about developmental stages, these are not absolute for all children. Some children develop faster in one area and may be slower to develop in other areas. Regardless of their developmental stage, all children must be approached in a kind, gentle, and age-appropriate manner. This is important for the long-term dental health of the child and the smooth functioning of the dental practice.

A child's development can be viewed in terms of different stages:

- *Chronological age.* This is the child's age in years and months. Dental development is closely tied to chronological age.
- *Mental age.* This is the child's level of intellectual development. There is a fairly wide range of "normal" for a given chronological age, but in general, children experience a predictable order of development stages.
- *Emotional age.* This is the child's maturity level. Emotional age can vary widely, depending on that child's natural personality and life experiences.

Some children may also have special needs, such as mental, physical, or emotional disabilities. These patients should be treated in a manner that is appropriate for their specific needs, with input from their guardians to ensure they are receiving compassionate and effective dental care. This topic is covered in greater depth in Chapter 22, Patients with Special Needs.

Childhood Stages of Development

Behavioral and educational experts have developed a basic model to describe the various stages of normal development for most children, based on chronological age.

- *Birth through age two.* During early development, children are acquiring the basic motor and social skills needed to navigate the world. They are learning to walk, talk, identify familiar people, and play and interact with other children and adults. Children of this age are frequently apprehensive around strange adults, but they are often able to follow instructions, even if they do not understand the basic idea of dentistry. They are also very responsive to smiling adults and enjoy little games such as hide and seek. Children this age frequently need to be accompanied by a parent or trusted guardian during dental appointments.
- *Three to five years.* Age-appropriate children of this stage are able to speak and communicate and follow simple directions such as "sit still" and "open up." Although they still may be apprehensive around adults, they are also working to establish their own autonomy and will respond to positive, supporting statements, such as, "You're being very brave! Mommy and Daddy will be very proud of you!" Children at this age need boundaries and typically enjoy pleasing adult figures of authority. Fear of dentists may be increasing if the child has previously had an uncomfortable procedure or associates the dentist with a doctor from whom they likely have received shots.
- *Six to twelve years.* This vast age range includes children of very different developmental stages. Six year olds are just beginning their primary education and learning to adapt to an environment where they are expected to follow instructions without direct, constant supervision. They may be very active, curious, eager to please, and unrestrained emotionally. This is the period when children begin their socialization, learning to relate to the world beyond their family units. As they grow, children gain considerable independence and experience. By the time they reach 12 years old, they are much better at rational and critical thinking, and they are able to work through complex problems and emotions, such as fear of dentistry. The key to working effectively with older preteens is to maintain your role as an authority figure while also showing the child respect and making your expectations clear.

Patients with Special Needs

The above stages of development apply to age-appropriate children. However, many children with special needs present with challenges that can be emotional, mental, or physical (or some combination). Some points to remember include:

- A child with special physical needs may be age-appropriate in every other way, capable of understanding and following instructions. In these cases, allowances may need to be made for medical equipment, such as wheelchairs or breathing devices, but the dental visit can proceed as with any age-appropriate child.
- Children with mental disabilities may exhibit uneven development. They may be able to comprehend what is being asked, but remain fearful. You should work closely with the child's guardians to develop a treatment approach that will work. This may include the use of premedication or restraints as necessary.
- Dental offices are increasingly seeing children with emotional and mental conditions including autism spectrum

disorders. These children may not be socialized and may be difficult to control. They often avoid eye contact, have sensory integration issues, and frequently dislike being touched. Some patients with these conditions are prone to tantrums that can be highly disruptive. Again, work with the child's guardians to develop an effective treatment approach.

Besides autism, special needs patients include children with Down syndrome and cerebral palsy. This topic is covered in greater depth in Chapter 22, Patients with Special Needs.

CHECKPOINTS

43-3 What are the three ways to measure a child's developmental age?

43-4 At what age are children typically able to follow simple instructions?

Pediatric Behavior Management

Behavior management is one of the distinguishing features of pediatric dentistry. Adult patients may be afraid of the dentist, but they are much less likely to have a tantrum in the reception area, and there is less need to coax reluctant patients through a procedure.

Behavior management for children takes on a special significance because these early visits set the tone for the child's perception of dentistry in general. This, in turn, will inform their oral health decisions as adults, so it is not an overexaggeration to say that a lifetime of healthy teeth and gingiva might depend on effective behavior management.

The Frankl Scale

Developed by Dr. Spencer Frankl, the Frankl scale is used to rate a child's behavior on a scale of 1 to 4. The ratings are:

1. Strongly negative behavior; refuses treatment; crying and tantrums; extreme fear; lashing out behavior
2. Negative behavior; only accepts treatment with reluctance; not cooperative, but not completely withdrawn; evidence of noncompliance, without actual noncompliance
3. Positive; accepts treatment, despite some minor misgivings; willingly complies with directions
4. Strongly positive; establishes open communication with dentists and other dental professionals; exhibits an interest in the procedures and even the instruments used during procedures; enthusiastic and smiling

Many pediatric dentists use this scale to record the child's behavior at each dental visit. The rating is entered on the patient's chart and can be used to anticipate a child's behavior during treatment.

Behavior Management Techniques

The Academy of Pediatric Dentistry has developed a number of methods dentists and dental professionals can use to help modify behavior, including:

- *Tell-show-do*. This technique involves the assistant explaining what is about to happen (tell), then showing the child the procedure, which might include allowing them to hold hand instruments such as the mouth mirror (show). Finally, the procedure is performed exactly as specified (do), so the child is reassured.
- *Distraction*. Children can sometimes be distracted away from the dental procedure, which makes them more compliant. Offices may be equipped with televisions, artwork, or other media to keep the child focused on something other than the dental procedure.
- *Modeling*. Modeling involves showing the child how other children act during a procedure. Open-bay dental offices are designed so that children model good behavior to each other because few children want to be seen as poorly behaved.
- *Voice control*. Your voice says a lot about your position of authority. Speak calmly, but firmly, to communicate that you are the authority. Do not ask the child's permission constantly by adding modifiers like "OK?" on the end of every sentence.
- *Facial control*. Children respond to smiling faces. Use facial expressions to show you are proud of the child's behavior by smiling to reward good behavior.
- *Hand over mouth*. Hand over mouth is a technique used to establish control and compliance with children who are exhibiting fearful behaviors or avoidance. During this procedure, the dentist places his or her hand over the child's mouth and then explains the procedure and what to expect and what kind of behavior is expected from the child. This technique should only be used with prior consent from guardians and, as a result, is not used very frequently.
- *Restraints*. Restraints are used only for patients who might suffer injury because of inappropriate movement. This movement might be related to behavior or to a physical condition that causes loss of control over limb movement. Restraints are used to protect both the patient and the operator. The most common physical restraint is the **papoose board**. This device restrains the child's arms, hands, and legs with Velcro straps attached to a board. Consent is required before restraints are used.
- *Pharmacological sedation*. Pharmacological sedation involves the use of a drug to calm or even completely sedate a child before the procedure. This may be recommended for children who are extremely anxious or fearful but who are not appropriate candidates for restraints. Conscious sedation can be accomplished with nitrous oxide or other drugs, and complete sedation can only be administered by a qualified professional, usually a nurse anesthetist or anesthesiologist. Prior consent is required for any sedation.

CHECKPOINTS

43-5 What does a 4 on the Frankl scale mean?

43-6 What does the hand-over-mouth behavior control technique entail? When can it be used?

Pediatric Treatments

Children are first introduced to the dentist usually around age two, when they are brought in for an initial exam. This first office visit is designed mainly to introduce the child to the dental office and treatment chair, as well as provide an opportunity for the dentist and dental staff to educate the parents about proper oral hygiene. After this appointment, children should return every 6 months for a routine dental exam.

As in adult dentistry, pediatric dental offices perform both preventive and restorative procedures. It is essential that all pediatric dental assistants know the various stages of tooth development and the details of any procedure performed.

Parental or legal consent is typically required before dental procedures can be performed on children and minors under 18 years of age. The dental office should have consent forms available, and dental assistants should be able to explain the procedure to adults during consent meetings.

Medical and Dental History

A pediatric medical and dental history is an updated record of the child's physical and oral health. New patients should also have a complete medical and dental history taken, or a previous record should be updated. Parents and guardians usually provide the information for the medical and dental history.

A complete medical and dental history includes existing conditions, prior conditions and treatments, allergies, habits or practices that might affect the teeth, and the general well-being of the child. This record should be updated, including charting teeth, after the patient arrives at the office and before dental treatment.

The Examination

The dental exam is the foundation for preventive oral care and healthy oral hygiene for children and pediatric patients. The examination is very similar to the adult dental exam, and any changes in status are noted. Additionally, dental radiographs may be obtained and the teeth cleaned. Dental charts should be updated during every examination to reflect the child's maturing dentition.

Pediatric Radiographs

Dental radiographs are used for pediatric patients to assess and diagnose gingival and tooth disease. The American Association for Pediatric Dentistry (AAPD) recommends that children at high risk of developing dental caries have updated radiographs every six months. Although this is more frequent that the recommendations for adult patients, children are more vulnerable to caries because of their rapidly developing teeth.

Pediatric dental radiography is covered in greater detail in Chapter 30, Producing Intraoral Dental Radiographs.

The Examination

During a pediatric examination, the dentist evaluates the patient's external profile to make sure the child is developing normally. This means assessing the bone structure in the face and the symmetry of the nose, eyes, ears, and mouth.

An internal examination is conducted to carefully inspect the teeth as well as gingival and oral mucosa tissues. These exams are usually conducted with a mouth mirror and explorer, although some children may balk if an explorer is used. For these children, it may be possible for the dentist to conduct an examination with fingers alone. During the exam, the position of teeth should be noted, including malocclusions, spacing, and crowding. A referral to an orthodontist may be appropriate.

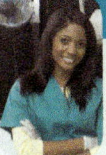

Voice of Experience

Here is a little tip you don't usually see in textbooks: Always be prepared with an emesis basin in case a child vomits. New dental assistants are often surprised how many kids throw up when they are scared or nervous. If you have an emesis basin handy, it makes cleanup much easier! Remember that vomit is considered a body fluid; be sure to follow the proper procedures for cleaning up a contaminated spill.

Preventive Dentistry

Education is a major component of preventive pediatric dentistry. Routine examinations present a perfect opportunity to talk about proper brushing and flossing, fluoride, diet, and other aspects of preventive dentistry.

Oral Hygiene

Comprehensive oral hygiene is the foundation of preventive self-care. Pay careful attention to teaching proper oral hygiene techniques during office visits (Figure 43-1), including:

- *Brushing techniques.* Effective brushing should be modeled and the patient given a chance to demonstrate during the exam.

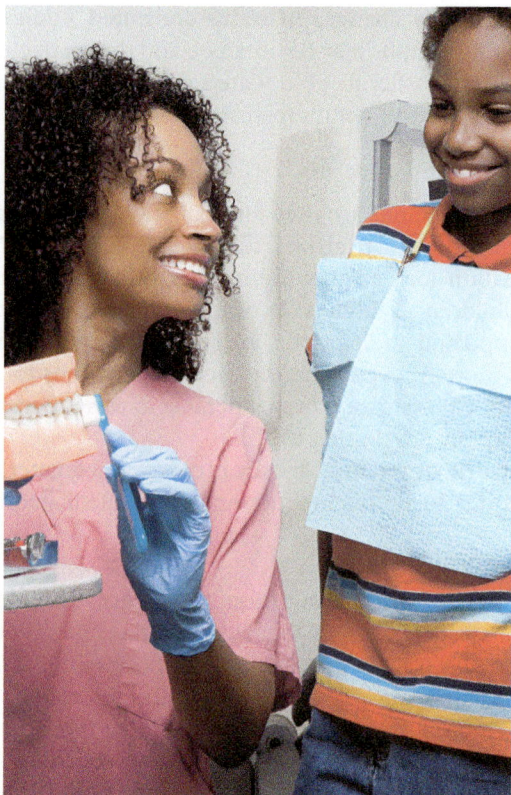

Figure 43–1 Oral hygiene. Demonstrate effective brushing for pediatric patients.

■ *Flossing*. Like brushing, flossing is a mainstay of oral care. A variety of products are available to make flossing easier and more palatable for pediatric patients, such as flavored floss and floss sticks instead of string.
■ *Fluoride*. Some parents have concerns about fluoridation. However, fluoride is a safe and essential component of healthy tooth development—at the correct levels. In pediatric dentistry, fluoride is used during fluoride rinses and varnishes, as well as during some sealing procedures. It is also available in many cities' drinking water and in toothpastes and mouthwashes. Dental assistants should know how much fluoride is safe for children and communicate that information clearly to parents.

Chapter 10, Prevention of Caries and Periodontal Disease, covers all aspects of oral hygiene in greater detail, including additional information about fluoride.

Diet

Diet, and especially consumption of sugary foods and drinks like soda, has a major effect on tooth health. Parents and guardians, and the patients themselves, should be aware of the dangers posed by drinking too many sugary drinks and eating candies and other foods that promote dental caries. If diet may be having a negative impact on a pediatric patient's oral health, it is important to talk with the parents about vitamin and mineral intake and its effect on developing teeth. This topic is covered in greater detail in Chapter 11, Nutrition.

Mouth Guards

Mouth guards are important tools to help prevent traumatic injury to children who play sports. Many states and cities require mouth guards for children who play contact sports, but even if they are not required, mouth guards can prevent damage or loss of teeth and trauma to sensitive oral structures. Mouth guards come in several varieties. They can be purchased as is, custom-made in the dental office with vacuum-formed models, or fabricated at home from do-it-yourself kits.

Coronal Polishing

Coronal polishing is accomplished with a rubber cub and a polishing paste that is applied to the crowns of the teeth during exams. Some pediatric patients may need supra-gingival and subgingival scaling prior to a coronal polishing. Coronal polishing removes extrinsic stains and plaque from tooth enamel. Coronal polishing is usually performed by dental hygienists, but in states with expanded functions dental assistants, it can be performed by dental assistants with additional training. See Chapter 44, Coronal Polishing, and Chapter 37, Expanded Clinical Functions, for more information on coronal polishing.

Preventive Orthodontics

Preventive orthodontics begins as early as the child's first visit to the dentist. Pediatric dentists chart and track the child's development, watching out for malocclusions, crowding, or crooked teeth, as well as other problems caused by habits such as thumb sucking or tongue thrusting, both of which can cause misalignment in primary teeth.

Treatment of problems depends on the nature of the issue. In some cases, a pediatric dentist can handle the problem in his or her office; in others, a referral to an orthodontist is appropriate.

Some of the techniques used in preventive orthodontics include:

■ *Space maintainer.* This device is a spacer that is inserted between teeth to hold an open space for permanent teeth (Figure 43-2). They are either cemented in place as

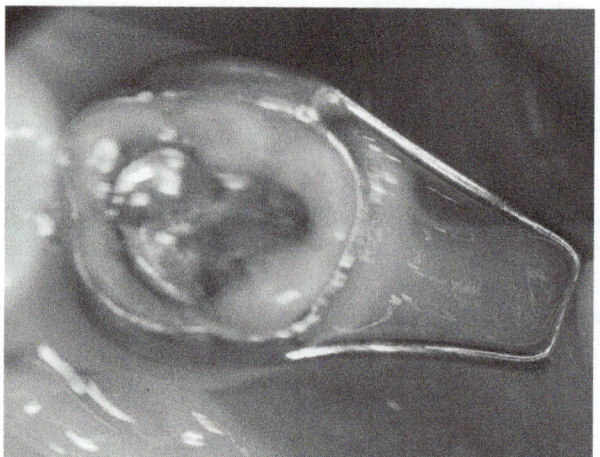

Figure 43–2 Space maintainer.

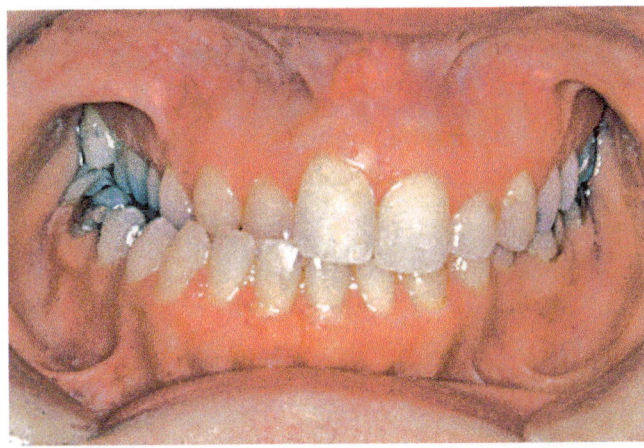

Figure 43–3 Crossbite. Untreated developmental crossbite.

fixed appliances or designed as removable appliances. Space maintainers are used when a primary tooth is lost prematurely and there is a risk of crowding as permanent teeth erupt. They are removed when the permanent tooth erupts.

- *Correcting oral habits.* Although the treatment of thumb sucking is controversial among dentists and orthodontists, devices are sometimes used to prevent children from sucking their thumb. Called habit breakers, cribs, or rakes, these devices are made up of wires and supporting bands that affix to the molars and extend to the back of the maxillary central incisors, making thumb sucking difficult. The devices are cemented into place and are typically worn for 6 months. Most dentists do not start treating thumb sucking until a child is 5 years of age and there is a risk of damage to the permanent teeth.
- *Occlusion issues.* Pediatric dentists use removable or fixed appliances to correct crossbites, which can affect occlusion permanently (Figure 43-3).

Pit and Fissure Sealants

Pit and fissure sealants, also called enamel sealants, are used to prevent dental caries in the pits and fissures of posterior teeth. Despite good diet and brushing habits, and adequate fluoridation, children are still susceptible to caries in these areas. More than three-fourths of dental caries in children form in these pits and fissures, which are hard to brush clean and often too deep for fluoride to reach.

Pit and fissure sealants, however, prevent caries from forming in these areas and can dramatically reduce the risk of caries. Children who have pit and fissure sealant treatments often pass through childhood without a single restoration.

Pit and fissure sealants are applied in the dental office.

Indications for Sealants

Sealants are used as part of a prevention program, so they are appropriate for most children and even some adults. Typically, dentists apply sealants to teeth that have erupted within the previous 4 years, before caries have formed in deep pits and fissures.

Sealants are placed by dentists or dental hygienists. In states with expanded functions dental assistants, they may be placed by dental assistants with additional training.

Contraindications for Sealants

In certain situations sealants are not recommended. Posterior teeth that have very smooth occlusal surfaces that exhibit shallow pits and fissures do not require dental sealants. Teeth that have been caries-free for more than 4 years also fall into this category. Since these teeth have remained caries-free this long, the chances of caries occurring is minimal. Posterior teeth that have not fully erupted and still have a flap of tissue on the occlusal surface should not be sealed until the occlusal surface has fully erupted.

Sealant Materials

The sealant material is a thin coating that prevents food and bacteria from collecting in pits and fissures. The idea is to seal the pit or fissure, so it is crucial that the material forms a smooth, solid surface. If the sealant is improperly applied or its surface is broken, the seal is compromised and decay is possible.

Sealant materials are composite materials that are either self-cured or light-cured. Self-cured materials must be placed within about 2 minutes of mixing the composite to prevent it from setting early. Light-cured sealants are cured by the operator with a light source. These sealants do not require mixing but are available in a premixed syringe. Light-cured sealants are more commonly used because there is no time constraint, making them easier to apply.

Additionally, sealants are either *filled* or *unfilled*. Unfilled sealants have just the composite material, while filled sealants have an additional material added to make it more resistant to wear. There is no difference in their performance, but some dentists prefer filled sealants because they believe it allows less wear on occlusal surfaces.

Finally, some sealants contain fluoride that is released after the composite is polymerized and set.

Placement of sealants is a detail-oriented process. The child must be able to follow instructions and remain still during placement. It is important to isolate the teeth being sealed and keep them absolutely dry. The number one reason for sealant failure is operator technique. Sealant placement is covered in Procedure 43-1.

Procedure 43–1 Assisting with Application of Pit and Fissure Sealants

Some states allow qualified dental assistants to perform this procedure; in other states the dental assistant assists the dentist during the procedure. Check the regulations governing your state for more information about the specific duties dental assistants are allowed to perform. See Procedure 37-1 in Chapter 37, Expanded Clinical Functions, for this procedure as performed by the dental assistant.

Materials needed (Figure P43-1-1):

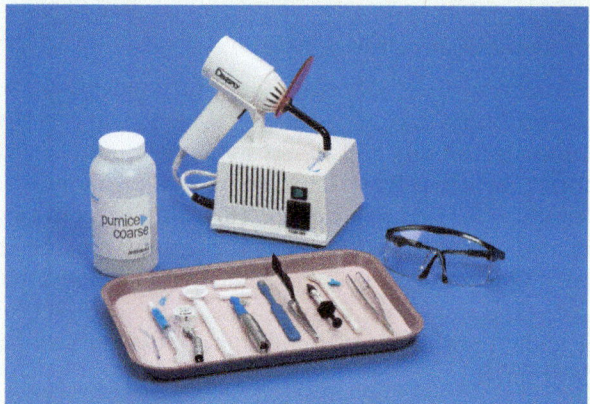

Figure P43-1-1

- Protective eyewear for patient and operators
- Dental dam, cotton rolls, and/or dry angles
- Basic setup
- Cotton tip applicator
- Sealant material
- Etching agent, gel or liquid
- Pumice and water
- Prophy brush
- Prophy angle
- Applicator device or syringe
- High-volume evacuator (HVE)
- Saliva ejector
- Air-water syringe
- Curing light with appropriate shield
- Articulating paper and holder
- Low-speed dental handpiece
- Round white stone, latch type
- Materials for occlusal adjustments, when filled resin product is used
- Dental floss

1. Put on appropriate PPE.
2. The dentist prepares the teeth with pumice and water. Standard tooth polish is not used because it may contain fluoride, flavors, and oils that can interfere with the sealant. Air polishers can also be used. If a sodium bicarbonate polisher is used, the dentist cleanses the teeth with hydrogen peroxide after cleaning to neutralize the sodium bicarbonate, and then thoroughly rinses the teeth with water.

3. Assist with the transfer of instruments and use the HVE to remove excess saliva and fluids.
4. The dentist checks the fissures with an explorer to make sure they are clear, then rinses and dries again with the air-water syringe.
5. The dentist isolates and dries the teeth using a dental dam, cotton rolls, and/or dry angles (Figure P43-1-2).

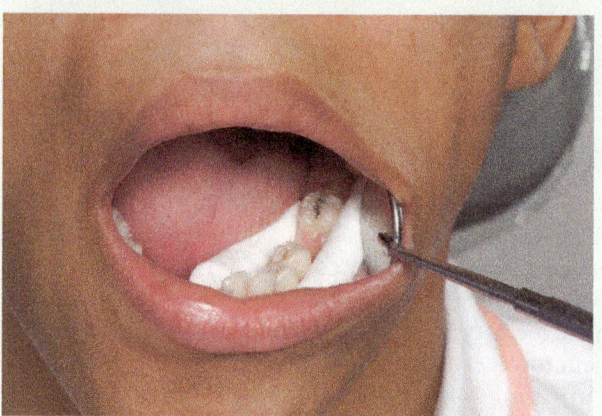

Figure P43-1-2

6. The dentist dries the teeth with the air-water syringe.
7. Transfer the etchant to the dentist. Be prepared to evacuate the area and provide instruments to the dentist as needed.
8. The dentist applies the etchant, following the manufacturer's directions, extending the margin of the etched area just beyond the margin of the area to be sealed (Figure P43-1-3). The dentist etches the teeth for between 15 and 30 seconds for permanent dentition, depending on the product, or between 50 and 60 seconds for primary dentition, but not for more than 60 seconds in either circumstance.

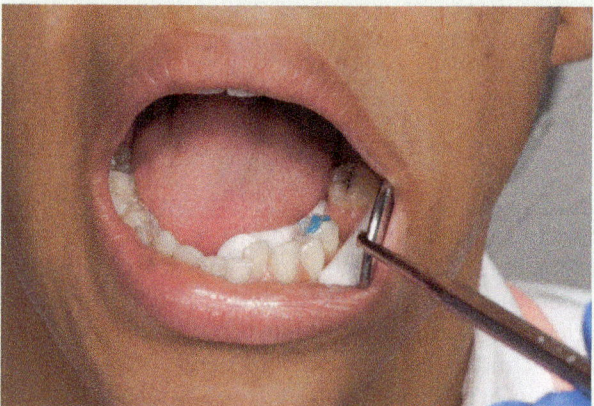

Figure P43-1-3

9. Use the evacuator to remove any excess etchant, and then rinse the area to completely remove all the etchant. Suction away water immediately.
10. Dry the tooth again, and replace the cotton rolls if they were used. Properly etched areas will be a frosty white (Figure P43-1-4).

Procedure 43-1 Assisting with Application of Pit and Fissure Sealants (Continued)

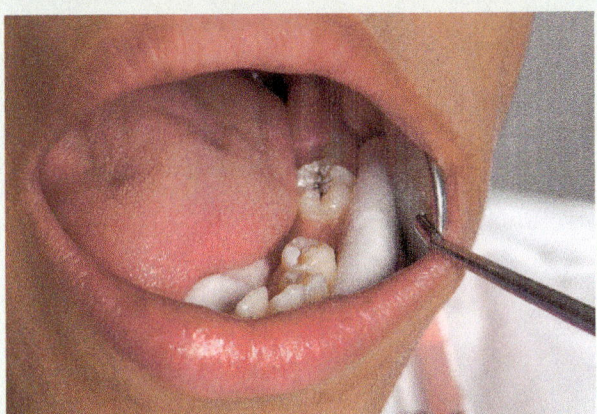

Figure P43-1-4

11. Transfer the sealant to the dentist. Be prepared to evacuate the area and provide instruments to the dentist as needed.

12. The dentist applies the sealant according to the manufacturer's directions, making sure the sealant does not flow beyond the etched areas (Figure P43-1-5). The dentist checks the sealed areas with an excavator to make sure the tooth is completely sealed. If there are gaps in coverage, more sealant is applied as long as no saliva has contacted the area. If saliva has contacted the unsealed area, it must be etched first.

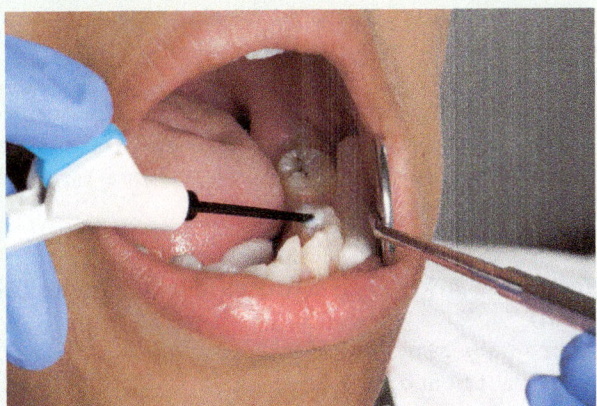

Figure P43-1-5

13. The dentist cures the sealant if necessary, according to the manufacturer's instructions.

14. The dentist checks the sealant again with an excavator and fills in any gaps in coverage.

15. The dentist removes the moisture control devices and checks the interproximal areas with dental floss to make sure that no extra sealant is obstructing the space.

16. The dentist wipes the hardened sealant with a cotton applicator to remove the haze (Figure P43-1-6).

17. Record the procedure in the patient's record and provide the patient with instructions.

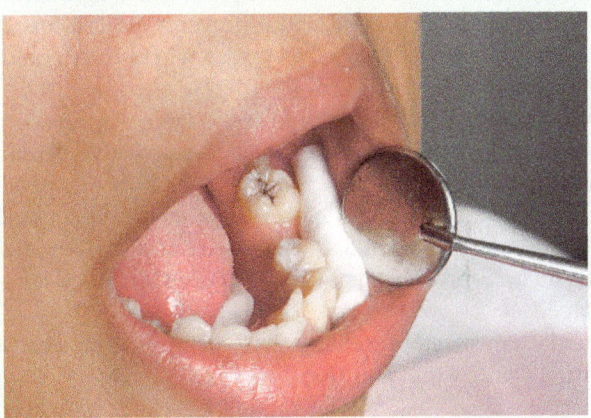

Figure P43-1-6

Restorative Procedures

Pediatric restorative dentistry is very similar to adult restorative dentistry. The same materials and procedures are generally used. The main difference is in the instrumentation—pediatric instruments are often smaller to fit more easily into a child's mouth. Smaller instruments include handpieces, forceps, dental dams, and dental clamps.

As with restorations in adults, dentists use amalgam and composite resins in primary and permanent teeth when pediatric restorations are needed. Additionally, pediatric patients can be fitted with appliances such as stainless steel crowns.

Pediatric Matrices

In adult dentistry, the most common matrix system is the Tofflemire matrix. However, in pediatric dentistry, the two most common matrices are the T-band matrix and spot-welded matrix band. These are custom matrices that can be used on primary teeth.

T-band matrices are made from pliable metal strips that can be adjusted to fit primary teeth. They do not require retainers. T-band matrices are available in various sizes for pediatric patients.

Spot-welded matrix bands are made in the office with a spot-welding machine that welds the matrix material to fit primary teeth.

Matrices are covered in greater depth in Chapter 36, Assisting in Restorations.

Pediatric Dental Dams

Dental dams are very useful during pediatric procedures, including the application of sealants. A properly fitted dental dam prevents the child from exploring the treatment area with his or her tongue, and it prevents materials and liquids from entering the child's throat, where they could be aspirated.

Pediatric dental dams function in the same way as adult dental dams, although they are smaller. A pediatric dental dam typically measures 5 × 5 inches. The holes in pediatric dams are smaller and closer together to reflect the smaller dentition. Dental dam clamps are also smaller and might include projections to help secure the dental dam in place.

Dental dams are covered in greater depth in Chapter 27, Moisture Control and Isolation.

Endodontic Procedures

Pulp Therapy

Pulp therapy is used to help rejuvenate teeth that have suffered from trauma or have extremely deep caries. Three therapies are used; the choice depends on the extent of the damage to the pulp and whether it is exposed or not. Pulp damage is assessed during an examination and with dental radiographs. Pain and tooth mobility are also useful indicators of the extent of a lesion.

Pulp therapies include:

- *Indirect pulp treatment* (IPT). This is used when the pulp is not yet exposed. In this procedure, the restoration site is prepared but a thin layer of dentin is left over the pulp (carious and non-carious pulp may be used). A medication is placed in the site and a temporary restoration is placed. After a healing period of 6 to 8 weeks, the temporary restoration is removed and a permanent restoration can be placed.
- *Direct pulp capping* (DPC). This is used when the pulp has been exposed, but the dentist feels there is a chance the pulp can regenerate. In this procedure, the restoration site is prepared and a medicated liner is applied directly to the pulp. A temporary restoration may be placed, or a permanent restoration put in place.

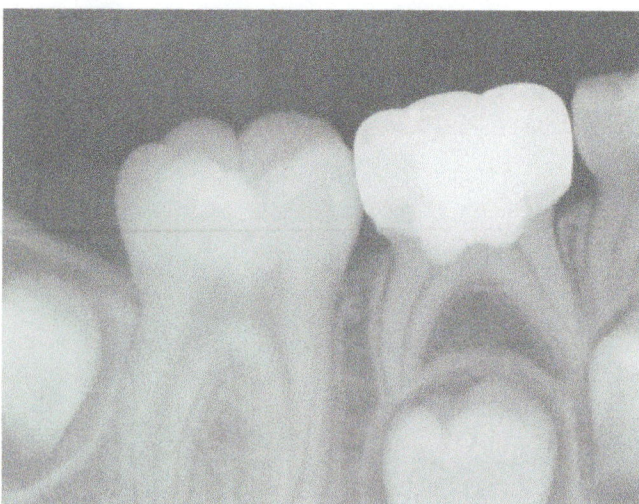

Figure 43–4 Radiograph of deciduous tooth with a pulpotomy and stainless steel crown. (Courtesy of Dr. Glenn Boyles, Fairmont, W.V.)

- *Pulpotomy*. A pulpotomy is indicated if the pulp is permanently damaged and has to be partially removed (Figure 43-4). During this procedure, the coronal pulp is removed, leaving healthy canal pulp. This treatment can help save newly erupted permanent teeth by allowing the roots to fully develop.

Prosthodontic Procedures

The most common prosthodontic procedure performed on primary teeth is the placement of **stainless steel crowns**. These crowns may be indicated in a variety of situations, including:

- Severe caries or carious lesions
- Teeth that lack sufficient calcification (hypocalcified teeth)
- After a pulpotomy
- After placement of a space maintainer
- After trauma

Stainless steel crowns are well tolerated by children and are an economical alternative to placement of restorations and can usually be placed in a single appointment. They are available in a variety of sizes. There are two types of stainless steel crowns:

- *Pretrimmed crowns*. These crowns have straightened sides and must be contoured prior to placement (**festooned**) to follow the natural contours of healthy, normal gingival tissue.
- *Precontoured crowns*. These have been contoured already and may only need additional minor trimming to fit the tooth.

Procedure 43-2 Assisting with Stainless Steel Crown Placement

Materials needed (Figure P43-2-1):

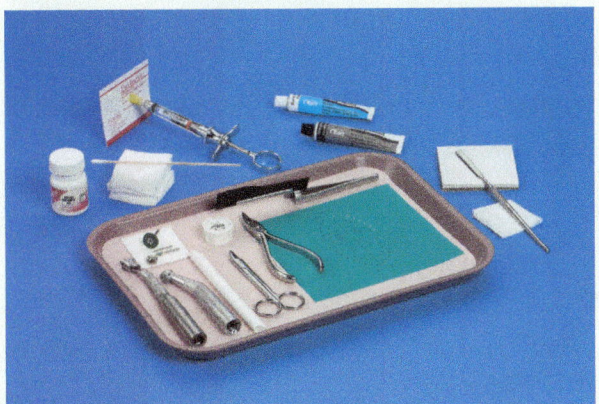

Figure P43-2-1

- Anesthetic supplies
- High-speed handpiece and low-speed handpiece
- Selected burs
- Green stone
- Rubber abrasive wheel
- High-volume evacuator (HVE)
- Dental dam
- Selection of stainless steel crowns
- Crown and collar scissors
- Articulating paper
- Dental floss
- Crimping pliers
- Cement supplies
- Spatula
- Mixing pad

1. Put on appropriate PPE.
2. Assist with the administration of local anesthetic and the placement of the dental dam.
3. Transfer the high-speed handpiece to the dentist during the tooth preparation. The most common bur is the tapered diamond bur.
4. The dentist reduces both the height and the circumference of the tooth.
5. The dentist makes sure that all areas of dental caries are removed.
6. The crown is selected that fits the tooth. It should fit tightly around the tooth circumference, with both mesial and distal contact.

7. The dentist adjusts the occlusal and gingival height of the crown with the crown and collar scissors (Figure P43-2-2). The occlusal surface should be level with the adjacent teeth and the gingival margin should extend one millimeter beyond the preparation margin.

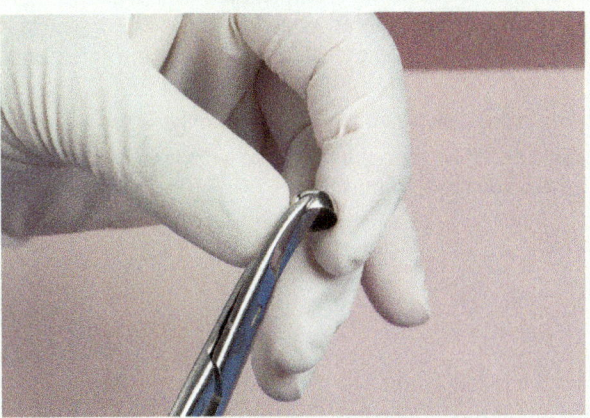

Figure P43-2-2

8. The dentist uses a green stone to smooth the rough edges of the crown where it was trimmed. The crown margin is then polished with a rubber abrasive wheel.
9. The dentist places the crown on the tooth and checks the occlusion with articulating paper. The dentist also checks the contacts with floss. Any necessary adjustments are made. The dentist then removes the crown.
10. The dentist contours and crimps the crown with the crimping pliers (Figure P43-2-3). The crown is crimped near the cervical margin toward the tooth.

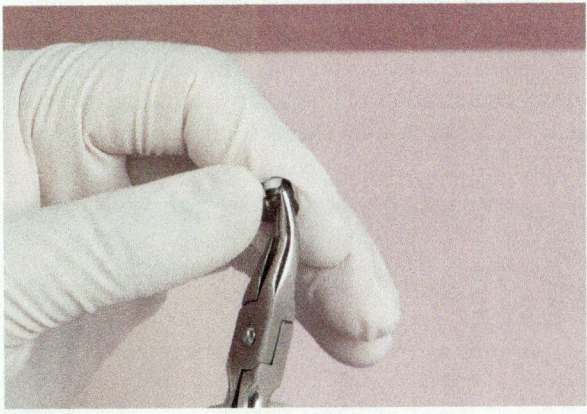

Figure P43-2-3

Procedure 43-2 **Assisting with Stainless Steel Crown Placement (Continued)**

11. Dry the tooth completely after the crown is removed.

12. Mix the cement according to the manufacturer's instructions and apply it to both the tooth and the crown.

13. Transfer the crown to the dentist for placement.

14. The dentist places the crown and removes excess cement from the crown with an explorer (Figure P43-2-4). Floss is used to remove excess cement from the interdental contacts.

15. Rinse the crown with the air-water syringe.

16. Document the procedure in the patient's record and provide the patient with instructions.

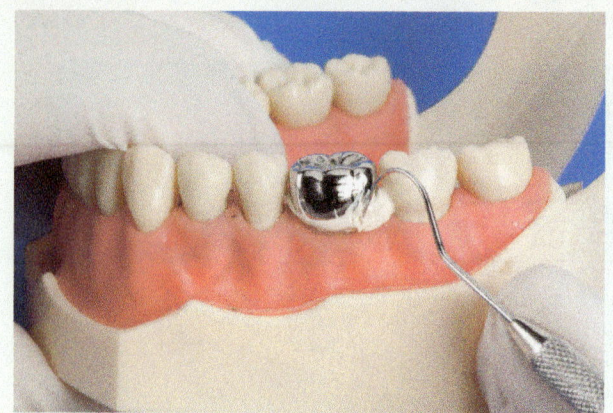

Figure P43-2-4

Treatment of Dental Trauma

Dental emergencies are relatively common in children, especially in the toddler years when children are learning how to walk and may be unsteady on their feet. Other causes of dental trauma include vehicular accidents (automobile and bicycle), sports injuries, and child abuse.

Dental trauma in primary teeth is important because of potential damage to the underlying permanent teeth.

Fractured Teeth

The teeth most commonly fractured are maxillary anterior teeth, which are usually damaged in an accident or a blow to the face (Figure 43-5). Children with fractured teeth should see the dentist as soon as possible. The office visit should include documentation of the injury, including its cause, a clinical examination, pulp vitality testing, and radiography.

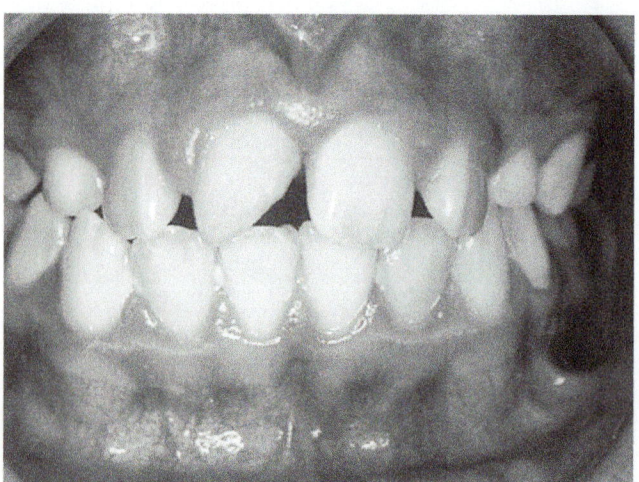

Figure 43-5 Fractured pediatric tooth.

Treatment for fractured teeth depends on the extent of the injury. In the initial assessment, the dentist determines the extent of the injury and if the pulp is injured. In mild injuries, where only the enamel is involved, treatment may be limited to smoothing the rough edges of the fractured tooth. If the crown is fractured and the pulp is exposed, however, a root canal followed by placement of a crown might be indicated. In many cases, the dentist delays treatment of the fracture to give the pulp time to recover on its own. A temporary restoration may be placed during this time.

Traumatic Intrusion

Traumatic intrusion occurs when one or more teeth are driven into the alveolus, leaving only a portion of the crown visible. Traumatic intrusion can occur with either primary or permanent teeth.

Treatment for traumatic intrusion of a primary tooth is to let the tooth re-erupt on its own. Later treatment may be required. In some cases, traumatic intrusion of a primary tooth causes damage to the underlying permanent tooth, but it is impossible to know the extent of this damage until the permanent tooth erupts.

Tooth Displacement

Tooth displacement occurs when teeth are shifted from their positions. These types of injuries are known as *extrusion* or *luxation* injuries. The displacement is often accompanied by extensive damage to the periodontal ligaments.

Treatment of tooth displacement among permanent teeth is to reposition the teeth as soon as possible. Splints may be placed for two to four weeks to stabilize the teeth. After treatment, the teeth should be monitored to see if they need endodontic treatment.

Avulsed Teeth

An avulsed tooth is a tooth that has been completely removed from the socket as a result of trauma. Primary teeth are not replaced after avulsion, while permanent teeth can be replaced with varying degrees of success. The key to success with permanent tooth replacement is speed: the tooth should be replaced as soon as possible. If parents replace the tooth in the socket, it increases the odds of a successful placement. If the tooth cannot be immediately replaced, it should be wrapped in a moistened gauze or placed in a container of milk, water, or saliva, and the patient and the tooth should be taken to the dentist immediately. Avulsed teeth should not be rinsed.

CHECKPOINTS

43-7 How frequently should pediatric patients have a routine dental exam?

43-8 How often should children at high risk of caries have their radiographs updated?

43-9 What is recommended to help prevent traumatic dental injury to children who play sports?

43-10 What procedure can help prevent the development of caries in posterior teeth?

Child Abuse and Reporting Laws

Child abuse is a serious societal issue that health care workers may encounter when working frequently with children. There are many types of abuse, including physical and sexual. Health care workers are mandated by law to report suspected child abuse. This includes physicians, nurses, dentists, orthodontists, dental hygienists, and dental assistants. All health professionals should be aware of the signs of child abuse and know the proper protocol for reporting suspected abuse.

Signs of possible child abuse include:

- Missing or chipped teeth with no explanation or an explanation inconsistent with the observed trauma
- Frequent and repetitive injuries
- Bruises around the mouth or anywhere else on the body

- Torn labial frena
- Lack of hygiene or appropriate clothing for the season
- Extensive caries and lack of parental concern
- Parental defensiveness
- Bite or tooth marks
- Injuries at various stages of healing
- Blackened eyes
- Broken nose

A child with any of these injuries has not necessarily been abused, since children are prone to injury from playing. But dental professionals should take cues from the parent's behavior. Are the parents or guardians evasive? Do they appear genuinely concerned? Does their story match with the child's explanation? Is the explanation consistent with the injuries?

Reporting suspected child abuse is a serious matter that brings a family into the legal system. Nevertheless, dental professionals are legally obligated to report suspected abuse. The legal term for this is mandated reporters, or people who face fines and legal action if they do not report suspected child abuse.

Suspected or validated child abuse must be reported by phone or in person to a state's child protective services agency, followed by a written report, usually within 72 hours, although reporting requirements vary from state to state. Typical requirements include:

- The nature of the injury or injuries
- A detailed description of the injury or injuries
- Diagnostic and lab work, such as radiographs or test results
- Personal information on the child, such as age, sex, address, and date of birth
- Personal information on the parents, such as address and names
- Name of the family physician, if available
- The explanations for the injury offered by the family

When confronted with a potential case of child abuse, it is important to remember that the reporting laws are there for the child's safety. Even if no abuse is found, mandated reporter laws are designed to identify and stop abuse that has lifelong consequences for its young victims. If you suspect a patient is a victim of abuse, speak to the dentist in private immediately.

CHECKPOINT

43-11 What happens if a dental professional does not report a case of suspected abuse?

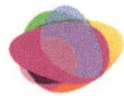

Chapter Highlights

✦ Pediatric dentistry focuses on children and some adults with special needs.

✦ Pediatric dental offices should be designed to put children at ease and keep them busy during office visits.

✦ Children's emotional and mental ages may differ from their chronological age.

✦ The Frankl scale rates behavior on a scale of 1 to 4. A 1 rating indicates the child behaves negatively, while a 4 rating indicates the child is strongly positive and behaves cooperatively.

✦ Behavior management techniques to help control children include tell, show, and do; distraction; modeling; voice and face control; restraints; and pharmacological sedation.

✦ Pediatric office visits include an exam, instruction in oral hygiene, polishing, radiographs, possibly fluoride treatments, and other procedures that will help instill a lifelong appreciation of dental care.

✦ Pit and fissure sealants are used to dramatically reduce the risk of caries in pediatric posterior teeth. The application of pit and fissure sealants is an expanded function in some states

✦ Pediatric restorative dentistry is similar to adult dentistry, only with smaller instrumentation and equipment such as matrices and dental dams.

✦ Pulp therapy is designed to rejuvenate pulp in a damaged tooth. Various procedures are used to allow the pulp to heal on its own.

✦ Stainless steel crowns may be placed on children with serious caries, with hypocalcification, after a pulpotomy or placement of a space maintainer, or after trauma.

✦ Dental trauma is a relatively common occurrence in children. Injuries include fractured teeth, displaced teeth, traumatic intrusion, and avulsed teeth.

✦ All suspected cases of child abuse must be reported by law to the state agency for child protection.

Review Questions

1. When does socialization usually start?

   a. Birth through age 2

   b. 3 to 5 years of age

   c. 6 to 12 years of age

   d. 12 to 15 years of age

2. Which supports positive modeling?

   a. Speaking in a firm voice

   b. Using props to demonstrate techniques

   c. Open-bay treatment areas

   d. None of the above

3. Pharmacological sedation

   a. Can only be used with prior consent.

   b. Can be either partial or total.

   c. Can be administered in the dental office.

   d. All of the above.

4. How often should children at risk of caries have updated radiographs?

   a. Yearly

   b. Every 6 months

   c. Every 2 years

   d. Every 3 months

5. Mouth guards are used

   a. To prevent thumb sucking.

   b. To correct grinding.

   c. To correct crossbite.

   d. To protect teeth during sports.

6. Pit and fissure sealants are indicated

   a. For children at risk for extensive caries.

   b. As a preventive measure for healthy children.

   c. For children with deep pits and fissures.

   d. All of the above.

7. Filled sealants

   a. Create a smooth chewing surface.

   b. Are made from amalgam.

   c. Contain additives to resist wear.

   d. Are putty-like.

8. Which matrix is often used in pediatric patients?

   a. Universal

   b. Tofflemire

   c. T-band

   d. Rubber loop

9. During direct pulp capping
   a. The tooth is removed.
   b. Medication is applied to an exposed pulp cavity.
   c. Medication is applied to an intact pulp cavity.
   d. The pulp is partially removed.

10. What might require placement of a stainless steel crown?
    a. Tooth avulsion
    b. Severe caries
    c. Traumatic intrusion
    d. Risk of premature eruption

11. What is done for traumatic intrusion of a primary tooth?
    a. Tooth removal
    b. Placement of bands to aid eruption
    c. Antibiotics and fluoride to prevent caries and infection
    d. Time to let tooth re-erupt

12. Who is a mandated reporter for suspected child abuse?
    a. Dental assistant
    b. Dental hygienist
    c. Dentist
    d. All of the above

Active Learning Exercises

1. Imagine that a 6-year-old child presents to the dental office with a severe toothache. Never having undergone treatment before, the child is scared and apprehensive about the visit. What behavior modifications or techniques can the dental team use to help manage this patient most effectively?

2. When a child presents as an emergency patient with several fractured teeth, what type of tray setup may be necessary? What are the initial steps the dentist may recommend before any treatment is administered?

3. What are the current laws in your state regarding the reporting of suspected child abuse or neglect? What are the differences between child abuse and neglect? Provide some examples.

Application Activities

1. Select one of the behavioral management techniques described in the chapter and write a specific strategy you could use to help calm a child who is exhibiting negative behavior during a procedure.

2. Practice explaining good oral hygiene practices in language that children can understand.

3. Describe a variety of common dental instruments in terms that children can understand. For example, the x-ray tube head is a "camera."

4. Practice explaining various dental procedures in language that children can understand.

5. Role-play a dental assistant explaining the importance of the primary teeth to a parent. Be sure to emphasize *why* it is important to take care of the primary teeth.

PREPARING FOR CERTIFICATION EXAMS

Review the following topics in this chapter to prepare for the Dental Assisting National Board (DANB) exam:

- **Pediatric Behavior Management**
- **Pediatric Treatments**
- **Pit and Fissure Sealants**

Coronal Polishing

CHAPTER OUTLINE

CHAPTER CHECKLIST

On completion of this chapter, students will be able to:

☑ Discuss the use of coronal polishing, including its indications and contraindications.

☑ Identify the types of stains and deposits that can be removed by coronal polishing.

☑ Identify and describe the equipment commonly used for coronal polishing.

☑ Identify the various types of abrasive agents and describe their function.

☑ Explain the role of the dental assistant in providing support during polishing procedures.

KEY TERMS

abrasion – the wearing away of a surface by an abrasive agent

coronal (KORE-uh-nul) polishing – removal of stains and plaque from the clinical crown

endogenous (en-DOJ-uh-nus) stain – a stain that occurs within the tooth's structure

exogenous (ek-SOJ-uh-nus) stain – a stain that is caused by external factors, such as food, drink, and tobacco

extrinsic stain – adherence of bacteria or discoloring agents to dental enamel that causes discoloration

intrinsic strain – discoloration of internal tooth structure due to external agents that have been absorbed into the tooth's structure

posteruptive stain – a stain that occurs after the tooth erupts and can include stains caused by amalgam and root canal therapy

preeruptive stain – a stain that occurs while the teeth are still forming and can include stains caused by medicines, fluoride in drinking water, and inherited conditions

prophylaxis angle – angled instrument that holds the rubber cup and brush bristles used in coronal polishing; also called a prophy angle

selective polishing – an approach to coronal polishing wherein only stained teeth are polished

Introduction

Coronal polishing is the removal of stains and plaque from the area of the tooth that is visible—called the clinical crown. However, there is an important difference between a dental prophylaxis, or cleaning, and coronal polishing. Polishing uses **abrasion**, or the wearing away of a surface by an abrasive agent, to remove soft deposits and stains from the outer surface of the tooth. In some states, this procedure can be performed by an expanded functions dental assistant. A dental prophylaxis involves removal of soft and hard deposits from the crown and roots of the teeth using instruments with cutting edges. Only a licensed dentist or registered dental hygienist is allowed to perform this procedure.

As a dental assistant you should understand the types of deposits and stains that can be removed with coronal polishing and the equipment and procedures used during the process.

Purposes for Coronal Polishing

Coronal polishing is used for several purposes, including:

- To reduce adhesion: smooth surfaces are harder for materials to stick to, which reduces the likelihood of stains and plaque
- To make the surface feel smoother: teeth that are smooth to the touch are more comfortable for patients
- To improve appearance: smooth, polished teeth are more attractive than stained, unpolished teeth
- To prepare the coronal portion of a tooth for a restoration or fixed appliance

Individuals who receive restorations often undergo coronal polishing before placement of the restoration. Such restorations include placement of dental sealants, crowns, bridges, and orthodontic bands.

Although coronal polishing is used to create a smooth surface, using abrasive material that is too coarse and strong can create grooves and scratches on the surface of the tooth. This causes the tooth surface to be uneven, actually increasing the likelihood of future plaque and stains. Table 44-1 outlines some guidelines for minimizing adverse effects when performing coronal polishing.

Contraindications for coronal polishing include the following:

- Lack of stains on tooth surfaces
- Sensitive teeth
- Exposed cementum or dentin
- Restored tooth surfaces
- Newly erupted teeth
- Implant abutments
- Areas of demineralization
- Gingiva that is enlarged, spongy, or soft or bleeds easily

TABLE 44-1 Dos and Don'ts of Coronal Polishing

DO...	DON'T...
Remember that all abrasive materials can potentially harm the surface of the tooth	Apply abrasives to gingival tissue
Apply abrasives slowly, using light-to-medium pressure	Apply quickly or produce too much heat when applying abrasives
Recognize that cementum and dentin abrade much easier than tooth enamel	Forget that polishing can damage the root surface
Use high-polish, low-abrasion prophy pastes	Use overly abrasive prophy pastes
Take a selective polishing approach	Polish every tooth simply because the patient asked you to; determine what does and does not need polishing and discuss with the patient

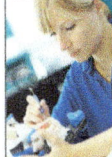

Voice of Experience

Some patients insist on undergoing coronal polishing even though their teeth do not need to be polished. It can be very difficult to convince these patients that the procedure is not needed. Before starting the polishing process, I find it helpful to educate patients on what procedures are considered "essential," such as a prophylaxis, and which are not always needed, such as polishing. I try to emphasize what can happen if teeth are polished unnecessarily—such as wearing down of enamel. This usually helps clear up any misconceptions and reassures patients that we are not neglecting their needs.

CHECKPOINT

45-1 Describe the difference between a dental prophylaxis and coronal polishing.

Deposits and Stains

Tooth stains can occur for a variety of reasons, and although they may not harm the health of the tooth, they can make teeth appear unattractive and unhealthy. Some stains can be removed using over-the-counter products, while tougher stains often must be removed by dental professionals. The stain removal process depends in part on the type of stain.

Cultural Diversity

Many cultures follow practices that ultimately lead to hard tissues stains. For example, in West Africa many people chew the seed of the *kola nut,* and in East Africa and some parts of the Middle East, many chew *khat* leaves. The remnants of these seeds and leaves create a very dark brown or black discoloration of the teeth. The *betel nut* is popular in many Asian and South Pacific countries, and those who chew it may develop a dark brown to black tarlike coating covering the teeth. Their lips may also turn deep red. Knowing about these prevalent practices can help you demonstrate your acceptance of patients from these cultures.

Types of Stains

The two main types of coronal stains are endogenous and exogenous. **Endogenous stains** occur within the tooth structure and include (Figure 44-1):

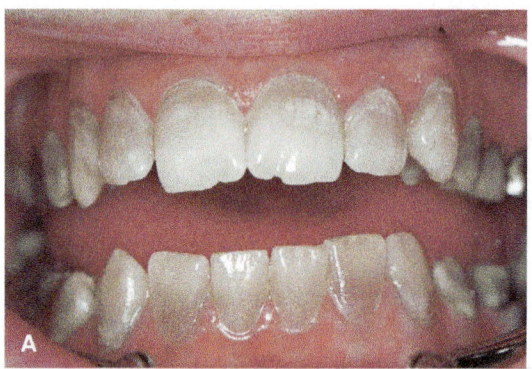

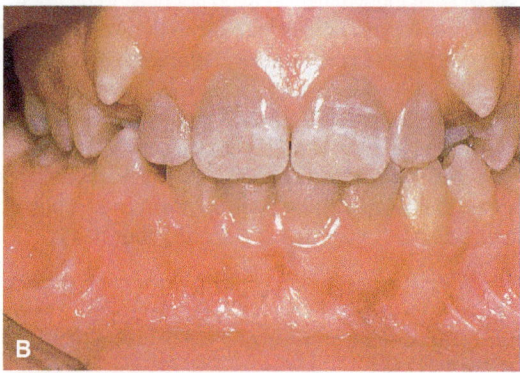

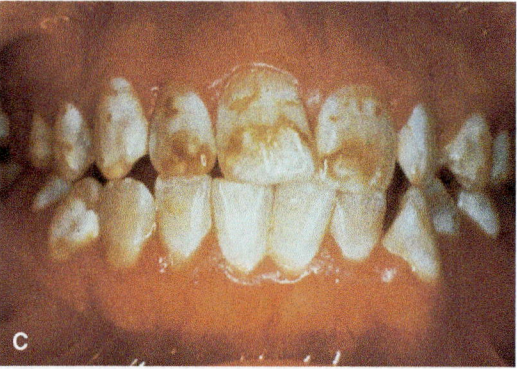

Figure 44–1 **Endogenous stains**. (**A**) Dentinogenesis imperfecta. (**B**) Tetracycline staining. (**C**) Fluorosis.

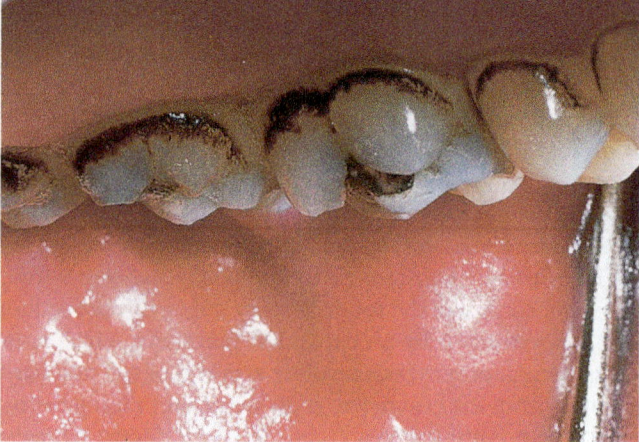

Figure 44–2 **Exogenous stains**. Caused by tobacco and coffee.

- **Posteruptive stains**: occur after the tooth erupts; include stains caused by silver amalgam, dental caries, and root canal therapy
- **Preeruptive stains**: occur while teeth are still forming and before they erupt; include stains caused by tetracycline antibiotics, high levels of fluoride in drinking water, and inherited conditions, such as dentinogenesis imperfecta and amelogenesis imperfecta

Exogenous stains are caused by external factors and are categorized as (Figure 44-2):

- **Extrinsic stains**: exist only on the outside of the tooth and are often caused by food and drinks, such as coffee, tea, and smoking and chewing tobacco; can sometimes be removed or reduced by over-the-counter whitening agents, but often must be removed in the dentist's office through scaling and coronal polishing
- **Intrinsic stains**: caused by external factors that have become absorbed into the structure of the tooth; frequently result from tobacco use

Types of Deposits

Dental deposits, which include plaque and bacteria, not only create an unattractive appearance and can cause halitosis, but they can also lead to dental caries and gingivitis. Deposits are categorized based on whether the deposited material is soft or hard in texture.

Soft Deposits

Soft deposits include materials that result in plaque, such as food particles. Soft deposits are removed during coronal polishing procedures.

Calculus

Hard deposits, also called calculus or tartar, form when plaque builds up over time and mineralizes. It is usually yellow or brown depending on the location of the calculus. Hard deposits result from unremoved plaque mixing with minerals and salts in saliva, causing the soft deposits to mineralize. Calculus does not cause gingival disease but it is a leading contributing factor. The outer surface of calculus is very rough and allows easy attachment for plaque. The dentist or dental hygienist removes any hard deposits from the patient's teeth before polishing takes place.

CHECKPOINTS

45-2 Name the two main types of coronal stains.

45-3 The use of tetracycline antibiotics while teeth are forming can cause what kind of stain?

Polishing Equipment

A variety of polishing equipment can be used to remove soft deposits and stains. Table 44-2 provides an overview of commonly used polishing equipment.

Using a Handpiece with a Prophylaxis Angle

The **prophylaxis angle**, or prophy angle, is an angled instrument that holds the rubber cup or brush bristles (Figure 44-3). It attaches to a low-speed handpiece through interlocking parts.

Prophy angles come in two types: reusable and disposable. A reusable prophy angle must be sterilized after every use, while a disposable prophy angle is used only once and then discarded. For infection control purposes, many offices use disposable prophy angles.

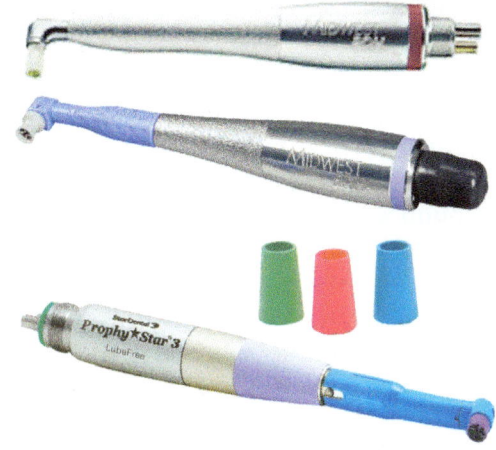

Figure 44–3 Prophy angle. Shown with a selection of cups and brushes. (Top two images courtesy of Dentsply Professional, www.prevent.dentsply.com. Bottom image courtesy of DentalEZ Group, www.dentalez.com/stardental/.)

The prophy angle and handpiece are held using the pen grip, with the handpiece resting between the thumb and index finger. Holding the prophy angle and handpiece correctly is important for avoiding hand strain. The handpiece itself should rotate at no more than 20,000 revolutions per minute. The speed of the handpiece can be controlled by pressing on the rheostat with the toe of the foot. When using the prophy angle and handpiece, the operator uses intermittent pressure and applies strokes in a circular motion. Steady pressure can cause excess heat, which can damage the tooth and cause pain for the patient. The rheostat should be released as soon as the prophy angle and handpiece is no longer touching the tooth; otherwise, it can cause the polishing material to splatter.

One key to ensuring proper use of a polishing instrument is the fulcrum, or finger rest. When using the handpiece, the operator's third finger usually acts as the fulcrum—just as when writing with a pencil. The fulcrum must be in the same arch and the same quadrant as the treatment area. The use of a fulcrum helps keep the instrument steady and prevents the hand and wrist from becoming tired or injured. The fulcrum may need to be repositioned as the prophy angle and handpiece are moved around the mouth. Avoid using a polishing instrument with a coiled cord, which can pull against your arm. The cord should be supported with your little finger or over the shoulder.

Abrasives

Abrasives are the materials that polish a surface. In dentistry, abrasive materials may be bound together on burs, disks, stones, wheels, or strips, or they may be used with liquids to form a paste. Single-use, premeasured prophy paste mixes are commonly used. Table 44-3 provides an overview of some commonly used dental abrasives.

TABLE 44-2 Commonly Used Polishing Equipment	
EQUIPMENT	**DESCRIPTION**
Air-powder	A handpiece that delivers a high-pressure stream of air, water, and sodium bicarbonate powder
Rubber cup	Attached to a low-speed handpiece and used with abrasive materials; the most popular type of polishing equipment used today
Bristle brush	Used to remove stains from deep grooves in the teeth; may be rough and stiff and must be used with care to avoid causing gingival bleeding

TABLE 44-3 Types of Abrasive Materials

TYPE	DESCRIPTION	FUNCTION
Chalk	■ A mineral form of calcite ■ Also called whiting or calcium carbonate ■ A mild abrasive	■ Used to polish teeth, gold and amalgam restorations, and plastic materials
Flour of pumice	■ Made from volcanic glass ■ An ingredient in "Lava Soap" and in pumice stones	■ Used to polish enamel, gold foil, and dental amalgam ■ Also used for finishing acrylic denture bases in the dental laboratory
Sand	■ A form of quartz ■ Comes in different colors ■ Typically bonded to special paper disks	■ Used for grinding metal and plastic
Silex	■ A commercial product ■ Supplied as a powder and mixed with liquid to form a paste	■ Used directly in the mouth as an abrasive material
Zirconium silicate	■ Powder form of the mineral zircon	■ Used to remove stains from enamel, composites, and gold restorations
Tin oxide	■ Supplied as a white powder ■ Extremely fine in texture ■ Used as a paste, similar to Silex	■ Used for polishing teeth and amalgams
Prophylaxis paste	■ Comes in several different colors, grits, flavors, and textures depending on the brand ■ May contain fluoride	■ Used to polish enamel

The operator must remember that coronal polishing with an abrasive always removes a microscopic layer of enamel. A variety of factors determine the amount of removal, including the speed of the handpiece, the pressure on the tooth, the amount of the abrasive used, the type of abrasive used, and the moisture content of the abrasive.

Commercially prepared prophy pastes and flour of pumice are available in a variety of grits or grades of abrasive particles. Grits can range from coarse to very fine. The choice of grit depends on the amount of stain and soft deposits to be removed. If the stain and soft deposit build-up is minimal, a fine or very fine grit is used. If the stains are heavier, a coarser grit is used. Therefore, the same grit is not used for all patients, since each patient's stain and soft deposit accumulation varies.

Tray Setup for Polishing Procedures

When setting up for polishing, make sure the tray includes these key pieces of equipment:

■ Mouth mirror
■ Explorer
■ Cotton gauze, rolls, and tips
■ Saliva ejector
■ Air-water syringe tip
■ Low-speed handpiece
■ Prophy angle
■ Rubber cups and brushes
■ Prophy paste
■ Disclosing solution
■ Dental floss

Patient and Operator Positioning

For the polishing procedure to be successful, both the patient and the operator must be seated in the proper position. Positioning for both is summarized in Table 44-4.

Selective Polishing

Most dental professionals perform **selective polishing**. This simply means that polishing is performed only in areas where it is necessary, since polishing areas of the tooth that are not stained may cause damage. It is not unusual for a patient to insist on polishing even if the teeth do not appear overly stained. It is important to explain to patients when polishing is and is not necessary, and how unnecessary polishing can contribute to the permanent removal of microscopic amounts of enamel.

TABLE 44-4 Proper Positions for Coronal Polishing

POSITIONING FOR THE PATIENT	POSITIONING FOR THE OPERATOR
Keep the chair in the supine position, with the head and knees even	Keep the seat close to the patient and low enough so that the thighs are parallel to the floor
For accessing the maxillary arch, tilt the chin upward	Elbows should be even with the patient's mouth
For accessing the mandibular arch, tilt the chin downward, toward the chest	For ideal positioning, imagine a clock, with the patient seated at the 12 o'clock position. Left-handed dental assistants should sit at the 2 to 3 o'clock position, while right-handed dental assistants should sit at 8 to 9 o'clock; occasionally the 12 o'clock position is recommended

Polishing Procedures

When polishing, the same procedure is used across all selected teeth, including the order in which teeth are polished and the area of the tooth surface that is polished. This helps ensure that all selected teeth are polished and done so in a correct manner. Polishing typically begins with the buccal surface and proceeds from the right side of the mouth to the left, moving across the mandibular arch. After all of the mandibular teeth are polished, work proceeds in the opposite direction, from left to right, focusing on the lingual surface. Next the teeth of the maxillary arch are polished in the same order and in the same manner.

Table 44-5 details a suggested order for rubber cup polishing.

Extra Patient Care

Offer patients lubricant for their lips and corners of their mouth. Prophylaxis and polishing procedures can cause the mouth to become very dry. Chapstick, Vaseline, or other lubricants can help patients feel more comfortable throughout the process.

CHECKPOINT

45-4 Why do many dental professionals use selective polishing rather than polishing all areas of a tooth?

TABLE 44-5 Rubber Cup Polishing Sequence

QUADRANT	OPERATOR POSITION	RETRACTION	FULCRUM
Maxillary right posterior, buccal aspect	8-9 o'clock	Cheek	Maxillary right incisors
Maxillary right posterior, lingual aspect	8-9 o'clock	Tongue	Lower incisors
Maxillary anterior, facial aspect	8-9 o'clock	None	Incisal edge
Maxillary anterior, lingual aspect	8-9 o'clock	None	Incisal edge
Maxillary left posterior, buccal aspect	9 o'clock	Cheek	Occlusal surface, buccal side
Maxillary left posterior, lingual aspect	8-9 o'clock	None	Maxillary left posterior teeth, buccal surface
Mandibular left posterior, buccal aspect	8-9 o'clock	Cheek	Mandibular left anterior teeth, incisal surface
Mandibular left posterior, lingual aspect	9 o'clock	Tongue	Mandibular anterior teeth
Mandibular anterior, facial aspect	8-9 o'clock	Lip	Incisal edge
Mandibular anterior, lingual aspect	8 o'clock	Tongue	Mandibular cuspid incisal edge
Mandibular right, buccal aspect	8 o'clock	Lip and cheek	Lower incisors
Mandibular right, lingual aspect	8 o'clock	Tongue	Lower incisors
Mandibular right, lingual aspect	8-9 o'clock	Tongue	Lower incisors

Procedure 44-1 Performing Rubber Cup Polishing

In some states, dental assistants are allowed to perform rubber cup polishing as an expanded function after meeting additional training and licensing requirements. In states that do not support expanded functions dental assistants, the dental assistant may assist while the dentist or dental hygienist performs this procedure.

Materials needed:

- Protective eyewear for patient and operators
- Rubber cups and brushes
- Disclosing solution
- Prophy paste
- Low-speed handpiece equipped with a prophy angle
- Saliva ejector or high-volume evacuator (HVE)
- Dental floss

1. Put on appropriate PPE.
2. Prepare the patient in the treatment chair with a neck napkin and protective eyewear. Explain the procedure and advise the patient on what to expect.
3. Use a disclosing solution to identify areas of heavy plaque concentration.
4. Begin polishing teeth. Use a set sequence to ensure that all teeth are polished in an efficient manner. Figures P44-1-1A through P44-1-1L show the position of the polishing cup and the proper fulcrum for different points within the oral cavity.

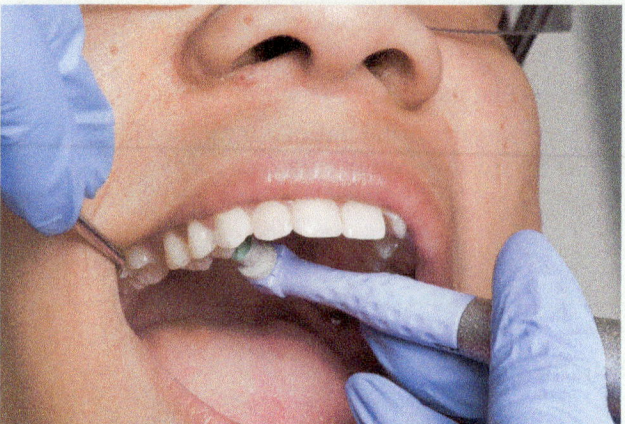

Figure P44-1-1B Polishing cup on maxillary right quadrant, lingual aspect, demonstrating fulcrum on mandibular incisors.

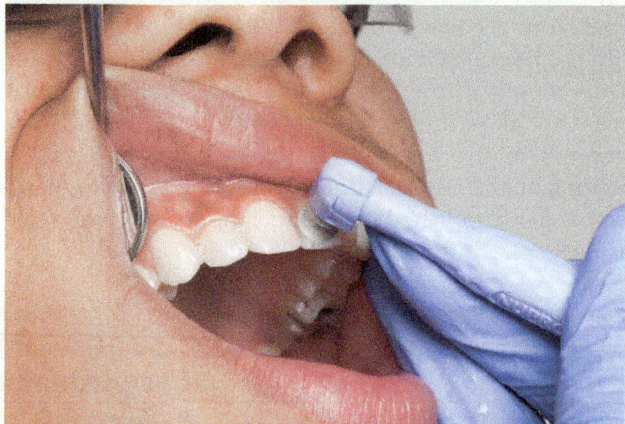

Figure P44-1-1C Polishing cup on maxillary anterior teeth, buccal aspect, demonstrating fulcrum on adjacent maxillary incisors.

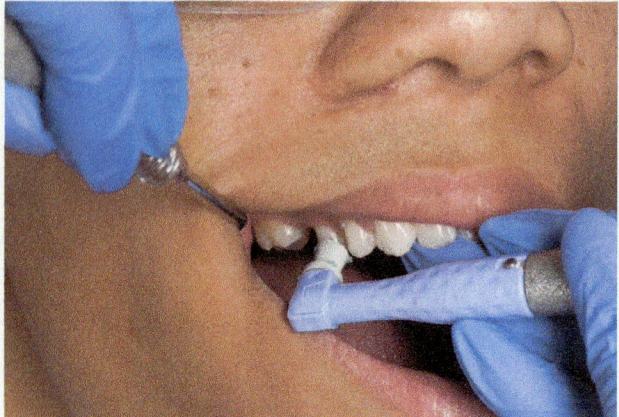

Figure P44-1-1A Polishing cup on maxillary right quadrant, buccal aspect, demonstrating fulcrum on maxillary right incisors.

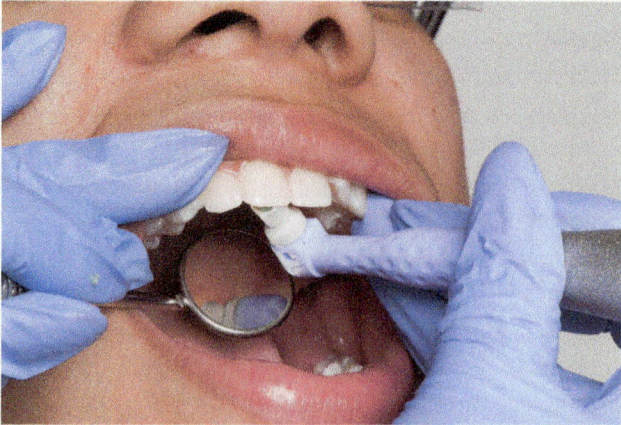

Figure P44-1-1D Polishing cup on maxillary anterior teeth, lingual aspect, demonstrating fulcrum on adjacent maxillary incisors.

Procedure 44-1 Performing Rubber Cup Polishing (Continued)

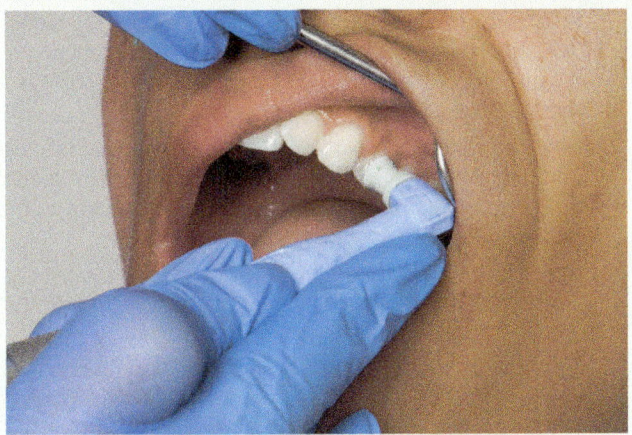

Figure P44-1-1E Polishing cup on maxillary left quadrant, buccal aspect, demonstrating fulcrum on mandibular premolars.

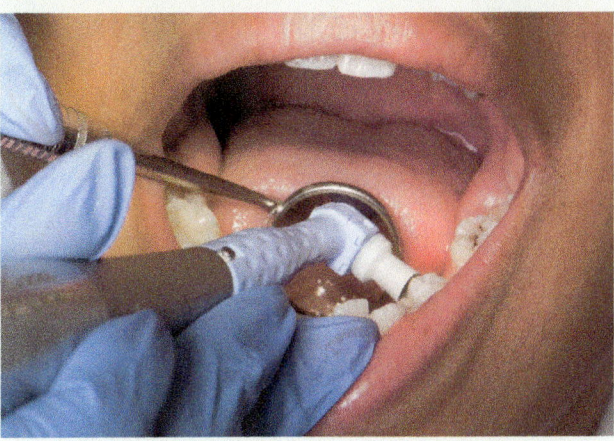

Figure P44-1-1H Polishing cup on mandibular left quadrant, lingual aspect, demonstrating fulcrum on mandibular anterior teeth.

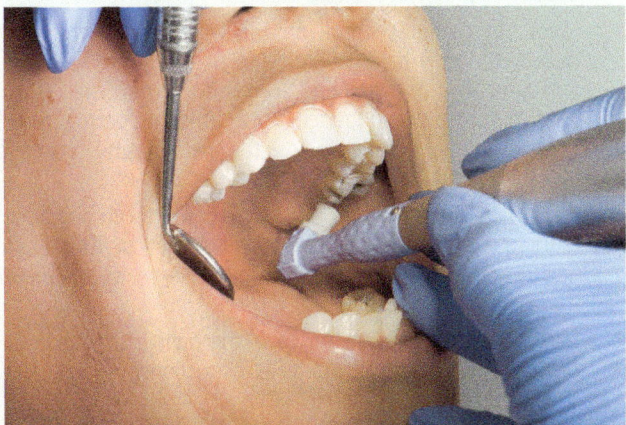

Figure P44-1-1F Polishing cup on maxillary left quadrant, lingual aspect, demonstrating fulcrum on mandibular left teeth.

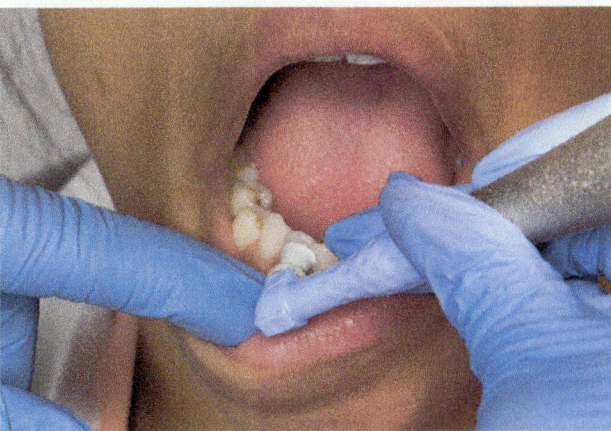

Figure P44-1-1I Polishing cup on mandibular anterior teeth, facial aspect, demonstrating fulcrum on adjacent anterior teeth.

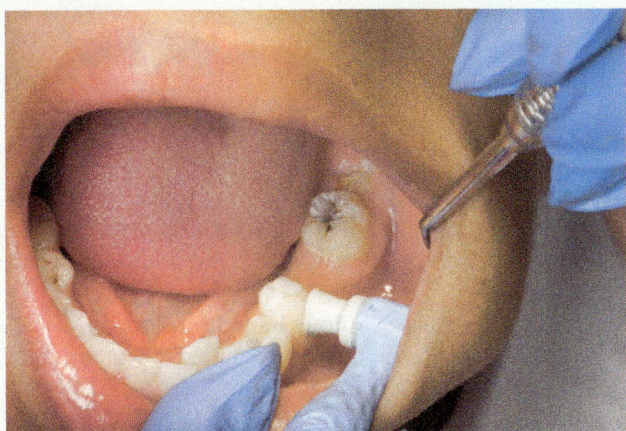

Figure P44-1-1G Polishing cup on mandibular left quadrant, buccal aspect, demonstrating fulcrum on mandibular left anterior teeth.

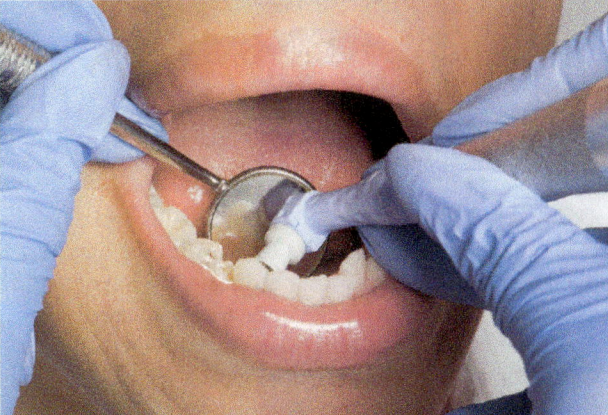

Figure P44-1-1J Polishing cup on mandibular anterior teeth, lingual aspect, demonstrating fulcrum on mandibular canine.

Procedure 44-1 **Performing Rubber Cup Polishing (Continued)**

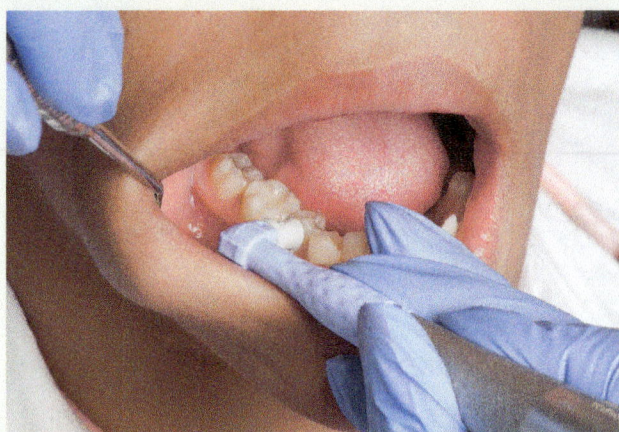

Figure P44-1-1K Polishing cup on mandibular right quadrant, buccal aspect, demonstrating fulcrum on mandibular anterior teeth.

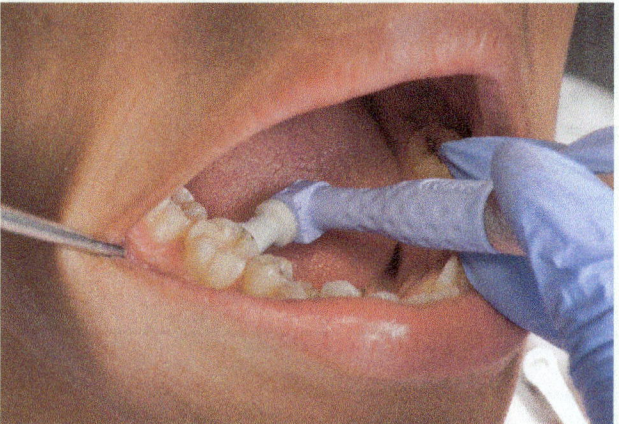

Figure P44-1-1L Polishing cup on mandibular right quadrant, lingual aspect, demonstrating fulcrum on mandibular anterior teeth.

5. Polish each tooth for approximately 3–5 seconds. Note that the cup should not remain on the tooth surface continuously for this amount of time, but rather, use light intermittent pressure and a sweeping motion.

6. Be sure to direct the polishing strokes from the cervical area down to the incisal or occlusal area. Never polish up into the cervical area, since this may cause the abrasive to be lodged under the tissue and become an irritant.

7. Use enough pressure on the tooth to see the rubber cup flare slightly. This flaring will enable you to polish to the gingival margin without causing tissue damage.

8. To polish the occlusal surfaces, use a bristle brush on the prophy angle or a disposable prophy angle with a bristle brush attached.

9. Once all teeth have been polished, rinse the patient's mouth with water and use the saliva ejector or high-volume evacuator to remove excess water and prophy paste.

10. Floss the patient's entire mouth, making sure that any debris that may have fallen between the teeth has been removed. To remove stains from the interproximal areas, apply prophy paste to the teeth or apply some prophy paste onto the dental floss, then floss the area, making sure that the abrasive paste is used on the stained areas.

11. Inspect all of the teeth to ensure that each tooth has been completely polished. Apply disclosing solution, then rinse and dry the teeth. If necessary, apply polish to any areas that still show debris.

12. Make a note of the procedure in the patient's record and provide the patient with self-care instructions.

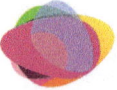 **Chapter Highlights**

✦ Coronal polishing is used to remove stains and deposits from the clinical crown of a tooth. Abrasive agents are used to make teeth smoother, reduce adhesion of plaque and stains, and improve the appearance of teeth.

✦ Tooth stains can be exogenous, occurring on the outside of the tooth, or endogenous, occurring within the structure of the tooth. Exogenous stains are often caused by food, drinks, and tobacco use, and can often be removed with polishing and whitening agents. Endogenous stains, however, are not easily removed.

✦ Soft deposits are removed during coronal polishing; hard deposits (called calculus) must first be removed with scaling.

✦ Commonly used polishing equipment includes air-powder equipment, rubber cups, bristle brushes, and the prophylaxis angle. When using polishing equipment, such as the prophylaxis angle, always use a fulcrum to ensure hand stability.

✦ Proper polishing technique includes using a low-speed handpiece, using a circular sweeping motion, avoiding applying steady pressure to the tooth, and using a fulcrum.

✦ Abrasive agents wear away at the surface of the tooth, resulting in a polished surface. There are numerous types of abrasives, each with a specific function.

✦ Most dentists today use a selective polishing approach, meaning that they only polish teeth that are stained and need to be polished. Although some patients request coronal polishing of all teeth, polishing teeth unnecessarily can cause a microscopic layer of enamel to be lost.

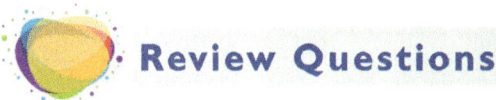

Review Questions

1. Coronal polishing
   a. Should be completed every time a patient comes in for a prophylaxis.
   b. Can improve the appearance of teeth and help make them healthier.
   c. Is needed only for front teeth that are visible.
   d. Is not needed for patients who use over-the-counter whitening products.

2. Which are less likely to be improved by coronal polishing?
   a. Soft deposits from food and drinks
   b. Dentinogenesis imperfecta
   c. Extrinsic tobacco stains
   d. Intrinsic tobacco stains

3. The most commonly used piece of equipment in coronal polishing is the
   a. Rubber cup and prophy angle.
   b. Air-powder handpiece.
   c. Bristle brush and prophy angle.
   d. Prophy angle and dental scaler.

4. When performing coronal polishing,
   a. Apply steady pressure with the rubber cup to ensure the stain is completely removed.
   b. Use a high-speed handpiece on tough stains.
   c. Use an up-and-down motion.
   d. Allow the third finger to act as a fulcrum.

5. All of the following abrasive materials are used for polishing teeth except
   a. Emery.
   b. Chalk.
   c. Silex.
   d. Prophylaxis paste.

6. Selective polishing
   a. Is used at the request of the patient.
   b. Is mandatory in some states but not mandatory in others.
   c. Ensures that teeth are not polished unnecessarily.
   d. Can reduce costs for patients without dental insurance.

Active Learning Exercises

1. Identify the types of stains that can be removed with coronal polishing. What is the method and pressure used to remove stains?

2. Most patients expect to have all of their teeth polished after they have had a dental scaling; however, in some cases, polishing is not indicated. Give some examples of when and why polishing would not be indicated.

3. List the states that allow dental assistants to perform coronal polishing.

Application Activities

1. Using the instruments and equipment your instructor provides (including a dental model), practice the correct polishing techniques, including the correct grasp of the prophy handpiece, using a fulcrum, and positioning of the hand as you work around the mouth. Develop a systematic procedure for ensuring that all teeth are polished as needed.

2. Suppose a patient insists on receiving coronal polishing even though stains are not present. How can you go about educating the patient without making it seem as though you are overlooking his or her needs? If a patient is insistent, what do you do? Do you perform the procedure even though it is not needed?

PREPARING FOR CERTIFICATION EXAMS

Review the following topics in this chapter to prepare for the Dental Assisting National Board (DANB) exam:

● **Tray Setup for Polishing Procedures**

● **Polishing Procedures**

Orthodontics

CHAPTER OUTLINE

CHAPTER CHECKLIST

On completion of this chapter, students will be able to:

- ☑ Identify the members of an orthodontic team and describe their responsibilities.
- ☑ Describe the characteristics of normal occlusion.
- ☑ Identify types of malocclusion and misalignment.
- ☑ Describe the steps of developing an orthodontic treatment plan.
- ☑ Identify and describe the various instruments used in orthodontic procedures.
- ☑ Identify and describe common fixed and removable appliances.
- ☑ Explain the role of the dental assistant in providing support during common orthodontic treatments.
- ☑ Describe important aspects of patient education and self-care for patients receiving orthodontic treatment.

KEY TERMS

buccoversion (buck-oh-VER-zhun) – malposition of a posterior tooth from the normal line of occlusion toward the cheek

crossbite – abnormal relationship of one or more teeth of one arch to the opposing tooth or teeth of the other arch due to labial, buccal, or lingual deviation of tooth position, or abnormal jaw position

crowding – a condition in which the teeth are crowded and in altered positions such as bunching, overlapping, displacement in various directions, and torsiversion

distoversion (dis-toe-VER-zhun) – malposition of a tooth distal to normal, in a posterior direction following the curvature of the dental arch

labioversion (lay-bee-oh-VER-zhun) – malposition of an anterior tooth from the normal line of occlusion toward the lips

linguoversion (ling-gwo-VER-zhun) – malposition of a tooth lingual to the normal position

mesioversion (mee-zee-oh-VER-zhun) – malposition of a tooth mesial to the normal position, in an anterior direction following the curvature of dental arch

open bite – a large intraoral distance in which the maxillary anterior teeth do not occlude with the mandibular anterior teeth

overbite – vertical overlap of teeth

overjet – horizontal overlap of teeth

supraversion – the position of a tooth when it is out of the line of occlusion in an occlusal direction

torsiversion (tor-sih-VER-zhun) – malposition of a tooth in which it is rotated on its long axis

traction – act of drawing or pulling, as by an elastic or spring force

transposition – misplacement of teeth from the normal sequence in the arch

transversion – eruption of a tooth in a position normally occupied by another

Introduction

Orthodontics is the branch of dentistry concerned with malocclusion and abnormalities in the alignment of facial structures, including teeth, jaws, and face. The most common orthodontic patient is a younger person with developing dentofacial structures, but orthodontic treatment is also becoming more common among adults. Orthodontics focuses on preventing irregularities and correcting existing problems. Dental assistants, especially those with additional training for expanded functions in those states that allow dental assistants to perform additional procedures, have an important role in orthodontic dentistry.

The Orthodontic Practice

The orthodontic practice is similar to the dental office, except it is headed by an orthodontist instead of a dentist. Orthodontic offices usually work closely with dental offices to provide complete treatment for patients.

In addition to the orthodontic assistant, a typical staff in an orthodontic office includes:

- *Orthodontist:* An orthodontist has an additional 2 to 3 years of schooling in an accredited orthodontic program after dental school. Orthodontists are highly trained in the anatomy and development of facial structures, as well as new technologies and procedures to correct irregularities.
- *Laboratory technician:* Orthodontics relies on the use of casts and molds. The laboratory technician is the staff member who pours the molds and creates casts, as well as fabricates appliances.
- *Treatment coordinator:* Serving as a liaison between the orthodontist and the patient, the treatment coordinator provides support and guidance to patients throughout the treatment process. Responsibilities include handling patient correspondence, discussing treatment options, understanding patient needs, scheduling appointments, and answering patient questions.
- *Office staff:* An orthodontic office is staffed with many of the same support personnel as a dental office, including a receptionist, office or business manager, and perhaps other personnel, depending on the size of the practice.

The Role of the Orthodontic Assistant

Orthodontic assistants function in a similar capacity to dental assistants: They provide a crucial link between the patient and the orthodontist; they help transition patients into the treatment area; and they assist with numerous procedures. Their exact responsibilities vary from state to state. In some states, expanded functions dental assistant laws allow orthodontic assistants with additional training to play a more direct role in procedures. In other states, the orthodontic assistant helps the orthodontist.

Orthodontic assistants who pass the Dental Assisting National Board in Orthodontic Assisting receive the certified orthodontic assistant (COA) designation. Many states have additional titles and licenses for orthodontic assistants.

Typical duties for an orthodontic assistant include:

- Take dental impressions
- Pour, trim, and finish diagnostic models
- Obtain dental radiographs when necessary
- Assist with chairside procedures
- Sterilize equipment and instruments
- Maintain inventory
- Provide patient education
- Give post-procedure instructions to patients on appliance care and maintenance
- Perform expanded functions where allowed, such as prefitting bands and placing and removing arch wires and ligatures

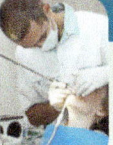

Voice of Experience

We don't require this from our new orthodontic assistants, but it always helps if a new assistant actually wore braces as a child or young adult. It's so much easier to talk to patients about their experience if you've experienced it yourself—and it helps put patients at ease and makes them more comfortable to know that their own orthodontic professionals had braces, too!

CHECKPOINT

45-1 Which staff member in an orthodontic office is typically responsible for guiding patients through the treatment process?

Occlusion and Malocclusion

Occlusion describes the relationship of the mandibular arch and the maxillary arch. In general, orthodontics is concerned with maintaining or achieving a normal occlusion, which promotes even tooth wearing, causes less stress on facial and jaw structures, and presents an aesthetically pleasing appearance.

Normal Occlusion

Normal occlusion describes the correct orientation between the maxillary and mandibular arches (Figure 45-1). Normal occlusion is characterized by:

- Mandibular teeth that are in fullest possible contact with maxillary teeth, with no rotation or open spaces
- Maxillary teeth that overlap the incisal edge of the mandibular teeth by about 2 mm
- Maxillary posterior teeth that are just distal to corresponding mandibular posterior teeth
- The mesial buccal groove of the maxillary first permanent molar occludes in the buccal groove of the first mandibular molar

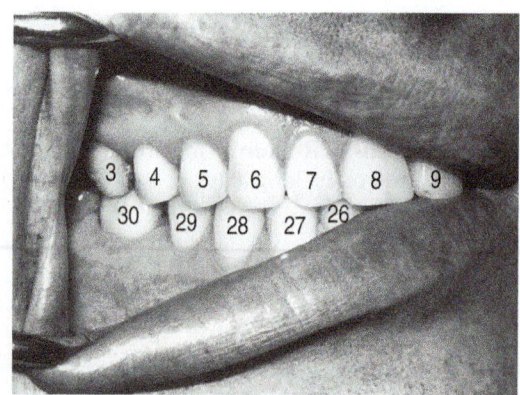

Figure 45–1 **Normal occlusion.** In the ideal tooth alignment, the center axis of the tooth types in the maxillary arch are aligned just distal to the center axis of the same type of tooth in the mandibular arch. For example, look at the two opposing canines: no. 6 is just distal to no. 27.

- If the first molars are not present, the positioning of the maxillary canine can be used to determine occlusion. The pointed tip of the maxillary canine is positioned between the mandibular canine and the mandibular first premolar if the teeth are in normal occlusion.

TABLE 45-1	Angle's Classification of Malocclusion and Facial Profiles		
CLASS	**DESCRIPTION**	**FACIAL PROFILE**	**ILLUSTRATION**
Neutroclusion or Class I	Normal occlusion except for individual or groups of teeth out of position	Mesognathic	**Class I**
Distoclusion or Class II Class II division I Class II division II	There are two divisions: 1. Maxillary incisors are in labioversion (pointing toward lips) 2. Maxillary central incisors are positioned inward while the maxillary lateral incisors are flared	Retrognathic	**Class II, Division 1** **Class II, Division 2**
Mesioclusion or Class III	Mandibular teeth are mesial to normal orientation (bulldog)	Prognathic	**Class III**

Malocclusion

Malocclusion occurs when the teeth deviate from the normal occlusion outlined above. Malocclusion can affect a single tooth or the entire jaw. Because there are so many types of malocclusion, in 1899, Edward Angle created a system known as Angle's Classification of Malocclusion and Facial Profiles. This system is still in use today to describe malocclusion. See Table 45-1 for a description of Angle's Classification.

There are a number of ways teeth can be maloccluded, as detailed in Table 45-2, and many patients will exhibit one or more of these (Figure 45-2).

Malocclusion is caused a variety of circumstances and conditions, including any of the following:

- *Habits.* Oral habits such as tongue thrusting, thumb and finger sucking, bruxism (grinding the teeth), and mouth breathing can all affect the normal orientation of teeth. Note, however, that thumb sucking and finger sucking are normal during early development and usually have little effect on tooth position. If the habit persists into the years of permanent dentition, however, it may affect occlusion.
- *Developmental abnormalities.* Developmental abnormalities can have a profound or a subtle effect on dentition. Conditions such as cleft palates and cleft lips have a dramatic effect on teeth position. However, more subtle conditions such as congenitally missing teeth, supernumerary teeth, malformed teeth, impaction, and ectopic eruption are much more common and need orthodontic intervention.
- *Genetic abnormalities.* Genetic abnormalities are usually caused by an inherited discrepancy in the size of the jaw versus the size of the teeth. Missing teeth can also be an inherited condition.
- *Environmental factors.* Environmental factors fall into two categories: birth injuries and trauma. Birth injuries typically occur when pressure is placed on the quickly developing oral structures, either as the infant passes through the birth canal or during forceps delivery. Trauma can affect occlusion by altering tooth position, especially when primary teeth are still present.

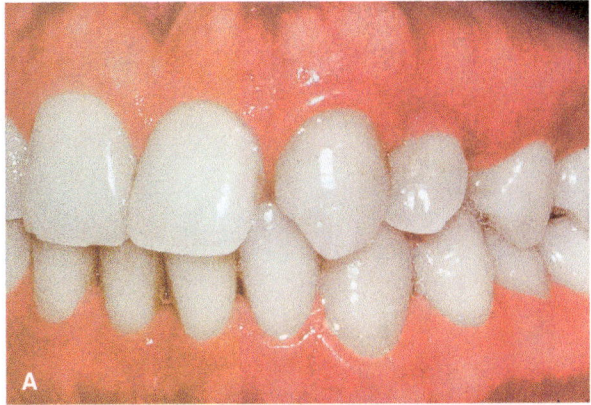

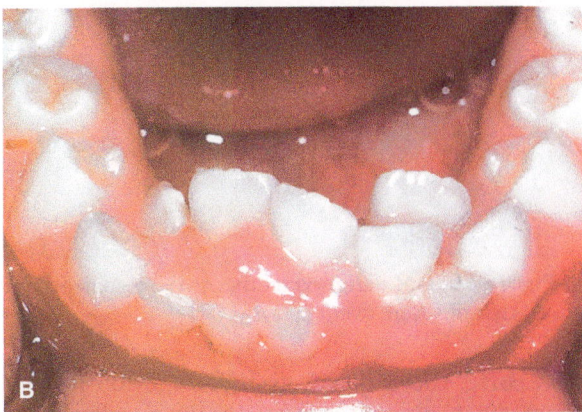

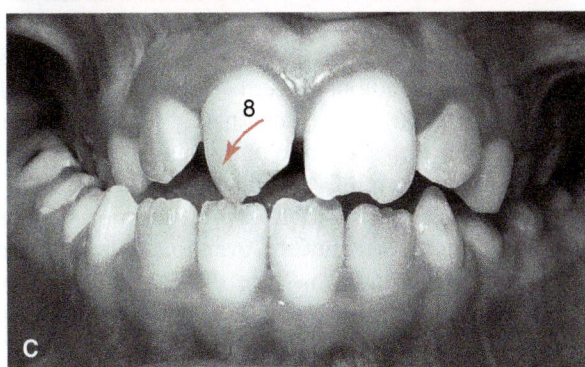

Figure 45–2 Malocclusions. (A) Transposition of maxillary canine and lateral. **(B)** Ectopic eruption, axial tilting, and rotated teeth. **(C)** Torsiversion (twisting) of tooth no. 8. Also notice that the posterior teeth on the patient's right side (left side of photo) are in crossbite.

Malaligned Teeth

Malalignment differs from malocclusion because the teeth may be in normal occlusion, but their alignment within the mandibular or maxillary arch is incorrect (Figure 45-3). Types of malalignment include:

- **Crossbite.** Teeth are not correctly aligned with their opposing teeth (see Figures 45-2C and 45-3A). This can occur with anterior or posterior teeth.
- **Open bite.** The maxillary and mandibular teeth do not meet in their normal occlusion when the jaw arches are closed; instead, an open space remains (Figure 45-3B).

TABLE 45-2 Malocclusion	
TYPE	**TOOTH IS...**
Transposition/ transversion	Out of order in the dental arch
Supraversion	Extended above the normal occlusive line
Labioversion/ buccoversion	Oriented toward the lip or cheek
Linguoversion	Positioned toward the tongue
Distoversion	Distal to its normal position
Mesioversion	Mesial to its normal position
Torsiversion	Turned or rotated in its normal position

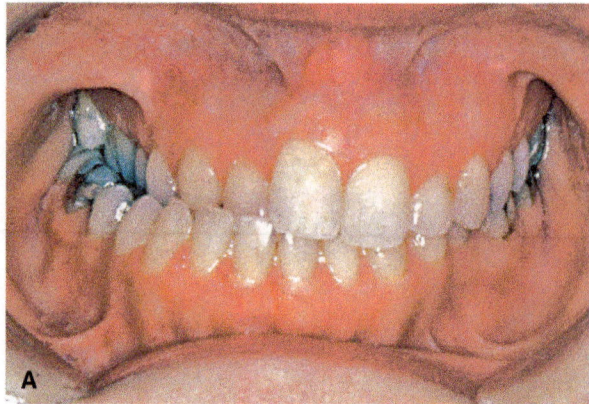

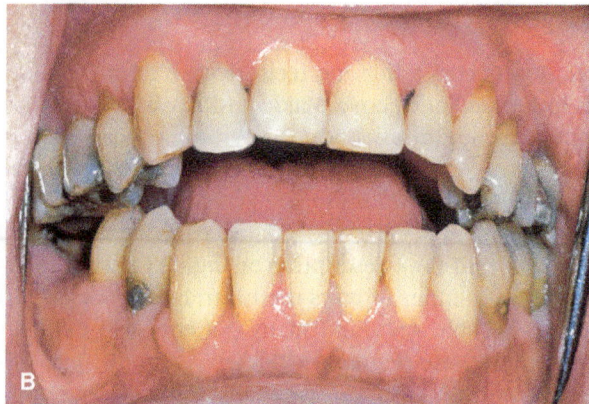

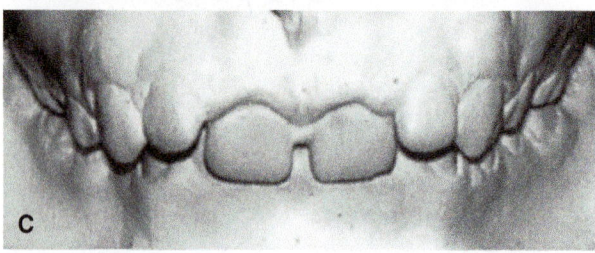

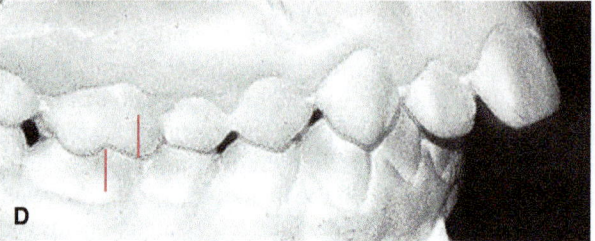

Figure 45–3 Malaligned teeth. (**A**) Developmental crossbite. (**B**) Anterior open bite. (**C**) Cast of severe overbite. (**D**) Cast of severe overjet.

- **Overbite**. The maxillary teeth extend too far downward and do not correctly overlap the mandibular teeth (Figure 45-3C). In their normal orientation, the maxillary teeth should cover about one-third of the incisal edge of the mandibular teeth. With an overbite, the mandibular anterior teeth can barely be seen because of excessive vertical overlap of the maxillary teeth over the mandibular teeth.

- **Overjet**. The maxillary incisors protrude too far beyond the mandibular teeth, but the overlap is otherwise normal (Figure 45-3D). In this case, there is an inappropriate space between the lingual surface of the maxillary teeth and the facial surface of the mandibular teeth. Excessive horizontal overlap occurs between the maxillary anterior teeth and the mandibular anterior teeth. The orthodontist measures the amount of overlap with a periodontal probe.

- **Crowding**. Crowding occurs when teeth are too close together in the arch (see Figure 45-2B). It can affect several teeth and is a very common cause of orthodontic intervention.

CHECKPOINTS

45-2 Define the following terms: transposition, supraversion, linguoversion, and mesioversion.

45-3 Is thumb-sucking a concern in a 3-year-old patient? What about a 6-year-old?

45-4 Describe the three main classes of malocclusion in Angle's system.

Orthodontic Treatments

Orthodontic treatments include two general groups: preventive procedures and corrective procedures. The goal of all orthodontic treatments is to establish a normal occlusion and alignment in the teeth and jaw structures. This prevents problems associated with incorrect alignment, improves the aesthetics of the face, and, depending on the age of the patient, allows development to progress normally.

Preventive Orthodontics

The goal of preventive orthodontics is to identify potential problem areas and correct them early before they worsen. This is sometimes called interceptive orthodontics. In many cases, preventive orthodontic treatments can be handled by a general dentist or pediatric dentist. However, in some more complex cases, orthodontic treatment by an orthodontist might be necessary.

Some common conditions that may warrant preventive orthodontic treatment include:

- Restorations used to prevent premature tooth loss
- Space maintainers used to reserve space for a missing tooth
- Abnormal growth patterns and development that might affect occlusion or alignment
- Habits such as excessive thumb sucking
- Tooth extraction to prevent overcrowding, especially concerning the third molars
- Early removal of primary teeth to clear space for permanent teeth

Corrective Orthodontics

Corrective orthodontics involves correcting occlusion and alignment issues once they have developed. This is most often performed by an orthodontist, using a variety of instruments, including fixed appliances that exert force on the bones and structures of the face and jaws. Common corrective procedures include:

- Placement of fixed appliances, including "braces," wires, brackets, bands, and other appliances that are fixed to the teeth and cannot be removed by the patient
- Removable appliances to maintain orthodontic treatments; these can be removed by the patient
- Orthognathic surgery for cases when other means are not sufficient

CHECKPOINTS

45-5 What are the two main types of orthodontic treatments?

45-6 What is the overall goal of all orthodontic treatments?

Treatment Planning

Orthodontic treatment may be preceded by one or more visits to the orthodontist's office. The purpose of these visits is to acquaint the orthodontist with the patient, chart the patient's development, and identify and diagnose conditions that need correction.

During these appointments, the orthodontist will build a patient record that can be used for comparison during and after treatment. Any number of steps might be involved in treatment planning—orthodontic treatment is often a multi-year process that involves several appliances and stages and relies on the patient's compliance. In the case of minors, the entire family may be involved in the treatment plan.

Medical and Dental History

Treatment begins with a thorough medical and dental history. Even though the patient has medical and dental histories on record at the dentist's office, the orthodontist's office still needs to take both histories. Some conditions can potentially affect orthodontic treatment that might not pertain to general dentistry, so it is important that the patient begin with a thorough history.

During the history, in addition to medical conditions, the orthodontist assesses:

- *Physical growth.* Orthodontics is related closely to a child's physical growth, so the orthodontist asks questions about recent growth spurts, growth patterns, and other factors that might affect physical growth. This may accelerate or delay the need for treatment.

- *Social and behavioral growth.* Orthodontics typically requires enthusiastic and cooperative patients. The orthodontist assesses their motivation for treatment and their enthusiasm level for following the plan, sometimes over the course of years. With children, the decision to pursue treatment is often made by the parents, but it is still important that the child understands the reasons for and benefits of orthodontic treatment. Adult patients typically seek treatment themselves and may have a clearer idea of their motivation and goals. In either case, patients should be prepared to follow the plan and understand the benefits of treatment.

Examination and Diagnosis

During the treatment planning period, the orthodontist also evaluates a number of physical characteristics. Any or all of the following might be part of the initial diagnosis period:

- *Clinical exam.* The orthodontic exam evaluates the face, teeth, and jaws for development, alignment, symmetry, proportion, and proper occlusion. The patient may be assessed using the Angle Classification System. Additionally, the patient's oral cavity is examined for signs of inadequate oral health, which may be an impediment to orthodontic treatment.

- *Radiography.* Radiographs are usually included in the patient record before treatment begins. Typical radiographs obtained before treatment include panoramic radiographs, cephalometric radiographs, and standard radiographs. Cephalometric images, in particular, are helpful. These extraoral images show a lateral image of the patient's head, including the jaws and teeth. From there, the orthodontist can map the patient's jaws and head by using cephalometric landmarks marked on the image. This map is used to analyze growth patterns and make predictions about treatment. Radiography techniques are covered in greater depth in Part VII, Dental Radiography.

- *Photographs.* Photographs are an important part of orthodontic treatment. Both intraoral and extraoral photographs are used to capture the color, size, shape, and character of structures before, during, and after treatment. Extraoral photographs include frontal and profile views. Intraoral photographs are taken from a variety of angles. Tissue retraction is important during intraoral photography so that the teeth are clearly visible. These photographs are included in the patient's orthodontic record.

- *Diagnostic models.* Sometimes called study models or diagnostic casts, diagnostic models are three-dimensional models of the patient's teeth, oral cavity, and arches. Diagnostic models are useful because they show actual distances and proportion of the patient's teeth and arches. They are made from alginate impressions and are included in the patient's orthodontic record. For more information about the materials and techniques used to create diagnostic models, see Chapter 35, Laboratory Materials and Techniques.

TABLE 45-3 Common Orthodontic Instruments

INSTRUMENT	USE
Howe pliers	Used to manipulate arch wires; they have a rounded, flat tip with serrations
Pin cutter	Used to cut wires; shaped like small wire cutters
Ligature cutter	Used to cut ligatures; shaped like small wire cutters
Ligature director	Used to tuck the small, twisted ligature ends into the interproximal space or around the bracket
Ligature tying needles	Used to tie ligatures; they have narrow beaks with fine serrations to make ligature tying easier
Mathieu needle holder	Used to tie ligature wire and place elastic ligature
Band driver	Used to push the band into place
Band seater	Used to seat posterior metal bands firmly into place
Bite block with band seater	A combination instrument with a bite block and band seater that relies on occlusal force to seat a band into place
Band contouring pliers	Used to fit and contour bands before placement
Band-removing pliers	Used to remove posterior bands
Bird-beak pliers	Used to form and bend wires and form springs
Bracket forceps	Used to carry and place brackets during bonding to the tooth surface
Three-prong pliers	Used to close and adjust clasps
Weingart utility pliers	Used in placement of arch wires; they have very fine, sharply serrated beaks that are good for use anywhere in the oral cavity
Tweed-loop pliers	Used to form loops and springs in wire
Distal end-cutting pliers	Used to cut the distal end of arch wires

> **CHECKPOINT**
> **45-7** How are photographs and diagnostic models used in orthodontics?

Orthodontic Instruments

Orthodontic instruments differ significantly from dental instruments. Orthodontic assistants are required to know all the various instruments used and their purpose (see Table 45-3 and Figure 45-4).

> **CHECKPOINT**
> **45-8** What are the following instruments used for: ligature cutters; band seater; bird-beak pliers; and three-prong pliers?

Orthodontic Appliances

Orthodontic appliances fall into two broad categories: fixed appliances and removable appliances. Both types of appliances are frequently used in the same patient at different times in the long-term treatment plan.

Self-care is an essential part of orthodontics, especially oral hygiene, which can be challenging when appliances are present. Orthodontic assistants are frequently the staff members who teach patients oral self-care techniques, so it is important that assistants can easily explain these techniques, in language that all patients can understand, and demonstrate how to perform them.

Fixed Appliances

Fixed appliances are permanently attached to the teeth and cannot be removed by the patient. Sometimes called braces, fixed appliances consist of brackets, bands, and wires and auxiliary appliances that are used to apply constant, gentle pressure to the teeth to move them into the correct positions. Fixed appliances may be worn anywhere from a few months to a few years, depending on the patient. Removable appliances are often used before and after placement of fixed appliances.

> **Extra Patient Care**
>
> New fixed appliances, no matter how perfectly they are fitted, will sometimes cause tissue aggravation. Always send your patients home with some rope wax and instructions on how to use it on sore spots to ease the discomfort. Your patients will really appreciate it!

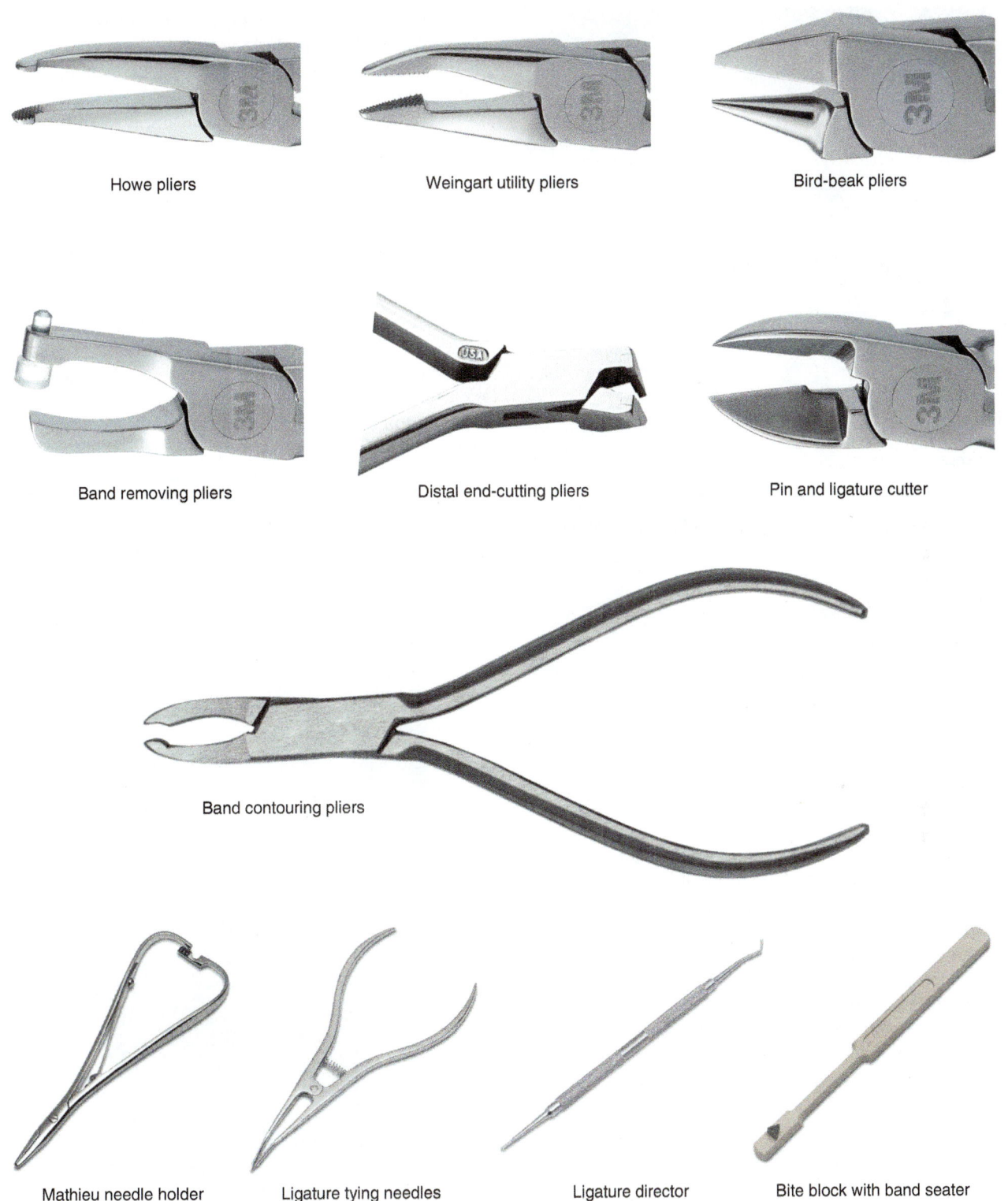

Howe pliers

Weingart utility pliers

Bird-beak pliers

Band removing pliers

Distal end-cutting pliers

Pin and ligature cutter

Band contouring pliers

Mathieu needle holder

Ligature tying needles

Ligature director

Bite block with band seater

Figure 45–4 Orthodontic instruments.

Bands

Bands are thin, stainless steel loops that are placed on the patient's posterior teeth (usually the first and second molars) and cemented into place (Figure 45-5). They are often presized and fitted before placement, using the patient's model, although they can be selected and fitted chairside. A number of appliances can be fastened to the bands, including buccal tubes, brackets, or other auxiliaries.

For more detail on placing bands, see Procedure 45-5, Assisting with Cementing Orthodontic Bands.

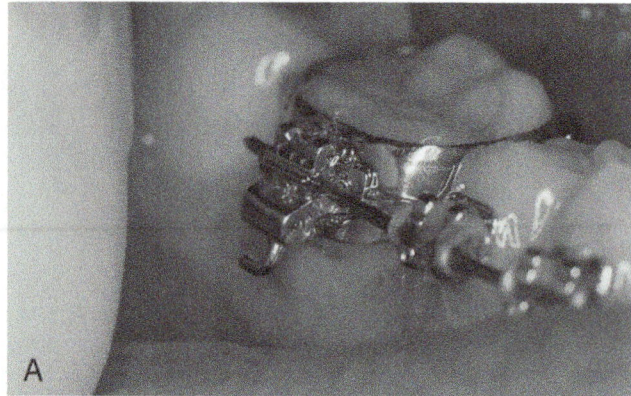

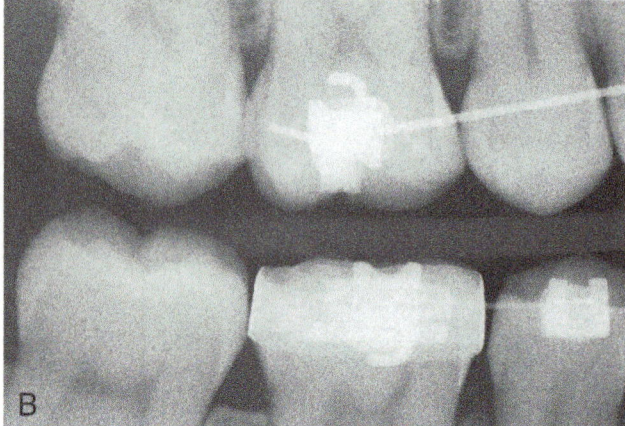

Figure 45–5 **Bands.** (**A**) Photograph of a band on a molar with a buccal tube. (**B**) Posterior bitewing of the same area. Notice that the mandibular tube uses a band and the maxillary tube is directly bonded to the molar.

Separators

Separators are used prior to band placement to widen tight interdental spaces, making it possible to insert bands into the narrow openings. Three main varieties of separators are available: steel springs, brass wire, or elastomeric. All styles of separators share a similar purpose and design: they are wedged into narrow interdental spaces to gradually force teeth apart.

For more detail on placing separators, see the procedures later in the chapter that describe placing and removing various types of separators.

Band Cements

Band cements are used to hold bands in place. These are generally the same cements used in restorations, and they may include fluoride. Band cements must attach only to enamel but they must provide the long-term strength and stability to hold the band in place during treatment. The most common cements used include glass ionomer, polycarbonate, or zinc phosphate cement.

Bonded Brackets

Brackets are used to hold the arch wires. Posterior brackets are typically welded directly to the band, while anterior brackets are bonded or cemented directly to the tooth (Figure 45-6). Brackets are designed so the arch wire is placed in the bracket's wings and then tied, or ligated, in place with ligating wire. This allows the force of the arch wire to be transmitted to the tooth, causing it to shift position according to the treatment plan.

Several types of brackets are available, including stainless steel, ceramic, and acrylic. Many patients prefer natural-colored ceramic brackets because they are nearly invisible on the teeth and more aesthetically pleasing. Some patients, however, favor brightly colored brackets. Lingual brackets are an alternative to traditional brackets. Because they are attached to the lingual surface of the teeth, they are less noticeable than posterior brackets. Although aesthetically pleasing, lingual brackets can interfere with tongue movement and may be more difficult for patients to maintain. The Damon system is another type of bracket that is self ligating. The bracket has a tiny slide on it that holds the wire in place, hence the term self ligating.

For more information on placing brackets, see Procedure 45-6, Assisting with Direct Bonding of Orthodontic Brackets.

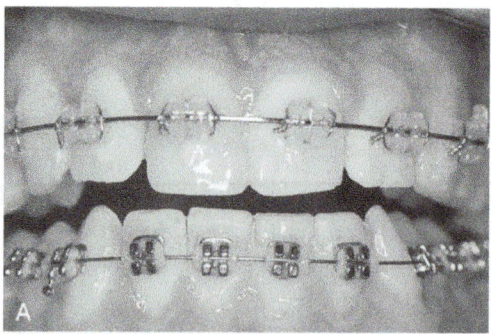

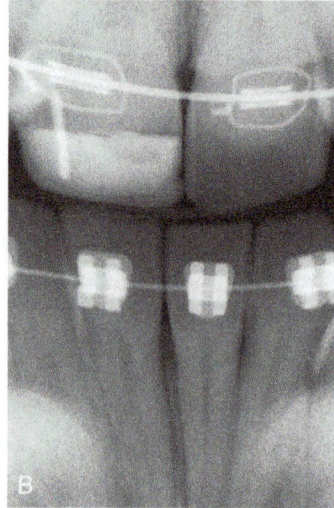

Figure 45–6 **Bonded brackets.** (**A**) Orthodontic fixed appliance consisting of polycarbonate brackets with metal ligatures and rectangular wire on the upper arch and stainless-steel brackets with elastic ties and a round wire on the lower arch. (**B**) Radiograph showing the same appliance. Note the composite restoration retained by a pin.

Arch Wires

Arch wires are U-shaped wires that are tied to the brackets and used to transmit force to the teeth to move them (see Figures 45-5 and 45-6). In the posterior teeth, arch wires are anchored in buccal tubes. Arch wires are held in place with ligature ties and wires. Arch wires are available in a number of shapes and sizes, to accommodate a wider variety of patients and treatment phases, including round, square, and rectangular.

Additionally, arch wires can be made from various materials including nickel titanium, stainless steel, beta titanium, and Optiflex. The type of material affects how much force the wire can deliver, so a single patient might have several different types of wire placed during a long-term treatment plan.

Ligature Ties and Wires

Ligature ties and wires are used to hold the arch wire in place against the bracket (see Figure 45-6). Ligature ties are thin wires that are wrapped around the arch wire and then twisted to hold the arch wire in place against the bracket. Ligature wire is available in spools or precut lengths. In situations in which the orthodontist wants to move several teeth as a group, or push teeth together, a single ligature wire can be shaped into a figure-eight that covers several teeth.

There are a few alternatives to ligature wires, depending on the situation. These include plastic rings, or elastomeric ties, that are slipped over the top of the bracket and around the ligature wire. Rings are also available in chains that are used similar to a figure-eight ligature wire.

For more information, see Procedure 45-8, Assisting with Placing and Removing Ligature Ties.

Buccal Tubes

Buccal tubes are attached to the molar bands on the buccal surface (see Figure 45-5). They are used to anchor the arch wire to the posterior teeth. Alternatively, headgear tubes are also sometimes welded to the first molar bands. These tubes are used to attach the inner bow of a headgear, or facebow, appliance.

Space Maintainers

Space maintainers consist of a band and wire loop soldered together into a single unit. The band is placed around a permanent tooth while the wire loop extends into the empty space next to the permanent tooth. The purpose of the device is to hold the empty space open until a permanent tooth can erupt and fill the position in the correct alignment. Without space maintainers in place, adjacent teeth would drift into the open space, compromising position for both the newly erupted tooth and the existing tooth. Space maintainers are cemented into position.

Palatal Separators

Palatal separators are used to widen the palatal vault to accommodate teeth in the arches. These devices are made from acrylic that is shaped to fit the palatal vault, then split down the middle and fitted with a tiny screw-like device. They are cemented to the posterior teeth and the screw is turned twice a day or according to the orthodontist's instructions. As the screw is turned, the device gradually expands, forcing the mid-palatal suture apart. New bone tissue forms in the opening.

Palatal spreading usually takes a few weeks, and it may be slightly uncomfortable as the patient feels the palatal vault spreading. However, spreading is permanent once bone fills the open mid-palatal suture.

Elastics

Elastics are rubber appliances used to connect teeth in the same arch, or from one arch to the other, to apply specific pressure. They are often referred to as *rubber bands*.

Removable Appliances

Removable appliances are designed to be removed and maintained by the patient, after instruction from the office staff. They are often used before or after treatment with fixed appliances to "lock in" gains. The most common removable appliances include headgear and traction devices, retainers, and tooth positioners.

Headgear and Traction Devices

Headgear includes a **traction** device that fits securely around the patient's head and applies pressure to the teeth through a *facebow* that attaches to permanent appliances fixed to the teeth (Figure 45-7). Headgear is used to control and affect tooth movement and growth and position of craniofacial bones.

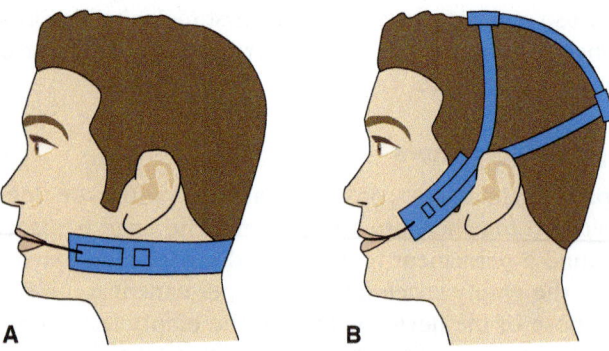

Figure 45–7 Headgear and traction. (**A**) Cervical traction is used to exert force parallel to the occlusal plane. (**B**) High-pull headgear hooks to the maxillary molar buccal tubes to exert traction.

There are several types of traction devices available, depending on each patient's individual needs. Some fit only around the patient's neck, while others extend to the crown of the head. The facebow typically attaches to buccal tubes inside the mouth.

Headgear is worn for a certain number of hours each day. It is the patient's responsibility to make sure he or she wears the headgear for the appropriate number of hours.

Retainers

After the permanent appliance is removed, many patients are fitted with a retainer (Figure 45-8) to make sure their teeth do not "drift" with time. Retainers also help by allowing gingival tissue to adapt to its new position and control new growth.

Retainers are custom devices made from plastic to conform to the patient's anatomy. The most common device is the Hawley retainer, which is a passive device. Retainers are usually worn for a specific amount of time each day or overnight. Some orthodontists cement the retainer on the lingual surfaces of the maxillary or mandibular teeth. This is typically performed for patients who have trouble wearing a removable retainer.

Oral hygiene is an important component of retainer use, and patients should be instructed in retainer care when they receive their device.

Tooth Positioners

Tooth positioners are clear plastic devices that somewhat resemble athletic mouth guards. They are worn over the crowns of all teeth and help to retain the teeth in position after treatment with permanent appliances. They are often prescribed before a retainer is issued, or while the retainer is being made.

Tooth Aligners

In recent years, clear plastic tooth aligners have become very popular among adults who want to fix orthodontic

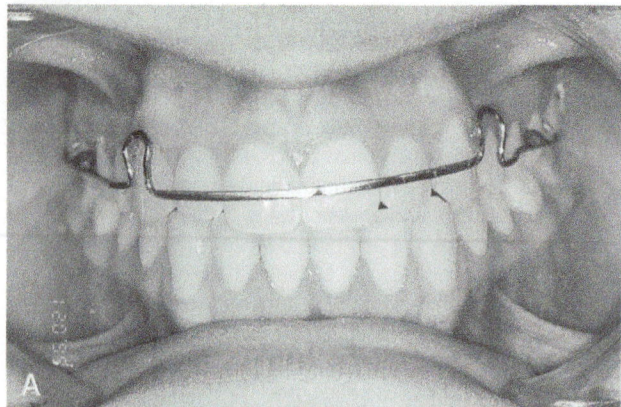

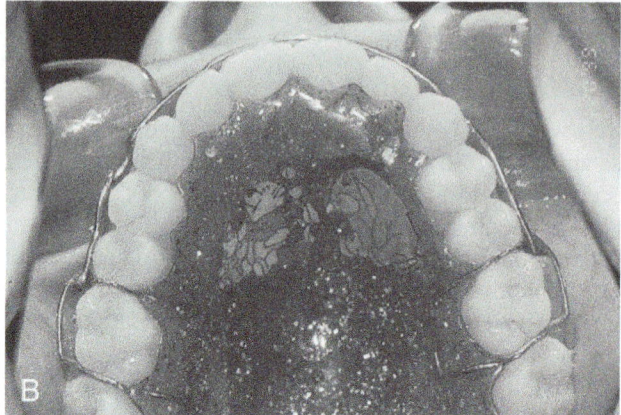

Figure 45–8 Retainer. (**A**) Facial view and (**B**) occlusal view of a maxillary retainer. (Courtesy of Dr. Daniel Foley, Beckley, W.V.)

issues but do not want permanent appliances. These devices are nearly invisible when worn correctly; they fit over the crowns of teeth and gently reposition them. Progressive aligners are worn in succession over the course of weeks to achieve results. They are usually removed only for eating, brushing, and flossing.

Aligners are offered through the dentist's office. One common brand is Invisalign. They are included as part of a comprehensive treatment plan. In addition to being nearly invisible, aligners make it easy to maintain oral hygiene because they are removable.

CHECKPOINTS

45-9 Which teeth are bands typically fastened to?

45-10 How are brackets usually attached to anterior teeth?

Orthodontic Procedures

Procedures 45-1 through 45-11 detail common procedures performed in the orthodontic office.

Procedure 45–1 **Preparation Appointment**

Some states allow qualified orthodontic assistants to perform some of the clinical procedures during the appointment; in other states the orthodontic assistant assists the orthodontist during the procedures. Check your state's regulations for more information about the specific duties orthodontic assistants are allowed to perform.

1. Before seating the patient in the treatment area, obtain an updated orthodontic, dental, and medical history.

2. Take intraoral and extraoral photos of the patient.

3. Expose any necessary radiographs.

4. Take impressions of the patient's teeth to create a cast for use during treatment.

5. Assist the orthodontist with the exam as needed.

6. Assist in explaining the intended procedures to the patient and the ultimate goal of treatment.

Procedure 45–2 **Placing and Removing a Wire Separator**

Some states allow qualified orthodontic assistants to perform this procedure; in other states the orthodontic assistant assists the orthodontist during the procedure. Check your state's regulations for more information about the specific duties orthodontic assistants are allowed to perform.

Materials needed:

- Brass wire
- Hemostat
- Ligature wire cutter

Placing a Wire Separator

1. Put on appropriate PPE.

2. Bend the brass wire separator into a J-hook shape.

3. Using the hemostat, slide the hooked end of the wire through the interproximal space from the lingual side (Figure P45-2-1).

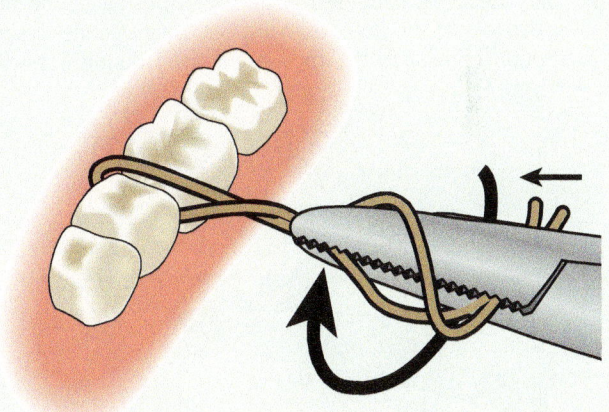

Figure P45-2-2

5. Using the ligature cutter, cut the twisted wire to within 3 mm of the teeth. Bend the remaining spoke of wire back toward the interproximal space to prevent damage to sensitive buccal tissues.

6. Make a note of the procedure in the patient's record and provide the patient with self-care instructions. Wire separators are typically left in place for 5–7 days.

Removing a Wire Separator

1. Put on appropriate PPE.

2. Carefully cut the wire using the ligature wire cutter.

3. Use the hemostat to slide or gently pry the wire from the interdental space.

4. Note the procedure in the patient's record and provide the patient with self-care instructions.

Note that, in most cases, the orthodontic bands are cemented immediately after the separators are removed. Refer to Procedure 45-5 for detailed steps on Assisting with Cementing Orthodontic Bands.

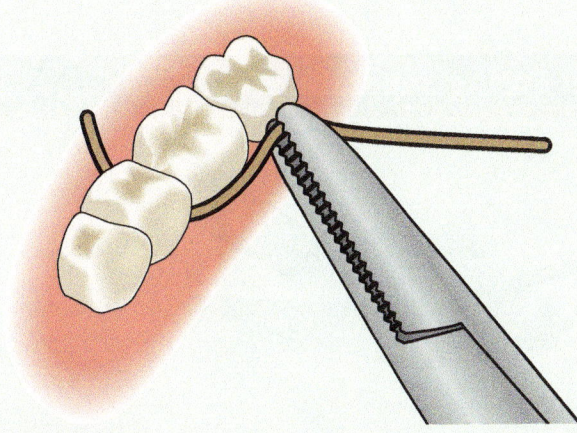

Figure P45-2-1

4. Loop the wire back over the contact and twist slightly (Figure P45-2-2).

Procedure 45-3 **Placing and Removing an Elastic Separator**

Some states allow qualified orthodontic assistants to perform this procedure; in other states the orthodontic assistant assists the orthodontist during the procedure. Check your state's regulations for more information about the specific duties orthodontic assistants are allowed to perform.

Materials needed:

- Elastic separator
- Separating pliers
- Dental floss
- Explorer

Placing an Elastic Separator

1. Put on appropriate PPE.
2. Prepare the elastic separator by placing it over the beaks of the separating pliers.
3. With the pliers squeezed in the open position, slide the separator into the interproximal space using a gentle rocking motion (similar to the movement used during flossing) (Figure P45-3-1).

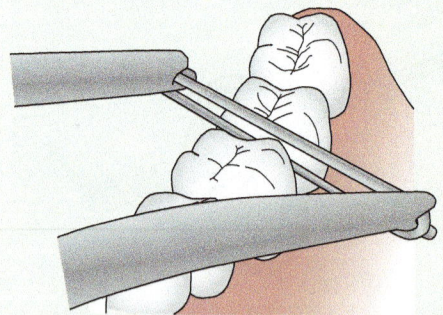

Figure P45-3-1

4. Release the separator pliers and remove them.
5. Alternatively, place two pieces of floss in the separator. Fold each piece over in half. Stretch the separator by pulling on the floss, then gently slide the separator into the interproximal space and remove the floss.
6. Make a note of the procedure in the patient's record and provide the patient with self-care instructions. Elastic separators remain in place 5–7 days.

Removing an Elastic Separator

1. Put on appropriate PPE.
2. To remove the separator, slide an explorer under the elastic band and place a finger over the separator so it does not snap inside the patient's mouth.
3. Gently remove the separator using steady pressure.
4. Note the procedure in the patient's record and provide the patient with self-care instructions.

Note that, in most cases, the orthodontic bands are cemented immediately after the separators are removed. Refer to Procedure 45-5 for detailed steps on Assisting with Cementing Orthodontic Bands.

Procedure 45-4 **Placing and Removing a Steel Spring Separator**

Some states allow qualified orthodontic assistants to perform this procedure; in other states the orthodontic assistant assists the orthodontist during the procedure. Check your state's regulations for more information about the specific duties orthodontic assistants are allowed to perform.

Materials needed:

- Steel spring separator
- Bird-beak pliers
- Scaler

Placing a Steel Spring Separator

1. Put on appropriate PPE.
2. Grasp the steel spring along the shorter leg with the bird-beak pliers (Figure P45-4-1).

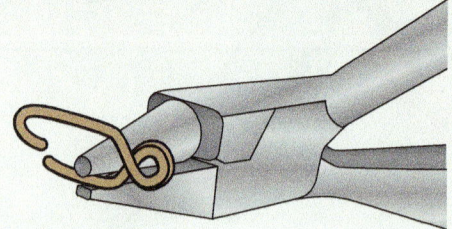

Figure P45-4-1

3. From the lingual side, place the hooked side of the spring into the contact. Open the spring with the pliers so the shorter end slides into the contact from the lingual side.
4. Slide the spring fully into place with the coil on the facial side.

Procedure 45-4 Placing and Removing a Steel Spring Separator (Continued)

5. Note the procedure in the patient's record and provide the patient with self-care instructions. Steel spring separators typically stay in place for 3–5 days.

Removing a Steel Spring Separator

1. Put on appropriate PPE.
2. Place your hand or finger over the spring to prevent it from springing into soft tissue (Figure P45-4-2).

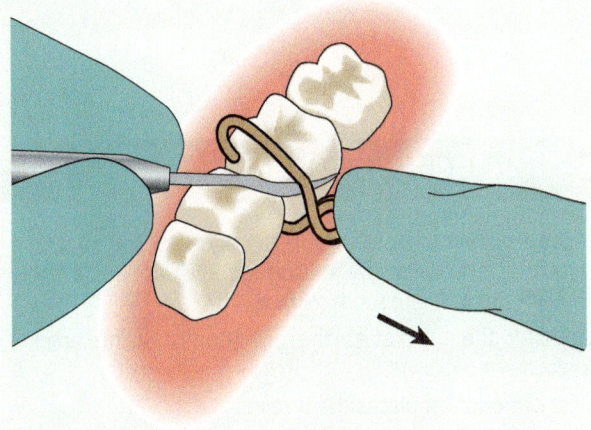

Figure P45-4-2

3. Slide a scaler into the coil and lift upward until the longer arm is free and visible.
4. Lift the separator out of the contact using a backward-rocking motion to slide the short end from the interproximal space.
5. Note the procedure in the patient's record and provide the patient with self-care instructions.

Note that, in most cases, the orthodontic bands are cemented immediately after the separators are removed. Refer to Procedure 45-5 for detailed steps on Assisting with Cementing Orthodontic Bands.

Procedure 45-5 Assisting with Cementing Orthodontic Bands

Some states allow qualified orthodontic assistants to perform this procedure; in other states the orthodontic assistant assists the orthodontist during the procedure. Check your state's regulations for more information about the specific duties orthodontic assistants are allowed to perform.

Materials needed:

- Orthodontic bands
- Cement supplies
- Spatula
- Band seater
- Band pusher
- Explorer
- Dental floss
- Scaler

1. Put on appropriate PPE.
2. Prepare the bands by placing them all on the working surface with their gingival margins facing up, in the order they will be placed.

3. Assist with isolating and drying the teeth.
4. Mix the cement according to the manufacturer's directions.
5. Load the cement into the first band with a spatula, making sure the inside of the band is coated with cement (Figure P45-5-1).

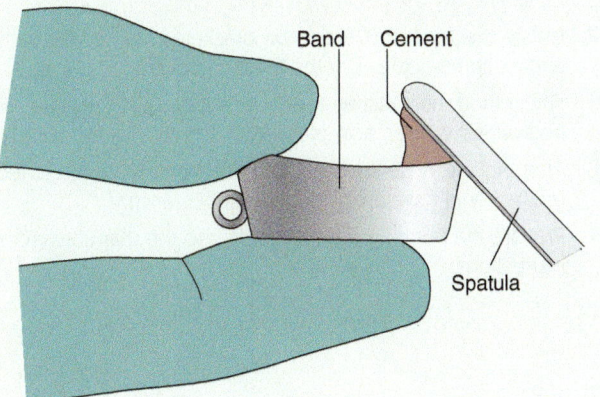

Band   Cement

Spatula

Figure P45-5-1

Procedure 45-5 Assisting with Cementing Orthodontic Bands (Continued)

6. Transfer the band to the orthodontist.

7. The orthodontist seats the band on the tooth.

8. Transfer the band seater to the orthodontist, who places it on the buccal margin of the band. The patient is instructed to bite gently on the band seater, which will help seat the band firmly in the middle third of the tooth.

9. Repeat steps 5–8 until all the bands are placed. Make sure the bands are transferred in the order they will be placed.

10. After the bands are placed, allow the excess cement to set.

11. The orthodontist removes the excess cement with an explorer or scaler.

12. Rinse the patient's mouth and floss the patient's teeth to remove any excess cement.

13. Note the procedure in the patient's record and provide the patient with self-care instructions.

Procedure 45-6 Assisting with Direct Bonding of Orthodontic Brackets

Some states allow qualified orthodontic assistants to perform this procedure; in other states the orthodontic assistant assists the orthodontist during the procedure. Check your state's regulations for more information about the specific duties orthodontic assistants are allowed to perform.

Materials needed:

- Rubber cups and brushes
- Prophy paste
- Low-speed handpiece equipped with a prophy angle
- Air-water syringe
- Cotton rolls or lip retractors
- Etching supplies
- Bonding supplies
- Brackets
- Bracket placement tweezers
- Scaler

1. Put on appropriate PPE.

2. The facial surfaces of the teeth receiving the brackets are polished with a rubber cup and prophy paste.

3. Rinse and dry the patient's mouth.

4. Isolate the teeth that are to be bracketed with cotton rolls and/or lip retractors. Dry the teeth thoroughly.

5. The orthodontist etches the facial surfaces of the teeth to be bonded with an acid etchant.

6. After etching, rinse the teeth and dry them. Properly etched teeth should have a chalky white appearance.

7. Prepare the bonding agent according to the manufacturer's instructions.

8. Apply a small amount of bonding agent to the back of a bracket. Simultaneously, the orthodontist applies a liquid sealant agent to the tooth surface.

9. Transfer the bracket to the orthodontist using bracket placement tweezers.

10. The orthodontist places the bracket.

11. Transfer a scaler to the orthodontist, who removes any excess bonding agent (Figure P45-6-1).

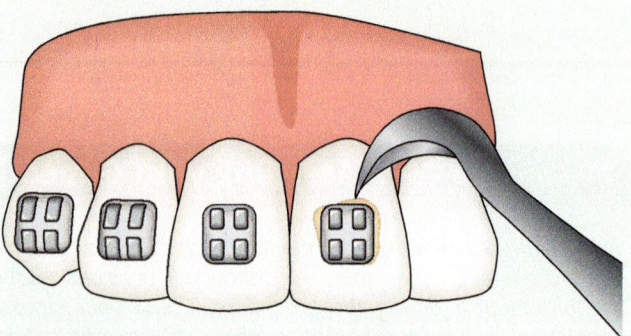

Figure P45-6-1

12. The orthodontist holds the bracket in place while the bonding agent is allowed to set or is light-cured.

13. Repeat steps 8–12 until all brackets are bonded into place.

14. Remove the isolation materials from the patient's mouth.

15. Note the procedure in the patient's record and provide the patient with self-care instructions.

Procedure 45-7 Placing Arch Wires

Some states allow qualified orthodontic assistants to perform this procedure; in other states the orthodontic assistant assists the orthodontist during the procedure. Check your state's regulations for more information about the specific duties orthodontic assistants are allowed to perform.

Materials needed:

- Arch wires
- Patient's model
- Weingart pliers
- Distal-end cutting pliers

1. Put on appropriate PPE.
2. Prepare preformed wires by measuring the wires against the patient's model before placement. The wires should extend beyond the buccal tubes on the last molar bands, but not so long that they cause injury. Trim with the distal-end cutting pliers as needed.
3. Locate the center of one arch wire.
4. Position the wire against the brackets in the patient's mouth with the center mark midway between the central incisors.
5. Slide the wire into the buccal tubes.
6. Using Weingart pliers, slide the wire in on both sides of the arch and position in the bracket slots.

7. Double-check to make sure the wire is not so long that it will cause injury (Figure P45-7-1).

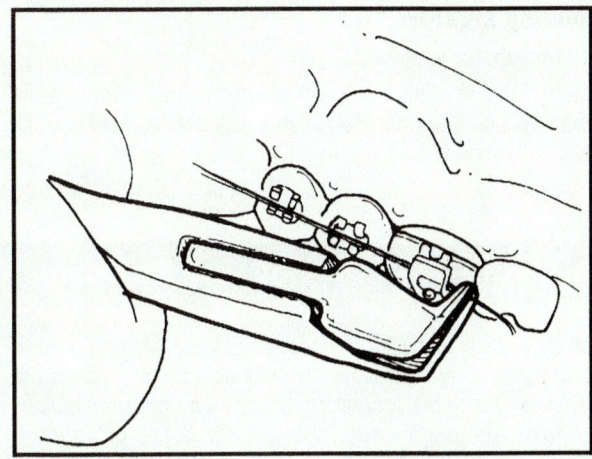

Figure P45-7-1

8. Repeat steps 3–7 for the other arch.
9. Note the procedure in the patient's record and provide the patient with self-care instructions.

Procedure 45-8 Placing and Removing Ligature Ties

Some states allow qualified orthodontic assistants to perform this procedure; in other states the orthodontic assistant assists the orthodontist during the procedure. Check your state's regulations for more information about the specific duties orthodontic assistants are allowed to perform.

Materials needed:

- Ligature ties
- Ligature director
- Hemostat
- Ligature cutters

Placing Ligature Ties

1. Put on appropriate PPE.
2. With the tie gripped in your thumb and index finger, wrap it around the bracket wings, then push the tie against the wings with the ligature director.
3. Braid the ends of the ligature tie together with the hemostat, twisting it tightly so the tie fits snugly against the arch wire and holds it in place (Figure P45-8-1).
4. Repeat steps 2–3 until all ligature ties are in place.

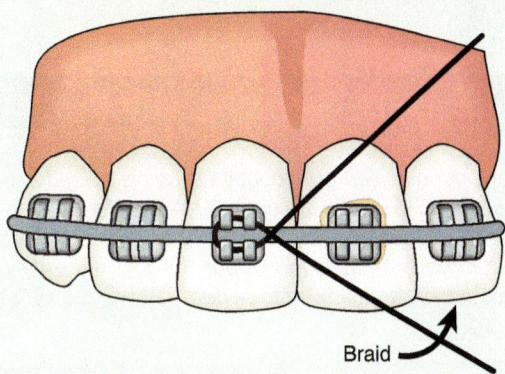

Braid

Figure P45-8-1

5. Trim off excess wire from the braids with the ligature cutters, leaving about 4 mm.
6. Using the ligature director, bend the remaining pigtail braid under the arch wire. Repeat with all ligature ties.
7. Check the arch by running your finger along the arch to make sure no sharp metal ends are protruding that could cause tissue injury.

Procedure 45–8 **Placing and Removing Ligature Ties (Continued)**

8. Note the procedure in the patient's record and provide the patient with self-care instructions.

Removing Ligature Ties

1. Put on appropriate PPE.
2. Using ligature cutters, snip off the pigtail end of the ligature tie. Make sure to hold the cut end so it does not fall into the patient's mouth.

3. Remove the tie carefully. Do not tug, twist, or pull on the tie. If it is still stuck, continue cutting—always careful to remove any bits of metal—until you can work it free.
4. Repeat steps 2–3 until all ligature ties are removed.
5. Note the procedure in the patient's record and provide the patient with self-care instructions.

Procedure 45–9 **Placing and Removing Elastomeric Ties**

Some states allow qualified orthodontic assistants to perform this procedure; in other states the orthodontic assistant assists the orthodontist during the procedure. Check your state's regulations for more information about the specific duties orthodontic assistants are allowed to perform.

Materials needed:

- Elastomeric ties
- Locking pliers
- Orthodontic scaler or an explorer

Placing Elastomeric Ties

1. Put on appropriate PPE.
2. Place the elastomeric tie on the locking pliers' beaks, then lock the pliers.
3. Slip the tie over the occlusal end of the bracket's wing, then slide the tie under the bracket. Hold it in place with your finger.

4. Once under the bracket, pull the tie over the tie wing, then down the other tie wing.
5. Release the pliers.
6. Repeat steps 2–5 until all ties are placed.
7. Note the procedure in the patient's record and provide the patient with self-care instructions.

Removing Elastomeric Ties

1. Put on appropriate PPE.
2. Using an orthodontic scaler or an explorer, place the instrument tip between the bracket wings and pull the tie up and back from the occlusal surface.
3. Remove the tie from the gingival direction.
4. Repeat steps 2–3 until all ties are removed.
5. Note the procedure in the patient's record and provide the patient with self-care instructions.

Procedure 45–10 **Assisting with the Removal of Orthodontics After Treatment**

Some states allow qualified orthodontic assistants to perform this procedure; in other states the orthodontic assistant assists the orthodontist during the procedure. Check your state's regulations for more information about the specific duties orthodontic assistants are allowed to perform.

Materials needed:

- Hemostat
- Ligature cutter
- Bracket and adhesive-removing pliers
- Band-removing pliers
- Scaler
- Ultrasonic scaler
- Rubber cups and brushes
- Prophy paste
- Low-speed handpiece equipped with a prophy angle

1. Put on appropriate PPE.
2. Remove all ligature ties and arch wires from the brackets.

3. The orthodontist will remove the bands by breaking the cement bond and lifting the band from the tooth with the band-removing pliers (Figure P45-10-1).

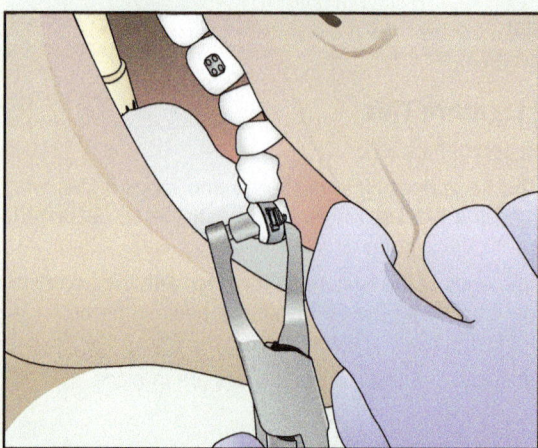

Figure P45–10–1 (Image modified from University of Kentucky.)

Procedure 45–10 Assisting with the Removal of Orthodontics After Treatment (Continued)

4. The orthodontist will remove the brackets by breaking the resin used to bond the bracket to the tooth surface with the bracket and adhesive-removing pliers.

5. The orthodontist will remove any excess bonding material or cement with a scaler; an ultrasonic scaler may also be used to remove excess cement.

6. The facial surfaces of the teeth that had brackets are polished with a rubber cup and prophy paste.

7. Note the procedure in the patient's record and provide the patient with self-care instructions.

Procedure 45–11 Final Appointment

Some states allow qualified orthodontic assistants to perform some of the clinical procedures involved in the final appointment, such as taking an alginate impression. In other states, the orthodontic assistant assists the orthodontist with the clinical procedures. Check your state's regulations for more information about the specific duties orthodontic assistants are allowed to perform.

1. With the appliances fully removed, take an alginate impression of both arches for the patient's record. These impressions are also used to create retainers, if necessary.

2. Take photos, both intraoral and extraoral.

3. Schedule an appointment for delivery of the retainer, if necessary.

4. Note the procedure in the patient's record and provide the patient with self-care instructions.

CHECKPOINTS

45-11 How long are wire separators typically left in place?

45-12 Which instrument is typically used to place arch wires?

Patient Education

Removal of fixed appliances is a big day for many patients, who have sometimes been fitted with appliances for several years—or at least a period of months. However, it is important to emphasize that treatment may not be completely over, even if the fixed appliances are being removed. Retainers may be prescribed, and it is very important for the patient to follow instructions and wear the retainer exactly as instructed so the teeth do not shift.

Additionally, patients who have been providing oral care for teeth with brackets and wires may need a refresher course on brushing and flossing techniques. These can be demonstrated on the patient, and the patient should have an opportunity to demonstrate proficiency.

Retainer instructions are typically given at the follow-up appointment, in conjunction with delivery of the retainer. Patients should be instructed in care for the appliance itself, as well as oral self-care techniques.

CHECKPOINT

45-13 Why is it important for a patient to wear a retainer as instructed once a fixed appliance is removed?

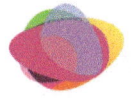

Chapter Highlights

+ Orthodontics is the practice of preventing or correcting malocclusions and maladjustments in both primary and permanent teeth of children and adult patients.

+ Orthodontic assistants fill many of the same roles as dental assistants and need in-depth knowledge of orthodontic practices.

+ Malocclusion occurs when teeth deviate from the normal occlusion; the traditional method for identifying malocclusion, called the Angle Classification of Malocclusion and Facial Profiles, was developed in 1899 by Edward Angle.

♦ Malocclusion can be caused by a number of factors, including habits and developmental, genetic, and environmental factors.

♦ Misaligned teeth are not oriented correctly in their arches, even if the occlusion is correct.

♦ Photographs and diagnostic models are routinely used during orthodontics to help track the patient's progress and growth.

♦ Orthodontic instruments are specifically designed for use in orthodontics and differ from dental instruments.

♦ Fixed appliances are attached directly to teeth and cannot be removed by patients; they may be worn for months or years. Fixed appliances include a system of bands, brackets, and wires that apply force to teeth and cause them to move.

♦ Removable appliances can be removed by the patient and are often used before and after treatment with fixed appliances. Removable appliances include retainers, headgear, and tooth positioners.

♦ Tooth aligners are a new system of orthodontics that use a series of custom-designed trays to apply pressure to teeth and move them; they are removable and nearly invisible when the patient is wearing them.

 **Review Questions**

1. Which of the following terms describes a tooth that extends above the normal occlusive line?

   a. Infraversion

   b. Supraversion

   c. Distoversion

   d. Torsiversion

2. What does neutroclusion mean in the Angle Classification?

   a. Normal occlusion except for individual or groups of teeth out of position

   b. Maxillary teeth are pointing toward the lips

   c. Mandibular teeth are mesial to normal orientation

   d. None of the above

3. What is an overjet?

   a. Teeth are not correctly aligned with their opposing teeth

   b. Maxillary teeth extend too far forward and do not correctly overlap mandibular teeth

   c. Maxillary incisors extend too far beyond mandibular teeth, but the overlap is otherwise normal

   d. Teeth appear bunched and crowded in the arch

4. When might removable appliances be used?

   a. Before a fixed appliance

   b. After a fixed appliance

   c. In place of a fixed appliance

   d. All of the above

5. On which teeth are bands placed?

   a. Molars

   b. Incisors

   c. Anterior

   d. None of the above

6. What are buccal tubes used for?

   a. To protect cheek tissue

   b. To distribute pressure to molars

   c. To anchor arch wire

   d. To help tie ligature wires

7. What is the name for the part of headgear that extends across the face and helps distribute pressure to the teeth?

   a. Arch wire

   b. Traction

   c. Facebow

   d. Sling

Active Learning Exercises

1. Other than providing an esthetically pleasing smile, list four other reasons why a patient may require orthodontic treatment.

2. How does the Invisalign technology used in orthodontics differ from that of traditional teeth banding or bracketing? Identify an ideal patient for Invisalign. What type of patient would not be a candidate for Invisalign? Why not?

3. Besides toothbrushing, list three other types of home-care aids a fully bracketed orthodontic patient can use. How and where are they used? Where can the patient purchase these items?

Application Activities

1. Draw each of the types of malocclusion and misalignment that are described in the chapter.

2. Practice giving oral self-care instructions for patients with fixed appliances.

chapter 46

Cosmetic Dentistry

CHAPTER OUTLINE

CHAPTER CHECKLIST

On completion of this chapter, students will be able to:

- ☑ Identify and describe the common characteristics of teeth that are assessed before developing a treatment plan for a cosmetic procedure.
- ☑ Discuss important aspects of working with patients undergoing cosmetic procedures.
- ☑ Describe the role of oral photography in cosmetic procedures.
- ☑ Identify and describe common cosmetic procedures, including whitening, contouring, use of cosmetic restorations, and occlusion procedures.
- ☑ Explain the role of the dental assistant in common cosmetic procedures.
- ☑ Identify and describe common forms of oral personalization and possible side effects on dental health.
- ☑ Explain the steps, risks, and post-care for oral piercings.

KEY TERMS

carbamide peroxide – a whitening agent that acts through oxidation of tooth enamel to lighten the enamel

contouring – shaping of the tooth

dental ornamentation – a type of oral personalization that includes dental tattoos and jewelry

front – a tooth cover that makes the teeth appear to be covered in metal, usually gold or silver; can be removable or permanent

hydrogen peroxide – unstable compound readily broken down to water and oxygen, used as a tooth whitening agent

lingual frenum (LING-gwul FREE-num) – the fold of tissue connecting the bottom of the tongue to the floor of the mouth

occlusal equilibration – a bite adjustment procedure that reduces pressure on the jaws and allows the bite to be more even

oral personalization – techniques used to alter the oral cavity and teeth for self-expression

sodium perborate (per-BORE-ate) – a tooth whitening agent

tongue bifurcation – a type of oral personalization that involves surgically splitting the tongue in two

uvula (YOO-vyuh-luh) – the tissue that hangs down from the maxillary posterior palatal area

Introduction

In addition to maintaining the health of teeth, more and more patients are interested in improving the appearance of their teeth. Having healthy looking teeth can make a person feel attractive and confident. As a result, cosmetic dentistry is growing in popularity. Dentists usually learn cosmetic procedures through specialized courses and training sessions and can become accredited on completion of an examination.

Cosmetic dentistry, also called aesthetic dentistry, uses procedures designed to improve the outer appearance of teeth. This includes a wide variety of procedures, such as:

- Teeth whitening
- Teeth straightening
- Placement of bridges, crowns, and veneers
- Removal of gingival tissue to lengthen teeth
- Closing spaces between teeth
- Repairing chipped, broken, or fractured teeth
- Oral personalization and oral piercing

Cosmetic Characteristics of Teeth

Before a cosmetic procedure is performed, the patient's teeth are examined for certain characteristics, including tooth color, shape, and position. The dentist can then decide what procedures can be helpful and, with the patient, formulate a treatment plan.

Color

Tooth color is very important and one of the first things other people notice about your teeth (Figure 46-1). There are several characteristics of color that dentists must consider when performing cosmetic procedures:

- Hue, or the actual color
- Intensity, or quality of the hue
- Brightness
- How well the color reflects light

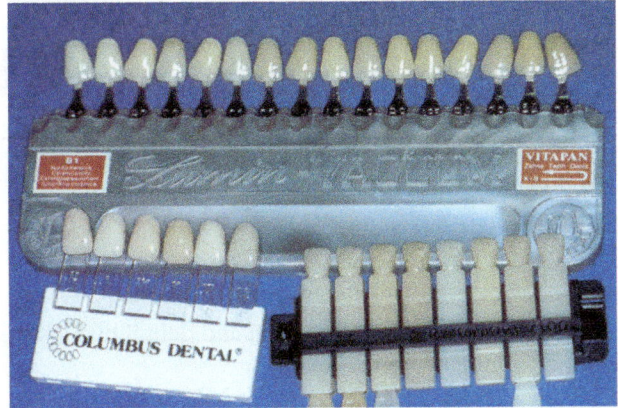

Figure 46–1 Shade guides. Photograph of several shade guides.

Shape

Cosmetic dentistry can change the shape of teeth by removing part of the tooth (e.g., shortening the tooth) or removing part of the gingival tissue (e.g., lengthening the tooth). Shaping the tooth, called **contouring**, can impact both the tooth's height and width. This can make teeth that are misshapen look more natural and similar in shape to the surrounding teeth. Contouring can also be used to restore shape to teeth that are chipped, broken, or crooked.

Position

Few people are lucky enough to be born with perfectly straight teeth. For many individuals, teeth may grow in crooked or may shift position over time. As a result, their occlusion may not be even. Cosmetic dentistry can use crowns, veneers, and bonding to make crooked or protruding teeth return to a natural and straight position (Figure 46-2). These same cosmetic techniques can also be used to reduce an excessive space between teeth, called a diastema, especially with anterior teeth.

✓ CHECKPOINT

46-1 What important tooth characteristics are assessed when planning a cosmetic procedure?

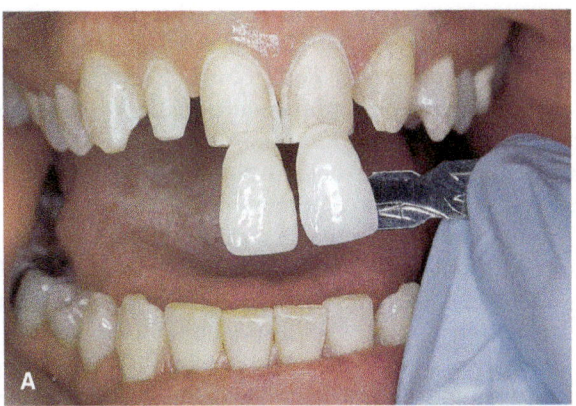

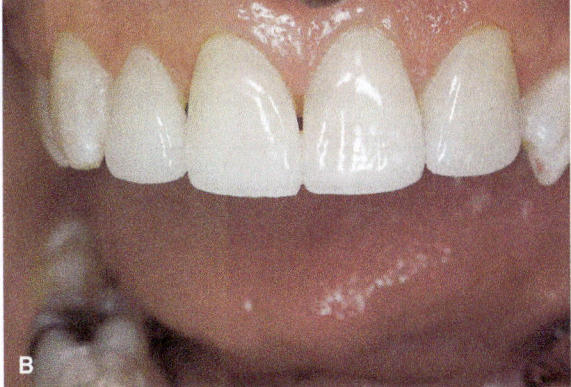

Figure 46–2 Veneers. (A) Teeth prepared for indirect veneers. **(B)** Veneers cemented in place. (Courtesy of Ultradent Products, Inc.)

Working with the Patient

The decision to undergo cosmetic dental procedures is personal and varies from patient to patient. Some patients feel that these techniques will improve their self-esteem and allow them to feel more confident in their appearance. Other patients may have cultural, religious, or spiritual reasons for undergoing such techniques. Remember that the role of the dental professional is to educate and maintain the health and safety of the patient. You may not agree with a patient's desire to undergo cosmetic dentistry, but as long as the procedure is safe and the patient is aware of any potential risks, the decision is up to the patient. All patients should feel that their dental team understands and respects their feelings.

It is important to help patients have realistic expectations for the outcome. This is where patient education becomes highly important. Patients often see pictures in magazines or see celebrities in movies or television and come to expect that their own smile too can look a certain way. Such expectations are sometimes reasonable, but other times they are not. The dental assistant plays a key role in helping patients understand their likely outcome.

The American Academy of Cosmetic Dentistry (AACD) provides accreditation for cosmetic dentists who attend specialized training classes and pass examinations in cosmetic dentistry skills. Some cosmetic dentists specialize in only one or two techniques, while others may provide a wide variety of cosmetic services. The AACD maintains a website (www.aacd.com) where the public can find accredited members near their home. In addition, many patients ask their general dentist for a referral.

Before undergoing any procedures, patients should meet with a cosmetic dentist for a consultation (see Table 46-1). This provides an opportunity to discuss the procedure they are interested in and to determine whether the dentist can perform the service. Patients may also ask to view "before" and "after" photographs of other patients who have undergone the same procedure so they can see how the dentist has treated that particular situation in the past.

Finally, dental professionals should always discuss legal issues with the patient and document their agreement. These documents can protect the dentist from legal action in the event that the patient is unhappy with the results. For example, explain the procedure in detail, including the steps involved, the benefits, the treatment plan, and the potential side effects and risks. After answering any of the patient's questions, have the patient sign a consent form stating that he or she understands the procedure and its risks and has had all questions answered. Make sure the patient is aware that cosmetic procedures can never be guaranteed to work effectively. Legal documents also include statements about the various fees and costs to the patient, the appointment schedule, and the consequences if the patient does not follow postprocedure self-care instructions.

CHECKPOINT

46-2 What important information should legal documents for cosmetic dentistry contain?

Oral Photography

Oral photography provides a better idea of what the teeth look like before as well as after a procedure. Digital photography can be used with a special computer software program, such as AlterImage or DENTRIX Clarity, to allow photographs to be manipulated, providing a preview of what the patient may look like after the procedure. This is particularly helpful for teeth whitening and repositioning procedures (for example, closing a space, straightening the teeth).

Extraoral photographs taken outside of the oral cavity are needed to show how the patient's teeth and mouth appear from the side and looking straight-on. Intraoral photographs are taken inside the oral cavity to show how the teeth appear on the maxillary arch and the mandibular arch.

Soft Tissue Contouring

Soft tissue contouring, which involves removing or restructuring the gingival tissue, is a cosmetic procedure that can enhance the overall shape of a tooth. It is typically used

TABLE 46-1 Reminders for Patients and Dentists	
PATIENTS SHOULD. . .	**DENTISTS SHOULD. . .**
Ask to see photographs of other patients who have had the same procedure	Maintain accreditation and not engage in procedures for which they have not been trained
Ask to see any licenses or certifications that show a dentist is properly trained and approved to perform cosmetic procedures	Review all of the details of the procedure with the patient and obtain written consent after answering all questions
Be sure to ask any questions that come to mind—no question is too small!	Review the patient's complete medical and dental history before performing any procedures

when excess gingival tissue covers a tooth. Dentists use a laser to reshape the tissue while ensuring that the tooth remains functional.

Occlusal Equilibration

Uneven occlusion can lead to uneven pressure on the hinges of the jaw, which can be painful. **Occlusal equilibration** is a bite adjustment procedure that can make the pressure of the bite more even. It also helps restore the appearance of the jaw when biting down. Occlusal equilibration is performed by reducing and reshaping the tops of select teeth, thereby allowing the jaw to close properly.

Cosmetic Restorations

Cosmetic restorations include veneers, crowns, and implants. (See Chapter 38, Fixed Prosthodontics, for a detailed discussion of veneers, crowns, and implants.) The materials used in fabricating these restorations vary depending on the function of the restoration and the health of the teeth. These materials are reviewed in Table 46-2.

CHECKPOINT

46-3 What cosmetic procedure might be used if a patient has an excess amount of gingival tissue covering a tooth?

Tooth Whitening

Tooth whitening, sometimes called tooth bleaching, has rapidly become one of the most requested procedures in dental offices. It can be accomplished with in-office treatments, professionally supervised at-home treatments, or over-the-counter products.

Dental assistants often manage tooth whitening for patients. In many practices, the dental assistant is the key source of patient information for tooth whitening, and may counsel the patient about the benefits and risks of the procedure, take before and after photos, match shades for the procedure, and document the procedure. During the procedure, dental assistants take impressions for whitening trays, fabricate and trim trays, and provide instructions on how to use the materials.

Tooth Discoloration

Teeth naturally discolor as people age, but a number of other factors also cause discoloration. Dentists distinguish between endogenous stains and exogenous stains, which are further categorized as intrinsic strains and extrinsic stains (see Chapter 44, Coronal Polishing).

Some patients also have naturally grey or yellow enamel. These patients are also candidates for whitening procedures. The choice of whitening procedure depends to some degree on the type of stain present, as later described in greater depth.

Whitening Materials

Materials used to whiten teeth include **hydrogen peroxide**, **carbamide peroxide**, and **sodium perborate**. These are applied to the surface of the tooth and left on for a prescribed time. These treatments work by *oxidizing* tooth enamel, or allowing oxygen to penetrate the enamel.

Hydrogen Peroxide

Hydrogen peroxide is a common whitener. It works by breaking down into water and oxygen within the tooth enamel, which interacts with pigments in the tooth and produces a whitening effect.

TABLE 46-2 Types and Functions of Cosmetic Restorations

MATERIAL/TYPE	USED FOR	CHARACTERISTICS
Porcelain restorations	■ Crowns (anterior) ■ Veneers	■ Good for making teeth appear whiter and more natural-looking ■ Brittle material that is prone to fracture
Composite resin restorations	■ Bonded veneers ■ Tooth-colored restorations that may be used to close spaces	■ Can be light-cured to make the appearance natural-looking ■ Stronger and more durable than porcelain ■ Stains more easily than porcelain
Porcelain-fused-to-metal restorations	■ Bridges ■ Crowns	■ Contains both metal and porcelain, making it high in strength ■ Natural-looking in appearance

Hydrogen peroxide can be used on both intrinsic and extrinsic stains. It is used in both in-office treatments and over-the-counter formulations. The main difference among the various hydrogen peroxide whiteners is the strength and mode of application. Peroxide whiteners vary from 5% to 35% solutions and are available as pastes or gels.

The most common side effect of hydrogen peroxide whiteners is tooth sensitivity. This increases with increased exposure and higher concentrations. It can also irritate nonoral tissues, such as eyes, mucus membranes, and skin, and it can discolor clothes. During application, the patient's clothing and skin should be well protected.

Carbamide Peroxide

Carbamide peroxide is formed through the combination of urea and hydrogen peroxide. Like hydrogen peroxide, it is an oxidizing agent, but it is weaker than hydrogen peroxide and more stable. A 10% carbamide solution has 3% hydrogen peroxide. Tooth whitening solutions are either 10% or 20% carbamide peroxide.

Carbamide peroxide is available as a liquid or gel. It is available for both in-office treatments and over-the-counter treatments. Like hydrogen peroxide, carbamide can irritate tissues, causing sensitivity in the teeth or gingiva. However, because it is weaker, it takes longer exposure to produce significant side effects.

Sodium Perborate

Sodium perborate is an oxidizing agent like hydrogen peroxide or carbamide peroxide. (The same ingredient is used in non-bleaching laundry detergents.) Sodium perborate is sometimes used during a root canal to bleach teeth from the inside out. It is available as a gel or liquid. Like other whitening agents, sodium perborate is a skin irritant.

Tooth Whitening Methods

Three major methods are available for tooth whitening. Two of them are performed under the supervision of a dentist, and one is controlled by the patient.

- *In-office whitening.* Whiteners are applied in the office and typically accelerated through the use of a light source or heat. Treatments can last up to 1 hour and whiten teeth by up to five shades.
- *At-home whitening.* The patient is supplied with a custom tray and a whitening gel. The treatment may last a few weeks and whiten teeth by up to six shades.
- *Over-the-counter whitening.* Numerous products are available with whitening agents, including toothpastes and rinses, trays, and strips. These products contain the same ingredients as professional whiteners, but at much lower concentrations and will not provide the same results.

In-Office Whitening

In-office whitening procedures are very common in modern dentistry. In many offices, dental assistants are the key contact with patients for whitening information. If a patient inquires, more often than not, it is the dental assistant who shows the patient how whitening works and what to expect.

Because this form of whitening uses the strongest whiteners, extra precautions must be taken to protect the patient. The teeth to be whitened have to be perfectly isolated before application of the whitener (Figure 46-3). This usually means placement of a dental dam, although a protective gel is sometimes used.

After the teeth are isolated, the whitener is applied. The exact method differs, depending on the product used, but in most cases, the product is brushed on to the teeth and left there for 10 to 15 minutes. Many whiteners are cured

Dental Facts

The seed of modern tooth whitening was planted when dentists discovered in the 1970s that they could mix materials in a glycerol gel that would adhere to the teeth for an extended period of time. This gave rise to early whitening systems, which used hydrogen peroxide mixed in a glycerol base and applied with trays. These systems allowed the peroxide to oxidize the stains in the enamel layer of the tooth, thus dissolving the discoloration without harming the tooth. Unfortunately, they did not last very long. Today, tooth whiteners still use hydrogen peroxide and other oxidizing agents, but their effectiveness is greatly enhanced through better delivery systems and accelerators such as the Zoom light system. These newer whiteners can sometimes whiten teeth by eight shades and provide a whitening effect for up to 6 months or 1 year.

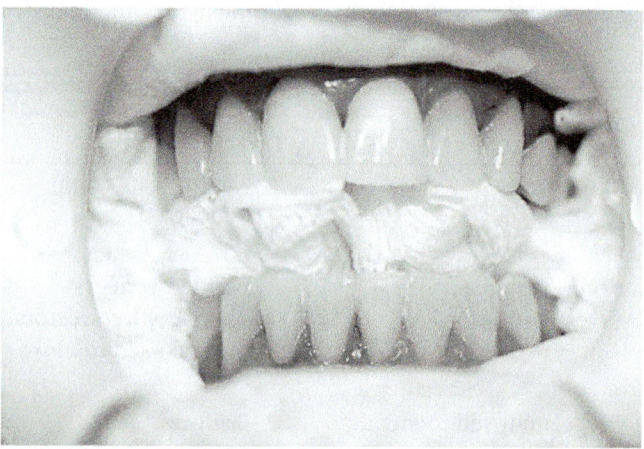

Figure 46-3 Tooth whitening. Retraction and isolation prior to whitening procedure.

with a laser light during application to enhance and speed up their whitening action. In between applications, the old whitener is rinsed off and evacuated, then another layer is applied. It usually requires three or four applications to achieve the desired results. The patient is sent home with a whitening tray and gel to apply over the next couple of days to compensate for any relapse in color.

In-office whitening has several advantages. It is the fastest method and requires the least follow-through on the patient's part. In an hour, the patient can experience significant whitening of his or her teeth.

However, there is increased risk of tooth sensitivity with in-office whitening. Not only are the whiteners stronger, the laser light used to cure the whiteners can, in some very rare circumstances, damage the tooth pulp and cause sensitivity.

At-Home Whitening

At-home whitening requires the use of custom-fitted trays that are filled with the whitening agent and applied by the patient at home. Many products are available, and their exact use depends on the manufacturer and the strength of the solution. Whiteners used for at-home applications include hydrogen peroxide and carbamide peroxide.

At-home whitening requires several appointments. At the first appointment, impressions are taken for a custom tray; the trays and bleaching agent are delivered during the second appointment. At home, the patient must follow the instructions exactly to achieve the desired effect. Some products are used overnight, while others are used once or twice a day. The overall length of treatment might be several weeks.

The major advantage to at-home whitening is its effectiveness and cost. Assuming the patient follows directions, he or she can experience a dramatic whitening of the teeth. The major disadvantage is the lack of direct oversight. Patients are in charge of their own regimen over the course of several weeks. During that time, the dentist or dental assistant cannot know whether the patient is following the procedures correctly. Also, as with in-office whitening, the whiteners can cause sensitivity.

Nonvital Whitening

Nonvital whitening is performed in the office, often after endodontic treatment. During endodontic treatment, teeth are sometimes discolored because of the presence of blood, debris, or materials used during a root canal.

During this procedure, after the root canal is opened up and treated, the target tooth is isolated with a dental dam and the root canal is sealed with a protective cement or light-cured ionomer to protect the tooth pulp from the whitening agent. Next, there are two options:

- A thick paste of whitener is applied to the crown and sealed with cement. The patient can leave the office

and return in three to five days. Multiple applications may be required to achieve the desired shade. This is known as *walking whitening*.
- The tooth chamber is exposed to a whitening gel in three increments of 10 minutes. In some cases, the whitener will be activated with heat or light-cured to achieve the desired results.

Multiple appointments may be required to adequately whiten the teeth. If the patient is unsatisfied with the final shade, a veneer might be required.

Over-the-Counter Whitening

Over-the-counter whitening products have become immensely popular with consumers over the past decade. These products are generally based on the same materials used by dental professionals, but at weaker concentrations. As a result, patients will not see the same results as they would with professional tooth-whitening. Also, in many cases, it takes much longer to achieve results, during which time the patient must follow the product directions exactly.

These products carry the same side effects as professional tooth whiteners, including tooth sensitivity and gingival irritation. The American Dental Association recommends that, even if patients choose over-the-counter products, they consult with their dentist beforehand about which product might work the best, as well as possible side effects. Patients with multiple crowns, restorations, and/or deep stains might achieve inconsistent results.

There are many forms of over-the-counter tooth whiteners, including:

- *Whitening enhanced toothpaste and rinses.* Whitening toothpastes and rinses are commonplace. Depending on the product, they contain hydrogen peroxide, sodium perborate, and even sodium bicarbonate. In general, because the concentration of whiteners in these products is extremely low to reduce the risk of side effects, many patients are not satisfied with their results, even with daily use.
- *Whitening gel.* Whitening gel is designed to be painted onto the facial surface of teeth and left in place. These gels typically contain a weak carbamide peroxide. Again, the concentration of whitening agents in these products is very low, and they are among the least effective whiteners on the market.
- *Whitening strips.* Whitening strips have been shown to be more effective than either pastes or paint-on gels. These products are very thin plastic strips that adhere directly to the facial surface of teeth. They have been treated with a weak hydrogen peroxide solution (typically 10% or less). The strips should be applied properly and worn for the specified amount of time, depending on the manufacturer's recommendations.

These strips can provide lightening in 30 days, depending on the product and as long as patients exactly adhere to the product directions. Patients should be aware that side effects are somewhat more common with strips than paint-on gels and pastes, and they might achieve inconsistent whitening of restorations.

- *Tray systems.* Over-the-counter tray systems are very similar to the ones offered by dental offices, and they have become very popular. Provided patients follow the system carefully, good results can be achieved. There are several types of trays, including simple preformed trays or plastic trays that must be boiled until softened, then fitted exactly to the teeth. To whiten, a peroxide-based gel is applied to the tray and worn for the prescribed amount of time. Although these trays are the best of the over-the-counter systems, patients should also be aware

that care should be taken to find well-fitted trays, and that exposure of gingival tissue to the whitening agent can result in gingival sensitivity. Use should be discontinued if the patient experiences pain.

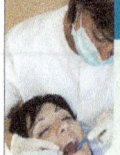

Voice of Experience

According to the American Dental Association, tooth whitening is the fastest-growing segment of modern dentistry—and the dental assistant is a key part of bringing this service to patients. In our office, dental assistants handle all the patient education and critical documentation for tooth whitening. Not only are we helping patients feel better about their smiles in a safe way—which is the most important objective of any aesthetic procedure—we're helping build a lucrative and healthy dental practice.

Procedure 46-1 At-Home Tooth Whitening

Materials needed (Figure P46-1-1):

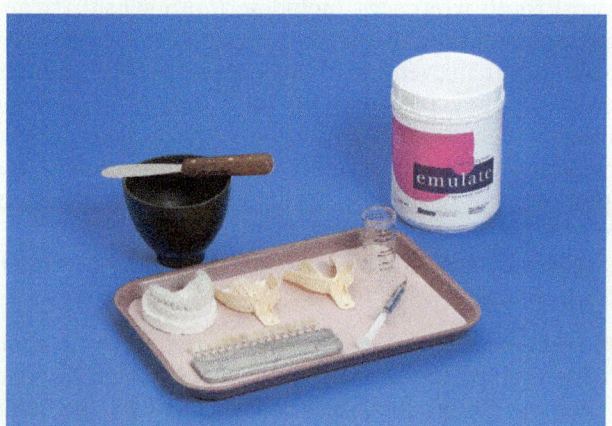

Figure P46-1-1

- Shade matching cards
- Dental camera
- Alginate impression materials
- Custom-fitted trays
- Peroxide-based gel

First appointment

1. Explain the benefits and risks of whitening to the patient, including the expected degree of whitening, the risk of tooth sensitivity, and the general procedure used.
2. Shade match the patient (Figure P46-1-2).

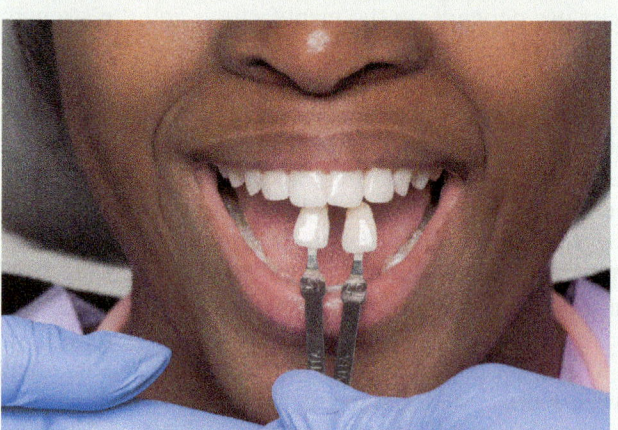

Figure P46-1-2

3. Take "before" photos of the patient's teeth.
4. Take an alginate impression of each arch. The alginate impressions are later poured into stone and prepared and then used to create custom-fit, vacuum-formed trays.
5. Record the procedure in the patient's record and schedule the patient for a second appointment.

Second appointment

1. Check the fit of the custom trays.
2. Give the patient complete instructions on how to use the trays, including how to place the gel (Figure P46-1-3), how long to wear them, and what to look for in terms of side effects.

Procedure 46–1 At-Home Tooth Whitening (Continued)

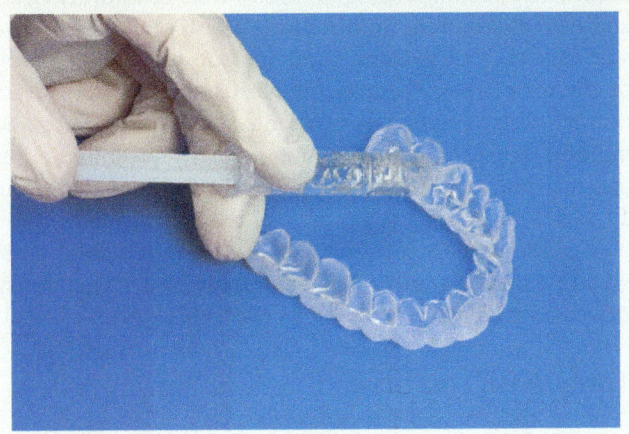

Figure P46-1-3

3. Have the patient perform the first bleaching in the office to confirm he or she understands the instructions.

4. Record the appointment in the patient's record and provide the patient with self-care instructions. Schedule a follow-up appointment for 2 weeks later to examine progress and tooth sensitivity if this is your office's policy.

Abuse of Tooth Whitening

In general, tooth whitening is a very safe, effective, and popular cosmetic dental procedure. Side effects tend to be mild and temporary; only in rare circumstances does permanent damage result.

However, some patients can develop an unhealthy attraction to tooth whitening, usually in their desire to have very bright, white teeth. This is especially problematic among younger patients. In patients under 18 years of age, whitening can cause discoloration because the tooth enamel is still forming. In patients in their 20s and early 30s, frequent whitening can eventually thin the enamel, leaving the tooth grey and pearly translucent. Ideally, patients should restrict themselves to once or twice a year for professional tooth whitening.

If a patient desires very frequent or extreme tooth whitening, gently remind the patient of the risks involved, including the risk of permanent tooth discoloration. Although it is an elective procedure, it is the responsibility of dental professionals to inform patients of possible risks.

CHECKPOINTS

46-4 What is the most common side effect associated with hydrogen peroxide whiteners?

46-5 What are the three primary methods of tooth whitening?

Oral Personalization

Just like body piercings and skin tattoos, **oral personalization** is becoming a popular way for people to express their creativity and style. This includes outfitting teeth with ink tattoos and jewelry, giving the mouth a unique and eye-catching appearance. Oral personalization also includes the piercing of different parts of the oral cavity, such as the tongue, uvula, and frenum. Ornamentation and piercings are especially popular among some celebrities. Younger patients often request personalization techniques as a way of imitating the celebrities they admire.

Ornamentation

Dental ornamentation includes tooth and gingival tattoos as well as dental jewels. All forms of dental ornamentation should always be applied by a licensed dentist or orthodontist in a clean environment, such as a dental office. While dental jewels can be ordered on the Internet, patients should never try to place these themselves. Similarly, dental tattoos should be applied only in a clean environment, such as a dental laboratory that offers this type of service. For dental jewels, encourage patients to be mindful of brushing the area around the jewel. Food and other bacteria can get caught around the edges of the jewel, leading to dental caries. Patients should not avoid brushing around the jewel for fear that it will come off. The jewels are bonded in much the same way that orthodontic brackets are bonded, and everyday brushing should not cause them to come loose. When taken care of properly, dental jewels can last anywhere from 6 months to 3 years.

Although dental ornamentation is generally considered safe when applied by a licensed dentist, always educate patients about possible risks that can occur. Dental tattoos have very few known risks, other than infection if the design is not applied by a licensed dentist in a dental lab. Following are possible side effects patients should be aware of when considering dental jewelry:

- Chips or fractures in the teeth
- Gingival infections, which, if untreated, can spread to other parts of the body, including the brain
- Accidental swallowing of jewels, leading to possible abdominal infection or suffocation during sleep
- Allergic reaction to the metals in the jewelry
- Swelling and recession of gingival tissue away from the teeth

Crown Tattoos and Designs

Similar to skin tattoos, ink designs can be placed on teeth. However, unlike traditional tattoos, no needle is used, and ink is not injected into the enamel of the tooth the way ink is injected into the skin for a traditional tattoo. Rather, dental tattoos are usually painted onto porcelain crowns in a dental laboratory and sealed to ensure that the design stays in place. Designs can be customized to fit the patient's personal taste, including the option of pictures, words, or popular symbols and logos. If the patient later no longer wants the tattoo, it can be removed from the crown by grinding down the surface of the restoration. This will not harm the crown and allows the restoration to continue protecting the tooth.

Twinkles

Twinkles is a European company that makes tooth jewelry from actual jewels, including gold and diamonds. The settings are temporarily bonded to the tooth and can be easily removed without causing damage to the enamel. Twinkles are nontoxic and generally considered safe. However, it is always important to review the patient's medical history for evidence of any metal allergies that might make jewelry placement potentially hazardous.

ToothJewelry

ToothJewelry is another brand of dental ornamentation that offers gold and diamond settings for teeth. Designs can be jewel-shaped but can also be ordered in custom forms, such as hearts, stars, and crosses. The jewels have a flat backing that allows them to adhere easily to the tooth with cement bonding. They can be applied to natural teeth as well as porcelain teeth.

Grillz

Grillz, also called **fronts**, are tooth covers made from gold, silver, and other metals. They are especially popular among hip-hop and rap musicians. Grillz snap on to cover one or more teeth; they are usually removable but can be permanently cemented in place. Grillz are relatively new,

and more research is needed to determine their safety. The American Dental Association (ADA) currently considers them safe but encourages patients to wear temporary Grillz and to remove them from time to time. Potential negative side effects from wearing Grillz include possible irritation or allergic reaction from the metals used in their construction. As with dental jewels, patients with Grillz need to be mindful of brushing and flossing properly. Food and other bacteria can become trapped under the fronts, making dental caries and infection of gingival tissue more likely. One way to reduce this is to remove Grillz before eating. Even when practicing good oral hygiene, patients with Grillz may experience gingival infections or wearing away of enamel.

Tongue Bifurcation

Another form of oral personalization involves surgically splitting the tongue into two sections—known as **tongue bifurcation**. During the bifurcation process, a surgeon uses a scalpel to split the tongue down the middle, starting from the tip and cutting toward the base until the tongue has a "forked" appearance. The split usually takes 1 to 2 weeks to heal. A number of negative side effects can occur with tongue bifurcation, including excessive bleeding and pain, swelling, damage to nerves, numbness, infection, loss of taste, and difficulty speaking, eating, and drinking.

There is some controversy about whether tongue bifurcation is safe or healthy, and as a result, many oral surgeons will not perform the procedure. The ADA warns that some patients have used improper techniques to achieve tongue splitting, such as allowing an unlicensed, unskilled individual to perform the procedure; undergoing tongue splitting without anesthesia; and pulling on the split, preventing it from healing correctly. The ADA does not recommend that oral professionals perform tongue bifurcation. For patients who insist on undergoing this procedure, the ADA emphasizes the importance of educating patients on the numerous risks associated with tongue splitting.

CHECKPOINT
46-6 Can patients safely apply dental jewels or tooth tattoos at home?

Oral Piercing

Oral piercing, including piercing the tongue, uvula, and frenum, is another form of oral ornamentation (see Figure 12-23 in Chapter 12). Patients often seek help from their dentist when they have questions about or problems with their piercing. Therefore, it is important for dental assistants to be aware of the different types of oral piercings and potential side effects of undergoing this type of procedure (see Table 46-3).

TABLE 46-3 Common Risks of Oral Piercing

LOCATION	POSSIBLE SIDE EFFECTS
Oral cavity and tongue	■ Excessive bleeding ■ Infection ■ Inability to speak, eat, or drink without pain or difficulty ■ Increased saliva production ■ Development of scars ■ Development of allergies to the metal ■ Excessive tongue swelling, leading to difficulty breathing or swallowing ■ Accidental swallowing and possible choking on jewelry
Teeth and gingival tissue	■ Infection of gingival tissues ■ Receding gingival tissue (moving away from the teeth) ■ Damage to teeth, restorations, and prostheses, such as fracturing, that can occur during the piercing procedure ■ Increased pulpal sensitivity ■ Difficulty for oral professionals to read x-ray images properly because of jewelry
Other parts of the body	■ Oral infections that are not treated can spread to all parts of the body, including the brain, heart, and liver ■ Unsafe piercing practices (for example, using unclean equipment) have been associated with blood-based diseases that are potentially fatal, including HIV and hepatitis B, C, and D ■ Blood clots can occur and travel to other parts of the body, such as the brain and lungs, possibly resulting in death

In 2004, the ADA released an official statement‡ describing the organization's opinion on oral piercing and tongue bifurcation. In this statement, the ADA declared:

■ "The National Institutes of Health has identified piercing as a possible vector for blood borne hepatitis (hepatitis B, C, D, and G) transmission."

■ "Secondary infection from oral piercing can be serious."

■ "Because of its potential for numerous negative sequelae, the American Dental Association opposes the practice of intraoral/perioral piercing and tongue splitting."

‡American Dental Association Statement on Intraoral/Perioral Piercing and Tongue Splitting. Available online at: http://www.ada.org/prof/resources/positions/statements/piercing.asp

Tongue Piercings

Tongue piercing is typically achieved by vertically inserting a needle through the thick center of the tongue. The tongue jewelry, which is barbell-shaped, is pulled through the hole and stays in place using balls that screw onto each end. There are numerous variations of tongue piercing. In some instances, a person may have the tongue pierced horizontally through the sides of the tongue, rather than vertically through the top. Others may have single, double, triple, or even quadruple and quintuple piercings in their tongue. Tongue piercings usually take 4 to 6 weeks to heal, as long as patients follow proper post-piercing care instructions.

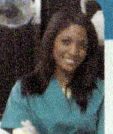

Voice of Experience

It can be unpleasant, when you ask a patient to remove a piece of oral jewelry, to find that it has not been cleaned by the patient. The jewelry is often caked with calculus that must be cleaned, either with ultrasonic equipment or with scaling instruments. This can be an important opportunity to educate patients about the importance of cleaning their jewelry and the effects of not doing so. This is also why it is important for dental assistants to become familiar with piercings and how best to advise patients on caring for them and for the health of their oral cavity.

Uvula Piercing

Piercing of the **uvula**, the tissue that hangs at the back of the maxillary palate, is not common, mainly because the area is hard to reach, making it difficult to pierce and apply jewelry. Due to its location near the opening of the throat, individuals who undergo uvula piercing are at an increased risk for gagging, accidental swallowing of jewelry, and possible choking.

Maxillary and Mandibular Frenum Piercing

The frenum is the band of skin that attaches the upper and lower lip to the maxillary and mandibular jaw bones. These piercings—also called "smileys" because they can be seen when the person smiles—are fairly simple because the frenum tissue is so thin and easily pierced. However, because the tissue contains many blood vessels, it is prone to excessive bleeding. Healing times for this type of piercing are usually between 6 and 8 weeks.

Lingual Frenum Piercings

The **lingual frenum** is the strip of tissue connecting the bottom of the tongue to the floor of the mouth. As with the maxillary and mandibular frenum, lingual frenum piercing, also known as "web piercing," is relatively easy because the tissue is so thin. Because of its location, individuals who undergo this type of piercing may be prone to irritation of the mouth floor and the underside of the tongue.

Post-Piercing Care

Dental assistants should be aware of the steps necessary for taking care of oral piercings. Patients often come to their dental office with questions or when problems occur. Basic guidelines to offer patients to maintain good oral hygiene after piercing include:

- Regularly brushing and rinsing with a saline solution (salt water) or a nonalcoholic mouthwash after every meal—at least 3 times per day

- Using a new, soft-bristled toothbrush
- Always remembering to wash hands before touching any piercing

More detailed steps to proper post-piercing care can be found in Table 46-4.

> ### Extra Patient Care
>
> If you have many patients with oral piercings, your office may want to provide a brochure to teach patients how to properly care for their oral cavity. Two examples of brochures you can supply can be found from the Association of Professional Piercers (downloadable from their Web site at www.safepiercing.com) and the ADA (the brochure, "Oral Piercing: Is It Worth It?" [#W284] is available by calling (800) 947-4746 or from adacatalog.org).

CHECKPOINT

46-7 What are some potential negative nonoral side effects from undergoing oral piercing?

TABLE 46-4 Common Dos and Don'ts of Post-Piercing Care

Do…	■ Take small bites when eating and let the molars do most of the chewing
	■ Eat cold foods and drink cold drinks, which can soothe swelling; try sucking on ice cubes for relief when piercings are sore
	■ For tongue piercings, try to keep the tongue level while eating; moving the tongue around too much can move the tongue jewelry around excessively
	■ Keep the phone number of your piercer and dentist nearby in case any questions or problems come up
	■ Take it easy and keep stress levels low
Don't…	■ Eat hot foods, spicy foods, or soft, mushy foods, like oatmeal, which can stick to the piercing
	■ Talk excessively
	■ Chew tobacco, gum, fingernails, or other objects (for example, pencils)
	■ Share silverware, plates, and drinking glasses with other people
	■ Use aspirin, alcohol, or caffeine if experiencing bleeding or swelling
	■ Swim in pools, lakes, or other large bodies of water
	■ "Play" with or pull on jewelry until the piercing is completely healed
	■ Use mouthwash containing alcohol, which can delay healing
	■ Engage in oral sexual contact during healing, including kissing, until completely healed (usually several weeks)

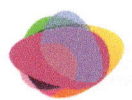

Chapter Highlights

- Cosmetic dentistry uses procedures to improve the appearance of teeth, including tooth whitening, straightening, placement of restorations, removal of gingival tissue, closing space between teeth, and repairing broken or fractured teeth.
- When working with patients, be sensitive to the personal reasons they may have for wanting cosmetic dental procedures.
- Before beginning any procedure, the steps involved, treatment, costs, and potential negative side effects should be outlined in a legal consent form, which should be explained to and signed by the patient.
- Oral photography promotes an understanding of how the teeth look before the procedure, and new computerized photography can approximate what the patient may look like after the procedure.
- Common procedures include soft tissue contouring, restorations, occlusal equilibration, and teeth whitening.
- Cosmetic restorations can be fabricated from porcelain, composite resin, or combinations of porcelain and metal.

- Tooth whitening can be accomplished in the office, under professional supervision at home, or with over-the-counter products. Common tooth whiteners include hydrogen peroxide and carbamide peroxide.
- Oral personalization is becoming an increasingly popular way for people to express themselves creatively. Such techniques include dental tattoos, gingival tattoos, dental jewelry, and oral piercing. All types of dental ornamentation carry potential risks to the patient's health, including infection, tooth destruction, or choking.
- Tongue bifurcation carries some significant risks, including pain; swelling; nerve damage; infection; and difficulty speaking, eating, and drinking.
- Oral piercing can occur in the tongue, frenum, uvula, and other parts of the oral cavity. Dental assistants should be aware of the risks of oral piercing, as patients often come to the dental office with questions or complications post-piercing.

Review Questions

1. All of the following are characteristics the cosmetic dentist must consider when performing cosmetic procedures, except
   a. Color.
   b. Contour.
   c. Texture.
   d. Position.

2. When working with patients interested in undergoing cosmetic dentistry,
   a. Be sure that they have cultural or religious reasons for wanting the procedure.
   b. Always explain the potential negative side effects that can occur.
   c. Do not show photographs of other patients, as this violates confidentiality laws.
   d. Offer your professional opinion on whether or not you think the patient really needs the procedure.

3. Excess gingival tissue can be removed, giving the teeth a longer and more natural appearance, during which procedure?
   a. Soft tissue equilibration
   b. Soft tissue extraction

   c. Soft tissue contouring
   d. Soft tissue repair

4. Which of the following procedures can make the pressure of the bite more even?
   a. Occlusal equilibration
   b. Occlusal contouring
   c. Occlusal ornamentation
   d. Occlusal bifurcation

5. Which type of cosmetic restoration is the most brittle?
   a. Ceramometal
   b. Composite resin
   c. Light-cured resin
   d. Porcelain

6. Which type of dental ornamentation has fewest known health risks?
   a. Grillz
   b. Dental tattoos
   c. Tongue bifurcation
   d. Dental jewelry

7. Oral piercings
   a. Can make it difficult for dental professionals to read x-rays.
   b. Are generally opposed by the American Dental Association.
   c. Have numerous risks, including pain, swelling, and infection that can spread throughout the body.
   d. All of the above.

8. After undergoing tongue piercing, patients should
   a. Rinse with an alcohol-based mouthwash several times per day.
   b. Rotate the piercing daily to speed the healing process.
   c. Eat and drink both hot and cold foods as normal.
   d. Suck on ice cubes for pain control.

9. Which is the strongest tooth whitening agent?
   a. Hydrogen peroxide
   b. Carbamide peroxide
   c. Sodium perborate
   d. Bleach

10. Which is an example of an intrinsic staining agent?
    a. Tobacco
    b. Wine
    c. Tetracycline antibiotics
    d. Cranberry juice

Active Learning Exercises

1. Tooth whitening products may be purchased over the counter and used by virtually anyone. What explanation could you give to the patient who does not understand the differences between over-the-counter and professionally applied products?

2. Think about the tooth whitening process and the chemical changes that take place. What are the differences between using carbamide peroxide versus hydrogen peroxide? What are their common solution percentages?

3. Imagine that a patient with a recent tongue piercing presents with sensitivity in the lower anterior teeth. Upon clinical examination, the enamel reveals numerous craze lines (fracture lines in the enamel that do not necessarily extend through the tooth). What may be causing damage to the enamel, and what other damage and oral manifestations may accompany an oral piercing?

Application Activities

1. Suppose a patient who has undergone a cosmetic procedure, such as tooth whitening, is unhappy with the results. He complains that his teeth do not look the way he thought they would, and he is asking for his money back. How do you handle this situation? Is there anything you can say to calm the patient? How does this relate to the importance of reviewing consent forms with patients? Might this situation make you do anything different when reviewing consent forms in the future?

2. Make a patient information sheet that describes self-care instructions to be followed after undergoing an oral piercing.

3. Do some research to find some cosmetic dentists in your area. What procedures do they specialize in? What membership or credentials do they hold? For each, is there anything of importance you should note, such as insurance information or weekend and evening office hours? Is there any cosmetic procedure that does not appear to be covered by any of your local cosmetic dentists?

PREPARING FOR CERTIFICATION EXAMS

Review the topic "Whitening Materials" in this chapter to prepare for the Dental Assisting National Board (DANB) exam.

Dental Practice

Office Management

CHAPTER OUTLINE

CHAPTER CHECKLIST

On completion of this chapter, students will be able to:

- ☑ Describe the major areas of staff responsibility in a dental office.
- ☑ Describe professional conduct in phone calling, collections, and other interactions.
- ☑ Describe various strategies for managing patient records.
- ☑ Describe how to order and stock supplies.
- ☑ Identify personnel policies that are covered in a typical office manual.
- ☑ Describe how to keep track of expenses and costs.
- ☑ Identify and describe the basic communication tools in a dental office.
- ☑ Explain the role of the dental assistant in performing basic office procedures.
- ☑ Develop a marketing strategy for a dental practice.

KEY TERMS

capitation – a type of insurance program in which a dentist agrees to provide services to enrolled patients in the program on a per capita rather than a fee-based system

carrier – insurance company

dependent – a person who receives dental benefits under a policy held by a primary subscriber

disbursement – payment

reorder point – the point at which quantities of a supply are running low and should be reordered

subscriber – the primary policyholder in dental insurance

Introduction

Dental office management relies on the teamwork of a number of professionals who manage patients, beginning with their first office visit. Many patients will continue with the same dental office for years, so it is essential to have an efficient system for scheduling, billing, medical records, and other facets of modern dental care. The overall patient experience is enhanced when every dental professional involved in the office knows each member's role and can help the office run smoothly. Office management often also involves tasks related to inventory, personnel policies, financial management and accounting, office communications, and dental practice marketing.

Office Staff Roles

Some office staff are not directly involved with patient treatment but nonetheless play a critical role in the office's success. Patients may not always be able to recognize quality dental care immediately, but almost every patient will instantly notice pleasant, well-trained, highly efficient office staff. Professional staff thus help cement patient loyalty.

Reception

The reception area is where first impressions of the office are formed. Reception areas vary from office to office, but a positive reception experience typically includes the following features:

- A friendly greeting for the patient, including eye contact
- Reliable information about waiting time, such as, "The dentist will be able to see you in 10 minutes."
- Activities to occupy patients while waiting, such as watching TV and reading current magazines or that day's newspaper. Pediatric offices may also have toys, books, and video games.

The reception area should also reflect the overall philosophy of the dental office. For example, some dental offices are set up as "dental spas" where it is appropriate to offer coffee or beverages to patients in the reception area. Additional information on elective procedures offered at the dental office can also be available in this area. A simple display with tooth whitening information might answer some questions and pique interest in these procedures.

In many practices, dental assistants are frequent visitors to the reception area as they greet patients and take them back to the treatment area. In these situations, you should display a confident, friendly professionalism and address any immediate concerns or questions the patients might have before treatment begins.

Scheduling Appointments

Scheduling is a basic yet fundamental part of a well-run dental practice. Scheduling is typically handled by the receptionist or a patient coordinator. Because scheduling is frequently the first contact a new patient has with a dental office, it is very important that scheduling is handled with professionalism and courtesy. Proper scheduling requires strong interpersonal and organizational skills and can make a huge difference in the quality of the patient experience.

The Appointment Book

An appointment book is a paper system used to keep track of daily appointments. It is a large book that lies flat and allows the scheduler to see an entire week or several days at a glance. Each day is divided into 10- or 15-minute increments, or units, that are filled with patient names (Figure 47-1).

The actual format of the appointment book depends on the needs of the practice. Large practices with many dentists need more columns in their daily book; solo practitioners can rely on a book that has only three columns for each day. Additionally, some books allow for separate scheduling for dental hygienist appointments.

When scheduling an appointment, the scheduler blocks off the number of units required for the particular procedure. For instance, a dental prophylaxis appointment might require three units, while a crown placement might require as many as five. Again, this depends on the practice itself, and there should be clear guidelines for how long each procedure will take and how many units should be allocated for each type of procedure.

The Schedule Matrix

The next step from a daily and weekly appointment book is a schedule matrix. The schedule matrix allows planning up to a year in advance. This book is where such events as holidays, vacations, and staff absences are recorded. Long-term follow-up treatment plans are recorded here as well. For example, a crown replacement might require several appointments over the space of months; these appointments are recorded in the schedule matrix.

Changes in the Schedule

In even the best-run offices, the schedule can change frequently as patients cancel or miss appointments, unexpected delays in treatment occur, and emergencies arise. Appointment books and matrices are kept in pencil to allow for frequent changes to the schedule. Additionally, some offices leave some "buffer time" open during the week to allow for scheduling emergencies.

Several strategies can be used to reduce the likelihood of cancellations:

- Do not schedule young children during morning nap times or lunch times. Children are more likely to be uncooperative during these times, which may make it difficult to adhere to the schedule.

THURSDAY, APRIL 11

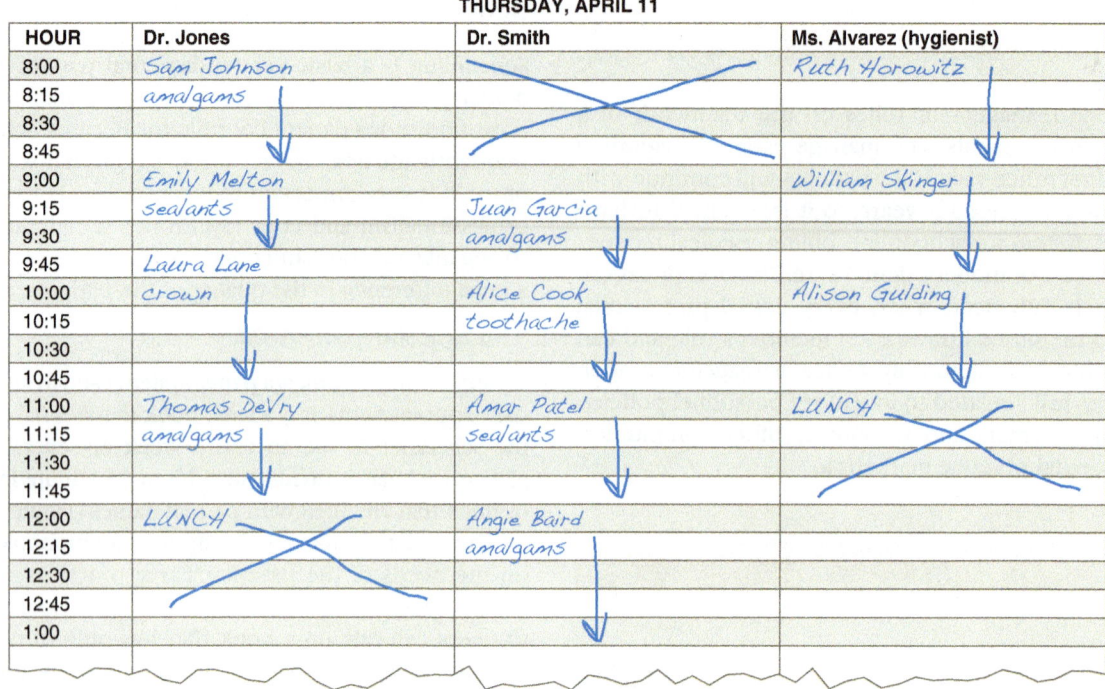

HOUR	Dr. Jones	Dr. Smith	Ms. Alvarez (hygienist)
8:00	Sam Johnson		Ruth Horowitz
8:15	amalgams		
8:30			
8:45			
9:00	Emily Melton		William Skinger
9:15	sealants	Juan Garcia	
9:30		amalgams	
9:45	Laura Lane		
10:00	crown	Alice Cook	Alison Gulding
10:15		toothache	
10:30			
10:45			
11:00	Thomas DeVry	Amar Patel	LUNCH
11:15	amalgams	sealants	
11:30			
11:45			
12:00	LUNCH	Angie Baird	
12:15		amalgams	
12:30			
12:45			
1:00			

Figure 47–1 Paper appointment book.

- When dealing with older patients, morning appointments often work better because many older adults prefer doctors' visits in the morning.
- Be aware of patients' health concerns that might impact scheduling, such as hypoglycemia and diabetes. These patients should not be scheduled for long periods of time and may need multiple visits to complete treatment.
- Be aware of the dentist's preferences. Many dentists prefer to have more complicated procedures scheduled in the morning.

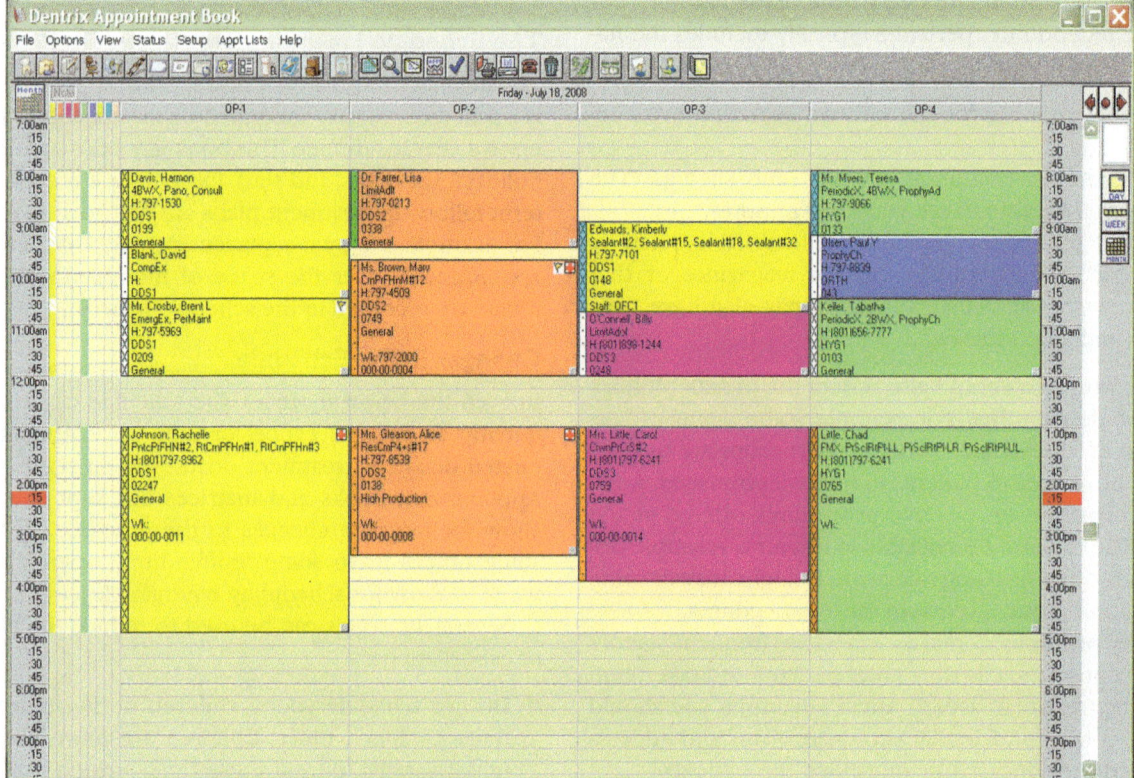

Figure 47–2 Computerized daily scheduling system. Dentrix image courtesy of Henry Schein Practice Solutions, American Fork, UT.

Computer Scheduling Systems

Although paper systems have been used for many decades, they are rapidly being replaced by computerized scheduling software (Figure 47-2). These systems enable daily, weekly, monthly, and yearly scheduling and can generate automatic reminders for patient appointments.

Computer scheduling offers several advantages over traditional scheduling. Handwriting is not an issue, and there is no need for erasing on paper. The computer can also automatically search for open appointment times and instantly provide a list of possible appointments.

Computer scheduling programs are more expensive than paper systems and require training and experience before the user becomes proficient. Nevertheless, computer scheduling is becoming more common.

Recare Scheduling

Recare, or recall, scheduling is the practice of having patients return to the office for routine oral care. Many patients are on a 6-month schedule, while others may be seen more frequently depending on their needs. Routine visits allow the dentist to examine the patient for signs of disease and provide an opportunity for the dental team to reinforce oral health techniques. Recommendations can be made regarding procedures, and the patient can have any questions answered.

Recare appointments can be automatically scheduled at the patient's current visit. Since the appointment is often many months away, some practices mail a reminder card as the appointment approaches (Figure 47-3). Some patients may not know their schedule so far in advance and prefer to fill out a recare card that prompts them to call to schedule an appointment. The card is then mailed to them when they are due to return. If the office uses a computerized system, the computer can automatically generate a recare card. Either way, the staff should make a confirmation call reminding the patient of the upcoming appointment.

Whatever system a dental office uses for recare appointments, it is important to understand how critical it is for

building and maintaining a successful dental practice. Patients who understand the value of regular dental care are more likely to report positive interactions with their dentists, just as they are more likely to have regular checkups. Ultimately, recall appointments are the foundation of preventive dentistry and allow the dentist to provide better care and the patient to experience the best possible oral care.

Patient Coordinating

A patient coordinator is a relatively new position in many dental offices. This position involves scheduling appointments and gives the patient a single contact to call with questions regarding scheduling concerns. The patient coordinator is also responsible for recare scheduling.

Telephoning

When the telephone is answered at the dental office, this might be the first connection in a long-term relationship between a new patient and the dental office. It is impossible to overestimate the value of positive phone interactions.

Basic Phone Etiquette

Dental offices use a variety of different phone systems, but basic phone etiquette has changed remarkably little over the past decade. Use the following tips to present a professional image:

- Answer the phone promptly
- Identify yourself when answering the phone
- Be friendly, enthusiastic, and polite
- Make sure you are speaking clearly
- Stay focused on the caller
- Do not eat, drink, or chew gum while you are talking
- Do not talk too quietly or loudly, or too fast
- Do not type, read email, or read journals and magazines while you are on the phone
- Do not surf the Internet or watch TV while you are on the phone
- Be respectful of both the patient's privacy and others within earshot of the conversation
- Ask for clarification if you cannot understand something
- Do not interrupt
- Take messages when appropriate and make sure calls are returned

Phone Systems

Many phone systems are available for small- and medium-size businesses such as dental offices. The choice of a system depends on several factors, including how many lines are needed, voice mail and calling options, and other automated or optional features.

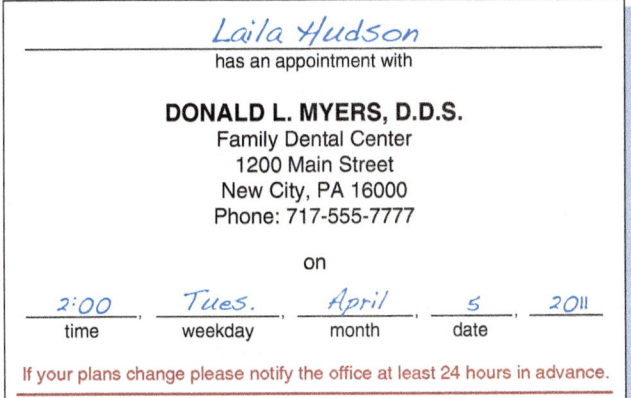

Laila Hudson
has an appointment with

DONALD L. MYERS, D.D.S.
Family Dental Center
1200 Main Street
New City, PA 16000
Phone: 717-555-7777

on

2:00	*Tues.*	*April*	*5*	*2011*
time	weekday	month	date	

If your plans change please notify the office at least 24 hours in advance.

Figure 47–3 Recare card.

Whatever particular phone system is used, the staff should be thoroughly trained in it. Most phone system companies also offer in-office training or make training materials available. Everyone who works with the phone system should be able to answer calls, place outgoing phone calls, place callers on hold, retrieve and store voice mail, forward calls, and use the intercom feature.

Voice mail, too, is an increasingly important part of dental practices. In the past, dental offices relied on answering machines to take after-hours phone calls from patients. However, a voice mail box dedicated to after-hours phone calls is now much more common. The receptionist should check this box every morning because patients frequently leave schedule changes here, making the phone system an integral part of proper scheduling.

Outgoing and Incoming Phone Calls

Incoming phone calls should be answered by a person—rather than voice mail—whenever possible. If the receptionist is consistently too busy to answer the phone during business hours, that person's job responsibilities may need to be reevaluated to ensure that phone calls are answered by staff as quickly as possible.

Patients call into a dental office for a variety of reasons, including scheduling changes, questions about their treatment plans, and questions and advice about dental problems, including dental emergencies. A receptionist should know how to handle each of these calls appropriately.

- *Scheduling calls.* The receptionist should be able to easily and efficiently schedule most dental appointments.
- *Questions about dental care.* The receptionist should get all relevant information from the caller and pass it along to the proper dental team member. These calls should not be routinely transferred to the treatment area to interrupt ongoing procedures. When collecting information, the receptionist should always be aware of privacy concerns and the need for confidentiality.
- *Dental emergencies.* Every office should have a system in place for dealing with dental emergencies, including a way to gain access to the dentist in a true emergency.

From the Dentist's Perspective

We get all kinds of calls from our patients, but some of the hardest to handle are patients seeking advice over the phone. They might be calling just after a procedure, or even before a procedure, and want to ask me a few questions. If possible, I will take the call, but often I rely on experienced dental assistants to talk to the patient and help with routine concerns, such as swelling after a bridge procedure. A good dental assistant knows how to rate pain and discomfort, how to determine if a patient needs to be seen again, and how to provide valuable oral-care advice to help my patients better understand their treatments.

When making outgoing calls, always be prepared with all the information you need before placing the call, including patient and insurance information. Having the patient's record in front of you helps ensure this. Identify yourself, state the reason for your call, and be courteous.

Long Distance Calls, Time Zones, and International Calls

It is sometimes necessary to place calls across time zones, or even place international calls. Calls to distant time zones should be placed during business hours *in that time zone.* There is a 3-hour difference between the Eastern and Pacific Time Zones, with four time zones in the continental United States. Take this into account before calling.

The same rules apply to international phone calls, where the time may differ by as many as 12 hours. Always take into account the local time and make the phone call during the appropriate time.

Long distance phone service is generally reliable, although not always inexpensive. However, calling technology is changing rapidly, and newer voice-over-Internet services are often used for calls over great distances for little or no charge. These services are not always as reliable as traditional phone service, but if your practice is frequently in contact with people or businesses at great distances, it might be worth investigating newer Internet-based technologies.

Making Collection Calls

Making collection calls can be difficult for all businesses, and dental offices are no exception. In most offices, collection calls are made not by the receptionist but by an office or business manager—if they are made at all from the office. Some dental practices hire collection services to pursue late payments. Alternatively, late notices can be sent through the mail.

Considering the complexity of dental insurance and treatment financing options available at some practices, patients often have questions, concerns, or objections about payments. How these are handled depends on the protocol in the dental office. In some smaller practices, the receptionist doubles as an office manager and can look up financial records and answer questions directly. In others, these questions should be referred to an insurance coordinator or the billing department.

CHECKPOINTS

47-1 What is a scheduling matrix?

47-2 What is a recare appointment?

47-3 Name five tasks you need to be able to perform using the phone system.

Filing and Records Management

Records management is a crucial part of the successful dental practice. It allows the practice to deliver better dental services, and dental offices are required by law to maintain certain patient records. Finally, record management must include the privacy requirements laid out in the Health Insurance Portability and Accountability Act (HIPAA), which governs patient confidentiality. See Chapter 4, Ethics and Law, for a detailed description of HIPAA requirements for handling patient records.

Filing Materials

Dental files are traditionally kept in fireproof filing cabinets in the dental office (Figure 47-4). A typical patient record includes a medical history, a clinical examination form (including dental chart), radiographs, treatment notes, and other documents related to patient care. For a detailed description of the components and organization of the patient record, see Chapter 21, The Patient Record.

Filing systems vary among dental offices. Some dental offices use color-coded file folders for patient records. Others use envelopes with patient's names and identifying information printed on the outside, such as color-coded tabs, patients' initials, and date of birth.

Filing cabinets too vary in style. Most dental offices use vertical file cabinets with doors that swing outward and up, exposing all the files at once. This design makes it easier to access alphabetized files quickly.

Patient records are usually organized in the filing cabinet alphabetically by patient last name. The color coding system usually divides patients by last name. For example, red files might include patients whose last names begin with letters A through D. This method makes it easier to quickly identify files and locate them. Some dental offices, however, use alternative organizational systems to maintain files, including numerical and subject files.

When returning materials to a patient's record, always place them back in the correct order.

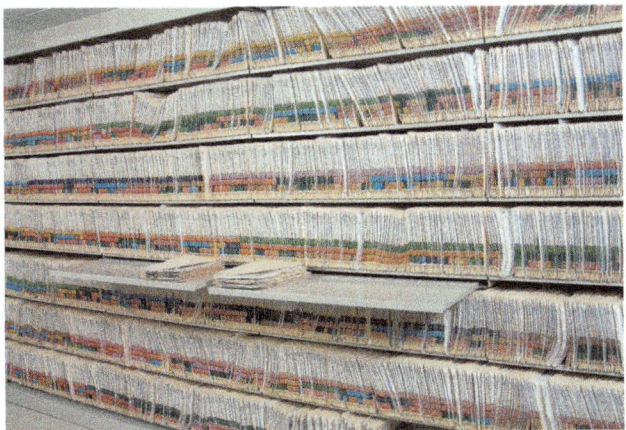

Figure 47–4 Dental files. Patient records are traditionally kept in fireproof horizontal filing cabinets that are color coded.

Patient Privacy

Patient confidentiality must be protected at all times. The rules and laws governing patient confidentiality (the HIPAA laws) are covered in Chapter 4, Ethics and Law. Use and access to patient files, including the transfer of files, is strictly regulated under these rules.

Patient records should never be left in a public area where they can be seen by other patients or by anyone without correct legal access. This also applies to the Internet—patient information should not be posted online where it can be accessed by others. Dental offices must also ensure confidentiality when communicating by email and fax.

Inventory Management

Inventory management is an important function that requires cooperation from the entire staff. Adequate supplies of inventory allow the office to function smoothly and prevent unnecessary situations arising due to lack of supplies (Figure 47-5).

Inventory management is typically delegated to one person in the office. This person is responsible for ordering supplies. However, the inventory management system requires the cooperation of all staff to identify when an item is running low and bring it to the attention of the person in charge.

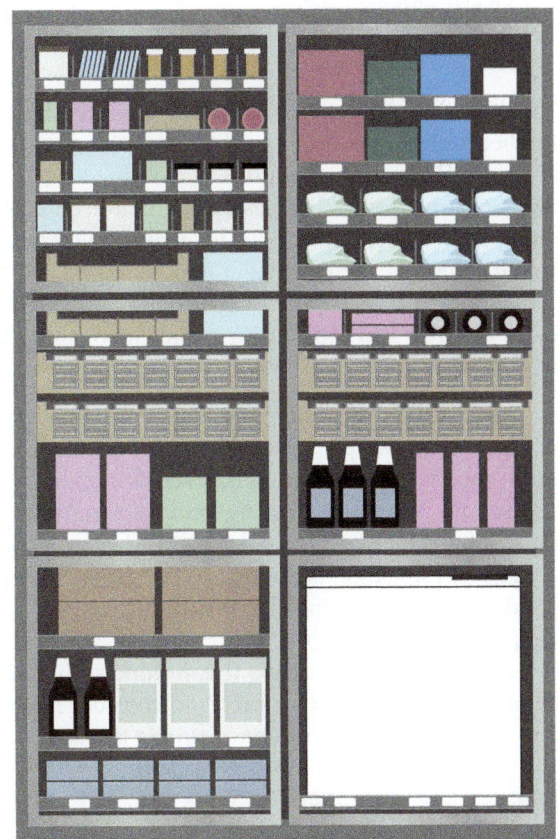

Figure 47–5 Inventory storage area.

In general, there are two classes of supplies in a dental office:

- *Expendable supplies.* These include supplies like cotton rolls, local anesthetics, disposable syringes, radiography supplies, restorative and impression materials, and paper goods that are used quickly and replaced frequently.
- *Nonexpendable supplies.* These include items such as instruments that remain in the office for a long time.

Elements of an Inventory System

An efficient inventory system includes a way to recognize when dental supplies are running low, a procedure for ordering them, and a system for storing them when they arrive. Such a system can use a software program designed for inventory management or be managed on paper.

When dental supplies are required, an order can be placed through a sales representative of a dental supply company, by phone from a catalog, or over the Internet. In addition to helping supply dental practices, a sales representative can be an important resource for offices by providing samples of new products as well as information about new technologies.

Finally, dental supplies should always be kept in a central location. This eliminates the need to search multiple areas to locate supplies and makes it easier to track supply levels. Some dental practices keep supplies in storage cabinets or clearly labeled bins.

When to reorder, and in what quantity, depends on several factors, including:

- *Quantity.* Supplies can be ordered as single items or bundled units, or in the case of high-volume expendable supplies, in bulk quantities.
- *Delivery time.* Some supplies can be delivered quickly, while others take more time to arrive; delivery time should always be factored in.
- *Consumption rate.* Supplies that are used quickly need to be ordered and stocked in sufficient quantities to prevent a gap in the supply.

These various factors determine the **reorder point** for any particular supply. This is the point at which new supplies should be ordered. Whatever system a dental office uses for stocking, ordering, and tracking supplies, every supply should have a clearly marked reorder point that triggers restocking. Many offices use bright red tags attached to products to indicate when it is time to order new supplies (Figure 47-6).

All staff members who use the products should be aware of the reorder point for each and consider it part of their responsibility to help monitor supply levels.

Exchanges and Replacements

Even in the smoothest inventory management system, products sometimes need to be replaced for a variety of

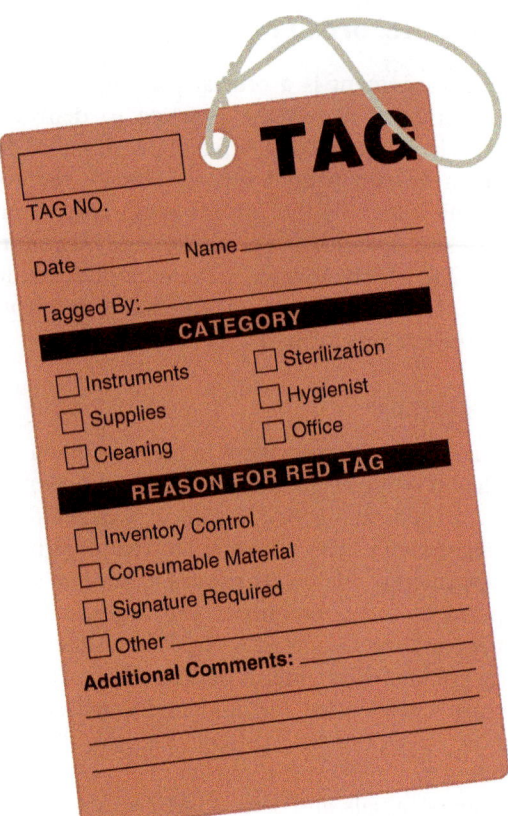

Figure 47–6 Reorder point. Many dental offices use red tags to indicate when it is time to order new supplies.

reasons. Perhaps the wrong item was ordered, the quantity was wrong, or the wrong item was shipped. As well, items are sometimes broken or damaged during shipment.

Exchanges and replacements are usually handled through the supplier or sales agent that sold the product. If the product was purchased through the sales representative of a dental supply company, the representative can also handle the replacement. If it was ordered through a catalog or direct from a supplier, then the inventory manager can handle it through one of these avenues.

Equipment Repair

Equipment repair is not necessarily an inventory issue, but it is often managed by the same person who tracks inventory. Dental equipment often requires regular servicing from a qualified technician to maintain good working condition. Additionally, radiography units require inspection from state agencies to guarantee they are safe and in excellent working condition. Even with adequate servicing, however, equipment sometimes breaks and requires repair.

With these myriad needs, it helps to maintain detailed records for every piece of equipment in the dental office. An equipment record should include:

- When the equipment was purchased
- The manufacturer or manufacturer's agent
- Warranty information

- Serial number
- Model number
- Manuals and instructions supplied by the manufacturer
- Repair log

Some larger pieces of equipment have service contracts. A service contract functions like a warranty but often includes additional services. A service contract might include regular maintenance, repairs, and even upgrades for a specified period of time. Service contracts are usually purchased along with the equipment for a fixed cost.

When a call for service is made regarding a piece of equipment, a repair log with detailed records should be kept outlining the nature of the problem, previous attempts to repair it, and the result of the call. This is true for equipment covered by a service contract as well as equipment that is not covered. Service calls can be expensive, so before calling in a service technician the problem needs to be well documented, along with the model and serial number of the equipment.

CHECKPOINTS
47-4 Give examples of expendable supplies.

47-5 Define reorder point.

47-6 What is a service contract?

Personnel Policies

Personnel policies are the rules and regulations that govern employees in the office. Every dental office should have a detailed office manual that explains the rights and responsibilities of all employees in the office. All employees should receive the manual along with an overview of personnel policies during their initial orientation.

Personnel policies in the manual should include:

- Vacation and time-off policies
- Nondiscrimination and equal opportunity employer statements
- Payment schedule
- Grievance systems
- Performance review policies
- Reprimand and dismissal procedures
- Mission statement, if applicable
- Any other policies relating to office functions

CHECKPOINT
47-7 At what stage in the hiring process should an employee receive an office manual outlining personnel policies?

Financial Management and Accounting

Accurate financial management of a dental practice is essential. Financial management issues include the money coming into the dental office (accounts receivable) and the money being paid out of the office (accounts payable), as well as insurance issues, payroll and staffing, and taxes.

Day-to-day financial issues at most small practices are handled by a bookkeeper or an office manager. These professionals keep track of money coming in and money being paid out, write checks and pay bills, and ensure that records are kept properly. Larger, more complicated financial issues may be handled by an accountant, who is a financial expert trained in the running of a business, including tax issues. Some large dental practices might have accountants on staff.

Dental assistants are not usually expected to handle financial issues directly, but like any employee, they should know how the company is managed and be able to keep appropriate records.

Patient Fees and Accounts

On a patient's first visit to a dental office, the patient enters into a financial arrangement with the business. Patients who are filling out paperwork for their initial visit are expected to provide financial information, including proof of dental insurance when they have it.

Fees charged for treatments depend on the type of treatment. An office visit is less expensive than a restoration, and restorations are less expensive than procedures such as root canal therapy. Some types of treatment, such as implants, can be very expensive, costing thousands of dollars.

Fees are generally explained to patients before treatment begins. For patients with insurance, the insurance plan dictates how much the insurance company will pay for a particular procedure. If the fee exceeds the level of insurance coverage, the patient is responsible for the difference. For that reason, it is very important to make sure the patient understands in advance the full financial implications of treatment.

Accounts Receivable and Billing

Accounts receivable tracks the amount of money owed to the dental practice and records incoming funds. In most practices, there are two forms of payments:

- *Private*, which are payments made directly from the patient with cash, by check, or by credit card
- *Insurance*, which are payments made by a patient's insurance company on behalf of the patient

When any payment comes in, it should be entered into the accounts receivable system.

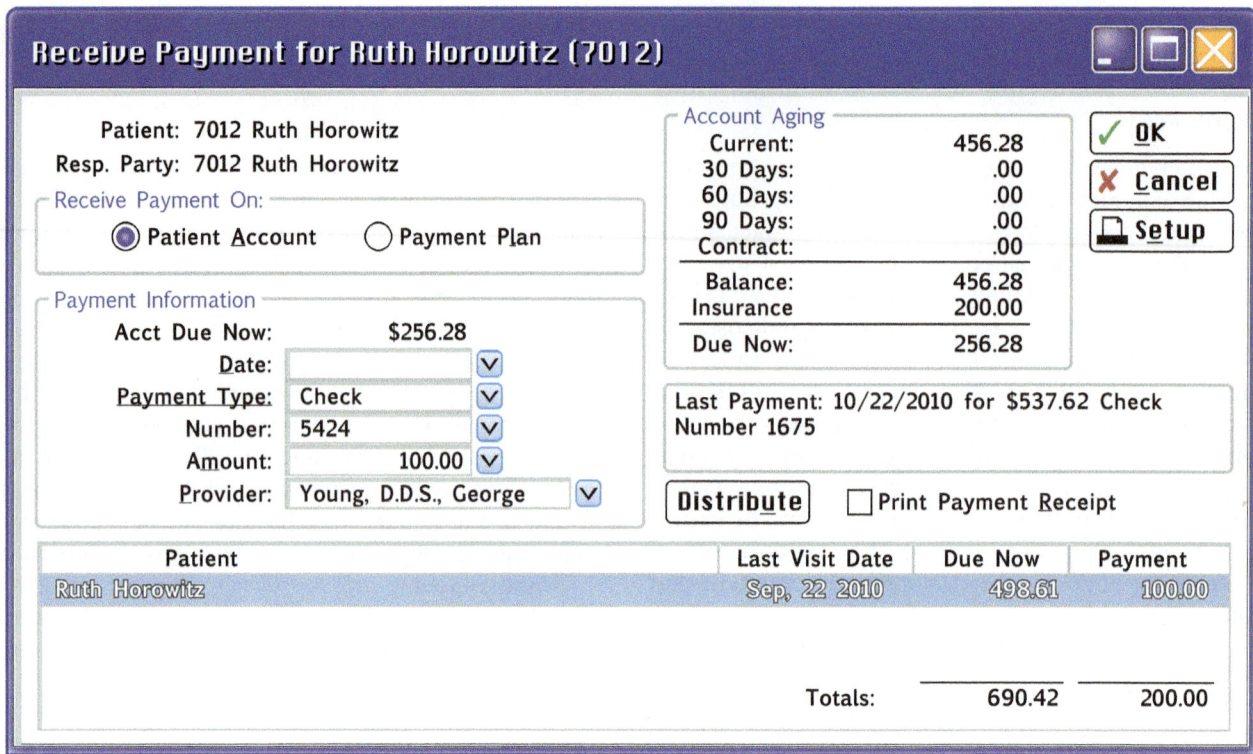

Figure 47–7 Computerized patient account.

Types of Accounts Receivable Systems

There are several types of accounts receivable systems, but all of them have the same basic purpose: to track incoming payments. The choice of system is a matter of personal preference and history within the practice. The two most common systems are the pegboard system and the computerized system.

Pegboard System

This manual system is known as the "one write" or "write it once" system. In the pegboard system, a ledger is kept every day of money coming in. The ledger has carbonized paper that enables multiple copies of each entry to be made the first time it is entered. Thus, the bookkeeper can generate an office record, a patient record, and a receipt by entering the figure only once.

Entries are made to the pegboard system by transferring billing data from the customer's ledgers cards onto a day sheet that simultaneously shows charges, receipts, and deposits, as well as what kind of service was performed. These are running totals, maintained on a daily basis. At the end of the month, the totals are transferred to a final sheet. These totals—including money owed to the practice and money obtained by the practice—should match the ledger cards or individual patient records exactly.

Because of the work associated with daily bookkeeping, many dental practices have switched to computerized accounts receivables.

Computerized Systems

Computerized systems remove much of the manual work from bookkeeping. These programs have gained widespread acceptance because of their ease of use. In a computerized system, daily totals are entered into the appropriate fields, which keep track of office visits, services provided, and procedure codes (Figure 47-7). Once the information is entered, the program automatically updates the patient's accounts with current balance information. These systems can easily generate an overview of each patient's account.

Professional Courtesy

Dentists have the option to adjust their fee schedules for colleagues or members of their families. This is known as *professional courtesy*. These discounts are usually noted directly on the chart by the dentist after treatment is complete and should be reflected in the final accounting of the procedure. The treatment is usually billed at its normal fee and then discounted.

Insurance

Dental insurance is an important source of accounts receivable for most dental offices and is often the single largest source of revenue. Thus, it is important to file insurance claims quickly and correctly to ensure payment to the dental practice.

Dental insurance is a service by which a patient pays a third-party company (the **carrier**) to cover part or all of the costs associated with dental care. The person who holds the policy is known as the **subscriber**; family members covered on the same policy are known as **dependents**. There are several ways patients can obtain dental insurance:

- *Private insurance.* Patients may purchase insurance themselves directly from an insurance company. These insurance premiums are usually higher, and the benefits lower, than in group insurance.
- *Group insurance.* Group insurance is typically offered through an employer and may cover a whole family. Group insurance is also offered through other groups such as professional associations and trade organizations. These premiums typically cost less and offer better benefits than private insurance.

Types of Dental Insurance

There are several forms of prepaid dental insurance. The type of insurance determines the payment schedule offered to the dental office. Dental offices are typically free to determine which type of insurance they accept, and from which insurance companies. If a patient's insurance is not accepted by a dental office, the patient must be made aware of that *before* any treatment begins.

Within the various categories of dental insurance, there are many different options and payment plans.

Traditional Insurance

This is the most common form of dental insurance. This is a fee-for-service insurance in which the dentist is reimbursed by the insurance company based on the type of procedure performed. The amount paid by the insurance company is often not the same as the actual fee for the service, and any difference is made up by the patient. There are a number of ways dentists measure their fees:

- *Usual fee.* The usual fee is the standard, typical fee charged by that dental practice for that service. Dentists typically provide a list of their usual fees to insurance carriers to help the insurance company determine reimbursement rates in that region.
- *Customary fee.* The customary fee is the usual fee for a treatment by dentists in a particular region or practice area. Customary fees are not necessarily averages, but they represent a range of what most dentists are charging for particular procedures.
- *Reasonable fee.* Reasonable fees are used to calculate reimbursement for complicated or specialized procedures. Dentists might charge reasonable fees for procedures that require above-average resources and time, but the insurance company usually asks for written justification for the higher fee.

The amount the insurance company pays may or may not cover the total cost of the procedure, depending on the unique circumstances of each region, the procedure, and the insurance carrier.

Fixed-Fee Programs

In fixed-fee programs, participating dentists accept a predetermined fixed fee for each patient. A number of fixed-fee options are available, and they are growing as more people seek to control the cost of dentistry. Perhaps the most well-known example of a fixed-fee program is the government Medicare program, which pays certain fees for procedures and forbids dentists from charging the difference to patients.

Fixed-fee options include:

- *Capitation.* In **capitation** programs, the dentist agrees to provide all the covered services in exchange for a fixed, per-capita fee based on the number of people in the program. The best-known examples of capitation programs are health maintenance organizations (HMOs) or dental maintenance organizations (DMOs). Dentists enroll in these groups and accept the fee schedule in exchange for the large pool of patients in the program. In exchange, patients can choose only from dentists enrolled in the program. Preferred provider organizations (PPOs) are a popular variation of this system. In PPOs, the dentist joins a PPO and the patients are offered reduced fees for services, but there may be increased out-of-pocket patient expenses in exchange for access to a greater number of dentists.
- *Direct reimbursement.* Direct reimbursement is a form of prepaid dental program that usually does not involve insurance companies. In these programs, the patient pays for dental services and is then directly reimbursed by the plan administrator, usually an employer. In these programs, the patient is limited to dentists enrolled in the program, but the benefits list may be limited by the plan administrator.

Managed Care

Managed care plans resulted from growing efforts to control and contain medical costs, including dental care. The original concept behind managed care was to encourage preventive dentistry and medical services at a reduced cost in exchange for limits or restrictions on the number and type of physicians a patient can see, and which types of procedures are covered fully or partially. Under this model, it was thought that the medical and dental communities could offer basic services to a greater pool of people at a reduced cost.

The success of managed care is a hotly debated topic among health care professionals. HMOs and PPOs are both forms of managed care. Although these groups have grown quickly and offer many people access to medical and dental services, costs have continued to rise. Even more troublesome in dentistry is the trend away from dental coverage. Many employers and individuals are dropping dental coverage, arguing that it is too expensive. When people do not have dental insurance, however, they are less likely to make regular visits to the dentist and are more likely to suffer from dental problems.

There is no easy solution to the rising expense of medical and dental treatment, but new solutions will likely be developed as health care providers strive to offer affordable and excellent patient care.

Dental Benefits

The amount of insurance paid depends on the type of insurance and the benefits outlined in the policy. For most group and private insurance policies, benefits are spelled out in the benefits booklet, which is provided when the insurance policy is first activated. Benefits are typically defined by:

- *Coverage*. Insurance coverage may vary from policy to policy, depending on how much insurance the subscriber or the group has purchased. Additionally, many insurance policies limit their pay-outs based on a concept known as *least expensive alternative treatment*. According to this concept, the insurance carrier pays only for the least expensive option to treat a certain condition. If, for example, a restoration can be performed, but the patient wants an extraction and bridge, the insurance carrier typically pays only the rate for a restoration. The patient has to pay the difference.

  Some patients are also covered by more than one plan. Known as dual coverage, this affects how insurance claims are submitted and processed. In these cases, the primary carrier covers the initial expenses, and the secondary carrier covers additional expenses up to 100% of the treatment cost. Pay-outs cannot exceed 100% of the cost of the treatment. Dual coverage is most common with two working spouses who both receive insurance through their employers. In this case, the patient's primary insurer is the one he or she subscribes to directly; the spouse's carrier is the second insurer.

  Children typically receive coverage on their parent's policies, and again, they may be covered by more than one policy. To determine the primary carrier in this situation, carriers follow the "birthday rule." According to this rule, the child's primary carrier is the policy carried by the parent whose birthday (month and day) is closest to the child's.

- *Benefits*. Benefits are determined by the policy and premium. Some plans, however, carry an automatic exemption known as *benefit-less benefit*. Under this provision, the insurance carrier is not liable for claims that are covered by any other insurance plan. If payment is still allowed, it is limited to the higher amount covered by

either plan, as opposed to 100% of the treatment fee. For example, if a treatment costs $100, and the primary carrier allows $70 and the secondary carrier allows $90, then the primary carrier will pay $70 for the service and the secondary will pay $20, totaling $90 (the highest of either plan). The patient will then be responsible for the remaining $10.

Extra Patient Care

Patients often assume that the dental staff automatically knows everything about their insurance policy, which can lead to misunderstandings and hurt feelings at billing time. If patients seem confused about their benefits, ask them to bring in their benefits booklet and help them figure out what their benefits, deductible, and limitations are before treatment begins. Not everybody understands that dental policies differ greatly.

Submitting Insurance Claims

Insurance claims are usually submitted on behalf of the patient by the dental office. To submit an insurance claim, patients must supply their name, address, ID number, and policy number, and the dental office supplies the office's identification and a description of the services rendered.

For consistency, dental procedures are identified by a uniform code known as the Code of Dental Procedures and Nomenclature, which is published in *Current Dental Terminology* (CDT) by the American Dental Association (ADA). CDT codes are the backbone of the billing process. Every dental service is identified by a five-digit code that is universally recognized throughout the dental industry. These codes are updated regularly by the ADA and interested groups.

Complete insurance claims include patient signatures in the *assignment of benefits* section and *release of information* section. The release of information signature allows the dentist's office to share confidential treatment information with the insurance company for the purpose of payment. The assignment of benefits signature allows the insurance company to pay the dental office directly, instead of sending a check to the patient. If this area is not signed, the check will be mailed to the patient.

Many dental offices handle the assignment of benefits and release of information by keeping a patient *signature on file*. This blanket permission is signed during the patient's introduction paperwork and allows the dental office to share information and collect payments.

Insurance claim forms are available from the ADA—they are standardized to most insurance carriers. A complete insurance claim includes two copies. One is sent to the insurance company, and the other is retained in the patient's record.

CDT Codes

Dental codes are made up of five characters, each yielding a piece of information. The first character is always a D, which stands for "Dental." The second character, a number, denotes the category of service, while the third and fourth designate the class and subclass of service. The fifth character, also a number, is open for expansion. A list of the most common dental codes includes:

CATEGORY	CODES	PROCEDURES
Diagnostic	D0100–D0999	Examinations, radiographs, biologic tests, biopsies
Preventive	D1000–D1999	Prophylaxis, fluoride treatments, preventive instructions, space maintainers
Restorative	D2000–D2999	Restorations, gold and porcelain procedures
Endodontics	D3000–D3999	Pulp capping, pulp therapy, apicoectomy
Periodontics	D4000–D4999	Gingivectomy, gingivoplasty, scaling and root planing, crown extensions, osteoplasty
Prosthodontics	D5000–D5899	Dentures (complete, partial, immediate)
Maxillofacial prosthetics	D5900–D5999	Prosthetics, surgery on jaw, surgical splinting
Implants	D6000–D6199	Endosteal, subperiosteal, transosteal
Prosthodontics, fixed	D6200–D6999	Crown, bridge, overdenture prosthesis
Oral surgery	D7000–D7999	Extraction, alveoplasty, fractures, trauma surgery
Orthodontics	D8000–D8999	Preventive, interceptive, and corrective orthodontics
Adjunctive general services	D9000–D9999	Anesthesia, diagnostic consultation, pharmaceutical support, cosmetic bleaching, and behavior management

Filing Electronic Claims

Claims processing has been streamlined with the introduction of automatic electronic claim processing. This allows dental offices to file claims directly from their computers. Claims processing software automatically checks the claims to make sure they are complete and provides the patient's information from the master file. This makes filing claims less labor intensive, more accurate, and faster, thus streamlining payment to the dental office. In some cases, electronic claims are filed to a third-party clearinghouse, which forwards the claim to the appropriate insurance carrier. These clearinghouses are covered by the release of information signature on the patient form and do not conflict with HIPAA privacy laws.

Electronic claims frequently can be monitored remotely so the dental office can see where the claim is in the processing system. This feature allows dental offices to obtain better information on whether claims have been accepted for payment and when payment will be released.

Insurance Payments

When the insurance carrier has processed a set of claims, it releases checks to the dental office. The checks should be accompanied by a statement explaining which claims have been paid and in what amounts. If a claim has been denied or only partially paid (an *underpayment*), there should be some explanation why the benefit was denied. If the dental office or patient feels this was made in error, the underpayment can be appealed to the insurance company and the carrier might readjust the payment.

Checks should be entered into the bookkeeping system in the appropriate patient account. Any outstanding balance should either be appealed to the insurance company or passed along to the patient, with an explanation that the insurance company did not cover the complete fee.

Overpayment

Overpayments occur when the patient pays for a procedure and the insurance company pays for the same procedure. This might happen when the insurance company is slow with payment or denies payment, only to reverse itself later and pay the claim after the patient has already settled the account. If this happens, the following steps are taken:

1. Process the check as you would any other payment. This ensures that the reporting will be consistent between the insurance carrier and the dental office. Uneven balances can potentially alert the Internal Revenue Service (IRS) and trigger an audit.
2. Credit the overpayment to the patient's account, creating a credit. The amount of this credit is refunded to the patient and listed as a business expense. This prevents the business from being taxed on this income.
3. Deduct the payment to the patient from the account again as an expense so it balances out.

Collections

Some degree of delinquency is inevitable when it comes to collecting fees for services. Thus, all dental offices have a collections mechanism to collect as many fees as possible.

This process must be handled delicately. Some patients may have every intention of paying but fall upon hard financial times and lose the means to pay their bills.

The goal of any collections effort is to collect the outstanding balance, not to punish late patients. This is best done when late balances are pursued quickly and patients are given every possible opportunity to pay their balance, including incremental payments and installment payments. No one wins when the patient is unable to pay.

The Fair Debt Collection Practice Act

The Fair Debt Collection Practice Act is designed to protect consumers, including patients, from overly aggressive collections efforts. Whether a dental practice pursues its own collections or hires a collection agency for seriously late accounts, the act covers all efforts. According to the law, people attempting to make collections are not allowed to:

- Call at inconvenient hours, such as the middle of the night
- Use threats of violence or obscene language
- Lie or use deception to obtain information
- Contact employers other than to gain information on employment status

Collection Tools

Businesses use two primary tools to collect outstanding bills: letters and phone calls.

- *Collection letters.* Collection letters are printed on the dental office's letterhead and sent to patients who cannot be reached by other means (Figure 47-8).

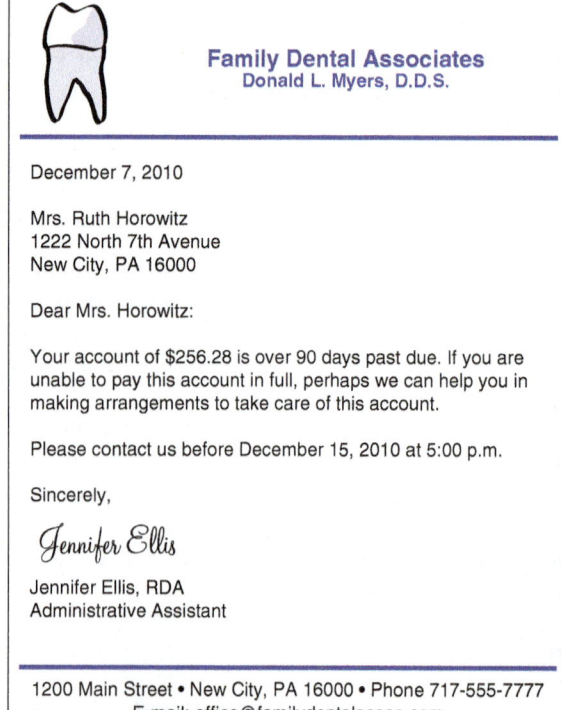

Family Dental Associates
Donald L. Myers, D.D.S.

December 7, 2010

Mrs. Ruth Horowitz
1222 North 7th Avenue
New City, PA 16000

Dear Mrs. Horowitz:

Your account of $256.28 is over 90 days past due. If you are unable to pay this account in full, perhaps we can help you in making arrangements to take care of this account.

Please contact us before December 15, 2010 at 5:00 p.m.

Sincerely,

Jennifer Ellis

Jennifer Ellis, RDA
Administrative Assistant

1200 Main Street • New City, PA 16000 • Phone 717-555-7777
E-mail: office@familydentalassoc.com

Figure 47–8 Sample collection letter.

Some dental offices send registered letters in order to establish a record of collections attempts. Registered letters have to be accepted with a signature, so the office can prove the patient received the letter if the need arises. In some cases, after a few letters have been sent, patients may be referred to a collections agency. Collections agencies are outside services that specialize in collecting outstanding bills, usually for a fee of about one-third of the outstanding cost. Collections agencies typically use a series of letters and phone calls to obtain payment, and they report past-due accounts to credit bureaus. Once the patient has paid the bill, the account should be marked as current.

- *Phone calls.* Phone calls are more personal and often more effective—it is harder to dismiss or ignore a real person than a letter. If a dental office employee is making the phone call, the employee should speak only with the patient about the collection efforts. Never leave a message with potentially private information on an answering machine or voice mail. During collections conversations, the dental office employee should remain calm and respectful, allowing the patient to explain why the payment is late and when it will arrive. Take notes during the conversation in case the information is needed for later collections efforts.

Accounts Payable

Accounts payable is the mirror image of accounts receivable. It describes all the money flowing from the dental office, including expenses and **disbursements**. Every business incurs expenses as the cost of operation. These include everything from rent to utilities to supplies and professional services. The money used to pay these expenses is known as disbursements. All expenses and disbursements should be tracked carefully to control costs and make sure the practice is current with all its bills.

Office Overhead

Office overhead refers to the costs of running a dental practice. Office overhead is a blanket term that covers everything from the cost of paper clips to the office space and building insurance. Overhead is typically divided into two categories:

- *Fixed overhead.* Fixed overhead is repeating, standard costs. This includes rent, utilities, salaries, insurance, and licensing fees. These costs seldom change and are usually paid on a regular, predictable schedule from the practice's cash flow.
- *Variable overhead.* Variable overhead is costs that are flexible and nonrepeating. This includes the cost of independent contractors and outside professional services, office supplies, dental supplies, fees, and other incidental costs.

Disbursements

Well-managed dental practices pay their bills within the time they are due and keep scrupulous records of disbursements. The easiest way to track disbursements is with a company checkbook for larger disbursements. Most practices also maintain a small petty cash supply for lesser expenses. Most businesses have a limit for petty cash expenditures, such as $50, and only one employee—the office manager, perhaps—is in control of the petty cash drawer.

Receipts and invoices should be obtained for any expense related to the dental practice and saved for the year-end accounting. If a receipt or invoice is not provided with any service or shipment, one should be requested.

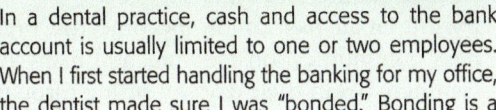

Voice of Experience

In a dental practice, cash and access to the bank account is usually limited to one or two employees. When I first started handling the banking for my office, the dentist made sure I was "bonded." Bonding is a form of insurance that protects the practice from dishonest acts such as theft, fraud, or embezzlement by employees who have access to money. Bonding is good for the business, but it is also good for employees—my job prospects are enhanced because it shows that I can be trusted with money.

Records

Larger expenses, such as a mortgage on the office building, are relatively easy to track. In many cases, these expenses are automated through online accounts and automatic withdrawals can be set up to make disbursement easier. For smaller, variable expenses, however, the dental practice needs to have a system of entering and tracking invoices so they are paid on time.

The most common accounts payable systems rely on expense categories to help track costs. For example, expenses might be classified as "professional development," "lab fees," or "supplies." These categories can be customized in most available bookkeeping software programs.

Payment Methods

Accounts payable are handled with regularity by the office or business manager. Outstanding invoices are usually paid on a monthly or biweekly basis, depending on the nature of the bill. The most common payment methods include:

- *Checks.* Checks are written drafts that promise the bearer funds withdrawn from the payee checking account. All dental practices maintain a business checking account against which checks can be written. Checks should always be filled out in full and dated on the day they were written, not pre- or postdated. In busy practices with extensive accounts payable, automated accounts payable systems can generate checks on a printer, thus reducing the labor and expense of writing them by

hand. All checks should be assigned a category so the accounts payable division can keep track of costs.
- *Automatic withdrawal.* For fixed overhead expenses, such as insurance and mortgage payments, many practices set up automated withdrawal systems whereby money is directly withdrawn from the practice's checking account on a regular schedule. This has the advantage of guaranteeing that the payments are never forgotten, but reduces flexibility because the payments are always withdrawn on the same day every month.
- *Cash.* Smaller expenditures can be handled from petty cash. Receipts should always be collected, and petty cash should be balanced every month against receipts to make sure all money is accounted for. If petty cash runs low, it can be replenished from the general checking account, with the expense always documented in the system.

Payroll

Payroll is typically the largest single expense in any dental practice. Payroll includes the salaries of all employees, from the dentist to the front office staff and receptionist. Payroll checks are usually issued weekly or biweekly, depending on the company's preference. Many practices are able to automatically deposit payroll checks into employees' bank accounts.

Payroll is subject to certain payroll deductions. The federal government maintains a list of deductions that are mandatory and must be subtracted from every employee's paycheck. The amount of the paycheck prior to deduction is known as the gross pay, or pretax total. Once deductions are figured in, the remaining amount is the net pay, or take-home pay. Pay stubs show the gross pay as well as all deductions so employees can see what money was deducted from their paycheck.

A list of the federal deductions is available through the *Employer's Tax Guide* published by the IRS. This publication does not cover state deductions, such as state income taxes. These are available through each state. When setting up a payroll, it is advisable to have an accountant assist with federal and state deductions.

Finally, not all payroll deductions are mandatory. Many practices have established retirement programs for long-term employees, such as 401k investment plans. These are typically deducted from the paycheck also, but this deduction is voluntary.

Careful records, including pay rate, deductions, and current personal information, must be maintained for every employee.

Federal Deductions

The following federal deductions must be taken from every paycheck:

- *Income Tax Withholding.* Income taxes are determined by the federal government based on the pay rate. These rates are available in the IRS's *Employer's Tax Guide*.

Income taxes deducted from each employee's paycheck are sent directly to the IRS. At the end of the year, the business issues each employee a W-2 form that shows how much money was deducted from the employee's paycheck throughout the year. It is used during income tax preparation. The amount of taxes withheld should roughly approximate the employee's overall tax rate. Employees can control how much money is deducted every pay period through the number of exemptions they claim.

- *Federal Insurance Contributions Act.* The Federal Insurance Contributions Act (FICA) consists of deductions for the federal Social Security program. Social Security deductions from the employee are matched by the employer and are not subject to exemptions. The amount of money deducted from the employee's paycheck is determined by his or her salary. The Social Security Administration keeps a record of each employee's lifetime contribution—these are used to figure benefits. Social Security is a mandatory government program designed to provide an income for older adults.

CHECKPOINTS

47-8 What happens if the fee for a dental procedure is more than what the insurance company will cover?

47-9 What is the pegboard system of accounts receivable?

47-10 What is "professional courtesy"?

47-11 What are the three types of fees used by insurance companies to determine payouts in traditional insurance?

47-12 What is capitation insurance? Give an example.

47-13 What is a CDT and what is it used for?

Office Communications

Smooth and complete office communications are essential to the functioning of a dental practice. At the same time, because dental practices deal in confidential medical information, any sensitive communication should be conducted in a way that does not violate patient privacy. (A more complete discussion of the HIPAA privacy laws is included in Chapter 4, Ethics and Law.)

Like all modern businesses, dental practices face a bewildering array of communications technologies. The most important consideration is a reliable system that meets the office's needs, rather than a system with a wealth of features that sound interesting and novel but have little practical application in a dental office.

Some of the basic communication tools include:

- *Mail and package delivery.* The United States Postal Service (USPS) has been joined in recent years by private package delivery services such as United Parcel Service (UPS), Federal Express (FedEx), DHL, and others. The USPS is still the largest mail carrier in the country, delivering mail to most areas in the United States within a few days for a nominal fee. For larger packages and express delivery, shop among the major express services, including USPS Express service. Overnight service is expensive and should be used only when the need warrants. In many cases, images and other documents can be sent faster and more efficiently over the Internet.
- *Phone.* Every dental practice needs a dedicated phone system that offers voice mail, call forwarding, hold, conference calling, and other services.
- *Email.* Email has rapidly become the preferred business communication medium, and many professionals routinely begin their days by sifting through dozens or even hundreds of emails. Email is a very fast and efficient way to communicate, but email security can be very lax. Emails are very easy to forward and duplicate, and it is not difficult for experienced hackers to gain access to almost any email account. All emails sent from a dental office should have a Confidentiality Notice attached, and senders should be cautious about sending sensitive information in email.
- *Fax.* Fax machines remain in heavy use in dental offices, despite the rise of email. They are used to secure permissions and signatures, as well as send and receive lab information and other paper documents. As with emails, privacy is a concern with faxes, and all faxes should be accompanied by a cover sheet that includes a confidentiality notice.

CHECKPOINT

47-14 What is a possible alternative to sending documents by overnight delivery?

Dental Practice

Marketing is the practice of advertising or raising awareness for a dental practice. The extent to which any dental practice engages in marketing activities depends on the size of the practice, the desire for new patients, and the budget. Some dental practices engage in extensive marketing, while others do very little marketing.

The best form of marketing is word of mouth. Dental practices that deliver consistently superior service to their patients are likely to attract new patients through their reputation for excellence.

Other marketing options include:

- *Television advertising.* This is one of the least common methods of marketing for dental practices. Television advertising can be prohibitively expensive and requires hiring professionals to shoot and create commercials, and most dentists have found that television advertising does not provide an adequate return on the investment.
- *Print advertising.* Print advertising is very common. Dentists often run small, business card–size ads in local newspapers, magazines, circulars, and other print publications. New patient specials, which offer a discount on the initial visit, can be used to attract new patients. Print ads are much less expensive to design and purchase than television ads, but still require the help of outside professionals to design and write the ads.
- *Radio advertising.* Radio advertising is less expensive than television, but more expensive than print. Larger dental practices sometimes advertise on the radio. Once again, external professionals should be hired to create a radio ad "script" and help record and produce a professional ad. Also, dental offices should be aware of when their ad will run. "Morning drive" shows are excellent ways to reach large numbers of commuters as they drive to work, but these shows vary widely in their content and some may be offensive to some listeners.
- *Outdoor advertising.* This category includes billboards and bench ads, which are both good ways to alert large numbers of local people to the presence of a dental practice. Billboards and bench ads are designed by advertising companies and usually contracted to run for a specific amount of time. Often, they can be bundled together, so the dentist will be buying ad space on a number of benches throughout a city. As with all advertising, these ads should prominently display contact information, such as a 1-800 phone number.
- *Websites.* Websites are frequently used to advertise dental practices and increase patient services. Websites offer an advantage that traditional advertising lacks: interactivity. For example, dentists can post forms online to reduce patient waiting times and allow patients to schedule appointments through email. Websites should be professional looking, which means hiring a web design company to produce and maintain the site.
- *Social media.* Social media includes websites such as Facebook and Twitter, which allow for extensive online networking. One advantage of using social media is cost: most social media websites are free and, if handled well, allow a practice to reach a large number of people. The downside, however, is time. Maintaining a social media site is time consuming, and it often takes months or even years to build up a large enough following to generate significant business.

- *Sponsoring sports teams.* Dental offices have been sponsoring children's sporting teams for decades, supplying uniforms and equipment with the office's name prominently displayed. This is a great way to reach parents in the community, build up good will, and attract new patients. Additionally, sponsorship is usually relatively inexpensive compared to other forms of advertising.
- *Free screenings.* Free screenings are sometimes offered at clinics or schools, with children receiving a rapid exam from a qualified professional. Children or patients who need additional treatment can be referred to the practice for more extensive therapy. Free screenings are often welcomed by many organizations and are inexpensive. Additionally, they provide a valuable service to the community. It is best to schedule screenings at a time that will not impact the dental practice.
- *Public relations.* Public relations is the practice of influencing media outlets to write or say positive things about a dental practice. Public relations professionals are people who specialize in generating good press coverage. Examples of public relations efforts include news articles or profiles of dentists who offer free services to low-income patients, or a dentist who appears as an expert on a local news segment. The best way to reach media outlets is through press releases or story proposals, which should be written in such a way as to attract media attention and trigger a positive story. Positive press coverage can help a business attract new patients, but it can be very difficult to place stories. Most dental offices do not engage in large-scale public relations campaigns, but alert the press when there is something happening that seems newsworthy.
- *Giveaways.* Giveaways include pens, pencils, refrigerator magnets, and other objects that include the dental practice's address, phone number, and website. These are inexpensive and a good way to make it easy for patients to find the office.

CHECKPOINT

47-15 What are some benefits websites have over traditional advertising?

Check Your Ethics

Mary Ellen is a patient at a busy dental practice. Recently, however, she fell upon hard times and is worried she'll no longer be able to pay for dental care for her family. At a quiet moment, she pulls you aside and asks you to help her out by providing a reduced fee for her exam and radiographs. You know she needs the help. What do you do?

Procedure 47-1 Preparing for the Day

Materials needed:

- Patient records
- Daily patient schedule

1. Pull the records for that day's patients, if they were not pulled the day before. Make them available to the dental staff.
2. Confirm that all lab work is ready for that day's patients.
3. Review the patient accounts and make notations on the patient records.

4. Note any premedications needed that day.
5. Assemble and distribute the daily patient schedule to dentist(s), hygienists, and assistants. Also, post the schedule in the appropriate place.
6. A "huddle meeting" is conducted before business begins. Subjects discussed at the huddle meeting include payment issues, lab work, and any personal issues that affect patient care, such as patients who require special care due to phobias.

Procedure 47-2 Day Sheet Preparation

Day sheets should be prepared before the first patient arrives. In manual systems, this sheet is used to track daily expenditures. In computerized systems, this procedure is not necessary.

Materials needed:

- Pegboard
- Day sheet
- Charge and receipt slips
- Ledger cards

1. Place a new day sheet on the pegboard.
2. Line up the charge and receipt slips and attach them on the corresponding lines.
3. Label the day sheet with the page number and date.
4. Carry over the previous day's information and fill in the appropriate columns.
5. Locate the ledger cards for that day's patients and have them available.

Procedure 47-3 Posting Charges and Payments

This procedure covers posting charges and payments to a pegboard manual bookkeeping system. The procedure for posting charges to a computerized bookkeeping system varies according to the software program used and will be covered in the software's operating instructions.

Materials needed:

- Pegboard
- Day sheet
- Ledger cards
- Patient records, including charts
- Charge and receipt slips

1. Place the patient's ledger card on the correct line of the pegboard, underneath the charge sheet.
2. Write in the date, the patient's name and insured's name, and the previous balance and credits in the appropriate places on the charge and receipt slips. This information should be automatically duplicated on the ledger card and day sheet.

3. Remove the charge sheet from the pegboard and attach it to the patient's chart. The chart is now ready for the dental team to use during treatment.
4. After the chart is completed with the procedure and charge sheet, it goes back to the reception area while the patient is dismissed.
5. Return the charge slip to the pegboard in the correct spot, then insert the patient's ledger card under the charge slip. Enter the charges and payments onto the charge sheet. They will automatically copy onto the ledger card.
6. Balance the patient's account by adding together the charges with the outstanding balances (if any) and subtracting payments. Place the final charges in the appropriate column.
7. The charge slip can now be removed. The first copy goes into the patient's record, and the second copy is provided to the patient as a receipt. The third copy is used for insurance reimbursement.

Procedure 47-4 Balancing Day Sheets and End-of-Month Figures

This procedure is performed to ensure that the bookkeeping is accurate. Computerized bookkeeping programs do this automatically.

Materials needed:

- Pegboard
- Day sheets for one month
- Ledger cards for one month

1. On the pegboard, total all the columns and write the totals in the "Total This Page" sections.
2. Add these column totals to the "Previous Page" totals that were carried forward from the day before. These numbers are then transferred to the "Month to Date" section to provide a running tally of the numbers. If there is a mistake later, this method helps identify where it happened.
3. Verify these totals against the "Proof of Posting" box, following the instructions provided with the pegboard.
4. When the proof of posting is complete and the numbers verified, total the accounts receivable.
5. Balance the month-end figures by totaling the amounts on the ledger cards using an adding machine with a tape. Check the figures on the tape against the ledger cards to eliminate transposition errors.
6. If the ledger card totals are equal to the total on the day sheets, the accounts receivable figure is correct. If it is not the same, go back and double-check all the figures to find the mistake.
7. Once the accounts are balanced, send out the statements.

Procedure 47-5 Preparing a Deposit Slip

Deposit slips are used to prepare checks for deposit into the practice's bank accounts. Deposits are done regularly, daily or weekly, depending on the size of the practice and the preferences of the dentist.

Materials needed:

- Deposit slip (Figure P47-5-1)

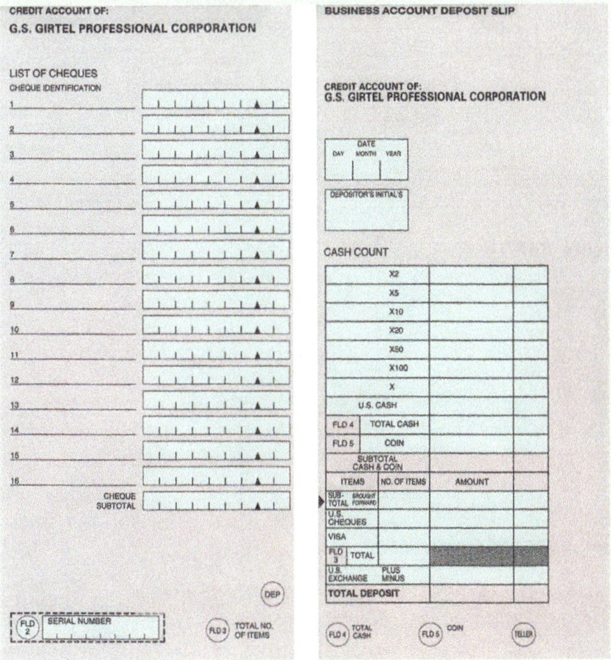
CREDIT ACCOUNT OF:
G.S. GIRTEL PROFESSIONAL CORPORATION
LIST OF CHEQUES
CHEQUE IDENTIFICATION
1 2 3 4 5 6 7 8 9 10 11 12 13 14 15 16
CHEQUE SUBTOTAL
FLD 2 SERIAL NUMBER
DEP
FLD 3 TOTAL NO. OF ITEMS

BUSINESS ACCOUNT DEPOSIT SLIP
CREDIT ACCOUNT OF:
G.S. GIRTEL PROFESSIONAL CORPORATION
DATE
DAY MONTH YEAR
DEPOSITOR'S INITIALS
CASH COUNT
X2
X5
X10
X20
X50
X100
X
U.S. CASH
FLD 4 TOTAL CASH
FLD 5 COIN
SUBTOTAL CASH & COIN
ITEMS | NO. OF ITEMS | AMOUNT
SUB-TOTAL BROUGHT FORWARD
U.S. CHEQUES
VISA
FLD 3 TOTAL
U.S. EXCHANGE PLUS MINUS
TOTAL DEPOSIT
FLD 4 TOTAL CASH
FLD 5 COIN
TELLER

Figure P47-5-1

- Currency and checks being recorded
- Day sheet indicating payments being recorded

1. Obtain a deposit slip and date it.
2. Separate the deposit into currency and checks.
3. Add the coins and enter the amount into the appropriate space on the deposit slip.
4. Add the paper currency and enter the amount into the appropriate space on the deposit slip.
5. List the checks singly in the appropriate space on the deposit slip. This is usually on the back, although there may be space on the front for a few checks.
6. Total the checks and transfer this total to the box labeled "checks" on the slip.
7. Total the coins, paper currency, and checks and enter this number in the "Total" box on the deposit slip. This should be the same number as the total cash and check payments received on the day sheet.
8. Enter the amount of the deposit into the checkbook stub.

Procedure 47-6 Reordering Supplies

Dental supplies can be ordered through a variety of avenues, including sales reps, catalogs, and the Internet. Ordering should be coordinated so multiple orders are not placed for the same items.

Materials needed:

- Red flags from the inventory system
- Inventory tracking system
- Ordering information for each item
- Telephone or computer

1. Collect red flags from the inventory system to see what needs to be reordered.
2. Gather ordering information for each item, including the part number and number of units needed.
3. Indicate in the inventory system that the item has been ordered and is awaiting delivery. Orders can be placed by telephone, in person, automatically with a wand/bar code system, or over the Internet.
4. After the item has arrived and been stocked, remove the indicator from the inventory system to reflect that no shipments are expected. Replace the red flag on the minimum number of the item to trigger another reordering.

Procedure 47-7 Reconciling a Bank Statement

Bank statements are reconciled at the end of every month, when they arrive. This procedure ensures that the accounting is accurate, both in the office and at the bank. If you are using computerized bookkeeping programs, reconcile using the program.

Materials needed:

- Checkbook
- Bank statement
- Calculator

1. Confirm that all deposits are recorded in the checkbook.
2. Subtract the bank service fees from the total in the checkbook.
3. Compare the bank statement to the checkbook to ensure that every check was entered in the correct amount and all the deposits are accounted for.
4. Carry forward the ending balance from the bank statement to the worksheet on the back of the statement (Figure P47-7-1) and enter it in the ending balance box.
5. Record all the checks that have not cleared the bank yet in the appropriate column on the worksheet.
6. Record all the deposits that have not yet been received by the bank in the appropriate column on the worksheet.
7. Total both the checks not cleared and the deposits not yet received by the bank. Subtract the checks not cleared from the ending balance and add the deposits not yet received by the bank to the ending balance. This number should equal the checkbook balance.

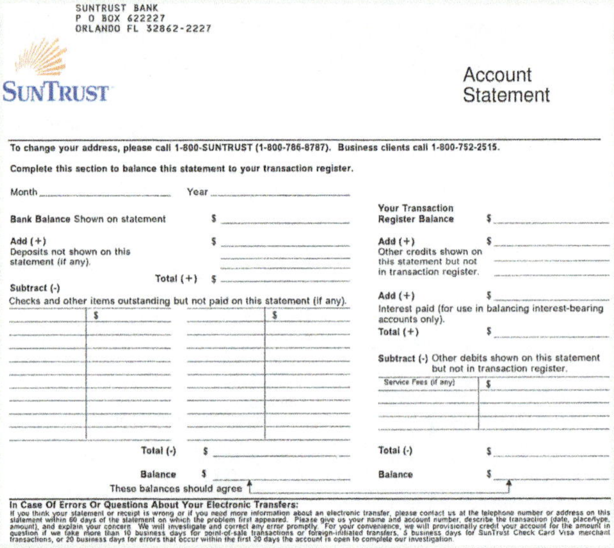
SUNTRUST BANK
P O BOX 622227
ORLANDO FL 32862-2227

SunTrust

Account Statement

To change your address, please call 1-800-SUNTRUST (1-800-786-8787). Business clients call 1-800-752-2515.

Complete this section to balance this statement to your transaction register.

Month ______ Year ______

Bank Balance Shown on statement $ ______

Add (+) Deposits not shown on this statement (if any). $ ______

Total (+) $ ______

Subtract (-) Checks and other items outstanding but not paid on this statement (if any).

	$		$

Total (-) $ ______

Balance $ ______

These balances should agree

Your Transaction Register Balance $ ______

Add (+) Other credits shown on this statement but not in transaction register. $ ______

Add (+) Interest paid (for use in balancing interest-bearing accounts only).

Total (+) $ ______

Subtract (-) Other debits shown on this statement but not in transaction register.

Service Fees (if any)	$

Total (-) $ ______

Balance $ ______

In Case Of Errors Or Questions About Your Electronic Transfers:
If you think your statement or receipt is wrong or if you need more information about an electronic transfer, please contact us at the telephone number or address on this statement within 60 days of the statement on which the problem first appeared. Please give us your name and account number, describe the transaction (date, place/type, amount), and explain your concern. We will investigate and correct any error promptly. For your convenience, we will provisionally credit your account for the amount in question if we take more than 10 business days for point-of-sale transactions or foreign-initiated transfers, 5 business days for SunTrust Check Card Visa merchant transactions, or 20 business days for errors that occur within the first 30 days the account is open to complete our investigation.

Figure P47-7-1

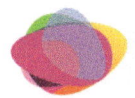

Chapter Highlights

✦ Efficient office management includes office communications, bookkeeping, and inventory management. These duties are often under the control of one person, but all professionals in the dental office might participate to ensure the office runs smoothly.

✦ Dental appointments are scheduled in units of time in the appointment book; each procedure should be allotted enough units of time to enable its completion. Appointment management also includes handling cancellations and recall appointments.

✦ Privacy is a concern in all dental office communications; phone conversations pertaining to private medical information should not be conducted in public and outgoing faxes and emails should all include confidentiality notices.

✦ Patient files are usually filed alphabetically and color-coded.

✦ Inventory consists of expendable items that are consumed quickly and frequently reordered, and nonexpendable items like machinery and equipment that are rarely replaced. The inventory system includes a mechanism for reordering.

✦ It is important to keep detailed records on large equipment, including purchase date, manufacturer and product information, warranty information, and service and repair information.

✦ All patients should have a separate account in the office's bookkeeping system, whether it is a pegboard system or a computerized bookkeeping system.

✦ There are many types of dental insurances and prepaid programs. Make sure patients understand their benefits and limitations at the outset of treatment.

✦ Dental offices receive payments both from private patients and insurance companies. Insurance claims are submitted with a standard insurance claim form or electronically using CDT codes.

✦ Insurance payments may cover the whole procedure or only part of it, depending on the policy; the difference is passed along to the patient.

✦ Collections efforts include letters and phone calls; always follow the law during collections efforts.

✦ Accounts payable include bills, payroll, and inventory expenses associated with running the practice.

✦ Payroll deductions are dictated by the IRS and state revenue laws, if any.

✦ Dental practice marketing takes many forms, including advertising, establishing an online presence, giveaways, local team sponsorships, and other avenues to reach out to the community.

Review Questions

1. When scheduling recare patients, how do you handle patients who do not want to schedule an appointment 6 months in advance?

    a. Schedule it anyway and tell them to cancel and set a new appointment when the time comes.

    b. Ask them to call the office when it is time.

    c. Mark the schedule a month before their recall to generate a call or reminder card.

    d. None of the above.

2. The pace at which supplies are used and need to be ordered is known as the

    a. Price.

    b. Break-even point.

    c. Reorder point.

    d. Consumption rate.

3. What is an advantage of computerized bookkeeping?

    a. More accurate

    b. Less labor

    c. Easier to generate records

    d. All of the above

4. What is the most common source of group insurance?

    a. Trade associations

    b. Employers

    c. Government

    d. Individuals

5. The "usual fee" is defined as

    a. A typical range of fees for a treatment in any particular region.

    b. The fee for friends and family.

    c. The fee that practices normally charge.

    d. A reasonable-sounding fee for that service.

6. What does the concept of least expensive alternative treatment mean in insurance?

   a. That dentists should choose only the least expensive treatments

   b. That the least expensive treatment yields better results

   c. That the insurance company will pay only for the least expensive treatment that yields satisfactory results

   d. That patients should be offered only the least expensive options

7. What is the birthday rule?

   a. That children are automatically dropped from their parent's insurance on their 18th birthday

   b. That if a child is covered by both parents, the policy belonging to the parent with the closer birthday will be billed first

   c. That children are eligible for dental insurance only through a parent's policy after their permanent teeth come in

   d. None of the above

8. What two signatures are required on file before insurance claims are considered complete?

   a. The assignment of benefits and release of information

   b. The release of information and indemnity clause

   c. The primary insured release and the assignment of benefits

   d. The indemnity and the benefit approval release

9. Which is part of the Fair Debt Collection Practice Act?

   a. The collection person cannot lie to obtain information

   b. The collection person cannot call an employer other than to confirm employment status

   c. The collection person cannot call in the middle of the night

   d. All of the above

10. A salary is an example of

   a. Variable overhead.

   b. Fixed-cost accounting.

   c. Fixed overhead.

   d. A negative disbursement.

11. Which is a mandated federal deduction?

   a. Value-added sales taxes

   b. 401k program

   c. FICA deductions

   d. Profit-sharing

Active Learning Exercises

1. Insurance companies have many different rules according to the plan type. What is the "birthday rule" and how does it apply to a family in which both husband and wife have dental insurance?

2. A dental assistant notices that the office is running low on many office supplies, such as cotton rolls, bibs, and gauze. What is the term used to denote that it is time to order supplies? Whose responsibility is it in the office to order the supplies?

Application Activities

1. Practice setting up the pegboard with a new day sheet and posting charges to a ledger card.

2. Practice filling out deposit slips, balancing end-of-month figures, and reconciling a bank statement.

3. Practice posting accounts receivable and updating patient records.

PREPARING FOR CERTIFICATION EXAMS

Review the following topics in this chapter to prepare for the Dental Assisting National Board (DANB) exam:

- **Scheduling Appointments**

- **Inventory Management**

- **Patient Fees and Accounts**

chapter 48

Employment and Career Issues

CHAPTER CHECKLIST

On completion of this chapter, students will be able to:

- ☑ Identify resources and strategies that can be used for career planning.
- ☑ Identify the various employment opportunities within the dental profession.
- ☑ State the purpose and basic components of a resume.
- ☑ Describe the purpose and basic components of a cover letter.
- ☑ Describe basic strategies for preparing for a job interview.

KEY TERMS

cover letter – a letter sent with a resume or job application
letter of recommendation – a letter written by a person in a position of authority to recommend someone for his or her experience, skills, or character; used during a job search
references – a list of individuals who can provide information about a job seeker's qualifications
resume – a short document listing a person's relevant job experience and education

Introduction

A career as a dental assistant can be a long, fulfilling professional career. Dental assistants are needed in every major city and place where dentistry is practiced—there is always opportunity in the field for those who approach their careers professionally. Successful career planning begins well before you send out your first resume. Networking to make connections in the field and doing thorough research to identify employment options that best suit your strengths are essential groundwork for a successful job search.

Understanding how to present your skills and qualifications in a resume and cover letter and developing strong job search skills will help you explore a variety of employment opportunities. Knowing how to properly present yourself in an interview and being prepared to answer common interview questions are also key to a successful job search.

Career Planning and Preparation

It is never too early to begin planning your career as a dental assistant. A thoughtful and organized approach to career planning while you are still a student will greatly increase your chances of finding a satisfying position once you graduate. Students have excellent opportunities to build professional contacts and gain hands-on experience that will prove invaluable when looking for a job.

Networking

Networking is one of the oldest career strategies. The old saying, "It's not *what* you know but *who* you know" may be less applicable than in the past, and professional knowledge and skills are certainly essential, but forming good professional connections will also help you throughout your career. The best way to do this is to network.

Networking is the act of seeking out other people in your profession and forming relationships with them. Once you identify possible contacts, you can ask for information and advice about the dental profession, and, later, about career opportunities in the field. There are many ways to network, but all of them involve becoming active in the dental profession in your area and seeking out people who are in your chosen field. Students, instructors, and your own dentist are possible networking contacts. Networking opportunities also come from joining professional organizations, taking on internships or externships, volunteering, and attending seminars and other educational events.

Voice of Experience

I can't recommend it highly enough: if you want to have the best career experience in dental assisting, join the American Dental Assistants Association (ADAA). The ADAA gives you an invaluable opportunity to meet other professionals, network, and even find a great job. Many dental assistants land their dream jobs from contacts gained in the ADAA.

Letters of Recommendation

A **letter of recommendation** is a letter written by a person in a position of authority to recommend someone based on his or her experience, skills, or character. Even before you begin your job search, plan ahead and start gathering letters of recommendation. Appropriate people to ask for recommendations include professors, teachers, and previous employers. In some cases, letters can also come from prominent members of the community, such as managers of volunteer organizations or even religious figures. Ideally, however, letters of recommendation come from someone in the dental field.

A good letter of recommendation addresses your strengths as a potential employee and, depending on the writer, might touch on your experience and character (Figure 48-1). Approaching someone in authority who is likely to write a good letter of recommendation is a good start. In some cases, people may decline to write a letter of recommendation if they feel it is not justified or they do not know you well enough.

Employers routinely request **references**, including letters of recommendation. When you receive a letter of recommendation, it is also a good idea to ask if you can use the writer as a reference on job applications. Some dental offices call all of an applicant's references; some do not. But almost all employers require references.

Gaining Experience

In the early stages of a career in the dental profession, it is a good idea to gain exposure to as many options as possible in order to discover what particular roles in dental assisting you like best. There are many types of dental practices (covered later in this chapter), as well as research facilities and other companies that support the dental profession, such as dental supply companies.

Students have the unique opportunity of beginning at square one: it is much easier for a student to select a career path than it is for an experienced clinician to turn his or her back on years of experience and start something new. Internships and externships are excellent ways to learn how different parts of the profession operate and to form relationships with different offices.

SMILE BRIGHT DENTISTRY
6919 Beech Avenue
Clarksville, MD 20012

February 20, 2011

Maryalice Stewart
Family Dentistry
72 Forrest Avenue
Jamesville, Maryland 21001

Dear Ms. Stewart:

I am writing to recommend Emily Brown to you for the position of Dental Assistant. Emily has been working for me at Smile Bright Dentistry for the past 6 months while my regular Dental Assistant was on maternity leave.

I have found Emily to be a benefit to my practice. She is efficient and eager to learn the procedures and workings of our office. She is punctual, bright, and always willing to chip in when help is needed.

Emily has been especially helpful in clearing out a backlog of billing that had been nagging the staff.

I would highly recommend you consider Emily as your new dental assistant. If you have any further questions, please do not hesitate to call me.

Sincerely,

Anne Harris

Anne G. Harris, DDS

Figure 48–1 Sample letter of recommendation.

While you are working on this, think about the type of work environment you hope to find. Some questions you might want to consider are:

- Do you like a routine, or do you want varied, unpredictable workdays? A dental practice tends to be more routine, while working in a hospital is faster paced.
- Do you want to work with adults or children?
- Do you want to work with older adults in a practice that sees high numbers of older patients?
- Are you interested in oral surgery or another dental speciality?
- Do you want to work with special needs patients?
- Do you like a smaller practice, such as a solo practice, or the hustle and bustle of a larger, multi-dentist practice?

The best way to find the perfect job is to experience as many types of settings as possible. This may even help your employment prospects—job candidates who know what they want and can clearly articulate why are more attractive job candidates than those who are unsure of what type of work they prefer.

Volunteering

Volunteerism can be a powerful addition to your background. The dental industry is a "people profession"—dental assistants interact with people all day, including some people who are frightened and under great stress. Volunteering indicates a compassion that is crucial for success.

Volunteering opportunities can be found in the dental profession, even for students. For example, nursing homes might need someone to help with denture care, or hospital wards might appreciate volunteers who can work with young patients on oral health.

CHECKPOINTS

48-1 What activities can you pursue for networking opportunities?

48-2 Who can you ask to provide letters of recommendation?

Employment Options

Types of Dental Practices

Within the wide range of different dental practices, there are many options for potential employment. Ideally, students and new dental assistants will gain early on a sense of what type of practice they want to work in; this will make it easier to build a long-term career in the specialty of their choice. Make an effort to observe many different types of practices so you can determine which one would be best for you.

Solo Private Practice

The traditional dental office is a small business owned and operated by a single dental practitioner with a small support staff and two or three dental hygienists on staff. Although solo practices are self-contained entities, this does not mean all solo practitioners work in isolated offices. Increasingly, solo dentists work in shared medical buildings to help reduce fixed overhead costs, such as rent and utilities. If a solo dentist becomes very busy, he or she might hire an associate dentist. This is usually a younger dentist who agrees to work as an employee of the owner of the practice. In some cases, an associate dentist may be offered the opportunity to buy into the practice after a period of time, thus becoming a partner.

Partnerships

A partnership is created when two dentists join in an equal arrangement to build a practice together. In partnerships, both dentists share financial responsibilities. Partnerships are somewhat larger and busier than solo practices, with more dental staff members. Front office duties and scheduling, however, are usually handled by a small staff to hold costs down.

Group Practices

Group practices include a larger number of dentists in a correspondingly larger practice. There are many varieties of group practices. Some have several dentists working from a single location, while others operate almost as franchises with multiple dentists working from multiple locations, all under the same name.

The complexity and size of a group practice varies and depends on how many dentists work in the practice and how many patients are seen. There are certain advantages to working in a group practice. Dentists and their associates are able to talk over cases with one another; back-office functions like accounting and payroll are often consolidated in one place, thus reducing costs; the business may be large enough to offer a more attractive benefits package and health insurance; and there is often opportunity for advancement into a management position.

Specialty Practices

Specialty practices are dedicated to particular populations. Examples of specialty practices include pediatric practices, which only treat children, or cosmetic dentists, which specialize in cosmetic procedures. Other types of specialty practices include oral surgery, endodontics, orthodontics, periodontics, prosthodontics, and public health. These practices can be any size or configuration; the main criteria for a successful work experience is enjoying the population served by the practice.

Other Employment Options

Job opportunities in the dental field are not limited to dental practices. In fact, there are a variety of opportunities you can pursue, depending on where you want to work and what type of work environment appeals to you.

Hospitals

Most dental procedures are performed in private offices, but sometimes a hospital is required, such as when general anesthesia is necessary or a full surgical suite is needed for a complicated procedure. In some cases, hospitals employ dental assistants to help with visiting dentists or oral surgeons. A hospital provides a very different working experience from a dental clinic and may offer less predictability and a greater variety of cases.

Dental Schools

Experienced and qualified dental assistants are sometimes hired by dental schools to work with students and provide hands-on training. Dental assistants in schools work on four-handed dentistry with students, assist in the laboratory with lab procedures, and sometimes teach and lecture.

Dental Research Centers

Dental research centers are devoted to initiating and performing clinical studies, writing grants, attracting research money, and publishing the results of their research. Funding for these centers comes from a variety of public and private sources, and employees are expected to be on the cutting edge of their fields. These jobs are excellent for those who enjoy research and can analyze large amounts of data.

Insurance Companies

Dental insurance companies need qualified, experienced dental assistants to help analyze claims and process payments. These positions offer excellent opportunities to advance into corporate management, but there is no significant interaction with patients. This type of job may be ideal for the qualified dental assistant who enjoys a business atmosphere.

Dental Supply Companies

Dental supply companies include manufacturers that sell directly to practices and sales agencies in which representatives sell products from multiple manufacturers. Dental assistants, with their knowledge of dental procedures and an insider perspective, often make excellent sales people. These jobs do not involve interaction with patients, as dental assistants travel from practice to practice to supply products and help dentists stay current on the latest dental technology and products.

Manufacturing Companies

Manufacturing companies create the products used by dentists. They sometimes hire dental assistants as sales representatives or to work in research and development. These positions do not use chairside skills but may allow for advancement, career flexibility, and the chance to work in a fast-paced, technological field.

Public Health Programs

A number of organizations provide dental services to low-income people or those who otherwise qualify for services. These organizations range from government-supported agencies to private charities and community organizations. Dental assistants in these roles often have more responsibility for direct patient care and may work as part of an integrated team of nurses, physicians, and dentists who serve the community.

CHECKPOINTS

48-3 What is the difference between a partnership and a group practice?

48-4 Name four examples of specialty practices.

48-5 Give an example of a public health program.

Seeking Employment

Job hunting skills are essential for anyone seeking to build a career in a professional field. A comprehensive job hunt yields several benefits. First, the job seeker hones his or her presentation skills, including interview and writing skills, which are always important. Second, the job seeker has an opportunity to learn more about the field by speaking to people active in the industry. And finally, a thorough job search is more likely to lead to a job that suits the candidate's goals and skills.

Finding Job Openings

In decades past, finding a job meant using personal connections, searching through classified ads, and perhaps visiting an employment office. Today, these are often still part of a job hunt, but there are many new ways for people to find the perfect job.

Classified Advertisements

Classified ads are still the mainstay of job hunting, but they have evolved considerably since the advent of the Internet. Today, there are several places classified ads are published:

- *Newspapers.* Local newspapers print classified ads, usually weekly.
- *Online job sites.* Several large job sites, such as Monster.com, Craigslist.org, and CareerBuilder.com, have classified ads from across the country, including ads that have appeared in local newspapers. These sites also allow

you to sort results by region, salary, and other criteria, and to post your resume for potential employers.

- *Trade magazines.* Magazines aimed specifically at the dental market are known as trade magazines. These magazines often feature classified ads with job openings.

Online sources should be checked daily. In reality, competition may be fierce for jobs at desirable practices or in desirable locations. Applicants who are prepared to respond early may have a better chance of landing an interview.

Employment Agencies

Employment agencies are companies that specialize in matching job applicants with potential employers. They often specialize in certain industries, so it is best to find an employment agency that specializes in medical and dental fields.

Reputable agencies are paid by the employer, not the employee. When you register with an employment agency, there should be no fees associated with its services. Instead, it will collect a fee from the employer if a successful hire is made. Employment agencies have the advantage of knowing the local job market and may have inside information about some jobs. However, because of their expense, some employers prefer not to work with employment agencies.

Campus Advisor or Placement Office

Students have access to campus placement offices that can help graduating students find work. Placement officers are frequently very knowledgeable about the local job market and can provide excellent advice and recommendations. In many cases, dental practices seeking new assistants contact the placement office.

Temporary Agencies

A temporary agency supplies employees on a contract or temporary basis to businesses with a short-term need. Like employment agencies, temporary agencies often specialize in particular industries, so a medical or dental temporary agency is recommended for work in the dental industry.

People who work as temporary workers are actually employed under contract by the agency, not the dental office. The dental office, in turn, has a contract arrangement with the temporary agency. Temporary work may lead to full-time employment, however, especially if the dental office and the assistant are well matched.

Professional Organizations

Professional organizations, such as the ADAA, can be an excellent resource for job seekers. Active membership in these organizations gives you access to local professionals, as well as resources such as a newsletter or job board. Dental offices can place classified ads with professional organizations, and in some cases, employers prefer applicants to be a member of such professional groups.

Writing a Resume and Cover Letter

As you compile a list of job search resources, it is time also to put together the materials you will send to prospective employers. This typically includes a resume and a cover letter.

The Resume

A **resume** is an important document that includes your education, experience, and any other qualifications that employers might be interested in, such as membership in professional organizations, awards, and volunteer work (Figure 48-2). In most cases, your resume is what creates that all-important first impression. The goal of a resume is to:

- Quickly communicate your qualifications
- Impress the reader
- Make you stand out as an exceptionally qualified job candidate

Because of the pace of hiring, your resume needs to accomplish these goals very quickly. A hiring manager may spend only a few seconds reviewing an individual resume.

Resumes follow a general format that makes it easier for managers to compare applicants. Resumes that depart dramatically from the accepted format are at risk of being disregarded because they force managers to work at deciphering the format, rather than instantly evaluating the information. In general, a resume should be a single page, well organized, and free from any spelling or grammatical errors.

The following elements should be part of a resume:

- *Name and Contact Information.* Your name should appear at the top of your resume, in a larger typestyle than the rest of the resume. It may be centered or set against the left margin as part of the overall header. Your personal contact information belongs near your name, either directly underneath it or alongside it. Your contact information should be smaller than your name, but still easy to read; this includes your street address, phone number, and email address.
- *Employment History.* This is typically the longest section of your resume and includes a list of your work history, beginning with the most recent position first. Your list of previous employers should include your title and responsibilities at each position, your beginning and ending date of employment, the full name of the employer, and basic information such as the city of

---

Resume

Emily Brown
100 Main Street
Hagerstown, Maryland 21200
410-426-0001
Emily.brown@dentmail.com

Employment:
June, 2010 to present:
    Smile Bright Dentistry as a dental assistant.
    Responsibilities included but were not limited to appointment confirmation, billing, patient interaction, instrument preparation, and taking x-rays.
March, 2008-October, 2010:
    Red Leaf Orchard as a tour guide and customer service representative.

Education:
January, 2011
    Passed the Radiation Health Safety Exam given by the Dental Assisting National Board, Inc. Scheduled to take Infection Control Exam in July 2011.
June, 2010
    Graduated from Loganville Technical Institute, Loganville, MD.
September, 2005–June, 2008:
    Graduated from Hagerstown High School. Member of the National Honor Society 2006-2008.

Volunteer:
2006-2008:
    Volunteered at Hagerstown Fire Department doing general volunteer work including setting up dances and taking tickets.

Additional Skills:
    I am experienced at working in Word and Excel. I am comfortable working with scanners and fax machines.

References:
    Available upon request.

Figure 48–2 Sample resume.

operation. Include a description of your responsibilities for each position. Keep your statements brief but active and descriptive, such as, "Managed accounts payable."

- *Education.* Your resume includes all of your educational experiences, with the most recent at the top. You should include the name of the school, the program, and the degree you received. You can also list achievements, such as Honors College and other academic designations. If you have a college degree, it is generally not necessary to list your high school experience. Do not list your grade point average on your resume.

- *Activities and Volunteer Experience.* If you have extensive volunteer experience in dentistry, or you have worked with nonprofit agencies or other organizations in the dental industry, these should also be included on your resume.

- *Additional Skills.* Certification, computer skills, and any special projects related to the field can be detailed in this section.

References generally are not included on your resume. Instead they are listed in a separate document and provided to a potential employer on request.

Check Your Ethics

When it comes time to put together a resume, always be factual and do not exaggerate the truth! Even if you do not list the director of your school's DA program as a reference, many dentists will call anyway and ask for a recommendation or confirmation that you have graduated. If you list incorrect graduation information or grades, you might be jeopardizing your career before it even gets started.

The Cover Letter

A **cover letter** accompanies your resume as part of the job application. Cover letters should be well written and thorough, but should not simply repeat the information on your resume. The main goal when writing a cover letter is to connect the skills and background outlined on your resume specifically to the position you are applying for. Like the resume, cover letters include standard elements and follow a standard business-letter format, which includes a return address, the date, the address of the recipient, and a salutation. Most word-processing programs have business letter templates that can be used to correctly format a cover letter (Figure 48-3).

January 12, 2011

Emily Brown
100 Main Street
Hagerstown, Maryland 21200

Maryalice Stewart
Family Dentistry
72 Forrest Avenue
Jamesville, Maryland 21001

Dear Ms. Stewart:

I am responding to your recent ad on Monster.com for a dental assistant. Smile Bright Dentistry has employed me, in a temporary capacity, as a dental assistant while the regular assistant was on maternity leave. She is returning in two weeks.

I have enjoyed my job here very much and am eager to find a new position as a dental assistant. I completed the dental assisting program at Loganville Technical Institute in June of 2010. I have since passed the Radiation Health Safety Exam.

While employed at Smile Bright Dentistry, I have been responsible for appointment confirmation, billing, patient interaction, instrument preparation, and x-rays. Although I enjoy all aspects of the job, billing has been my favorite function.

I have attached my resume for your consideration. I would be delighted to discuss this job opportunity face to face. Please call me so that we can schedule an interview.

Sincerely,

Emily

Emily Brown
410-426-0001
Emily.brown@dentmail.com

Figure 48–3 Sample cover letter.

The cover letter should include this content:

- Immediately identify the position you are applying for and name the source you used to find out about the opening. For example, it might begin, "I'm responding to your ad seeking a dental assistant, as advertised in *The Chronicle* on March 4."
- Identify yourself as a highly qualified applicant in a few sentences. You can mention relevant educational and job experience, and directly address any qualities mentioned in the ad. Additionally, you can give specific reasons you are interested in the open position, such as geography, reputation, or specialty.
- Request a callback or interview. The letter should close with an invitation to call you and should express your willingness to come in for an interview. Ultimately, the goal of your cover letter and resume is to land an interview.

A cover letter should be included with every resume you send out. It is best to personalize cover letters to fit each ad, rather than use the same standard letter each time. All cover letters should be addressed to a person (if a name is given in the ad) and directed to the company itself.

Online Applications

In recent years, online job applications have gained popularity. This method allows employers to post classifieds on websites and collect resumes from applicants over the Internet. There are two main ways you can apply online:

- *Electronic resume.* An electronic resume is an electronic version of your paper resume. These resumes can be emailed to potential employers, along with a cover letter included in the body of the email.
- *Online application.* Online applications can also be sent through forms that ask for information such as education, experience, and qualifications. These forms also typically include a box for a cover letter, or a space where you can "cut and paste" your resume and/or cover letter. When filling out an online application, make sure to check and double-check your work so the spelling and grammar is correct. It is just as important to present a professional image in an online application as it is in a paper resume.

In addition, some online job search sites allow applicants to post their resumes and manage job searches from the site itself. Once you have finalized your resume and created an electronic version, it is a good idea to post it to as many sites as possible. Most of these are free services.

Privacy Concerns

In all online communication, privacy should be a concern, especially when you are dealing with personal information, such as your home address and phone number. Never post personal information to message boards or forums that are public to any viewer. Post online resumes only on reputable websites that protect your private information.

Finally, be aware of your *complete* online presence. In recent years, social media sites such as Twitter and Facebook have exploded in popularity, and many people maintain pages for their friends and family. When you are job hunting, however, be aware that material you (or your friends) post online may be available to anyone using a search engine—and employers are increasingly doing online checks of prospective employees. This means you should not post anything online that might be embarrassing or unprofessional.

Preparing for an Interview

Once you have sent out resumes and cover letters, you hope for an invitation for a personal interview. Employers first narrow the pool of applicants to the strongest few. Since it is time consuming to conduct interviews, if you are called in for an interview you can assume you have a real chance of landing the job. As a result, approach interviews with considerable preparation, enthusiasm, and the utmost professionalism.

Personal Presentation

Personal presentation is a very important part of the interview process. This is the first time your future employer will see you in person, so you want to present a professional appearance. Clothing should be business casual, not jeans or formal wear. Do not wear anything revealing, ill-fitting, or wrinkled. It is a good idea, in fact, to have an interview outfit cleaned and pressed and ready to go at a moment's notice; this way, if you are called in for an interview on little notice, you do not have to worry about what to wear (Figure 48-4). Accessories, too, should be appropriate. Many dental offices have rules about piercings, length of nails, and even length of hair. During interviews, do not wear multiple piercings and be aware that factors such as the length of your nails will be noticed.

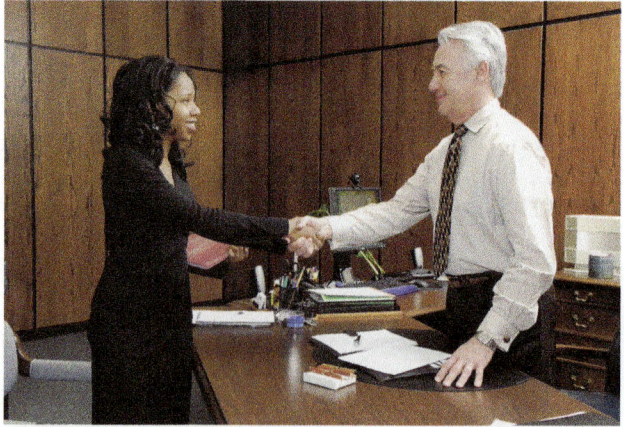

Figure 48–4 Personal presentation. Dress in business casual clothes that fit well and wear minimal accessories.

What to Bring

Do not walk into a job interview empty-handed. Pack your briefcase or document case with the following items:

- Extra copies of your resume
- A blank pad of paper for notes
- Pens and pencils
- List of references
- Academic transcripts, if necessary

During the Interview

Leave early to ensure you are on time for the interview. When you arrive, remember to shake everyone's hands, introduce yourself, and make eye contact immediately. Make note of people's names and use them throughout the interview.

During the interview, you will likely meet with the office manager, dentist, and other dental assistants. Each will have questions for you. Try to answer questions completely and concisely, and always be truthful. If you are nervous about the interview process, try to imagine what questions you might be asked and practice interviewing with a friend, colleague, or family member beforehand. Try to think of all the possible questions you might be asked and practice providing thoughtful, comprehensive answers. Common interview questions include the following:

- What can you tell me about yourself?
- What are your greatest strengths and weaknesses?
- Do you work better alone or as a team?
- Why do you want this position?
- How would a former supervisor describe you?
- What are your long-term goals in this field?

Remember that the interview also is an opportunity for you to ask questions of a potential employer. Before the interview, think about the types of questions you want answered. This might include questions such as:

- What are the typical work hours?
- Do assistants work weekends and nights?
- Is there opportunity for advancement here? To what type of position?
- How do you handle employee reviews?
- How are raises determined?
- Are there performance bonuses? Profit-sharing bonuses?
- What health and retirement benefits are available?
- How do you handle sick days?
- What is the vacation policy?
- What responsibilities will I have beyond chairside functions?
- Are there uniforms? Am I expected to buy my own uniform?
- Is there a staff room?

Do not worry about asking too many questions. A poor match between dental assistant and dental practice can be a wrenching experience for everyone involved. Make sure you get as much information as possible.

This also means paying attention to the office itself. When you arrive, note how the reception area is maintained and how you are greeted. Look for simple, small things. Is coffee or water available in the waiting room? Are the staff courteous? During the interview, pay attention to unspoken signals. A dentist who takes three or four non-emergency phone calls during your job interview is likely to be a distracted employer later on. An office manager who seems domineering early on will likely be difficult to deal with in a work context. All of these are potential clues to the working environment.

The Working Interview

Working interviews are common among dental assistants. The relationship between a dentist and a dental assistant is very close—they work together wordlessly and seamlessly, providing patient care to people who may be nervous or even frightened. Thus, to determine a good match, many dentists call prospective assistants back in for a working interview. This usually consists of a few hours or a shift of direct chairside experience.

A working interview is a chance for both the interviewer and the interviewee to get to know each other. Just as the dentist will be evaluating your performance, you should pay attention to the dentist's interactions with other staff and patients. This will provide important clues for how you will be received should you get a job offer.

After the Interview

After the interview process, usually a short time passes while the dentist evaluates candidates before finally extending a job offer. During this period, it is advisable to send a short note to the dentist thanking him or her for the interview and again briefly restating why you think you are a good candidate for the job (Figure 48-5). If possible, personalize the note with observations from the interview itself. For example, you could write, "I was very impressed with the staff's professional attitude and your philosophy of patient care. It's exactly the kind of work environment I am looking for, and I think I would be a strong asset to an office that so closely matches my own personal philosophy."

Follow-up phone calls are generally discouraged immediately after the interview. However, if a significant amount of time passes, feel free to place a call to the office to inquire how the candidate search is progressing.

An Employment Offer

An employment offer is a formal offer from the dental office to join the staff. Although this is a significant achievement, there are still things you need to work out before accepting the job. Most employment offers come with a salary

January 23, 2011

Emily Brown
100 Main Street
Hagerstown, Maryland 21200

Maryalice Stewart
Family Dentistry
72 Forrest Avenue
Jamesville, Maryland 21001

Dear Ms. Stewart:

I enjoyed meeting you recently to discuss the Dental Assistant's job. I was very impressed with the other employees and the offices themselves. Everyone seemed to be committed to taking care of the patients' needs.

Family Dentistry and I seem to be a good match. My experience in billing, patient care, and x-rays seem tailor made for the position of Dental Assistant.

I would be happy to talk with you again to answer any remaining questions.

Sincerely,

Emily

Emily Brown
410-426-0001
Emily.brown@dentmail.com

Figure 48–5 Sample thank-you note.

offer. Before accepting the salary offer, research dental assistant salaries in your area to determine if the pay is fair. If the salary seems considerably below the market rate in your area, it is acceptable to raise that as an issue and try to negotiate for a better salary.

Any other issues that might affect your employment should also be worked out before you accept the offer. This might include, for example, previously scheduled travel commitments or medical issues relating to your work life.

Continuing Professional Success

Dental assistants provide dental care and education to patients who need it. You will have the opportunity to work with highly trained professionals, often specialists in their fields, while caring for a great number of patients. Additionally, the field of dentistry is always evolving, always presenting new challenges. Dental assistants who thrive will find a highly rewarding career.

To succeed in this environment, be sure to maintain a professional attitude throughout all stages of your career.

Beginning Your Job

Your first few days on the job are critical in forming a lasting, positive impression with your new employer. It is a good idea to show up early for your first day of work prepared to help in whatever way possible and absorb as much information as you can. Remain focused on the work at hand. Leave your cell phone in a purse or jacket pocket, and only take calls that are emergencies. In the first few days, you will probably meet with staff to go over personnel policies, pay and benefits packages, and other new employee issues. Take notes during these sessions and ask questions if anything is not clear. The better your job starts, the more likely it is to be successful.

Employee Longevity

Longevity refers to the length of time you stay with any particular employer. This is important for employers. Because it costs money to hire and train employees, employees who leave after a few months end up costing the business. Most employers look for employees who are able and willing to commit to long-term employment.

The following guidelines can help you maintain a long-term positive relationship with your employer:

- Ensure there are periodic reviews and pay raises. Larger offices often have an automatic system of performance reviews and pay raises. Smaller practices, however, may be run more informally, without such a structure in place. If a year goes by without a performance review or raise, do not hesitate to politely bring the topic up and request a review and/or raise. The alternative—to let the issue fester until it becomes a morale problem—is a lose/lose situation for the dentist and you.

- Keep your skills up. Even in states without certification requirements, you should stay current in your skills. This means being active in the ADAA and other professional organizations, staying current with dental technology and trends, and, when appropriate, seeking out new challenges and specialties. This topic is covered in greater depth in Chapter 2, Professionalism, and Chapter 3, The Dental Office Team.

- Accept new responsibilities. Over time, doing the same tasks month after month may become repetitive. Always keep an eye open for new challenges you can add. This helps increase your job satisfaction and makes you a more valuable employee.

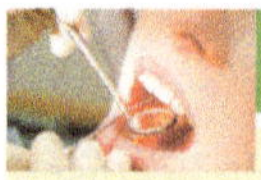

From the Dentist's Perspective

My patients expect me to offer the very best care possible, which means staying current with all the latest techniques and materials. So naturally, I require the same thing from my assistants. The more we know, the better patient care we can provide—and the better patient care we provide, the more successful our practice. That's why I tell all my assistants: stay current!

Employment Changes

In any career, less-than-ideal employment situations may require a change. There are many reasons a job might not work out, ranging from personality issues to disagreements over responsibilities and pay or staff changes. Whatever the reason, recognizing when a situation becomes unacceptable is an important part of managing a career. Similarly, navigating an involuntary termination (such as getting fired) will help you remain gainfully employed in the field.

If you leave a job, try to do so under the best possible circumstances. Remember that individuals employed in the dental profession frequently share knowledge—especially in smaller markets, they are all part of the same community. A bad reputation can make it very hard to find new work. When leaving a job, the following steps are recommended:

- Give at least two weeks' notice. If you are on good terms, you can give a longer notice and offer to help find and train your replacement.
- Always give logical reasons for leaving. (If the reason, however, is a personality conflict with the dentist, try to find a more diplomatic approach.)
- Never mention quitting as a negotiating tool; it destroys the trust bond.
- Leave your work area, desk, or locker in good condition.

A Lifetime Career

Dental assistants are a vital part of the dental profession. Patients remember and appreciate dental assistants who helped with their treatment, and dental offices place great value on professional assistants who are skilled and enthusiastic. The key to a long, fruitful career in dental assisting is to maintain good relationships with your patients, your employer, and other staff; to keep your skills current and fresh; and to continue to grow in your profession. Remember that everyone on the dental team is united in the desire to provide excellent patient care.

CHECKPOINTS

48-6 Name several resources for locating job openings.

48-7 What are the main goals of a resume?

48-8 How long should a typical resume be?

48-9 What is the main goal of a cover letter?

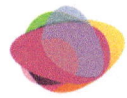

Chapter Highlights

- You should ideally start planning your dental career before graduating by learning about as many options in the field as possible and beginning to network within the profession.
- Letters of recommendation can be provided by former employers, teachers, professors, and other authority figures who are able to comment on your character, experience, and skills.
- Volunteering demonstrates a community-minded spirit and also provides opportunities to network.
- Solo private practices are run by one dentist, while partnerships are two dentists joined in a practice. Group practices have more dentists and may operate across multiple locations.
- In addition to dental practices, dental assistants are sometimes hired by hospitals, dental schools, dental research centers, insurance companies, dental supply companies, manufacturing companies, and public health programs.

- The best job searches use multiple outlets to find job opportunities, including classified ads, Internet sites, employment agencies, and professional organizations.
- A resume should be limited to a single page and follow a standard resume format. Resumes may be posted online on job search sites.
- Resumes should always be accompanied by a simple cover letter introducing yourself and explaining why you are interested in the job.
- Always dress appropriately for interviews in professional clothing; do not wear excessive jewelry and keep your fingernails short and tidy. Enter the interview prepared to answer questions about yourself and your career goals; also, keep a list of questions you want to ask.
- Some dentists call prospects back for working interviews.
- If you have to leave a job in the future, try to leave on the best possible terms and give two weeks' notice.

Review Questions

1. When should you start planning your dental career?
   a. As soon as possible
   b. After graduation
   c. After you get your first job
   d. After you leave your first job

2. Seeking out other dental professionals and discussing industry news and other items related to the profession is an example of
   a. Studying.
   b. Networking.
   c. Volunteering.
   d. Applying.

3. Where can you find ads for dental practices seeking assistants?

   a. Newspapers

   b. Online job websites

   c. Trade magazines

   d. All of the above

4. How long should a typical resume be?

   a. One or two paragraphs

   b. One page

   c. Two to three pages

   d. Four to five pages

5. Which of the following items should be included on your resume?

   a. A list of the classes you took in high school

   b. A description of your volunteer work assisting at a community clinic

   c. A link to your Facebook page

   d. A detailed description of your favorite hobby

6. Which of the following items should *not* be included on your resume?

   a. Social Security number

   b. Home address

   c. Home phone

   d. Email address

7. A successful cover letter should contain

   a. Only generic content so it can be used for all positions.

   b. A listing of all the coursework you have completed.

   c. An outline describing all the jobs you have had over the past 10 years.

   d. Material that is tailored to fit a specific position.

8. Which of the following actions should you take to prepare for a job interview?

   a. Purchase a new pair of jeans to wear to the interview.

   b. Practice answering questions commonly asked during an interview.

   c. Write a second cover letter describing your qualifications for the position.

   d. Think of ways to make it sound like you have more experience than you actually do without outright lying.

9. After a job interview, what should you send to the people who interviewed you?

   a. A more detailed version of your resume

   b. A copy of your original cover letter

   c. A short thank-you note

   d. A small gift

10. How much notice should you give when you quit a job?

   a. None

   b. As long as the employer wants

   c. Two weeks

   d. A month

Active Learning Exercises

1. Other than working in a dental office as an assistant, what other career opportunities does a qualified dental assistant have? Make a list of other employment options.

2. What would the ideal employment interview include? What should and should not be discussed during an interview? What are your thoughts about sharing personal information if asked for it?

3. Continuing education is essential for the qualified dental assistant. What are the requirements for continuing education in your state? Do any of the local colleges offer a degree in dental assisting? Are there any available online degree granting programs available?

Application Activities

1. Write a sample resume in a proper format.

2. Using some of the job search strategies outlined in the chapter, assemble a list of five appealing job opportunities.

3. Using the Internet or the library for research, compile a list of 25 questions typically asked during a job interview. Create sample answers for each one so you will be prepared if the question is asked during an interview.

Professional Organizations and Resources

Academy of Dental Materials
21 Grouse Terrace
Lake Oswego, OR 97035
503-636-0861
http://academydentalmaterials.org

Academy of General Dentistry (AGD)
211 East Chicago Ave., Ste. 900
Chicago, IL 60611
888-AGD-DENT (888-243-3368)
www.agd.org

American Academy of Periodontology (AAP)
737 N. Michigan Ave., Suite 800
Chicago, IL 60611
312-787-5518
www.perio.org

American Association of Orthodontists (AAO)
401 N. Lindbergh Blvd.
St. Louis, MO 63141
800-424-2841 or 314-993-1700
www.aaomembers.org

American Academy of Cosmetic Dentistry (AACD)
402 W. Wilson St.
Madison, WI 53703
800-543-9220 or 608-222-8583
www.aacd.com

American Academy of Oral and Maxillofacial Radiology (AAOMR)
PO Box 231422
New York, NY 10023
www.aaomr.org

American Academy of Pediatric Dentistry (AAPD)
211 East Chicago Ave., Suite 1700
Chicago, IL 60611
312-337-2169
www.aapd.org

American Association of Endodontists
211 E. Chicago Ave., Suite 1100
Chicago, IL 60611
800-872-3636
www.aae.org

American Association of Oral and Maxillofacial Surgeons (AAOMS)
9700 West Bryn Mawr Avenue
Rosemont, IL 60018
847-678-6200 or 800-822-6637
www.aaoms.org

American Association of Women Dentists (AAWD)
216 W. Jackson Blvd., Suite 625
Chicago, IL 60606
800-920-2293
www.aawd.org

The American Board of Oral and Maxillofacial Surgery
625 North Michigan Avenue, Suite 1820
Chicago, Illinois 60611
312-642-0070
www.aboms.org

The American College of Prosthodontists
211 E. Chicago Ave., Suite 1000
Chicago, IL 60611
312-573-1260
www.prosthodontics.org

American Dental Assistants Association (ADAA)
35 East Wacker Drive, Suite 1730
Chicago, IL 60601
1-877-874-3785 or 312-541-1550
www.dentalassistant.org

American Dental Association (ADA)
211 East Chicago Ave.
Chicago, IL 60611
312-440-2500
www.ada.org

American Dental Education Association
1400 K Street, NW, Suite 1100
Washington, DC 20005
Tel: 202-289-7201
Fax: 202-289-7204
www.adea.org

American Dental Hygienists' Association (ADHA)
444 North Michigan Avenue, Suite 3400
Chicago, IL 60611
312-440-8900
www.adha.org

American Dental Society of Anesthesiology (ADSA)
211 E. Chicago Ave, Ste. 780
Chicago, IL 60611
877-255-3742 or 312-664-8270
www.adsahome.org

American Latex Allergy Association (ALAA)
PO Box 198
Slinger, WI 53086
1-888-972-5378 or 262-677-9707
www.latexallergyresources.org

American National Standards Institute
25 West 43rd Street, 4th floor
New York, NY 10036
212-642-4900
www.ansi.org

The American Society for Dental Ethics (ASDE)
c/o Ethics Center
Loma Linda University
Centennial Plaza 3227 Q
24760 Stewart Street
Loma Linda, CA 92350
909-651-5025
www.dentalethics.com

ASTM International
100 Barr Harbor Drive
PO Box C700
West Conshohocken, PA 19428
610-832-9500
www.astm.org

Centers for Disease Control and Prevention
1600 Clifton Rd.
Atlanta, GA 30333
800-CDC-INFO (800-232-4636)
www.cdc.gov

Children's Dental Health Project
1020 19th Street NW, Suite 400
Washington, DC 20036
202-833-8288
www.cdhp.org

Dental Assisting National Board, Inc. (DANB)
444 N. Michigan Ave., Suite 900
Chicago, Illinois 60611
1-800-FOR-DANB or 312-642-3368
www.danb.org

Environmental Protection Agency (EPA)
Ariel Rios Building
1200 Pennsylvania Avenue, NW
Washington, DC 20460
(202) 272-0167
www.epa.gov

Hispanic Dental Association
3085 Stevenson Dr., Ste. 200
Springfield, IL 62703
800-852-7921 or 217-529-6517
www.hdassoc.org

International Association for Dental Research
1619 Duke Street,
Alexandria, VA 22314
703-548-0066
www.dentalresearch.org

MedlinePlus
U.S. National Library of Medicine
8600 Rockville Pike,
Bethesda, MD 20894
www.nlm.nih.gov/medlineplus

National Association of Dental Laboratories (NADL)
325 John Knox Rd #L103
Tallahassee, FL 32303
800-950-1150 or 850-205-5626
www.nadl.org

National Institute of Dental and Craniofacial Research (NIDCR)
National Institutes of Health
Bethesda, MD 20892
301-496-4261
www.nidcr.nih.gov

Occupational Safety & Health Administration (OSHA)
U.S. Department of Labor
200 Constitution Ave., NW
Washington, DC 20210
800-321-OSHA (or 800-321-6742)
www.osha.gov

The Oral Cancer Foundation
3419 Via Lido #205
Newport Beach, CA, 92663
949-646-8000
http://oralcancerfoundation.org

Oral Health America
410 North Michigan Ave., Suite 352
Chicago, IL 60611
312-836-9986
http://oralhealthamerica.org

Organization for Safety, Asepsis and Prevention
2530 Riva Road, Ste. 309
Post Office Box 6297
Annapolis, MD 21401
800-298-6727 or 410-571-0003
www.osap.org

U.S. Food and Drug Administration (FDA)
10903 New Hampshire Ave.
Silver Spring, MD 20993
1-888-INFO-FDA (1-888-463-6332)
www.fda.gov

References and Resources

American Academy of Pediatric Dentistry. *Guideline on Management of Dental Patients with Special Health Care Needs*. Chicago: American Academy of Pediatric Dentistry; 2008.

A healthy smile may promote a healthy heart. American Academy of Periodontology. Web site. http://www.perio.org/consumer/healthy-heart.htm. January 8, 2008.

Aging Statistics. Administration on Aging. Web site. http://www.aoa.gov/AoARoot/Aging_Statistics/index.aspx. Updated June 30, 2010.

AlgiNot. Kerr. Sybron Dental Specialties. Web site. http://www.kerrdental.com/index/kerrdental-impressionmaterial-alginot-2.

AlterImage Cosmetic Simulation. Web site. http://www.seattlesoftwaredesign.com/.

American Academy of Cosmetic Dentistry Membership. Web site. http://www.aacd.com/index.php?module=aa cd&cmd=memberreferral.

American Dental Association. Intraoral/Perioral Piercing and Tongue Splitting. www.ada.org/1891.aspx.

American Dental Association. Oral Health Topics: Antibiotic Prophylaxis. www.ada.org/2985.aspx?currentTab=1.

American Dental Association. Oral Health Topics: Diet and Oral Health. www.ada.org/2984.aspx?currentTab=1.

American Dental Association. Oral Health Topics: Infective Endocarditis. www.ada.org/3565.aspx?currentTab=1.

Andujo E. *Prentice Hall Health's Complete Review of Dental Assisting: Success Across the Boards*. 2nd Ed. Upper Saddle, NJ: Pearson Prentice Hall; 2004.

Bedford DJ, Allen MM. *Visual Atlas of Medical Assisting Skills*. Philadelphia: Lippincott Williams & Wilkins; 2007.

Beers MH. *Merck Manual of Medical Information,* 2nd edition. Gallery: Whitehouse Station, NJ: 2003.

Biber JT. Oral piercing: The hole story. *Northwest Dent*. 2003: 82:6. http://www.mndental.org/archive/january/features/article_6/. Accessed February 10, 2010.

Bird DL, Robinson DS. *Torres and Ehrlich Modern Dental Assisting*. 9th ed. Philadelphia: Elsevier; 2008.

Buchman M. *Medical Assisting Made Incredibly Easy*. Clinical Competencies. Baltimore: Lippincott Williams & Wilkins; 2007.

Cluett J. How to Lift; About.com Orthopedics. Web site. http://orthopedics.about.com/cs/backpain/ht/lift.htm. Updated June 8, 2010.

Cohen BJ, Taylor JJ. *Memmler's Structure and Function of the Human Body*. 9th ed. Baltimore: Lippincott Williams & Wilkins; 2009.

Cohen BJ. *Memmler's The Human Body in Health and Disease*. 10th ed. Baltimore: Lippincott Williams & Wilkins; 2005.

Colquhoun J. Child dental health differences in New Zealand. *Community Health Stud*. 1987;11:85–90.

Colquhoun J. Is there a dental benefit from water fluoride? *Fluoride* 1994;27(1):13–22.

CompuDent Instrument. Milestone Scientific. Web site. http://milesci.com/dental_compudent.html.

Crosta P. What is Scurvy? What Causes Scurvy? *Medical News Today*. Web site. http://www.medicalnewstoday.com/articles/155758.php. June 30, 2009.

DeBate RD, Tedesco LA, Kerschbaum WE. Knowledge of oral and physical manifestations of anorexia and bulimia nervosa among dentists and dental hygienists. *J Dent Educ*. 2005 Mar;69(3):346–354.

Dental MadaJet XL product literature. Available at Mada Medical. Web site. http://www.madamedical.com/library_madajet_xl.htm.

Dentistry for the disabled child and adult. Our-Kids. Web site. http://our-kids.org/Archives/dentistry_disabled.html. Updated June 1, 2002.

Dentrix Clarity. Web site. http://clarity.dentrix.com/.

Diseases and Conditions database. Mayo Clinic. Web site. http://www.mayoclinic.com/health/DiseasesIndex/DiseasesIndex.

Durley CC, Koch L, Brown K, Capper D. *DANB's Glossary of Dental Assisting Terms: A Guide to Applied Practical and Clinical Dental Terminology*. 2nd ed. Chicago, IL: Dental Assisting National Board; 2005.

Durley CC, Koch L, Brown K, Capper D. *The DANB Review*. 3rd ed. Chicago, IL: Dental Assisting National Board; 2005.

eMedicine/Medscape database. Web site. http://emedicine.medscape.com/

Escudero-Castaño N, Perea-García MA, Campo-Trapero J, Cano-Sánchez, Bascones-Martínez A. Oral and perioral piercing complications. *Open Dent J*. 2008;2:133-136.

Esthetic teeth - cosmetic dental treatments. Dentist-Planet. Web site. http://www.dentist-planet.com/esthetic-teeth.php. Accessed February 9, 2010.

Fagin D. Second thoughts on fluoride. *Scientific American Magazine*. http://www.scientificamerican.com/article.cfm?id=second-thoughts-on-fluoride. December 16, 2007.

FAQs - tongue splitting. Pennsylvania Dental Association. Web site. http://www.padental.org/AM/Template.cfm?Section=Resource_Center&Template=/CM/HTMLDisplay.cfm&ContentID=12611. Accessed February 9, 2010.

Fauci AS, Braunwald E, Kasper DL, et al. *Harrison's Principles of Internal Medicine*. 17th ed. New York: McGraw-Hill Professional; 2008.

Ferracane JL. *Materials in Dentistry: Principles and Applications*. 2nd ed. Baltimore: Lippincott Williams & Wilkins; 2001.

Finkbeiner BL, Johnson CS. *Mosby's Comprehensive Review of Dental Assisting*. St. Louis, MO: Mosby; 1997.

Fluoride Action Network. Web site. http://www.fluoridealert.org/health/.

Foster S, Johnson RL. *Desk Reference to Nature's Medicine*. Washington, DC: National Geographic Society; 2006.

Frequently asked questions about root canals. American Association of Endodontists. Web site. http://www.aae.org/Patients/Endodontic_Treatments/Frequently_Asked_Questions.aspx. Accessed January 8, 2010.

Frommer HH, Stabulas-Savage J. *Radiology for the Dental Professional*. 8th ed. St. Louis, MO: Mosby; 2005.

Gladwin MA, Bagby M. *Clinical Aspects of Dental Materials: Theory, Practice, and Cases*. 3rd Ed. Baltimore: Lippincott Williams & Wilkins; 2008.

Gohsman R. *Medical Assisting Made Incredibly Easy: Law & Ethics*. Baltimore: Lippincott Williams & Wilkins; 2008.

Guideline on management of dental patients with special health care needs. American Academy of Pediatric Dentistry Reference Manual. 2008;32(6):132-136. http://www.aapd.org/media/policies_guidelines/g_shcn.pdf

Hallucinogens—LSD, peyote, psilocybin, and PCP. Fact Sheet. National Institute on Drug Abuse. National Institutes of Health. Web site. http://www.nida.nih.gov/Infofacts/hallucinogens.html. Revised June 2009. Accessed June 2009.

Hiatt JL, Gartner LP. *Textbook of Head and Neck Anatomy*. 3rd ed. Philadelphia: Lippincott Williams & Wilkins; 2002.

Hildebrandt G, Larson TD. Management of rampant caries. *Northwest Dent*. Jan-Feb 2009. http://www.mndental.org/features/2009/02/02/93/management_of_rampant_caries. 2009.

Hydroplastic. TAK Systems. Web site. http://www.taksystems.com/hydroplastic.html.

Iannucci JM, Howerton LJ. *Dental Radiography: Principles and Techniques,* 3rd ed. St. Louis, MO: Saunders Elsevier; 2005.

Impression Materials - Regisil. Dentsply International. Web site. http://www.dentsply.com/default.aspx?pageid=177

Intellectual Disability. Centers for Disease Control and Prevention. Web site. http://www.cdc.gov/ncbddd/dd/ddmr.htm. Updated October 29, 2005.

Johnson ON, Thomson EM. *Essentials of Dental Radiography for Dental Assistants and Hygienists*. 8th ed. Upper Saddle, NJ: Pearson Prentice Hall; 2008.

Kaiser K. The Driving Force. RDH. Web site. http://www.rdhmag.com/display_article/184868/56/none/none/Feat/The-Driving-Force. August 1, 2003.

Kale-Smith G. *Medical Assisting Made Incredibly Easy: Administrative Competencies*. Baltimore: Lippincott Williams & Wilkins; 2007.

Kasper DL, Braunwald E, Hauser S, Longo D, Jameson JL, Fauci AS. *Harrison's Principles of Internal Medicine*, 16th ed. New York: McGraw-Hill Professional; 2004.

Kohn WG, Collins AS, Cleveland JL, Harte JA, Eklund KJ, Malvitz DM. CDC guidelines for infection control in dental healthcare settings. *MMWR*. 2003:52(RR17);1-61. www.cdc.gov/mmwr/preview/mmwrhtml/rr5217a1.htm.

Kronenberger J, Durham LS, Woodson D. *Comprehensive Medical Assisting*, 3rd ed. Philadelphia: Lippincott, Williams & Wilkins; 2008.

Langland OE, Langlais RP, Preece JW. *Principles of Dental Imaging*. 2nd ed. Philadelphia: Lippincott Williams & Wilkins; 2002.

Lawton L. Providing dental care for special patients: Tips for the general dentist. *J Am Dent Assoc*. 2002; 133(12):1666-1670. http://jada.ada.org/cgi/context/full/133/12/1666.

Little JW. Eating disorders: dental implications. *Oral Surg Oral Med Oral Pathol Oral Radiol Endod*. 2002 Feb;93(2):138-143. Review.

Lo Russo L, Campisi G, Di Fede O, Di Liberto C, Panzarella V, Lo Muzio L. Oral manifestations of eating disorders: a critical review. *Oral Dis*. 2008 Sep;14(6):479-484. Review.

Logan BL, Reynolds PA, Hutchings RT. *McMinn's Color Atlas of Head and Neck Anatomy*. 3rd ed. London: Mosby Elsevier; 2004.

Marshall J. *Medical Assisting Made Incredibly Easy: Professionalism*. Baltimore: Lippincott Williams & Wilkins; 2009.

McConnell TH. *The Nature of Disease: Pathology for the Health Professions*. Baltimore: Lippincott Williams & Wilkins, 2006.

Medical Dictionary. Medline Plus. National Library of Medicine. National Institutes of Health. Web site. http://www.nlm.nih.gov/medlineplus/mplusdictionary.

Medical Encyclopedia. MedlinePlus. National Library of Medicine. National Institutes of Health. Web site. http://www.nlm.nih.gov/medlineplus/ency.

MedlinePlus. National Library of Medicine. National Institutes of Health. Web site. http://www.nlm.nih.gov/medlineplus/.

Melfi RC, Alley KE. *Permar's Oral Embryology and Microscopic Anatomy*. 10th ed. Philadelphia: Lippincott Williams & Wilkins; 2000.

Model Plans and Programs for the OSHA Bloodborne Pathogens and Hazard Communications Standards.

Occupational Safety and Health Administration. http://www.osha.gov/Publications/osha3186.pdf.

Moynihan PJ. The relationship between nutrition and systemic and oral well-being in older people. *J Am Dent Assoc.* 2007;138(4):493–497.

National Guideline Clearinghouse. Agency for Healthcare Research and Quality. US Department of Health and Human Services. Web site. http://www.guideline.gov/.

Netter FH. *Atlas of Human Anatomy.* 3rd ed. Teterboro, NJ: Icon Learning Systems; 2004.

NFPA 704 FAQs. National Fire Protection Association. Web site. http://www.nfpa.org/faq.asp?categoryID=928.

Nield-Gehrig JS. *Fundamentals of Periodontal Instrumentation & Advanced Root Instrumentation.* 6th ed. Baltimore: Lippincott Williams & Wilkins; 2007.

Nield-Gehrig JS, Willmann DE. *Foundations of Periodontics for the Dental Hygienist.* 2nd ed. Philadelphia: Lippincott Williams & Wilkins; 2008.

Obikoya G. Fluoride Benefits. The Vitamins & Nutrition Center. Web site. http://www.vitamins-nutrition.org/vitamins/fluoride.html.

Oral Health Topics. American Dental Association. Web site. http://www.ada.org/286.aspx.

Organic foods: Are they safer? More nutritious? Mayo Clinic. Web site. http://www.mayoclinic.com/health/organic-food/nu00255. Updated December 18, 2010.

Perim S, Perez-Mera M. Periodontal Disease Part I: How Oral Health Affects the Body. *Healthcare Traveler.* Dec 1, 2002. http://healthcaretraveler.modernmedicine.com/healthcaretraveler/Clinical+Topics/Periodontal-Disease-Part-I-How-Oral-Health-Affects/ArticleStandard/Article/detail/46399.

Periodontal examination and probing. Simple Steps to Better Dental Health. Reviewed by the Faculty of Columbia University College of Dental Medicine. http://www.simplestepsdental.com/SS/ihtSS/r.WSIHW000/st.32477/t.32587/pr.3.html. Updated January 9, 2009. Accessed September 20, 2009.

Periodontitis. The New York Times Health Guide. Web site. http://health.nytimes.com/health/guides/disease/periodontitis/risk-factors.html. Reviewed January 22, 2009.

Phinney DJ, Halstead JH. *Delmar's Handbook of Essential Skills and Procedures for Chairside Dental Assisting.* Clifton Park, NY: Delmar Cengage Learning; 2002.

Phinney DJ, Halstead JH. *Dental Assisting: A Comprehensive Approach.* 3rd ed. Clifton Park, NY: Delmar Cengage Learning; 2007.

Pickett FA, Terézhalmy GT. *Dental Drug Reference with Clinical Applications.* 2nd ed. Baltimore: Lippincott Williams & Wilkins; 2009.

PVS Bite Technique Guide. Aligntech Institute. Web site. http://www.aligntechinstitute.com/GetHelp/Documents/pdf/PVSBiteRegistrationGuide.pdf.

Reynolds T, Dombeck M. American Association on Mental Retardation diagnostic classification. Austin Travis County Integral Care. Web site. http://resources.atcmhmr.com/poc/view_doc.php?type=doc&id=10349.

Roach SS, Zorko J. *Pharmacology for the Health Professionals.* Philadelphia: Lippincott Williams & Wilkins; 2005.

Scanlon VC, Sanders T. *Essentials of Anatomy and Physiology.* 5th ed. Philadelphia: FA Davis; 2007.

Scheid RC. *Woelfel's Dental Anatomy: Its Relevance to Dentistry.* 7th ed. Philadelphia: Lippincott Williams & Wilkins; 2007.

Schreiner K. *Medical Assisting Made Incredibly Easy: Therapeutic Communications.* Baltimore: Lippincott Williams & Wilkins; 2009.

Sroda R. *Nutrition for a Health Mouth.* 2nd ed. Baltimore: Lippincott Williams & Wilkins; 2009.

Stedman's Medical Dictionary for the Dental Professions. 2nd ed. Baltimore: Lippincott Williams & Wilkins; 2012.

Stedman's Medical Dictionary for the Health Professions and Nursing. 6th ed. Baltimore: Lippincott Williams & Wilkins; 2007.

Steelink C, Fowler M, Osborn M, et al. *Findings and Recommendations of Subcommittee on Fluoridation.* City of Tucson, AZ: City of Tucson; 1992.

Study finds direct association between cardiovascular disease and periodontal bacteria. NIH News. National Institutes of Health. Web site. http://www.nih.gov/news/pr/feb2005/nidcr-07.htm. February 7, 2005.

Teotia SPS, Teotia M. Dental caries: A disorder of high fluoride and low dietary calcium interactions (30 years of personal research). *Fluoride.* 1994;27(2)59–66.

The WebMD Portion Size Plate. WebMD. Web site. http://www.webmd.com/diet/healthtool-portion-size-plate.

Thomson EM. *Exercises in Oral Radiography Technique: A Laboratory Manual.* 2nd ed. Upper Saddle, NJ: Pearson Prentice Hall; 2006.

Touyz SW, Liew VP, Tseng P, Frisken K, Williams H, Beumont PJ. Oral and dental complications in dieting disorders. *Int J Eat Disord.* 1993 Nov;14(3):341–347.

Up To Date medical database. Web site. http://www.uptodate.com/.

Waldman HB, Perlman SP. Evolving realities of dental practice: Care for patients with special needs. *The Dental Assistant.* September 1, 2005. http://goliath.ecnext.com/coms2/gi_0199-4918971/Evolving-realities-of-dental-practice.html

Wayne DB, Trajtenberg CP, Hyman DJ. Tooth and periodontal disease: A review for the primary-care physician. *Sound Med J.* 2001;94(9). http://www.medscape.com/viewarticle/410839_3

What are dental implants? Colgate Oral & Dental Health Basics. Web site. http://www.colgate.com/app/Colgate/US/OC/Information/OralHealthBasics/Checkups DentProc/DenturesAndDentalImplants/WhatAre DentalImplants.cvsp. Accessed November 29, 2009.

Wilkins EM. *Clinical Practice of the Dental Hygienist.* 10th ed. Baltimore: Lippincott Williams & Wilkins; 2009.

Yiamouyiannis J. Water fluoridation and tooth decay: Results from the 1986–1987 National Survey of U.S. Schoolchildren. *Fluoride*. 1990;23(2):55-67.

Your dental visit: What to expect. Consumer Information Sheet. Simple Steps to Better Dental Health. Reviewed by Columbia University College of Dental Medicine. http://www.simplestepsdental.com/SS/ihtSS/r.WSIHW000/st.31855/t.32270/pr.3.html. Updated October 8, 2007. Accessed May 31, 2009.

abandonment – to withdraw protection, support, or help (Ch. 4)

abdominal cavity – part of the ventral cavity; contains the digestive tract and related organs and structures (Ch. 5)

abrasion – the wearing away of a surface by an abrasive agent (Ch. 44)

abscess – a sac filled with purulent material and surrounded by inflamed tissue that forms as a result of localized infection (Ch. 12)

abutment (uh-BUT-munt) – a tooth or implant used for the support or retention of a fixed or removable prosthesis (Ch. 39)

accuracy – being true, correct, or exact (Ch. 2)

acidity – the amount of acid that is present in a substance (Ch. 33)

active listening – a form of listening that involves giving full attention to the sender and the message communicated (Ch. 23)

acute hepatitis – the initial stage of infection with the hepatitis virus; acute hepatitis may or may not convert into chronic hepatitis, depending on the strain of the virus and other, unknown factors; acute hepatitis ranges in severity from a mild, cold-like illness to a severe illness requiring hospitalization (Ch. 13)

acute toxicity – a medical condition caused by exposure to high levels of a toxic substance such as a chemical; acute toxic reactions typically occur within minutes of exposure and can include a range of symptoms from minor to life-threatening (Ch. 15)

adaptability – the quality of being adaptable; able to adjust oneself to changing circumstances (Ch. 2)

adhesion – the joining together of two objects (Ch. 33)

adjacent – directly next to (Ch. 8)

administrator – one who manages a business or agency (Ch. 2)

advocate – one who defends or acts on behalf of an individual or cause (Ch. 2)

aerobic – living in air; requiring oxygen to live (Ch. 13)

air-water syringe – a dental device that provides focused streams of air and water, or a combination of both to produce water spray (Ch. 27)

ala (A-luh) – rounded outside tip of each nostril (Ch. 6)

ALARA – when dealing with radiation, using the lowest amount of radiation possible to achieve the objective; stands for As Low As Reasonably Achievable (Ch. 29)

Albucasis (al-byuh-KA-sis) – noted Islamic physician (936–1013). In addition to his accomplishments as a surgeon, he identified tartar on the teeth as a major cause of gingival disease and wrote detailed instructions on how dentists could effectively scrape it away using special dental instruments he had designed (Ch. 1)

alginate (AL-juh-nate) – an irreversible hydrocolloid material used to obtain impressions of teeth and soft tissues (Ch. 35)

alloy (AL-oi) – a combination of two or more metals (Ch. 34)

alveolar (al-VEE-uh-lur) bone – the bone that forms the sockets of the upper and lower jaw to support and protect the roots of the teeth (Ch. 7)

alveolar crest – the peak-like portion of the alveolar bone that is closest to the tooth crown (Ch. 7)

alveolar process – bony ridge on either side of the upper and lower jaw; contains sockets for teeth (Ch. 6)

alveolar sacs – grape-like clusters of alveoli within the lungs (Ch. 5)

alveoli (al-VEE-oh-lie) – small, thinly walled sacs within the lungs that facilitate respiration and the exchange of oxygen and carbon dioxide (Ch. 5)

alveolitis (al-vee-oh-LIE-tis) – inflammation of a tooth socket (Ch. 42)

alveoplasty (al-vee-oh-PLAS-tee) – surgical preparation of the alveolar ridges for the reception of dentures; reshaping and smoothing of socket margins after extraction of teeth (Ch. 42)

Alzheimer disease – a progressive disease that develops slowly and causes a decline in cognitive functioning; affects memory, movement, language, behavior, judgment, and reasoning (Ch. 22)

amalgam (uh-MAL-gum) – a restorative dental material composed of an alloy mixed with mercury, primarily of two types: silver-tin alloy, containing small amounts of copper, zinc, and perhaps other metal, and a second type containing more copper by weight; amalgams are used in restoring teeth and making dies (Ch. 34)

amalgam carrier – an instrument used to transfer mixed amalgam into a cavity preparation until the restoration is completely filled (Ch. 26)

amalgamator (uh-MAL-guh-ma-tur) – a device for combining mercury with a metal or an alloy to form a new alloy; also used for some newer dental materials that come prepared in a premeasured capsule (Ch. 34)

Ambroise Paré (AME-brohz pah-RA) – 16th-century French surgeon who is considered the Father of Surgery. He wrote extensively on dental procedures, particularly extraction and reimplantation, in his *Complete Works* (Ch. 1)

ameloblasts (uh-MEL-oh-blasts) – specialized cells of the enamel organ that produce enamel (Ch. 7)

American Dental Assistants Association (ADAA) – professional organization representing dental assistants on a national level (Ch. 1)

American Dental Association (ADA) – the world's largest and oldest professional organization dedicated to dentistry and dental health issues (Ch. 1)

American Dental Hygienists Association (ADHA) – largest professional organization representing the interest of dental hygienists (Ch. 1)

Americans with Disabilities Act (ADA) – enacted in 1990; prohibits discrimination against those with disabilities and ensures equal access to employment, education, public accommodations, transportation, telecommunications, and all levels of government service (Ch. 4)

amphetamine – stimulant; some are used to treat narcolepsy and attention deficit disorder (Ch. 16)

anaerobic – living without oxygen (Ch. 13)

analgesic – a drug used to relieve pain (Ch. 16)

analog – in radiography, a non-digital image that is comprised of continuous shades of grey obtained by traditional x-ray film (Ch. 29)

anaphylaxis – rare, potentially life threatening allergic reaction to a drug (Ch. 16)

anaphylaxis (an-uh-fih-LAK-sis) – an immediate, transient immunologic (allergic) reaction characterized by contraction of smooth muscle and dilation of capillaries due to release of pharmacologically active substances (histamine, bradykinin, serotonin), classically induced by the combination of antigen (allergen) and antibody (Ch. 14)

anatomic crown – the part of the tooth covered by enamel (Ch. 7)

anatomic root – the part of the tooth covered by cementum (Ch. 7)

anatomical position – the position the body assumes when discussing bodily planes and directions (Ch. 5)

anchor tooth – during placement of a dental dam, the tooth the clamp is fastened to as well as another tooth used to keep the dam material in place (Ch. 27)

anesthesia – a temporary loss of feeling induced by medication (Ch. 28)

anesthetic – a drug used to prevent or control the perception of pain (Ch. 16)

angina (an-JIE-nuh) – recurrent short episodes of chest pain due to restricted blood flow to the heart caused by arteries narrowed due to build up of plaques containing cholesterol and other substances (Ch. 22)

angle former – a hand instrument with angled and beveled blades used to create line angles inside the cavity preparation (Ch. 26)

angle of the mandible – lower portion of the mandibular ramus nearest the ear (Ch. 6)

ankylosis – a stiffening or fixation of a joint as the result of a disease process, with fibrous or bony union across the joint (Ch. 31)

anode (AN-ode) – the positively charged end of an x-ray tube containing the tungsten focal spot where x-rays are generated after being bombarded with electrons from the cathode end (Ch. 29)

anorexia nervosa (an-oh-REK-see-uh ner-VOH-suh) – an eating disorder in which an individual refuses to eat and/or exercises excessively in order to maintain a very low body weight; often simply called anorexia (Ch. 11)

antecubital (an-tee-KYOO-bih-tul) space – the inside fold of the arm, opposite the elbow (Ch. 17)

anterior – located toward the front of the body (Ch. 5)

anterior teeth – refers to teeth at the front of the mouth; canine to canine (Ch. 20)

antibiotic – a drug used to treat infections (Ch. 16)

anticholinergic (an-tee-koh-lih-NUR-jik) – a drug that inhibit secretions; used in dentistry to inhibit saliva production (Ch. 16)

antihistamine – a drug used to relieve allergy symptoms, such as a runny nose or watery eyes (Ch. 16)

antihypertensive – a drug that reduces blood pressure (Ch. 16)

anxiolytic (ang-zee-oh-LIT-ik) – a medication to relieve anxiety (Ch. 28)

aorta – major artery ascending from the heart with blood to supply branch arteries throughout the body (Ch. 6)

apex (A-peks) – the tip of the root (Ch. 8)

apex finder – an electronic device that helps determine the length of the root of the tooth by measuring the distance to the tooth apex; also called an apex locator (Ch. 40)

apexification (a-pek-sih-fih-KAY-shun) – placement of a paste to aid a root in closing; placed after an apicoectomy (Ch. 40)

apexogenesis (a-pek-suh-JEN-eh-sis) – a procedure used to close an open tooth apex (Ch. 40)

aphthous (AF-thus) ulcer – stomatitis characterized by intermittent episodes of painful oral ulcers that are covered by gray exudate, are surrounded by a halo, and range from several mm to 2 cm in diameter; they are limited to oral mucosa membranes; sometimes called a canker sore (Ch. 12)

apical curettage (AP-ih-kul kyur-ih-TAZH) – removal of apical tissue (Ch. 40)

apical foramen (AP-ih-kul fuh-RAY-mun) – the small opening at the apex where nerves and blood vessels enter the root to connect with the tooth pulp (Ch. 8)

apical periodontitis (per-ee-oh-don-TI-tis) – inflammation of the periapical tissue (Ch. 40)

apicoectomy (ap-ih-koh-EK-tuh-mee) – a surgical procedure that removes a small amount of the root apex, usually 1 to 3 mm (Ch. 40)

armamentarium – the instruments, equipment, and materials used for a procedure (Ch. 3)

arthritis – a condition characterized by pain and stiffness caused by inflammation in joints including the knees, wrists, or spinal column. Although there are some 22 different types of arthritis, the two main types are osteoarthritis and rheumatoid arthritis. (Ch. 22)

articulating forceps – a device used to hold articulating paper for the patient to bite down on (Ch. 26)

articulating paper – used to determine tooth contacts when the patient bites on it; synonymous with occluding paper or carbon paper (Ch. 26)

articulator (ar-TIK-yoo-lay-ter) – device built to resemble the temporomandibular joint and human jaw to which casts of the mandibular and maxillary arches may be attached (Ch. 35)

aspirating syringe – the most commonly used type of syringe in a dental practice, it allows the dental professional to ensure the needle has not been placed in a blood vessel (Ch. 28)

assistive device – a device or modification that helps a person overcome or remove a disability (Ch. 22)

asthma – a condition that occurs when airways in the lungs become inflamed and constricted and produce extra mucus; symptoms range from mild wheezing to severe attacks (Ch. 22)

atoms – basic units of matter, atoms are made of electrons orbiting a nucleus (Ch. 29)

atrophy – to decrease in size and strength, and deteriorate in condition (Ch. 5)

autism spectrum disorders – disorders including autistic disorder, pervasive developmental disorder, and Asperger syndrome that cause significant impairment in communication, social interaction, and unusual interests and behaviors; often begins in early childhood and lasts throughout a person's life (Ch. 22)

autoimmune disorder – a mistaken destructive response by the immune system to the body's own organs and tissues (Ch. 5)

autoimmune response – the immune system's response to foreign cells, bacteria, viruses, and other substances (Ch. 5)

automatic processing – in dental radiography, the use of a machine to transform the latent images on exposed x-ray films to visible images for interpretation and diagnosis, as opposed to manual processing (Ch. 32)

autonomy (aw-TON-ah-mee) – ethical principle of a patient's personal independence (Ch. 4)

avulsed (uh-VULST) tooth – a tooth that has been forcibly removed from its socket; such a tooth can often be resituated and retained if given prompt medical attention (Ch. 18)

axial (AK-see-ul) wall – the internal wall of a cavity running parallel to the tooth's long axis (Ch. 36)

axial skeleton – one of the two main divisions of the skeleton; corresponds to the axial region of the body and includes the bones of the cranium, face, ribs, spinal column, and sternum (Ch. 5)

axillary thermometer – an instrument that is placed inside the armpit to measure temperature (Ch. 17)

bacilli (buh-SIL-lie) – a genus of aerobic or facultatively anaerobic, spore-forming, ordinarily motile bacteria containing gram-positive rods (Ch. 13)

barbiturate – a sedatives derived from barbituric acid (Ch. 16)

basal cell carcinoma – one of the two most common types of skin cancer (Ch. 5)

basal metabolism – the amount of energy (or calories) the body needs to maintain important functions while at rest, such as cellular function, body temperature, respiration, and heart beat (Ch. 11)

base metal – metal, such as iron, tin, and zinc, known for their hardness (Ch. 35)

baseplate – the rigid acrylic resin structure, representing the base of a denture, used to fit a full denture (Ch. 39)

bell stage – the fourth stage of tooth development (Ch. 7)

beneficence (buh-NIHF-ih-senz) – ethical principle of the habit, intention, or practice of doing good (Ch. 4)

bicuspid (bi-KUS-pid) – a tooth with two cusps (Ch. 8)

bifurcated (BI-fur-kay-tid) – split into two (Ch. 8)

bifurcation (bi-fur-KAY-shun) – the area where the tooth roots separate into two (Ch. 8)

binging – eating an excessively large amount of food in a single sitting, usually more than one individual would normally eat; a behavior seen in individuals with bulimia nervosa (Ch. 11)

biofilm – thin coating of microorganisms that forms on a body surface, especially the surface of a tooth (Ch. 14)

biopsy – the process of removing tissue from a patient for diagnostic examination (Ch. 12)

bisecting (bi-SEKT-ing) technique – a dental x-ray technique in which the primary x-ray beam is directed at a perpendicular angle to an imaginary plane created by bisecting the plane of the long axis of the teeth and the film (Ch. 30)

bisector – a line that divides an angle into two even, smaller angles, for example, a 90-degree angle into two 45-degree angles; used in radiography to determine the angulation of the primary x-ray beam in the bisecting technique (Ch. 30)

bitewing exposure – a radiograph that includes the crowns of teeth on both the mandible and maxillary bone (Ch. 30)

blade – the working end of an instrument with special shapes or designs used to create and cut lines or grooves on or in a tooth surface (Ch. 26)

blister – a fluid-filled, thin-walled structure under the epidermis or within the epidermis (Ch. 12)

blood pressure – the pressure of blood against the walls of the arteries as the heart pumps and relaxes (Ch. 17)

Bloodborne Pathogen Standard – OSHA regulation for reducing the risk of transfer of disease-producing microorganisms transmitted by means of blood, tissue, and body fluids (Ch. 14)

body mechanics – the study and use of proper muscle movement in daily activities (Ch. 19)

bonding – the process of using a substance to create adhesion (Ch. 33)

bonding agent – a material used to obtain a strong seal between the tooth surface and a restoration material (Ch. 34)

bone grafting – adding bone or bone substitute to an area (Ch. 41)

brachial (BRAY-kee-ul) artery – a blood vessel located in the upper arm that can be felt at the antecubital space (Ch. 17)

brand name – the name assigned to a drug by its manufacturer (Ch. 16)

bridge – a restoration used to replace one or more missing teeth (Ch. 38)

bronchi (BRONG-kee) – also known as bronchial tubes; connect the trachea, or "windpipe," to the lungs (Ch. 5)

bronchioles (BRONG-kee-ole) – small tubes that funnel air from the bronchi into the alveolar sacs of the lungs (Ch. 5)

bruxism (BRUK-sihz-uhm) – the habit of grinding or gritting the teeth; particularly during sleep or times of stress (Ch. 6)

buccal (BUK-ul) – near the cheek (Ch. 8)

buccal surface – the facial surface of the posterior teeth that is near the cheek (Ch. 8)

buccinator (BUK-suh-nay-ter) muscle – a thin, broad muscle of facial expression; forms the wall of the cheek (Ch. 6)

buccoversion (buck-oh-VER-zhun) – malposition of a posterior tooth from the normal line of occlusion toward the cheek (Ch. 45)

bud stage – the second stage of tooth development (Ch. 7)

bulimia nervosa (buh-LEE-mee-uh ner-VOH-suh) – an eating disorder in which individuals binge and purge in order to control their weight; often simply called bulimia (Ch. 11)

bulla (BUL-uh) – a fluid-filled blister greater than 1 cm in diameter appearing as a circumscribed area of separation of the epidermis from the subepidermal structure or as a circumscribed area of separation of epidermal cells caused by the presence of serum (Ch. 12)

burnisher – an instrument for smoothing and polishing surfaces or margins of a dental restoration (Ch. 26)

calcium hydroxide (high-DROK-side) – a dental material used for lining (Ch. 33)

calculus (KAL-kyoo-lus) – a mineralized bacterial plaque, covered on its external surface by nonmineralized, living bacterial plaque (Ch. 9)

calorie – scientifically, the amount of heat needed to raise the temperature of 1 kg of water 1 degree Celsius; also a measure of the amount of energy contained in a given food (Ch. 11)

cancellous (KAN-suh-luhs) bone – mesh-like networks of light-weight intersecting bone called trabeculae; also called spongy bone (Ch. 5)

canine (cuspid) – a sharply pointed anterior tooth distal to the lateral incisors (Ch. 8)

canthus (KAN-thus) (inner) – fold of tissue at the inner corner of the eyelid (Ch. 6)

canthus (outer) – fold of tissue at the outer corner of the eyelid (Ch. 6)

cap stage – the third stage of tooth development (Ch. 7)

capitation – an insurance program in which a dentist agrees to provide services to enrolled patients in the program on a per capita rather than a fee-based system (Ch. 47)

carbamide peroxide – a whitening agent formed from the combination of hydrogen peroxide and urea; acts through oxidation of tooth enamel to lighten tooth enamel (Ch. 46)

carbohydrate – sugar and starch nutrient (Ch. 11)

carcinoma – any of the various types of malignant neoplasm derived from epithelial cells, chiefly glandular (adenocarcinoma) or squamous cell carcinoma (Ch. 12)

cardiopulmonary resuscitation (CPR) – restoration of cardiac output and pulmonary ventilation following cardiac arrest and apnea using artificial respiration and manual or mechanical closed chest compression (Ch. 18)

caries (KARE-eez) – infectious disease of teeth caused by acidogenic bacteria with dissolution of enamel and dentin or cementum and dentin (Ch. 9)

carotid (kuh-ROT-id) artery – a major blood vessel located in the neck, under the jaw bone about halfway between the chin and the ear (Ch. 17)

carotid artery (external) – branches from the common carotid artery to supply blood to the face and mouth (Ch. 6)

carotid artery (internal) – branches from the common carotid artery to supply blood to the brain (Ch. 6)

carpal tunnel syndrome – a condition in which a nerve in the carpal tunnel area of the wrist is compressed and loses blood supply; caused by repeatedly extending and holding the wrist in the same position over long periods of time (Ch. 19)

carrier – insurance company (Ch. 47)

cartilage – a particularly strong kind of connective tissue that lacks any blood vessels; found where bones join and in parts of the nose and ears (Ch. 5)

carver – a dental hand instrument, available in a wide variety of end shapes, used to form and contour wax as well as temporary and permanent restoration materials (Ch. 26)

cassette – a device used in extraoral radiography that holds the screen film and two intensifying screens in a light-safe environment during exposure (Ch. 31)

cast – a positive reproduction of the patient's mouth; three-dimensional representation of the teeth and other tissues of the oral cavity; also called a model (Ch. 35)

casting – indirect restoration formed by pouring molten material into a previously obtained mold (Ch. 35)

cathode – the negatively charged end of an x-ray tube where electrons are created by heating a tungsten filament before being shot across the vacuum tube to the anode end (Ch. 29)

cavitation (ka-vih-TAY-shun) – 1. the production by ultrasound of small, vapor-containing bubbles in a liquid (Ch. 14); 2. the formation of a cavity in the enamel of a tooth, the final stage in the caries process. (Ch. 9)

cavity liner – a dental material used to seal the dentin and to protect the pulp of the tooth being restored (Ch. 33)

cavity varnish – a dental material used as a liner to create a protective seal over the dentin and pulp of the tooth being restored (Ch. 33)

cavity wall – the internal surface of the restoration (Ch. 36)

cavosurface (kay-voh-SUR-fus) margin – the intersection between the cavity and the healthy surface of a tooth (Ch. 36)

cell senescence (sih-NES-ens) – cell death (Ch. 29)

cellulitis – inflammation of subcutaneous, loose connective tissue (Ch. 12)

cement base – a dental material placed under a restoration to protect the pulp of the tooth being restored; can protect, insulate, and/or sedate the pulp (Ch. 33)

cementoblasts – cells that produce cementum (Ch. 7)

cementoclasts – cells that resorb cementum (Ch. 7)

cementodentinal (sim-en-toe-DEN-tun-ul) junction – the area within the root of the tooth where the cementum lining meets the dentin (Ch. 7)

cementoenamel (sim-en-toe-ee-NAM-ul) junction (CEJ) – where the anatomic crown (enamel) joins the anatomic root (cementum) (Ch. 7)

cementum – the outer layer of the anatomic root (Ch. 7)

central air compressor – provides the compressed air needed to operate air-driven handpieces and the air-water syringe (Ch. 24)

central groove – developmental groove at the center of the occlusal surface (Ch. 8)

cephalometer – an instrument used to position the head to produce oriented, reproducible lateral and posteroanterior head films; also called cephalostat (Ch. 31)

cephalometric (sef-uh-loh-MEH-trik) film – a radiograph of the jaws and cranium that allows their measurement and diagnosis of conditions (Ch. 29)

ceramic casting – restoration made of clay-like material topped by a metallic glaze (Ch. 35)

cerebellum – region of the brain coordinating unconscious and conscious movement (Ch. 5)

cerebral palsy – a group of disorders that affect a person's ability to move and to maintain balance; caused by an abnormality in the part of the brain that controls muscle tone; characterized by spasticity, which involves stiff muscles and awkward movement (Ch. 22)

cerebrum – region of the brain known as the "seat of consciousness"; origin of uniquely human reasoning and thought (Ch. 5)

certified dental assistant (CDA) – designation earned by dental assistants who have successfully completed the DANB certification examination and complete continuing education offerings annually as required (Ch. 2)

certified dental technician (CDT) – credentialed by passing written and clinical examinations offered through the Dental Assisting National Board (Ch. 3)

certified orthodontic assistant (COA) – designation earned by orthodontic assistants who have successfully completed the DANB certification examination and complete continuing education offerings annually as required (Ch. 2)

chain of infection – the required conditions for an infectious microorganism to transfer from one host to another host (Ch. 14)

chairside dental assistant – works on the opposite side of the chair from the dentist; mixes materials, exchanges instruments, and manages oral evacuation during procedures (Ch. 3)

chisel – a single beveled end-cutting blade instrument with a straight or angled shank used for cutting or splitting dentin and enamel (Ch. 26)

chromosomes – large strands of DNA within the cell nucleus, susceptible to radiation damage (Ch. 29)

chronic hepatitis – infection with the hepatitis virus that causes long-term and sustained live inflammation; chronic hepatitis ranges in severity from mild inflammation with no symptoms to severe inflammation that leads to cirrhosis of the liver (Ch. 13)

chronic obstructive pulmonary disease (COPD) – a group of lung diseases, including emphysema and chronic bronchitis, that restricts airflow and makes breathing difficult; can cause shortness of breath, wheezing, fatigue, chronic cough, and headaches (Ch. 22)

chronic toxicity – a medical condition caused by exposure to lower levels of a toxic substance over time; chronic toxic reactions often take years to become apparent and are often characterized by diffuse symptoms and organ damage such as cancer or kidney or liver failure (Ch. 15)

cingulum (SING-you-lum) – a small bump located on the cervical third of the lingual surface of the anterior teeth (Ch. 8)

circulating assistant – assists in whatever ways are needed in the office (Ch. 3)

civil law – includes laws that address wrongful acts that are not crimes, for which the guilty party may have to pay a monetary amount (Ch. 4)

clarification – an understanding of the message communicated (Ch. 23)

clinical crown – the part of the anatomic crown that is visible in the oral cavity (above the gingiva) (Ch. 7)

clinical examination form – generated during clinical examinations, this form records exam results, diagnoses, and treatments (Ch. 21)

clinical root – the part of the anatomic root that is not visible in the oral cavity (below the gingiva) (Ch. 7)

clinician – health professional who examines and helps care for patients (Ch. 2)

cocci (KOK-sigh) – a bacterium of round, spheroid or ovoid form (Ch. 13)

code of ethics – a set of rules or principles to be followed voluntarily by members of a profession. Often based in part on a moral code of right and wrong (Ch. 4)

coin test – a test used to measure safe lights in radiology dark rooms (Ch. 30)

collimator (KOL-uh-may-ter) – a lead-based safety device in the x-ray tubehead that focuses and targets the x-ray beam as it emerges from the x-ray tube (Ch. 29)

colony-forming unit – the measure of unit used to gauge water safety; colony-forming units are made up of coliform bacteria, which at high enough concentrations can cause illness (Ch. 14)

commission (act of) – the act of professional negligence and performing a treatment incorrectly on a patient or committing a wrongful act on a patient (Ch. 4)

commitment – the act of promising to engage in a particular act or course of action (Ch. 2)

common carotid artery – branches from the aorta to supply blood to the head (Ch. 6)

communication – the ways information is sent, received, and responded to (Ch. 23)

compact bone – the hardest bone found in the body; also known as dense bone (Ch. 5)

composite resin – a dental material used for permanent cementing of restorations such as crowns, bridges, inlays, and onlays (Ch. 33)

computed tomography – a form of x-ray imaging that uses multiple sensors placed around the patient and a computer program to yield high-quality diagnostic images of thin slices of tissue or organs; this same principle is used in panoramic dental radiography (Ch. 31)

computer-aided design/computer-aided manufacture (CAD/CAM) – a special method of fabricating prosthodontic restorations using computerized systems (Ch. 38)

concave – a surface curved inward (Ch. 8)

condylar neck – condyles located in the neck bones (Ch. 31)

condyle – a rounded articular surface at the extremity of a bone (Ch. 31)

condyloid (KON-duh-loyd) joint – one of six types of synovial joints (Ch. 5)

cone cut – section of a radiograph that appears clear due to improper alignment between the film and the PID (Ch. 30)

confidentiality – legally protected right and responsibility of health professionals not to disclose information gained during consultation with or treatment of a patient (Ch. 4)

congenital condition – existing at birth, referring to certain mental or physical traits, anomalies, malformations, diseases, and like findings, which may be either hereditary or due to an environmental influence (Ch. 12)

congestive heart failure – a condition characterized by the heart not being able to pump as much blood as the body needs; can be caused by conditions that weaken the heart, including long-term high blood pressure, coronary artery disease, and diabetes (Ch. 22)

conscious sedation – a state of sedation in which patients remain awake, relaxed, responsive, reflexive, and able to cooperate (Ch. 28)

contact area – where the proximal surfaces of adjacent teeth touch (Ch. 8)

contact dermatitis (der-muh-TIE-tis) – inflammatory rash marked by itching and redness resulting from cutaneous contact with a specific allergen (allergic contact dermatitis) or irritant (irritant contact dermatitis) (Ch. 14)

contouring – shaping of the tooth (Ch. 46)

contract – voluntary agreement between two parties from which each party benefits (Ch. 4)

contraindication – a condition or instance in which a particular drug should not be used (Ch. 16)

contrast – describes the quality of a radiograph; contrast is determined by the different densities of the areas radiographed, with denser areas showing up as white or grey and less dense areas as black (Ch. 29)

control panel – a component on a dental x-ray machine where the operator can control the unit's kilovoltage (kV), milliamperage (mA), and other settings; control panels vary by manufacturer and type of machine (Ch. 29)

convenience form – alterations in the shape of a cavity preparation to allow removal of decay and to enable proper instrumentation for the cavity preparation and insertion of a dental restoration (Ch. 36)

convex – a surface curved outward (Ch. 8)

core buildup – a retention technique that provides support for a crown and helps restore the natural shape of the tooth; involves using amalgam or composites to replace damaged or missing parts of a tooth prior to crown placement (Ch. 38)

coronal (KORE-uh-nul) polishing – removal of stains and plaque from the clinical crown (Ch. 44)

corrosion – a breakdown in metal caused by a chemical reaction from metal mixing with water (Ch. 33)

cortical (KOR-tik-ul) bone – part of the alveolar bone that forms the hard outer wall of the upper and lower jaws, surrounds the lamina dura, and supports the sockets (Ch. 7)

cosmetic dentistry – branch of dentistry that deals with improving the appearance of otherwise healthy teeth (Ch. 1)

cover letter – a letter sent with a resume or job application (Ch. 48)

cranial nerves – operate between the brain and organs and structures of the head and neck (Ch. 5)

cranium – the portion of the skull that encloses the brain (Ch. 6)

crepitus (KREP-uh-tis) – the sound or sensation of grating or clicking (Ch. 42)

crests – the length between the peaks on a wave; x-rays are short-wavelength waves and thus high-energy, penetrating energy (Ch. 29)

criminal law – includes laws that address wrongs committed against a person or society as a whole for which the guilty party may go to jail (Ch. 4)

crossbite – abnormal relationship of one or more teeth of one arch to the opposing tooth or teeth of the other arch due to labial, buccal, or lingual deviation of tooth position, or abnormal jaw position (Ch. 45)

crowding – a condition in which the teeth are crowded, assuming altered positions such as bunching, overlapping, displacement in various directions, and torsiversion (Ch. 45)

curette (kyu-RET) – instrument used to perform gingival curettage; also used to remove calculus from the teeth, mainly subgingival calculus (Ch. 41)

curing – the process by which dental material sets and hardens (Ch. 33)

curing light – used to cure (set or harden) light-cured dental materials (Ch. 24)

curve of Spee – anterior-to-posterior curvature that follows the line of the incisal edges and cusp tips (Ch. 8)

curve of Wilson – side-to-side curvature that follows the cusp tips of the posterior teeth (Ch. 8)

cusp – peak on the incisal surface of the canines or on the occlusal surface of premolars and molars (Ch. 8)

cusp of Carabelli – nonfunctional fifth cusp that often forms on the mesiolingual cusp of the maxillary first molar (Ch. 8)

cuspid (canine) – a sharply pointed anterior tooth distal to the lateral incisors (Ch. 8)

custom tray – an impression tray specially constructed for an individual patient (Ch. 35)

cyst – an abnormal sac containing gas, fluid, or a semisolid material, with a membranous lining (Ch. 12)

dappen dish – a heavy, double-ended glass dish or plastic disposable cup device with a variety of uses in dentistry (Ch. 26)

DEA number – the identifying number assigned to medical professionals who prescribe controlled substances (Ch. 16)

débridement (day-BREDE-mahnt) – a procedure that involves scaling and ultrasonic instrumentation of the root surfaces of the teeth to attain healthy gingival tissue (Ch. 41)

deciduous teeth – the primary teeth, which are lost or shed (Ch. 8)

definition – describes the clarity of a radiograph; determined by the film speed and motion (Ch. 29)

demineralization (dee-mhin-uh-rih-lih-ZAY-shun) – major stage in the dental caries process in which minerals, primarily calcium and phosphorous, are dissolved from tooth structure by acids formed by acidogenic bacteria, primarily mutans streptococci and lactobacilli (Ch. 9)

density – the compactness of a substance; in radiography, it describes the opacity of an object to x-rays, with denser objects more opaque (Ch. 29)

dental assistant – dental professional trained to provide support to a dentist by performing a multitude of tasks ranging from clerical work and assistance at chairside to laboratory work, infection control, and possibly additional enhanced functions (Ch. 1)

Dental Assisting National Board (DANB) – agency that administers the national examination to certify dental and orthodontic assistants (Ch. 1)

dental chair – the chair in which the patient sits during treatment (Ch. 24)

dental chart – a graphical representation of the teeth that is included as part of the dental record; it includes areas for notations regarding exam results and lesions; alternatively, the term is sometimes used to encompass the entire dental record (Ch. 21)

dental dam – a device consisting of a frame and sheet of thin, pliable material that is used to isolate teeth during dental procedures (Ch. 27)

dental equipment technician – repairs and maintains dental equipment (Ch. 3)

dental floss – twisted or untwisted thread made of fine, short silk or synthetic fibers, frequently waxed; used for cleaning the interproximal spaces and between the contact areas of the teeth (Ch. 10)

dental flow – changes in the shape of dental materials, such as waxes, due to pressure or force; also called creep (Ch. 33)

dental history – a patient history of dental care and habits, medications, and lifestyle factors that might affect oral health (Ch. 21)

dental hygienist (hi-JEN-ist) – licensed, professional auxiliary in dentistry who is both an oral health educator and clinician, and who uses preventive, therapeutic, and educational methods for the control of oral diseases (Ch. 1)

dental implant – a metal fixture typically made of titanium which is surgically embedded into the jaw. The implant acts as the root and allows for an abutment or prosthesis to be attached to it, such as a crown, bridge, or denture attachment (Ch. 1)

dental laboratory – a well-ventilated area where various dental devices are trimmed, adjusted, or fabricated outside of the patient's mouth (Ch. 24)

dental laboratory technician – dental professional who provides support to dental practices by filling prescriptions from dentists for crowns, bridges, dentures, and other dental prosthetics (Ch. 1)

dental lamina (LAM-uh-nuh) – specialized cell layer of the oral epithelium from which the tooth buds develop (Ch. 7)

dental ornamentation – a type of oral personalization that includes dental tattoos and jewelry (Ch. 46)

dental papilla (puh-PIL-uh) – cells of the mesenchyme that form within the cap-shaped enamel organ (Ch. 7)

dental practice act – title given to each set of state laws that regulate the dental profession (Ch. 4)

dental public health – dental specialty emphasizing prevention and control of dental diseases and promotion of dental health through community efforts (Ch. 3)

dental sac – an enclosure of the mesenchyme around the enamel organ and dental papilla (Ch. 7)

dental stimulator – device used to massage and increase blood flow in the gingival tissue, frequently made from rubber or wood (Ch. 10)

dental supply person – represents one or more dental supply companies; takes orders and provides product information (Ch. 3)

dental tape – a wide thread similar to dental floss, composed of fine, short silk or synthetic fibers; used for cleaning interproximal spaces and between contact areas of teeth (Ch. 10)

dental unit – provides the electrical and air-operated components needed to utilize the air-water syringe, dental handpieces, saliva ejector, high-volume evacuator, and ultrasonic scaler (Ch. 24)

dentifrice (DEN-tuh-fris) – any preparation used to cleanse teeth, e.g., a tooth powder, toothpaste, or tooth wash (Ch. 10)

dentin – yellow-colored tissue that covers the pulp (Ch. 7)

dentinal (DEN-tun-ul) tubule – a tube or canal in the dentin that extends out from the pulp to the dentinoenamel and cementodentinal junctions (Ch. 7)

dentinal (DEN-tun-ul) wall – an external wall that includes dentin (Ch. 36)

dentinoenamel (den-tuh-no-ee-NAM-ul) junction – where the enamel joins the dentin, on the inner surface of the tooth (Ch. 7)

dentistry – the science and art concerned with the prevention, diagnosis, and treatment of deformities, diseases, and injuries to the teeth, gingiva, mouth, and jaws (Ch. 1)

dentition (den-TIH-shun) – the set of natural teeth on a dental arch (Ch. 8)

dependable – worthy of trust; reliable (Ch. 2)

dependent – a person who receives dental benefits under a policy held by a primary subscriber (Ch. 47)

depressant – a drug or agent that slows the speed of bodily processes and physical reactions (Ch. 16)

detail person – representative of a specific company; takes orders and provides information about that company's services and products (Ch. 3)

developer – the first chemical used in the processing of dental films; developer reduces the silver halide on dental films, leaving behind silver specks that correspond to dark areas on the final x-ray image (Ch. 32)

developmental groove – distinct linear depression formed while the tooth was developing that separates major features of the tooth or lobes on the occlusal surface of a posterior tooth (Ch. 8)

diabetes – a metabolic disease in which the body does not produce sufficient insulin or use it adequately to process the glucose in the blood, leaving high levels of glucose in the blood, resulting in symptoms ranging from chronic hyperglycemia and infection to water and electrolyte loss, ketoacidosis, and coma (Ch. 18)

diagnosis – the practice of identifying diseases, abnormalities, or pathologies based on the information in a radiograph; only dentists are allowed to make diagnoses (Ch. 32)

diagnostic cast or study model – positive replica of the form of the teeth and tissues made from an impression; used to study the size and position of the oral tissues (Ch. 24)

diastema (di-uh-STEE-muh) – space between adjacent teeth of the same arch that have no point of contact (Ch. 8)

diastolic (die-uh-STOL-ik) pressure – the pressure of blood on the walls of the arteries as the heart relaxes and fills up with blood (Ch. 17)

digastric muscle – one of the muscles of the floor of the mouth; assists in swallowing (Ch. 6)

diplococci (dih-ploh-KOK-sigh) – spheric or ovoid bacteria linked together in pairs (Ch. 13)

direct supervision – supervision provided by a dentist who is in the treatment area with the operator/dental assistant (Ch. 37)

disbursement – payment (Ch. 47)

disclosure – the act of telling a patient the reasons, risks, and benefits of a procedure, including radiography; disclosure is a legal requirement to obtain informed consent (Ch. 29)

disinfectant – an agent capable of destroying pathogenic microorganisms or inhibiting their growth (Ch. 14)

disinfection – destruction of pathogenic microorganisms or their toxins or vectors by direct exposure to chemical or physical agents (Ch. 14)

distal (DIS-tul) – farther from the midline (Ch. 8)

distal surface – the side surface of a tooth that is farther from the midline (Ch. 8)

distortion – a change in the dimensions of an impression that has already set; also changes that occur during removal of an impression from a patient's mouth (Ch. 35)

distoversion (dis-toe-VER-zhun) – malposition of a tooth distal to normal, in a posterior direction following the curvature of the dental arch (Ch. 45)

dorsal – toward the back half of the body (Ch. 5)

double image – results from accidentally exposing the same dental x-ray film twice, so it shows one image laid over the top of another (Ch. 30)

Down syndrome – a type of mental retardation caused by a chromosomal defect; often accompanied by identifiable physical characteristics, including a flattened back of the head, slanted eyes, and depressed bridge of the nose (Ch. 22)

Drug Enforcement Agency – federal agency within the Department of Justice; enforces controlled substance laws (Ch. 16)

drug interaction – occurs when one drug alters the effect of another (Ch. 16)

ductility (duk-TIL-uh-tee) – how much a material stretches out or lengthens when under stress (Ch. 33)

duplicating film – special film used in a film duplicator to make exact duplicates of radiographs; duplicate film has emulsion only on one side (Ch. 32)

early childhood caries (ECC) – the presence of one or more decayed, missing, or filled tooth surfaces in any primary tooth in a child before 6 years of age (Ch. 9)

eating disorders – psychological disorders in which people take extreme actions to control their weight or eating habits (Ch. 11)

ecchymosis (eh-kuh-MOH-sis) – a discoloration of the skin caused by extravasation of blood into the skin, differing from petechiae only in size (i.e., larger than 3 mm in diameter) (Ch. 12)

ectoderm (EK-toe-durm) – the outermost layer of embryonic cells (Ch. 7)

edentulous (ee-DEN-chuh-lus) – without teeth (Ch. 30)

educator – trained teacher or other individual who plans, directs, or engages in education (Ch. 2)

efficacy (EF-ih-kuh-see) – the effectiveness of a drug in accomplishing its intended purpose (Ch. 16)

efficiency of motion – minimizing the size and the number of motions made in order to optimize benefits to the body (Ch. 25)

elasticity – the ability of dental material to change shape when force is applied and return to its original shape when force is removed (Ch. 33)

elastomeric – having a rubbery elastic quality (Ch. 35)

electrocardiogram – a test that measures the patterns of electrical activity and determines whether the heart is beating regularly or irregularly (Ch. 17)

electromagnetic energy spectrum – the array of electromagnetic radiation, organized by wavelength, and including gamma rays, radio waves and visible light, and x-rays (Ch. 29)

electrons – a negatively charged subatomic particle that orbits a nucleus as part of atom; flowing electrons constitute electricity and are used to generate the energy that creates x-rays (Ch. 29)

elongated (ee-LONG-gate-ed) image – an x-ray image in which the teeth appear stretched in relation to their roots; results from insufficient vertical angulation in the bisecting technique (Ch. 30)

embrasure (em-BRAY-zhur) space – triangular spaces that surround the contact area of two adjacent teeth (Ch. 8)

embryo – the human organism from the second to eighth week of development (Ch. 7)

embryology – the study of an organism's development from conception to birth (Ch. 7)

emotional disability – a condition not explicable by intellectual, sensory, or health factors and that is characterized by an inability to maintain satisfactory interpersonal relationships, inappropriate behavior or feelings under normal circumstances, and a persistent feeling of unhappiness or depression (Ch. 22)

empathy – identifying with and understanding another person's situation or feelings (Ch. 2)

enamel – the white outer surface of the anatomic crown (Ch. 7)

enamel erosion – the wearing away of the outer enamel of the tooth; common in patients with bulimia nervosa who regularly make themselves vomit (Ch. 11)

enamel hypoplasia (hi-poh-PLAY-zhuh) – developmental disturbance of teeth characterized by deficient or defective enamel matrix formation (Ch. 10)

enamel lamellae (luh-MEL-ee) – leaf-like projections from the surface of the enamel to the dentinoenamel junction (Ch. 7)

enamel tuft – projection from the dentinoenamel junction into the enamel caused by a defect in mineralization (Ch. 7)

enamel wall – an external wall that includes enamel (Ch. 36)

encephalitis (en-sef-uh-LIE-tis) – inflammation of the membrane surrounding the brain (Ch. 13)

endoderm (EN-doe-durm) – the outermost layer of embryonic cells (Ch. 7)

endodontics (en-doh-DON-tiks) – dental specialty concerned with diseases of and injuries to the pulp (Ch. 3)

endodontics (en-doh-DON-tiks) – a branch of dentistry that deals with the functions of and problems with the tooth pulp and surrounding tissues (Ch. 40)

endogenous (en-DOJ-uh-nus) stain – a stain that occurs within the tooth structure (Ch. 44)

endosteal (en-DOS-tee-ul) implant – an implant that is inserted directly into the alveolar bone of the maxillary or mandibular jawbone (Ch. 38)

energy – in physics, defined as the ability to perform work; energy has no mass (Ch. 29)

epidermis – the top-most layer of skin (Ch. 5)

epilepsy – a chronic disorder characterized by some alteration of consciousness; clinical manifestations of the attack may vary from complex abnormalities or behavior, including generalized or focal convulsions, to momentary spells of impaired consciousness (Ch. 18)

ergonomics (er-goh-NOM-iks) – the study of how work environments and work tasks can be made safe and comfortable for people on the job (Ch. 19)

erosion – tooth loss due to chemical or unknown factors; also a shallow ulcer in the mucosa, with no penetration of the mucosa (Ch. 12)

erythroplakia (ih-rith-roh-PLAY-kee-uh) – a red, velvety, plaquelike lesion of mucous membrane that often represents a malignant change (Ch. 12)

etchant (ETCH-unt) – acid-based dental material used to improve the bond between a restoration and the tooth (Ch. 33)

ethics – principles or guidelines for determining proper behavior or conduct and standards of practice (Ch. 4)

ethmoid (ETH-moid) bone – thinly walled bone with a honeycomb-like structure; sits in the center of the skull between the eye sockets and helps form parts of the nasal and orbital cavities (Ch. 6)

etiologic (ee-tee-uh-LOJ-ik) agent – the specific cause of a disease, such as a bacteria or virus (Ch. 13)

etiology (ee-tee-OL-uh-jee) – the science and study of causes of disease and their mode of operation (Ch. 12)

excavator – a dental hand instrument, generally a small, spoon-shaped instrument used for cleaning out and shaping a carious cavity preparatory or other materials from a tooth or restoration (Ch. 26)

exfoliation – the loss of the primary teeth (Ch. 8)

exogenous (ek-SOJ-uh-nus) stain – a stain that is caused by external factors, such as food, drink, and tobacco (Ch. 44)

exothermic (ek-so-THER-mik) reaction – a chemical reaction that causes heat to be released (Ch. 33)

expanded functions dental assistant – a dental assistant who is able to provide additional specific chairside duties after meeting state requirements, which typically include taking additional course work in a state-approved or CODA-accredited program and passing an examination (Ch. 3)

explorer – a slender instrument, sharply pointed at one or both ends, used to detect imperfections in the enamel and to determine the condition of restorations (Ch. 20)

external wall – the surface of the cavity that extends to the tooth surface; usually identified by its location, such as medial, distal, lingual, facial, and gingival (Ch. 36)

extraoral – outside the oral cavity (Ch. 20)

extraoral radiography – a technique of obtaining dental radiographs in which the film is placed outside the patient's oral cavity during exposure (Ch. 31)

extrinsic stain – adherence of bacteria or discoloring agents to dental enamel that causes discoloration (Ch. 44)

fabrication – in dentistry, the ways in which restorations are manufactured and assembled (Ch. 38)

facial – toward the face (Ch. 8)

facial surface – the surface of the crown on the outer side of the dental arch, nearest to the face (Ch. 8)

facultative anaerobe (FAK-ul-tay-tiv AN-uh-robe) – an anaerobe that grows in the presence of air or under conditions of reduced oxygen tension (Ch. 13)

fat – a nutrient that provides energy and helps the body use vitamins properly; includes both oils and solid fats (Ch. 11)

feedback – the response to the message communicated (Ch. 23)

female athlete triad – three conditions that girls and young women who exercise vigorously or play sports intensely are at risk for; include disordered eating, loss of menstrual period, and weakening of the bones (Ch. 11)

femoral artery – a major blood vessel in the thigh, located inside the crease between the groin and the inner thigh (Ch. 17)

festooned (fes-TOONDE) – sculpting of a crown or other restoration to follow the natural contours of the gingival tissue (Ch. 43)

fetus – the human organism from the ninth week of development until birth (Ch. 7)

fever – a complex physiological response to disease that is characterized by a rise in core temperature, generation of acute phase reactants, and activation of immunologic systems (Ch. 13)

fiber – a type of complex carbohydrate that the body cannot digest; found in fruit, vegetables, beans, and whole grains (Ch. 11)

fibroblasts – spindle-shaped cells that form the collagen fibers within the pulp (Ch. 7)

fibromyalgia – a chronic condition characterized by widespread pain and stiffness of connective tissues (Ch. 5)

field block anesthesia – one of the three most common dental injections, this type of local infiltration anesthesia is injected near the apex of the tooth, near larger terminal nerve branches, to prevent impulses from passing from the tooth to the central nervous system (Ch. 28)

film badge – a device worn by employees in dental offices to measure exposure to radiation (Ch. 29)

film duplicator – a device used to make exact duplicates of radiographs (Ch. 32)

film-holding device – special device that is designed to hold film steady in a patient's mouth during radiography; reduces exposure to radiation by preventing the need to manually hold film (Ch. 29)

fissure (FIH-shur) – narrow slit that forms deep within a groove during tooth development when enamel fails to fuse along the groove (Ch. 8)

fistula (fis-CHOO-luh) – an abnormal passage from one epithelial surface to another (Ch. 12)

fixed bridge – a fixed, nonremovable prosthesis used to fill the gap where one or more teeth are missing (Ch. 38)

fixed prosthesis – a prosthodontic restoration that cannot be removed from the oral cavity; includes crowns, inlays, onlays, bridges, and veneers (Ch. 38)

fixer – the second chemical used in the processing of dental films; fixer solution stops the chemical reaction started by the developer solution and hardens to emulsion to fix the image onto the final film (Ch. 32)

flange (FLANJ) – the part of a denture that extends from the cervical margin to the border of the prosthesis (Ch. 39)

floss threader – a flexible device resembling a large needle used to transport floss under fixed bridges or behind appliances such as orthodontic wires (Ch. 10)

fluoresce – to glow or emit light, in this case under the influence of radiation (Ch. 31)

fluorosis (fluh-ROH-sis) – a condition caused by an excessive intake of fluoride (2 ppm or more in drinking water), characterized mainly by mottling, staining, or hypoplasia of the tooth enamel (Ch. 10)

focal spot – the spot in the anode where x-rays are generated after being hit with a stream of electrons; the focal spot is made from tungsten and precisely aimed to direct the x-ray beam out of the x-ray tube (Ch. 29)

focal trough – in panoramic radiography, the curved, narrow region where the x-ray beam is focused to yield clear images; it is created by the movement of the x-ray tubehead in relation to the film (Ch. 31)

focusing cup – a component in an x-ray tube head, made from molybdenum; a heated tungsten filament creates an electron cloud that remains within the focusing cup until the exposure button is pressed, at which time the electron cloud shoots across the vacuum to a tungsten target called a focal spot, thus creating x-rays (Ch. 29)

fomites (FOH-mie-teez) – objects such as clothing, towels and utensils that may harbor a disease agent and are capable of transmitting it (Ch. 14)

foramen magnum – the natural opening in the base of the occipital bone through which the spinal cord passes (Ch. 6)

foreshortened image – an x-ray image in which the teeth appear shortened with rounded roots; results from excessive vertical angulation in the bisecting technique (Ch. 30)

fossa (FOS-uh) – a small depression located between the marginal ridges on the lingual surfaces of anterior teeth and on the occlusal surfaces of posterior teeth (Ch. 8)

four-handed dentistry – the method of providing dental treatment in which the operator and the assistant work together as a team while both are seated in specific positions near the patient; by working as a team, four hands are available to perform one procedure. This method increases the efficiency and productivity of the dental team, while reducing the stress, strain, and fatigue on the members of that team; also known as team dentistry (Ch. 25)

Frankfort plane – an imaginary plane that extends from the orbital ridge directly under the eye to the top of the ear canal (Ch. 31)

frena (FREE-nuh) (singular: frenum) – folds of skin or a mucous membrane that are positioned between a more stationary and a more flexible part or organ, which restricts movement (Ch. 6)

frenectomy (fruh-NEK-tuh-mee) – surgical removal of the frenum (Ch. 41)

front – a tooth cover that makes the teeth appear to be covered in metal, usually gold or silver; can be removable or permanent (Ch. 46)

frontal bone – the forward-most bone of the cranium; shapes the forehead and forms most of the top of the eye sockets, or orbits (Ch. 6)

frontonasal process – area of facial development where the forehead, eyes, and nose form (Ch. 7)

fulcrum (FUL-krum) – a finger rest that allows the muscles of the hand to relax and remain steady (Ch. 19)

full denture – a prosthesis that replaces all the teeth in a single dental arch; also called a complete denture (Ch. 39)

fungicide (FUN-juh-side) – agent that destroys fungus (Ch. 14)

furcal (FUR-kul) region – the area between two or more roots (Ch. 8)

furcation (fur-KAYshun) – place where the root trunk branches off into separate roots (Ch. 8)

galvanism (GAL-vuh-nih-zum) – the process by which two metals connect to one another by electric shock when the metals mix with water (Ch. 33)

gauge – thickness of a needle (Ch. 28)

general anesthesia – a medication-induced state in which the patient loses feeling and enters an unconscious state (Ch. 28)

general dentist – dentist practicing all phases of dentistry; often refers cases to specialists for specific treatment (Ch. 3)

generic – a drug identified by its nonproprietary name rather than by brand name (Ch. 16)

genetic cells – reproductive cells, or cells that carry half as many chromosomes as regular cells, and are very sensitive to radiation exposure; examples include sperm and egg cells (Ch. 29)

genioglossus (jee-nee-oh-GLAW-sus) muscle – one of the extrinsic muscles of the tongue; depresses the tongue and enables it to protrude (Ch. 6)

geniohyoid muscle – one of the muscles of the floor of the mouth; draws the hyoid bone and tongue forward (Ch. 6)

gingiva – the tissue that surrounds the necks of the teeth and covers the alveolar processes; also called *gums* (Ch. 6)

gingival (jin-JIH-vul) curettage – procedure to remove inflamed tissue and debris from the gingival lining of a periodontal pocket (Ch. 41)

gingival grafting – taking tissue from one area and replacing it where gingival tissue is missing (Ch. 41)

gingival margin trimmer – an angulated, chisel-like curved-blade instrument used to bevel the gingival margin of a tooth in cavity preparation (Ch. 26)

gingival retraction – the process of pulling the gingival tissue away from the tooth so that the entire area of the tooth surface can be molded for an accurate impression (Ch. 38)

gingival sulcus (SUL-kus) – the small space between the tooth and the free gingiva (Ch. 7)

gingival wall – the internal wall nearest the gingiva, running perpendicular to the long axis of the tooth (Ch. 36)

gingivectomy (jin-juh-VEK-tuh-mee) – surgical removal of diseased gingival tissue (Ch. 41)

gingivitis – a reversible condition; inflammation of the gingiva as a response to bacterial plaque on adjacent teeth; characterized by erythema, edema, and fibrous enlargement of the gingiva without resorption of the underlying alveolar bone (Ch. 9)

gingivoplasty (jin-juh-voh-PLAS-tee) – surgical reshaping and contouring of gingival tissues (Ch. 41)

glass ionomer (eye-ON-uh-mer) – a dental cement used for permanent cementing of restorations such as crowns, bridges, inlays, onlays, and orthodontic bands and brackets; also used as a base and a permanent liner (Ch. 33)

glossitis – inflammation of the tongue (Ch. 12)

gold alloy – a combination of gold with silver, copper, zinc, or other elements, which creates a restorative material that is hard and durable (Ch. 38)

Good Samaritan law – state laws protecting people from being sued if they help an injured victim in an emergency (Ch. 4)

gram-negative bacteria – refers to the inability to resist decolorization with alcohol after being treated with Gram crystal violet stain; however, following decolorization, these bacteria can be readily counterstained with safranin, imparting a pink or red color to the bacteria when viewed by light microscopy (Ch. 13)

gram-positive bacteria – refers to the ability of a bacterium to resist decolorization with alcohol after being treated with Gram crystal violet stain, imparting a violet color to the bacterium when viewed by light microscopy (Ch. 13)

granuloma – term applied to nodular inflammatory lesions, usually small or granular, firm, persistent, and containing compactly grouped modified phagocytes (Ch. 12)

grey scale – in digital imaging, the number of shades of grey that an image possesses; most computers recognize about 256 shades of grey, while the human eye recognizes about 32 shades of grey; the greater the number of shades of grey, the more detailed the radiograph (Ch. 29)

grid – in extraoral radiography, a device used to reduce the amount of scatter radiation produced during exposure (Ch. 31)

gutta percha (GUT-uh PUR-chuh) – a rubber-like substance used to fill a root canal; comes in the form of cones, called gutta percha points (Ch. 40)

gypsum (JIP-sum) – a form of calcium sulfate used in dental plasters, investments, and stone (Ch. 35)

halide (HAL-ide) crystals – used in the manufacture of dental x-ray film; halide crystals are suspended in a gelatin coating on the film surface, they are sensitive to x-rays and form a latent image when struck by x-rays during exposure (Ch. 29)

halitosis (hal-ih-TOH-sis) – malodorous breath caused chiefly by bacteria in the oral cavity, and exacerbated by various dietary choices or physical conditions; also called bad breath (Ch. 10)

handpiece – a hand-held powered dental instrument, used to hold rotary cutting, grinding, or polishing tips; can be low-speed or high-speed (Ch. 26)

hard palate – the bony anterior portion of the palate; forms the roof of the mouth (Ch. 6)

hardness – the ability of dental material to resist scratches or marks (Ch. 33)

hatchet – a dental instrument with a curved shank and a flat, single-beveled blade, used to smooth cavity walls in preparation for a restoration (Ch. 26)

Hazard Communication Standard – OSHA regulation concerned with alerting workers about exposure to possibly dangerous chemicals in the workplace (Ch. 14)

heart attack – see *myocardial infarction* (Ch. 18)

hematoma – localized mass of extravasated blood relatively or completely confined within an organ or tissue; blood is usually clotted or partly clotted; for example, a bruised area (Ch. 12)

hemisection (heh-mee-SEK-shun) – a procedure in which half of the entire tooth is removed (Ch. 40)

hemophilia – a genetic disease in which the body's blood-clotting ability is compromised (Ch. 22)

hemorrhage (HEM-er-ij) – an escape of blood through ruptured or unruptured vessel walls; internal or external bleeding (Ch. 18)

hemostat (HEE-moh-stat) – a locking, pliers-like instrument used during surgical procedures to hold tissue and objects (Ch. 42)

herringbone pattern – an x-ray image with an irregular pattern across the surface of the image, caused by reversing the film in the patient's mouth during exposure so the x-rays must pass through the embossed lead foil; a nondiagnostic image (Ch. 30)

high-volume evacuator (HVE) – a dental device that provides a strong suction, used to remove large amounts of fluid and debris from the oral cavity during dental procedures; also called an oral evacuator (Ch. 27)

HIPAA – Health Insurance Portability and Accountability Act of 1996. Specific regulations that ensure privacy and confidentiality of patient health care information (Ch. 2)

Hippocrates – ancient Greek physician (500 BCE) who is considered the father of modern medicine. Many fundamental concepts of modern medicine, including patient confidentiality and the ethical obligation to do no harm, can be traced to his early writings and teachings (Ch. 1)

histology – the study of the relationship between the structure and function of cells, tissues, and organs (Ch. 7)

Hittorf-Crookes (HIT-orf Kruks) tube – an early x-ray tube based on a cathode/anode design (Ch. 29)

Hodgkin disease – also known as Hodgkin lymphoma; a cancer of the lymph nodes (Ch. 5)

hoe – a single-beveled dental excavator, with a blade at an angle to the axis of the handle and a cutting edge perpendicular to the plane of the angle (Ch. 26)

homeostasis – the proper balance of conditions within the body necessary for its survival (Ch. 5)

horizontal angulation – the angle of the PID on a horizontal plane around the patient's head during exposure (Ch. 30)

hydrogen peroxide – unstable compound readily broken down to water and oxygen, a reaction catalyzed by various powdered metals and by the enzyme catalase; used as a tooth whitening agent (Ch. 46)

hygiene – practices that promote or preserve health (Ch. 2)

hyoglossus muscle – one of the extrinsic muscles of the tongue; retracts and pulls down the tongue (Ch. 6)

hyoid (HI-oyd) bone – suspended between the mandible and larynx; supports the tongue and other nearby muscles (Ch. 6)

hyperglycemia (hi-per-glie-SEE-mee-uh) – an elevated level of glucose in blood plasma, with symptoms and signs that include hunger and thirst, fatigue, weight loss, depressed wound healing function, impotence, or coma; when prolonged, damage to various systems of the body may result (Ch. 18)

hypertension – high blood pressure (Ch. 5)

hyperthyroidism (hi-per-THIE-roy-dih-zum) – an overactive thyroid that produces too much of the hormone thyroxine, with accompanying symptoms that may include increased appetite, heat intolerance and sweating, anxiety, fatigue, and depression (Ch. 22)

hyperventilating – greatly increased breathing rate that can cause carbon dioxide levels in the blood to drop below normal; may result in dizziness and confusion (Ch. 18)

hypoglycemia (hi-po-glie-SEE-mee-uh) – a reduced level of glucose in blood plasma, with symptoms and signs that include anxiety, shakiness, double vision, headache, numbness, paralysis, and coma (Ch. 18)

hypotension – low blood pressure (Ch. 5)

hypothyroidism – an underactive thyroid that does not produce enough hormones, with accompanying symptoms that may include fatigue, depression, cold intolerance, cramps, weight gain, and constipation (Ch. 22)

idiopathic – denoting a disease of unknown cause (Ch. 12)

imbibition (im-buh-BISH-un) – changes in a set alginate impression due to swelling or additional moisture (Ch. 35)

immediate denture – a removable dental prosthesis fabricated for placement immediately after the removal of a natural tooth or teeth (Ch. 39)

impacted tooth – a tooth that has been prevented from erupting normally (Ch. 42)

implied consent – principle that patient's consent has been given (implied) because the patient's action indicates he or she is accepting treatment (opening the mouth when the dentist sits down) (Ch. 4)

impression – an imprint or negative reproduction/likeness of the teeth or other tissues of the oral cavity (Ch. 35)

impression tray – a metal or plastic tray used in obtaining impressions (Ch. 35)

incipient lesion – beginning stage of caries, usually not visible upon examination (Ch. 9)

incisal (in-SI-zul) – toward the biting surface of an incisor or canine (Ch. 8)

incisal edge – the thin, flat incisal surface of an incisor (Ch. 8)

incisal surface – the biting surface of the incisors and canines (Ch. 8)

incisor, central – the tooth on either side of the midline at the front of the oral cavity (Ch. 8)

incisor, lateral – the tooth distal to the central incisors (Ch. 8)

indirect restoration – a restoration, such as a crown, that is created outside the patient's mouth (Ch. 35)

indirect supervision – supervision provided by a dentist who is in the office, but not the same treatment area, with the operator/dental assistant (Ch. 37)

infection – invasion of the body by organisms that have the potential to cause disease (Ch. 13)

infection control – measures taken to prevent infection (Ch. 13)

infective endocarditis (en-do-kar-DI-tis) – infection of the valves and lining of the heart (Ch. 16)

inferior – located below the transverse plane of the body, toward the legs and feet (Ch. 5)

infiltration anesthesia – one of the three most common dental injections, this method puts the anesthetic solution into tissues near the small terminal nerve branches (Ch. 28)

inflammation – a fundamental, stereotyped complex of reactions that occur in affected blood vessels and adjacent tissues in response to an injury or abnormal stimulation caused by a physical, chemical, or biologic agent (Ch. 13)

informed consent – principle that patients have the right to know about and understand any procedure that is to be performed; usually obtained in writing (Ch. 4)

inhalation – administering drugs or medications by inhaling them through the mouth or nose (Ch. 16)

initiative – possessing the readiness and ability to take action of one's own (Ch. 2)

intellectual disability – cognitive disability or mental retardation; may be characterized by a significantly below-average score on a test of intelligence and by limitations in functioning in areas such as communication, self-care, and socialization (Ch. 22)

intensifying screen – device used in extraoral radiography to convert x-ray beams into visible light, which is used to expose the screen film; an intensifying screen reduces the amount of radiation needed to create a diagnostic exposure (Ch. 31)

interferon – a class of small proteins produced in response to viral infection and other biological and synthetic stimuli; interferons bind to specific receptors on cell membranes; their effects include inducing enzymes, suppressing cell proliferation, inhibiting viral proliferation, and enhancing the immune system (Ch. 13)

intermediate restorative material (IRM) – reinforced zinc oxide eugenol; a dental material used to create provisional restorations, as well as liners, bases, and cements, and to create impressions; IRM restorations can only last for about a year in the oral cavity (Ch. 34)

internal wall – the wall of the cavity that does not extend to the tooth surface (Ch. 36)

interpretation – the act of reading the information on a radiograph, including anatomical structures, foreign objects, and caries, as distinct from formally diagnosing a patient based on the interpretation of a radiograph (Ch. 32)

interproximal (in-ter-PRAWK-sih-mul) brush – a brush with nylon bristles meant to penetrate the interproximal space to clean the tooth surface and stimulate the gingival tissue (Ch. 10)

interproximal (in-ter-PRAWK-suh-mul) decay – decay that occurs where adjoining teeth touch each other (Ch. 30)

interproximal radiograph – a radiograph that images the region where teeth come into contact with one another; used to diagnose interproximal decay (Ch. 30)

interproximal space – embrasure space cervical to the contact area, just above the interdental papilla (Ch. 8)

interseptal dam – in a dental dam, the part that is placed between the teeth (the area of the dam between the punched holes) (Ch 27)

intradermal administration – injecting drugs and medications beneath the epidermis (Ch. 16)

intramuscular administration – injecting drugs or medications into a muscle (Ch. 16)

intraoral – inside the oral cavity (Ch. 20)

intravenous administration – administering drugs directly into a vein (Ch. 16)

intrinsic strain – discoloration of internal tooth structure due to external agents that have been absorbed into the tooth structure (Ch. 44)

investment material – material used to envelope or cover an object during laboratory procedures, such as soldering, curing, or casting (Ch. 35)

ion (EYE-on) – an unstable atom in which one electron has been removed or added through exposure to energy, including x-rays; ions are attracted to surrounding atoms and can cause biological damage (Ch. 29)

ionization (EYE-uh-nih-ZAY-shun) – the process of creating an ion through exposure to energy (Ch. 29)

irrigant – water-based solution used to disinfect the canal system by killing bacteria and dissolving the pulp tissue (Ch. 40)

Isaac Greenwood – first American-born dentist (Ch. 1)

jurisprudence (juh-ris-PROO-denz) – the law as it relates to dentistry, professional malpractice, or the Dental Practice Act (Ch. 4)

key punch hole – in a dental dam, the largest hole in the dental dam, meant to be used with the bow on a dental clamp to securely hold the dental dam material in place (Ch. 27)

kilovolts (KIL-oh-vohlts) (kV) – a unit of electrical potential, equal to 10^3 volts; in dental radiography, a measure of the power of the dental x-ray unit (Ch. 29)

kinesics (kih-NEE-siks) – positioning of the body (Ch. 23)

labial – near the lips (Ch. 8)

labial commissures (KOM-ih-shorz) – corners of the mouth (Ch. 6)

labial mounting – a method of mounting radiographs in which the view is from the front, similar to the perspective of a viewer facing the patient (Ch. 32)

labial surface – the facial surface of the anterior teeth that is near the lips (Ch. 8)

labioversion (lay-bee-oh-VER-zhun) – malposition of an anterior tooth from the normal line of occlusion toward the lips (Ch. 45)

lacrimal (LAK-rih-muhl) bones – two small, thin bones at the corner of each orbit at the inner angle of the eye socket (Ch. 6)

lactobacilli (lak-to-buh-SIL-lie) – bacteria that produce lactic acid when they encounter dietary carbohydrates (Ch. 9)

lamina dura – thin layer of bone that lines the tooth socket and surrounds the tooth roots. (Ch. 7)

Langerhans (LANG-er-hanz) cells – found in the upper layer of the skin, they protect the body against invasive pathogens (Ch. 5)

latent image – a radiographic image stored on dental film after exposure but before processing; the latent image cannot be seen with the naked eye but is only visible after it has been processed (Ch. 29)

latent period – the period between radiation exposure and its biological effects; the latent period may be years (Ch. 29)

lathe (LAYTHE), dental – an appliance fitted with attachments for grinding, cutting, and polishing dental materials and appliances (Ch. 35)

law – set of rules established and enforced by local, state, and national officials (Ch. 4)

lead apron – a protective device used in dental offices to shield patients from excess radiation exposure during radiography; lead aprons extend from the neck to below the reproductive organs (Ch. 29)

leakage radiation – radiation that escapes from an improperly functioning x-ray tubehead; equipment should be regularly tested to guard against leakage radiation (Ch. 29)

lesion – wound or injury; any abnormal tissue (Ch. 12)

letter of recommendation – a letter written by a person in a position of authority to recommend someone for his or her experience, skills, or character; used during a job search (Ch. 48)

leukoplakia (loo-kuh-PLAY-kee-uh) – white patch of oral mucous membrane that cannot be wiped off and cannot be diagnosed clinically as any specific disease entity (Ch. 12)

line angle – 1. the intersection of two tooth surfaces along a line (Ch. 8); 2. in a cavity preparation, the angle formed when two walls or surfaces intersect (Ch. 36)

lingual – near the tongue (Ch. 8)

lingual frenum (LING-gwul FREE-num) – the fold of tissue connecting the bottom of the tongue to the floor of the mouth (Ch. 46)

lingual mounting – a method of mounting radiographs in which the view is from the tongue-side, or back, as if the viewer was located in the back of the patient's throat (Ch. 32)

lingual surface – the surface of the crown on the inner side on the dental arch that is near the tongue (Ch. 8)

linguoversion (ling-gwo-VER-zhun) – malposition of a tooth lingual to the normal position (Ch. 45)

local anesthetic – a liquid medication injected into the soft tissues that comes into contact with sensory nerve fibers and blocks sensations from registering a feeling of pain in the brain (Ch. 28)

local infections – infections that are confined to a specific region of the body (Ch. 13)

local-action drug – a drug applied to the skin or mucosa as an ointment, lotion, or gel; affects only the area of the body where it is directly applied. (Ch. 16)

long axis of the tooth – an imaginary line drawn from the end of the root to the incisal or occlusal surface of a tooth (Ch. 30)

luting (LOO-ting) agent – a dental material that is used as an adhesive to hold the tooth and restoration together; also helps create a barrier against microleakage by sealing any gaps between the tooth and restorative (Ch. 33)

lymph node – part of the lymphatic system; produces lymphocytes in response to disease and infection (Ch. 6)

lymph node (cervical) – lymph node in the neck; may be palpable when swollen (Ch. 6)

lymphadenopathy (lim-fad-uh-NOP-uh-thee) – swollen and enlarged lymph nodes that last for several months (Ch. 6)

macronutrient – a nutrient that the body needs large amounts of in order to function and survive; includes carbohydrates, protein, fat, water, and fiber (Ch. 11)

macule – a flat area, up to 1 cm in diameter, differing perceptibly in color from surrounding tissue; small discolored patch or spot on skin, neither elevated above nor depressed below skin's surface; for example, freckles (Ch. 12)

magnetic resonance imaging – a technique of medical imaging that uses powerful magnetic waves to create high-quality images of internal structures and organs (Ch. 31)

malignant melanoma – a particularly dangerous form of skin cancer (Ch. 5)

malocclusion (mal-uh-KLOO-zhun) – a condition in which opposing teeth do not meet in normal occlusal contact (Ch. 8)

malpractice – mistreatment of a patient through ignorance, carelessness, neglect, or criminal intent; professional negligence (Ch. 4)

mamelons (MAM-uh-lunz) – three small bumps often present on the incisal surface of a newly erupted incisor (Ch. 8)

mandible – long, strong bone that forms the lower jaw (Ch. 6)

mandibular arch – dental arch of the lower jaw (Ch. 8)

mandibular process – process of the mandibular arch that forms the lower jaw and structures of the lower lip and lower cheeks (Ch. 7)

mandibular ramus (man-DIB-yoo-ler RAY-mus) – the vertical portion on either side of the lower jaw that articulates with the skull (Ch. 6)

manual processing – in dental radiography, the practice of manually transferring exposed dental films from a developer solution to a water bath and then to a fixer solution, under controlled circumstances in terms of time and temperature, to produce diagnostic images (Ch. 32)

marginal ridge – mesial and distal edges of the lingual surfaces of incisors and canines (Ch. 8)

Maryland bridge – a bridge that has small, metal, wing-like extensions that are bonded to the lingual surface of the anterior teeth (Ch. 38)

masseter (mah-SEE-ter) muscle – one of four pairs of muscles of mastication (Ch. 6)

mastication – the act of chewing (Ch. 5)

matter – a substance that has form and shape and occupies space (Ch. 29)

maturity (muh-CHUR-uh-tee) – the state of being mature or fully developed (Ch. 2)

maxillae (mak-SIL-ee) – bones that form the upper part of the jaw and a part of the hard palate (Ch. 6)

maxillary arch – dental arch of the upper jaw (Ch. 8)

maxillary process – process of the mandibular arch that forms the upper jaw and structures of the upper lip and upper cheeks (Ch. 7)

maxillary tuberosity – large, rounded protuberance situated on the outer surface of the maxillary bones near the posterior teeth (Ch. 6)

maximum permissible dose (MPD) – according to the National Council on Radiation Protection and Measurements, the maximum permissible dose of radiation a body can receive in a given time frame without causing biological damage (Ch. 29)

meatus (mee-AY-tus) – the external opening of a bodily canal (Ch. 6)

medical history – a patient history of medical care, including past conditions, diagnoses, and treatments; medications and substances; and lifestyle factors that may affect health (Ch. 21)

medium – how communication takes place, such as face-to-face, over the telephone, or in writing (Ch. 23)

mental protuberance – a tuberosity of the mandible or lower jaw; commonly known as the chin (Ch. 6)

mental retardation – a disability characterized by significant limitations both in intellectual functioning and in adaptive behavior, as expressed in conceptual, social, and practical skills (Ch. 22)

mentalis (men-TAY-lus) – muscle of facial expression that moves the chin and lower lip (Ch. 6)

mesial (MEE-zee-ul) – closer to the midline (Ch. 8)

mesial surface – the surface of a tooth that is closer to the midline (Ch. 8)

mesioversion (mee-zee-oh-VER-zhun) – malposition of a tooth mesial to the normal position, in an anterior direction following the curvature of dental arch (Ch. 45)

mesoderm (MEZ-uh-durm) – the middle layer of embryonic cells (Ch. 7)

message – the information communicated (Ch. 23)

metabolism – a measure of the rate at which energy is released from cells (Ch. 11)

metastasize – the shifting of disease or its local manifestations from one part of the body to another; spread of a disease process from one part of the body to another, as in appearance of distant neoplasms in an area removed from the locale of the original neoplasm (Ch. 12)

microbiology – the science concerned with microorganisms, including fungi, protozoa, bacteria, and viruses (Ch. 13)

microleakage (my-kroh-LEE-kuj) – leakage of saliva or food particles into the small spaces between the tooth and a restoration (Ch. 33)

micronutrient – a nutrient that the body needs small amounts of in order to function and survive; includes vitamins and minerals (Ch. 11)

microorganisms – microscopic organisms (Ch. 13)

midline – the imaginary line that splits a dental arch in half between the central incisors (Ch. 8)

midsagittal plane – an imaginary line that divides the body into right and left halves, used in radiology to help determine angulation (Ch. 30)

milliamperage (mil-ee-AM-per-ej) (mA) – one thousandth of an amp; in dental radiography, a measure of how many electrons are contained in an x-ray beam (Ch. 29)

mineral – a chemical element needed to maintain body structure and body functioning (Ch. 11)

mitochondria (my-toh-KON-dree-uh) – a cell structure where energy is generated for use by the cell (Ch. 29)

mitosis (my-TOH-sis) – the process of cell division by which one cell is split into two exact copies of itself (Ch. 29)

mixed dentition – dentition consisting of both primary and permanent teeth (Ch. 8)

model trimmer – appliance used to trim away excess plaster or dental stone from models or casts (Ch. 35)

molar – a posterior tooth characterized by a broad crown, located at the back of the oral cavity (Ch. 8)

mold – a filamentous fungus, generally a circular colony that may be cottony, wooly, or glabrous, but with filaments not organized into large fruiting bodies, such as mushrooms (Ch. 13)

molecule – unit of matter comprised of atoms arranged in a predictable pattern; a water molecule, for example, includes two atoms of hydrogen and one atom of oxygen (Ch. 29)

morphology – the anatomical form and structure of a tooth (Ch. 8)

mouth mirror – used to see areas within the intraoral cavity that cannot be seen by direct vision (Ch. 20)

mouth rinse – a liquid used to clean the oral cavity and treat disorders of oral mucosa; also known as mouthwash (Ch. 10)

multiple sclerosis (skluh-ROH-sis) – an autoimmune disease in which the body's immune system destroys the protective sheath covering the nerves; can be debilitating and can cause numbness or weakness in the limbs, full or partial vision loss, pain or tingling, unsteady gait, tremors, fatigue, dizziness, and an inability to walk or talk (Ch. 22)

muscular dystrophy – a group of inherited muscle diseases that causes muscle fibers to be very susceptible to damage; muscles weaken progressively and, late in this disease, are replaced by fat and connective tissue (Ch. 22)

musculoskeletal (mus-kyuh-loh-SKEL-ih-tul) injuries – injuries to the skeleton and muscles of the body (Ch. 19)

mutans streptococci (MYOO-tanz strep-toh-KOK-sigh) – infectious bacteria (*Streptococci mutans*) primarily responsible for caries (Ch. 9)

myelin sheath (MI-uh-lihn) – soft white material, made up of protein and fatty substances, that surrounds and protects some nerves in the peripheral nervous system (Ch. 5)

mylohyoid muscle – one of the muscles of the floor of the mouth; forms the floor itself (Ch. 6)

myocardial infarction – sudden insufficiency of blood supply to an area of the heart muscle, usually as a result of blockage of a coronary artery; commonly called a heart attack (Ch. 18)

narcotic – any of a variety of opioid drugs, including opium and cocaine (Ch. 16)

naris (NAY-rihs), anterior – facial landmark; refers to the nostril (Ch. 6)

nasal bone – forms the bridge of the nose (Ch. 6)

nasal conchae (KONG-kee) – three bony projections that scroll inward from the ethmoid bone and form the nasal cavity; known as the *inferior*, *medial*, and *superior* nasal conchae (Ch. 6)

nasal septum – the bony and cartilaginous partition between the two nasal passages (Ch. 6)

nasion (NAY-zee-on) – facial landmark lying midway between the eyes, just below the eyebrows (Ch. 6)

nasolabial groove – runs from the ala of the nose to the corners of the mouth (Ch. 6)

natural killer cells – large granular lymphocytes that kill targeted cells using antibody-dependent cell-mediated cytotoxicity (Ch. 13)

natural radiation – environmental radiation caused by the sun and emitted from radon within the earth; exposure to natural radiation is unavoidable (Ch. 29)

negligence – failure to perform duties or activities with due diligence and attention or to meet the standards of regular care; the failure to use due care or the lack of due care (omission and commission) (Ch. 4)

neoplasm – abnormal tissue that grows by cellular proliferation more rapidly than normal and continues to grow after the stimuli that initiated the new growth cease (Ch. 12)

nerve block anesthesia – one of the three most common dental injections, this is given near a main nerve trunk to prevent pain sensation from passing to the brain; eliminates sensation over a large area; also known as mandibular block injection (Ch. 28)

neurological disorder – any disease or disorder that affects the nervous system; including Alzheimer disease, epilepsy, Parkinson disease, cerebral palsy, and multiple sclerosis (Ch. 22)

neutral position – best position to maintaining good posture while sitting, standing, or reaching; includes keeping the back straight, legs slightly apart, feet flat on the floor or footrest, lower back pressed against the chair, and ears, shoulder, and hips in a straight line (Ch. 19)

nib – the portion of a condensing instrument that comes into contact with the restorative material being condensed into the tooth; usually blunt and not bladed (Ch. 26)

nitrous oxide – an inhaled anesthetic used in dentistry (Ch. 16)

noble metal – metal such as gold, palladium, or platinum, known for resistance to tarnish and etching (Ch. 35)

nodule – a small node; in skin, a node up to 1 cm in diameter, solid, with palpable depth (Ch. 12)

nonmaleficence (non-mah-LEF-uh-senz) – ethical principle of doing no harm (Ch. 4)

nonregulated waste – waste that is not regulated by any government agency, including normal office waste and used barrier material (Ch. 15)

nonverbal communication – communication without words or language, including body gestures, facial expressions, and eye contact (Ch. 23)

nosocomial (nose-oh-KOH-mee-uhl) infection – an infection acquired in a hospital (Ch. 13)

NSAIDs – nonsteroidal anti-inflammatory drugs; includes commonly used over-the-counter analgesics (Ch. 16)

nucleus – a cell center; in a biological cell, the nucleus is home to the DNA; in a non-biological cell, the electrons orbit the nucleus in predictable patterns (Ch. 29)

nutrient – a food substance necessary for the body to live and function properly (Ch. 11)

nutrition – the study of what people eat and how the body uses food to function (Ch. 11)

oblique ridge – triangular ridges of the mesiolingual cusp and distobuccal cusp, which are diagonally across from each other, that meet along the occlusal surface (Ch. 8)

obturation – obstruction or occlusion (Ch. 40)

occipital bone – the lower-most bone of the skull; forms the back and base of the cranium (Ch. 6)

occipital protuberance – the raised and tangible lump in the base of the neck caused by the occipital bone, which is located in the back of the head (Ch. 31)

occlusal (uh-KLOO-zul) – toward the chewing surface of premolars or molars (Ch. 8)

occlusal equilibration – a bite adjustment procedure that reduces pressure on the jaws and allows the bite to be more even (Ch. 46)

occlusal exposure – an x-ray technique used to show large areas of the maxillary and mandibular arches (Ch. 30)

occlusal surface – the chewing surface of premolars and molars (Ch. 8)

occlusion (uh-KLOO-zhun) – when the incisal and occlusal surfaces of opposing maxillary and mandibular teeth come together (Ch. 8)

odontoblast (oh-DON-toe-blast) – cell that forms dentin (Ch. 7)

odontogenesis (oh-don-toe-JEN-uh-sis) – the process of tooth development (Ch. 7)

omission (act of) – the failure to perform a service that should be performed on a patient (Ch. 4)

open bite – large intraoral distance; the maxillary anterior teeth do not occlude with the mandibular anterior teeth (Ch. 45)

operating field – during a dental procedure, the imaginary area where the work will be performed, including the oral cavity and the transfer space where instruments are transferred between the operator and the dental assistant (Ch. 27)

operating light – a bright, moveable, overhead light used to light up the patient's oral cavity during a dental procedure (Ch. 24)

operating zones – specific areas around the patient designated for the different dental team members and equipment (Ch. 25)

operatory (OP-er-uh-tor-ee) – a treatment room in which dental work is performed on the patient (Ch. 24)

oral administration – administering drugs orally (Ch. 16)

oral and maxillofacial (mak-sihl-oh-FAY-shul) pathology – dental specialty concerned with diagnosis, causes, and treatment of diseases of the oral cavity (Ch. 3)

oral and maxillofacial radiology – dental specialty using imaging techniques to locate tumors, disorders, or other conditions affecting the head, jaw, and neck (Ch. 3)

oral and maxillofacial surgery – dental specialty concerned with diagnosis and surgical correction of defects, injuries, and diseases of the head, jaws, and teeth (Ch. 3)

oral embryology – the study of the formation of the oral cavity and its structures (Ch. 7)

oral histology – the study of the structure and function of teeth and their connective tissues (Ch. 7)

oral personalization – techniques used to alter the mouth and teeth for self-expression (Ch. 46)

oral photography – a method of photography that allows dentists and patients to view the teeth before and after a cosmetic procedure; includes intraoral and extraoral photography (Ch. 46)

oral thermometer – an instrument that is placed under the tongue to measure temperature (Ch. 17)

oral thrush – candidiasis of the mouth (Ch. 16)

orbicularis oris (or-bik-yoo-LAR-is OR-is) muscle – one of the muscles of facial expression; encircles and helps move the mouth (Ch. 6)

organic food – food that has been grown and processed in nontraditional ways, usually to reduce pollution or environmental waste, to reduce the use of chemicals, or to feed and raise livestock differently (Ch. 11)

orthodontics (or-thoh-DON-tiks) and dentofacial orthopedics (den-toh-FAY-shul or-thoh-PEE-diks) – dental specialty concerned with diagnosing and recommending treatment for all forms of poor alignment or malocclusion of the teeth or jaws (Ch. 3)

orthostatic (or-thoh-STAT-ik) hypotension – a form of low blood pressure that occurs when a seated patient quickly stands or suddenly changes position; accompanied by symptoms that may include lightheadedness, dizziness, obscured vision, and numbness; also called postural hypotension (Ch. 18)

osseointegration (os-ee-oh-in-tuh-GRAY-shun) – apparent direct attachment or connection of osseous tissue to an inert alloplastic material without intervening connective tissue, as with dental implants (Ch. 42)

osseous (AW-see-us) tissue – the connective tissue that makes up bone (Ch. 5)

ostectomy (os-TEK-tuh-mee) – removing bone (Ch. 41)

osteoblast (OS-tee-oh-blast) – bone-forming cell (Ch. 7)

osteoclast (OS-tee-oh-klast) – bone-resorbing cell (Ch. 7)

osteoplasty (OS-tee-oh-plas-tee) – contouring and shaping bone (Ch. 41)

outline form – the shape of the tooth surface area included within the cavosurface margins of a cavity preparation of a dental restoration (Ch. 36)

overbite – vertical overlap of teeth (Ch. 45)

overdenture – a removable prosthesis that rests on one or more remaining natural teeth, tooth roots, or dental implants (Ch. 39)

overdose – a lethal or toxic amount of a drug (Ch. 16)

overjet – horizontal overlap of teeth (Ch. 45)

overlapping image – a dental x-ray in which the images of teeth improperly overlap on the final image, obscuring the interproximal area; results from incorrect horizontal angulation (Ch. 30)

palatal – near the palate (Ch. 8)

palatal surface – the lingual surface of the maxillary teeth that is near the palate (Ch. 8)

palatine (PAL-uh-tine) bone – facial bone important to the structure of the mouth; forms the posterior portion of the roof of the mouth and the floor of the nose, along with the side walls of the nasal cavity (Ch. 6)

palatoglossus (pal-uh-toe-GLAW-sus) – one of the two major muscles of the soft palate (Ch. 6)

palatopharyngeus (pal-uh-toe-fa-RIHN-jee-us) – one of the two major muscles of the soft palate (Ch. 6)

palpate (PAL-pate) – to examine by feeling with the fingers or hands (Ch. 17)

panoramic radiograph – radiograph of the complete jaw structure (Ch. 29)

panoramic radiography – the practice of obtaining extraoral radiographs using a special x-ray unit that rotates around the head and visualizes both the maxilla and mandible in one large film (Ch. 31)

paper point – used to dry a root canal before it is filled (Ch. 40)

papoose board – a type of restraint made from a still board and Velcro straps that restrains a patient's arms and legs (Ch. 43)

papule – a circumscribed, solid elevation up to 1 cm in diameter on the skin (Ch. 12)

parallel technique – a dental x-ray technique in which the film is held parallel to the long axis of the tooth and the primary x-ray beam strikes the film at a perpendicular angle (Ch. 30)

paresthesia (par-us-THEE-zha) – a condition that occurs when numbness induced by local anesthesia does not wear off as it should; numbness may last for days, weeks, years, or permanently (Ch. 28)

parietal bone – found on each side of the cranium; forms its rounded back and upper sides (Ch. 6)

parotid (pah-ROT-id) duct – duct that carries saliva from the parotid gland to the mouth; also known as Stensen duct (Ch. 6)

parotid gland – the largest of the salivary glands; located on each side of the head just below and in front of the ear (Ch. 6)

partial denture – a removable prosthesis used to replace one or more missing teeth (Ch. 39)

partial image – a processing error resulting from the processing of x-ray film in tanks that are only partially filled (Ch. 32)

pathogen (PATH-uh-jin) – an agent, such as a bacterium or fungus, that causes disease (Ch. 2)

pathogenic (path-oh-JEN-ik) – causing disease or abnormality (Ch. 13)

pediatric dentistry – dental specialty concerned with the dental care and treatment of children (Ch. 3)

penumbra (pih-NUM-bruh) – a partial shadow around an object; in dental radiography, penumbra reduces detail in the image and can be reduced by a tight focal spot (Ch. 29)

percussion test – tapping the tooth with the handle of a dental mirror to determine whether pulpal damage is present (Ch. 40)

periapical (per-e-A-pih-kul) abscess – breakdown of the periapical tissue caused by a build up of purulent material and fluids in the tissue (Ch. 40)

periapical area – the area of the gingiva at the apex of the tooth (Ch. 40)

periapical (per-ee-AP-ih-kul) exposure – at or around the apex of a tooth; used in radiology to describe radiographs that show the tooth from its apex to its root (Ch. 30)

periodontal ligament – the fibrous tissue that connects the roots of the teeth to the alveolar bone (Ch. 7)

periodontal probe – instrument used to measure the depth of the sulcus (Ch. 20)

periodontics (per-ee-oh-DON-tiks) – dental specialty concerned with the treatment of abnormal conditions of the tissues surrounding the teeth (Ch. 3)

periodontitis – an irreversible condition; inflammatory disease of the periodontium occurring in response to bacterial plaque on adjacent teeth; characterized by gingivitis, destruction of alveolar bone and periodontal ligament, apical migration of the epithelial attachment resulting in formation of periodontal pockets, and possibly, if left untreated, eventual loosening and exfoliation of teeth (Ch. 9)

periodontium (per-ee-oh-DON-she-um) – tissues that surround and support the tooth (Ch. 7)

periosteal (per-ee-OS-tee-ul) elevators – a surgical instrument used to separate the attached periosteum from the underlying alveolar bone (Ch. 42)

peripheral nervous system – nerves outside the brain and spinal cord that transmit and receive stimuli from inside and outside the body. (Ch. 5)

permanent dentition – the set of thirty-two teeth that are ordinarily present throughout a person's life (Ch. 8)

personal characteristic – a trait that characterizes a person, such as honesty, tactfulness, adaptability, compassion (Ch. 2)

pestle (PES-ul) – rodlike instrument with one rounded and weighted extremity, used for mixing substances; in restorative dentistry, pestles are included within amalgam capsules to combine alloy and mercury during amalgamation (Ch. 34)

petechiae (pih-TEE-kee-ee) – minute (1-2 millimeter) hemorrhagic spots on mucosa or skin that do not blanch even when pressed (Ch. 12)

phagocytosis (fayg-oh-sigh-TOE-sis) – the process of ingestion and digestion by cells of solid substances (Ch. 13)

pharmacokinetics (far-muh-ko-kih-NET-iks) – how a drug is absorbed, distributed, and metabolized within the body (Ch. 16)

pharmacology – the study of drugs and their effect on living organisms (Ch. 16)

pharynx – the throat (Ch. 5)

philtrum (FIL-trum) – the ridge running from just under the nostrils to the middle of the upper lip (Ch. 6)

photoinitiator – a substance that, when exposed to light, acts as a catalyst to begin the hardening process of dental materials (Ch. 24)

physical disability – a disability (orthopedic, neuromuscular, cardiovascular, or pulmonary) that may cause a person to depend on a wheelchair, crutches, cane, or another assistive device for mobility; disability may be congenital or the result of an injury, disease or condition, or amputation; some physical disabilities are not apparent to others (Ch. 22)

***Physician's Desk Reference* (PDR)** – comprehensive reference work on drugs in current use (Ch. 16)

Pierre Fauchard (pe-Ar fo-SHARD) – 18th-century French physician who is known as the Father of Modern Dentistry. He described advanced techniques for cleaning the teeth and filling decay in his comprehensive textbook on dentistry, *Treatise on the Teeth* (1723) (Ch. 1)

pit – pointed depression in the enamel surface caused by faulty enamel calcification deep within a fossa (Ch. 8)

planing – procedure to smooth tooth surfaces by removing calculus and necrotic cementum that may be embedded in the root surface; this procedure is rarely performed in modern dentistry (Ch. 41)

plaque – 1. deposits on teeth, composed primarily of bacteria and acids (Ch. 9); 2. patch or small differentiated area on a body surface (Ch. 12)

plaster – a type of gypsum containing calcium sulfate hemihydrate and porous crystals that is used to make dental casts (Ch. 35)

pocket marker – tweezer-like dental instrument used to perforate gingival tissue with small markings, indicating locations for incisions (Ch. 41)

point angle – the intersection of three tooth surfaces at a point (Ch. 8)

polycarboxylate (pol-ee-kar-BOK-suh-late) – a dental cement used for permanent cementing of restorations such as crowns, bridges, inlays, onlays, and orthodontic bands and brackets; also used for temporary cementing of restorations and as a base (Ch. 33)

polyether (pol-ee-EH-thur) – material used to make elastomeric impressions for crowns and bridges (Ch. 35)

polymerization (pol-ih-mer-uh-ZAY-shun) – a process by which composite material hardens (Ch. 34)

polysulfide (pol-ee-SUL-fide) – synthetic elastic material used to make elastomeric dental impressions (Ch. 35)

pontic (PON-tik) – an artificial tooth that serves as a substitute for a missing tooth (or teeth) (Ch. 38)

porcelain – a commonly used dental ceramic (Ch. 35)

portal of entry – refers to the process whereby a pathogen enters the body, gains access to susceptible tissues, and causes disease or infection (Ch. 14)

portal of exit – refers to the process whereby a pathogen exits the mode of transmission and attempts to gain access to a new host (Ch. 14)

position indicator device (PID) – a device on the x-ray tubehead that aims the x-ray beam; PIDs are available in cylindrical and rectangular shapes, with rectangular shapes reducing radiation exposure (Ch. 29)

post dam – the seal at the posterior area of a maxillary denture that secures it in place; also called the posterior palatal seal (Ch. 39)

posterior – toward the back half of the body (Ch. 5)

posterior teeth – refers to teeth at the back of the mouth; premolars and molars (Ch. 20)

posteruptive stain – a stain that occurs after the tooth erupts and can include stains caused by amalgam and root canal therapy (Ch. 44)

preeruptive stain – a stain that occurs while the teeth are still forming and can include stains caused by medicines, fluoride in drinking water, and inherited conditions (Ch. 44)

premolar (bicuspid) – a double-cusp tooth located between canines and molars (Ch. 8)

primary dentin – dentin that begins forming during tooth development and continues until the root formation is finished (Ch. 7)

primary dentition – the first set of twenty teeth that erupt in a child's oral cavity (Ch. 8)

primary palate – triangle-shaped area of the palate located behind the upper four front teeth (Ch. 7)

primary radiation – direct exposure to x-ray beams from their source (Ch. 29)

prion (PRY-on) – small, infectious proteinaceous particle (Ch. 13)

process – a raised portion or projection along the surface of a bone; sometimes called a prominence (Ch. 6)

professional – an individual whose knowledge, training, skills, and conduct meet the standards of a chosen profession (Ch. 2)

prophylactic – a preventive measure; as when giving a drug to prevent rather than treat infection (Ch. 16)

prophylaxis angle – angled instrument that holds the rubber cup and brush bristles used in coronal polishing; also called a prophy angle (Ch. 44)

prosthodontics (pros-thuh-DON-tiks) – an area of dentistry that is focused on restorations that replace missing or broken teeth or parts of the tooth (Ch. 38)

protected health information (PHI) – includes all records that have information that could link their contents to a specific patient (Ch. 4)

protein – a nutrient made up of amino acids responsible for building, maintaining, and repairing all of the body's muscles and tissues; includes mostly animal meat, eggs, and milk products, but also some vegetables, legumes, and nuts (Ch. 11)

provisional coverage – a temporary prosthesis, such as a crown or bridge, that is placed while a permanent prosthesis is being fabricated (Ch. 38)

proximal – next to, adjacent (Ch. 8)

proximal surfaces – surfaces adjacent to other teeth (Ch. 8)

psychosocial problem – a problem, including depression, anxiety, bipolar disorder, dementia, addiction, and behavioral problems, that results from background, personality, and social factors and that creates difficulties in a person's external world. Some of these conditions are not at first apparent. (Ch. 22)

pterygoid (TER-ih-goyd) muscle (external) – one of four pairs of muscles of mastication (Ch. 6)

pterygoid muscle (internal) – one of four pairs of muscles of mastication (Ch. 6)

pulp – the soft inner core of the tooth that contains the tooth's nerves and blood vessel (Ch. 40)

pulp canal – the portion of the pulp cavity that extends into the root of the tooth (Ch. 7)

pulp cap – placement of a cement base underneath a restoration in order to provide extra protection of the pulp (Ch. 40)

pulp cavity – the area of the tooth that contains the pulp (Ch. 7)

pulp chamber – the part of the pulp cavity that extends into the crown of the tooth (Ch. 7)

pulp necrosis (neh-KROH-sis) – death of the tooth's pulp (Ch. 40)

pulpal (PUL-pul) wall – the internal wall that runs perpendicular to the long axis of the tooth, usually covering the tooth pulp; also called the floor or pulpal floor (Ch. 36)

pulpectomy (pul-PEK-tuh-mee) – removal of all pulp from both the crown and the root canal (Ch. 40)

pulpotomy (pul-POT-uh-mee) – removal of pulp from the crown of the tooth but not from the root canal (Ch. 40)

pulse – the expansion and relaxation of an artery; also called a pulsation (Ch. 17)

pulse oximeter (ok-SIM-ih-ter) – a device that attaches to the finger and measures the amount of oxygen in the blood; used for patients under anesthesia to monitor vital signs (Ch. 17)

pulse rate – the number of pulsations measured per minute (Ch. 17)

pulse rhythm – the pattern of pulsations (e.g., steady, skipping) (Ch. 17)

pulse volume – the force of pulsations (e.g., strong, weak) (Ch. 17)

purging – getting rid of food in the body; in bulimia nervosa, usually occurs after binging by forcing oneself to vomit by sticking a finger or object down the throat or using laxatives (Ch. 11)

purpura (PUR-pyur-uh) – a large area of skin discoloration caused by underlying bleeding (Ch. 12)

pustule – a circumscribed, superficial elevation of the skin, up to 1 cm in diameter, containing purulent material (Ch. 12)

quadrant – the four identical sections of the oral cavity: upper right, upper left, lower left, lower right (Ch. 8)

radial artery – a blood vessel located on the inside of the wrist, under the bone by the thumb (Ch. 17)

radiation absorbed dose (RAD) – a unit for measuring the dose of absorbed radiation; 100 RAD = 1 Gy (Ch. 29)

radiolucent (ray-dee-oh-LOO-sunt) – the quality of being penetrable by x-rays; radiolucent objects show up as dark areas on a radiograph (Ch. 29)

radiometer – a hand-held device that measures the intensity of a curing light (Ch. 24)

radiopaque (ray-dee-oh-PAKE) – the quality of being impenetrable by x-rays; radiopaque objects absorb x-ray energy and show up as lighter areas on a radiograph (Ch. 29)

radiosensitive – the quality of being sensitive to radiation; radiosensitivity of different organs varies, with reproductive organs, the thyroid gland, and non-specialized cells being more radiosensitive than other kinds of cells (Ch. 29)

ramus – a part of an irregularly shaped bone that forms an angle with the main body, e.g., ramus of the mandible (Ch. 31)

rebasing (re-BAY-sing) – a procedure in which the denture base is replaced (Ch. 39)

receiver – the person receiving the message from the sender (Ch. 23)

reciprocity (res-ih-PROS-uh-tee) – agreement between two states when each agrees to grant a license to practice dentistry to any person licensed by the other state (Ch. 4)

Recommended Dietary Allowances (RDAs) – guidelines that tell how much of a nutrient is needed for nearly all people (about 98%) to stay healthy, depending on age and gender (Ch. 11)

rectal administration – administering drugs and medications through the rectum (Ch. 16)

rectal thermometer – an instrument that is placed gently inside the rectum to measure temperature (Ch. 17)

references – a list of individuals who can provide information about a job seeker's qualifications (Ch. 48)

regulated waste – hazardous waste that falls under the jurisdiction of a government agency such as OSHA, EPA, or a local agency; regulated waste includes hazardous chemicals and potentially contaminated materials (Ch. 15)

relining – a procedure in which the tissue side of the denture base receives a new lining to improve fit and comfort (Ch. 39)

remineralization – healing process in which minerals are redeposited in the demineralized tooth structure; accomplished by the protective factors of the saliva and the action of fluoride to inhibit demineralization and interfere with the enzymatic requirements of bacteria (Ch. 9)

reorder point – the point at which quantities of a supply are running low and should be reordered (Ch. 47)

repetitive stress injuries – injuries that come from performing the same motion repeatedly, especially motions that are awkward for the body (Ch. 19)

res gestae **(REEZ JES-tee)** – "things done"; the facts that may be used in evidence in a legal case, such as words or statements said by the assistant during treatment (for example, "Oops!"). These statements can be admitted as legal evidence against the dentist (Ch. 4)

reservoir – living or nonliving material in or on which an infectious agent multiplies and develops and is dependent on for its survival in nature (Ch. 14)

resistance – the degree to which dental material can hold up under force or stress (Ch. 33)

resistance form – the shape given to a cavity preparation that enables a dental restoration to withstand masticatory forces (Ch. 36)

respiration – the movement of oxygen into and carbon dioxide out of the lungs (Ch. 17)

respiratory depth – amount of oxygen inhaled and carbon dioxide exhaled (Ch. 17)

respiratory rate – number of breaths per minute (Ch. 17)

respiratory rhythm – pattern of breaths (Ch. 17)

respondeat **(rih-SPON-dee-uht)** *superior* – legal principle that means the head of an organization can legally be held responsible for the actions of those who report to him or her; the dentist is responsible for any harm caused the patient by an employee (DA, RDH, etc.) while carrying out the requests or expectations of the dentist/employer (Ch. 4)

responsibility – being obliged to certain actions or outcomes (Ch. 2)

rest – a metal projections that is part of the framework of a removable partial denture and which comes into contact with the occlusal or lingual surface of the abutment teeth and aids in the support of the pontic tooth (Ch. 39)

restoration – a dental material used to restore the health and function of a damaged or missing tooth, such as crowns, bridges, inlays, and onlays (Ch. 33)

restorative dentistry – branch of dentistry that deals with restoring or replacing damaged or missing teeth (Ch. 1)

resume – a short document listing a person's relevant job experience and education (Ch. 48)

retainer – a clasp that comes into contact with abutment teeth and prevents a partial denture from moving (Ch. 39)

retention – the way in which dental material is held in place (Ch. 33)

retention form – the shape of a cavity preparation that prevents displacement of a dental restoration by lateral or tipping forces as well as masticatory forces (Ch. 36)

retention pin – a nail-like device placed into the dentin of the tooth and placed underneath a core buildup for strength (Ch. 38)

retention technique – a techniques used to make sure a prosthesis stays in place (Ch. 38)

retraction cord – used to move gingival tissue either by hand or by chemicals in the cord (Ch. 38)

retractor – an instrument for holding oral tissues away from the operating field or holding back structures adjacent to the operating field (Ch. 42)

Retzius striae (RET-see-us STRY-ee) (lines) – darkened concentric lines visible in a cross-section of the tooth enamel that indicate variations in calcification (Ch. 7)

rheostat (REE-oh-stat) – a round, disk-shaped, foot-operated power control that controls the speed of handpieces attached to the dental unit (Ch. 24)

rheumatoid arthritis – an autoimmune disorder characterized by swollen, painful, stiff, and sometimes degenerating joints. (Ch. 5)

risk management – practices in an office or business that minimize the potential for errors, or legal action (Ch. 4)

roentgen (RENT-gen) – a unit of measure for ionizing radiation, named after the discoverer of x-rays, Dr. Wilhelm Roentgen; one roentgen is the amount of radiation needed to ionize one cubic centimeter of dry air (Ch. 29)

roentgen equivalent man (REM) – a unit for measuring how much radiation was actually absorbed in a human; REM varies based on the kind of radiation and how easily it is absorbed into tissue; 100 REM = 1 Sv (Ch. 29)

root caries – a soft, progressive lesion of cementum and dentin that involves bacterial infection and invasion (Ch. 9)

rotational center – in panoramic radiography, the imaginary point around which the tubehead and film cassette rotate (Ch. 31)

saliva ejector – a dental device that provides low-strength suction and is meant to remove excess saliva during a procedure; it does not remove debris (Ch. 27)

sandblaster – small hand-held instrument used to roughen smooth surfaces for better adhesion (Ch. 35)

sarcoma – connective tissue neoplasm, usually highly malignant, formed by proliferation of mesodermal cells (Ch. 12)

saturated fat – a type of fat that generally comes from animals, such as in meat, eggs, and milk products, but also found in coconut, coconut oil, and palm oil (Ch. 11)

scaling – type of tooth surface debridement that removes plaque, calculus, and stains (Ch. 41)

scatter radiation – radiation caused when the primary radiation beam bounces of obstructing objects, such as bones and tissues; scatter radiation is weaker than primary radiation (Ch. 29)

screen film – film used in extraoral radiography; screen film is larger than intraoral films and must be exposed with intensifying screens enclosed in a cassette to yield a diagnostic image (Ch. 31)

secondary dentin – dentin formed by the pulp of the tooth after root formation is finished (Ch. 7)

secondary palate – the area of the palate formed behind the primary palate by the fusion of the palatal shelves (Ch. 7)

secondary radiation – radiation that has been deflected or leaked from a source other than the primary source; scatter radiation is a form of secondary radiation (Ch. 29)

sedative – a drug that reduces excitement, including anxiety (Ch. 16)

seizure disorder – see *epilepsy*

selective polishing – an approach to coronal polishing wherein only stained teeth are polished (Ch. 44)

semi-supine position – the position of the dental chair in which the back of the patient's chair is about 45 degrees from the floor; typically used when the operator is working on the mandibular arch, or when

the operator cannot put the patient back due to medical conditions (Ch. 25)

sender – the person communicating the message (Ch. 23)

septum – facial landmark; connective tissue that divides the nasal cavity into two passages (Ch. 6)

seroconversion (sir-oh-kun-VER-zhun) – the process by which, after exposure to an etiologic agent of a disease, the blood changes from a negative to a positive serum market for that specific disease (Ch. 13)

sextant – the six parts of the dentition; there are three sextants on each arch (Ch. 8)

shaft – the handle of an instrument (Ch. 26)

shank – the portion of the instrument that connects the cutting or functional portion to a handle; with rotary instruments, it connects burs and drills into the chuck of the handpiece (Ch. 26)

sharp – any medical/dental instrument or any disposable material that is sharp or may produce sharp pieces; should be disposed of in a biohazard container (Ch. 14)

sialolith (SIGH-uh-loe-lith) – salivary gland stone (Ch. 6)

side effect – an unintended result of drug use (Ch. 16)

sign – any abnormality indicative of a disease, discoverable on examination of a patient; an objective symptom of disease (Ch. 18)

silicone – material used in dentistry to make elastomeric impressions (Ch. 35)

simple carbohydrate – a sugar carbohydrate that is quickly digested and used by the body for energy; includes table sugar, fruit and sugar from fruit, molasses, and sugar from milk (Ch. 11)

sinus – in head and neck anatomy, an air-filled cavity within any of a number of the bones of the skull; usually communicates with the nostrils (Ch. 6)

six-handed dentistry – a variation of four-handed dentistry that includes the dentist and two chairside assistants, one on the dentist's right and one on the left (Ch. 25)

skull radiograph – an x-ray image of a portion of the skull (Ch. 31)

sodium perborate (per-BORE-ate) – a tooth whitening agent (Ch. 46)

solubility – the degree to which dental material dissolves and breaks apart when it is wet (Ch. 33)

somatic (soh-MAT-ik) cells – non-reproductive cells that contain 46 chromosomes and are present in tissues, organs, and other biological structures (Ch. 29)

sonic scaler – an electronically powered instrument attached to the dental unit that uses rapid energy vibrations of a powered instrument tip (3,000–8,000 cycles per second) to remove calculus (tartar) and other hard deposits from the surface of the teeth (Ch. 24)

spatula – a flat blade, like a knife blade without the sharp edge, used for mixing impression materials, cements, and plaster, as well as some ointments (Ch. 26)

spatula, mixing – a flat blade used for mixing plaster and other dental materials (Ch. 35)

spatula, wax – a double-ended flat blade used to shape wax (Ch. 35)

sphenoid (SFEE-noyd) bone – forms the anterior, or forward-most part, of the base of the skull (Ch. 6)

sphygmomanometer (sfig-moh-muh-NOM-ih-ter) – a device for measuring blood pressure that includes an arm cuff and gauge (Ch. 17)

sporicide (SPOR-uh-side) – any agent that kills bacterial spores (Ch. 14)

squamous (SKWAY-mus) cell carcinoma – one of the two most common types of skin cancer (Ch. 5)

stainless steel crowns – crowns made from stainless steel and used in pediatric dentistry during restorations (Ch. 43)

Standard of Care (SOC) – the diagnostic and treatment process that a health care provider should follow for a particular type of patient, illness, or circumstance (Ch. 2)

standard precautions – current guidelines for prevention of infectious diseases and nosocomial infections as established by the Centers for Disease Control; these precautions state that health care workers should avoid contact with all bodily fluids, including saliva and blood, regardless of a patient's diagnosis or possible infectious status (Ch. 14)

sterile – the condition of being aseptic, or free from all living microorganisms and their spores (Ch. 14)

sterilization – the destruction of all microorganisms in or about an object (Ch. 14)

stethoscope – an instrument used to listen to sounds in the heart, lungs, and other body organs; includes ear pieces that fit into the ear and a flat metal disc that is placed on the body and picks up sounds (Ch. 17)

stimulant – a drug or agent that increases the speed and efficiency of bodily processes (Ch. 16)

stock tray – a prefabricated impression tray intended to fit a wide variety of patients (Ch. 35)

stomatitis – inflammation of the mucous membrane of the mouth (Ch. 12)

stomodeum (stoh-muh-DEE-um) – primitive mouth of the embryo (Ch. 7)

strain – changes in the shape or function of dental material that are a result of being under stress (Ch. 33)

streptococci (strep-toe-KOK-sigh) – a genus of non-motile, non-spore-forming, aerobic to facultatively anaerobic bacteria containing gram-positive, spheric or ovoid cells that occur in pairs or short or long chains (Ch. 13)

stress – the force or pressure applied to dental material (Ch. 33)

stroke – any acute clinical event that impairs blood flow to the brain for longer than 24 hours (Ch. 18)

styloglossus (sti-loh-GLAW-sus) muscle – one of the extrinsic muscles of the tongue; retracts the tongue (Ch. 6)

stylohyoid (sti-loh-HI-oyd) muscle – one of the muscles of the floor of the mouth; assists in swallowing (Ch. 6)

subcutaneous administration – injecting drugs or medications just below the skin (Ch. 16)

sublingual (sub-LING-gwul) – below the tongue (Ch. 30)

sublingual administration – placing drugs beneath the tongue until they dissolve (Ch. 16)

sublingual duct – duct that transports saliva from the sublingual glands to the oral cavity; also known as Bartholin duct (Ch. 6)

sublingual gland – major salivary gland; located under the mucous membrane between the tongue and the mandible (Ch. 6)

submandibular duct – duct that transports saliva from the submandibular gland to the oral cavity; also known as Wharton duct (Ch. 6)

submandibular gland – major salivary gland; located on each side of the mouth inside and near the lower edge of the mandible (Ch. 6)

subperiosteal (sub-per-ee-OS-tee-ul) implant – an implant that is inserted into the gingival tissue but sits on top of the jawbone (Ch. 38)

subscriber – the primary policyholder in dental insurance (Ch. 47)

succedaneous (suk-sih-DAY-nee-us) teeth – the teeth that come after, or succeed, the primary teeth (Ch. 8)

sulcus (SUL-kus) – valley on the occlusal surface of a posterior tooth (Ch. 8)

superior – located above the transverse plane of the body, toward the head (Ch. 5)

supine position (su-PINE) – the position of the dental chair in which the patient's body is horizontal with the chest at the same level as the knees, toes, and the top of the patient's head at the top edge of the headrest; the most common position used during dental treatment (Ch. 25)

supplemental groove – smaller, less distinctive groove that is not located between lobes or other notable features of the tooth (Ch. 8)

supraversion – the position of a tooth when it is out of the line of occlusion in an occlusal direction (Ch. 45)

surgical asepsis (a-SEP-sis) – procedures used to ensure a sterile environment in the operating area (Ch. 42)

suture – the jagged articulation where bones, for example, of the skull, meet and form a fibrous joint that does not move (Ch. 6)

symptom – any adverse phenomenon or undesirable departure from structural, functional, or sensational norm experienced by a patient; a subjective sign of disease (Ch. 18)

syneresis (sih-NER-uh-sis) – changes in a set alginate impression due to dryness and loss of moisture resulting in shrinkage (Ch. 35)

synergistic effect – a drug interaction that occurs when drugs produce an effect that is greater than the sum of their separate actions (Ch. 16)

systemic fluoride – fluoride that is ingested and absorbed through the bloodstream (Ch. 10)

systemic infection – an infection that occur throughout the body (Ch. 13)

systolic pressure – the pressure of blood on the walls of the arteries as the heart pumps and send blood out to the rest of the body (Ch. 17)

tactfulness – avoiding giving offense; considerate in dealing with others (Ch. 2)

tactile sensation – using the sensation of touch to gain information when performing a dental stroke or procedure; "reading" the information gained by the touch (Ch. 26)

team – group working toward a common goal; members see themselves and their work as interdependent and are committed to each other's success (Ch. 3)

temperature – the measure of the balance between heat produced and lost by the body (Ch. 17)

template – a dental device that contains the imprint of the dental arch used for marking hole positions on the dental dam (Ch. 27)

temporal bone – found on each side of the cranium and surrounding the ear (Ch. 6)

temporal muscle – one of the four pairs of muscles of mastication (Ch. 6)

temporomandibular joint – a synovial articulation between the head of the mandible and mandibular fossa and articular tubercle of temporal bone; a fibrocartilaginous articular disc divides it into two cavities (Ch. 31)

temporomandibular joint dysfunction (TMJD) – joint inflammation and dysfunction caused largely by stress-induced clenching and grinding of the teeth (Ch. 6)

tensile strength – the amount of force or pulling dental material is able to resist without tearing or falling out of place (Ch. 33)

teratogen (TARE-uh-toh-jen) – any agent or factor that induces or increases the incidence of abnormal prenatal development (Ch. 12)

tertiary dentin – dentin that forms in response to damage to or irritation of the tooth (Ch. 7)

therapeutic – use of drugs to treat illness and disease (Ch. 16)

thermal conductivity – the speed at which dental material heats up (Ch. 33)

thermal expansion – the degree to which dental material expands when heated (Ch. 33)

thermoluminescent (thur-moh-loo-muh-NES-unt) device (TLD) – a device worn by employees in dental offices that measures radiation exposure; thermoluminescent devices emit light energy when exposed to radiation and are very accurate measures of exposure (Ch. 29)

thyroid collar – a protective device worn by patients during radiography to protect the thyroid gland in the neck; thyroid collars are made from lead and can be either separate devices or incorporated into a lead apron (Ch. 29)

tidal volume – the amount of air inhaled and exhaled with each breath (Ch. 28)

tinea (TIN-ee-uh) – a fungus infection (Ch. 13)

tinnitus (TIN-ih-tus) – a ringing in the ears (Ch. 42)

tomogram – an x-ray projection of the temporomandibular joint (Ch. 31)

tomography – the practice of obtaining tomograms (Ch. 31)

tongue bifurcation – a type of oral personalization that involves surgically splitting the tongue in two (Ch. 46)

tonsillitis (ton-suh-LIE-tihs) – an infection of the tonsils common in children (Ch. 5)

tooth morphology – study of a tooth's shape and structure (Ch. 8)

topical administration – administering drugs through lotions or gels applied to the skin (Ch. 16)

topical anesthetic – a solution that is applied to oral mucosa to numb the mucosa and nerve endings to prevent pain during injection (Ch. 28)

topical fluoride – fluoride that is applied directly to the tooth surface and that penetrates the outermost layer of enamel (Ch. 10)

topographic technique – an exposure technique used in occlusal imaging in which the primary x-ray beam is directed at a perpendicular plane created by bisecting the central axis of the teeth and the film (Ch. 30)

torsiversion (tor-sih-VER-zhun) – malposition of a tooth in which it is rotated on its long axis (Ch. 45)

tort (TORT) – wrongful acts or breach of contract for which damages can be obtained (Ch. 4)

toxicology – the scientific study of poisons and their effects (Ch. 16)

trabeculae (truh-BEK-yoo-lee) – the interior substance of spongy or cancellous bone; mesh-like in structure and sponge-like in appearance. (Ch. 5)

traction – act of drawing or pulling, as by an elastic or spring force (Ch. 45)

trade name – the brand name of a drug (Ch. 16)

tragus (TRAY-gus) – portion of the external ear lying anterior to the acoustic meatus (Ch. 6)

tranquilizer – a drug that relieves anxiety and promotes relaxation (Ch. 16)

transdermal administration – delivering medications through a skin patch (Ch. 16)

transfer zone – the space where instrument transfer occurs during four-handed dentistry, usually below the patient's chin and directly over the throat and upper chest (Ch. 26)

transient ischemic attack – any acute clinical event that impairs blood flow to the brain for shorter than 24 hours, producing a sudden focal loss of neurologic function with complete recovery (Ch. 18)

transillumination (tranz-ih-LOO-muh-NAY-shun) testing – pulpal testing using a fiber optic light to look for cracks or other signs of bacteria leakage that could cause pulp necrosis (Ch. 40)

transitional mixed dentition – describing the dentition of a child who has both primary and adult teeth (Ch. 30)

transposition – misplacement of teeth from the normal sequence in the arch (Ch. 45)

transverse ridge – two triangular ridges of cusps on opposite sides of the tooth that join at the depression in the occlusal surface (Ch. 8)

transversion – eruption of a tooth in a position normally occupied by another (Ch. 45)

traumatic intrusion – a condition in which newly erupted baby teeth are pushed back into their sockets as a result of trauma to the teeth (Ch. 18)

tray – a flat receptacle with a lipped edge and compartments; in the preset tray system, trays are organized with all the dental instruments and armamentarium needed for a particular procedure before the procedure begins (Ch. 26)

Trendelenburg position – the position of the dental chair in which the head is placed lower than the legs and feet. This position is not used very often; it is mostly used in emergency situations such as syncope. (Ch. 25)

triangular ridge – a ridge that runs from the cusp tip to the center of the occlusal surface (Ch. 8)

trifurcated (tri-fur-KAY-tid) – split into three (Ch. 8)

trifurcation (tri-fur-KAY-shun) – the area where the tooth roots separate into three (Ch. 8)

trigeminal nerve – Cranial Nerve V; serves as the primary source of innervation for the oral cavity (Ch. 6)

trituration (trit-yoo-RAY-shun) – mixing dental amalgam in a mortar and pestle or with a mechanical device (Ch. 34)

triturator (trit-yoo-RATE-ur) – a device used to triturate; another term for an amalgamator (Ch. 34)

tubehead – the portion of the x-ray unit containing the x-ray tube, collimator, and PID, where x-rays are actually generated (Ch. 29)

tympanic thermometer – an instrument placed inside the ear to measure body temperature (Ch. 17)

ulcer – a lesion through skin or mucous membrane resulting from loss of tissue, usually with inflammation (Ch. 12)

ultrasonic scaler – an electronically powered instrument attached to a portable unit with an electric generator that uses rapid energy vibrations of a powered instrument tip (18,000–42,000 cycles per second) to remove calculus (tartar) and other hard deposits from the surface of the teeth and to cleanse the environment of a periodontal pocket; some models use water (lavage) to cool the instrument while in use (Ch. 24)

universal distress signal – a posture assumed by patients who are choking; patients stand with their hands at their throats (Ch. 18)

universal precautions – a set of procedural directives and guidelines to prevent parenteral, mucous membranes, and nonintact skin exposures of health care workers to bloodborne pathogens; this term has generally been replaced by the term *standard precautions* (Ch. 14)

unsaturated fat – a type of fat that comes from plant sources; can be divided into monounsaturated fat, such as nuts, olives and olive oil, peanut oil, and avocados, and polyunsaturated fats, such as corn, flax seed, and canola oils (Ch. 11)

upright position – the vertical, seated position of the dental chair in which the back of the chair is tilted back slightly from a 90-degree angle; this position allows the patient easy entrance and exit of the dental chair (Ch. 25)

uvula (YOO-vyuh-luh) – the tissue that hangs down from the maxillary posterior palatal area (Ch. 46)

vacuum former – an appliance used to warm plastic and construct custom trays (Ch. 35)

vasoconstrictor (vay-zoh-kun-STRIK-ter) – a medication that narrows blood vessels in the area where the drug is administered; prolongs the effects of an anesthetic and slows down the flow of blood in that area (Ch. 28)

veneer (vuh-NERE) – a thin layer of acrylic, composite, or porcelain used to cover the facial (front) surface of badly stained teeth or to improve the shape of highly visible front teeth (Ch. 1)

ventral – toward the front of the body (Ch. 5)

ventral cavity – made up of the thoracic, abdominal, and pelvic cavities (Ch. 5)

ventricular fibrillation – an abnormal heart rhythm in which the main pumping chambers of the heart, the ventricles, quiver and beat far too fast, thus reducing the supply of freshly oxygenated blood to the body (Ch. 18)

verbal communication – communication using words or language (Ch. 23)

vermilion border – the border of the lips (Ch. 6)

vermilion zone – reddish portion of the lips (Ch. 6)

vertical angulation – the angle of the PID on a vertical plane around the patient's head during exposure (Ch. 30)

vesicle – a small bladder or bladder-like structure; a small, less than 1 cm, circumscribed skin elevation containing fluid; for example, a blister (Ch. 12)

vestibule (of the oral cavity) – space between the teeth and the inner lining of the cheeks and lips (Ch. 6)

vibrator – a platform used to agitate mixes (Ch. 35)

viroid – a fragment of RNA that is an infectious organism (Ch. 13)

virucide (VIE-ruh-side) – an agent active against virus infections (Ch. 14)

virulence (VIR-yuh-lunz) – the disease-evoking power of a pathogen (Ch. 14)

viscosity (vis-KOS-uh-tee) – how well a liquid moves and flows (Ch. 33)

vital signs – physical measures of body functioning that provide important information about the basic systems that keep a person alive, such as breathing and heart functioning (Ch. 17)

vitamin – a complex substance that aids digestion and allows cells to use food for fuel; may be fat soluble or water soluble (Ch. 11)

vomer (VOH-mer) – a single, flat bone that forms the base of the nasal septum (Ch. 6)

wavelength – in the electromagnetic spectrum, a measure of the length of each wave of energy; the shorter the wavelength, the more penetrating and higher energy the wave; x-rays have a very short wavelength and are very penetrating, high-energy waves (Ch. 29)

wettability (wet-uh-BIL-ih-te) – the degree to which a dental material can be wetted so it can spread across a solid surface (Ch. 33)

whitening – lightening of teeth to a whiter color by the use of dental bleaching materials (Ch. 1)

work group – group working toward a common goal; members generally focus on their own assigned tasks (Ch. 3)

work pan – a plastic tray used to hold ongoing laboratory work (Ch. 35)

working end – the part of an instrument used to perform a task or procedure (Ch. 26)

xerostomia (ze-roh-STOG-mee-uh) – an oral condition wherein the mouth is dry due to a lack of saliva (Ch. 10)

x-ray tube – the portion of the dental x-ray unit where the x-rays are generated; a vacuum tube containing the anode and cathode; x-ray beams are directed from the x-ray tube, through the PID, and toward the patient (Ch. 29)

xylitol (ZYE-lih-tol) – an sugar substitute that has been shown to help prevent dental caries (Ch. 10)

yeast – a general term denoting true fungi of the family *Saccharomycetaceae* that are widely distributed (Ch. 13)

zinc oxide eugenol (YOO-juh-nawl) (ZOE) – a dental cement used for temporary cementing of restorations such as crowns, bridges, inlays, and onlays; also used as a temporary restoration and a base (Ch. 33)

zinc phosphate (FOS-fate) – a dental cement used for permanent cementing of restorations such as crowns, bridges, inlays, onlays, and orthodontic bands and brackets; also used as a base (Ch. 33)

zygomatic arch – arch formed by temporal process of zygomatic bone that joins (Ch. 31)

zygomatic bone – also known as malar bone; helps form the prominence, or highest part, of each cheekbone and the side and bottom of each eye socket (Ch. 6)

zygomatic major – a muscle of facial expression that extends along the cheek to the mouth; important in laughter (Ch. 6)

zygote (ZIE-gote) – the fertilized egg (Ch. 7)

Figure Credits

Chapter 1

Figure 1-1. Courtesy of National Museum of Science & Industry, London, UK.

Figure 1-2. Courtesy of National Museum of Dentistry, Baltimore, MD.

Figure 1-4. Courtesy of University of Maryland Health Sciences & Human Services Library, Baltimore, MD.

Figure 1-5. Courtesy of Bird DL, Robinson DS. *Torres and Ehrlich Modern Dental Assisting*, 9th ed. Philadelphia: Saunders, 2009.

Chapter 2

Figure 2-4. Courtesy of American Dental Assistants Association.

Figure 2-5. Courtesy of Dental Assisting National Board.

Chapter 3

Figure 3-2. Bedford DJ, Allen MM. *LWW's Visual Atlas of Medical Assisting Skills*. Baltimore: Lippincott Williams & Wilkins, 2008.

Figure 3-3. Irlbacher-Girtel GS, Girtel G. *Dental Office Administration*. Baltimore: Lippincott Williams & Wilkins, 2010.

Chapter 4

Figure 4-5. Bedford DJ, Allen MM. *LWW's Visual Atlas of Medical Assisting Skills*. Baltimore: Lippincott Williams & Wilkins, 2008.

Chapter 5

Figure 5-1. From *Stedman's Medical Dictionary*, 27th ed. Baltimore: Lippincott Williams & Wilkins, 2000.

Figure 5-2. From Willis MC. *Medical Terminology: A Programmed Learning Approach to the Language of Health Care*. 2nd ed. Baltimore: Lippincott Williams & Wilkins, 2008.

Figures 5-3, 5-10, 5-11, 5-15, 5-16, 5-23, and 5-26. From Cohen BJ, Taylor JJ. *Memmler's Structure & Function of the Human Body*, 9th ed. Baltimore: Lippincott Williams & Wilkins, 2009.

Figures 5-4, 5-12, 5-17, 5-18, 5-19, 5-22, and 5-24. From Cohen BJ, Taylor JJ. *Memmler's The Human Body in Health and Disease*, 11th Edition. Baltimore: Lippincott Williams & Wilkins, 2009.

Figure 5-5. From Moore KL, Agur A. *Essential Clinical Anatomy*, 2nd ed. Philadelphia: Lippincott Williams & Wilkins, 2002.

Figures 5-6 and 5-13. From Oatis CA. *Kinesiology. The Mechanics and Pathomechanics of Human Movement*, 2nd ed. Baltimore: Lippincott Williams & Wilkins, 2008.

Figure 5-7. From Moore KL, Agur A. *Essential Clinical Anatomy*, 2nd ed. Philadelphia: Lippincott Williams & Wilkins, 2002.

Figure 5-8. Asset provided by Anatomical Chart Co.

Figure 5-9. Courtesy of Carl Allen, D.D.S., M.S.D.

Figure 5-14. From *Stedman's Medical Dictionary*, 28th ed. Baltimore: Lippincott Williams & Wilkins, 2006.

Figures 5-20 and 5-25. From Premkumar K. *The Massage Connection Anatomy and Physiology*. Baltimore: Lippincott Williams & Wilkins, 2004.

Figure 5-21. From McConnell TH. *The Nature of Disease Pathology for the Health Professions*. Baltimore: Lippincott Williams & Wilkins, 2007.

Chapter 6

Figures 6-1 and 6-17. From Clay JH, Pounds DM. *Basic Clinical Massage Therapy: Integrating Anatomy and Treatment*, 2nd ed. Baltimore: Lippincott Williams & Wilkins, 2006.

Figures 6-2, 6-11, and 6-24. Modified from Scheid RC, Weiss G. *Woelfel's Dental Anatomy: Its Relevance to Dentistry*, 7th ed. Philadelphia: Lippincott Williams & Wilkins, 2007.

Figures 6-3, 6-6, 6-7, 6-8, and 6-9. From Scheid RC, Weiss G. *Woelfel's Dental Anatomy: Its Relevance to Dentistry*, 7th ed. Philadelphia: Lippincott Williams & Wilkins, 2007.

Figures 6-4 and 6-10. Asset provided by Anatomical Chart Company.

Figure 6-5. From Cohen BJ, Taylor JJ. *Memmler's The Human Body in Health and Disease*, 11th Edition. Baltimore: Lippincott Williams & Wilkins, 2009.

Figures 6-12, 6-13, 6-28, 6-29, 6-30, 6-31, 6-32, 6-33, and 6-34. From Hiatt JL, Gartner LP. *Textbook of Head and Neck Anatomy*, 4th ed. Baltimore: Lippincott Williams & Wilkins, 2010.

Figure 6-14. From Oatis CA. *Kinesiology. The Mechanics and Pathomechanics of Human Movement*, 2nd ed. Baltimore: Lippincott Williams & Wilkins, 2008.

Figure 6-15. From Moore KL, Agur A. *Essential Clinical Anatomy*, 2nd ed. Philadelphia: Lippincott Williams & Wilkins, 2002.

Figure 6-19. Modified from Moore KL, Dalley AF. *Clinical Oriented Anatomy*, 4th ed. Baltimore: Lippincott Williams & Wilkins, 1999.

Figure 6-21. From Premkumar K. *The Massage Connection Anatomy and Physiology*. Baltimore: Lippincott Williams & Wilkins, 2004.

Figure 6-22. Courtesy of Dr. Martha Ann Keels.

Figure 6-23. From Fleisher GR, Ludwig W, Baskin MN. *Atlas of Pediatric Emergency Medicine*. Philadelphia: Lippincott Williams & Wilkins, 2004.

Figure 6-25. From Nield-Gehrig JS, Willmann DE. *Foundations of Periodontics for the Dental Hygienist*, 3rd ed. Baltimore: Lippincott Williams & Wilkins, 2011.

Chapter 7

Figure 7-1. From Cohen BJ, Taylor JJ. *Memmler's Structure & Function of the Human Body*, 9th ed. Baltimore: Lippincott Williams & Wilkins, 2009.

Figure 7-2. Neil O. Hardy, Westport, CT. From *Stedman's Medical Dictionary*, 27th ed. Baltimore: Lippincott Williams & Wilkins, 2000.

Figures 7-3, 7-4, 7-5A,B, and 7-8. From Hiatt JL, Gartner LP. *Textbook of Head and Neck Anatomy*, 4th ed. Baltimore: Lippincott Williams & Wilkins, 2010.

Figure 7-7. From DeLong L, Burkhart N. *General and Oral Pathology for the Dental Hygienist*. Baltimore, Lippincott Williams & Wilkins, 2008.

Figure 7-9. Modified from Anatomical Chart Co.

Figure 7-10. From *Stedman's Medical Dictionary for the Dental Professions*, 2nd ed. Baltimore: Lippincott Williams & Wilkins, 2012.

Figure 7-11. From Nield-Gehrig JS, Willmann DE. *Foundations of Periodontics for the Dental Hygienist*, 3rd ed. Baltimore: Lippincott Williams & Wilkins, 2011.

Figure 7-13. From Wilkins EM, Wyche C. *Clinical Practice of the Dental Hygienist*, 10th ed. Baltimore: Lippincott Williams & Wilkins, 2008.

Figure 7-14. From Bear MF, Connors BW, Parasido, MA. *Neuroscience - Exploring the Brain*, 2nd ed. Philadelphia: Lippincott Williams & Wilkins, 2001.

Chapter 8

Figure 8-1C. ©iStockPhoto/Bill Noll

Figure 8-2A,B. From Langlais RP, Miller CS, Nield-Gehrig JS. *Color Atlas of Common Oral Diseases*, 4th ed. Baltimore: Lippincott Williams & Wilkins, 2010.

Figure 8-3A,B. From DeLong L, Burkhart N. *General and Oral Pathology for the Dental Hygienist*. Baltimore, Lippincott Williams & Wilkins, 2008.

Figures 8-9 and 8-10. From Scheid RC. *Woelfel's Dental Anatomy: Its Relevance to Dentistry*, 7th ed. Philadelphia: Lippincott Williams & Wilkins, 2007.

Chapter 9

Figures 9-1, 9-3, 9-4, 9-7, 9-9, and 9-12. From Langlais RP, Miller CS, Nield-Gehrig JS. *Color Atlas of Common Oral Diseases*, 4th ed. Baltimore: Lippincott Williams & Wilkins, 2010.

Figures 9-2, 9-8, and 9-13. From Nield-Gehrig JS, Willmann DE. *Foundations of Periodontics for the Dental Hygienist*, 3rd ed. Baltimore: Lippincott Williams & Wilkins, 2011.

Figure 9-5. From Scheid RC, Weiss G. *Woelfel's Dental Anatomy: Its Relevance to Dentistry*, 7th ed. Philadelphia: Lippincott Williams & Wilkins, 2007.

Figure 9-6. Courtesy of KaVo Dental.

Figures 9-10 and 9-11. From Wilkins EM, Wyche C. *Clinical Practice of the Dental Hygienist*, 10th ed. Baltimore: Lippincott Williams & Wilkins, 2008.

Chapter 10

Figures 10-1, 10-2, 10-3, 10-4, 10-6, 10-7, 10-8, and 10-9. From Wilkins EM, Wyche C. *Clinical Practice of the Dental Hygienist*, 10th ed. Baltimore: Lippincott Williams & Wilkins, 2008.

Figure 10-5. Used with permission from the American Dental Association.

Figure 10-10. From Langlais RP, Miller CS, Nield-Gehrig JS. *Color Atlas of Common Oral Diseases*, 4th ed. Baltimore: Lippincott Williams & Wilkins, 2010.

Chapter 11

Figure 11-1. From Wilkins EM, Wyche C. *Clinical Practice of the Dental Hygienist*, 10th ed. Baltimore: Lippincott Williams & Wilkins, 2008.

Figure 11-2. From Kronenberger J, Durham LS, Woodson D. *Lippincott Williams & Wilkins' Comprehensive Medical Assisting*, 3rd ed. Baltimore: Lippincott Williams & Wilkins, 2008.

Figure 11-5. From Langlais RP, Miller CS, Nield-Gehrig JS. *Color Atlas of Common Oral Diseases*, 4th ed. Baltimore: Lippincott Williams & Wilkins, 2010.

Chapter 12

Figure 12-1. Photo provided by CDx Laboratories, Inc.

Figure 12-2. From Langland OE, Langlais RP, Preece J. *Principles of Dental Imaging*, 2nd ed. Philadelphia: Lippincott Williams & Wilkins, 2002.

Figures 12-3, 12-4, 12-5, 12-6, 12-7, 12-8, 12-9, 12-10, 12-11, 12-12, 12-13, 12-14, 12-15, 12-16, 12-18, 12-19, 12-20, 12-23, 12-24, 12-25, 12-26A, 12-27, 12-28, 12-29, 12-30, 12-31, 12-32, 12-34, 12-35, 12-36, 12-37, 12-38, 12-39. From Langlais RP, Miller CS, Nield-Gehrig JS. *Color Atlas of Common Oral Diseases*, 4th ed. Baltimore: Lippincott Williams & Wilkins, 2010.

Figures 12-17, 12-21, 12-22, 12-26B. From DeLong L, Burkhart N. *General and Oral Pathology for the Dental Hygienist*. Baltimore, Lippincott Williams & Wilkins, 2008.

Figure 12-22. Courtesy of Dr. Peter Jacobsen.

Figure 12-33. Courtesy of Dr. Harvey Kessler.

Chapter 13

Figures 13-1, 13-2, and 13-3. From Engelkirk PG, Duben-Engelkirk J. *Burton's Microbiology for the Health Sciences*, 9th ed. Baltimore: Lippincott Williams & Wilkins, 2010.

Figures 13-4 and 13-5. From Langlais RP, Miller CS, Nield-Gehrig JS. *Color Atlas of Common Oral Diseases*, 4th ed. Baltimore: Lippincott Williams & Wilkins, 2010.

Chapter 14

Figure 14-1. From Engelkirk PG, Duben-Engelkirk J. *Burton's Microbiology for the Health Sciences*, 9th ed. Baltimore: Lippincott Williams & Wilkins, 2010.

Figures 14-2, 14-7, and 14-9. From Molinari JA, Harte JA. *Cottone's Practical Infection Control in Dentistry*, 3rd ed. Baltimore: Lippincott Williams & Wilkins, 2009.

Figures 14-3A, B, and C. Courtesy of Crosstex, www.crosstex.com.

Figures 14-4 and 14-6. From Gladwin MA, Bagby M. *Clinical Aspects of Dental Materials: Theory, Practice, and Cases*, 3rd ed. Baltimore: Lippincott Williams and Wilkins, 2008.

Figure 14-5. From Mitchell M and Total Care Programming, Inc. *Dental Instruments: A Pocket Guide to Identification*, 2nd ed. Baltimore: Lippincott Williams and Wilkins, 2011.

Figure 14-8A. UltraClave® courtesy of Midmark Corporation.

Figure 14-8B. STATIM 2000 courtesy of SciCan, www.scican.com.

Figure 14-10. Used with permission from Dr. Thomas K. Lee, DDS.

Figures P14-1-1, P14-1-2, P14-1-3, P14-1-4, P14-1-5, P14-6-2, P14-6-3, P14-6-4, P14-6-5, and P14-6-6. Bedford DJ, Allen MM. *LWW's Visual Atlas of Medical Assisting Skills*. Baltimore: Lippincott Williams & Wilkins, 2008.

Figures P14-2-1, P14-2-2, P14-2-3, and P14-2-4. Craven RF, Hirnle CJ. *Fundamentals of Nursing: Human Health and Function*, 6th ed. Philadelphia: Lippincott Williams & Wilkins, 2008.

Figures P14-3-1, P14-3-2, and P14-3-3. From Kronenberger J, Durham LS, Woodson D. *Lippincott Williams & Wilkins' Comprehensive Medical Assisting*, 3rd ed. Baltimore: Lippincott Williams & Wilkins, 2008.

Chapter 15

Figures 15-1, and 15-3. From McCall RE, Tankersley CM. *Phlebotomy Essentials*, 5th ed. Baltimore: Lippincott Williams & Wilkins, 2011.

Figure 15-2. From Molinari JA, Harte JA. *Cottone's Practical Infection Control in Dentistry*, 3rd ed. Baltimore: Lippincott Williams & Wilkins, 2009.

Figure 15-4. From Kronenberger J, Durham LS, Woodson D. *Lippincott Williams & Wilkins' Comprehensive Medical Assisting*, 3rd ed. Baltimore: Lippincott Williams & Wilkins, 2008.

Figure 15-5. Courtesy Brevis Corp, Salt Lake City, UT.

Chapter 16

Figure 16-2. From Kronenberger J, Durham LS, Woodson D. *Lippincott Williams & Wilkins' Comprehensive Medical Assisting*, 3rd ed. Baltimore: Lippincott Williams & Wilkins, 2008.

Figure 16-3. From Langlais RP, Miller CS, Nield-Gehrig JS. *Color Atlas of Common Oral Diseases*, 4th ed. Baltimore: Lippincott Williams & Wilkins, 2010.

Chapter 17

Figures 17-1, 17-2, 17-3, and 17-4. From Kronenberger J, Durham LS, Woodson D. *Lippincott Williams & Wilkins' Comprehensive Medical Assisting*, 3rd ed. Baltimore: Lippincott Williams & Wilkins, 2008.

Figures P17-2-1, P17-3-2, and P17-3-3. From Nield-Gehrig JS. *Patient Assessment Tutorials: A Step-By-Step Guide for the Dental Hygienist*, 2nd ed. Baltimore: Lippincott Williams & Wilkins, 2009.

Chapter 18

Figure 18-1. Courtesy of Banyan International.

Figures 18-2, 18-3, 18-4, P18-1-2, P18-1-3, P18-1-4, and P18-1-5. From Kronenberger J, Durham LS, Woodson D. *Lippincott Williams & Wilkins' Comprehensive Medical Assisting*, 3rd ed. Baltimore: Lippincott Williams & Wilkins, 2008.

Figure 18-5. From Langland OE, Langlais RP, Preece J. *Principles of Dental Imaging*, 2nd ed. Philadelphia: Lippincott Williams & Wilkins, 2002.

Figures P18-2-1 and P18-2-2. LifeART image copyright © 2012 Lippincott Williams & Wilkins. All rights reserved.

Figure P18-3-1. From Taylor CR, Lillis C, LeMone P, Lynn P. *Fundamentals of Nursing: The Art and Science of Nursing Care*, 7th ed. Philadelphia: Lippincott Williams & Wilkins, 2011.

Figure P18-4-1. From Smeltzer SC, Bare BG. *Textbook of Medical-Surgical Nursing*, 9th Ed. Philadelphia: Lippincott Williams & Wilkins, 2000.

Chapter 19

Figure 19-1. From Wilkins EM, Wyche C. *Clinical Practice of the Dental Hygienist*, 10th ed. Baltimore: Lippincott Williams & Wilkins, 2008.

Figures 19-2 and 19-5. From Millar D. *Reinforced Periodontal Instrumentation and Ergonomics for the Dental Care Provider*. Baltimore: Lippincott Williams & Wilkins, 2008.

Chapter 20

Figures 20-2, 20-3, and 20-5. Images courtesy of Hu-Friedy, www.hu-friedy.com.

Figures 20-4 and 20-6. From Scheid RC, Weiss G. *Woelfel's Dental Anatomy: Its Relevance to Dentistry*, 7th ed. Philadelphia: Lippincott Williams & Wilkins, 2007.

Figures 20-11 and 20-12. From Wilkins EM, Wyche C. *Clinical Practice of the Dental Hygienist*, 10th ed. Baltimore: Lippincott Williams & Wilkins, 2008.

Figures P20-2-2, P20-2-3, P20-2-4, P20-2-5, P20-2-6, P20-2-7, P20-2-8, and P20-2-9A and B. From Nield-Gehrig JS. *Patient Assessment Tutorials: A Step-By-Step Guide for the Dental Hygienist*, 2nd ed. Baltimore: Lippincott Williams & Wilkins, 2009.

Chapter 21

Figures 21-1, 21-2, and 21-3. From Nield-Gehrig JS. *Patient Assessment Tutorials: A Step-By-Step Guide for the Dental Hygienist*, 2nd ed. Baltimore: Lippincott Williams & Wilkins, 2009.

Chapter 22

Figures 22-1, 22-2, 22-3, 22-4, and 22-5. From Wilkins EM, Wyche C. *Clinical Practice of the Dental Hygienist*, 10th ed. Baltimore: Lippincott Williams & Wilkins, 2008.

Figure 22-6. From Langlais RP, Miller CS, Nield-Gehrig JS. *Color Atlas of Common Oral Diseases*, 4th ed. Baltimore: Lippincott Williams & Wilkins, 2010.

Chapter 24

Figure 24-9. From Wilkins EM, Wyche C. *Clinical Practice of the Dental Hygienist*, 10th ed. Baltimore: Lippincott Williams & Wilkins, 2008.

Chapter 26

Figures 26-3, 26-17, and 26-26. Images courtesy of Miltex, www.miltex.com.

Figures 26-4, 26-5, 26-6, 26-8, 26-9, 26-11, 26-15A, 26-15C, and 26-37B. Images courtesy of Hu-Friedy, www.hu-friedy.com.

Figures 26-7, 26-10, 26-12, 26-13, 26-15B, 26-16, and 26-19. Images courtesy of Premier Dental Products, www.premusa.com.

Figure 26-18. Alginate bowls courtesy of Coltene-Whaledent, www.coltene.com.

Figure 26-20. Image courtesy of American Eagle Instruments®, Inc., www.am-eagle.com.

Figures 26-27C, 26-29A, 26-30, 26-35, and 26-36. Image courtesy of Dentsply Professional, www.dentsply.com.

Figures 26-28A and 26-32. Images courtesy of DentalEZ Group, www.dentalez.com/stardental/

Figure 26-31. Image courtesy of Aseptico, www.aseptico.com.

Figures 26-34 and 26-40. From Mitchell M and Total Care Programming, Inc. *Dental Instruments: A Pocket Guide to Identification*, 2nd ed. Baltimore: Lippincott Williams and Wilkins, 2011.

Figure 26-39. Image courtesy of Shofu Dental Corporation, www.shofu.com.

Figure 26-41. From Gladwin MA, Bagby M. *Clinical Aspects of Dental Materials: Theory, Practice, and Cases*, 3rd ed. Baltimore: Lippincott Williams and Wilkins, 2008.

Figure 26-42. Images courtesy of Danville Materials, www.danvillematerials.com.

Figure 26-43. From Millar D. *Reinforced Periodontal Instrumentation and Ergonomics for the Dental Care Provider*. Baltimore: Lippincott Williams & Wilkins, 2008.

Chapter 27

Figure 27-1. From Millar D. *Reinforced Periodontal Instrumentation and Ergonomics for the Dental Care Provider*. Baltimore: Lippincott Williams & Wilkins, 2008.

Figures 27-3, 27-9, and 27-10. From Mitchell M and Total Care Programming, Inc. *Dental Instruments: A Pocket Guide to Identification*, 2nd ed. Baltimore: Lippincott Williams and Wilkins, 2011.

Figure 27-5. Image courtesy of Miltex, www.miltex.com.

Figure 27-7. From Wilkins EM, Wyche C. *Clinical Practice of the Dental Hygienist*, 10th ed. Baltimore: Lippincott Williams & Wilkins, 2008.

Figures 27-11, 27-12, and 27-14. Images courtesy of Hu-Friedy, www.hu-friedy.com.

Chapter 28

Figure 28-1. From Mitchell M and Total Care Programming, Inc. *Dental Instruments: A Pocket Guide to Identification*, 2nd ed. Baltimore: Lippincott Williams and Wilkins, 2011.

Figure 28-2. Image courtesy of Miltex, www.miltex.com.

Figure 26-3. Image courtesy of Crosstex, www.crosstex.com.

Figure 28-6. From Wilkins EM, Wyche C. *Clinical Practice of the Dental Hygienist*, 10th ed. Baltimore: Lippincott Williams & Wilkins, 2008.

Chapter 29

Figures 29-2 and 29-4. From Cohen BJ, Taylor JJ. *Memmler's Structure & Function of the Human Body*, 9th ed. Baltimore: Lippincott Williams & Wilkins, 2009.

Figures 29-6 and 29-8. From Langland OE, Langlais RP, Preece J. *Principles of Dental Imaging*, 2nd ed. Philadelphia: Lippincott Williams & Wilkins, 2002.

Figure 29-7. Images courtesy of DENTSPLY Rinn, www.rinncorp.com.

Figures 29-9 and 29-15. Images courtesy of Air Techniques, Inc., www.airtechniques.com.

Figure 29-10. From Wilkins EM, Wyche C. *Clinical Practice of the Dental Hygienist*, 10th ed. Baltimore: Lippincott Williams & Wilkins, 2008.

Figure 29-12. Images courtesy of Carestream Health, Inc., www.kodakdental.com.

Figure 29-13. From Mitchell M and Total Care Programming, Inc. *Dental Instruments: A Pocket Guide to Identification*, 2nd ed. Baltimore: Lippincott Williams and Wilkins, 2011.

Figure 29-14. Images courtesy of Gendex Dental Systems, www.gendex.com.

Chapter 30

Figures 30-1 through 30-35, P30-2-4, P30-2-6, P30-2-8, P30-2-10, P30-2-13, P30-2-15, P30-2-17, P30-2-19, P30-3-10, P30-4-3, and P30-4-5. From Langland OE, Langlais RP, Preece J. *Principles of Dental Imaging*, 2nd ed. Philadelphia: Lippincott Williams & Wilkins, 2002.

Chapter 31

Figures 31-1, 31-6, and 31-12. Images courtesy of Gendex Dental Systems, www.gendex.com.

Figures 31-2, 31-3, 31-5, 31-7, 31-9, 31-10, 31-11, 31-14, 31-15, 31-16, and P31-1-1. From Langland OE, Langlais RP, Preece J. *Principles of Dental Imaging*, 2nd ed. Philadelphia: Lippincott Williams & Wilkins, 2002.

Figure 31-13. From Snell RS. *Clinical Anatomy by Regions*, 7th ed. Philadelphia: Lippincott Williams & Wilkins, 2003.

Chapter 32

Figures 32-4, 32-7, 32-8, 32-9. and 32-10. From Gladwin MA, Bagby M. *Clinical Aspects of Dental Materials: Theory, Practice, and Cases*, 3rd ed. Baltimore: Lippincott Williams and Wilkins, 2008.

Figure 32-6. Image courtesy of Carestream Health, Inc., www.kodakdental.com.

Figure P32-2-2. From Langland OE, Langlais RP, Preece J. *Principles of Dental Imaging*, 2nd ed. Philadelphia: Lippincott Williams & Wilkins, 2002.

Chapter 33

Figures 33-1, 33-2, and 33-3. From Gladwin MA, Bagby M. *Clinical Aspects of Dental Materials: Theory, Practice, and Cases*, 3rd ed. Baltimore: Lippincott Williams and Wilkins, 2008.

Chapter 34

Figures 34-1, 34-2, 34-5, 34-6, 34-7, 34-8, and 34-9. From Gladwin MA, Bagby M. *Clinical Aspects of Dental Materials: Theory, Practice, and Cases*, 3rd ed. Baltimore: Lippincott Williams and Wilkins, 2008.

Figures 34-3 and 34-4. From Ferracane JL. *Materials in Dentistry: Principles and Applications*, 2nd ed. Baltimore: Lippincott Williams and Wilkins, 2001.

Chapter 35

Figure 35-2A. Image courtesy of Hu-Friedy, www.hu-friedy.com.

Figures 35-2B, 35-3, and 35-4. From Mitchell M and Total Care Programming, Inc. *Dental Instruments: A Pocket Guide to Identification*, 2nd ed. Baltimore: Lippincott Williams and Wilkins, 2011.

Figure 35-5. Courtesy of DR Dental Resources, Inc.

Figure 35-6. From Scheid RC, Weiss G. *Woelfel's Dental Anatomy: Its Relevance to Dentistry*, 7th ed. Philadelphia: Lippincott Williams & Wilkins, 2007.

Figures 35-7 and 35-8. From Gladwin MA, Bagby M. *Clinical Aspects of Dental Materials: Theory, Practice, and Cases*, 3rd ed. Baltimore: Lippincott Williams and Wilkins, 2008.

Chapter 36

Figures 36-3, 36-7, 36-8. and 36-9. From Langlais RP, Miller CS, Nield-Gehrig JS. *Color Atlas of Common Oral Diseases*, 4th ed. Baltimore: Lippincott Williams & Wilkins, 2010.

Figures 36-4A and 36-6B. Images courtesy of Miltex, www.miltex.com.

Figure 36-5. Image courtesy of Dentsply, www.dentsply.com.

Figure 36-6A. Image courtesy of Hu-Friedy, www.hu-friedy.com.

Figure 36-6B. Image modified from University of Kentucky (568m-6).

Figures P37-9-2, P37-9-3, P37-9-4. From Nield-Gehrig JS, Willmann DE. *Foundations of Periodontics for the Dental Hygienist*, 3rd ed. Baltimore: Lippincott Williams & Wilkins, 2011.

Chapter 38

Figure 38-1. Image courtesy of Julie Holloway, D.D.S., M.S.

Figures 38-2 and 38-3. From Gladwin MA, Bagby M. *Clinical Aspects of Dental Materials: Theory, Practice, and Cases*, 3rd ed. Baltimore: Lippincott Williams and Wilkins, 2008.

Figure 38-4. Images courtesy of Sirona Dental Systems, www.sirona.com.

Figure 38-5. Courtesy of Dr. Roger A. Lawton, Olympia, WA, and Nobel Biocare, Yorba Linda, CA.

Figure 38-6. Image courtesy of Hu-Friedy, www.hu-friedy.com.

Figure 38-7. Courtesy of Ultradent Products, Inc.

Chapter 39

Figure 39-1. From Langlais RP, Miller CS, Nield-Gehrig JS. *Color Atlas of Common Oral Diseases*, 4th ed. Baltimore: Lippincott Williams & Wilkins, 2010.

Figures 39-2, 39-4, 39-8, and 39-10. From Wilkins EM, Wyche C. *Clinical Practice of the Dental Hygienist*, 10th ed. Baltimore: Lippincott Williams & Wilkins, 2008.

Figures 39-3, 39-5, 39-6, 39-7, and 39-9. From Gladwin MA, Bagby M. *Clinical Aspects of Dental Materials: Theory, Practice, and Cases*, 3rd ed. Baltimore: Lippincott Williams and Wilkins, 2008.

Chapter 40

Figures 40-2 and P40-1-7. From Langland OE, Langlais RP, Preece J. *Principles of Dental Imaging*, 2nd ed. Philadelphia: Lippincott Williams & Wilkins, 2002.

Figure 40-3. From Langlais RP, Miller CS, Nield-Gehrig JS. *Color Atlas of Common Oral Diseases*, 4th ed. Baltimore: Lippincott Williams & Wilkins, 2010.

Figures 40-4 and 40-6. Images courtesy of SybronEndo, www.sybronendo.com.

Figures 40-5, P40-1-4, and P40-1-6. From Mitchell M and Total Care Programming, Inc. *Dental Instruments: A Pocket Guide to Identification*, 2nd ed. Baltimore: Lippincott Williams and Wilkins, 2011.

Chapter 41

Figures 41-1, 41-6, 41-7, 41-8, 41-9, and P41-3-2A and B. From Nield-Gehrig JS, Willmann DE. *Foundations of Periodontics for the Dental Hygienist*, 3rd ed. Baltimore: Lippincott Williams & Wilkins, 2011.

Figures 41-2, 41-3, 41-4, and 41-5. Images courtesy of Hu-Friedy, www.hu-friedy.com.

Chapter 42

Figures 42-1, 42-2B, 42-3, 42-4, 42-5, 42-6, 42-7C and F, 42-8, 42-9A-D, 42-11A, 42-12, 42-13, 42-14B, and 42-15. Images courtesy of Hu-Friedy, www.hu-friedy.com.

Figure 42-2C. Image courtesy of Karl Schumacher Dental Instruments Company, Inc., www.karlschumacher.com.

Figures 42-7A, B, D, E, G, and H, 42-9E, 42-11B and C, and 42-16. Images courtesy of Miltex, www.miltex.com.

Figure 42-10. Image courtesy of Premier Dental Products, www.premusa.com.

Figure 42-14A. Image courtesy of Aseptico, www.aseptico.com.

Figures P42-8-2 and P42-9-1. From Nield-Gehrig JS, Willmann DE. *Foundations of Periodontics for the Dental Hygienist*, 3rd ed. Baltimore: Lippincott Williams & Wilkins, 2011.

Chapter 43

Figure 43-1. ©Image Source/The Dentist's Chair

Figures 43-2 and 43-4. From Gladwin MA, Bagby M. *Clinical Aspects of Dental Materials: Theory, Practice, and Cases*, 3rd ed. Baltimore: Lippincott Williams and Wilkins, 2008.

Figure 43-3. From Langlais RP, Miller CS, Nield-Gehrig JS. *Color Atlas of Common Oral Diseases*, 4th ed. Baltimore: Lippincott Williams & Wilkins, 2010.

Figure 43-5. From Fleisher GR, Ludwig S, Baskin MN. *Atlas of Pediatric Emergency Medicine*. Philadelphia: Lippincott Williams & Wilkins, 2004.

Chapter 44

Figures 44-1 and 44-2. From Langlais RP, Miller CS, Nield-Gehrig JS. *Color Atlas of Common Oral Diseases*, 4th ed. Baltimore: Lippincott Williams & Wilkins, 2010.

Figure 44-3A. Image courtesy of Dentsply Professional, www.dentsply.com.

Figure 44-3B. Image courtesy of DentalEZ Group, www.dentalez.com/stardental/.

Chapter 45

Figures 45-1, 45-2C, and 45-3C and D. From Scheid RC, Weiss G. *Woelfel's Dental Anatomy: Its Relevance to Dentistry*, 7th ed. Philadelphia: Lippincott Williams & Wilkins, 2007.

Figures 45-2A and B and 45-3A and B. From Langlais RP, Miller CS, Nield-Gehrig JS. *Color Atlas of Common Oral Diseases*, 4th ed. Baltimore: Lippincott Williams & Wilkins, 2010.

Figures 45-4A-G, I, and J. Images courtesy of 3M Unitek - © 2010 3M. All rights reserved., www.3MUnitek.com.

Figure 45-4H. Image courtesy of Hu-Friedy, www.hu-friedy.com.

Figure 45-4K. Image courtesy of Dentronix, www.dentronix.com.

Figures 45-5, 45-6, and 45-8. From Gladwin MA, Bagby M. *Clinical Aspects of Dental Materials: Theory, Practice, and Cases*, 3rd ed. Baltimore: Lippincott Williams and Wilkins, 2008.

Figure P45-3-1 and P45-7-1. From Mitchell M and Total Care Programming, Inc. *Dental Instruments: A Pocket Guide to Identification*, 2nd ed. Baltimore: Lippincott Williams and Wilkins, 2011.

Figure P45-10-1. Image modified from the University of Kentucky.

Chapter 46

Figures 46-1, 46-2, and 46-3. From Gladwin MA, Bagby M. *Clinical Aspects of Dental Materials: Theory, Practice, and Cases*, 3rd ed. Baltimore: Lippincott Williams and Wilkins, 2008.

Chapter 47

Figure 47-2. DENTRIX image courtesy of Henry Schein Practice Solutions, American Fork, UT.

Figure 47-4. From Kronenberger J, Durham LS, Woodson D. *Lippincott Williams & Wilkins' Comprehensive Medical Assisting*, 3rd ed. Baltimore: Lippincott Williams & Wilkins, 2008.

Chapter 48

Figure 48-4. From Kronenberger J, Durham LS, Woodson D. *Lippincott Williams & Wilkins' Comprehensive Medical Assisting*, 3rd ed. Baltimore: Lippincott Williams & Wilkins, 2008.

Index

Note: Page numbers in *italics* indicate figures; page numbers followed by t indicate tables; and P followed by a page number indicates a procedure.